CARDIOLOGY BOARD REVIEW AND SELF-ASSESSMENT: A COMPANION GUIDE TO HURST'S THE HEART

CARDIOLOGY BOARD REVIEW AND SELF-ASSESSMENT: A COMPANION GUIDE TO HURST'S THE HEART

For use with the 14th edition of HURST'S THE HEART

EDITED BY

MARK J. EISENBERG, MD, MPH
Professor of Medicine
Cardiology Division
Department of Medicine
Jewish General Hospital
McGill University
Montreal, Quebec, Canada

JONATHAN AFILALO, MD, MSc
Associate Professor of Medicine
Cardiology Division
Department of Medicine
Jewish General Hospital
McGill University
Montreal, Quebec, Canada

JACQUELINE E. JOZA, MD
Assistant Professor of Medicine
Cardiology Division
Department of Medicine
McGill University Health Centre
McGill University
Montreal, Quebec, Canada

RAVI KARRA, MD, MHS
Assistant Professor of Medicine
Cardiology Division
Department of Medicine
Duke University School of Medicine
Durham, North Carolina

PATRICK R. LAWLER, MD, MPH
Assistant Professor of Medicine
Peter Munk Cardiac Centre
Toronto General Hospital
University of Toronto
Toronto, Ontario, Canada

New York Chicago San Francisco Athens London Madrid Mexico City
Milan New Delhi Singapore Sydney Toronto

Cardiology Board Review and Self-Assessment: A Companion Guide to Hurst's The Heart

Copyright © 2019 by McGraw-Hill Education. All rights reserved. Printed in China. Except as permitted under the United States Copyright Act of 1976, no part of this publication may be reproduced or distributed in any form or by any means, or stored in a data base or retrieval system, without the prior written permission of the publisher.

1 2 3 4 5 6 7 8 9   DSS   23 22 21 20 19 18

ISBN 978-1-260-02615-3
MHID 1-260-02615-9

This book was set in Minion Pro by Cenveo® Publisher Services.
The editors were Karen G. Edmonson and Robert Pancotti.
The production supervisor was Catherine H. Saggese.
Project management was provided by Shivani Salhotra, Cenveo Publisher Services.
The cover designer was Randomatrix.

Library of Congress Cataloging-in-Publication Data

Names: Eisenberg, Mark J., editor. | Afilalo, Jonathan, editor | Joza,
   Jacqueline E., editor | Karra, Ravi, editor | Lawler, Patrick R., editor
Title: Cardiology board review and self-assessment: a companion guide to Hurst's the heart : for
   use with the 14th edition of Hurst's the heart / edited by Mark J.
   Eisenberg, Jonathan Afilalo, Jacqueline E. Joza, Ravi Karra, Patrick R.
   Lawler.
Other titles: Complemented by (work): Hurst's the heart. 14th edition.
Description: 14th edition. | New York : McGraw-Hill Education, [2019] |
   Complemented by: Hurst's the heart / editors, Valentin Fuster, Robert A.
   Harrington, Jagat Narula, Zubin J. Eapen. 14th edition. 2017. | Includes
   bibliographical references and index.
Identifiers: LCCN 2018010185| ISBN 9781260026153 (pbk. : alk. paper) | ISBN
   1260026159 (pbk. : alk. paper)
Subjects: | MESH: Cardiovascular Diseases | Examination Questions
Classification: LCC RC667 | NLM WG 18.2 | DDC 616.1—dc23
LC record available at https://lccn.loc.gov/2018010185

McGraw-Hill Education books are available at special quantity discounts to use as premiums and sales promotions or for use in corporate training programs. To contact a representative, please visit the Contact Us pages at www.mhprofessional.com.

CONTENTS

SECTION 4   SYSTEMIC ARTERIAL HYPERTENSION

CONTENTS

SECTION 8   VALVULAR HEART DISEASE

CONTENTS

CONTENTS

SECTION 14   DISEASES OF THE GREAT VESSELS AND PERIPHERAL VESSELS

SECTION 15 MISCELLANEOUS CONDITIONS AND CARDIOVASCULAR DISEASE

SECTION 16 POPULATIONS AND SOCIAL DETERMINANTS OF CARDIOVASCULAR DISEASE

CONTENTS

CONTRIBUTORS

MARIA L. ALCARAZ, BA
Clinical Research Assistant
Division of Clinical Epidemiology
Department of Medicine
Jewish General Hospital
McGill University
Montreal, Quebec, Canada

EMMANUEL E. EGOM, MD, MSc, PHD
Clinician-Lead for Heart Health Clinic and
    Hearts in Motion Program
Department of Medicine
St Martha's Regional Hospital
Antigonish, Nova Scotia, Canada

INNA ERMEICHOUK, MSc
Clinical Research Assistant
Division of Clinical Epidemiology
Department of Medicine
Jewish General Hospital
McGill University
Montreal, Quebec, Canada

CAROLINE FRANCK, MSc
Clinical Research Assistant
Division of Clinical Epidemiology
Department of Medicine
Jewish General Hospital/McGill University
Montreal, Quebec, Canada

SARAH B. WINDLE, MPH
Clinical Research Associate
Division of Clinical Epidemiology
Department of Medicine
Jewish General Hospital
McGill University
Montreal, Quebec, Canada

PREFACE

Cardiology Board Review and Self-Assessment is an all-inclusive study guide written to complement the 14th Edition of *Hurst's The Heart*. Edited by Drs. Valentin Fuster, Robert A. Harrington, Jagat Narula, and Zubin J. Eapen, the 14th Edition of *Hurst's The Heart* is an exhaustive and thorough state-of-the-art review of the entire field of cardiovascular medicine.

Cardiology Board Review contains over 1100 questions and answers presented in a multiple-choice format. Each of the 112 chapters of *Hurst's The Heart* is represented in *Cardiology Board Review* with 10 multiple-choice questions. Detailed answers are provided for each question including not only an explanation of why the correct answer is correct but also why incorrect answers are incorrect. Questions and answers correspond to appropriate sections of *Hurst's The Heart* and include tables, figures, and references. The more than 1100 questions presented in *Cardiology Board Review* span the depth and breadth of the fascinating field of cardiovascular medicine.

Cardiology Board Review is designed to be a study guide for individuals preparing to take the Subspecialty Examination in Cardiovascular Disease given by the American Board of Internal Medicine. Thus, *Cardiology Board Review* will be of particular interest to cardiology fellows preparing to take the board examination for the first time and for practicing cardiologists preparing to take the board examination as part of their recertification process. *Cardiology Board Review* will also be of interest to medical students, residents, fellows, practicing physicians, and other health care professionals who wish to advance their knowledge of cardiovascular medicine.

The current generation of health care professionals increasingly obtains their knowledge from nontraditional formats. To that end, *Cardiology Board Review and Self-Assessment* is available in multiple electronic formats in addition to the traditional print format. The book will be available in print, e-book, and online on McGraw-Hill Education's cardiology web site at www.AccessCardiology.com.

It has been my distinct pleasure to work with four coauthors while preparing *Cardiology Board Review*: Drs. Jonathan Afilalo, Jacqueline E. Joza, Ravi Karra, and Patrick R. Lawler. Each of us contributed original questions and answers corresponding to our particular areas of expertise. We would like to thank the members of the editorial and production departments at McGraw-Hill Education with whom we worked, including Karen Edmonson, Robert Pancotti, and Shivani Salhotra. We would also like to acknowledge the contributions and assistance of a number of other individuals, including Maria L. Alcaraz, Emmanuel E. Egom, Inna Ermeichouk, Caroline Franck, and Sarah B. Windle. Finally, on behalf of myself and my coauthors, we would like to express thanks to our families and colleagues for their encouragement and forbearance during the many months it took to prepare this study guide.

Taking care of patients with cardiovascular disease is an honor and a privilege. Many of these patients have life-threatening conditions that require advanced knowledge and highly technical skills. It is our responsibility, as health care professionals, to ensure that our knowledge and skills match the needs of our patients. It is our hope that you will find *Cardiology Board Review and Self-Assessment* to be an essential and valuable tool in your study of the ever expanding and always fascinating field of cardiovascular medicine.

Mark J. Eisenberg, MD, MPH

CREDITS FOR FIGURES AND TABLES

The following figures and tables have been used with permission from this McGraw-Hill Education publication:

Fuster V, Harrington RA, Narula J, Eapen ZJ, eds. *Hurst's The Heart.* 14th ed. New York: McGraw-Hill Education; 2017:

Chapter 9: Figure 9-1.
Chapter 11: Figures 11-1, 11-2, and 11-3.
Chapter 14: Figures 14-1, 14-2, 14-3, and 14-4.
Chapter 15: Figures 15-1, 15-2, 15-3, 15-4, 15-5, 15-6, 15-7, and 15-8.
Chapter 16: Figures 16-1, 16-2, 16-3, 16-4, and 16-5.
Chapter 17: Figures 17-1, 17-2, 17-3, 17-4, and 17-5.
Chapter 18: Figures 18-1 and 18-2.
Chapter 19: Figures 19-1, 19-2, 19-3, and 19-4.
Chapter 20: Figure 20-1.
Chapter 33: Figure 33-1.
Chapter 34: Figure 34-2.
Chapter 39: Figure 39-1 and Tables 39-1 and 39-2.
Chapter 40: Table 40-1.
Chapter 45: Table 45-1.
Chapter 55: Figure 55-2.
Chapter 59: Figure 59-1.
Chapter 61: Figure 61-1.
Chapter 63: Figure 63-1.
Chapter 66: Tables 66-1 and 66-2.
Chapter 72: Figure 72-1.
Chapter 74: Figure 74-1.
Chapter 76: Tables 76-1 and 76-2.
Chapter 78: Figure 78-1.
Chapter 80: Figure 80-1.
Chapter 82: Figure 82-1.
Chapter 86: Figure 86-1.
Chapter 89: Figure 89-1.
Chapter 94: Table 94-1.
Chapter 111: Figure 111-1.

Data from Fuster V, Alexander RW, O'Rourke RA, et al. *Hurst's The Heart.* 11th ed. New York: McGraw-Hill; 2004:

Chapter 5: Figure 5-1.

SECTION 1

Cardiovascular Disease: Past, Present, and Future

CHAPTER 1

A History of the Cardiac Diseases, and the Development of Cardiovascular Medicine as a Specialty

Mark J. Eisenberg

QUESTIONS

DIRECTIONS: Choose the one best response to each question.

1-1. All of the following were experimental questions asked by William Harvey *except*:

A. What is the relationship of the motion of the auricle to the ventricle?
B. Do the arteries distend because of the propulsive force of the heart?
C. What purpose is served by the orientation of the cardiac and venous valves?
D. How much blood is present, and how long does its passage take?
E. All were questions asked by William Harvey

1-2. What were the primary component(s) of the clinical examination until the 17th century?

A. Palpating the pulse
B. Palpating the pulse and inspecting the urine
C. Palpating the pulse and percussion
D. Palpating the pulse and auscultation
E. Palpating the pulse, percussion, and auscultation

1-3. Which physician received the Nobel Prize for his work in electrophysiology?

A. Albert von Kölliker
B. Heinrich Müller
C. Augustus Waller
D. Willem Einthoven
E. Thomas Lewis

1-4. Who performed the first cardiac catheterization in a human?

A. Werner Forssmann
B. Claude Bernard
C. Dickinson Richards
D. Etienne Jules Marey
E. André Cournand

1-5. From which Latin word is the term *angina* appropriated?

A. Pain
B. Stress
C. Strangulation
D. Anxiety
E. Discomfort

1-6. Before the defibrillator and coronary care units, the in-hospital mortality associated with acute myocardial infarction was approximately:

A. 10%
B. 15%
C. 20%
D. 30%
E. 40%

1-7. Who first described audible heart murmurs?

A. James Hope
B. John Mayow
C. William Cowper
D. René Laennec
E. Raymond Vieussens

1-8. Which procedure pioneered by Helen Taussig and Alfred Blalock was a pivotal breakthrough in thinking about congenital heart abnormalities?

A. Balloon atrial septostomy
B. Subclavian-pulmonary artery shunt
C. Closure of atrial septal defect
D. Closure of ventricular septal defect
E. Stenting of patent ductus arteriosus

1-9. Who invented the first device for measuring blood pressure?

A. Etienne Jules Marey
B. Jean Poiseuille
C. Scipione Riva-Rocci
D. Karl von Vierordt
E. Carl Ludwig

1-10. Which of the following statements about hypertension is *false*?

A. In 1913, Janeway showed that patients, once diagnosed with hypertensive heart disease and symptoms, lived an average of 4 to 5 years
B. Until the latter half of the 20th century, the asymptomatic state of most patients with hypertension and a prevalent view that lowering the blood pressure would be deleterious to the kidney and brain lulled most physicians into accepting the condition as being normally associated with aging
C. Effective oral treatment was available before President Franklin Roosevelt's death in 1945 from severe hypertension
D. In the 1970s, reports from the Framingham Heart Study showed hypertension to be a major contributing cause to stroke, heart attack, and heart and kidney failure
E. Richard Bright's 1836 discovery of the relationship of cardiac hypertrophy and dropsy to shrunken kidneys introduced the kidneys as a cause of heart failure long before hypertension was known

1-1. **The answer is E.** (*Hurst's the Heart, 14th Edition, Chap. 1*) Starting in 1603, Harvey dissected the anatomy and observed the motion of the cardiac chambers and the flow of blood in more than 80 species of animals. His experimental questions "to seek unbiased truth" can be summarized in the following questions: What is the relationship of the motion of the auricle to the ventricle? Which is the systolic and which is the diastolic motion of the heart? Do the arteries distend because of the propulsive force of the heart? What purpose is served by the orientation of the cardiac and venous valves? How does blood travel from the right ventricle to the left side of the heart? Which direction does the blood flow in the veins and the arteries? How much blood is present, and how long does its passage take? After many experiments and without knowledge of the capillary circulation of the lungs, which was not known until 1661, Harvey stated, "It must of necessity be concluded that the blood is driven into a round by a circular motion and that it moves perpetually; and hence does arise the action or function of the heart, which by pulsation it performs." This was published in 1628 as *Exercitatio Anatomica de Motu Cordis et Sanguinis in Animalibus.*[1] This revolutionary concept eventually became accepted in Harvey's lifetime and remains the foundation of our understanding of the purpose of the heart.

1-2. **The answer is B.** (*Hurst's the Heart, 14th Edition, Chap. 1*) Until the 17th century, the clinical examination consisted of palpating the pulse and inspecting the urine to reveal disease and predict prognosis. Percussion was first suggested in 1761 by Leopold Auenbrugger, a Viennese physician, who published a book proposing "percussion of the human thorax, whereby, according to the character of the particular sounds thence elicited, an opinion is formed of the internal state of that cavity."[2] It was reintroduced by Jean-Nicolas Corvisart in early 19th-century France and became an essential addition to the chest examination until it was mostly supplanted by the chest x-ray. While auscultation of the chest was first practiced by Hippocrates (460-370 BC), who applied his ear directly to the chest, it was not until the mid-19th century that the stethoscope (first invented by René Laennec in Paris in 1816) moved auscultation to the forefront of the clinical examination.[3,4]

1-3. **The answer is D.** (*Hurst's the Heart, 14th Edition, Chap. 1*) In 1856, von Kölliker and Müller demonstrated that the heart also produced electricity. Augustus Waller, with a capillary electrometer device (1887), detected cardiac electricity from the limbs, a crude recording that he called an "electrogram." Willem Einthoven, a physiologist in Utrecht, devised a more sensitive string galvanometer (1902), for which he received the Nobel Prize, and the modern electrocardiogram was born. Initially weighing 600 lb and requiring five people to operate, the three-lead electrocardiograph would eventually become portable, 12 leads, routine, and capable of providing both static and continuous recordings of cardiac rhythm.[5] With the electrocardiogram, the activation and sequence of stimulation of the human heart could now be measured, and the anatomic basis for the conduction system confirmed. Thomas Lewis in London was the first to realize its great potential, beginning in 1909, and his books on disorders of the heartbeat became essential for aspiring electrocardiographers.[2,6]

1-4. **The answer is A.** (*Hurst's the Heart, 14th Edition, Chap. 1*) Claude Bernard in 1844 was the first to insert a catheter into the hearts of animals to measure temperature and pressure.[2] In the early 1860s, Auguste Chauveau, a veterinary physiologist, and Etienne Jules Marey, inventor of the sphygmograph, collaborated to develop a system of devices called sounds, forerunners of the modern cardiac catheter, which they used to catheterize the right heart and left ventricle of the horse.[7] Cardiac catheterization in humans was thought an inconceivable risk until Werner Forssmann, a 29-year-old surgical resident in Germany, performed a self-catheterization in 1929.[8,9] Interested in discovering a method of injecting adrenaline to treat cardiac arrest, Forssmann passed a ureteral catheter into his antecubital vein and confirmed its right atrial position using x-ray. The next year he tried to image his heart using an iodide injection. However, he was reprimanded by superiors and did not experiment further.

Catheterization began in earnest in the early 1940s in New York and London. André Cournand and Dickinson Richards at Bellevue, interested in respiratory physiology, developed and demonstrated the safety of complete right heart catheterization, for which they shared the Nobel Prize with Forssmann in 1956.[7,10]

1-5. **The answer is C.** *(Hurst's the Heart, 14th Edition, Chap. 1)* On July 21, 1768, William Heberden presented "Some Account of a Disorder of the Breast" to the Royal College of Physicians, London: "But there is a disorder of the breast marked with strong and peculiar symptoms, considerable for the kind of danger belonging to it, and not extremely rare. The seat of it, and sense of strangling and anxiety with which it is attended, may make it not improperly be called angina pectoris."[2,11] Heberden appropriated the term *angina* from the Latin word for strangling. His classic account marks the beginning of our appreciation of coronary artery disease and myocardial ischemia. Edward Jenner and Caleb Parry were the first to suspect a coronary etiology, which Parry published in 1799. Allan Burns, in Scotland, likened the pain of angina pectoris to the discomfort brought about by walking with a tight ligature placed on a limb (1809), a prescient concept that remains relevant today.

1-6. **The answer is D.** *(Hurst's the Heart, 14th Edition, Chap. 1)* Before the defibrillator and coronary care units, the in-hospital mortality associated with acute myocardial infarction was approximately 30%. With the development of the defibrillator by William Kouwenhoven, Claude Beck and Paul Zoll were able to prove that rescue of cardiac arrest victims was possible. Beck's concept that "the heart is too good to die" instilled optimism into the care of coronary patients and aggressiveness into their providers. Myocardial infarction was no longer a disease to be watched but rather one that might benefit from aggressive therapeutic interventions. Zoll reported closed chest defibrillation in 1956 and cardioversion of ventricular tachycardia in 1960. The monitoring of patients in close proximity to skilled nursing personnel who could perform cardiopulmonary resuscitation was a logical next step suggested by Desmond Julian in 1961.

1-7. **The answer is D.** *(Hurst's the Heart, 14th Edition, Chap. 1)* Valvular pathology was described in the 17th and 18th centuries; however, Laennec was the first to describe audible heart murmurs, calling them "blowing, sawing, filing, and rasping."[3] Originally, he attributed the noises to actual valvular disease, but he later decided that they were caused by spasm or contraction of a cardiac chamber. James Hope in England was the first to classify valvular murmurs in *A Treatise on the Diseases of the Heart and Great Vessels* (1832).[12] He interpreted physical findings in early physiologic terms and provided detailed pathologic correlations.[13] Constriction of the mitral valve was recorded by John Mayow (1668) and Raymond Vieussens (1715); the latter also recognized that this condition could cause pulmonary congestion.[14] The presystolic murmur of mitral stenosis was described by Bertin (1824), timed as both early diastolic and presystolic by Williams (1835), and placed on firmer grounds by Fauvel (1843) and Gairdner (1861). Aortic stenosis was first described pathologically by Rivière (1663), and Laennec pointed out that the aortic valve was subject to ossification (1819).[15] Corvisart showed an astute grasp of the natural history of aortic stenosis (1809). Early descriptions of aortic regurgitation were by William Cowper (1706) and Raymond Vieussens (1715),[16] whereas Giovanni Morgagni recognized the hemodynamic consequences of aortic regurgitation (1761). In 1832, Corrigan provided his classic description of the arterial pulse and murmur of aortic regurgitation. Flint added that the presystolic murmur was sometimes heard with severe aortic regurgitation (1862).[4]

1-8. **The answer is B.** *(Hurst's the Heart, 14th Edition, Chap. 1)* The pivotal breakthrough in thinking about congenital abnormalities came from Helen Taussig and Alfred Blalock at Johns Hopkins Hospital with their "blue baby operation." Taussig had observed that patients with cyanotic heart disease worsened when their ductus arteriosus closed. She suggested creating an artificial ductus to improve oxygenation.[17] Blalock, assisted by Vivian Thomas, successfully created a shunt from the subclavian to the pulmonary artery in November 1944. This innovative operation, in which a blue baby was dramatically changed to a pink one—the Blalock-Taussig shunt—was highly publicized, and other operations soon followed. These include closure of atrial septal defects (1950s), closure of ventricular septal defects (1954), and tetralogy of Fallot repair (1954). In 1966, Rashkind introduced the balloon septostomy, a novel catheter therapeutic technique that bought time for severely cyanotic infants with transposition of the great arteries.[7] In the 1980s, catheters were adapted to dilate stenotic aortic and pulmonic valves as well as aortic coarctation. Today, transcatheter closure of patent ductus arteriosus (1971), atrial septal defects (1976), and ventricular septal defects (1987) has become routine. Indomethacin therapy to enable closure of a patent ductus in the premature infant (1976) and prostaglandin infusion to maintain ductal patency (1981) profoundly changed the medical management of fragile newborns. Stents now help keep the ductus open as well as alleviate right ventricular obstruction in tetralogy of Fallot.

1-9. **The answer is B.** (*Hurst's the Heart, 14th Edition, Chap. 1*) Stephen Hales, an English country parson, reported in his *Statical Essays* (1733) that the arterial blood pressure of the cannulated artery of a recumbent horse rose more than eight feet above the heart—the first true measurement of arterial pressure and the beginning of sphygmometry.[2,18,19] His pioneering efforts stood alone until 1828 when Jean Poiseuille introduced a mercury manometer device to measure blood pressure.[20,21] Over the next 60 years, various sphygmomanometric methods were developed—notably by Ludwig (1847), Vierordt (1855), and Marey (1863)—to refine the measurement of the arterial pressure. An inflatable arm cuff coupled to the sphygmograph, a device small enough to allow measurement outside the laboratory, was invented by Riva-Rocci (1896), who also noted the "white-coat effect" on blood pressure.[22] Nicolai Korotkoff, a Russian military surgeon, first auscultated brachial arterial sounds (1905), a discovery that marked the advent of modern blood pressure recording. This auscultatory approach eventually ensured its widespread use by the 1920s. In 1939, blood pressure recordings were standardized by committees of the American Heart Association (AHA) and the Cardiac Society of Great Britain and Ireland.

1-10. **The answer is C.** (*Hurst's the Heart, 14th Edition, Chap. 1*) President Franklin Roosevelt's death in 1945 from severe hypertension and stroke called international attention to the consequences of hypertension and its inadequate treatment—he had been managed with diet, digitalis, and phenobarbital. Effective oral treatment became possible in 1949, first with reserpine and then with hydrochlorothiazide.[23] Lumbar sympathectomy and adrenalectomy (1925), the last resort, was abandoned. Subsequently, β-adrenergic blockers, calcium channel blockers, ACE inhibitors, angiotensin receptor blocking agents, and direct renin inhibitors have brought antihypertensive relief to many. Severe salt restriction, as practiced earlier with the Kempner rice diet, has taken a lesser role, whereas the Dietary Approaches to Stop Hypertension (DASH) diet, exercise, and alcohol restriction are encouraged. Since 1973, recommendations published by the Joint National Committee (JNC) on Detection, Evaluation, and Treatment of High Blood Pressure have been very helpful.

References

1. Harvey W. *Anatomical Studies on the Motion of the Heart and Blood.* Leake CD, trans. Springfield, IL: Charles C Thomas; 1970.
2. Acierno LJ. *The History of Cardiology.* London, UK: Parthenon; 1994.
3. Duffin JM. The cardiology of RTH Laënnec. *Med Hist.* 1989;33:42-71.
4. Hanna IR, Silverman ME. A history of cardiac auscultation and some of its contributors. *Am J Cardiol.* 2002;90:259-267.
5. Burch GE, DePasquale NP. *A History of Electrocardiography.* Chicago, IL: Year Book; 1964.
6. Fleming P. *A Short History of Cardiology.* Amsterdam, Netherlands: Rodopi; 1997.
7. Bing RJ. *Cardiology: The Evolution of the Science and the Art.* Basel, Switzerland: Harwood; 1992.
8. Forssmann-Falck R. Werner Forssmann: a pioneer of cardiology. *Am J Cardiol.* 1997;79: 651-660.
9. Mueller RL, Sanborn TA. The history of interventional cardiology: cardiac catheterization, angioplasty, and related interventions. *Am Heart J.* 1995;129:146-172.
10. Fishman AP, Dickinson WR. *Circulation of the Blood: Men and Ideas.* Bethesda, MD: American Physiological Society; 1982.
11. Leibowitz JO. *The History of Coronary Heart Disease.* Berkeley, CA: University of California Press; 1970.
12. Flaxman N. The hope of cardiology: James Hope (1801–1841). *Bull Hist Med.* 1938;6:1-21.
13. Vander Veer JB. Mitral insufficiency: historical and clinical aspects. *Am J Cardiol.* 1958;2:5-10.
14. Rolleston H. The history of mitral stenosis. *Br Heart J.* 1941;3:1-12.

15. Vaslef SN, Roberts WC. Early descriptions of aortic valve stenosis. *Am Heart J*. 1993;125:1465-1474.

16. Vaslef SN, Roberts WC. Early descriptions of aortic regurgitation. *Am Heart J*. 1993;125:1475-1483.

17. Engle MA. Growth and development of state of the art care for people with congenital heart disease. *J Am Coll Cardiol*. 1989;13:1453-1457.

18. Willius FA, Dry TJ. *A History of the Heart and the Circulation*. Philadelphia, PA: Saunders; 1948.

19. Naqvi NH, Blaufox MD. *Blood Pressure Measurement: An Illustrated History*. New York, NY: Parthenon; 1998.

20. Dustan HP. History of clinical hypertension: from 1827 to 1970. In: Oparil S, Weber MA, eds. *Hypertension: A Companion to Brenner and Rector's The Kidney*. Philadelphia, PA: Saunders; 2000:1-4.

21. Ruskin A. *Classics in Arterial Hypertension*. Springfield, IL: Charles C Thomas; 1956.

22. Posten–Vinay N. *A Century of Arterial Hypertension: 1896-1996*. Chichester, UK: Wiley; 1996.

23. Piepho RW, Beal J. An overview of antihypertensive therapy in the 20th century. *J Clin Pharmacol*. 2000;40:967-977.

CHAPTER 2

The Global Burden of Cardiovascular Diseases

Mark J. Eisenberg

QUESTIONS

DIRECTIONS: Choose the one best response to each question.

2-1. How many deaths worldwide are caused each year by cardiovascular disease (CVD)?

A. 10 million
B. 15 million
C. 17 million
D. 20 million
E. 23 million

2-2. Which of the following statements about global cardiovascular disease (CVD) is *false*?

A. There has been a steady decrease in the age-specific death rate for CVD in both sexes over the past 20 years
B. Women represent 50% of CVD deaths worldwide
C. The total number of deaths from CVD increased more than 40% between 1990 and 2013
D. Increases in gross domestic product are well correlated with reductions in cardiovascular disease mortality
E. A continued increase in the number of CVD deaths is expected as a result of demographic changes worldwide

2-3. What proportion of ischemic heart disease (IHD) patients from low-income world regions are taking *none* of the standard secondary prevention medications?

A. 20%
B. 30%
C. 40%
D. 60%
E. 80%

2-4. Which noncommunicable disease (NCD) is the second most common cause of all disability globally?

A. Stroke
B. Ischemic heart disease
C. Chronic obstructive pulmonary disease
D. Lower back and neck pain
E. Depression

2-5. Which of the following cardiovascular diseases are more commonly diagnosed in men than in women worldwide?

A. Abdominal aortic aneurysm
B. Peripheral arterial disease
C. Atrial fibrillation
D. Both A and B
E. Both A and C

2-6. What is the most common complication of infective endocarditis?

A. Stroke
B. Embolization other than stroke
C. Heart failure
D. Intracardiac abscess
E. Intracardiac fistula

2-7. Which of the following statements about Chagas disease is *false*?

A. Chagas disease is primarily transmitted through the bites of the *Triatoma infestans* insect
B. No rapid diagnostic tests are available to detect the causative parasite
C. The acute phase immediately following infection is often asymptomatic, but it produces fever and malaise in up to 5% of people
D. More than 50% of those infected will not progress to chronic Chagas disease
E. Approximately 30% of those infected will develop chronic cardiovascular Chagas disease

2-8. What percentage of patients with acute rheumatic fever will develop rheumatic heart disease (RHD)?

A. 50%
B. 60%
C. 70%
D. 80%
E. 90%

2-9. Which modifiable cardiovascular risk factor is responsible for the most morbidity and mortality worldwide?

A. Low fruit intake
B. High body mass index
C. High sodium
D. High blood pressure
E. Smoking

2-10. In 2013, the WHO and all member states (194 countries) agreed to a Global Non-Communicable Disease (NCD) Action Plan, which aims to reduce the number of premature deaths from NCDs by 25% by 2025 through nine voluntary global targets. Which of the following is *not* one of the nine voluntary targets?

A. A 20% relative reduction in daily exposure to outdoor and indoor air pollution
B. A 30% relative reduction in the prevalence of current tobacco use in persons aged 15 years and over
C. A 25% relative reduction in the prevalence of raised blood pressure or else containing the prevalence of raised blood pressure, according to national circumstances
D. A halt in the rise of diabetes and obesity
E. At least 50% of eligible people receiving drug therapy and counseling (including glycemic control) to prevent heart attacks and strokes

2-1. The answer is C. *(Hurst's The Heart, 14th Edition, Chap. 2)* In 2013, more than 17 million people died from CVDs, with an estimated US $863 billion in direct health care costs and productivity losses worldwide.[1] As a result of the large populations in many low- and middle-income countries (LMICs), nearly 70% of CVD deaths occurred in LMICs. CVDs account for 50% of all NCD deaths in the world each year and represent a significant threat to human welfare and sustainable development. CVDs are the leading cause of death in every region of the world, with the exceptions of sub-Saharan Africa—where infectious diseases are still the leading cause of death—and South Korea and Japan, where cancers cause more deaths. The leading cause of CVD-related death was IHD, accounting for more than eight million deaths, followed by ischemic and hemorrhagic strokes, with more than three million deaths each. Rheumatic heart disease, although not the leading cause of death, was a significant contributor to the global burden and a leading cause of highly preventable death, with approximately 275,000 deaths in 2013.

2-2. The answer is D. *(Hurst's The Heart, 14th Edition, Chap. 2)* Despite the steady decrease in death rate for both sexes over the past 20 years, the total number of deaths is increasing as a result of population growth and aging, which disproportionately affects low- and middle-income countries (LMICs). Globally, the total number of CVD deaths increased from 12.3 to 17.3 million, a 41% increase between 1990 and 2013.[2] Women represent 50% of these deaths. Although most countries have seen an increased national income per capita over this time, the decrease in the number of CVD deaths cannot be entirely explained by economic growth. The decline in age-specific CVD mortality does not correlate well with increases in country income, except weakly in upper-middle income countries. Therefore, it appears unlikely that economic growth alone will improve a country's burden of CVD. Despite an overall decrease in the global age-specific CVD death rate, a continued increase in the number of CVD deaths is expected as a result of demographic changes. The United Nations estimated that the global population in 2015 was 7.3 billion and will increase to a total of 8.5 billion by 2025 and 9.7 billion by 2050. When population growth slows down as a result of a reduction in fertility, the population ages, and the proportion of older persons aged 60 or older increases over time. In 2015, about 10% of the population was aged 60 or older, and the number of adults in this age group is projected to more than double by 2050 and more than triple by 2100, with more than two-thirds of these older adults residing in LMICs.

2-3. The answer is E. *(Hurst's The Heart, 14th Edition, Chap. 2)* Ischemic heart disease is the leading cause of death worldwide, encompassing myocardial infarction and all other acute coronary syndromes as well as long-term sequelae of coronary heart disease, including angina pectoris and ischemic cardiomyopathy. Since the 1990s, the high-income regions, specifically Australasia, Western Europe, and North America, have seen dramatic declines in the age-standardized IHD mortality.[3] However, IHD mortality has increased in other regions, including Central Asia, South Asia, and East Asia. Although IHD burden falls largely on those aged older than 70 years in high-income regions, the age of IHD deaths is much lower in other regions, with a mean age of onset of IHD events before age 50 years in more than 29% of males and 24% of females in North Africa/Middle East and South Asia.[3,4] As more patients with IHD survive their initial event, the IHD death rate and case fatality will no longer be the sole public health benchmark for success; improved symptom control and overall quality of life and access to adequate treatment will be important secondary outcomes.[3] The mainstays of treatment include standard, low-cost medications that are insufficiently used in low- and middle-income countries (LMICs). The Prospective Urban Rural Epidemiological (PURE) study found that only 11% of patients from high-income countries were not taking standard secondary prevention medications, whereas 80% of low-income-region patients were taking none of the recommended medications.[5,6]

2-4. The answer is A. *(Hurst's The Heart, 14th Edition, Chap. 2)* Stroke was the second largest contributor to disability globally and in developing countries, whereas it was the third largest contributor to disability in developed countries (after IHD and lower back and neck pain).[7] Globally, the proportional contribution of stroke-related disability-adjusted life years (DALYs) as a proportion of all diseases increased from 3.5% in 1990 to 4.6% in 2013. The deaths caused by stroke also increased from 9.7% in 1990 to 11.8% in 2013. In order to reduce the rising burden of stroke worldwide, urgent prevention and management strategies are needed. Prevention of risk factors remains key to reversing the stroke pandemic, and universal access to organized stroke services must remain a priority, especially in LMICs.[8] In 2013, the top five noncommunicable causes of disability globally (from most to least) were: IHD, stroke, lower back and neck pain, chronic obstructive pulmonary disorder, and depression.[9]

2-5. **The answer is E.** (*Hurst's The Heart, 14th Edition, Chap. 2*) Abdominal aortic aneurysm (AAA) and atrial fibrillation (AF) are more commonly diagnosed in men than in women worldwide, while peripheral arterial disease (PAD) is equally common among men and women in developed countries, and it is more often diagnosed in women than in men in developing countries. AAA is a focal dilation of the abdominal aorta of at least 1.5 times the normal diameter or an absolute value of 3 cm or greater. Risk factors include male sex, smoking, hypertension, atherosclerosis, and history of AAA in a first-degree relative. In 2010, the age-specific prevalence rate per 100,000 ranged from 7.9 to 2274. Prevalence was higher in developed versus developing nations. The age-specific annual incidence rate per 100,000 ranged between 0.83 and 164.6.[10] AF and atrial flutter are irregular heart rhythms that often cause a rapid heart rate and can increase the risk of stroke, heart failure, and other heart-related complications. In 2010, the estimated age-standardized DALYs resulting from AF was 65 per 100,000 population in males and 46 in females, which was an increase of 18.8% and 19% for males and females since 1990, respectively.[11] Higher burden in men compared with women may reflect actual disease rates or poorer access to medical care among women in resource-poor settings. PAD is a circulatory problem in which narrowed arteries reduce blood flow to the limbs and cause symptoms of leg pain with walking (claudication). PAD is defined as an ankle brachial index lower than or equal to 0.90. In developed countries, among adults aged 45–49 years, the prevalence is similar for males and females and is around 5%. The prevalence increases to around 18% for males and females in those aged 85 to 89 years.[12] In developing countries, for the same age groups, the prevalence is around 6% for females and 3% for males and increases to 15% in females and 14% in males.[12]

2-6. **The answer is C.** (*Hurst's The Heart, 14th Edition, Chap. 2*) Infective endocarditis (IE) is an infection caused by bacteria, or other infectious pathogens, that enter the bloodstream and cause inflammation in the heart tissues, often on a valve. Because of the lack of direct blood supply, the heart valves are particularly susceptible to bacterial colonization and are neither protected by the typical immune response nor easily reached by antibiotics. IE is a serious illness, with up to 22% in-hospital and 40% five-year mortality rates.[13] A global collaboration was formed to assess the current characteristics of patients with IE via a large, prospective multicenter registry, called the International Collaboration on Endocarditis (ICE). ICE found that contemporary infective endocarditis is most often an acute disease with a high rate of infection with *Staphylococcus aureus* and involving the mitral (41.1%) and aortic (37.6%) valves. Common complications included stroke (16.9%), embolization other than stroke (22.6%), heart failure (32.3%), and intracardiac abscess (14.4%); these often required surgical intervention (48.2%). In-hospital mortality was high (17.7%).[14] Unfortunately, there were few sites in Asia and Africa included in the registry, which limits the ability to assess geographic differences in patient and microbiologic characteristics in these areas. IE is estimated to have resulted in 65,000 deaths and 1.9 million DALYs in 2013. More complete knowledge and improved surveillance are needed in all world regions.[15]

2-7. **The answer is B.** (*Hurst's The Heart, 14th Edition, Chap. 2*) Chagas disease is a disease of poverty and is localized to Latin America because it is primarily transmitted through bites from the nocturnal "kissing bug," *Triatoma infestans*, which is endemic to this region. The infection can be asymptomatic, but it can eventually lead to premature morbidity and mortality, especially in young women of childbearing age. There are rapid diagnostic tests that can detect the causative parasite, *Trypanosoma cruzi*, in serum and can diagnose chronic infections. Pesticides have been developed for vector control programs, but much is still unknown about this disease. In any case, prevention and elimination of the vector remain the keys to Chagas control. The disease has three phases: acute, indeterminate, and chronic. The acute phase immediately follows infection and is often asymptomatic, but it produces fever and malaise in up to 5% of people. The indeterminate phase is asymptomatic, with more than 50% of those infected remaining in this phase for life without any long-term sequelae. After a decade or more, approximately 30% of people will experience chronic cardiovascular Chagas disease, with symptoms including heart failure, arrhythmias, and thromboembolism.[16] Deaths are rare in the acute phase, and most deaths attributable to Chagas disease result from downstream cardiovascular sequelae. In addition, approximately 15%–20% of people will experience chronic gastrointestinal disease sequelae, including megaesophagus and megacolon. Between 5 and 18 million people are currently infected, and the infection is estimated to cause more than 10,000 deaths annually.[17]

2-8. **The answer is B.** *(Hurst's The Heart, 14th Edition, Chap. 2)* Rheumatic heart disease is an endemic disease that is common in settings of poverty. It is caused by group A streptococcus infection and leads to mitral stenosis and premature mortality, particularly in young, predominantly female, poorer individuals living in Oceania, South Asia, Central Asia, Africa, and the Middle East. Approximately 60% of all acute rheumatic fever cases will develop RHD, based on data from Aboriginal Australian populations, and 1.5% of patients with RHD will die each year.[18] Globally in 2010, RHD affected more than 34 million people, causing more than 345,000 deaths, almost all in LMICs.[19] The disease can progress to cause moderate to severe multivalvular disease, leading to congestive heart failure, pulmonary hypertension, or AF. RHD also contributes (3%–7.5%) to an estimated 144,000–360,000 incident strokes each year.

2-9. **The answer is D.** *(Hurst's The Heart, 14th Edition, Chap. 2)* Elevated blood pressure is estimated to be the single largest contributor to the global burden of disease and global mortality. There are gaps in the awareness, treatment, and control of hypertension globally. High blood pressure in populations appears to occur in tandem with economic development, but notably in the highest income countries, individuals with lower socioeconomic status are the group most likely to be untreated.[20,21] In Africa, hypertension is thought to be the leading cause of heart failure, whereas at global levels, hypertension is linked to the development of atherosclerotic vascular disease. In high-income countries, it is estimated to be responsible for 25% of deaths from stroke, 20% of deaths from IHD, and more than 17% of all global deaths.[22] The number of people with uncontrolled hypertension was 978 million in 2008, a substantial increase from 605 million in 1980, largely because of population growth and aging.[23] Other modifiable cardiovascular risk factors are: high body mass index, low fruit intake, smoking, high sodium, and high total cholesterol.[24]

2-10. **The answer is A.** *(Hurst's The Heart, 14th Edition, Chap. 2)* While a reduction in exposure to outdoor and indoor air pollution is not one of the nine targets, such pollution ranks as the largest single environmental health risk factor, with more than 2.9 million deaths attributed to outdoor air pollution and a similar number attributed to indoor air pollution.[25] Air pollution has been shown to increase preclinical cardiovascular risk factors such as atherosclerosis, endothelial dysfunction, and hypertension. The estimated excess risk of cardiovascular mortality rises 11% per 10 $\mu g/m^3$ rise in levels of particulate matter, with no threshold level below which long-term exposure to urban air pollution has no ill effect on cardiovascular health.[26] Answers B through E: Modeling studies have shown that significant reductions in premature CVD are possible by 2025 if multiple risk factor targets are achieved. Globally, the risk factor change that would lead to the largest reduction in premature mortality would be the decreased prevalence of hypertension, followed by tobacco smoking prevalence for men and obesity for women.

References

1. Bloom DE, Cafiero E, Jané-Llopis E, et al. The global economic burden of noncommunicable diseases. Program on the Global Demography of Aging, World Economic Forum, 2011.
2. Roth GA, Huffman MD, Moran AE, et al. Global and regional patterns in cardiovascular mortality from 1990 to 2013. *Circulation.* 2015;132:1667-1678.

3. Moran AE, Forouzanfar MH, Roth GA, et al. The global burden of ischemic heart disease in 1990 and 2010: the Global Burden of Disease 2010 study. *Circulation*. 2014;129:1493-1501.

4. Moran AE, Tzong KY, Forouzanfar MH, et al. Variations in ischemic heart disease burden by age, country, and income: The Global Burden of Diseases, Injuries, and Risk Factors 2010 study. *Glob Heart*. 2014;9:91-99.

5. Yusuf S, Islam S, Chow CK, et al. Use of secondary prevention drugs for cardiovascular disease in the community in high-income, middle-income, and low-income countries (the PURE Study): a prospective epidemiological survey. *Lancet*. 2011;378:1231-1243.

6. Khatib R, McKee M, Shannon H, et al. Availability and affordability of cardiovascular disease medicines and their effect on use in high-income, middle-income, and low-income countries: an analysis of the PURE study data. *Lancet*. 2016;387:61-69.

7. Barker-Collo S, Bennett DA, Krishnamurthi RV, et al. Sex differences in stroke incidence, prevalence, mortality and disability-adjusted life years: results from the Global Burden of Disease study 2013. *Neuroepidemiology*. 2015;45:203-214.

8. Feigin VL, Krishnamurthi R, Bhattacharjee R, et al. New strategy to reduce the global burden of stroke. *Stroke*. 2015 Jun;46(6):1740-1747.

9. Murray CJL, Barber RM, Foreman KJ, et al. Global, regional, and national disability-adjusted life years (DALYs) for 306 diseases and injuries and healthy life expectancy (HALE) for 188 countries, 1990–2013: quantifying the epidemiological transition. *Lancet*. 2015;386:2145-2191.

10. Sampson UK, Norman PE, Fowkes FG, et al. Estimation of global and regional incidence and prevalence of abdominal aortic aneurysms 1990 to 2010. *Glob Heart*. 2014;9:159-170.

11. Chugh SS, Roth GA, Gillum RF, Mensah GA. Global burden of atrial fibrillation in developed and developing nations. *Glob Heart*. 2014;9:113-119.

12. Fowkes FGR, Rudan D, Rudan I, et al. Comparison of global estimates of prevalence and risk factors for peripheral artery disease in 2000 and 2010: a systematic review and analysis. *Lancet*. 2013;382:1329-1340.

13. Bannay A, Hoen B, Duval X, et al. The impact of valve surgery on short- and long-term mortality in left-sided infective endocarditis: do differences in methodological approaches explain previous conflicting results? *Eur Heart J*. 2011;32:2003-2015.

14. Murdoch DR. Clinical presentation, etiology, and outcome of infective endocarditis in the 21st century: the International Collaboration on Endocarditis–Prospective Cohort Study. *Arch Intern Med*. 2009;169:463.

15. Chu VH, Park LP, Athan E, et al. Association between surgical indications, operative risk, and clinical outcome in infective endocarditis: a prospective study from the International Collaboration on Endocarditis. *Circulation*. 2015;131:131-140.

16. Nunes MC, Dones W, Morillo CA, Encina JJ, Ribeiro AL. Chagas disease: an overview of clinical and epidemiological aspects. *J Am Coll Cardiol*. 2013;62:767-776.

17. Stanaway JD, Roth G. The burden of Chagas disease. *Glob Heart*. 2015;10:139-144.

18. Carapetis JR, Steer AC, Mulholland EK, Weber M. The global burden of group A streptococcal diseases. *Lancet Infect Dis*. 2005;5:685-694.

19. Global, regional, and national age-sex specific all-cause and cause-specific mortality for 240 causes of death, 1990-2013: a systematic analysis for the Global Burden of Disease Study 2013. *Lancet*. 2015;385:117-171.

20. Chobanian AV, Bakris GL, Black HR, et al. The Seventh Report of the Joint National Committee on Prevention, Detection, Evaluation, and Treatment of High Blood Pressure: the JNC 7 report. *JAMA*. 2003;289:2560-2572.

21. Colhoun HM, Hemingway H, Poulter NR. Socio-economic status and blood pressure: an overview analysis. *J Hum Hypertens*. 1998;12:91-110.

22. Forouzanfar MH, Alexander L, Anderson HR, et al. Global, regional, and national comparative risk assessment of 79 behavioural, environmental and occupational, and metabolic risks or clusters of risks in 188 countries, 1990-2013: a systematic analysis for the Global Burden of Disease Study 2013. *Lancet*. 2015;386:2287-2323.

23. Danaei G, Finucane MM, Lin JK, et al. National, regional, and global trends in systolic blood pressure since 1980: Systematic analysis of health examination surveys and epidemiological studies with 786 country-years and 5.4 million participants. *Lancet*. 2011;377:568-577.

24. Institute for Health Metrics and Evaluation (IHME). GBD Compare. Seattle, WA: IHME, University of Washington, 2015. Available from http://vizhub.healthdata.org/gbd-compare (Accessed February 2, 2016).

25. GBD 2013 Risk Factors Collaborators. Global, regional and national comparative risk assessment of 79 behavioural, environmental/occupational and metabolic risks or clusters of risks in 188 countries 1990-2013: a systematic analysis for the GBD 2013. *Lancet*. 2015;5;386(10010):2287-3223.

26. Cosselman KE, Navas-Acien A, Kaufman JD. Environmental factors in cardiovascular disease. *Nat Rev Cardiol*. 2015;12:627-642.

CHAPTER 3

Assessing and Improving the Quality of Care in Cardiovascular Medicine

Mark J. Eisenberg

QUESTIONS

DIRECTIONS: Choose the one best response to each question.

3-1. Which of the following statements concerning health care expenditures in the United States is *false*?

A. Health care expenditures accounted for nearly 17.5% of the gross domestic product in 2014
B. The United States invested an estimated $3.0 trillion in health care in 2014
C. Expenditures related to cardiovascular disease were estimated to be $656 billion in 2015
D. The United States health system ranked lowest among 11 similar countries with respect to access, equity, quality, efficiency, and healthy lives, despite spending the most on health care
E. Increasing the use of expensive medical care is associated with better quality of care and patient outcomes

3-2. Which of the following factors influences the variability and appropriateness of health care delivery?

A. Patients' clinical status
B. Sociodemographic factors
C. Providers and facilities
D. Geographic location
E. All of the above

3-3. How many years, on average, does it take for guidelines to be incorporated into clinical practice?

A. 4 years
B. 10 years
C. 13 years
D. 17 years
E. 21 years

3-4. Which of the following is *not* generally considered a part of defining quality of care?

A. Cost of care
B. Evidence-based care
C. Improving outcomes
D. Patient satisfaction
E. All of the above are important for defining quality of care

3-5. Which constitute the primary domains of the Donabedian framework for quality assurance?

A. Structure, process, and outcome
B. Process, outcome, and evaluation
C. Research, guidelines, and implementation
D. Research, structure, and outcome
E. Research, outcome, and cost

3-6. Which of the following is *not* a principal thematic dimension in the Institute of Medicine (IOM)'s landmark report on quality improvement initiatives, *Crossing the Quality Chasm: A New Health System for the 21st Century*?

A. Safety
B. Cost
C. Timeliness
D. Efficiency
E. Equity

3-7. What is the specific function of clinical data standards?

A. To measure and improve access to evidence-based care
B. To enable the reproducible collection of data across hospitals and settings
C. To measure physician performance
D. To measure the quality of clinical trial data
E. To enable the assessment of standards of care

3-8. The ACC/AHA guidelines indicate that percutaneous aortic balloon dilation may be considered a bridge to surgical aortic valve replacement or transcatheter aortic valve replacement for symptomatic patients with severe aortic stenosis (Class IIb, level C).[23] A Class IIb level C recommendation could indicate that the intervention is:

A. Probably indicated, based on data from multiple randomized trials
B. Probably indicated, based on expert opinion
C. Probably indicated, based on case studies
D. Possibly indicated, based on expert opinion
E. Possibly indicated, based on a single randomized trial

3-9. Which of the following tools for improving the quality of cardiovascular care involves quantifying a range of health care processes and outcomes, identifying multiple points in the continuum of care for which clinical inertia (the failure to implement or titrate recommended therapies) can occur, and then selecting those with the strongest evidence and highest correlation with clinically meaningful outcomes?

A. Clinical practice guidelines
B. Clinical data standards
C. Performance measures
D. Appropriate use criteria
E. Procedural registries

3-10. Some of the most exciting opportunities to improve care come from the combination of registries and national coalitions to target significant gaps in care. A dramatic example of this is the Door-to-Balloon (D2B) initiative. Which of the following was *not* a performance recommendation in the D2B initiative?

A. Prompt data feedback to the emergency department and cath lab staff
B. Expectations of having the cath lab team assembled within 30 minutes
C. Targeted times to first ECG acquisition for chest pain patients within 15 minutes
D. Emergency medicine physician activates cath lab
E. Single-call activation of the cath lab

3-1. **The answer is E.** *(Hurst's the Heart, 14th Edition, Chap. 3)* In the United States, health care expenditures accounted for nearly 17.5% of the gross domestic product in 2014 (an estimated $3 trillion) and are expected to reach 19.6% by 2024.[1] Cardiovascular disease (CVD) remains the leading cause of death and disability,[2] with an estimated annual total cost of $656 billion in 2015.[3] In a recent report, the US health system ranked lowest among 11 countries with respect to access, equity, quality, efficiency, and healthy lives,[4] despite spending the most on health care.[5] It is often thought that high-quality health care is dependent on the continued discovery and delivery of novel diagnostic and therapeutic interventions. However, studies suggest that greater use of expensive medical care is actually associated with lower quality and worse outcomes.[6,7] Woolf and Johnson[8] have extended this concept to mathematically quantify the trade-off between the development of new interventions and the more consistent delivery of known therapies. They argue that despite tremendous scientific and technologic advancements, the failure to consistently deliver proven therapies dilutes and reduces the overall quality of a health care system. Thus, money spent on improving this actual delivery of care may be equally or even more critical than money spent on improving technology to result in improved quality of both routine and specialized health care.

3-2. **The answer is E.** *(Hurst's the Heart, 14th Edition, Chap. 3)* A critical goal of efforts to disseminate high-quality care is to ensure rational and efficient use of effective treatment to those who derive the most benefit.[9] Yet surveys evaluating processes of care have shown that, on an average, only one in two US adults receives recommended care when receiving health care services.[10] Several studies have suggested that there are marked variations in the use of evidence-based treatments of cardiovascular disease (CVD) based on gender, age, race, education, income, and insurance status.[10,11,12,13] A study examining differences in the treatment of myocardial infarction showed that although blacks lived closer than whites to hospitals with revascularization capability that were considered high-quality, they were less likely than whites to be admitted to revascularization-capable and high-quality hospitals.[14] Further emphasizing the need to monitor the quality of care has been the observation of marked variations in the processes of care by geographic region. Pioneering work from the Dartmouth Atlas series, a comprehensive evaluation of health care services provided to Medicare beneficiaries, has documented broad variation in the use of both diagnostic and treatment modalities in CVD as a function of the site of care.[15] Beyond concerns about overall disparities in care, there is emerging evidence that among the patients eligible for treatments, those with the least potential to benefit are preferentially treated, whereas those with the most to gain are systematically undertreated. This finding is referred to as the *risk-treatment paradox*. Many investigators have shown that high-risk patients—who would be expected to benefit more than lower-risk patients—are treated less aggressively, whereas lower-risk patients are treated more aggressively.[16,17]

3-3. **The answer is D.** *(Hurst's the Heart, 14th Edition, Chap. 3)* It is estimated that, on average, it takes about 17 years for guidelines to be incorporated into clinical practice,[9] even with an intervention as simple as aspirin use at the time of myocardial infarction (> 20 years for full adoption). There can be several levels of barriers to the effective implementation of clinical evidence and guidelines in routine practice. These exist at policy, societal, system/organizational, provider, and patient levels. These can be addressed through the use of frameworks for quality metrics and tools to improve quality of care in cardiovascular disease.

3-4. **The answer is E.** *(Hurst's the Heart, 14th Edition, Chap. 3)* Lohr and Schroeder broadly define quality of care as "the degree to which health services for individuals and populations increase the likelihood of desired health outcomes and are consistent with current professional knowledge."[18] The US Agency for Healthcare Research and Quality has proposed a similar definition: "Quality healthcare means doing the right thing at the right time in the right way for the right person and having the best results possible."[19] The Institute for Healthcare Improvement recommends that to improve the United States' health care system requires simultaneous pursuit of three aims, called the "Triple Aim"—improving the patient experience of care (including satisfaction), improving outcomes (of individuals and populations), and reducing the per capita cost of health care.[20] Achieving the best quality of care as marked by highest quality patient outcome and experience with the lowest possible cost is what a health care system usually strives to achieve. Although the concept of quality health care is intuitive and relatively easy to understand, to actually measure, monitor, and improve quality requires the use of a clear conceptual framework that encompasses important, relevant aspects of health care.

3-5. **The answer is A.** (*Hurst's the Heart, 14th Edition, Chap. 3*) One of the earliest approaches to conceptualizing the components of quality assurance was proposed by Donabedian.[21] This framework considers quality to comprise three main domains: structure, process, and outcome. Structure refers to the attributes of settings where care is delivered and includes aspects that exist independently of the patient. Examples of structural attributes include provider training and experience, the availability of specialized treatments, nurse-to-patient ratios, and treatment and discharge plans. Process refers to whether or not good medical practices are followed, and it incorporates concepts such as the medications given and the timing of their administration, the use of diagnostic and therapeutic procedures, and patient counseling. Outcome refers to tangible measures that capture the consequences of care and range from manifestations of disease progression (eg, mortality and hospitalizations) to patient-centered outcomes of health status and treatment satisfaction. As noted by Donabedian, these three components of quality are interdependent and are built on a framework that focuses mainly on linking the delivery of care to outcomes.

3-6. **The answer is B.** (*Hurst's the Heart, 14th Edition, Chap. 3*) The current driving force and roadmap for quality improvement initiatives in American health care is the Institute of Medicine (IOM)'s landmark report, *Crossing the Quality Chasm: A New Health System for the 21st Century.*[9] The IOM recognized the following principal thematic dimensions needed to guide QI in health care:

- Safety—avoiding injuries to patients from the care that is intended to help them
- Effectiveness—providing services based on scientific knowledge to those who could benefit while refraining from providing services to those not likely to benefit
- Patient-centeredness—providing care that is respectful of and responsive to individual patient preferences, needs, and values, and ensuring that patient values guide all clinical decisions
- Timeliness—reducing waits and sometimes harmful delays in care
- Efficiency—avoiding waste, including waste of equipment, supplies, ideas, and energy
- Equity—providing care that does not vary in quality because of personal characteristics such as sex, ethnicity, geographic location, and socioeconomic status

Cost is not one of the principal themes of the IOM report, but it is considered among the outcomes in the Donabedian framework for quality assurance.

3-7. **The answer is B.** (*Hurst's the Heart, 14th Edition, Chap. 3*) To measure and improve care, one first needs to know both how and what to measure. It is critical to have standardized data definitions that enable the reproducible collection of data across different hospitals and settings. To create the foundation for clear, explicit data capture, the ACC/AHA Clinical Data Standards were developed to serve as a foundation for implementing and evaluating the other ACC/AHA quality tools.[22] These data standards are a set of standardized definitions of particular conditions and treatments that can and should be applied in both QA/QI activities and, importantly, clinical trials. Inclusion in clinical trials is especially important to support both comparability across studies and their incorporation into guidelines, performance measures, and clinical care. In particular, standardized definitions support the consistent definition of symptoms, comorbidities, and outcomes in many areas of CVD (eg, acute coronary syndromes, congestive heart failure, PCI).[22] The more these data standards are used in clinical trials, observational registries, and QA/QI efforts, the greater the ability will be to translate the emerging knowledge from clinical research to clinical care.

3-8. **The answer is D.** *(Hurst's the Heart, 14th Edition, Chap. 3)* To distill the rapidly expanding body of cardiovascular literature, professional agencies, such as the AHA and ACC, have commissioned expert committees to synthesize the available evidence into clinical practice guidelines.[24-25] The creation of guidelines requires writing committees to systematically review the medical literature and to assess the strength of evidence for particular treatment strategies. This necessitates ranking the types of research from which knowledge is generated. Randomized controlled trials are given the highest weight. When these are not available, other study designs, including preintervention and postintervention studies, observational registries, and clinical experience are used. To transparently communicate the strength of a recommendation and the evidence on which it is generated, a class recommendation (Class I = strongly indicated, Class IIa = probably indicated, Class IIb = possibly indicated, or Class III = not indicated) and strength of the evidence (level A evidence [data derived from multiple randomized trials] through level C [data derived from expert opinion, case studies, or standard of care]) are provided.[25] An intervention that is probably indicated, based on data from multiple randomized trials (option A) is a Class IIa level A recommendation. An intervention that is probably indicated, based on expert opinion (option B) or probably indicated, based on case studies (option C) are both Class IIa level C recommendations. An intervention that is possibly indicated, based on a single randomized trial (option E), is a Class IIb level B recommendation.

3-9. **The answer is C.** *(Hurst's the Heart, 14th Edition, Chap. 3)* At times, the evidence supporting (or for avoiding) a particular diagnostic or therapeutic action is so strong that failure to perform such actions jeopardizes patients' outcomes. Performance measures represent that subset of the clinical practice guidelines (option A) for which the strongest evidence exists and for which their routine use (or avoidance) is felt to be an important advance to elevating quality.[26,27,28] Performance measures are often constructed as a set of measures that quantify a range of health care processes and outcomes; they are designed to identify multiple points in the continuum of care for which clinical inertia—the failure to implement or titrate recommended therapies—can occur.[28,29] Once the relevant domains are identified, then those guideline recommendations with the strongest evidence and highest correlation with clinically meaningful outcomes are selected for performance measure creation. Clinical data standards (option B) are a set of standardized definitions of particular conditions and treatments that can be applied in both quality assurance/improvement activities and clinical trials. Appropriate use criteria (option D) help identify what specific tests and procedures to perform and when and how often, based on estimates of the relative benefits and harms of a procedure or a test for a specific indication. Procedural registries (option E) support the prospective collection of data for assessing performance and guideline compliance within hospitals.

3-10. **The answer is C.** *(Hurst's the Heart, 14th Edition, Chap. 3)* First ECG acquisition for chest pain patients was recommended within 10 minutes. Launched in 2006, the Door-to-Balloon (D2B) initiative sought to increase the proportion of ST-segment elevation myocardial infarction patients receiving primary PCI within 90 minutes of hospital presentation from approximately 50% to more than 75%.[30] This program supplemented data collected through the NCDR CathPCI registry with explicit recommendations about how to improve performance,[31] including (1) activation of the catheterization laboratory (cath lab) by emergency department physicians, (2) single-call activation of the cath lab, (3) expectations of having the cath lab team assembled within 30 minutes, (4) prompt data feedback to the emergency department and cath lab staff, and (5) activation of the cath lab based on prehospital ECGs and targeted times to first ECG acquisition for chest pain patients within 10 minutes. Between January 2005 and September 2010, this effort led to a decline in median D2B time, from 96 minutes in December 2005 to 64 minutes in September 2010.[32] There were corresponding increases in the proportion of patients undergoing primary PCI within 90 minutes (from 44.2% to 91.4%), and within 75 minutes (from 27.3% to 70.4%). The declines in median times were greatest among groups that had the highest median times during the first period.[32]

References

1. Centers for Medicare & Medicaid Services. National health expenditure data. https://www.cms.gov/Research-Statistics-Data-and-Systems/Statistics-Trends-and-Reports/NationalHealthExpendData/NationalHealthAccountsProjected.html. Accessed December 8, 2015.

2. *NHLBI Morbidity and Mortality Chart Book: National Heart, Lung, and Blood Institute.* https://www.nhlbi.nih.gov/research/reports/2012-mortality-chart-book. Accessed December 9, 2015.

3. Mozaffarian D, Benjamin EJ, Go AS, et al. Heart disease and stroke statistics—2015 update: a report from the American Heart Association. *Circulation.* 2015;131(4): e29-322.

4. Davis K, Stremikis K, Suires D, Schoen C. Mirror, mirror on the wall, 2014 update: how the U.S. health care system compares internationally. *The Commonwealth Fund.* June 2014; http://www.commonwealthfund.org/publications/fund-reports/2014/jun/mirror-mirror. Accessed December 8, 2015.

5. Squires D, Anderson C. Health care from a global perspective: spending, use of services, prices, and health in 13 countries. *The Commonwealth Fund.* October 2015; http://www.commonwealthfund.org/publications/issue-briefs/2015/oct/us-health-care-from-a-global-perspective.

6. Skinner JS, Staiger DO, Fisher ES. Is technological change in medicine always worth it? The case of acute myocardial infarction. *Health Affairs (Project Hope).* 2006;25(2): w34-47.

7. Fisher ES, Bynum JP, Skinner JS. Slowing the growth of health care costs—lessons from regional variation. *N Engl J Med.* 2009;360(9):849-852.

8. Woolf SH, Johnson RE. The break-even point: when medical advances are less important than improving the fidelity with which they are delivered. *Ann Family Med.* 2005;3(6):545-552.

9. Committee on Quality of Health Care in America; Institute of Medicine. *Crossing the Quality Chasm: A New Health System for the 21st Century.* Washington, DC: National Academy Press; 2001.

10. Asch SM, Kerr EA, Keesey J, et al. Who is at greatest risk for receiving poor-quality health care? *N Engl J Med.* 2006;354(11):1147-1156.

11. Mody P, Gupta A, Bikdeli B, Lampropulos JF, Dharmarajan K. Most important articles on cardiovascular disease among racial and ethnic minorities. *Circ Cardiovasc Qual Outcomes.* 2012;5(4):e33-41.

12. Daly C, Clemens F, Lopez Sendon JL, et al. Gender differences in the management and clinical outcome of stable angina. *Circulation.* 2006;113(4):490-498.

13. Blomkalns AL, Chen AY, Hochman JS, et al. Gender disparities in the diagnosis and treatment of non-ST-segment elevation acute coronary syndromes: large-scale observations from the CRUSADE (Can Rapid Risk Stratification of Unstable Angina Patients Suppress Adverse Outcomes With Early Implementation of the American College of Cardiology/American Heart Association Guidelines) National Quality Improvement Initiative. *J Am Coll Cardiol.* 2005;45(6):832-837.

14. Popescu I, Cram P, Vaughan-Sarrazin MS. Differences in admitting hospital characteristics for black and white Medicare beneficiaries with acute myocardial infarction. *Circulation.* 2011;123(23):2710-2716.

15. The Center for the Evaluative Clinical Sciences, Dartmouth Medical School; The Center for the Evaluative Clinical Sciences, Maine Medical Center. *The Dartmouth Atlas of Cardiovascular Health Care.* Chicago, IL: AHA Press; 1999.

16. Spertus JA, Decker C, Gialde E, et al. Precision medicine to improve use of bleeding avoidance strategies and reduce bleeding in patients undergoing percutaneous coronary intervention: prospective cohort study before and after implementation of personalized bleeding risks. *BMJ.* 2015;350:h1302

17. Marso SP, Amin AP, House JA, et al. Association between use of bleeding avoidance strategies and risk of periprocedural bleeding among patients undergoing percutaneous coronary intervention. *JAMA.* 2010;303(21):2156-2164.

18. Lohr KH. *Medicare: A Strategy for Quality Assurance, Volume I.* Washington: National Academy of Sciences; 1990.

19. US Department of Health & Human Services, The US Agency for Healthcare Research and Quality Archive. *A Quick Look at Quality.* Available at: http://archive.ahrq.gov/consumer/qnt/qntqlook.htm. Accessed December 11, 2015.

20. Institute for Healthcare Improvement: The IHI Triple Aim. http://www.ihi.org/engage/initiatives/tripleaim/Pages/default.aspx. Accessed December 11, 2015.

21. Donabedian A. The quality of care. How can it be assessed? *JAMA.* 1988;260(12): 1743-1748.

22. Hendel RC, Bozkurt B, Fonarow GC, et al. ACC/AHA 2013 methodology for developing clinical data standards: a report of the American College of Cardiology/American Heart Association Task Force on Clinical Data Standards. *J Am Coll Cardiol.* 2014;63(21): 2323-2334.

23. Nishimura, et al. (2017). 2017 AHA/ACC focused update of the 2014 AHA/ACC guideline for the management of patients with valvular heart disease: a report of the American College of Cardiology/American Heart Association Task Force on Clinical Practice Guidelines. http://circ.ahajournals.org/content/early/2017/03/14/CIR.0000000000000503. Accessed April 7, 2017.

24. Gibbons RJ, Smith S, Antman E. American College of Cardiology/American Heart Association clinical practice guidelines: Part I: where do they come from? *Circulation.* 2003;107(23):2979-2986.

25. Halperin JL, Levine GN, Al-Khatib SM, et al. Further evolution of the ACC/AHA clinical practice guideline recommendation classification system: a report of the American College of Cardiology/American Heart Association Task Force on Clinical Practice Guidelines. *J Am Coll Cardiol.* 2016;67(13):1572-1574.

26. Bonow RO, Masoudi FA, Rumsfeld JS, et al. ACC/AHA classification of care metrics: performance measures and quality metrics: a report of the American College of Cardiology/American Heart Association Task Force on Performance Measures. *Circulation.* 2008;118(24):2662-2666.

27. Spertus JA, Eagle KA, Krumholz HM, Mitchell KR, Normand SL. American College of Cardiology and American Heart Association methodology for the selection and creation of performance measures for quantifying the quality of cardiovascular care. *J Am Coll Cardiol.* 2005;45(7):1147-1156.

28. Turner BJ, Hollenbeak CS, Weiner M, Ten Have T, Tang SS. Effect of unrelated comorbid conditions on hypertension management. *Ann Intern Med.* 2008;148(8):578-586.

29. Phillips LS, Twombly JG. It's time to overcome clinical inertia. *Ann Intern Med.* 2008;148(10):783-785.

30. Krumholz HM, Bradley EH, Nallamothu BK, et al. A campaign to improve the timeliness of primary percutaneous coronary intervention: Door-to-Balloon: an alliance for quality. *JACC Cardiovasc Interv.* 2008;1(1):97-104.

31. Bradley EH, Nallamothu BK, Herrin J, et al. National efforts to improve door-to-balloon time results from the Door-to-Balloon Alliance. *J Am Coll Cardiol.* 2009;54(25):2423-2429.

32. Krumholz HM, Herrin J, Miller LE, et al. Improvements in Door-to-Balloon Time in the United States: 2005-2010. *Circulation.* 2011;124(9):1038-1045.

SECTION 2

Foundations of Cardiovascular Medicine

CHAPTER 4

Functional Anatomy of the Heart

Jacqueline Joza

QUESTIONS

DIRECTIONS: Choose the one best response to each question.

4-1. Which of the following statements is *false*?

A. The main pulmonary artery, portions of both venae cavae, distal pulmonary veins, and nearly the entire ascending aorta are intrapericardial

B. The right and left pulmonary arteries are extrapericardial structures

C. The transverse sinus forms a tunnel-like passageway that separates the great arteries anteriorly from the great veins posteriorly

D. The oblique sinus lies posterior to the right atrium

E. The serous pericardium forms the inner lining of the fibrous pericardium; over the heart, it is referred to as the epicardium

4-2. A 35-year-old woman presents to your clinic for evaluation of a murmur. She describes intermittent regular palpitations that have been associated with lightheadedness. Auscultation reveals a midsystolic click and a crescendo systolic murmur. The S1-click distance increases with squatting and decreases with standing. Regarding this valve or valve defect, which statement is *true*?

A. The valve leaflets are characteristically thin

B. Annular dilatation is not typically present

C. Prolapse of the anterior leaflet occurs more frequently

D. The anterolateral papillary muscle is commonly single and usually has a dual blood supply from the left coronary circulation

E. The posteromedial papillary muscle usually has a single head and is most commonly supplied by the left anterior descending artery

4-3. Regarding Figure 4-1, select the statement that is *false:*

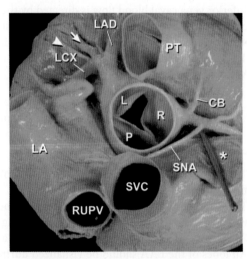

FIGURE 4-1 Superior view of the heart. (Reproduced with permission from McAlpine W. *Heart and Coronary Arteries: An Anatomic Atlas for Radiologic Diagnosis and Surgical Treatment.* New York: Spring-Verlag; 1975.)

A. The central structures labelled L, P, and R are supplied by the conus artery

B. The * depicts the right atrial appendage

C. The arrowhead points to a circumflex marginal branch

D. An ablation catheter positioned at P will reveal atrial electrogram signals

E. The oblique sinus is not visualized in this figure

4-4. All of the following are used to differentiate the right ventricle from the left ventricle *except*:

A. The presence of a moderator band
B. Free wall typically < 0.4 mm thick
C. A prominent arch-shaped muscular ridge known as the crista supraventricularis separates the tricuspid and pulmonary valves
D. The apex is thin and lacks trabeculation
E. The tricuspid valve always follows the morphological right ventricle

4-5. Which of the following statements regarding structures within the right atrium is *false*?

A. The cavotricuspid isthmus is targeted during typical right atrial flutter ablation
B. The cavotricuspid isthmus is a well-defined region of atrial tissue that is bordered by the eustachian ridge and valve posteriorly, and the tricuspid valve annulus anteriorly
C. The right atrial free wall is a very thin structure between pectinate muscles and can perforate during catheter positioning
D. Inferior vena caval blood flow is directed by the eustachian valve toward the foramen ovale, and superior vena caval blood is directed toward the tricuspid valve
E. The right atrial appendage abuts the left aortic sinus of Valsalva

4-6. A patient undergoes a transesophageal echocardiography (TEE) as workup for possible left atrial appendage (LAA) closure. Regarding the LAA, which of the following statements is *false*?

A. There is no known relationship between stroke and LAA morphology
B. There are four basic morphologic patterns to the LAA: windsock, cactus, cauliflower, and chicken wing
C. Age is not a determinant for the dimensions of an LAA
D. All lobes of the LAA should be visualized during TEE to rule out a thrombus
E. Both the right and the left atrial appendages are located close to the right ventricular outflow tract

4-7. All of the following are true statements *except*:

A. The left anterior descending artery courses within the epicardial fat of the anterior interventricular groove
B. The first septal perforating branch of the left anterior descending artery supplies the AV (His) bundle and proximal left bundle branch
C. Dominance is left in 70% of human hearts, right in 10%, and shared in 20%
D. A patient who presents acutely with an anterior ST elevation myocardial infarction secondary to a left anterior descending artery occlusion is at risk for a mechanical complication
E. The right coronary artery typically arises nearly perpendicularly from the aorta

4-8. In a typical right-dominant system, which of the following left ventricular segments would most likely *not* be affected in a patient with left anterior descending artery occlusion?

A. Mid anterior wall
B. Mid inferolateral wall
C. Basal anterior septum
D. Basal anterior wall
E. Mid anterolateral wall

4-9. Regarding the great vessels, which of the following statements is *true*?

A. Most coarctations occur just proximal to the left subclavian artery
B. When the eustachian or the adjacent thebesian valve of the coronary sinus is large and fenestrated, it is referred to as the ligamentum arteriosum
C. The ligamentum arteriosum represents the vestigial remnant of the fetal ductal artery, which, when patent, connects the proximal right pulmonary artery to the undersurface of the aortic arch
D. The ostium of the superior vena cava (SVC) is guarded by a crescent-shaped, often fenestrated flap of tissue called the eustachian valve
E. The ligament of Marshall is the vestigial remnant of the vein of Marshall, which forms the terminal connection between a persistent left SVC and the coronary sinus

4-10. Which of the following statements is *false* concerning the triangle of Koch?

A. It is bordered by the coronary sinus ostium, the septal tricuspid annulus, and the tendon of Todaro
B. The AV node is a subendocardial structure that is located within the upper portion of the triangle of Koch
C. The His bundle is located within the triangle of Koch. The apex of the triangle corresponds to the central fibrous body of the heart where the His bundle penetrates
D. The atrial end of the fast pathway in AV nodal reentrant tachycardia inserts near the ostium of the coronary sinus, while the slow pathway lies closer to the apex of the triangle near the AV node
E. AV node displacement occurs in Ebstein malformation and persistent left SVC

4-1. The answer is D. *(Hurst's The Heart, 14th Edition, Chap. 4)* The reflections along the pulmonary veins and venae cavae are continuous and form a posterior midline cul-de-sac known as the oblique sinus. The oblique sinus lies immediately posterior to the left atrium, *not* the right atrium (option D). The main pulmonary artery, portions of both venae cavae, distal pulmonary veins, and nearly the entire ascending aorta are intrapericardial (option A). The right and left pulmonary arteries are extrapericardial structures (option B). The transverse sinus forms a tunnel-like passageway that separates the great arteries anteriorly from the great veins posteriorly (option C). The serous pericardium forms the delicate inner lining of the fibrous pericardium and continues onto the surface of the heart and great vessels at the pericardial reflection.[1] Over the heart, it is referred to as the epicardium, and it contains the epicardial coronary arteries and veins, autonomic nerves, lymphatics, and a variable amount of adipose tissue (option E).

4-2. The answer is D. *(Hurst's The Heart, 14th Edition, Chap. 4)* The anterolateral papillary muscle is single and usually has a dual blood supply from the left coronary circulation (option D).[2] Mitral valve prolapse is characterized by *thickened* and redundant leaflets (option A), annular dilatation (with or without calcium) and thickened and elongated chordae tendineae (with or without rupture) (option B). Prolapse of the posterior leaflet occurs more often than that of the anterior leaflet (option C). The posteromedial papillary muscle usually has multiple heads and is most commonly supplied only by the dominant coronary artery (option E).[2] Small left atrial branches supply the most basal aspects of the mitral leaflets.[3]

4-3. The answer is A. *(Hurst's The Heart, 14th Edition, Chap. 4)* The figure shows a superior view of the heart, including the aortic and pulmonic valves, the origins of the left and right coronary arteries, the superior aspect of the left atrium, the SVC, and the right upper pulmonary vein. The aortic cusps (labeled L for left aortic cusp; P for posterior aortic cusp; and R for right aortic cusp) form pocketlike tissue flaps that are avascular (option A). The conus artery is the first branch of the right coronary artery in 50%–60% of persons; it supplies the right ventricular outflow tract and forms an important collateral anastomosis (circle of Vieussens) just below the pulmonary valve with an analogous branch from the left anterior descending coronary artery.[1-3] The * symbol (option B) represents the right atrial appendage, which is retracted by the rod to disclose the sinus node artery (SNA). The arrowhead (option C) is pointing to a marginal branch of the left circumflex artery. An ablation catheter positioned at the posterior (or noncoronary) cusp (option D) will reveal atrial electrogram signals due to its close proximity to the interatrial septum. The oblique sinus (option E) is not seen in this figure. It is formed from the reflections along the pulmonary veins and venae cavae that form a posterior midline cul-de-sac that lies posterior to the left atrium.

4-4. The answer is D. *(Hurst's The Heart, 14th Edition, Chap. 4)* The right ventricular apex is heavily trabeculated.[1,3] This apical trabecular zone extends inferiorly beyond the attachments of the papillary muscles toward the ventricular apex and about halfway along the anterior wall. This muscular meshwork is the usual site of insertion of transvenous ventricular pacemaker electrodes, and it is the preferred site for positioning the tip of an implantable cardioverter defibrillator lead. The moderator band (option A) forms an intracavitary muscle that connects the septal band with the anterior tricuspid papillary muscle. The right ventricular wall is thin in normal adults, usually less than 0.4 cm (regional variation between 0.2 and 0.7 cm) (option B). A prominent arch-shaped muscular ridge known as the crista supraventricularis separates the tricuspid and pulmonary valves. It is made up of three components (parietal band, infundibular septum, and septal band) that can appear as distinct structures or can merge together (option C).[1,3] The tricuspid valve always follows the morphological right ventricle, which is an important consideration when evaluating patients with congenital heart disease (option E).

4-5. The answer is E. *(Hurst's The Heart, 14th Edition, Chap. 4)* The right atrial appendage abuts the right aortic sinus of Valsalva and overlies the proximal right coronary artery (option E). The cavotricuspid isthmus, a frequent target of atrial flutter ablation, is a well-defined region of atrial tissue that is bordered by (1) the eustachian ridge and valve posteriorly and (2) the tricuspid valve annulus anteriorly (options A, B). The right atrial free wall is paper-thin between pectinate muscles and therefore can be perforated easily by stiff catheters (option C).[1-3] The atrial lead of a dual-chamber pacemaker is normally positioned within the trabeculations of the right atrial appendage. Inferior vena caval blood flow is directed by the eustachian valve toward the foramen ovale, and superior vena caval blood is directed toward the tricuspid valve (option D).[4]

4-6. The answer is A. *(Hurst's The Heart, 14th Edition, Chap. 4)* The left atrial appendage is usually multilobed and narrower than its right atrial counterpart, and it exhibits more variability in shape.[1-3,5] The chicken wing variety of LAA morphology has the *least* likelihood for embolic events (option A).[6] There are four basic morphologic patterns: windsock, cactus, cauliflower, and chicken wing (option B).[6] Age and sex are both determinants for LAA dimension (option C).[4] There may be multiple lobes in the LAA; all lobes must be visualized in order to rule out thrombus prior to planned cardioversion, electrophysiology or structural procedure, or percutaneous balloon valvuloplasty procedures (option D). Either atrial appendage may serve as a vantage point from which to access and ablate arrhythmias in the adjacent segment of the right ventricular outflow tract (option E).[7]

4-7. The answer is C. *(Hurst's The Heart, 14th Edition, Chap. 4)* Dominance is right in 70% of human hearts, left in 10%, and shared in 20%.[1-3] In patients with a congenitally bicuspid aortic valve, the incidence of left coronary dominance is 25% to 30%.[3] The left anterior descending artery (LAD) courses within the epicardial fat of the anterior interventricular groove (option A). The first septal perforating branch supplies the AV (His) bundle and the proximal left bundle branch (option B).[3] In patients with symptomatic hypertrophic obstructive cardiomyopathy, nonsurgical septal reduction by percutaneous transluminal occlusion of septal branches of the LAD is a therapeutic approach aimed at reducing the outflow gradient.[8] Anterior infarcts have been shown to be independent predictors of ventricular septal defects post myocardial infarction (option D). Whereas the right coronary artery arises almost perpendicularly from the aorta, the left arises at an acute angle (option E).[4]

4-8. The answer is B. *(Hurst's The Heart, 14th Edition, Chap. 4).* The midventricular inferolateral wall is typically supplied by the *circumflex artery*, not the left anterior descending artery (LAD). In a typical right-dominant system, the LAD supplies the midventricular and basal segments of the anterior (options A and D), anterolateral walls (option E) and anterior septum (option C) and all apical segments. The left circumflex artery supplies the midventricular and basal inferolateral segments, and the right coronary artery supplies the midventricular and basal inferior wall and inferior septum. In the setting of a large obtuse marginal branch of the circumflex artery, the anterolateral or inferior wall may not be supplied by the LAD. However, because the patterns of coronary distribution are so highly variable, these correlations between coronary blood flow and regional anatomy are not precise. For example, a hyperdominant right coronary artery can supply the apex, and a large, obtuse marginal branch of the circumflex artery can supply the anterolateral or inferior wall.[1-3] Ventricular septal defects are more common in the setting of a wrap-around LAD.

4-9. The answer is E. *(Hurst's The Heart, 14th Edition, Chap. 4)* The vein of Marshall forms the terminal connection between a persistent left SVC and the coronary sinus. Its vestigial remnant in normal adults is the ligament of Marshall; it is a potential source of arrhythmias and a common site for recurrences after pulmonary vein isolation (option E). Most coarctations occur just *distal* to the left subclavian artery (option A). The ostium of the inferior vena cava is guarded by a crescent-shaped, often fenestrated flap of tissue, the eustachian valve,[1-3] which is readily seen by echocardiography. Although generally small, the eustachian valve can become so large that it can produce a double-chambered right atrium.[2] Also, when either the eustachian or the adjacent thebesian valve of the coronary sinus is large and fenestrated, it is referred to as a Chiari network (option B).[1-3] The ligamentum arteriosum represents the vestigial remnant of the fetal ductal artery, which, when patent, connects the proximal *left* pulmonary artery to the undersurface of the aortic arch (option C). The ostium of the *inferior* vena cava (not the SVC) is guarded by the eustachian valve. It is an important structure during cavotricuspid isthmus ablation (option D).

4-10. **The answer is D.** *(Hurst's The Heart, 14th Edition, Chap. 4)* The atrial end of the fast pathway in AV nodal reentrant tachycardia inserts closer to the AV node at the apex of the triangle, whereas the slow pathway (target for radiofrequency ablation) inserts near the ostium of the coronary sinus (option D). The triangle of Koch is bordered by the coronary sinus ostium posteroinferiorly, the septal tricuspid annulus anteriorly, and the tendon of Todaro posteriorly (option A). The tendon of Todaro is a fibrous extension of the Eustachian valve (option B). The body of the AV node is found near the apex of the triangle. The His bundle, also located in the triangle of Koch, penetrates through the central fibrous body separating the atria and ventricles (option C). The bundle of His then bifurcates into right and left main bundle branches, which branch further to become Purkinje fibers that spread conduction to the ventricles. Differences in the conduction system primarily reside in the arrangement of the transitional and compact components of the AV node and in the length and route of the His bundle. In both Ebstein's anomaly and persistent left SVC syndrome with a grossly enlarged CS ostium, the size of the triangle of Koch is reduced, resulting in a shorter distance between the compact AV node and the CS ostium (option E).

References

1. Edwards WD. *Anatomy of the Cardiovascular System: Clinical Medicine.* Vol 6. Philadelphia, PA: Harper & Row; 1984:1-24.
2. Edwards WD. Cardiac anatomy and examination of cardiac specimens. In: Emmanouilides G, Reimenschneider T, Allen H, Gutgesell H, eds. *Moss & Adams' Heart Disease in Infants, Children, and Adolescents.* 5th ed. Baltimore, MD: Williams & Wilkins; 1995:70-105.
3. Edwards WD. Applied anatomy of the heart. In: Giuliani ER, Fuster V, Gersh BJ, et al, eds. *Cardiology Fundamentals and Practice.* Vol 1. 2nd ed. St Louis, MO: Mosby-Year Book; 1991:47-112.
4. Kitzman D, Edwards WD. Minireview: age-related changes in the anatomy of the normal human heart. *J Gerontol Med Sci.* 1990;45:M33-M39.
5. Veinot JP, Harrity PJ, Gentile F, et al. Anatomy of the normal left atrial appendage: a quantitative study of age-related changes in 500 autopsy hearts: implications for echocardiographic examination. *Circulation.* 1997;96:3112-3115.
6. Di Biase L, Santangeli P, Anselmino M, et al. Does the left atrial appendage morphology correlate with the risk of stroke in patients with atrial fibrillation? Results from a multicenter study. *J Am Coll Cardiol.* 2012;60(6):531-538.
7. Tabatabaei N, Asirvatham SJ. Supravalvular arrhythmia identifying and ablating the substrate. *Circ Arrhythm Electrophysiol.* 2009;2:316-326.
8. Naqueh SF, Lakkis NM, He ZX, et al. Role of myocardial contrast echocardiography during nonsurgical septal reduction therapy for hypertrophic obstructive cardiomyopathy. *J Am Coll Cardiol.* 1998;32:225-229.

CHAPTER 5

Normal Physiology of the Cardiovascular System

Ravi Karra

DIRECTIONS: Choose the one best response to each question.

5-1. Which of the following is *true* about Figure 5-1?

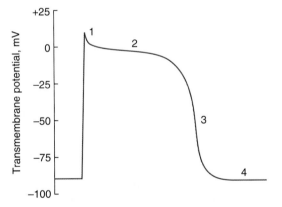

FIGURE 5-1 Phases of the action potential and major associated currents in ventricular myocytes.

A. Sodium influx during phase 1 depolarization is decreased by membrane depolarization
B. Sodium influx is limited after phase 1 by the closure of inactivation gates
C. The phase 2 plateau of the action potential is the result of a decrease in intracellular calcium through the L-type calcium channel
D. Phase 3 repolarization is the result of potassium influx into the cell through the funny channel (I_F)
E. Maintenance of the membrane potential during diastole is an energy-independent process

5-2. Please select the *true* statement about Figure 5-2.

A. Calcium-induced calcium release occurs by calcium influx through ion channel B with release of calcium from the sarcoplasmic reticulum via ion channel C
B. The magnitude of the calcium transient is, in part, determined by calcium influx into the cell via channels B and D
C. The decline in the calcium transient occurs via channel C and is energy-independent
D. Increased cytoplasmic calcium results in contraction, in part, by the binding of calcium to TnI
E. None of the above

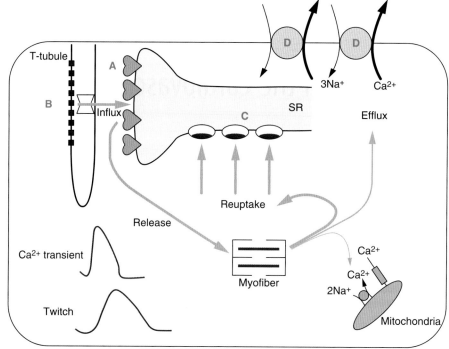

FIGURE 5-2 Major components of excitation–contraction coupling in cardiomyocytes. (Adapted with permission from Scoote M, Poole-Wilson PA, Williams AJ, et al. The therapeutic potential of new insights into myocardial excitation-contraction coupling. *Heart.* 2003 Apr;89(4):371-376.)

5-3. A 54-year-old woman was recently started on furosemide for pedal edema related to prolonged standing. Shortly after starting furosemide, she feels fatigued and confirms dizziness with standing. Her past medical history is notable for hypertension that had not been treated. Her blood pressure is 158/82 sitting and her heart rate is 85. Her physical exam is notable for flat neck veins, a nondisplaced apical impulse, and a soft S4. Which of the following is *not true* for this patient?

A. Discontinuation of her diuretic and increased fluid intake would increase the peak tension in her cardiac muscle fibers following muscle contraction

B. Increasing preload through hydration would increase cardiac output, in part by the increased sensitivity to calcium by myofilaments at longer sarcomere lengths

C. Increased heart rate would result in faster cardiac relaxation

D. Increasing afterload would increase myofilament shortening velocity

E. A cup of coffee could increase contractility

5-4. Which of the following is *true* regarding the cardiac cycle?

A. The *c* wave occurs during isovolumic contraction

B. The *v* wave occurs just after the QRS complex on the ECG, but before the T wave

C. The change in ventricular pressure during ventricular filling is a property of ventricular stiffness

D. Ventricular stiffness is constant during contraction and relaxation

E. The area enclosed within the pressure–volume loop (PVA) is proportional to myocardial oxygen consumption

Questions 5-5 through 5-7 relate to the following vignette.

A 54-year-old woman is brought to the catheterization laboratory to assess her hemodynamics for shortness of breath. A precatheterization echocardiogram revealed normal ventricular function. Moreover, her filling pressures are normal.

5-5. Which of the following is *not true* regarding ventricular function?

A. A modest volume challenge would be expected to increase stroke volume

B. Left ventricular (LV) compliance is determined entirely by the intrinsic elastic properties of the left ventricle

C. A bolus of norepinephrine would be expected to decrease the velocity of LV shortening

D. The rate of LV pressure development (dP/dt) is dependent on preload but relatively independent of afterload

E. Increasing the heart rate from 80 to 95 is unlikely to increase cardiac output

5-6. Which of the following is *true* regarding her diastolic function?

A. Ventricular relaxation is energy-independent

B. Tau, the time constant of LV relaxation, is increased with β-adrenergic receptor stimulation

C. The end-diastolic pressure–volume relationship is influenced by changes in intrathoracic pressure, pericardial constraint, and ventricular interaction

D. The sarcomeric protein titin does not meaningfully contribute to diastolic function

E. The PV relationship during systole reflects the lusitropic state of the heart

5-7. Right heart catheterization revealed a right atrial pressure of 5 mm Hg, a right ventricular (RV) pressure of 25/5 mm Hg, a pulmonary artery (PA) pressure of 25/10 mm Hg, and a wedge pressure of 10 mm Hg. The aortic pressure was 120/85 mm Hg, and heart rate was 85. The cardiac output was calculated to be 6 L/min. Which of the following is correct?

A. The mean arterial pressure (MAP) is 108 mm Hg
B. The mean PA pressure is 15 mm Hg
C. The systemic vascular resistance (SVR) is 14.5 Wood units
D. The pulmonary vascular resistance (PVR) is 2.5 Wood units
E. None of the above

5-8. Which of the following is *true* about the coronary circulation?

A. Collateral vessels around a coronary obstruction have myocardial blood flow during exercise similar to that of the native coronary artery
B. To meet the increased oxygen demands during exercise, the myocardium dramatically increases its extraction of oxygen from the blood
C. Adenosine is a major mediator of coronary autoregulation
D. Coronary vascular resistance is greater in the subendocardial coronary circulation than in the subepicardial coronary circulation
E. The principal endothelial derived relaxing factor is adenosine

5-9. Which of the following is *true* about control of the circulation?

A. Arterial pressure regulation is controlled primarily by the parasympathetic nervous system
B. One result of carotid baroreflex resetting is increased receptor firing for a given mean arterial blood pressure
C. The Bezold–Jarisch reflex occurs with a decrease in ventricular distension and results in bradycardia and hypotension
D. Endothelins constrict arterioles and decrease preload
E. Endocannabinoids increase contractility

5-10. With reference to the venous return curves in Figure 5-3, which of the following is *incorrect*?

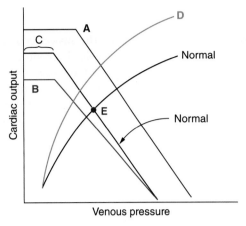

FIGURE 5-3 Venous pressure–cardiac output return curve.

A. Line A is the effect of volume loading or increasing venous pressure
B. Line B is the effect of arteriolar vasodilation
C. The flat portion of the curve in C represents the maximal cardiac output as venous return is reduced
D. The shift in the Frank–Starling curve to curve D is the effect of increased sympathetic tone
E. Point E is the equilibrium point where the ability of the venous system to provide enough return at a given pressure is matched by the ventricle's ability to pump that return when distended to that pressure

5-1. The answer is B. (*Hurst's The Heart, 14th Edition, Chap. 5*). Cardiomyocytes are specialized cells that couple membrane depolarization with cellular contraction. Phase 1 depolarization is the result of sodium influx through Na^+ channels. Sodium influx is *regenerative*, in that increasing membrane depolarization opens more Na^+ channels (option A). Rapid depolarization is limited by K^+ efflux but also by the closure of inactivation gates on Na^+ channels that prevent reopening of individual channels only after the membrane has been fully repolarized (option B). The phase 2 plateau is the result of balanced K^+ efflux and Ca^{2+} influx through L-type Ca^{2+} channels (option C). Phase 3 repolarization is the result of K^+ efflux primarily through the delayed outward K current (I_K). The funny current (I_F) is a specialized channel found in pacemaker cells that results in spontaneous depolarization of the cell during phase 4 and in automaticity (option D). Phase 4 occurs during diastole and requires the Na^+/K^+ ATPase to restore and maintain low intracellular Na^+ and high intracellular K^+ concentrations (option E).

5-2. The answer is B. (*Hurst's The Heart, 14th Edition, Chap. 5*). In Figure 5-2, channel A is the ryanodine receptor on the sarcoplasmic reticulum (SR). Channel B is the L-type Ca^{2+} channel on the sarcolemma. Channel C is the SERCA pump on the sarcoplasmic reticulum, and channel D is the Na^+/Ca^+ exchanged (NCX) on the sarcolemma. Calcium-uptake calcium release is the result of calcium release from the SR through the ryanodine receptor (A) after calcium influx into the cell through the L-type Ca^{2+} channel (B) (option A). The calcium transient is a result of (1) Ca^{2+} influx through the L-type Ca^{2+} channel and the *reverse mode* NCX; (2) the amount of calcium in the SR; (3) the amount of calcium released by the SR for a given calcium current; and (4) intracellular Ca^{2+} buffers. NCX can operate in the reverse mode during cellular depolarization, when the intracellular Na^+ content is high. The net effect is Na^+ extrusion and Ca^{2+} uptake. This is a minor contribution to the calcium transient (option B). The calcium transient declines largely because the SERCA ATPase sequesters calcium into the SR. This requires ATP and is energy-dependent (option C). Calcium concentrations are coupled to contraction. Calcium bound TnC essentially pulls TnI off actin. Thus, TnI can no longer inhibit the formation of myosin-actin crossbridges (option D).

5-3. The answer is D. (*Hurst's The Heart, 14th Edition, Chap. 5*) Options A and B reflect the Frank–Starling mechanism. A key property of healthy cardiac muscle is faster relaxation times with increasing heart rates (option C). This occurs by increased SERCA activity as a result of phospholamban phosphorylation. By the force–velocity relationship, the initial velocity of shortening is inversely related to afterload (option D). Caffeine is a calcium sensitizer and can result in an increased force of contraction (option E).

5-4. The answer is C. (*Hurst's The Heart, 14th Edition, Chap. 5*) The *c* wave is the result of increased atrial pressure as the mitral valve bulges into the atrium during isovolumic contraction (option A). The *v* wave occurs as the atrium fills during ventricular systole and atrial pressure falls with mitral valve opening. The *v* wave occurs after the T wave (option B). During ventricular filling, change in ventricular pressure is a function of ventricular compliance (option C). Isolated, perfused hearts have been instrumental in the development of our understanding of ventricular mechanics. These models have allowed for the determination that ventricular elastance increases during ventricular contraction and decreases with ventricular relaxation (option D). The PVA is proportional to the myocardial oxygen consumption but includes the area within the PV loop as well as the area between the end-systolic pressure relation and the end-diastolic P–V relation (option E).

5-5. The answer is B. (*Hurst's The Heart, 14th Edition, Chap. 5*) The woman in the vignette has a normal right heart catheterization and likely is short of breath for noncardiac reasons. Increasing preload is expected to increase stroke volume (option A). LV compliance in vivo is determined by pericardial pressure, right ventricular pressure and volume, coronary artery perfusion, and the intrinsic elastic properties of the LV (option B). An increase in afterload, such as with a bolus of norepinephrine, is expected to decrease stroke volume and the velocity of LV shortening (option C). Changes in heart rate from 60 to 160 beats per minute are unlikely to increase cardiac output because the small increase in contractility is offset by the decrease in diastolic filling time and the resulting preload (option E).

5-6.   **The answer is C.** *(Hurst's The Heart, 14th Edition, Chap. 5)* Ventricular relaxation is an energy-dependent process requiring ATP for SERCA sequestration of calcium into the sarcoplasmic reticulum, among other processes (option A). β-adrenergic stimulation leads to the activation of PKA and the phosphorylation of phospholamban, resulting in increased SERCA activity. Increased SERCA activity results in faster relaxation, and a decrease of Tau (option B). Chamber stiffness is affected by intrinsic LV factors and extrinsic factors such as pericardial constraint, atrial contraction, intrathoracic pressures, and ventricular interaction (option C). In addition to active relaxation, diastolic function is also related to the viscoelastic properties of the LV. LV recoil is affected by titin and the extracellular matrix (option D). The P–V relationship during diastole reflects the lusitropic state of the heart (option E).

5-7.   **The answer is B.** *(Hurst's The Heart, 14th Edition, Chap. 5)* The MAP is (120 + 2 * 85)/3 = 97 (option A). The PA pressure is (25 + 2 * 10)/3 = 15 (option B). SVR is (97 − 5)/6 = 15.33 Wood units (option C). The PVR is (15 − 10)/6 = 0.83 Wood units (option D).

5-8.   **The answer is C.** *(Hurst's The Heart, 14th Edition, Chap. 5)* Collateral vessels that become prominent with obstructive coronary disease cannot augment coronary flow similar to that of the native artery with stress or exercise (option A). Unlike skeletal muscle, the myocardium operates at nearly peak oxygen extraction at rest. Increased oxygen needs are met by increases in blood flow through the coronary circulation (option B). Adenosine levels increase with the breakdown of ATP, and adenosine is a potent coronary vasodilator. If coronary blood flow decreases, local adenosine levels increase, making adenosine an integral component of coronary autoregulation (option C). To maintain equal coronary flow throughout the myocardium, the subendocardial vessels have less resistance than the subepicardial vessels. This is important because subendocardial vessels have a limited ability to further vasodilate in time of stress, and subendocardial zones are more prone to ischemia (option D). The principal endothelial derived relaxing factor is nitric oxide (NO) (option E).

5-9.   **The answer is C.** *(Hurst's The Heart, 14th Edition, Chap. 5).* Parasympathetic nerves supply only a small portion of the resistance in vessels; the sympathetic nervous system is the primary regulator of vascular resistance (option A). Carotid baroreflex resetting results in decreased receptor firing for a given mean arterial blood pressure (option B). The Bezold–Jarisch reflex is mediated by ventricular C fibers, which are activated by hypovolemia. The net result is a paradoxical bradycardia and hypotension (option C). Endothelin constricts arterioles and venules. The effect on venules serves to increase preload (option D). Endocannabinoids decrease contractility (option E).

5-10.   **The answer is B.** *(Hurst's The Heart, 14th Edition, Chap. 5).* The venous return curve describes the relationship of cardiac output and venous pressure. Volume loading or venoconstriction shifts the curve up and to the right (option A). By contrast, arteriolar vasoconstriction shifts the curve down and to the left (option B). The flat portion of the curve in C represents the maximal cardiac output as venous return is reduced (option C). The Frank–Starling curve describes the effect of ventricular loading with cardiac output and moves up and to the left at higher levels of contractility (option D). The intersection of the Frank–Starling curve and the venous return curve represents the equilibrium point of venous return and ventricular performance (option E).

CHAPTER 6

Molecular and Cellular Biology of the Heart

Ravi Karra

QUESTIONS

DIRECTIONS: Choose the one best response to each question.

6-1. A 55-year-old man presents with exertional dyspnea and a 10 lb weight gain. His physical exam is notable for an elevated jugular venous pressure, a soft apical holosystolic murmur, and an S3 gallop. Echocardiography reveals a dilated left ventricle with an ejection fraction of 35%. Which of the following is most likely *true* regarding β-adrenergic signaling in this patient?

A. β2-adrenergic receptors (β2-AR) are the dominant type of β-adrenergic receptor in the heart
B. An increase in GRK2 activity contributes to β-adrenergic receptor desensitization
C. β1-AR density is increased in this patient's myocytes
D. This patient's heart is more sensitive to β-agonists now than before developing decompensated heart failure
E. β1-AR signaling is likely to protect against apoptosis in his cardiomyocytes

6-2. Which of the following is *incorrect* regarding excitation–contraction coupling?

A. Depolarization of the cardiomyocyte membrane results in the opening of L-type calcium channels
B. The SERCA ATPase functions to sequester calcium in the sarcoplasmic reticulum during relaxation
C. In a healthy heart, tachycardia results in decreased calcium in the cytoplasm of the cardiomyocyte and increased contractile force
D. PKA and CaMKII maintain SERCA activity by phosphorylating and inactivating phospholamban
E. The efficiency of the ryanodine receptor response to cytoplasmic calcium is dependent on the ryanodine receptor's proximity to the L-type calcium channel

6-3. A 54-year-old patient with a history of heart failure with reduced ejection fraction is admitted following 3 shocks from his internal cardiac defibrillator. Which of the following could contribute to a proarrhythmic state in this patient?

A. Hyperphosphorylation of the ryanodine receptor contributes to a calcium leak from the sarcoplasmic reticulum
B. Increased systolic calcium concentrations in myocytes
C. An increased force-frequency relationship
D. A shortened relaxation phase
E. Increased SERCA expression and activity

6-4. Which of the following is *not true* regarding signaling pathways in heart failure?

A. An increased intracellular concentration of calcium leads to increased activity of calcineurin in failing myocytes
B. CaMKII contributes to hypertrophy by phosphorylating transcription factors such as MEF2 and class II histone deacetylases
C. Prohypertrophic growth factors tend to work through heterotrimeric proteins of the Gq family
D. Mechanical stretch alone can induce many hypertrophic signaling pathways
E. Hallmarks of a fetal-gene expression program during hypertrophy include the expression of BNP, ANF, and α-MHC

Questions 6-5 through 6-7 refer to the following vignette.

A 52-year-old man presents to your office for a follow-up appointment. He has a long-standing history of hypertension. His ECG is suggestive of left ventricular hypertrophy, and his echocardiogram shows a left ventricular wall thickness of 1.4 cm.

6-5. Which of the following is *not true* regarding signaling pathways in this patient?

A. Protein synthesis is dramatically upregulated through the PI3K and mTOR pathways
B. Extracellular signal-related kinases (ERKs) are activated
C. GSK-3β activity is reduced in cardiomyocytes undergoing hypertrophic growth
D. Hypertrophic signaling has a strong overlap with factors known to broadly regulate organ size
E. mTORC1 has an important role in pathologic, but not physiologic hypertrophy

6-6. Which of the following is *not true* regarding microRNA signaling in this patient?

A. The miR212/132 family of microRNAs promotes hypertrophy by the inhibition of the antihypertrophic transcription factor FoxO3
B. MiR-133 levels are increased and promote hypertrophy and fibrosis
C. Anti-miRs are an approach to pharmacologically modulate microRNA signaling
D. MiRs that promote myocardial glucose utilization are investigational approaches to prevent the progression to heart failure
E. Exosomes secreted from the heart allow for the systemic circulation of miRNAs to other organ beds

6-7. Which of the following is *true* regarding lncRNAs in this patient?

A. The lncRNA CHAST is likely to be upregulated
B. LncRNAs, by definition, are not translated into protein products
C. LncRNAs exert their effects solely through the inhibition of complementary transcripts
D. LncRNAs are found only in intergenic regions
E. LncRNAs are highly conserved across phyla

6-8. Which of the following is *not true* regarding cell death in the development of heart failure?

A. Cytochrome C release marks cells about to undergo necrotic cell death in the failing heart
B. Prolonged ER stress can trigger cell death pathways
C. Apoptotic cell death is programmed cell death that does not typically result in an inflammatory response
D. Necrotic cell death is marked by a loss of membrane integrity, extrusion of intracellular contents, and inflammation
E. Apoptotic cell death is energy dependent, but necrotic cell death is energy independent

6-9. Which of the following is *not true* regarding cardiac fibroblasts?

A. Cardiac fibrosis is the result of collagen production in excess of collagen degradation
B. Cardiac fibroblasts differentiate into myofibroblasts that express contractile proteins
C. The main components of cardiac extracellular matrix are proteoglycans and elastin
D. Pathologic cardiac fibrosis is proarrhythmogenic, in part, because of electrical isolation of regions of the myocardium
E. Cardiac fibroblasts in the adult heart are primarily derived from resident fibroblasts

6-10. Which of the following is *true* regarding cardiac microRNAs?

A. The majority of transcripts in the genome encode proteins
B. MicroRNAs, PIWI-interacting RNAs, and endogenous short interfering RNAs are types of long ncRNAs
C. MiRNAs regulate gene expression by binding to mRNAs, resulting in degradation
D. The number of ncRNAs decreases with increasing complexity of the species
E. Long ncRNAs are more than 2000 base pairs long

6-1. **The answer is B.** (*Hurst's The Heart, 14th Edition, Chap. 6*) This patient presents with classic findings of heart failure with reduced ejection fraction. In the normal heart, 60% to 80% of β-adrenergic receptors are of the β1 subtype.[1] With heart failure, β1-AR is downregulated, and the β1-AR/β2-AR ratio nearly normalizes (options A and C).[2] A molecular hallmark of heart failure is the desensitization of the β-adrenergic signaling axis. A failing heart is less sensitive to exogenous β-AR ligands than is a normal heart (option D). At the molecular level, this occurs by a decreased density of β1-AR in cardiomyocytes and increased levels of GRK2. GRK2 phosphorylates β-ARs and reduces their sensitivity (option B).[3] Chronic β-AR signaling through the β1-AR is believed to contribute to cardiomyocyte apoptosis seen in heart failure (option E).[3]

6-2. **The answer is C.** (*Hurst's The Heart, 14th Edition, Chap. 6*) Following depolarization of the cardiomyocyte membrane, L-type calcium channels open, and calcium influxes into the cardiomyocyte (option A).[4] In response, ryanodine receptors release calcium from the sarcoplasmic reticulum. The net result is an increase in cytoplasmic calcium that leads to increased myofilament contractility. Activation of ryanodine receptors is more efficient when they are in close proximity to the calcium influx through L-type calcium channels (option E).[5] An increase in force with increasing heart rate is due to increased cytoplasmic calcium and is known as the force-frequency relationship (option C). The force-frequency relationship is an important feature of the healthy heart. During relaxation, cytoplasmic calcium is sequestered in the sarcoplasmic reticulum by the SERCA ATPase (option B). SERCA activity is negatively regulated by phospholamban.[6,7] PKA and CaMKII can phosphorylate and inactivate phospholamban, thus maintaining SERCA activity (option D).

6-3. **The answer is A.** (*Hurst's The Heart, 14th Edition, Chap. 6*) Intracellular calcium homeostasis is altered in the failing cardiomyocyte. Hallmarks of the failing cardiomyocyte include (1) decreased systolic calcium, (2) increased diastolic calcium, and (3) a prolonged relaxation phase (options B and D).[4] Additionally, the force-frequency relationship is altered such that contractile force decreases with increasing heart rate (option D). Biochemically, the L-type calcium channel does not activate the ryanodine receptor as efficiently, and hyperphosphorylation leads to an increased sensitivity of the ryanodine receptor.[8] Calcium leak from the ryanodine receptor can result in delayed afterdepolarizations, an important contributor to arrhythmogenesis (option A).[4,9] Finally, SERCA expression has been demonstrated to be reduced in animal and human models of heart failure, and the restoration of normal SERCA levels has been a focus of gene therapy efforts for patients with heart failure (option E).[7,8]

6-4. **The answer is E.** (*Hurst's The Heart, 14th Edition, Chap. 6*) Hypertrophic signaling results from complex inputs at the membrane and within the cell. Mechanical stretch alone can activate many of the signaling pathways involved in hypertrophy through surface-bound integrins and mechanically activated ion channels (option D).[10] Additionally, prohypertrophic growth factors such as angiotensin II work through heterotrimeric G-proteins (option C). The Gq family is particularly important because overexpression of Gq is sufficient to cause hypertrophy.[11] A key feature of hypertrophic signaling is an increase in intracellular calcium that binds to calmodulin, resulting in the activation of calcineurin and CaMKII (option A). Both calcineurin and CaMKII lead to the activation of transcription factors that promote hypertophic gene expression programs. CaMKII activates the transcription factors MEF2 and HDAC2 by phosphorylation (option B).[12] One result of hypertrophic signaling is re-expression of factors from cardiac development, such as BNP, ANF, and β-MHC (option E).[13]

6-5. **The answer is E.** (*Hurst's The Heart, 14th Edition, Chap. 6*) Hypertrophic cardiomyocytes have dramatic upregulation of protein synthesis via the PI3K and mTORC pathways (option A). Many stimuli that result in cardiac hypertrophy also activate PI3K signaling. mTORC1 signaling is one example of several growth pathways that are activated with cardiac hypertrophy.

mTORC1 appears to be broadly related to cardiac growth as inhibition compromises both physiologic and pathologic hypertrophy (options D and E).[14] Additionally, MAPK activity is thought to be increased and GSK-3β activity reduced during hypertrophy (option C).[15]

6-6. **The answer is B.** (*Hurst's The Heart, 14th Edition, Chap. 6*) The importance of microRNA signaling to the pathologic hypertrophy and the progression of heart failure is being increasingly recognized. MicroRNAs regulate multiple processes, such as hypertrophic signaling pathways, tissue fibrosis, vascular density, and cardiac metabolism (option D).[16] MiR-133 is downregulated with cardiac stress and has protective effects against hypertrophy and tissue fibrosis (option B).[17] By contrast, miR212/132 are increased with cardiac stress and promote hypertrophic signaling by repressing the antihypertrophic transcription factor FoxO3 (option A).[18-20] MicroRNAs are promising therapeutic targets and can be specifically targeted by modified nucleic acids that function as anti-miRs (option C). Finally, the systemic roles of cardiac microRNAs are being increasingly understood because cardiac microRNAs can be found in the circulation within small vesicles called exosomes (option E).[21]

6-7. **The answer is A.** (*Hurst's The Heart, 14th Edition, Chap. 6*) LncRNAs were originally defined as noncoding RNAs greater than 200 base pairs in length.[22] LncRNAs can be found within coding genes and intergenic regions (option D). LncRNAs have emerged as complex molecules with a diverse set of regulatory functions.[23] They can repress transcription by binding transcripts, and they directly interact with proteins to regulate their function (option C). More recently, some lncRNAs have been identified that encode small proteins, such as the protein DWORF that activates the SERCA pump (option B).[24] LncRNAs tend to be poorly conserved across phyla (option E). The lncRNA CHAST is an exception, and elevations have been identified in murine models of pressure overload and in hypertrophied human heart tissue (option A).[25]

6-8. **The answer is A.** (*Hurst's The Heart, 14th Edition, Chap. 6*) Cardiomyocyte cell death is an important contributor to the progression to heart failure. Cell death can occur via necrotic cell death following injuries to the heart or programmed apoptotic cell death. Necrotic cell death is an energy independent process that is marked by a loss of membrane integrity, resulting in extrusion of intracellular contents and inflammation (option D).[26] Apoptotic cell death, by contrast, is programmed and triggered by both intracellular and extracellular stimuli (options C and E). For example, prolonged ER stress can lead to the triggering of death pathways (option B). In failing hearts, some myocytes exhibit features of apoptotic cell death, such as mitochondrial cytochrome C release, but they can survive and maintain intact nuclei (option A).[27] These cells are thought to undergo reversible damage.

6-9. **The answer is C.** (*Hurst's The Heart, 14th Edition, Chap. 6*) In response to stress, the heart undergoes pathologic remodeling, with proliferation of resident fibroblasts to make more fibroblasts (option E).[28] These fibroblasts tip the balance of extracellular matrix turnover toward excess production compared to degradation (option A).[28,29] Extracellular matrix is a complex network of collagens, elastin, glycoproteins, and proteoglycans. However, type I collagen is the main component (option C).[30] Cardiac fibrosis stiffens the heart and can be proarrhythmic by electrically isolating parts of the myocardium (option D).[31,32] In addition to roles in maintaining the balance of cardiac extracellular matrix, cardiac fibroblasts can differentiate into myofibroblasts that express contractile proteins. Myofibroblasts play important roles in contracting the wound following injury (option B).[33]

6-10. **The answer is C.** (*Hurst's The Heart, 14th Edition, Chap. 6*) As a result of widespread sequencing, the vast number of ncRNAs has been recognized. It has now been determined that although about three-fourths of the mammalian genome is transcribed, less than 2% is ultimately translated into proteins (option A).[34] Short ncRNAs are < 200 bp in length and include micoRNAs, PIWI-interacting RNAs, and endogenous short interfering RNAs. By contrast, long ncRNAs are longer than 2 kb in length (options B and E).[35-38] MiRNAs can repress gene expression by binding to target mRNAs, resulting in degradation (option C). MiRNAs are increasingly recognized as important regulators of gene expression and cell identity. The number of ncRNAs increases with increasing organism complexity (option D).[39]

References

1. Triposkiadis F, Karayannis G, Giamouzis G, et al. The sympathetic nervous system in heart failure physiology, pathophysiology, and clinical implications. *J Am Coll Cardiol.* 2009;54(19):1747-1762.

2. Nikolaev VO, Moshkov A, Lyon AR, et al. Beta2-adrenergic receptor redistribution in heart failure changes cAMP compartmentation. *Science.* 2010;327(5973):1653-1657.

3. Sato PY, Chuprun JK, Schwartz M, Koch WJ. The evolving impact of g protein-coupled receptor kinases in cardiac health and disease. *Physiol Rev.* 2015;95(2):377-404.

4. Bers DM. Cardiac sarcoplasmic reticulum calcium leak: basis and roles in cardiac dysfunction. *Ann Rev Physiol.* 2014;76:107-127.

5. Zulkifli Amin H, Suridanda Danny S. Tolvaptan. A novel diuretic in heart failure management. *J Tehran Heart Cent.* 2016;11(1):1-5.

6. Gorski PA, Ceholski DK, Hajjar RJ. Altered myocardial calcium cycling and energetics in heart failure—a rational approach for disease treatment. *Cell Metab.* 2015;21(2):183-194.

7. Kranias EG, Hajjar RJ. Modulation of cardiac contractility by the phospholamban/SERCA2a regulatome. *Circ Res.* 2012;110(12):1646-1660.

8. Kho C, Lee A, Hajjar RJ. Altered sarcoplasmic reticulum calcium cycling—targets for heart failure therapy. *Nat Rev Cardiol.* 2012;9(12):717-733.

9. Marks AR. Calcium cycling proteins and heart failure: mechanisms and therapeutics. *J Clin Invest.* 2013;123(1):46-52.

10. Brancaccio M, Fratta L, Notte A, et al. Melusin, a muscle-specific integrin beta1-interacting protein, is required to prevent cardiac failure in response to chronic pressure overload. *Nat Med.* 2003;9(1):68-75.

11. Adams JW, Sakata Y, Davis MG, et al. Enhanced Galphaq signaling: a common pathway mediates cardiac hypertrophy and apoptotic heart failure. *Proc Natl Acad Sci U S A.* 1998;95(17):10140-10145.

12. Passier R, Zeng H, Frey N, et al. CaM kinase signaling induces cardiac hypertrophy and activates the MEF2 transcription factor in vivo. *J Clin Invest.* 2000;105(10):1395-1406.

13. van Berlo JH, Maillet M, Molkentin JD. Signaling effectors underlying pathologic growth and remodeling of the heart. *J Clin Invest.* 2013;123(1):37-45.

14. Zhang D, Contu R, Latronico MV, et al. MTORC1 regulates cardiac function and myocyte survival through 4E-BP1 inhibition in mice. *J Clin Invest.* 2010;120(8):2805-2816.

15. Antos CL, McKinsey TA, Frey N, et al. Activated glycogen synthase-3 beta suppresses cardiac hypertrophy in vivo. *Proc Natl Acad Sci U S A.* 2002;99(2):907-912.

16. el Azzouzi H, Leptidis S, Dirkx E, et al. The hypoxia-inducible microRNA cluster miR-199a~214 targets myocardial PPARdelta and impairs mitochondrial fatty acid oxidation. *Cell Metab.* 2013;18(3):341-354.

17. Care A, Catalucci D, Felicetti F, et al. MicroRNA-133 controls cardiac hypertrophy. *Nat Med.* 2007;13(5):613-618.

18. Thum T, Galuppo P, Wolf C, et al. MicroRNAs in the human heart: a clue to fetal gene reprogramming in heart failure. *Circulation.* 2007;116(3):258-267.

19. Ucar A, Gupta SK, Fiedler J, et al. The miRNA-212/132 family regulates both cardiac hypertrophy and cardiomyocyte autophagy. *Nat Commun.* 2012;3:1078.

20. Gupta SK, Thum T. Non-coding RNAs as orchestrators of autophagic processes. *J Mol Cell Cardiol.* 2016;95:26-30.

21. Gupta SK, Bang C, Thum T. Circulating microRNAs as biomarkers and potential paracrine mediators of cardiovascular disease. *Circ Cardiovasc Genet.* 2010;3(5):484-488.

22. Batista PJ, Chang HY. Long noncoding RNAs: cellular address codes in development and disease. *Cell.* 2013;152(6):1298-1307.

23. Thum T, Condorelli G. Long noncoding RNAs and microRNAs in cardiovascular pathophysiology. *Circ Res.* 2015;116(4):751-762.

24. Nelson BR, Makarewich CA, Anderson DM, et al. A peptide encoded by a transcript annotated as long noncoding RNA enhances SERCA activity in muscle. *Science.* 2016;351(6270):271-275.

25. Viereck J, Kumarswamy R, Foinquinos A, et al. Long noncoding RNA Chast promotes cardiac remodeling. *Sci Transl Med.* 2016;8(326):326ra22.

26. Pasparakis M, Vandenabeele P. Necroptosis and its role in inflammation. *Nature.* 2015;517(7534):311-320.

27. Narula J, Pandey P, Arbustini E, et al. Apoptosis in heart failure: release of cytochrome c from mitochondria and activation of caspase-3 in human cardiomyopathy. *Proc Natl Acad Sci U S A.* 1999;96(14):8144-8149.

28. Moore-Morris T, Guimaraes-Camboa N, Banerjee I, et al. Resident fibroblast lineages mediate pressure overload-induced cardiac fibrosis. *J Clin Invest.* 2014;124(7):2921-2934.

29. Kong P, Christia P, Frangogiannis NG. The pathogenesis of cardiac fibrosis. *Cell Mol Life Sci.* 2014;71(4):549-574.

30. Camelliti P, Borg TK, Kohl P. Structural and functional characterisation of cardiac fibroblasts. *Cardiovasc Res.* 2005;65(1):40-51.

31. Azevedo CF, Nigri M, Higuchi ML, et al. Prognostic significance of myocardial fibrosis quantification by histopathology and magnetic resonance imaging in patients with severe aortic valve disease. *J Am Coll Cardiol.* 2010;56(4):278-287.

32. Nguyen TP, Qu Z, and Weiss JN. Cardiac fibrosis and arrhythmogenesis: the road to repair is paved with perils. *J Mol Cell Cardiol.* 2014;70:83-91.

33. Brilla CG, Maisch B, Zhou G, and Weber KT. Hormonal regulation of cardiac fibroblast function. *Eur Heart J.* 1995;16 Suppl C:45-50.

34. Derrien T, Johnson R, Bussotti G, et al. The GENCODE v7 catalog of human long noncoding RNAs: analysis of their gene structure, evolution, and expression. *Genome Res.* 2012;22(9):1775-1789.

35. Tay Y, Rinn J, and Pandolfi PP. The multilayered complexity of ceRNA crosstalk and competition. *Nature.* 2014;505(7483):344-352.

36. Mitra SA, Mitra AP, and Triche TJ. A central role for long non-coding RNA in cancer. *Front Genet.* 2012;3:17.

37. Li T, Mo X, Fu L, Xiao B, and Guo J. Molecular mechanisms of long noncoding RNAs on gastric cancer. *Oncotarget.* 2016;7(8):8601-8612.

38. Saxena A, and Carninci P. Long non-coding RNA modifies chromatin: epigenetic silencing by long non-coding RNAs. *Bioessays.* 2011;33(11):830-839.

39. Taft RJ, Pheasant M, and Mattick JS. The relationship between non-protein-coding DNA and eukaryotic complexity. *Bioessays.* 2007;29(3):288-299.

CHAPTER 7

Biology of the Vessel Wall

Ravi Karra

DIRECTIONS: Choose the one best response to each question.

7-1. Which of the following is *true* about vascular development?

A. A bipotent hemangioblast is capable of giving rise to endothelial cells and blood cells
B. The primitive vasculature arises from coalesced blood islands
C. Postnatal vasculogenesis requires angioblasts that are active in the adult
D. Collateral arteries that form in the presence of obstructive coronary artery disease are the result of bone-marrow-derived progenitor cells
E. VEGF is a potent inhibitor of angiogenesis

7-2. Which of the following is *incorrect* regarding the role of endothelial cells?

A. The endothelium serves as a prothrombotic surface
B. The endothelium regulates the inflammatory response by affecting leukocyte recruitment and margination
C. The endothelium helps to regulate vascular tone
D. The endothelium regulates signaling by allowing for the selective passage of molecules across the barrier
E. The endothelium serves as a barrier to circulating blood constituents

7-3. Which of the following is *not true* about signaling in endothelial cells?

A. Inflamed endothelium produces tissue factor, which creates a procoagulant surface
B. Water-soluble molecules are transported across the endothelium via caveolae

C. L-selectin, P-selectin, and VCAM-1 are important to the capture of leukocytes by the endothelium during inflammation
D. NO acts as a vasoconstrictor by increasing levels of cGMP, which reduces intracellular calcium concentrations and results in the dephosphorylation of MLCK in smooth muscle
E. PGI2 is made by the endothelium and promotes vascular relaxation by increasing cAMP levels in smooth muscle cells

7-4. Which of the following *do not* promote the conversion of vascular smooth muscle to a synthetic phenotype?

A. PDGF
B. FGF
C. TGF-β
D. NO
E. IGF-1

7-5. Which of the following is *not true* regarding the vascular extracellular matrix (ECM)?

A. Degradation of the ECM is one of the earliest events during angiogenesis
B. Matrix metalloproteinases degrade the ECM
C. Increased MMP activity has been noted in abdominal aneurysms
D. Increased MMP activity is found in the shoulder of an atherosclerotic plaque
E. Secreted MMPs are inactivated by plasmin

7-6. Which of the following is *not* a characteristic of endothelial dysfunction?

A. Endothelial dysfunction is associated with cardiovascular risk factors such as diabetes, smoking, and a family history of atherosclerotic disease
B. A hallmark of dysfunctional endothelium is increased NO production
C. Dysfunctional endothelium recruits monocytes and macrophages to the vessel wall
D. Endothelial dysfunction precedes the morphological presence of atherosclerotic plaque
E. All of the above

7-7. A 64-year-old man is admitted with an anterior ST elevation myocardial infarction. He is taken to the cardiac catheterization laboratory and undergoes successful percutaneous intervention with a drug-eluting stent. Which of the following is *not true* regarding the stent?

A. Drug-eluting stents inhibit intimal smooth muscle proliferation
B. Smooth muscle proliferation is the cause of in-stent restenosis
C. Restenosis occurs in 5% to 10% of older generation drug-eluting stents
D. Newer generation drug-eluting stents with thicker struts and improved drug delivery have worse reendothelialization than older drug-eluting stents
E. None of the above

7-8. Which of the following is *true* about vascular progenitor cells?

A. Endothelial progenitor cells are found only in the bone marrow
B. Pericytes share properties with mesenchymal stem cells
C. Adventitial stem cells give rise to cardiomyocytes
D. Vascular smooth muscle progenitors, unlike other smooth muscle cells within the vascular wall, are proliferative
E. B and C

7-9. A 43-year-old woman presents with progressive shortness of breath. Physical exam reveals elevated neck veins, a right ventricular (RV) lift, and a loud P2. Echocardiography shows normal left ventricular function but elevated pulmonary artery pressures. Right heart catheterization shows a normal pulmonary capillary wedge pressure but markedly elevated pulmonary artery pressures. Which of the following is *not true* regarding therapies for pulmonary hypertension?

A. Epoprostenol, iloprost, and treprostinil result in vasodilation of the pulmonary vasculature
B. Sildenafil and tadalafil cause vasodilation by increasing NO levels
C. Bosentan affects endothelin receptors on smooth muscle cells and endothelial cells
D. Ambrisentan and macicentan are selective ET-A antagonists that inhibit smooth muscle vasoconstriction
E. All of the above are true

7-10. Which of the following is *true* regarding signaling pathways in vascular smooth muscle cells?

A. IP3 increases cytoplasmic calcium by direct inhibition of SERCA
B. DAG inhibits muscle contraction via PKC
C. The initial phase of smooth muscle contraction is the result of the latch-bridge state
D. Rho activation desensitizes MLC to intracellular calcium
E. None of the above

ANSWERS

7-1. The answer is B. (*Hurst's The Heart, 14th Edition, Chap. 7*) The notion that a bipotent hemangioblast gives rise to endothelial cells and blood cells has recently been challenged. Instead, blood cells probably develop from hemogenic endothelial cells residing in specialized vascular niches (option A).[1] Early blood vessels are derived from blood islands, which are clusters of mesodermal progenitor cells. These islands are marked by central hematopoietic progenitor cells and peripheral angioblasts (option B). Unlike during development, postnatal vasculogenesis does not rely on angioblasts, but instead occurs by the sprouting of new vessels from preexisting vessels. In the adult, vasculogenesis may be limited. However, in scenarios such as the development of collateral vasculature with obstructive coronary artery disease, arteriogenesis occurs. Arteriogenesis occurs by the sprouting of new vessels from preexisting capillaries or arterio-arterio anastomoses (option C).[2] Much work has gone into understanding cytokines that stimulate vasculogenesis. The prototypical angiokine is VEGF.[3] In fact, VEGF inhibitors are used clinically as anticancer agents to inhibit tumor-related angiogenesis (option E).

7-2. The answer is A. (*Hurst's The Heart, 14th Edition, Chap. 7*) Among its many functions, the endothelium is of particular importance for maintaining and protecting the integrity and function of the vascular wall, with specific roles. These include (1) functioning as a metabolic tissue that actively secretes vasoactive factors governing vascular tone (option C); (2) acting as an anticoagulant and antithrombotic surface (option A); (3) serving as a barrier to most circulating blood constituents (option E); (4) regulating the transendothelial passage of specific molecules, proteins, and cells across this barrier (option D), and (5) participating in the inflammatory response via active leukocyte recruitment and facilitation of leukocyte margination from the lumen into the vessel wall and adjacent tissues (option E).

7-3. The answer is D. (*Hurst's The Heart, 14th Edition, Chap. 7*) As a part of its barrier function, the endothelium regulates the transport of molecules from the vascular lumen to tissues. Water-soluble molecules, in particular, are transported across endothelial cells in vesicles called caveolae.[4] The endothelium generally serves as an antithrombotic surface. However, when inflamed, the endothelium expresses tissue factor, factor VIII, PAI-1, and factor Va, which create a procoagulant milieu (option A).[5] The endothelium has important roles in regulating inflammation. These include capture, adhesion, and migration of leukocytes (option C).[6] NO and PGI2 are vasodilators (options D and E).

7-4. The answer is D. (*Hurst's The Heart, 14th Edition, Chap. 7*) Conversion of a vascular smooth muscle cell from a quiescent, differentiated phenotype to a proliferative, synthetic phenotype is a hallmark of pathologic states such as neointimal hyperplasia. Agents such as NO, prostacyclin, and heparin inhibit growth and promote a differentiated phenotype (option D).[7-9] By contrast, growth factors such as PDGF, FGF, and IGF-1 promote smooth muscle cell migration and hyperplasia (options A, B, and E).[10] TGF-β can promote either the differentiated or synthetic phenotype, depending on the context (option C).

7-5. The answer is E. (*Hurst's The Heart, 14th Edition, Chap. 7*) MMPs are a diverse class of proteins that degrade the ECM (option B). TIMPs antagonize MMPs and stabilize the ECM. MMPs allow for the growth and proliferation of new blood vessels (option A). Importantly, TIMPs and MMPs play a pivotal role in the pathology of atherosclerotic plaques and aneurysms (option C).[11,12] MMPs are highly expressed in the shoulder regions of atherosclerotic plaques and predispose to plaque rupture (option D).[13] MMPs can either be membrane-spanning or secreted. Secreted MMPs are secreted as zymogens and are activated after cleavage by plasmin (option E).

7-6. The answer is B. (*Hurst's The Heart, 14th Edition, Chap. 7*) Endothelial dysfunction precedes the development of atherosclerotic plaque (option D). Dysfunctional endothelium has an impaired capacity for NO production (option B) and upregulates inflammatory markers that lead to the recruitment of inflammatory cells (option C).[14,15] These inflammatory cells infiltrate the vessel wall and oxidize LDL, triggering atheroma formation.[16] Endothelial dysfunction has been correlated to many clinical factors associated with coronary athero-sclerotic disease (option A).[17-19]

7-7. **The answer is D.** (*Hurst's The Heart, 14th Edition, Chap. 7*) Percutaneous interventions with balloon angioplasty and bare metal stents were plagued with high rates of restenosis. Acute arterial injury results in smooth muscle proliferation. This proliferation is a major feature of restenosis (option B). Stents eluting antiproliferative drugs prevent smooth muscle pro-liferation, leading to reduced rates of restenosis (option A). Unfortunately, these drugs also prevented reendothelialization of the stents and are associated with acute stent thrombosis. Newer generation drug-eluting stents, with thinner struts and better drug delivery, are asso-ciated with less stent thrombosis and have better reendothelialization (option D). In the contemporary era of drug-eluting stents (DES), clinically significant restenosis arises in only 5% to 10% of treated.

7-8. **The answer is B**. (*Hurst's The Heart, 14th Edition, Chap. 7*) Endothelial progenitor cells (EPCs) expand and proliferate to make new endothelial cells. Recent work has identified a local source of EPCs within the vessel wall (option A).[2] Pericytes can differentiate into adipocytes, chondrocytes, and osteocytes and share properties with mesenchymal stem cells (option B).[2,22] Adventitial stem cells are still under investigation but appear to give rise to smooth muscle cells, endothelial cells, and myofibroblasts (option C).[23] The presence of VSMCs in the vessel wall is controversial. Both putative VSMCs and mature SMCs can proliferate (option D).[24,25]

7-9. **The answer is B.** (*Hurst's The Heart, 14th Edition, Chap. 7*). Epoprostenol, iloprost, and treprostinil are all prostacyclin analogs and result in pulmonary vasodilation (option A).[26] Sildenafil and tadalafil inhibit phosphodiesterase and increase cGMP levels, leading to vasodilation. They do not directly increase NO levels (option B).[26] Bosentan, ambrisentan, and macicentan are endothelin receptor antagonists. Endothelin causes smooth muscle-mediated vasoconstriction via the ET-A receptor and endothelial cell-mediated vasodilation via the ET-B receptor (option C). Bosentan is a mixed ET-A/ET-B antagonist, but the newer agents ambrisentan and macicentan are more selective for the ET-A receptor (option D).[26,27]

7-10. **The answer is B.** (*Hurst's The Heart, 14th Edition, Chap. 7*). Vasoactive agents lead to the hydrolysis of phosphoinositides by phospholipase C. As a result, inositol triphosphate (IP3) and diacylglycerol (DAG) are produced.[28] IP3 binds to IP3 receptors on intracellular organelles to increase intracellular levels of calcium (option A).[29] Increased DAG levels lead to increased PKC activity. PKC works to stimulate contraction in the presence of increased intracellular calcium levels (option B).[30] While the initial phase of smooth muscle cell contraction depends on increased intracellular calcium, the sustained phase is related to the latch-bridge state (option C). Essentially, myosin is dephosphorylated when bound to actin. Although the myosin will not actively cycle, it can maintain tension through its association with actin.[31] The GTPase Rho activates Rho kinase, leading to inactivation myosin phosphatase, type I.[32] As a result, MLC remains phosphorylated and is more sensitive to intracellular calcium (option D).[33]

References

1. Sandler VM, Lis R, Liu Y, et al. Reprogramming human endothelial cells to haematopoietic cells requires vascular induction. *Nature*. 2014;511(7509):312-318.
2. Kovacic JC, Moore J, Herbert A, et al. Endothelial progenitor cells, angioblasts, and angiogenesis—old terms reconsidered from a current perspective. *Trends Cardiovasc Med*. 2008;18(2):45-51.
3. Shalaby F, Rossant J, Yamaguchi TP, et al. Failure of blood-island formation and vasculogenesis in Flk-1-deficient mice. *Nature*. 1995;376(6535):62-66.
4. Zhang Y, Zhang L, Li Y, Sun S, and Tan H. Different contributions of clathrin- and caveolae-mediated endocytosis of vascular endothelial cadherin to lipopolysaccharide-induced vascular hyperpermeability. *PLoS One*. 2014;9(9):e106328.

5. Snow SJ, Cheng W, Wolberg AS, and Carraway MS. Air pollution upregulates endothelial cell proco-agulant activity via ultrafine particle-induced oxidant signaling and tissue factor expression. *Toxicol Sci.* 2014;140(1):83-93.

6. Zarbock A, Ley K, McEver RP, and Hidalgo A. Leukocyte ligands for endothelial selectins: specialized glycoconjugates that mediate rolling and signaling under flow. *Blood.* 2011;118(26):6743-6751.

7. Newby AC, Southgate KM, and Assender JW. Inhibition of vascular smooth muscle cell proliferation by endothelium-dependent vasodilators. *Herz.* 1992;17(5):291-299.

8. Ettenson DS, Koo EW, Januzzi JL, and Edelman ER. Endothelial heparan sulfate is necessary but not sufficient for control of vascular smooth muscle cell growth. *J Cell Physiol.* 2000;184(1):93-100.

9. Ueba H, Kawakami M, and Yaginuma T. Shear stress as an inhibitor of vascular smooth muscle cell proliferation. Role of transforming growth factor-beta 1 and tissue-type plasminogen activator. *Arterioscler Thromb Vasc Biol.* 1997;17(8):1512-1516.

10. Krishnan P, Purushothaman KR, Purushothaman M, et al. Relation of internal elastic lamellar layer disruption to neointimal cellular proliferation and type III collagen deposition in human peripheral artery restenosis. *Am J Cardiol.* 2016;117(7):1173-1179.

11. Zhang XJ, He C, Tian K, et al. Ginsenoside Rb1 attenuates angiotensin II-induced abdominal aortic aneurysm through inactivation of the JNK and p38 signaling pathways. *Vascul Pharmacol.* 2015;73:86-95.

12. Galis ZS, and Khatri JJ. Matrix metalloproteinases in vascular remodeling and atherogenesis: the good, the bad, and the ugly. *Circ Res.* 2002;90(3):251-262.

13. Galis ZS, Sukhova GK, Lark MW, and Libby P. Increased expression of matrix metalloproteinases and matrix degrading activity in vulnerable regions of human atherosclerotic plaques. *J Clin Invest.* 1994;94(6):2493-2503.

14. Xu S, Ha CH, Wang W, et al. PECAM1 regulates flow-mediated Gab1 tyrosine phosphorylation and signaling. *Cell Signal.* 2016;28(3):117-124.

15. Huang Q, Qin L, Dai S, et al. AIP1 suppresses atherosclerosis by limiting hyperlipidemia-induced inflammation and vascular endothelial dysfunction. *Arterioscler Thromb Vasc Biol.* 2013;33(4):795-804.

16. Lu Z, Zhang X, Li Y, Lopes-Virella MF, and Huang Y. TLR4 antagonist attenuates atherogenesis in LDL receptor-deficient mice with diet-induced type 2 diabetes. *Immunobiology.* 2015;220(11):1246-1254.

17. Clarkson P, Celermajer DS, Donald AE, et al. Impaired vascular reactivity in insulin-dependent diabetes mellitus is related to disease duration and low density lipoprotein cholesterol levels. *J Am Coll Cardiol.* 1996;28(3):573-579.

18. Woo KS, Robinson JT, Chook P, et al. Differences in the effect of cigarette smoking on endothelial function in Chinese and white adults. *Ann Intern Med.* 1997;127(5):372-375.

19. Clarkson P, Celermajer DS, Powe AJ, et al. Endothelium-dependent dilatation is impaired in young healthy subjects with a family history of premature coronary disease. *Circulation.* 1997;96(10):3378-3383.

20. Bangalore S, Toklu B, Amoroso N, et al. Bare metal stents, durable polymer drug eluting stents, and biodegradable polymer drug eluting stents for coronary artery disease: mixed treatment comparison meta-analysis. *BMJ.* 2013;347:f6625.

21. Park SJ, Ahn JM, Kim YH, et al. Trial of everolimus-eluting stents or bypass surgery for coronary disease. *N Engl J Med.* 2015;372(13):1204-1212.

22. Pierantozzi E, Badin M, Vezzani B, et al. Human pericytes isolated from adipose tissue have better differentiation abilities than their mesenchymal stem cell counterparts. *Cell Tissue Res.* 2015;361(3):769-778.

23. Passman JN, Dong XR, Wu SP, et al. A sonic hedgehog signaling domain in the arterial adventitia supports resident Sca1+ smooth muscle progenitor cells. *Proc Natl Acad Sci U S A.* 2008;105(27):9349-9354.

24. Tang Z, Wang A, Yuan F, et al. Differentiation of multipotent vascular stem cells contributes to vascular diseases. *Nat Commun.* 2012;3:875.

25. Nguyen AT, Gomez D, Bell RD, et al. Smooth muscle cell plasticity: fact or fiction? *Circ Res.* 2013;112(1):17-22.

26. Galie N, Humbert M, Vachiery JL, et al. 2015 ESC/ERS Guidelines for the diagnosis and treatment of pulmonary hypertension: The Joint Task Force for the Diagnosis and Treatment of Pulmonary Hypertension of the European Society of Cardiology (ESC) and the European Respiratory Society (ERS): Endorsed by: Association for European Paediatric and Congenital Cardiology (AEPC), International Society for Heart and Lung Transplantation (ISHLT). *Eur Heart J.* 2016;37(1):67-119.

27. Liu C, Chen J, Gao Y, Deng B, and Liu K. Endothelin receptor antagonists for pulmonary arterial hypertension. *Cochrane Database Syst Rev.* 2013;(2):CD004434.

28. Berridge MJ, and Irvine RF. Inositol trisphosphate, a novel second messenger in cellular signal transduction. *Nature.* 1984;312(5992):315-321.

29. Yamamoto H, and van Breemen C. Inositol-1,4,5-trisphosphate releases calcium from skinned cultured smooth muscle cells. *Biochem Biophys Res Commun.* 1985;130(1):270-274.

30. Nishizuka Y. The role of protein kinase C in cell surface signal transduction and tumour promotion. *Nature.* 1984;308(5961):693-698.

31. Roman HN, Zitouni NB, Kachmar L, et al. Unphosphorylated calponin enhances the binding force of unphosphorylated myosin to actin. *Biochim Biophys Acta.* 2013;1830(10):4634-4641.

32. Mills RD, Mita M, Nakagawa J, et al. A role for the tyrosine kinase Pyk2 in depolarization-induced contraction of vascular smooth muscle. *J Biol Chem.* 2015;290(14):8677-8692.

33. Kitazono T, Ago T, Kamouchi M, et al. Increased activity of calcium channels and Rho-associated kinase in the basilar artery during chronic hypertension in vivo. *J Hypertens.* 2002;20(5):879-884.

CHAPTER 8

Molecular and Cellular Development of the Heart

Ravi Karra

DIRECTIONS: Choose the one best response to each question.

8-1. Which of the following is *not true* about the specification of cardiac precursors during gastrulation?

A. Cardiac precursors are derived from mesoderm following gastrulation
B. The fates of cardiac progenitor cells are already determined at the epiblast stage
C. The fates of progenitor cells are determined by the sequence and intensity of external signals encountered during gastrulation
D. A precursor cell's position within the epiblast determines the complement of external signals it receives
E. Mesoderm is the result of epithelial-to-mesenchymal transition (EMT) in the epiblast

8-2. Which of the following is *true* about the specification of mesoderm that gives rise to cardiac cells?

A. Cells that migrate from the anterior primitive streak give rise to lateral mesoderm
B. Cardiac progenitors are found in the lateral plate mesoderm
C. The heart and liver are the last mesoderm to be produced by the embryo
D. Retinoic acid gradients are important for separating cardiac and forelimb fields, but they do not have a role in determining whether cardiac precursors give rise to atrial cells or ventricular cells
E. The first cardiac cells formed in the lateral plate mesoderm are atrial cells

8-3. You see a 2-year-old child for episodes of cyanosis ameliorated by squatting. She is found to have Tetralogy of Fallot. Tetralogy of Fallot most likely results from defects in:

A. The proliferation of cells in the first heart field
B. Fusion of the primordial heart tubes
C. The addition of cells from the second heart field to the heart tube
D. Cardiac specification during gastrulation
E. Specification of atrial and ventricular cardiomyocytes

8-4. Which of the following is *not true* about signaling pathways during cardiac development?

A. Increased levels of nodal and canonical Wnt signaling promote cardiac specification of pluripotent stem cells to cardiac progenitors
B. Endoderm-derived BMP2 promotes the differentiation of cardiac mesoderm to cardiomyocytes
C. Noncanonical Wnt signaling restricts the differentiation of cardiac progenitors to cardiomyocytes, but canonical Wnt signaling promotes cardiac differentiation
D. Both cardiac progenitors and differentiated cardiomyocytes are equally proliferative
E. The differentiation and expansion of the second heart field occurs by a fine balance of canonical Wnt signaling, Notch signaling, and BMP signaling

8-5. Which of the following is *true* about the transcriptional control of cardiac differentiation?

A. Tbx5 is present mostly in cells from the second heart field
B. Pitx2 is important to anterior-posterior patterning
C. Nkx2.5, in coordination with Isl1, regulates the differentiation of cardiac progenitors to cardiomyocytes
D. Association of p300/CBP with cardiac transcription factors leads to histone deacetylation and the activation of transcription
E. Tissue-specific variants of chromatin complexes are not essential to cardiac differentiation

8-6. Which of the following is *true* about cardiac chamber morphogenesis?

A. The fetal heart begins to approximate the morphology of the adult heart by 6 weeks
B. Cardiac jelly is secreted by the endocardium and prevents blood flow until the valves are functional
C. Tbx2 and 3 are required for chamber maturation, whereas Tbx20 represses chamber maturation
D. Chamber formation and proportion are unrelated to localized regions of proliferation
E. Noncompaction results from the lack of the trabecular myocardium to be packed into the compact myocardium

8-7. A 67-year-old woman presents with right-sided hemiparesis. During her evaluation, she is noted to have a patent foramen ovale (PFO). Which of the following is *true* about atrial septation and her PFO?

A. Her foramen primum failed to close
B. Her septum primum did not migrate properly
C. Her septum primum and septum secundum failed to fuse
D. Her left sinus venosus remains linked to her left atrium
E. Her membranous ventricular septum failed to develop

8-8. An infant presents within 1 week of birth with poor feeding, intermittent cyanosis, and respiratory distress. Her exam is notable for a hyperdynamic precordium, bounding peripheral pulse, and a single S2. Echocardiography reveals a diagnosis of truncus arteriosus. Which of the following is *true* about cardiac development in this patient?

A. Failure to form a truncus could result from defects in neural crest migration or in second heart field precursors
B. There is persistence of the fifth pair of aortic arch artery pairs
C. The left sixth branchial arch artery failed to give rise to the trunk of the pulmonary artery
D. There is persistence of the right sixth branchial arch artery
E. There is persistence of the ductus arteriosus

8-9. Which of the following is *not true* of the epicardium?

A. The epicardium is a mesothelial sheet that covers the heart and has epithelial properties
B. The epicardium is multipotent with contributions to cardiac endothelium, fibroblasts, and coronary artery smooth muscle cells
C. In the adult heart, the epicardium is inert
D. The epicardium arises from the coelomic epithelium, which forms the proepicardium
E. The epicardium is a heterogeneous group of cells

8-10. Which of the following is *true* about cardiac development and homeostasis?

A. Cardiomyocyte renewal does not occur in the adult heart
B. The SA node has contributions from both the first and second heart fields
C. Cardiac innervation occurs independently of coronary vasculogenesis
D. The coronary endothelium has a single source of cells
E. Purkinje cardiomyocytes have more mitochondria than other cardiomyocytes in the ventricle

8-1. The answer is B. *(Hurst's The Heart, 14th Edition, Chap. 8)* After gastrulation, the cardiogenic area, containing cardiac precursors, is formed by early gastrulating mesoderm (option A). It is located within the mesodermal component of the splanchnopleural layer of the anteriormost lateral plate.[1,2] Mesoderm itself is formed by EMT of cells at the central-posterior position in the epiblast (option E).[3] Although different regions of the epiblast give rise to specific cell types, the fates of the precursor cells themselves at this stage are not yet determined (option B).[4] Transplantation studies have shown, for example, that epiblast regions fated to produce brain transplanted to the cardiac-forming region will form the heart, and vice versa. Ultimately, the history of external signals cells receive during their journey through gastrulation determines the differentiation pathway of precursor cells (option C). The sequence of signals received is determined by the location of precursor cells within the epiblast (option D).[3]

8-2. The answer is B. *(Hurst's The Heart, 14th Edition, Chap. 8)* Cells migrate out of the primitive streak, such that the anteriormost cells form the axial mesoderm and the posterior cells form the lateral mesoderm (option A). The cardiac fields are found in the lateral plate mesoderm, and along with the hepatic mesoderm they are among the first types of mesoderm specified (options B and C). The first cardiac mesoderm specified gives rise to the septum transversus (option E). Like with gastrulation, local signaling gradients drive differentiation. Retinoic acid gradients, in particular, have been shown to contribute to the separation of cardiac and forelimb fields in addition to the specification of subtypes of cardiac cells, such as atrial and ventricular cardiomyocytes (option D).[5]

8-3. The answer is C. *(Hurst's The Heart, 14th Edition, Chap. 8)* Tetralogy of Fallot is classically characterized by pulmonary atresia, a VSD, an overriding aorta, and right ventricular hypertrophy. Following cardiac specification in the lateral plate mesoderm, two heart fields emerge (options D and E). The first heart field gives rise to the left ventricle and most of the atria (option A). The second heart field is adjacent to the first heart field and gives rise to the right ventricle, the outflow tract, and parts of the atria and inflow tract.[2,6,7] Cells from the first heart field differentiate and contribute to the primitive heart tubes (option B). Cells from the second heart tube differentiate somewhat later and are sequentially added. In humans and chicks, there are two primordial heart tubes that must fuse at the midline to form a single heart tube.[8,9] Defects observed in tetralogy of Fallot are associated with structures derived primarily from the second heart field (option C).

8-4. The answer is C. *(Hurst's The Heart, 14th Edition, Chap. 8)* Pluripotent cells are fated to cardiac progenitors by canonical Wnt signaling (option A).[2,10] As cardiac mesoderm, cardiac progenitors differentiate into cardiomyocytes in response to BMP signaling from the extraembryonic tissues and endoderm adjacent to cardiac mesoderm (option B).[1] Progenitor cells are proliferative and tend to expand to cardiac fields, while differentiated cells are less proliferative (option D). In general, canonical Wnt/FGF/Shh signaling promote the specification of cells to cardiac progenitors, while BMP and noncanonical Wnt signaling promote differentiation into cardiomyocytes (options C and E).[10,11]

8-5. The answer is C. *(Hurst's The Heart, 14th Edition, Chap. 8)* The molecular regulation of cardiomyocyte specification and differentiation has been the subject of intense study. Different transcription factors are important to regional specification of the heart. For example, Tbx5 is present in anterior heart field cells (option A), Hand2 in second heart field cells, and Tbx1 in cells of the outflow tract.[12,13] More broadly, Gata, Nkx, and Isl factors are important for cardiomyocyte identity. Nkx2.5 is thought to promote cardiomyocyte differentiation, and the balance of a progenitor state versus a differentiated state is maintained by Nkx2.5 competing with Isl1 and Meis factors (option C).[14,15] In addition, *Pitx2c* is expressed in the left side of the SHF, as part of its general role in left-right patterning of lateral plate derivatives in the embryo (option B).[16] While transcription factors can trigger gene expression, access to a locus occurs at the chromatin level. Recent work has highlighted the role of HDACs to deacetylate chromatin, leading to the repression of expression at a locus. Conversely, p300/CBP acetylate histones lead to gene activation (option D). Further, tissue-specific isoforms, such as the Mel1 isoform of PRC1, are important for dictating tissue-specific gene expression programs (option E).[17]

8-6. **The answer is E.** (*Hurst's The Heart, 14th Edition, Chap. 8*) Cardiac morphogenesis starts at 3.5 weeks. In the 12th week, outflow tract subdivision and complete interventricular and atrial septation lead to a heart bearing the gross morphological organization of a definitive adult heart (option A).[8] The heart initially starts as a tube with an inner endocardium. Cardiac jelly is secreted by cardiomyocytes, and it prevents blood flow through the heart tube until the valves are competent (option B). Localized regions of proliferation lead to chamber ballooning. Tbx2 and 3 are important repressors of differentiation, but Tbx20 is required for chamber maturation (option C).[1,18] Following looping, chamber formation results from localized proliferation and ballooning of the chambers (option D).[19,20] The trabecular myocardium initially preserves cardiac output but is incorporated into the compact myocardium during compaction (option E).

8-7. **The answer is C.** (*Hurst's The Heart, 14th Edition, Chap. 8*) Cardiac septation occurs during the seventh week with the growth of a muscular ventricular septum between the right and left ventricles (option E). Later, a membranous septum grows between the muscular septum and the mesenchyme that contains the AV cushions. Atrial septation occurs first with a septum primum that grows between the atria, but that leaves a foramen primum between the septum primum and the AV cushions (option B). As the foramen primum is closed, a second foramen secundum develops in the septum primum (option A). A second septum secundum develops and occludes the foramen secundum. However, the septum secundum contains the foramen ovale, which allows for right-to-left blood flow but not the reverse. The foramen ovale closes due to fusion of the septum primum and secundum. Failure to fuse can lead to a persistent PFO (option C).[21]

8-8. **The answer is A.** (*Hurst's The Heart, 14th Edition, Chap. 8*) The aortic arch and pulmonary artery result from extensive remodeling of the embryonic aortic arch arteries. The six aortic arch artery pairs develop into five pairs of branchial arch arteries. The fifth aortic arch artery pair undergoes involution and does not contribute to a branchial arch artery pair (option B). The first two pharyngeal artery pairs and the right VI artery regress and do not produce any definitive contribution to the adult aorta (option D). The left VI artery forms the pulmonary trunk and pulmonary arteries (option C). The III pair of arteries forms the common carotid arteries, and the IV pair of arteries makes small contributions to the right subclavian artery and aortic arch. The pulmonary trunk remains attached to the aorta through the ductus arteriosus, which closes and involutes at birth (option E). Outflow tract septation results from the contribution of migrating neural crest and second heart field precursors (option A).[22] Defects can lead to truncus arteriosus.

8-9. **The answer is C.** (*Hurst's The Heart, 14th Edition, Chap. 8*) The epicardium is the outer mesothelial layer of the heart that makes important contributions to the noncardiomyocyte cells of the heart. The epicardium is an epithelial sheet that covers the heart and can undergo EMT to become smooth muscle cells or fibroblasts (option A). The epicardium is heterogeneous, and some subsets may contribute to the endocardium and coronary endothelium (options B and E).[23-25] The epicardium forms from the proepicardium, which derives from the coelomic epithelium (option D).[26] In the adult heart, the epicardium is activated following injury. The epicardium proliferates and invades the injured area (option C).[27,28]

8-10. **The answer is B.** (*Hurst's The Heart, 14th Edition, Chap. 8*) Cardiomyocytes are originally added to the developing heart by the expansion and differentiation of progenitor cells. Over time, additional cardiomyocytes are added to the heart by symmetric division of cardiomyocytes. The capacity for cardiomyocyte proliferation wanes with time, but recent work has suggested a low grade of cardiomyocyte proliferation and renewal in the adult heart (option A).[29] The conduction system is a set of specialized cells that coordinate ordered chamber contraction. Cells of the conduction system, such as the Purkinje cells, have less contractility than the working myocardium. They have decreased numbers of mitochondria and disorganized sarcomeres (option E). The cellular origins of the conduction systems are diverse. For example, the SA node is derived from both first and second heart field progenitors (option B).[30,31] The coronary endothelium starts to develop as cardiac muscle thickens. The coronary endothelium has diverse cellular origins, including the sinus venosus endothelium, the ventricular endocardium, and potentially a subset of epicardial cells (option D).[23,32-36] Finally, coronary development is also important for the innervation pattern of the heart (option C).

References

1. Rana MS, Christoffels VM, and Moorman AF. A molecular and genetic outline of cardiac morphogenesis. *Acta Physiol (Oxf)*. 2013;207(4):588-615.
2. Buckingham M, Meilhac S, and Zaffran S. Building the mammalian heart from two sources of myocardial cells. *Nat Rev Genet*. 2005;6(11):826-835.
3. Tam PP, Loebel DA, and Tanaka SS. Building the mouse gastrula: signals, asymmetry and lineages. *Curr Opin Genet Dev*. 2006;16(4):419-425.
4. Tam PP, and Behringer RR. Mouse gastrulation: the formation of a mammalian body plan. *Mech Dev*. 1997;68(1-2):3-25.
5. Waxman JS, Keegan BR, Roberts RW, Poss KD, and Yelon D. Hoxb5b acts downstream of retinoic acid signaling in the forelimb field to restrict heart field potential in zebrafish. *Dev Cell*. 2008;15(6):923-934.
6. Cai CL, Liang X, Shi Y, et al. Isl1 identifies a cardiac progenitor population that proliferates prior to differentiation and contributes a majority of cells to the heart. *Dev Cell*. 2003;5(6):877-889.
7. Galli D, Dominguez JN, Zaffran S, et al. Atrial myocardium derives from the posterior region of the second heart field, which acquires left-right identity as Pitx2c is expressed. *Development*. 2008;135(6):1157-1167.
8. Sylva M, van den Hoff MJ, and Moorman AF. Development of the human heart. *Am J Med Genet A*. 2014;164A(6):1347-1371.
9. Moreno-Rodriguez RA, Krug EL, Reyes L, et al. Bidirectional fusion of the heart-forming fields in the developing chick embryo. *Dev Dyn*. 2006;235(1):191-202.
10. Paige SL, Plonowska K, Xu A, and Wu SM. Molecular regulation of cardiomyocyte differentiation. *Circ Res*. 2015;116(2):341-353.
11. Cohen ED, Miller MF, Wang Z, Moon RT, and Morrisey EE. Wnt5a and Wnt11 are essential for second heart field progenitor development. *Development*. 2012;139(11):1931-1940.
12. Devine WP, Wythe JD, George M, Koshiba-Takeuchi K, and Bruneau BG. Early patterning and specification of cardiac progenitors in gastrulating mesoderm. *Elife*. 2014;3.
13. Tsuchihashi T, Maeda J, Shin CH, et al. Hand2 function in second heart field progenitors is essential for cardiogenesis. *Dev Biol*. 2011;351(1):62-69.
14. Watanabe Y, Zaffran S, Kuroiwa A, et al. Fibroblast growth factor 10 gene regulation in the second heart field by Tbx1, Nkx2-5, and Islet1 reveals a genetic switch for down-regulation in the myocardium. *Proc Natl Acad Sci U S A*. 2012;109(45):18273-18280.
15. Dupays L, Shang C, Wilson R, et al. Sequential binding of MEIS1 and NKX2-5 on the Popdc2 gene: a mechanism for spatiotemporal regulation of enhancers during cardiogenesis. *Cell Rep*. 2015;13(1):183-195.
16. Campione M, Ros MA, Icardo JM, et al. Pitx2 expression defines a left cardiac lineage of cells: evidence for atrial and ventricular molecular isomerism in the iv/iv mice. *Dev Biol*. 2001;231(1):252-264.
17. Morey L, Santanach A, Blanco E, et al. Polycomb regulates mesoderm cell fate-specification in embryonic stem cells through activation and repression mechanisms. *Cell Stem Cell*. 2015;17(3):300-315.
18. Greulich F, Rudat C, and Kispert A. Mechanisms of T-box gene function in the developing heart. *Cardiovasc Res*. 2011;91(2):212-222.
19. Kelly RG, Buckingham ME, and Moorman AF. Heart fields and cardiac morphogenesis. *Cold Spring Harb Perspect Med*. 2014;4(10).
20. de Boer BA, van den Berg G, de Boer PA, Moorman AF, and Ruijter JM. Growth of the developing mouse heart: an interactive qualitative and quantitative 3D atlas. *Dev Biol*. 2012;368(2):203-213.
21. Anderson RH, Spicer DE, Brown NA, and Mohun TJ. The development of septation in the four-chambered heart. *Anat Rec (Hoboken)*. 2014;297(8):1414-1429.
22. Kirby ML, Gale TF, and Stewart DE. Neural crest cells contribute to normal aorticopulmonary septation. *Science*. 1983;220(4601):1059-1061.
23. Perez-Pomares JM, Carmona R, Gonzalez-Iriarte M, et al. Origin of coronary endothelial cells from epicardial mesothelium in avian embryos. *Int J Dev Biol*. 2002;46(8):1005-1013.
24. Mikawa T, and Gourdie RG. Pericardial mesoderm generates a population of coronary smooth muscle cells migrating into the heart along with ingrowth of the epicardial organ. *Dev Biol*. 1996;174(2):221-232.

25. Gittenberger-de Groot AC, Vrancken Peeters MP, Mentink MM, Gourdie RG, and Poelmann RE. Epicardium-derived cells contribute a novel population to the myocardial wall and the atrioventricular cushions. *Circ Res.* 1998;82(10):1043-1052.

26. Perez-Pomares JM, and de la Pompa JL. Signaling during epicardium and coronary vessel development. *Circ Res.* 2011;109(12):1429-1442.

27. Balmer GM, Bollini S, Dube KN, et al. Dynamic haematopoietic cell contribution to the developing and adult epicardium. *Nat Commun.* 2014;5:4054.

28. Smart N, Risebro CA, Melville AA, et al. Thymosin beta4 induces adult epicardial progenitor mobilization and neovascularization. *Nature.* 2007;445(7124):177-182.

29. Bergmann O, Zdunek S, Felker A, et al. Dynamics of cell generation and turnover in the human heart. *Cell.* 2015;161(7):1566-1575.

30. Christoffels VM, Mommersteeg MT, Trowe MO, et al. Formation of the venous pole of the heart from an Nkx2-5-negative precursor population requires Tbx18. *Circ Res.* 2006;98(12):1555-1563.

31. Mommersteeg MT, Brown NA, Prall OW, et al. Pitx2c and Nkx2-5 are required for the formation and identity of the pulmonary myocardium. *Circ Res.* 2007;101(9):902-909.

32. Mikawa T, and Fischman DA. Retroviral analysis of cardiac morphogenesis: discontinuous formation of coronary vessels. *Proc Natl Acad Sci U S A.* 1992;89(20):9504-9508.

33. Katz TC, Singh MK, Degenhardt K, et al. Distinct compartments of the proepicardial organ give rise to coronary vascular endothelial cells. *Dev Cell.* 2012;22(3):639-650.

34. Arita Y, Nakaoka Y, Matsunaga T, et al. Myocardium-derived angiopoietin-1 is essential for coronary vein formation in the developing heart. *Nat Commun.* 2014;5:4552.

35. Red-Horse K, Ueno H, Weissman IL, and Krasnow MA. Coronary arteries form by developmental reprogramming of venous cells. *Nature.* 2010;464(7288):549-553.

36. Wu B, Zhang Z, Lui W, et al. Endocardial cells form the coronary arteries by angiogenesis through myocardial-endocardial VEGF signaling. *Cell.* 2012;151(5):1083-1096.

CHAPTER 9

Genetic Basis of Cardiovascular Disease

Ravi Karra

QUESTIONS

DIRECTIONS: Choose the one best response to each question.

9-1. A 23-year-old woman presents with a long history of muscle weakness. Her past medical history is notable for "hypertrophic" cardiomyopathy (HCM), cryptogenic stroke, and optic neuritis. She was told that she had a dilated cardiomyopathy prior to developing a hypertrophic cardiomyopathy. Physical examination, in addition to findings of HCM, are remarkable for short stature and hearing loss. Labs are notable for an elevated CPK. Her family history includes multiple family members with cardiac problems. Her pedigree is shown in Figure 9-1. Her brother has a similar constellation of findings of similar severity. Her mother, her maternal grandmother, and her maternal uncle also have a similar set of findings but with milder severity. Based on the presentation and pedigree, what is the likely mode of inheritance?

A. Autosomal recessive
B. Spontaneous somatic mutation
C. X-linked
D. Mitochondrial inheritance
E. Spontaneous chromosomal translocation

9-2. Which of the following is *true* of heritable cardiomyopathies?

A. About 1 in 500 people carry a gene associated with HCM
B. Patients with sarcomeric mutations can have either a hypertrophic, dilated, or restrictive cardiomyopathy
C. Most heritable cardiomyopathies are autosomal recessive
D. Heritable cardiomyopathies are rare
E. Patients with heritable cardiomyopathies only have mutations in sarcomeric genes

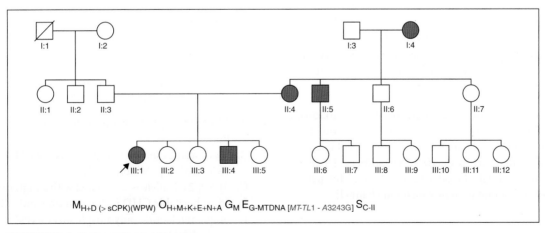

FIGURE 9-1 Pedigree for question 9-1.

9-3. A 38-year-old man is admitted with acute aortic dissection. Upon inquiry, he is noted to have a strong family history of aortic disease with dissection. Which of the following is *not true* about heritable thoracic aortic diseases?

A. Genetic disorders with increased risk for thoracic aortic dissection are associated with mutations in genes related to extracellular matrix proteins and TGF-β signaling

B. Patients with bicuspid aortic valves are at increased risk for aortic dilation

C. He most likely has an autosomal dominant genetic syndrome

D. A bifid uvula would suggest a diagnosis of Marfan syndrome

E. Translucent skin would suggest a diagnosis of Ehlers–Danlos syndrome

9-4. A 28-year-old woman is sent to you for evaluation of shortness of breath. Her examination reveals elevated neck veins, a right ventricular (RV) heave, and a loud P2. Echocardiography confirms the presence of pulmonary hypertension (PH). Family history is notable for multiple members with PH. Which of the following is *true* about heritable PH?

A. Familial PH is classified as type 2 PH

B. The most common form of heritable PH is associated with a mutation in *BMPR2*

C. Less common mutations in PH include mutations in *FBN1*

D. The presence of multiple telangiectasias would suggest a diagnosis of Gaucher disease

E. Mutations in *BMPR2* are only associated with familial PH

9-5. Which of the following is *not true* of inherited atrial diseases?

A. Mutations of *NPPA* are associated with an autosomal recessive atrial dilated cardiomyopathy

B. Mutations in *SCN5A* are associated with heritable sick sinus syndrome, LQT3, and Brugada syndrome

C. Mutations of *HCN4* are associated with heritable sick sinus syndrome

D. Mutations in the gene *Shugosin-like 1* are associated with chronic atrial and intestinal dysrhythmia (CAID)

E. Having a parent with atrial fibrillation has no effect on one's risk for developing atrial fibrillation

9-6. A 28-year-old man is admitted for syncope following exercise. He has no other prior medical history, and physical examination is normal. Family history is notable for a history of sudden cardiac death. ECG shows evidence of a long QT interval with broad-based T waves. This patient most likely has a mutation in which ion channel?

A. *NPPA*
B. *SCN5A*
C. *KCNQ1*
D. *KCNH2*
E. *HCN4*

9-7. A 34-year-old man presents after resuscitation following cardiac arrest. He is otherwise healthy. ECG shows ST elevation in the anterior precordial leads. Which of the following is *not true* about Brugada syndrome?

A. Brugada syndrome is more common in Southeast Asia

B. Brugada syndrome is associated with mutations in *RYR2*

C. The ECG manifestations of Brugada syndrome can be variable, but they are induced with drugs like ajmaline

D. Arrhythmia can be exacerbated by fevers

E. Arrhythmia can be exacerbated by interactions with certain drugs

9-8. A 35-year-old man presents with atrial arrhythmias. He has a past medical history of thyroid tumors. The physical exam is notable for pigmented skin lesions. Echocardiogram shows the presence of an atrial myxoma. Which of the following is *true* of his syndrome?

A. His syndrome is associated with mutations in the *PTCH1* gene

B. His syndrome is associated with an increased incidence of pancreatic tumors

C. Histologically, the myocytes are round and vacuolated

D. His myxoma will likely respond to rapamycin

E. He is at increased risk for medulloblastoma

9-9. A 21-year-old female presents to you for evaluation of chest pain. She has had recurring bouts of chest pain since she was 8 years old. Her chest pain is worse when lying supine and improves when sitting upright. Her chest pain is also made worse with deep inspiration. In addition to chest pain, she has abdominal pain and fevers during these episodes. The episodes are self-limited and have no specific trigger. Family history of a similar disorder is not known. Which of the following is *true* of familial Mediterranean fever (FMF)?

A. FMF is autosomal dominant

B. FMF is the result of a mutation in the *G6PD* gene

C. The chest pain and abdominal pain are part of a pan-serositis

D. The disease is most common in Western European populations

E. Heterozygous patients are not at risk for the periodic fever syndrome

9-10. Which of the following is *true* about the genetic basis of coronary heart disease (CHD)?

A. Most of the genetic variants that contribute to CHD are known

B. Twin studies show a decreased risk of CHD if the other twin died of premature CHD

C. The 9p21-3 allele is associated with a high risk for CHD

D. Most heritable CHD is due to monogenic disorder

E. Single nucleotide polymorphisms (SNPs) that contribute to CHD are uncommon

9-1. **The answer is D.** *(Hurst's The Heart, 14th Edition, Chap. 9)* The patient has a syndrome of mitochondrial encephalomyopathy with lactic acidosis and strokelike episodes (MELAS). MELAS patients can have a dilated cardiomyopathy that transitions to a HCM.[1] MELAS is a mitochondrial myopathy and often is the result of a mutation in transfer RNA (option D). The pedigree shows the phenotype in every generation. Spontaneous mutations would not be in each generation (options B and E). Autosomal recessive mutations skip every generation (option A). Similarly, X-linked mutations tend to involve males because males have a single X chromosome (option C). Autosomal dominant mutations result in affected family members in each generation, but this is not a choice. Mitochondrial DNA is maternally derived, so the disease can only be passed by females. The penetrance of the disease is related to the amount of abnormal mitochondrial DNA that is inherited.

9-2. **The answer is B.** *(Hurst's The Heart, 14th Edition, Chap. 9)* Hypertrophic cardiomyopathy is the most common heritable cardiomyopathy. One in 500 young adults are affected, and 1 in 200 people carry a mutation that is associated with HCM (option A).[2] While patients with HCM primarily have mutations of sarcomeric proteins, sarcomeric mutations can result in either a hypertrophic, dilated, or restrictive cardiomyopathy (option B).[3] While the full complement of mutations leading to heritable cadiomyopathies remains unknown, up to 80% of heritable cardiomyopathies are autosomal dominant (options C and E).[4] Furthermore, heritable cardiomyopathies are common, with more than 50% of patients with dilated cardiomyopathy having evidence for an underlying genetic cause (option D).[4]

9-3. **The answer is D.** *(Hurst's The Heart, 14th Edition, Chap. 9)* Heritable thoracic aortic aneurysm and dissection (TAAD) includes more than 40 genetically different disorders. The genetic basis for these disorders is diverse, and many involve mutations in genes related to extracellular matrix proteins and TGF-β signaling (option A). For example, Marfan syndrome is associated with mutations in the extracellular matrix protein *FBN1*, and mutations of *TGFBR1* and *TGBFR2* cause Loeys–Dietz syndrome type 1 (LDS1) and Loeys–Dietz syndrome type 2 (LDS2), respectively.[5] In 25% of cases, patients with bicuspid aortic valves have dilation of the ascending aorta (option B).[6] Most heritable thoracic aortic aneurysm disorders (TAAD) are autosomal dominant (option C). Different TAAD syndromes are associated with other clinical features. Patients with Marfan syndrome have typical skeletal traits. LDS1 patients have craniofacial traits, including a bifid uvula and craniosynostosis (option D). Patients with Ehlers–Danlos type IV (EDSIV) have a typical skin and face morphology. Facial features include a thin nose, thin lips, prominent eyes, hollow cheeks, a small chin, and lobeless ears. The skin is very thin and nearly translucent, allowing for visualization of the underlying blood vessels (option E).

9-4. **The answer is B.** *(Hurst's The Heart, 14th Edition, Chap. 9)* The WHO classifies PH in five groups.[7] Group 1 includes idiopathic PH, heritable PH, drug-induced PH, CHD with PH, pulmonary veno-occlusive disease, and pulmonary capillary hemangiomatosis. Group 2 includes PH related to left heart disease (option A). Group 3 includes PH secondary to lung disease. Group 4 includes chronic thromboembolic PAH. Group 5 PH includes miscellaneous disorders that can affect the pulmonary vasculature with unclear or multifactorial mechanisms. Up to 80% of patients with familial autosomal dominant PH have mutations in *BMPR2* (option B).[8] Similarly, up to 20% of sporadic PH is associated with acquired mutations of *BMPR2* (option E). Mutations in *FBN1* are associated with Marfan syndrome (option C). While Gaucher disease can be associated with PH, telangiectasias are associated with Osler–Weber–Rendu syndrome (option D).

9-5. **The answer is E.** *(Hurst's The Heart, 14th Edition, Chap. 9)* Atrial dilated cardiomyopathy (ADCM) is a rare autosomal recessive disease that manifests as biatrial dilation with progression to electrical standstill of the atria. ADCM is associated with mutation of the

NPPA gene (option A).[9] *SCN5A* encodes a key sodium channel within the heart, and different mutations of *SCN5A* are associated with various arrhythmias, including sick sinus syndrome, LQT3, and Brugada syndrome (option B).[10-14] Mutations of *HCN4* are also associated with a heritable sick sinus syndrome (option C). CAID is associated with mutations in the *Shugosin-like 1* gene and manifests with atrial dysrhythmias and chronic intestinal pseudo-obstruction (option D). The genetic basis for familial atrial fibrillation is not as clear for other arrhythmias, but having an affected parent increases a person's risk for developing atrial fibrillation by 85% (option E).[15]

9-6. **The answer is C.** *(Hurst's The Heart, 14th Edition, Chap. 9)* This patient has LQT1. LQT1 manifests with exercise-induced arrhythmias. ECG shows broad T waves with a prolonged QT interval. LQT1 involves mutations in *KCNQ1*, and it can be treated with beta blockade (option C). Mutations in *NPPA* are associated with heritable atrial dilated cardiomyopathy (option A). Mutations in *SCN5A* are associated with LQT3, SSS, and Brugada syndrome (option B). Mutations in *KCNH2* are associated with LQT2 (option D). Mutations in *HCN4* are associated with heritable sick sinus syndrome (option E).

9-7. **The answer is B.** *(Hurst's The Heart, 14th Edition, Chap. 9)* Brugada syndrome is a genetic syndrome that is associated with increased risk for sudden cardiac death. Brugada syndrome is heritable, most commonly involving mutations of *SCN5A*, and it tends to occur most commonly in patients from Southeast Asia (options A and B).[16] The ECG typically has ST elevations in the anterior precordial leads. However, these findings are not always readily apparent. Drugs like ajmaline can elicit a more classical pattern in such patients (option C). Arrhythmias can occur with sensitizing factors like fever or drugs (options D and E).

9-8. **The answer is B.** *(Hurst's The Heart, 14th Edition, Chap. 9)* This patient has Carney syndrome. Type I Carney complex is associated with mutations in the *PRKAR1A* gene (option A). As many as 2.5% of patients with Carney syndrome have pancreatic tumors (option B).[17] Purkinje cell hamartomas, not atrial myxomas, are associated with round and vacuolated myocytes (option C). mTOR inhibitors are used to treat rhabdomyomas associated with tuberous sclerosis (option D).[18] Medulloblastoma is associated with cardiac fibromas and Gorlin

9-9. **The answer is C.** *(Hurst's The Heart, 14th Edition, Chap. 9)* Familial Mediterranean fever is a rare autosomal recessive disorder, most common in patients of Eastern European ancestry (options A and D).[19] FMF is most commonly caused by a mutation in the *MEFV* gene that encodes pyrin, a component of the cellular inflammasome (option B). Patients typically present with abdominal pain and chest pain indicative of serositis (option C). Heterozygous patients can also manifest the disease during stresses, or they can alternatively present with other inflammatory syndromes

9-10. **The answer is C.** *(Hurst's The Heart, 14th Edition, Chap. 9)* Coronary heart disease is a prototypical complex genetic disease (option D). The genetic basis for CHD has been supported by twin studies showing an increased risk for CHD in the second twin when the first twin dies of CHD (option B).[23] Large-scale, genome-wide association studies have identified multiple common SNPs associated with CHD (option E). Together, these SNPs account for about 10% of the heritable basis for CHD (option A).[24] Each SNP generally has a small effect. However, the 9p21-3 allele, in particular, is considered a high risk for CHD (option C).[25,26]

References

1. El-Hattab AW, Adesina AM, Jones J, Scaglia F. MELAS syndrome: clinical manifestations, pathogenesis, and treatment options. *Mol Genet Metab.* 2015;116(1-2):4-12.
2. Semsarian C, Ingles J, Maron MS, Maron BJ. New perspectives on the prevalence of hypertrophic cardiomyopathy. *J Am Coll Cardiol.* 2015;65(12):1249-1254.
3. Haas J, Frese KS, Peil B, et al. Atlas of the clinical genetics of human dilated cardiomyopathy. *Eur Heart J.* 2015;36(18):1123-1135a.

4. Arbustini E, Narula N, Tavazzi L, et al. The MOGE(S) classification of cardiomyopathy for clinicians. *J Am Coll Cardiol.* 2014;64(3):304-318.

5. Andelfinger G, Loeys B, Dietz H. A decade of discovery in the genetic understanding of thoracic aortic disease. *Can J Cardiol.* 2016;32(1):13-25.

6. Prakash SK, Bosse Y, Muehlschlegel JD, et al. A roadmap to investigate the genetic basis of bicuspid aortic valve and its complications: insights from the International BAVCon (Bicuspid Aortic Valve Consortium). *J Am Coll Cardiol.* 2014;64(8):832-839.

7. Simonneau G, Gatzoulis MA, Adatia I, et al. Updated clinical classification of pulmonary hypertension. *J Am Coll Cardiol.* 2013;62(25 Suppl):D34-D41.

8. McLaughlin VV, Archer SL, Badesch DB, et al. ACCF/AHA 2009 expert consensus document on pulmonary hypertension: a report of the American College of Cardiology Foundation Task Force on Expert Consensus Documents and the American Heart Association developed in collaboration with the American College of Chest Physicians; American Thoracic Society, Inc.; and the Pulmonary Hypertension Association. *J Am Coll Cardiol.* 2009;53(17):1573-1619.

9. Disertori M, Quintarelli S, Grasso M, et al. Autosomal recessive atrial dilated cardiomyopathy with standstill evolution associated with mutation of natriuretic peptide precursor A. *Circ Cardiovasc Genet.* 2013;6(1):27-36.

10. Monfredi O, Boyett MR. Sick sinus syndrome and atrial fibrillation in older persons—a view from the sinoatrial nodal myocyte. *J Mol Cell Cardiol.* 2015;83:88-100.

11. Benson DW, Wang DW, Dyment M, et al. Congenital sick sinus syndrome caused by recessive mutations in the cardiac sodium channel gene (*SCN5A*). *J Clin Invest.* 2003;112(7):1019-1028.

12. Kodama T, Serio A, Disertori M, et al. Autosomal recessive paediatric sick sinus syndrome associated with novel compound mutations in *SCN5A. Int J Cardiol.* 2013;167(6):3078-3080.

13. Abe K, Machida T, Sumitomo N, et al. Sodium channelopathy underlying familial sick sinus syndrome with early onset and predominantly male characteristics. *Circ Arrhythm Electrophysiol.* 2014;7(3):511-517.

14. Detta N, Frisso G, Limongelli G, et al. Genetic analysis in a family affected by sick sinus syndrome may reduce the sudden death risk in a young aspiring competitive athlete. *Int J Cardiol.* 2014;170(3):e63-e65.

15. Chetaille P, Preuss C, Burkhard S, et al. Mutations in *SGOL1* cause a novel cohesinopathy affecting heart and gut rhythm. *Nat Genet.* 2014;46(11):1245-1249.

16. Watanabe H, Minamino T. Genetics of Brugada syndrome. *J Hum Genet.* 2016;61(1):57-60.

17. Gaujoux S, Tissier F, Ragazzon B, et al. Pancreatic ductal and acinar cell neoplasms in Carney complex: a possible new association. *J Clin Endocrinol Metab.* 2011;96(11):E1888-E1895.

18. Hoshal SG, Samuel BP, Schneider JR, Mammen L, Vettukattil JJ. Regression of massive cardiac rhabdomyoma on everolimus therapy. *Pediatr Int.* 2016;58(5):397-399.

19. Heller H, Sohar E, Sherf L. Familial Mediterranean fever. *AMA Arch Intern Med.* 1958;102(1):50-71.

20. The International FMF Consortium. Ancient missense mutations in a new member of the RoRet gene family are likely to cause familial Mediterranean fever. *Cell.* 1997;90(4):797-807.

21. Jeru I, Hentgen V, Cochet E, et al. The risk of familial Mediterranean fever in MEFV heterozygotes: a statistical approach. *PLoS One.* 2013;8(7):e68431.

22. Hentgen V, Grateau G, Stankovic-Stojanovic K, Amselem S, Jeru I. Familial Mediterranean fever in heterozygotes: are we able to accurately diagnose the disease in very young children? *Arthritis Rheum.* 2013;65(6):1654-1662.

23. Brown DW, Giles WH, Burke W, Greenlund KJ, Croft JB. Familial aggregation of early-onset myocardial infarction. *Community Genet.* 2002;5(4):232-238.

24. Bjorkegren JL, Kovacic JC, Dudley JT, Schadt EE. Genome-wide significant loci: how important are they? Systems genetics to understand heritability of coronary artery disease and other common complex disorders. *J Am Coll Cardiol.* 2015;65(8):830-845.

25. Fan M, Dandona S, McPherson R, et al. Two chromosome 9p21 haplotype blocks distinguish between coronary artery disease and myocardial infarction risk. *Circ Cardiovasc Genet.* 2013;6(4):372-380.

26. Munir MS, Wang Z, Alahdab F, et al. The association of 9p21-3 locus with coronary atherosclerosis: a systematic review and meta-analysis. *BMC Med Genet.* 2014;15:66.

CHAPTER 10

Stem Cells and the Cardiovascular System

Ravi Karra

QUESTIONS

DIRECTIONS: Choose the one best response to each question.

10-1. Which of the following is *not true* about mechanisms of cell therapy?

A. Transdifferentiation is when a differentiated cell type commits to becoming a new cell type

B. Angiogenesis is the formation of new blood vessels

C. Bone marrow cell therapy is likely to promote ventricular recovery by transdifferentiation into cardiomyocytes

D. Dedifferentiation likely confers a protective effect for injured cardiomyocytes

E. Transplanted bone marrow cells are transiently retained in the heart following cardiac injury

10-2. Which of the following is *true* of stem cell delivery approaches to the heart?

A. Intracoronary injection of stem cells results in better engraftment of cells than transendocardial injection

B. Transendocardial injection does not require adjunctive imaging modalities to target injured myocardium

C. Intravenous administration of stem cells is a promising approach because stem cell populations evaluated thus far are efficient in their homing to injured myocardium

D. Transepicardial injection of stem cells requires adjunctive imaging modalities to target injured myocardium

E. Activation of resident stem cells has been evaluated in human studies after acute myocardial infarction (MI)

10-3. Which of the following limits the clinical application of skeletal myoblasts to improve cardiac function following injury?

A. Skeletal myoblasts do not share contractile properties with cardiomyocytes

B. Skeletal myoblasts are difficult to isolate

C. Skeletal myoblasts are difficult to expand

D. Skeletal myoblasts do not readily adapt to a hypoxic environment

E. Skeletal myoblasts do not electrically couple to the myocardium and may increase the risk for arrhythmia

10-4. A 54-year-old man presents to your office asking for stem cell therapy. He recently had a large anterior infarct with residual left ventricular (LV) dysfunction. He has read about bone marrow mononuclear cell (BMMNC) therapy and would like some guidance. Which of the following can you tell him?

A. The cells responsible for improving LV function in preclinical models are hematopoietic progenitor cells

B. Early clinical studies after acute MI demonstrate an unequivocal increase in LV function after treatment with BMMNCs

C. BMMNCs can be administered relatively safely, but their efficacy is not proven following acute MI or for chronic heart failure

D. Treatment with BMMNCs improves functional status but not ventricular function

E. None of the above

10-5. The patient from question 10-4 returns to your clinic and is now asking about treatment with mesenchymal stem cells (MSCs). Which of the following can you tell him?

A. Unlike BMMNCs, allogeneic MSCs require immunosuppression

B. MSCs are more effective than BMMNCs for improving ventricular function following acute MI

C. MSCs can differentiate into cardiac progenitors in vivo

D. MSCs from different sources, such as the bone marrow or Wharton's jelly, are equivalent

E. Preliminary data on MSCs for the treatment of cardiovascular disease are promising, but additional studies are needed before routine use can be recommended

10-6. Which of the following is *not true* about angiogenic progenitor cells (APCs)?

A. APCs give rise primarily to endothelial cells
B. Intracoronary injection of CD34$^+$ APCs can reduce angina, but they are associated with small elevations of cardiac biomarkers
C. APCs for the treatment of heart failure have had mixed results
D. Patients with nonischemic heart failure have normally functioning APCs
E. Early studies do not suggest a benefit of APCs for peripheral arterial disease (PAD)

10-7. Which of the following is *true* of adipose stem cells?

A. MSCs derived from adipose tissue are attractive for cell therapy because they are more easily obtained than bone marrow MSCs
B. Adipose-derived MSCs can be differentiated to cardiomyocytes in vivo
C. Adipose tissue can be transdifferentiated to endothelium in vivo
D. The number of adipose-derived MSCs is related to glucose sensitivity
E. Adipose-derived MSCs are limited by adverse events in early clinical trials

10-8. A 65-year-old woman presents to your clinic for advice about stem cell therapy. She brings in a brochure for the use of cardiac stem cells and wants to know your thoughts on stem cell therapy for the heart. She has a nonischemic cardiomyopathy with reduced LV function (LVEF 25%) and class III heart failure symptoms. Her ECG reveals a left bundle branch block with a QRS duration of 150 ms. She has been taking guideline-directed medical therapy for her heart failure and has an implantable defibrillator. She is very intent on going to a stem cell clinic. Which of the following can you use to advise her?

A. Cardiac stem cells are known to promote heart regeneration in preclinical models
B. Current approaches to isolate resident cardiac stem cells include harvest from peripheral blood
C. A resident stem cell population in the heart has been clearly identified, but work regarding clinical efficacy is still preliminary
D. She is more likely to benefit from an upgrade of her ICD to a biventricular pacing system
E. Cardiac progenitor cells are a promising approach to treat heart failure and should be sought out to the best of one's ability

10-9. Which of the following is *not* a limitation to using embryonic stem (ES) cells for cardiac cell therapy?

A. Obtaining ES cells for cell therapy is limited by ethical controversies
B. ES cells would be used as an autologous cell source, requiring immunosuppression after transplantation
C. ES cells are potentially tumorigenic
D. Protocols for robustly differentiating ES cells into cardiomyocytes are lacking
E. Evidence is lacking for the clinical efficacy of ES cells for heart regeneration

10-10. Which of the following is *not true* regarding induced pluripotent stem cells (iPSCs)?

A. iPSCs can be used to generate autologous cardiomyocytes for cell therapy
B. The generation of iPSCs from somatic cells has the potential for tumorigenesis
C. iPSCs can be used to model genetic diseases
D. Like ES cells, the generation of iPSCs remains controversial
E. iPSCs can provide a human model system for fundamental mechanistic work

10-1. **The answer is C.** *(Hurst's The Heart, 14th Edition, Chap. 10)* Multiple groups have tested the efficacy of bone marrow cell therapy after MI. Bone marrow cells in preclinical models rarely transdifferentiate into cardiomyocytes (options A and C), are transiently retained in the heart (option E), and most likely exert their beneficial effects on cardiac function through a paracrine mechanism that stimulates new blood vessels through angiogenesis (option B).[1-4] Lastly, a novel concept in cardiac repair is modulation of dedifferentiation. Dedifferentiation is the process by which cardiomyocytes take on a gene and protein expression profile that is more similar to fetal. This phenotype occurs more often in acute and chronic injury of the heart and seems to confer a potential survival advantage of these cardiomyocytes (option D).

10-2. **The answer is A.** *(Hurst's The Heart, 14th Edition, Chap. 10)* While additional work is needed for cell therapy to be considered a treatment modality, the science of stem cell delivery has rapidly developed. Current approaches include intravenous delivery, but this is limited by poor retention of stem cells in the myocardium (option C). Intracoronary injection of stem cells can be done during percutaneous coronary intervention, but stem cell retention is not as good as with transendocardial injection (option A).[4,5] Transendocardial injection can also be done in the catheterization laboratory, but it requires advanced imaging to identify target areas for injection (option B). Transepicardial injection may be of similar value, but it requires direct visualization of the heart (option D).[6] An alternative to intracardiac injection is activation of resident stem cells, but this approach remains in preclinical investigation (option E).

10-3. **The answer is E.** *(Hurst's The Heart, 14th Edition, Chap. 10)* Skeletal myoblasts are skeletal muscle precursor cells derived from skeletal muscle satellite cells. Interest in this population was supported by similarity to adult cardiomyocytes, the potential for autologous utilization, ease of expansion in vitro, and resistance to hypoxic environment (options A through D). However, the MAGIC clinic trial and other pilot studies showed an increased risk for arrhythmia.[7] Functionally, skeletal muscle fails to couple with endogenous cardiac muscle (option E).[8]

10-4. **The answer is C.** *(Hurst's The Heart, 14th Edition, Chap. 10)* Several preclinical studies showed an improvement in ventricular function after MI with infusion of BMMNCs.[9,10] However, these findings have since proven controversial. Key questions remain as to the mechanism of action and the cell type responsible for the reverse remodeling that has been observed (option A). Nonetheless, human trials have been taking place for nearly two decades. These have been mostly small trials of variable design, and meta-analyses for treatment following acute MI or for ischemic cardiomyopathy have shown mixed results for improving ventricular function or functional status (options B and D).[11] While the science of BMMNCs is still developing, methods of delivery have evolved, and catheter-based delivery of BMMNCs has proven to be relatively safe (option C).

10-5. **The answer is E.** *(Hurst's The Heart, 14th Edition, Chap. 10)* MSCs are a promising source for cell therapy. MSCs arise from diverse sources and can be differentiated into multiple cell types, including cardiomyocytes, in vitro (option C).[12,13] Unlike BMMNCs, MSCs are thought to be immune privileged, raising the possibility for allogeneic transplantation without immunosuppression (option A). The POSEIDON trial evaluated MSCs in patients with ischemic cardiomyopathy. Interestingly, the autologous MSC group showed improved 6-minute walk distances and Minnesota Living with Heart Failure Questionnaire scores, whereas the allogeneic MSCs group showed a reduction in LV end-diastolic dimension. Both groups showed a reduction in infarct size (option B).[14] MSCs from different sources may have differing efficacies, but MSCs from different sources have yet to be tested for comparative efficacy (option D). Finally, like BMMNCs, clinical studies for MSCs are small, and additional studies are needed before MSCs can be recommended therapeutically (option B).

10-6. **The answer is D.** (*Hurst's The Heart, 14th Edition, Chap. 10*) APCs are a population of progenitor cells that mainly give rise to endothelial cells (option A).[15] Patients with nonischemic heart failure have functionally impaired APCs (option D). Vrtovec et al. conducted one of the largest randomized trials, with 110 nonischemic cardiomyopathy patients randomized to receive either CD34+ intracoronary infusion or standard therapy. At 12 and 60 months, the CD34+ treatment group showed a significant improvement in LVEF and 6-minute walk distance.[16] However, injection of CD133+ cells led to improved myocardial perfusion but resulted in a lower LVEF, and no difference in functional capacity.[17] This study contradicted findings from prior nonrandomized studies that investigated CD133+ cells (option C).[18] APCs are promising for the treatment of chronic angina, but intracoronary infusion has been associated with small elevations of cardiac biomarkers (option B).[19,20] Patients with nonischemic heart failure have abnormally functioning APCs (option D).[21] Multiple studies have examined the role of APCs in the treatment of PAD, with most showing an excellent safety profile with marginal to no benefit (option E).[19,22-24]

10-7. **The answer is A.** (*Hurst's The Heart, 14th Edition, Chap. 10*) Adipose tissue harbors a heterogeneous set of progenitor cells, mostly MSCs. These MSCs are attractive because they can be obtained from liposuction, which is easier than bone marrow biopsy (option A). The study of adipose-derived stem cells is still early. MSC cell fates in vivo are still being explored, and conditions for generating MSCs are still being optimized (options B through D). Initial clinical work suggests safety, but additional studies are needed to evaluate efficacy (option E).[25,26]

10-8. **The answer is D.** (*Hurst's The Heart, 14th Edition, Chap. 10*) Despite nearly two decades of preclinical research, cardiac progenitor cells remain very controversial. Beyond issues of identity, whether the postnatal heart harbors a population of resident progenitor cells has been hotly debated (options A and C).[27,28] Several groups have pushed forward with putative cardiac stem cells. These groups rely on harvest of stem cells from the heart for expansion and then retransplantation (option B).[29,30] Early results are promising, but definitive results for clinical efficacy remain. This patient is the ideal candidate for cardiac resynchronization therapy, and upgrading her device to a biventricular pacing system should be strongly recommended before pursuing less proven approaches (options D and E).

10-9. **The answer is D.** (*Hurst's The Heart, 14th Edition, Chap. 10*) The isolation and expansion of human ES cells was a formidable scientific achievement. Many groups have used this model to understand mechanisms of development and to develop protocols for robustly differentiating ES cells into specific cell types, such as cardiomyocytes. Current protocols allow for differentiation, expansion, and isolation of cardiomyocytes with greater than 90% purity (option D).[31,32] However, widespread use of ES cells to make new cardiomyocytes remains limited by controversy in obtaining new lines of ES cells, concerns for the tumorigenic potential of transplanted ES cells, and the possible need for immunosuppression after the transplantation of ES cells (options A, B, and C).[33] Initial clinical trials testing ES cells in patients with ischemic cardiomyopathy are underway (option E).

10-10. **The answer is D.** (*Hurst's The Heart, 14th Edition, Chap. 10*) The ability to transform somatic cells to pluripotency was a major scientific achievement. The delivery of a cocktail of factors can generate ES-cell–like cells from somatic cellular sources, including fibroblasts and urinary epithelial cells. Thus, iPSCs can be developed to represent individual patients without the ethical concerns surrounding ES cells (option D). As with ES cells, however, concerns remain about the tumorigenic potential of transplanted iPSC cells (option B). Unlike ES cells, because a patient's own cells can be reprogrammed to cardiomyocytes, the possibility exists for autologous cell therapy not requiring immunosuppression (option A). Over the past decade, iPSCs have been used to model genetic cardiovascular diseases and to create platforms for assessing drug safety. Further, iPSC-derived models of disease are being used to better understand the mechanisms that underlie many genetic disorders (option E). Disease modeling is primarily limited to heritable, cell-autonomous disorders (option C).

References

1. Balsam LB, Wagers AJ, Christensen JL, et al. Haematopoietic stem cells adopt mature haematopoietic fates in ischaemic myocardium. *Nature.* 2004;428(6983):668-673.
2. Alvarez-Dolado M, Pardal R, Garcia-Verdugo JM, et al. Fusion of bone-marrow-derived cells with Purkinje neurons, cardiomyocytes and hepatocytes. *Nature.* 2003;425(6961):968-973.
3. Nygren JM, Jovinge S, Breitbach M, et al. Bone marrow-derived hematopoietic cells generate cardiomyocytes at a low frequency through cell fusion, but not transdifferentiation. *Nat Med.* 2004;10(5):494-501.
4. Kinnaird T, Stabile E, Burnett MS, et al. Local delivery of marrow-derived stromal cells augments collateral perfusion through paracrine mechanisms. *Circulation.* 2004;109(12):1543-1549.
5. Sheng CC, Zhou L, Hao J. Current stem cell delivery methods for myocardial repair. *Biomed Res Int.* 2013;2013:547902.
6. Campbell NG, Suzuki K. Cell delivery routes for stem cell therapy to the heart: current and future approaches. *J Cardiovasc Transl Res.* 2012;5(5):713-726.
7. Veltman CE, Soliman OI, Geleijnse ML, et al. Four-year follow-up of treatment with intramyocardial skeletal myoblasts injection in patients with ischaemic cardiomyopathy. *Eur Heart J.* 2008;29(11):1386-1396.
8. Leobon B, Garcin I, Menasche P, et al. Myoblasts transplanted into rat infarcted myocardium are functionally isolated from their host. *Proc Natl Acad Sci U S A.* 2003;100(13):7808-7811.
9. Mouquet F, Pfister O, Jain M, et al. Restoration of cardiac progenitor cells after myocardial infarction by self-proliferation and selective homing of bone marrow-derived stem cells. *Circ Res.* 2005;97(11):1090-1092.
10. Orlic D, Kajstura J, Chimenti S, et al. Mobilized bone marrow cells repair the infarcted heart, improving function and survival. *Proc Natl Acad Sci U S A.* 2001;98(18):10344-10349.
11. Fisher SA, Zhang H, Doree C, Mathur A, Martin-Rendon E. Stem cell treatment for acute myocardial infarction. *Cochrane Database Syst Rev.* 2015(9):CD006536.
12. Toma C, Pittenger MF, Cahill KS, Byrne BJ, Kessler PD. Human mesenchymal stem cells differentiate to a cardiomyocyte phenotype in the adult murine heart. *Circulation.* 2002;105(1):93-98.
13. Amado LC, Schuleri KH, Saliaris AP, et al. Multimodality noninvasive imaging demonstrates in vivo cardiac regeneration after mesenchymal stem cell therapy. *J Am Coll Cardiol.* 2006;48(10):2116-2124.
14. Hare JM, Fishman JE, Gerstenblith G, et al. Comparison of allogeneic vs autologous bone marrow-derived mesenchymal stem cells delivered by transendocardial injection in patients with ischemic cardiomyopathy: the POSEIDON randomized trial. *JAMA.* 2012;308(22):2369-2379.
15. Asahara T, Murohara T, Sullivan A, et al. Isolation of putative progenitor endothelial cells for angiogenesis. *Science.* 1997;275(5302):964-967.
16. Patel AN, Geffner L, Vina RF, et al. Surgical treatment for congestive heart failure with autologous adult stem cell transplantation: a prospective randomized study. *J Thorac Cardiovasc Surg.* 2005;130(6):1631-1638.
17. Nasseri BA, Ebell W, Dandel M, et al. Autologous CD133$^+$ bone marrow cells and bypass grafting for regeneration of ischaemic myocardium: the Cardio133 trial. *Eur Heart J.* 2014;35(19):1263-1274.
18. Stamm C, Kleine HD, Choi YH, et al. Intramyocardial delivery of CD133$^+$ bone marrow cells and coronary artery bypass grafting for chronic ischemic heart disease: safety and efficacy studies. *J Thorac Cardiovasc Surg.* 2007;133(3):717-725.
19. Losordo DW, Henry TD, Davidson C, et al. Intramyocardial, autologous CD34$^+$ cell therapy for refractory angina. *Circ Res.* 2011;109(4):428-436.
20. Wang S, Cui J, Peng W, Lu M. Intracoronary autologous CD34$^+$ stem cell therapy for intractable angina. *Cardiology.* 2010;117(2):140-147.
21. Valgimigli M, Rigolin GM, Fucili A, et al. CD34$^+$ and endothelial progenitor cells in patients with various degrees of congestive heart failure. *Circulation.* 2004;110(10):1209-1212.
22. Perin EC, Silva G, Gahremanpour A, et al. A randomized, controlled study of autologous therapy with bone marrow-derived aldehyde dehydrogenase bright cells in patients with critical limb ischemia. *Catheter Cardiovasc Interv.* 2011;78(7):1060-1067.
23. Szabo GV, Kovesd Z, Cserepes J, et al. Peripheral blood-derived autologous stem cell therapy for the treatment of patients with late-stage peripheral artery disease-results of the short- and long-term follow-up. *Cytotherapy.* 2013;15(10):1245-1252.
24. Raval AN, Schmuck EG, Tefera G, et al. Bilateral administration of autologous CD133$^+$ cells in ambulatory patients with refractory critical limb ischemia: lessons learned from a pilot randomized, double-blind, placebo-controlled trial. *Cytotherapy.* 2014;16(12):1720-1732.
25. Lee HC, An SG, Lee HW, et al. Safety and effect of adipose tissue-derived stem cell implantation in patients with critical limb ischemia: a pilot study. *Circ J.* 2012;76(7):1750-1760.
26. Bura A, Planat-Benard V, Bourin P, et al. Phase I trial: the use of autologous cultured adipose-derived stroma/stem cells to treat patients with non-revascularizable critical limb ischemia. *Cytotherapy.* 2014;16(2):245-257.

27. Karra R, Poss KD. Redirecting cardiac growth mechanisms for therapeutic regeneration. *J Clin Invest.* 2017;127(2):427-436.

28. Smith RR, Barile L, Cho HC, et al. Regenerative potential of cardiosphere-derived cells expanded from percutaneous endomyocardial biopsy specimens. *Circulation.* 2007;115(7):896-908.

29. Makkar RR, Smith RR, Cheng K, et al. Intracoronary cardiosphere-derived cells for heart regeneration after myocardial infarction (CADUCEUS): a prospective, randomised phase 1 trial. *Lancet.* 2012;379(9819):895-904.

30. Chugh AR, Beache GM, Loughran JH, et al. Administration of cardiac stem cells in patients with ischemic cardiomyopathy: the SCIPIO trial: surgical aspects and interim analysis of myocardial function and viability by magnetic resonance. *Circulation.* 2012;126(11 Suppl 1):S54-S64.

31. Burridge PW, Matsa E, Shukla P, et al. Chemically defined generation of human cardiomyocytes. *Nat Methods.* 2014;11(8):855-860.

32. Burridge PW, Keller G, Gold JD, Wu JC. Production of de novo cardiomyocytes: human pluripotent stem cell differentiation and direct reprogramming. *Cell Stem Cell.* 2012;10(1):16-28.

33. Lee AS, Tang C, Rao MS, Weissman IL, Wu JC. Tumorigenicity as a clinical hurdle for pluripotent stem cell therapies. *Nat Med.* 2013;19(8):998-1004.

SECTION 3

Evaluation of the Patient

CHAPTER 11

The History, Physical Examination, and Cardiac Auscultation

Patrick R. Lawler

QUESTIONS

DIRECTIONS: Choose the one best response to each question.

11-1. All of the following findings would suggest a diagnosis of hypertrophic cardiomyopathy *except*:

A. Paradoxically split S2
B. Bifid pulse
C. "Triple ripple" apical impulse
D. S4
E. Fixed split S2

11-2. A 35-year-old man with a history of intravenous drug abuse and known bicuspid aortic valve presents with increasing shortness of breath, fevers, and lethargy. All of the following physical examination findings would suggest a diagnosis of aortic insufficiency complicating infective endocarditis *except*:

A. Bisferiens pulse
B. A high-pitched, "cooing," diastolic murmur
C. A middiastolic rumble
D. Diastolic murmur best heard over the second right intercostal space
E. Arterial pulse that is increased in amplitude

11-3. A 59-year-old man presents with several episodes of substernal chest pressure of 15 minutes' duration, which was brought on by an argument with his neighbor. His pain is relieved by nitroglycerine. According to the Forrester and Diamond chest pain classification, this patient's angina would be described as:

A. Noncardiac chest pain
B. Atypical angina
C. Typical angina
D. Dyspnea
E. Walk-through angina

11-4. A 76-year-old woman with severe aortic stenosis presents with dyspnea and worsening functional class in the setting of new-onset atrial fibrillation. Which of the following auscultatory findings would *not* be expected?

A. A late-peaking crescendo-decrescendo systolic murmur
B. A soft S2
C. An apical systolic murmur
D. Delayed and weak carotid upstroke
E. An S4

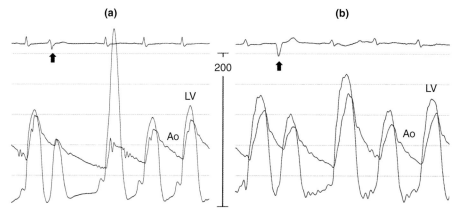

(a)

(b)

200

LV

Ao

LV

Ao

FIGURE 11-1 Simultaneous aortic and left ventricular pressure tracings taken from two patients (*a* and *b*).

11-5. The simultaneous left ventricular and aortic pressure tracings (Figure 11-1) are obtained from two different patients undergoing cardiac catheterization for dyspnea. Which of the following diagnoses are suggested in Figure 11-1(*a*) and Figure 11-1(*b*), respectively?

A. Aortic stenosis and hypertrophic obstructive cardio-myopathy (HOCM), respectively
B. Hypertrophic obstructive cardiomyopathy and aortic stenosis, respectively
C. Mitral stenosis and aortic stenosis, respectively
D. Mitral regurgitation and mitral stenosis, respectively
E. Hypertrophic obstructive cardiomyopathy and mitral stenosis, respectively

11-6. A 25-year-old woman is referred for a murmur. Trans-thoracic echocardiography demonstrates mitral valve prolapse. Which of the following is *true* about the click accompanying mitral valve prolapse?

A. This usually occurs in early systole
B. Upon standing, the click will occur earlier in systole
C. It decreases in intensity with inspiration and moves closer to S1
D. This is a lough, high-pitched sound
E. Upon Valsalva maneuver, the click will occur later in systole

11-7. A 34-year-old man presents with a family history of bicuspid aortic valve disease. On auscultation, a loud murmur is heard at the upper sternal border. No thrill is palpable. How should this murmur be graded?

A. Grade I
B. Grade II
C. Grade III
D. Grade IV
E. Grade V or Grade VI

11-8. A 45-year-old woman is referred for a murmur. Which finding on physical examination would be suggestive of a diagnosis of HOCM?

A. A decrease in the intensity of the systolic murmur upon standing
B. A midsystolic click
C. A decrease in the systolic ejection murmur with inspiration
D. A palpable P2
E. An apical holosystolic murmur

11-9. An 18-year-old asymptomatic man is referred for a murmur. The murmur is continuous, present in systole and diastole, and is characterized by a "to-and-fro" sound. The differential diagnosis should include all of the following *except*:

A. Ruptured sinus of Valsalva aneurysm
B. Arteriovenous fistula
C. Patent ductus arteriosus
D. Severe coarctation of the aorta
E. Mixed aortic valve disease (aortic stenosis and aortic regurgitation)

11-10. A 67-year-old woman presents with three days' duration stuttering chest pressure radiating to her jaw and arm. ECG demonstrates inferior ST-segment elevations. In the emergency room, she suddenly develops worsening shortness of breath. Which of the following physical exam findings could help distinguish acute mitral regurgitation from acute ventricular septal rupture?

A. Assessment of dyspnea in supine and upright positions
B. Soft systolic murmur
C. Cool extremities
D. Increased jugular venous pressure
E. S3

11-1. The answer is E. *(Hurst's The Heart, 14th Edition, Chap. 11)* Fixed splitting of S2 is classically found in ostium secundum atrial septal defect, where wide splitting of S2 is present at baseline with minimal or no change in the A2-P2 interval during inspiration. Conversely, paradoxical splitting of the S2 is more common in obstructive hypertrophic cardiomyopathy, suggesting severe dynamic left ventricular outflow obstruction. Hypertrophic cardiomyopathy with obstruction is a cause of a bifid pulse, caused by the occurrence of obstruction starting in midsystole. This is seen as a spike-and-dome pattern on aortic pressure tracing. Patients with HOCM might also have a classic apical impulse—the so-called triple ripple—corresponding to the presence of palpable systolic impulse in early and midsystole, separated by withdrawal of the apical impulse related to dynamic outflow obstruction; a palpable atrial contraction corresponds to the third impulse. An S4 is often heard in patients with abnormalities of ventricular relaxation, such as hypertropic cardiomyopathy.

11-2. The answer is D. *(Hurst's The Heart, 14th Edition, Chap. 11)* Aortic regurgitation murmurs heard over the second right intercostal space result from annular dilatation, whereas murmurs heard over the third left intercostal space result from a valvular process. When mixed aortic valve disease is present and the aortic regurgitation is the predominant lesion, an arterial contour with increased amplitude and two palpable systolic peaks can be present—the bisferiens pulse (option A is incorrect). The murmur of aortic regurgitation is a high-pitched "cooing" sound resulting from the high pressure difference between the aorta and left ventricular pressures during diastole (option B is incorrect). A middiastolic rumble, the Austin-Flint murmur, may be heard in aortic regurgitation when an eccentric jet hits the anterior leaflet of the mitral valve, causing it to reverberate and generating the apical rumble (option C is incorrect). In aortic regurgitation, the combination of increased stroke volume and the regurgitation itself gives rise to an arterial pulse that is increased in amplitude ("bounding"), which also collapses very quickly—the so-called water hammer pulse (option E is incorrect).

11-3. The answer is C. *(Hurst's The Heart, 14th Edition, Chap. 11)* Forrester and Diamond categorized chest pain into typical angina (all three criteria were present), atypical angina (two criteria), and noncardiac chest pain (only one criterion). They based this classification on whether the pain (1) was substernal and pressure-like, (2) was precipitated by exertion or emotional stress, and (3) was relieved by rest or nitroglycerin and lasted less than 30 minutes. In certain patient populations (eg, elderly men), this approach yielded such a high pretest probability of coronary artery disease that stress testing was unnecessary for the diagnosis of coronary atherosclerosis. This continues to be of value in clinical practice, particularly for male patients. It is commonly said that women often present with atypical symptoms, and the diagnosis of myocardial ischemia may be missed using these classic criteria. However, data suggest that anginal symptoms might be similar in men and women and that the idea that women often present with atypical symptoms might be misleading.[1] Rarely, patients will report that angina improves with continued exercise (walk-through angina).

11-4. The answer is E. *(Hurst's The Heart, 14th Edition, Chap. 11)* In the early phases of diastolic dysfunction, abnormal (prolonged) ventricular relaxation impairs early diastolic ventricular filling, decreasing the amount of filling in early diastole with a compensatory enhanced atrial contribution of diastolic filling.[2] An audible left heart fourth heart sound (S4) represents this prominent, forceful left atrial contraction into a noncompliant left ventricle. Therefore, although often present in patients with aortic stenosis and sinus rhythm, it is *never* present in atrial fibrillation (due to the loss of the *a* wave). When present, a left-sided S4 is a low-pitched sound, typically only heard at the apex with the bell and easily missed if auscultation in the left lateral decubitus position is not performed. Among the other findings, a late-peaking crescendo-decrescendo systolic murmur, a soft S2, and delayed and weak carotid upstroke (pulsus tardus and parvus) are all signs of *severe* aortic stenosis (options A, B, and D are incorrect). The murmur of aortic stenosis can radiate and, in fact, increase in intensity toward the apex—the Gallavardin phenomenon (option C is incorrect).[3]

11-5. **The answer is B.** *(Hurst's The Heart, 14th Edition, Chap. 11)* In patients with systolic murmur, attention should be paid to the change in intensity of the murmur on the postectopic beats. There is an increase in ventricular contractility and a decrease in afterload on the postectopic beat; thus, there will be an increase in the intensity of the murmur with both fixed (aortic stenosis) and dynamic (hypertrophic cardiomyopathy) left ventricular outflow tract obstruction. This response is much more striking in the setting of obstructive hypertrophic cardiomyopathy because there will also be an increase in the degree of obstruction (Figure 11-1). Alternatively, in patients with mitral regurgitation, there will be no change in the intensity of the murmur on the postectopic beat due to the decrease in afterload. Aortic and left ventricular pressure tracings illustrate the postectopic beat (arrow) response in dynamic outflow tract obstruction (left) versus fixed aortic stenosis (right). Although systolic gradients increase in both diseases, the response is much more exuberant in hypertrophic cardiomyopathy (the Brockenbrough-Braunwald-Morrow phenomenon).

11-6. **The answer is B.** *(Hurst's The Heart, 14th Edition, Chap. 11)* Systolic clicks can arise from valvular and nonvalvular structures (eg, the great arteries). The two most common (and more relevant) clicks are the ones heard in bicuspid aortic valve and mitral valve prolapse. Although the former is typically described as an ejection click and the latter a nonejection click, a description based on timing is more appropriate. The systolic click associated with mitral valve prolapse usually occurs in mid-to-late systole (option A is incorrect), when there is full excursion of the prolapsed mitral leaflet(s) into the left atrium. The click can be single or multiple (salvo of clicks). The timing of the click of mitral valve prolapse occurring later in systole helps to differentiate it from clicks arising from semilunar valves. With increased preload (squatting, supine) the click occurs later in systole, whereas decreased preload (Valsalva maneuver, standing) has the opposite effect (Figure 11-2; option E is incorrect).

Conversely, the click of a bicuspid aortic valve (and sometimes of other congenitally abnormal aortic valves such as unicuspid valves) is secondary to the doming of the valve cusps in early systole as the aortic valve opens. The sound is high-pitched (higher than S1)

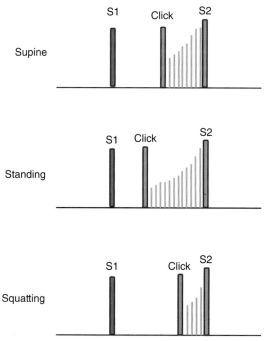

FIGURE 11-2 Positional changes in the systolic click and murmur of mitral valve prolapse. S1, first heart sound; S2, second heart sound.

and sometimes quite loud; it should not be confused with a loud split S1 (two components of the same pitch and intensity) or an S4 (low-pitched sound that vanishes if the bell is firmly pressed against the skin) (option D is incorrect). Doming of the cusps is also seen in valvular pulmonary stenosis, and an early systolic click is also typical. As in bicuspid aortic valve, the click of pulmonary stenosis introduces the systolic murmur. However, the click noted in pulmonary stenosis has a unique and important characteristic: it decreases in intensity with inspiration and moves closer to S1 (option C is incorrect). This is the only right-sided auscultatory finding that diminishes with inspiration. Early systolic clicks can also arise from dilated great vessels (aorta or pulmonary artery).

11-7. **The answer is C.** *(Hurst's The Heart, 14th Edition, Chap. 11)* Systolic murmurs are graded I to VI, as in the following table:

Grade I	Faint murmur; heard only after a few seconds of auscultation
Grade II	Moderately loud murmur heard immediately
Grade III	Loud murmur; not associated with a thrill
Grade IV	Loud murmur associated with a thrill
Grade V	Very loud; can be heard if only the edge of the stethoscope is in contact with the skin
Grade VI	Loudest possible; can be heard with the stethoscope just removed from the chest and not touching the skin

11-8. **The answer is C.** *(Hurst's The Heart, 14th Edition, Chap. 11)* The simultaneous left ventricular and aortic hemodynamic pressure tracings from a patient with HOCM shown in Figure 11-3 demonstrate characteristic respirophasic hemodynamic changes. Inspiration leads to increased left ventricular afterload; as a result, the systolic gradient between the left ventricle and the aorta decreases with inspiration. At the bedside, this is manifested by a decrease in the systolic ejection murmur noted with inspiration. The presence of this finding suggests dynamic instead of fixed outflow tract obstruction as the source of the murmur. Standing decreases preload and worsens obstruction in HOCM, which will make the murmur louder (option A is incorrect). A midsystolic click is not characteristic of HOCM (option B is incorrect); the approach to a click is reviewed in question 11-6. A palpable P2 can be observed in patients with advanced pulmonary hypertension; although secondary pulmonary hypertension (Group 2) can result from HOCM, this finding is not specific to HOCM (option D is incorrect). An apical holosystolic murmur suggests mitral regurgitation, and it is not specific to HOCM (option E is incorrect).

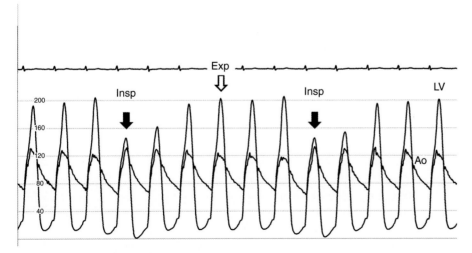

FIGURE 11-3 Simultaneous left ventricular and aortic hemodynamic pressure tracings from a patient with hypertrophic obstructive cardiomyopathy demonstrate characteristic respirophasic hemodynamic changes.

11-9. **The answer is E.** *(Hurst's The Heart, 14th Edition, Chap. 11)* The continuous murmur is characterized by a to-and-fro sound with no interruption between systole and diastole. The pitch should be similar, but the intensity can vary throughout the cardiac cycle. By definition, the continuous murmur envelops the heart sounds. This is distinctly different from a systolic and diastolic murmur, as noted in mixed aortic valve disease. In that case, one will hear a harsh, diamond-shaped systolic murmur, a second heart sound (which might be single), and a diastolic murmur. These murmurs will have two distinctly different pitches.

The most common continuous murmur seen in current practice is secondary to iatrogenic arteriovenous fistulas (for hemodialysis), which is generally appreciated in the region of the clavicle on the respective side (option B is incorrect). Other causes of continuous murmurs are rare and include patent ductus arteriosus (best heard over the left infraclavicular area), ruptured sinus of Valsalva aneurysm, coronary fistula, intrathoracic arteriovenous fistulae, severe coarctation of the aorta, and a surgically created shunt (eg, Blalock-Taussig, Potts, Waterston) (options A, C, and D are incorrect). The venous hum is a continuous murmur heard on auscultation of the neck. It results from a high flow in the internal jugular vein, which most likely causes a vibration of the venous wall. It is most commonly heard in young, otherwise healthy individuals and is not associated with pathology. The venous hum will disappear with the supine position or with compression of the vein itself.

11-10. **The answer is A.** *(Hurst's The Heart, 14th Edition, Chap. 11)* In acute severe mitral regurgitation secondary to papillary muscle rupture or mitral valve dehiscence, the left atrium is not accustomed to the severe volume overload. A very large *v* wave is generated because of lack of atrial compliance, and left ventricular and left atrial pressures essentially equalize in systole. The auscultatory result is a very short, early systolic murmur or even absence of a murmur. Accordingly, color-flow and continuous-wave Doppler findings are also often very brief, making the diagnosis of acute mitral regurgitation challenging. Patients with acute severe mitral regurgitation are in frank pulmonary edema and are therefore sitting upright, whereas patients with ventricular septal defect can tolerate the supine position. A soft murmur, cool extremities, increased jugular venous pressure, and an S3 are not specific to either mitral regurgitation or a ventricular septal defect.

References

1. Kreatsoulas C, Shannon HS, Giacomini M, Velianou JL, Anand SS. Reconstructing angina: cardiac symptoms are the same in women and men. *JAMA Intern Med.* 2013;173(9):829-831.
2. Nishimura RA, Tajik AJ. Evaluation of diastolic filling of left ventricle in health and disease: Doppler echocardiography is the clinician's Rosetta Stone. *J Am Coll Cardiol.* 1997;30(1):8-18.
3. Giles TD, Martinez EC, Burch GE. Gallavardin phenomenon in aortic stenosis. A possible mechanism. *Arch Intern Med.* 1974;134(4):747-749.

CHAPTER 12

Surface Electrocardiography

Jacqueline Joza

QUESTIONS

DIRECTIONS: Choose the one best response to each question.

12-1. Which of the following technical errors may result in an electrocardiogram with farfield signals in lead II?

A. Interchanging of the right arm and right leg leads
B. Interchanging of the right arm and left arm leads
C. Interchanging of the left arm and left leg leads
D. Interchanging of the right arm and left leg leads
E. Interchanging of the right leg and left leg leads

12-2. Which of the following is strongly suggestive of an *atypical* right bundle branch block (RBBB) on electrocardiogram?

A. QRS of at least 0.12 seconds with midfinal slurring
B. RSr' in lead V_1
C. qRS in V_6 with S wave slurring and a positive T wave
D. T wave with an opposite polarity to the QRS slurring
E. QR in aVR with R wave slurring and a negative T wave

12-3. A 42-year-old woman presents to the emergency department with a 12-hour history of worsening dyspnea and weakness. She describes a recent business trip to India. Which of the following represent the *least* likely electrocardiographic sign to be observed in this clinical situation?

A. Right bundle branch block
B. aVL + SV_3 > 20 mm
C. Sinus tachycardia
D. Normal sinus rhythm
E. McGinn-White pattern

12-4. A 24-year-old male with a history of palpitations presents to the emergency department. The following electrocardiographic findings may be observed in a patient with Wolff-Parkinson-White syndrome, *except*:

A. Absence of a right bundle branch pattern in a patient with Ebstein's anomaly
B. Preexcited atrial fibrillation
C. A normal PR interval in the setting of a left-lateral accessory pathway
D. Prolongation of the PR interval
E. A narrow QRS tachycardia with a mid-RP interval

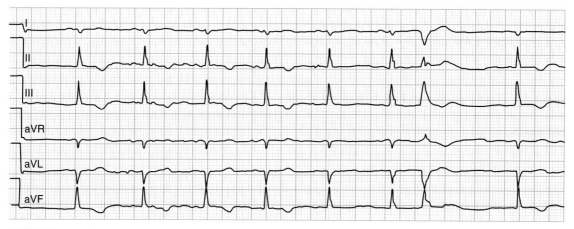

FIGURE 12-1 Electrocardiogram of a 35-year-old woman with syncope.

12-5. See Figure 12-1. A 35-year-old woman presents with syncope. The origin of negative T waves in the inferior leads on the electrocardiogram may include which of the following?

A. Hyperkalemia
B. Left ventricular hypertrophy
C. Acute pericarditis
D. Advanced atrioventricular block
E. Mitral valve prolapse

12-6. A 75-year-old female presents with nausea and vomiting to the emergency department. Her EKG reveals ST elevation in the inferior leads. Which of the following findings is most likely to suggest the presence of an accompanying right ventricular infarct?

A. Negative T wave in V_4R
B. ST elevations in lead I
C. ST elevations lead II > III
D. ST elevations in lead V_4R
E. ST depression in V_4R

12-7. A 35-year-old woman with a history of rheumatic fever presents to your office in consultation for intermittent palpitations and worsening dyspnea. A physical exam reveals a diastolic murmur over the apex. Thyroid studies are within normal limits. Which of the following ECG findings is *least* likely to be observed in this patient?

A. Atrial fibrillation
B. Atrial tachycardia
C. Biphasic positive-negative p wave in V_1
D. R wave in V_1
E. T-wave inversions in II, III, aVF

12-8. Causes of pathologic Q waves *not* secondary to myocardial infarction include all of the following *except*:

A. Amyloidosis
B. Dilated cardiomyopathy
C. Wolff-Parkinson-White syndrome
D. Cardiac transplant
E. Acute myocarditis

12-9. You are consulted on a 21-year-old female who requires a cardiac workup following a small right middle cerebral artery stroke. She has no other significant past medical history. On questioning, she admits to having a history of breathlessness with maximal exertion for as long as she can remember. All of the following findings may be observed on her electrocardiogram *except*:

A. Leftward QRS axis
B. Left bundle branch block (LBBB)
C. Atrial fibrillation
D. Negative P waves in II, III, aVF
E. Presence of an rsR' in V_1 with a QRS < 0.12 seconds

12-10. All of the following are associated with a dominant R in V_1 on electrocardiogram *except*:

A. Athlete's heart
B. Ebstein's anomaly
C. Arrhythmogenic right ventricular dysplasia
D. Wolff-Parkinson-White electrocardiographic pattern
E. Lateral wall myocardial infarction

ANSWERS

12-1. **The answer is A.** *(Hurst's The Heart, 14th Edition, Chap. 12)* Interchanging of the right arm and right leg leads would result in farfield signals (diminished signals) in lead II. Interchanging of the right arm and left arm leads would result in a pattern of negative P, negative QRS, and negative T waves in lead I (and positive in aVR) (option B). A normal pattern of R wave progression from V_1 to V_6 would argue against dextrocardia in this instance if the leads were placed correctly. Interchanging left arm and left leg leads would result in reversal of leads aVL and aVF, reversal of leads I and II, and inversion of lead III (option C). Interchanging right arm and left leg leads would result in inversion of leads I, II, and III, and reversal of leads aVR and aVF (option D). Interchanging of the right and left leg leads will not result in a different ECG recording compared to one obtained with standard electrode placement (option E).

12-2. **The answer is B.** *(Hurst's The Heart, 14th Edition, Chap. 12)* The first upward deflection (R) of the QRS should always be shorter than the second upward deflection (r′) in a typical RBBB. Options A, C, D, and E represent diagnostic criteria for a typical RBBB.

12-3. **The answer is B.** *(Hurst's The Heart, 14th Edition, Chap. 12)* The cause of the patient's dyspnea is most likely secondary to a pulmonary embolus in the context of recent travel. Commonly, the presenting ECG is normal (option D), however the most valuable diagnostic findings for a large pulmonary embolus, which are poorly sensitive but highly specific, are as follows: (1) the McGinn-White pattern (S_I, Q_{III}, negative T_{III} pattern) (option E); (2) RBBB (option A) (3) a rightward-directed QRS axis (typically > 30° to the right of its usual position); (4) negative T wave in right precordial leads; and (5) sinus tachycardia (option C), which is common except in elderly patients or in those with sinus node dysfunction. (Option B) aVL + SV_3 > 20 mm in a woman and > 28 mm in a man (Cornell voltage criterion) is highly specific for left ventricular hypertrophy, which this patient has no indication of having.

12-4. **The answer is D.** *(Hurst's The Heart, 14th Edition, Chap. 12)* Shortening, as opposed to prolongation of the PR interval is observed in patients with Wolff-Parkinson-White pattern on their resting electrocardiogram. The absence of an RBBB pattern in a patient with Ebstein's anomaly is highly suggestive of the presence of an accessory pathway (option A). In a recent PACES/HRS expert consensus document on the treatment of asymptomatic young WPW subjects, it is recommended that ablation should be considered in subjects between 8 and 21 years with asymptomatic WPW pattern if they have RR intervals shorter than 250 ms during atrial fibrillation due to increased risk of sudden cardiac death (option B).[1] Preexcitation suggesting antidromic conduction in WPW syndrome may still be present with a normal PR interval if the accessory pathway is far from the sinus node (eg, left lateral pathway) (option C). An orthodromic AV reciprocating tachycardia using a retrograde accessory pathway can typically present as a narrow complex tachycardia with either a mid or a long RP (option E).

12-5. **The answer is E.** *(Hurst's The Heart, 14th Edition, Chap. 12)* Although an infrequent finding, an electrocardiogram with mitral valve prolapse will typically reveal T-wave inversions in the inferior leads and/or V_5 and V_6. This patient had bileaflet mitral valve prolapse with moderate mitral valve regurgitation. She presented after three episodes of high-risk syncope, and she was diagnosed with malignant mitral valve syndrome. The origin of the PVC was from the anterolateral papillary muscle. Hyperkalemia classically causes peaked T waves (option A) (in contrast, hypokalemia may cause T-wave flattening). Left ventricular hypertrophy would cause a more positive than normal T wave (option B). Acute pericarditis would be more likely to show more positive T waves (option C). Advanced atrioventricular block would demonstrate tall and peaked T waves in the narrow QRS complex escape rhythm (option D).

12-6. The answer is D. *(Hurst's The Heart, 14th Edition, Chap. 12)* ST elevations in V_4R would be highly suggestive of a right ventricular infarct. Options A, B, C, and E are more suggestive that the left circumflex is the culprit artery.

12-7. The answer is E. *(Hurst's The Heart, 14th Edition, Chap. 12)* The patient presents with a history and a physical exam suggestive of mitral stenosis (note: a palpable S1 may be noted in mitral stenosis, thyrotoxicosis, anxiety, and in the setting of a short PR interval). Atrial fibrillation (option A), atrial tachycardia (option B), biphasic positive-negative p wave in V_1 (option C), and an R wave in V_1 (option D) are classical electrocardiographic findings of mitral stenosis. T-wave inversions in the inferior leads are not specific for mitral stenosis, but they may be observed in a patient with mitral valve prolapse (option E).

12-8. The answer is D. *(Hurst's The Heart, 14th Edition, Chap. 12)* Pathologic Q waves are not typically seen in a transplanted heart. Patients with cardiac transplant are often observed to have the P wave of both the donor and the recipient on the same ECG. Generally the donor P wave is of a higher rate than the recipient P wave because there is no vagal control on the donor heart. A pathologic Q wave is wide (≥ 0.04 seconds) and typically exceeds 25% of the following R wave. The presence of abnormal Q waves suggests myocardial necrosis, but it may also be observed in other circumstances, such as amyloidosis (option A), dilated cardiomyopathy (option B), Wolff-Parkinson-White syndrome (option C), and acute myocarditis (option E). Other causes of pathologic Q waves include recording artifacts, normal variants (Q in aVL in a vertical heart, and Q in III in the dextrorotated and horizontal heart), QS in V_1 in septal fibrosis, emphysema, the elderly, and chest abnormalities, some types of right ventricular hypertrophy (chronic cor pulmonale) or left ventricular hypertrophy (QS in V_1-V_2 with a slow increase in the R wave through the precordial leads), left bundle branch conduction abnormalities, infiltrative processes (sarcoidosis, tumors, chronic myocarditis), coronary vasospasm, pheochromocytoma, and congenital heart diseases (coronary artery abnormalities or dextrocardia).

12-9. The answer is B. *(Hurst's The Heart, 14th Edition, Chap. 12)* The question points toward an atrial septal defect (ASD) as a potential etiology for the patient's stroke. An LBBB would not specifically be seen in the presence of an ASD (option B). A leftward QRS axis may be observed in a primum ASD, whereas a normal or rightward axis is more typical of a secundum ASD (option A). Atrial fibrillation, associated with or independent of an ASD, may be the cause of stroke in this patient (option C). Negative P waves in the inferior leads suggest a low/ectopic atrial pacemaker, which can be seen in sinus venosus/SVC defects (option D). A partial or complete RBBB, not an LBBB, may be seen in combination with an ASD (option E).

12-10. The answer is A. *(Hurst's The Heart, 14th Edition, Chap. 12)* An athlete's heart is not typically associated with a dominant R in V_1. Options B through E are all causes of a dominant R in V_1. Ebstein's anomaly and arrhythmogenic right ventricular dysplasia present as atypical RBBB. Other causes of a dominant R in V_1 on electrocardiogram include incorrect lead placement, chest anomalies, abnormal variants (post-term infants, scant Purkinje fibers in the anteroseptal region), typical RBBB, Brugada syndrome, and right ventricular or biventricular enlargement.

Reference

1. Cannon BC, Davis AM, Drago F, et al. PACES/HRS Expert Consensus Statement on the Management of the Asymptomatic Young Patient with a Wolff-Parkinson-White (WPW, Ventricular Preexcitation) Electrocardiographic Pattern. Heart Rhythm 2012;9:1006-1024.

CHAPTER 13

Electrocardiographic Exercise Testing

Jacqueline Joza

QUESTIONS

DIRECTIONS: Choose the one best response to each question.

13-1. What are the determinants of myocardial oxygen uptake?

A. Minute ventilation and the fraction of ventilation extracted by the tissues
B. Cardiac output and the peripheral arteriovenous oxygen difference
C. Intramyocardial wall tension, contractility, and heart rate
D. Stroke volume and heart rate
E. The maximal heart rate and the maximal systolic blood pressure

13-2. A 65-year-old male is referred to you for evaluation of possible coronary artery disease. He gives a 4-week history of chest discomfort with climbing two flights of stairs, where he had previously been able to climb several flights without difficulty. He denies any dyspnea, orthopnea, paroxysmal nocturnal dyspnea, or syncope. Two weeks ago, he was started on isosorbide mononitrate 30 mg po daily, metoprolol 25 mg po twice daily, and aspirin 80 mg po daily by his primary care physician. Physical exam is within normal limits. You plan to perform an exercise stress test. Which of the following sets of instructions is *false*?

A. Instruct the patient to hold metoprolol for at least 24 hours prior to the test
B. Instruct the patient to avoid vigorous exercise the day of the test
C. Instruct the patient to hold his morning dose of isosorbide mononitrate the day of the test
D. Instruct the patient to continue all medications
E. Instruct the patient to avoid caffeine in the event that a vasodilator stress will be performed at the same time

13-3. A 48-year-old female presents to the emergency department with central chest pain and dyspnea that now occurs after walking one block. The chest pain began six months ago, but the symptoms have become more frequent and occur with even less exertion. She describes an episode of syncope without prodrome. Her family history is significant for a brother having undergone a cardiac surgery at age 52. A systolic ejection click with an associated systolic murmur is noted on exam. Serial troponins are negative. What is the next best course of action?

A. Book an exercise stress test
B. Proceed with transthoracic echocardiography
C. Proceed with coronary angiography
D. Consult cardiac surgery
E. Start a beta blocker and discharge home with follow-up in clinic

13-4. Which of the following is *not* an absolute contraindication to exercise stress testing?

A. Severe mitral stenosis
B. Unstable angina
C. Acute pericarditis
D. Stable, sustained monomorphic VT
E. > 3 mm ST segment depression at rest

13-5. Which of the following statements about exercise stress testing is *false*?

A. The formula MPHR = 220 – age results in an underestimation of maximum heart rate, particularly in older patients
B. The formula MPHR = 220 – age was originally developed to be used for patients' exercise prescriptions
C. The exercise stress test may be terminated when the maximal predicted heart rate reaches 85%
D. Achieving either maximum effort or an ischemic endpoint is crucial for exercise testing performed with or without imaging
E. The maximum predicted heart rate is best achieved by using the formula MPHR = 208 – 0.7 × age

Questions 13-6, 13-7, and 13-8 relate to the following vignette:

A 42-year-old man with diabetes mellitus type II and dyslipidemia is referred for an exercise stress test from the emergency department. He began to complain of dull left shoulder pain 2 weeks prior to presentation. The pain has worsened in the last few days, and it is precipitated by walking up stairs. He remarks that he thinks he may have hurt his shoulder during snow shoveling 2 weeks ago. A physical exam reveals a blood pressure of 138/78 HR 84 regular, oxygen saturation 98% on room air, and respiratory rate of 14. He is afebrile. Normal heart sounds are auscultated, and no murmurs are present. Serial troponins are negative.

13-6. In this patient, all of the following resting electrocardiographic findings may cause reconsideration of an exercise stress test as the primary investigation, *except*:

A. Presence of preexcitation
B. Presence of an LBBB
C. Presence of a paced rhythm
D. Atrial fibrillation with a rapid ventricular response
E. Intraventricular conduction delay

13-7. All of the following parameters should usually prompt exercise stress test termination *except*:

A. 1 mm ST elevation in the anterior precordial leads
B. A decrease in the systolic blood pressure by 10 mm Hg
C. Patient would like to terminate the test
D. Isolated premature ventricular contractions
E. Mobitz type 1 second-degree heart block

13-8. Which of the following results would constitute the worst prognosis?

A. 1 mm of slow upsloping ST depression at 5 METS, with resolution upon termination of exercise
B. 0.5 mm of slow downsloping ST depression at 7 METS, with persistence into 2 minutes of recovery
C. 1.5 mm of horizontal ST depression at 5 METS, with resolution upon termination of exercise
D. 1.5 mm of horizontal ST depression at 5 METS, with persistence into 2 minutes of recovery
E. 1.5 mm of downsloping ST depression at 7 METS, with resolution upon termination of exercise

13-9. Which of the following patients performing an exercise stress test would be identified as a moderate risk for cardiovascular death or nonfatal myocardial infarction over 5 years follow-up?

A. A 45-year-old male performs 7 minutes on EST, limited by chest pain with 2 mm ST depressions during exercise in the inferior leads
B. A 55-year-old female performs 7 minutes on EST, and she stops due to fatigue with 1 mm of horizontal ST depressions into recovery in the anterior precordial leads
C. A 64-year-old female performs 8 minutes on EST, and she stops as a result of leg pain with 0.5 mm ST depressions in the inferior leads during exercise only
D. A 55-year-old female performs 4 minutes on EST, and she stops due to dyspnea, with 3 mm of horizontal ST depressions in the anterior precordial leads during exercise
E. A 70-year-old male performs 7 minutes on EST, limited by leg cramping, with no ST deviation

13-10. Select the *false* statement about EST:

A. Digoxin can produce ST segment depression during exercise even if the effect is not evident on the resting ECG
B. Exercise-induced ST segment elevation is nonspecific for the territory of myocardial ischemia and the coronary artery involved
C. The expected lower sensitivity and specificity traditionally observed in women may be explained by differing CAD prevalence and severity
D. Submaximal exercise testing in which exercise is stopped at a predetermined end point, such as a peak heart rate of 120 beats/min, 70% of MPHR, or a peak MET level of 5, can be used as a class I indication 4 to 7-plus days post-MI for evaluation of medical therapy, prognostic assessment, or development of an activity prescription
E. Exercise-induced ST segment depression does not localize the site of myocardial ischemia, nor does it indicate which coronary artery is involved

13-1. **The answer is C.** *(Hurst's The Heart, 14th Edition, Chap. 13)* The determinants of myocardial oxygen uptake are intramyocardial wall tension (left ventricular pressure and end-diastolic volume), contractility, and heart rate (option C). Myocardial oxygen uptake can be estimated by the product of heart rate and systolic blood pressure (the double product or rate pressure product). This information is valuable clinically because exercise-induced angina often occurs at the same myocardial oxygen demand and thus double product. The higher the double product achieved, the better the myocardial perfusion and prognosis. VO_2 max is determined by the maximal amount of ventilation (volume of expired gas [VE]) moving into and out of the lung and by the fraction of this ventilation that is extracted by the tissues: $VO_2 = VE \times (FiO_2 - FeO_2)$ where VE is the minute ventilation and FiO_2 and FeO_2 are the fractional concentration of oxygen in the inspired and expired air, respectively (option A). The determinants of volume oxygen consumption [VO_2] are cardiac output and the peripheral arteriovenous oxygen difference. Because maximal arteriovenous difference behaves more or less as a constant, maximal oxygen uptake serves as an indirect estimate of maximal cardiac output (option B). The product of stroke volume and heart rate is the cardiac output (option D). The rate pressure product is the product of the maximal heart rate (bpm) and the maximal systolic blood pressure (mm Hg), and it represents the internal workload or hemodynamic response (option E).

13-2. **The answer is D.** *(Hurst's The Heart, 14th Edition, Chap. 13).* The exercise stress test is being performed to determine if the patient has coronary artery disease. Antianginal medications should be held to minimize their anti-ischemic impact (hold beta-blockers for 24 hours [option A] and hold nitrates and calcium channel blockers the day of the study [option C]). If medications are not held, the test sensitivity may be decreased either by the patient's medical regimen or by the fact that the ischemia was not seen at the level of exertion or double product achieved. If the test is being performed for prognostic reasons (that is, if coronary disease is known to be present), then medications do *not* need to be held. Avoiding vigorous exercise on the day of exercise testing is appropriate to enhance the patient's ability to achieve maximum exercise on the test (option B). Caffeine is a competitive antagonist of adenosine receptors and thus blocks the effect of dipyridamole, adenosine, and regadenoson. It should be withheld for at least 12 hours if there is a possibility of the patient undergoing a vasodilator stress the same day (option E).

13-3. **The answer is B.** *(Hurst's The Heart, 14th Edition, Chap. 13)* The patient has a probable diagnosis of a stenotic bicuspid aortic valve. Her symptoms are suggestive of a high degree of valve stenosis with possible concomitant coronary artery disease. A transthoracic echocardiogram would be the best first choice (option B). Exercise stress testing would be an absolute contraindication in a patient with possible severe aortic stenosis (option A). Proceeding directly with coronary angiography (option C) or cardiac surgery (option E) would be premature. The patient's symptoms, and particularly that of syncope, are worrisome enough to keep the patient in the hospital until at least a transthoracic echocardiogram is performed (option E).

13-4. **The answer is E.** *(Hurst's The Heart, 14th Edition, Chap. 13)* >3 mm ST segment depression at rest is a *relative* contraindication to exercise stress testing. Options A through D are all absolute contraindications to exercise stress testing. Other absolute contraindications include patients with acute myocardial infarction, acute myocarditis, Mobitz type 2, second or third degree heart block, known severe left main disease, acutely ill patients, patients with locomotive problems, severe aortic or other valve stenosis, acute pulmonary embolus, and uncontrolled symptomatic heart failure.

13-5. **The answer is C.** *(Hurst's The Heart, 14th Edition, Chap. 13)* Stopping exercise prematurely once 85% of an estimated maximal heart rate is achieved decreases exercise testing sensitivity and minimizes the opportunity to assess ischemia electrocardiographically and with adjunctive imaging (option C). Bairey and coworkers compared patients undergoing exercise myocardial perfusion imaging with a normal perfusion scan relative to whether they achieved 85% of MPHR. The annual event rate of death, nonfatal MI, or late revascularization was 1.9% for those who reached ≥ 85% MPHR compared to 8.6% for those who achieved < 85%.[1] The formula of MPHR = 220 – age results in an underestimation of maximum heart rate, particularly in older patients (option A), and was originally developed for use in patients' exercise prescriptions (option B). Further, achieving either maximum effort or an ischemic endpoint is crucial (option D). In a meta-analysis of 351 studies involving 18,712 patients, Tanaka and colleagues found that the formula of 208 – 0.7 × age best predicted the maximum heart rate.[2] The formula was predictive in men and women and independent of habitual activity level (option E).

13-6. **The answer is E.** *(Hurst's The Heart, 14th Edition, Chap. 13)* Exercise stress testing will be difficult to interpret in the presence of a delta wave (option A), LBBB (option B), ventricular pacing (option C), > 1 mm of resting ST depressions, or any atrial arrhythmia with an uncontrolled ventricular response (option D). Accompanying myocardial perfusion imaging, stress echocardiography, or calcium scoring would be other tests of choice.

13-7. **The answer is D.** *(Hurst's The Heart, 14th Edition, Chap. 13)* The 2002 ACC/AHA guidelines state that exercise should be terminated when premature ventricular contractions occur in pairs with increasing frequency as exercise increases, or when at least three-beat ventricular tachycardia occurs. Other causes for termination include, but are not limited to: ST elevation > 1 mm in precordial or inferior leads that do not have a resting Q wave; onset of Mobitz type 1 or 2 second-degree or third-degree heart block; any decrease in systolic blood pressure during exercise, particularly if accompanied by another indication of ischemia; ST depression ≥ 2 mm; atrial tachycardia, atrial fibrillation, or atrial flutter; patient dyspnea; fatigue or lightheadedness; moderate musculoskeletal pain; patient becomes pale or clammy; and anginal pain increasing to moderate severity.

13-8. **The answer is D.** *(Hurst's The Heart, 14th Edition, Chap. 13)* The ACC/AHA 2002 exercise testing guidelines classify an abnormal result as ≥ 1 mm of horizontal or downsloping ST depression. In the 2013 AHA scientific statement on exercise standards for testing and training, ≥ 1 mm of slow upsloping is defined as equivocal. There is sufficient evidence to conclude, however, that slow upsloping ST depressions of ≥ 1.5 mm should be included as a criterion for a positive exercise test in addition to the conventional criterion of ≥ 1 mm of horizontal or downsloping ST depression.[3] The earlier during exercise that ST depression occurs, and the lower the rate pressure product of this depression, and the longer it lasts during recovery, the more severe the coronary artery disease, as manifested by the incidence of multivessel and left main disease on coronary angiography.

13-9. **The answer is B.** *(Hurst's The Heart, 14th Edition, Chap. 13)* This patient's Duke Treadmill score is 2, which falls into the moderate risk category. Duke Treadmill Score (DTS) = Exercise time in minutes on the standard Bruce protocol – 5 × ST deviation (depression or elevation measured in mm in the lead with the greatest degree of ST deviation) – 4 × exercise angina index, where 0 = no angina on the treadmill, 1 = angina occurred, 2 = angina caused termination of exercise. A DTS of +5 or greater constitutes the lowest risk; a DTS of +4 to −10 constitutes a moderate risk; and a DTS of −11 or lower constitutes the highest risk. Option A has a DTS of −11 (high risk). Option C has a DTS of 5.5 (low risk). Option D has a DTS of −11 (high risk). Option E has a DTS of 7 (low risk).

13-10. **The answer is B.** *(Hurst's The Heart, 14th Edition, Chap. 13)* Unlike ST segment depression, ST segment elevation during exercise in contiguous leads with an R wave localizes to the coronary artery involved. Although ST depression is consistent with subendocardial ischemia, ST elevation is most consistent with transmural ischemia. Options A and C through E are true.

References

1. Bairey CN, Rozanski A, Maddahi J, Resser KJ, Berman DS. Exercise thallium-201 scintigraphy and prognosis in typical angina pectoris and negative exercise electrocardiography. *Am J Cardiol.* 1989;64:282-287.
2. Tanaka H, Monahan KD, Seals DR. Age-predicted maximal heart rate revisited. *J Am Coll Cardiol.* 2001;37:153-156.
3. Ellestad MH. Stress testing: principles and practice. Philadelphia, PA: Davis; 1975.

CHAPTER 14
Cardiac Radiography
Jonathan Afilalo

QUESTIONS

DIRECTIONS: Choose the one best response to each question.

14-1. Radiographic assessment of the lung can often reflect the underlying pathophysiology of diseases of the heart. Which of the following statements regarding the normal radiographic appearance of the pulmonary vasculature of an upright human being is *false*?

A. The pressure differential between the apex and the base of the lung is approximately 22 mm Hg in adult men
B. The number of vessels and their length are more important than their caliber
C. Pulmonary blood volume can be assessed by comparing the size of the pulmonary artery with that of the accompanying bronchus
D. There is caudalization of the pulmonary vascularity because of gravity
E. None of the above

14-2. A 55-year-old man, with no prior cardiac history, presented to the emergency department complaining of acute dypsnea. His chest x-ray revealed cephalad redistribution of the pulmonary vascularity. In which of the following conditions does cephalization *not* occur?

A. Mitral stenosis
B. Pulmonic stenosis associated with ventricular septal defect
C. Aortic stenosis
D. Left ventricular (LV) failure
E. Severe mitral regurgitation (MR)

14-3. A 25-year-old immigrant, with no prior medical history, is referred to your clinic for further evaluation of an abnormal chest radiography, which was discovered incidentally after a positive tuberculin skin test (Mantoux test). Otherwise she had no chest pain, dyspnea, or other specific signs or symptoms. Her chest x-ray is illustrated in Figure 14-1. Which of the following is the most likely radiographic diagnosis?

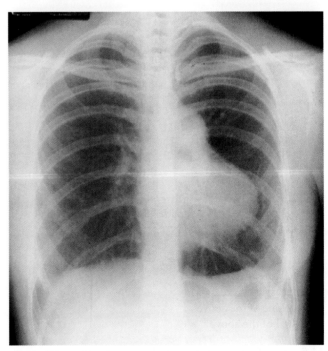

FIGURE 14-1 The heart is normal; however, the cardiac contour is markedly abnormal with elevation of the heart and in particular the cardiac apex. There is a broad band of lucency between the inferior cardiac border and the left hemidiaphragmatic silhouette, caused by normal left lung parenchyma beneath the heart that moves into place below the heart.

A. Congenital absence of the pericardium
B. Late presentation of tetralogy of Fallot
C. Left ventricular aneurysm
D. Severe rheumatic mitral stenosis with tricuspid regurgitation
E. None of the above

14-4. A 64-year-old man, with a 40 pack-year history of tobacco smoking, was admitted to the emergency department with a chief complaint of progressive worsening dyspnea on exertion. A chest radiography was performed, illustrated in Figure 14-2, and was reported as overaeration of the lungs, centralized flow pattern, and a small heart size. Besides chronic obstructive pulmonary disease, which of the following conditions may also present with a smaller-than-average heart on a chest radiography?

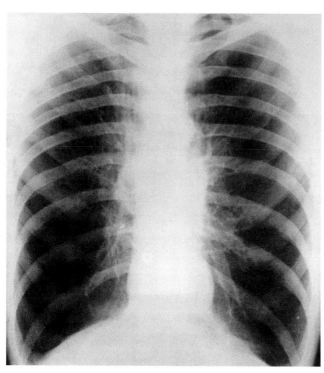

FIGURE 14-2 Severe obstructive emphysema showing overaeration of the lungs, centralized flow pattern, and a small heart size.

A. Addison disease
B. Anorexia nervosa
C. Starvation
D. None of the above
E. All of the above

14-5. A 75-year-old woman underwent a routine preoperative chest radiography prior to surgery for a carcinoma of the sigmoid colon. Her past medical history is significant for type 2 diabetes and arterial hypertension. Her chest x-ray shows linear calcifications within the aortic arch knob. Which of the following statements regarding radiologically detectable calcification in the heart is *false*?

A. Calcification of the coronary artery is almost always associated with flow-limiting luminal stenosis
B. Calcification of the coronary artery is almost always atherosclerotic in nature
C. The extent of valvular calcification tends to be proportionate to the severity of the valve stenosis
D. Mitral annular calcification is rarely indicative of significant disease
E. None of the above

14-6. A 25-year-old man sustained a severe stab wound to the left anterior hemithorax while attempting to break up a domestic fight. On presentation at the emergency department, he was hemodynamically stable. After a left-sided thoracostomy tube was inserted, the patient had a chest x-ray, which showed abnormal lucent areas around the heart. Which of the following conditions may cause abnormal lucent areas in and around the heart?

A. Displaced subepicardial fat stripes
B. Pneumopericardium
C. Pneumomediastinum
D. None of the above
E. All of the above

14-7. A 44-year-old woman with no prior medical history presented to the emergency department complaining of chest pain and palpitations. The admitting physician incidentally noted that the patient had heart sounds on the right side of the chest with no added sounds. A chest x-ray was performed and is illustrated in Figure 14-3. Which of the following diagnoses is consistent with the chest radiography findings?

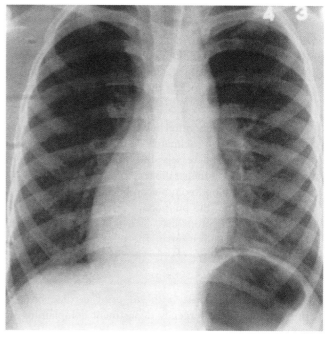

FIGURE 14-3 Note that the aortic arch and the stomach air bubble are both on the left and the apex of the ventricles is pointing to the right inferiorly. This patient had the typical combination of congenitally corrected transposition of the great arteries, ventricular septal defect, and pulmonary stenosis. He was cyanotic. The pulmonary vascularity appears decreased.

A. Dextrocardia with situs inversus
B. Dextrocardia with situs solitus
C. Levocardia with situs inversus
D. Levocardia with situs solitus
E. Cardiac malpositions with situs ambiguus

14-8. The abnormal size and distribution of both the pulmonary and systemic vessels may give important clues to the presence of certain conditions. In which of the following conditions is the prominence of the pulmonary trunk reliably correlated with the degree of enlargement of the right ventricle (RV)?

A. Tetralogy of Fallot
B. Idiopathic dilatation of the pulmonary artery
C. Patent ductus arteriosus
D. Straight-back syndrome
E. None of the above

14-9. A 47-year-old man was admitted to the emergency department complaining of increasing fatigue and dyspnea on exertion. His past medical history is significant for dyslipidemia and poorly controlled hypertension despite being on three antihypertensive medications, including a diuretic. Physical examination was significant for bilateral femoral pulses that were palpable but weak and delayed, as compared with the brachial pulses. The magnified view of the left upper thorax of the chest radiography is illustrated in Figure 14-4. With regard to the radiographic appearance, which of the following statements is *true*?

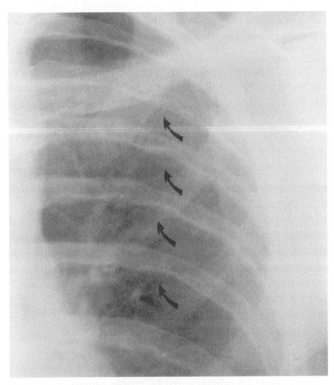

FIGURE 14-4 Magnified view of the left upper thorax showing multiple areas of rib notching (arrows).

A. Rib notching provides important clues to the diagnosis of coarctation of the aorta
B. Notching of the ribs has many origins
C. Superior vena cava (SVC) syndrome can produce a similar radiographic appearance
D. Neurofibromatosis can produce rib notching
E. All of the above

14-10. Cardiac fluoroscopy explores the dynamic features of the heart that are discernible in motion. Which of the following statements regarding cardiac fluoroscopy is *false*?

A. It has been largely displaced by other imaging techniques for the precise evaluation of cardiac size and function
B. It can assess the function of radiodense and echodense prosthetic valves during cardiac catheterization
C. It can be used to guide the positioning of pacemakers or ICDs in the cardiac catheterization laboratory
D. It is routinely used during transcatheter aortic valve implantation to guide the deployment of the prosthesis
E. None of the above

ANSWERS

14-1. **The answer is B.** *(Hurst's The Heart, 14th Edition, Chap. 14)* In the evaluation of pulmonary vasculature, the caliber of the vessels is more important than the length or the number (option B). As long as the pulmonary blood flow pattern remains normal, with a greater amount of flow to the bases than to the apices, the volume of the flow is proportional to the caliber of the pulmonary arteries. Options A, C, and D are correct.

14-2. **The answer is B.** *(Hurst's The Heart, 14th Edition, Chap. 14)* Patients with pulmonic stenosis and associated ventricular septal defect (VSD) often show decreased pulmonary vascularity with smaller and shorter pulmonary arteries and veins and more radiolucent lungs. Cephalization tends to occur instead in (1) left-sided obstructive lesions—for example, mitral valvular or aortic valvular stenosis (options A and C); (2) LV failure (option D)—for example, coronary heart disease or cardiomyopathies; and (3) severe MR even before pump failure of the LV occurs (option E).[1] Option B is therefore the correct answer.

14-3. **The answer is A.** *(Hurst's The Heart, 14th Edition, Chap. 14)* An elevated cardiac silhouette with lucency between the inferior cardiac border and the left hemidiaphragmatic silhouette is characteristic of congenital absence of the pericardium (option A). A coeur en sabot, a "boot-shaped heart," is characteristic of tetralogy of Fallot (option B). A bulge along the left cardiac border with a retrosternal double density is virtually diagnostic of LV aneurysm (option C). A markedly widened right cardiac contour with a straightened left cardiac border is often seen in patients with severe MS leading to tricuspid regurgitation (option D).

14-4. **The answer is E.** *(Hurst's The Heart, 14th Edition, Chap. 14)* The cardiothoracic ratio remains the simplest yardstick for assessing cardiac size. A smaller-than-average heart is encountered in patients with chronic obstructive pulmonary disease, Addison disease (option A), anorexia nervosa (option B), and starvation (option C). However, an abnormally small heart size is difficult to define except retrospectively after successful treatment of the underlying pathology.

14-5. **The answer is A.** *(Hurst's The Heart, 14th Edition, Chap. 14)* Any radiologically detectable calcification in the heart may be clinically important. In general, the heavier the calcification, the more significant it becomes; however, calcification does not imply luminal stenosis, and oftentimes calcification visualized in the coronary arteries is not obstructive (option A). Mitral annular calcification, a commonly encountered cause of cardiac calcification, is rarely indicative of significant disease (option D), but it has been associated with an increased risk of atherosclerotic cardiovascular disease.[2] The extent of valvular calcification tends to be proportionate to the severity of the valve stenosis regardless of the other radiographic signs of the disease (option C).[3-6] Calcification of the coronary artery is almost always atherosclerotic in nature (option B).

14-6. **The answer is E.** *(Hurst's The Heart, 14th Edition, Chap. 14)* The abnormal lucent areas in and around the heart include (1) displaced subepicardial fat stripes caused by effusion or thickening of the pericardium (option A), (2) pneumopericardium (option B), and (3) pneumomediastinum (option C). Pneumomediastinum is differentiated from pneumopericardium in that the former shows a superior extension of the air strip beyond the confines of the pericardium.

14-7. **The answer is B.** *(Hurst's The Heart, 14th Edition, Chap. 14)* Dextrocardia with situs solitus represents an anomaly with normal situs but a right-sided heart. Radiographically, normal situs (situs solitus) is a certainty when both the aortic knob and the gastric air bubble are on the left side. Situs solitus also means that both the abdominal viscera and the atria are in the normal positions. Dextrocardia with situs inversus indicates the mirror image of normal (option A). Levocardia with situs inversus is a mirror image of dextrocardia with situs solitus (option C). Levocardia with situs solitus is entirely normal (option D). In Cardiac malpositions with situs ambiguus, the patient's heart can be on either the left or right side, but the site is ambiguous because the aortic arch and the stomach are not on the same side (option E).

14-8. **The answer is E.** *(Hurst's The Heart, 14th Edition, Chap. 14)* Prominence of the pulmonary trunk is a reliable secondary sign of RV enlargement, with the following exceptions: (1) Tetralogy of Fallot with RV hypertrophy but pulmonary trunk hypoplasia (option A); (2) idiopathic dilatation of the pulmonary artery (option B); (3) patent ductus arteriosus with dilated pulmonary trunk but normal RV size (option C); and (4) straight-back syndrome (option D), pectus excavatum, and scoliosis with narrowed AP diameter of the chest. Under the latter conditions, the heart is compressed, displaced, and rotated to the left, giving rise to a falsely enlarged pulmonary artery.

14-9. **The answer is E.** *(Hurst's The Heart, 14th Edition, Chap. 14)* Rib notching provides important clues to the diagnosis of coarctation of the aorta (option A).[7,8] Notching of the ribs has many origins (option B). Basically, any of the three major intercostal structures can enlarge, compress, and erode the lower borders of the ribs, producing areas of notching. They are intercostal arteries, veins, and nerves. Coarctation of the aorta represents the most common cause of rib notching as a result of dynamic dilatation and tortuosity of the arteries. SVC syndrome can produce a similar radiographic appearance (option C), albeit through long-standing venous dilation. Neurofibromatosis also can produce rib notching through the compressive effect of numerous intercostal neurofibromas (option D).

14-10. **The answer is E.** *(Hurst's The Heart, 14th Edition, Chap. 14)* Cardiac fluoroscopy has been largely displaced by other imaging techniques (option A), particularly two-dimensional echocardiography, MRI, and CT, and its use is limited to the cardiac catheterization laboratory, where it can assess the function of radiodense and echodense prosthetic valves (option B) and can guide the positioning of pacemakers or ICDs (option C). With the emergence of transcatheter aortic valve replacement therapy, cardiac fluoroscopy has experienced a resurgence at some centers, where it is commonly used to guide the positioning of the prosthesis (option D).

References

1. Milne ENC, Pistolesi M. *Reading the Chest Radiograph: A Physiologic Approach.* St. Louis, MO: Mosby; 1993:164-241, 343-369.
2. Koza Y. Mitral annular calcification and cardiovascular diseases: does correlation imply causation? *Angiology.* 2016;67(6):505-506.
3. Chen JT. *Essentials of Cardiac Imaging.* Philadelphia, PA: Lippincott-Raven Press; 1997.
4. Chen JT. The plain radiograph in the diagnosis of cardiovascular disease. *Radiolog Clin North Am.* 1983;4:609-621.
5. Applegate KE, Goske MJ, Pierce G, Murphy D. Situs revisited: imaging of the heterotaxy syndrome 1. *Radiographics.* 1999;19:837-852.
6. Margolis JR, et al. The diagnostic and prognostic significance of coronary artery calcification. A report of 800 cases. *Radiology.* 1980;137:609-616.
7. Juhl JH, Grummy AB. *Essentials of Radiologic Imaging.* Philadelphia, PA: Lippincott-Raven Press; 1993:1065-1138.
8. Figley MM. Accessory roentgen signs of coarctation of the aorta. *Radiology.* 1954;62:671-687.

CHAPTER 15

Echocardiography

Jonathan Afilalo

QUESTIONS

DIRECTIONS: Choose the one best response to each question.

15-1. High-quality echocardiographic images require optimal resolution, that is, the ability to distinguish two individual objects separated in space. Which of the following will *not* yield high-resolution images?

A. Short wavelengths
B. High-frequency signal
C. Low-frequency signal
D. Small beam width
E. All of the above

15-2. There has been a great deal of interest in using mitral inflow velocity patterns to evaluate left ventricular diastolic properties. Which of the following variables is *not* capable of influencing transmitral filling velocities?

A. Age
B. Heart rate
C. Respiration
D. Position of the Doppler sample volume
E. None the above

15-3. A 55-year-old woman with no prior cardiac history was admitted to the emergency department complaining of a 6-month history of dyspnea. On physical examination, she had jugular venous distension, distended abdomen secondary to hepatomegaly and tense ascites, severe bilateral lower limbs pitting edema, and an S3 gallop. After an initial management she was referred to the cardiologist, who performed an echocardiography, and some of the images are illustrated in Figure 15-1. Based on the echo's findings, which of the following is the most likely diagnosis?

A. Constrictive pericarditis
B. Amyloid-induced cardiomyopathy
C. Hypereosinophilic cardiomyopathy
D. Endomyocardial fibrosis
E. Idiopathic restrictive cardiomyopathy

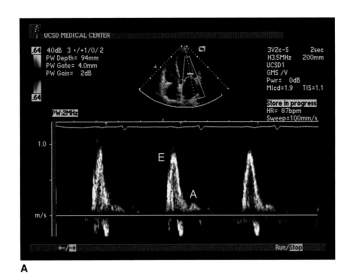

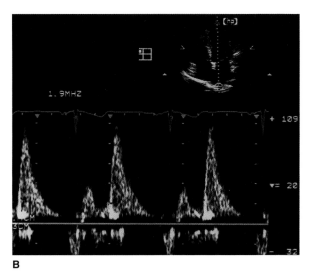

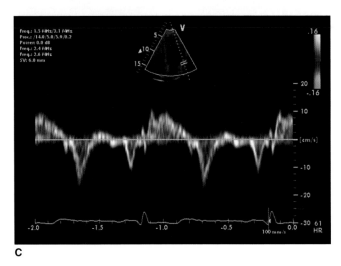

FIGURE 15-1 (A) Pulsed-wave Doppler (PWD) tracing. (B) PWD recording of pulmonary venous flow. The S wave is small, whereas the D wave is prominent. (C) Tissue Doppler recording of lateral mitral annular motion (apical transducer position). Peak early diastolic annular velocity is 17 cm/s.

15-4. A 54-year-old woman with no prior cardiac history was admitted to the emergency department complaining of a 2-week history of progressive chest discomfort and dyspnea. On physical examination, she had a 3/6 holosystolic murmur radiating to the axilla. The initial blood tests, ECG, and chest radiography were all unremarkable. A transthoracic echo showed mitral valve prolapse with a flail posterior leaflet. Transesophageal echo was performed, and some of the images are illustrated in Figure 15-2. Measurements derived from the size of the turbulent jet recorded by color Doppler are often used in clinical practice to assess the severity of mitral regurgitation. Which of the following technical factors *cannot* influence jet size?

A. Instrument gain
B. Angle of incidence of the interrogating beam
C. Frequency and pulse repetition rate of the transducer
D. The temporal sampling rate
E. None of the above

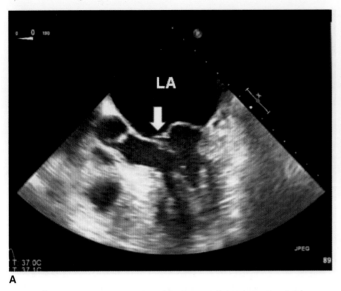

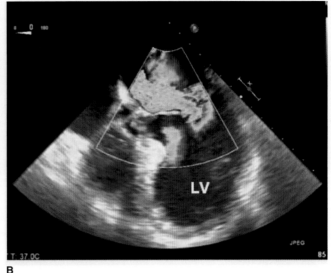

A

B

FIGURE 15-2 Transesophageal echocardiography image (five-chamber view) demonstrating a flail posterior leaflet of the mitral valve (arrow), and the corresponding color Doppler showing severe mitral regurgitation into the left atrium (LA). LV, left ventricle.

15-5. An 11-year-old woman was referred to the cardiology clinic for further evaluation of a diastolic murmur. Her past medical history was significant for a surgically closed patent ductus arteriosus at the age of 7 and recurrent chest infections since she was one year old. On general inspection, she appeared thin and slender, and she had an anterior chest deformity as well as a disproportionately long arm span compared to her height. An echo was performed, and a parasternal long-axis view is illustrated in Figure 15-3. Which of the following conditions is the most likely underlying cause associated with this patient's aortic regurgitation (AR) murmur?

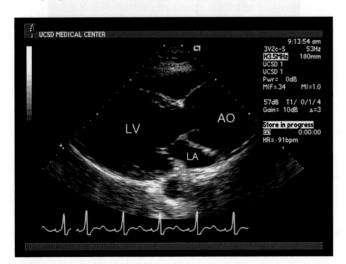

FIGURE 15-3 Parasternal long-axis view. AO, Aorta; LA, left atrium; LV, left ventricle.

A. Marfan syndrome
B. Sinus of Valsalva aneurysm
C. Supravalvular aortic stenosis
D. Coarctation of the aorta
E. None of the above

15-6. A 92-year-old man with a prior history of dyslipidemia, type 2 diabetes, and hypertension was admitted to the emergency department complaining of dyspnea and chest pain. On physical examination, he had a grade 1/6 systolic murmur. An echo was performed, and a continuous-wave Doppler (CW) tracing (from the apical transducer position) through the aortic valve is illustrated in Figure 15-4. Which of the following factors is *not* a potential source of error in the estimation of the transvalvular aortic gradient by CW Doppler recordings?

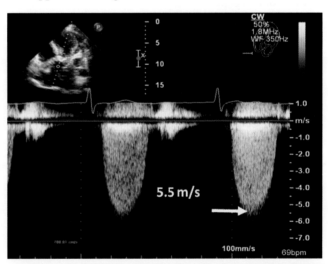

FIGURE 15-4 Continuous-wave Doppler tracing (from the apical transducer position) through the aortic valve in a case of severe aortic stenosis. The peak systolic velocity is 5.5 m/s, corresponding to a maximal instantaneous gradient of 121 mm Hg; the mean gradient is 80 mm Hg.

A. Angle of incidence of the interrogating beam greater than 20 degrees
B. Narrow ascending aorta
C. Concomitant dynamic LV outflow obstruction
D. None of the above
E. All of the above

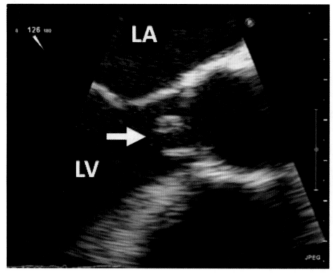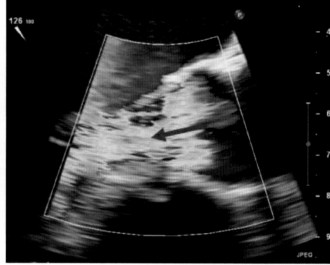

FIGURE 15-5 Transesophageal view depicting the anomaly (white arrow). Color Doppler shows severe aortic regurgitation, with the color jet occupying all of the left ventricle outflow tract. LA, left atrium; LV, left ventricle.

15-7. A 35-year-old man with no known past medical history was admitted to the emergency department complaining of a 2-day history of acute dyspnea. Upon further questioning, the patient had not been feeling well for the past 2 weeks with fever, malaise, and headaches. On physical examination, he had a diastolic murmur, best heard at the left sternal border, which was confirmed to be AR on transthoracic echo. The patient subsequently underwent a transesophageal echo, and some images are illustrated in Figure 15-5. Which of the following is the most likely cause of this patient's AR?

A. Bicuspid aortic valve
B. Aortic dissection
C. Aortitis secondary to vasculitis
D. Aortitis secondary to syphilis
E. Infectious endocarditis

15-8. A 19-year-old man with no personal or family history of sudden cardiac death was admitted to the emergency department following a collapse while playing soccer. On cardiac auscultation, there was a grade 3/6 systolic murmur best heard over the apex. After unremarkable blood tests, ECG, and chest radiography, an echo was performed. An apical four-chamber view is illustrated in Figure 15-6. In which of the following conditions does systolic anterior motion of the mitral valve (SAM) *not* occur?

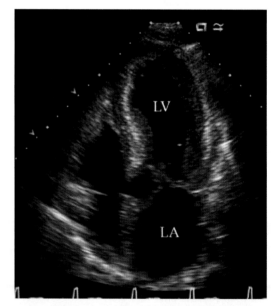

FIGURE 15-6 Apical four-chamber view during systole, demonstrating systolic anterior motion of the mitral valve. LA, left atrium; LV, left ventricle; RA, right atrium.

A. Hypertrophic cardiomyopathy (HCM)
B. Anemia
C. Dehydration
D. Following mitral annuloplasty surgery with a rigid ring
E. None of the above

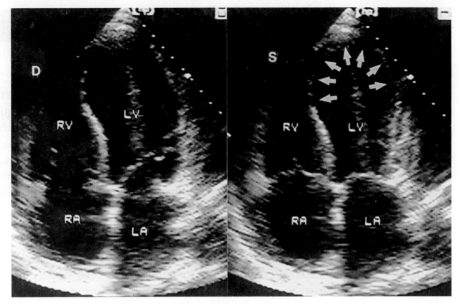

FIGURE 15-7 Apical four-chamber view. Diastole (D) is displayed on the left, systole (S) on the right. During systole, the base of the ventricle contracts, but the apex is dyskinetic (arrows). LA, left atrium; LV, left ventricle; RA, right atrium; RV, right ventricle.

15-9. An asymptomatic 47-year-old man with a recent history of anterior STEMI was referred to the cardiology clinic by his family doctor because of a persistent ST-segment elevation in the anterior leads. An echo was performed, and an apical four-chamber view is illustrated in Figure 15-7. Based on the echo's findings, which of the following is the most likely diagnosis?

A. LV aneurysm
B. LV pseudoaneurysm
C. Apical ballooning syndrome
D. LV noncompaction
E. Dilated cardiomyopathy

15-10. A 55-year-old woman with a prior history of a modified radical mastectomy for a left breast adenocarcinoma was admitted to the emergency department complaining of acute dyspnea. Chest radiography showed cardiomegaly and left pleural effusion. An echo was performed, and the apical four-chamber view is illustrated in Figure 15-8. With regard to cardiac tamponade, which of the following statements is *false*?

A. Right atrium (RA) collapse during atrial systole is the most specific sign of tamponade
B. Diastolic collapse of the right ventricular (RV) free wall is the most sensitive sign of tamponade

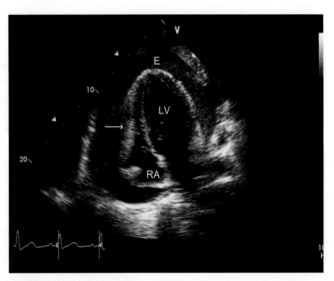

FIGURE 15-8 Right ventricular compression (arrow) in cardiac tamponade (apical four-chamber plane).

C. Left ventricular outflow tract obstruction (LVOT) velocities increase significantly with inspiration
D. Transmitral diastolic gradient during inspiration increases significantly
E. All of the above

15-1. **The answer is C.** *(Hurst's The Heart, 14th Edition, Chap. 15)* Short wavelengths yield excellent resolution in echo imaging (option A) because the shorter the cycle length, the smaller the object that will reflect the signal and be detected by the echo scanner. Because wavelength is inversely related to frequency, transducers that emit a high-frequency signal (≥ 3.5–7.0 MHz) yield high-resolution images (option B). Because ultrasonic beams diverge as they propagate away from the transducer, the width of the beam can become sufficiently great to encompass multiple targets and decrease resolution (option D). The degree of beam divergence is also less with high-frequency sonic energy than with low-frequency signals.

15-2. **The answer is E.** *(Hurst's The Heart, 14th Edition, Chap. 15)* The abnormal mitral inflow patterns are often useful in suggesting the presence and severity of diastolic dysfunction. Several variables other than diastolic function, however, are capable of influencing transmitral filling velocities. Transmitral Doppler filling dynamics are affected by the age of the patient (option A), concomitant mitral regurgitation, high-flow states, changes in heart rate (option B),[1] respiration (option C), and the position of the Doppler sample volume within the mitral valve orifice (option D).[2]

15-3. **The answer is A.** *(Hurst's The Heart, 14th Edition, Chap. 15)* Transmitral flow demonstrates a restrictive pattern, with an abnormally high E/A ratio and a markedly shortened E wave deceleration time (see Figure 15-1*a*). Concomitant pulmonary venous tracings show a very low S velocity and elevated D velocity (S << D) (see Figure 15-1*b*) and a prolonged atrial reversal wave, thus predicting elevated left atrial pressure.[3] In severe LV diastolic dysfunction, tissue Doppler imaging (TDI) of the mitral annulus should show marked blunting of both Em and Am velocities. An exception to this occurs in constrictive pericarditis, where Em is relatively normal at the medial mitral annulus and only mildly reduced at the lateral mitral annulus. Thus when transmitral and pulmonary venous Doppler suggest severe diastolic dysfunction, this TDI pattern suggests constrictive rather than restrictive physiology (amyloid-induced cardiomyopathy [CM], hypereosinophilic CM, endomyocardial fibrosis, and idiopathic restrictive CM).

15-4. **The answer is E.** *(Hurst's The Heart, 14th Edition, Chap. 15)* A number of technical factors can influence jet size, including instrument gain, the angle of incidence of the interrogating beam, the frequency and pulse repetition rate of the transducer, and the temporal sampling rate.[4] Therefore, measurements derived from the size of the turbulent jet recorded by color Doppler are at best semiquantitative and should not be expected to correlate with the volume of blood contained in the flow disturbance.

15-5. **The answer is A.** *(Hurst's The Heart, 14th Edition, Chap. 15)* Echocardiography is routinely used to assess aortic pathology in patients with Marfan syndrome. The aortic pathology is characterized by symmetrical dilatation of the annulus, sinuses of Valsalva, and aorta (Figure 15-3). Aortic leaflet coaptation may be compromised, leading to AR. In sinus of Valsalva aneurysm, the lesion causes asymmetric dilatation of the aorta. Supravalvular aortic stenosis is recognized as an hourglass narrowing or a discrete fibrous ridge just superior to the aortic valve leaflets, whereas coarctation of the aorta presents a more localized, abrupt luminal reduction in the descending aorta or distal portion of the aortic arch; both of these conditions tend to cause more of a systolic than a diastolic murmur.

15-6. **The answer is D.** *(Hurst's The Heart, 14th Edition, Chap. 15)* Several potential sources of error exist in the estimation of the transvalvular aortic gradient by CW Doppler recordings. It is imperative that Doppler signals from the stenotic jet be obtained with an angle of incidence of less than 20 degrees so as not to underestimate the velocity or gradient. For this purpose, and because two-dimensional techniques rarely reveal the precise direction of the jet, each Doppler examination must use all possible windows and angulations, and the window that provides the highest velocity is chosen. Also, one must be careful to account for the proximal flow velocity in the Bernoulli equation if it is 1.5 m/s or greater. In the adult, CW Doppler can occasionally overestimate peak systolic pressure gradients, especially in patients with narrow ascending aortas (due to pressure recovery). Lastly, in patients with concomitant dynamic LV outflow obstruction, it is usually difficult to separate the increased velocity caused by each of these conditions.

15-7. **The answer is E.** *(Hurst's The Heart, 14th Edition, Chap. 15)* Perhaps the most important contribution of echocardiographic imaging to the assessment of AR is in identifying its etiology and adaptation of the LV to the volume overload. Aggressive vegetations can cause perforation or distortion of the affected leaflet, leading to varying degrees of valvular regurgitation. AR caused by infectious endocarditis can be identified by the presence of valvular vegetations (Figure 15-5), whereas functional AR caused by diseases of the aorta can be identified by anatomic changes of the aortic root or dissection.

15-8. **The answer is E.** *(Hurst's The Heart, 14th Edition, Chap. 15)* SAM is not pathognomonic for HCM, and it can occur in other conditions involving hyperdynamic LV function (eg, hypovolemia/dehydration, anemia) or anterior displacement of the annulus (eg, use of a rigid mitral ring in mitral valve repair).

15-9. **The answer is A.** *(Hurst's The Heart, 14th Edition, Chap. 15)* Echocardiography is of great value in assessing complications associated with acute myocardial infarction (AMI).[5] Postinfarction LV aneurysms are recognized as wide-mouthed, thin-walled myocardial segments that display dyskinetic expansion during systole (option A). Pseudoaneurysms (most often secondary to a free wall rupture, which is subsequently sealed off by clot and pericardial inflammation) is distinguished from a true aneurysm by the presence of a narrow neck, multilayered thrombi, and characteristic Doppler flow signals at the junction with the ventricle.[6] Because the risk of rupture is high, accurate diagnosis and prompt surgical repair of pseudoaneurysms is important (option B). Takotsubo cardiomyopathy (also called stress cardiomyopathy or apical ballooning syndrome) is a syndrome of sudden-onset chest pain associated with significant LV dysfunction but no occlusive coronary disease and only minor troponin elevations.[7] Echocardiography is well suited for evaluation in this setting and often shows dramatic apical ballooning with preservation (or hyperkinesis) of the LV basal segments (option C). LV noncompaction is a form of cardiomyopathy that is characterized by a prominent noncompacted layer of myocardium lining the cavity of the left ventricle.[8] A ratio of > 2.0 between the systolic thicknesses of the noncompacted and compacted myocardial layers is suggestive of noncompaction (option D).[9] The echocardiographic findings in dilated cardiomyopathy include an increased LV end-diastolic diameter and decreased ejection fraction, in the absence of other features specifically associated with other etiologies (option E).

15-10. **The answer is E.** *(Hurst's The Heart, 14th Edition, Chap. 15)* Because diastolic pressures are slightly lower in the right heart than in the left, the RA and RV are usually the first chambers to exhibit evidence of increased intrapericardial pressure. High intrapericardial pressure can cause compression or collapse of right heart chambers. Invagination of the RA wall during atrial systole is a sensitive (but not specific) sign of tamponade. Diastolic collapse or buckling of the RV free wall is a more specific sign of tamponade. Doppler echocardiographic recordings in patients with tamponade demonstrate an exaggeration of the normal respiratory variation in ventricular inflow and outflow. Thus transmitral and LVOT velocities decrease significantly with inspiration, most likely because of enhanced ventricular interdependence and a marked decrease in the transmitral diastolic gradient during inspiration. The latter is caused both by high intrapericardial pressure and by leftward motion of the interventricular septum from increased RV filling.

References

1. Harrison MR, Clifton GD, Pennell AT, DeMaria AN. Effect of heart rate on left ventricular diastolic trans-mitral flow velocity patterns assessed by Doppler echocardiography in normal subjects. *Am J Cardiol.* 1991;67:622-627.

2. Dittrich HC, Blanchard DG, Wheeler KA, McCann HA, Donaghey LB. Influence of Doppler sample volume location on the assessment of changes in mitral inflow velocity profiles. *J Am Soc Echocardiogr.* 1990;3:303-309.

3. Nishimura RA, Housmans PR, Hatle LK, Tajik AJ. Assessment of diastolic function of the heart: background and current applications of Doppler echocardiography. Part I. Physiologic and pathophysiologic features. *Mayo Clin Proc.* 1989;64:71-81.

4. Matsumura M, Wong M, Omoto R. Assessment of Doppler color flow mapping in quantification of aortic regurgitation—correlations and influencing factors. *Jap Circulation J (English E).* 1989;53:735-746.

5. Flachskampf FA, Schmid M, Rost C, Achenbach S, DeMaria AN, Daniel WG. Cardiac imaging after myocardial infarction. *Eur Heart J.* 2011;32:272-283.

6. Lindner JR, Case RA, Dent JM, Abbott RD, Scheld WM, Kaul S. Diagnostic value of echocardiography in suspected endocarditis. An evaluation based on the pretest probability of disease. *Circulation.* 1996;93:730-736.

7. Hurst RT, Prasad A, Askew JW III, Sengupta PP, Tajik AJ. Takotsubo cardiomyopathy: a unique cardiomyopathy with variable ventricular morphology. *JACC Cardiovasc Imaging.* 2010;3:641-649.

8. Petersen SE, Selvanayagam JB, Wiesmann F, et al: Left ventricular non-compaction: insights from cardiovascular magnetic resonance imaging. *J Am Coll Cardiol.* 2005;46:101-105.

9. Jenni R, Oechslin E, Schneider J, Attenhofer JC, Kaufmann PA. Echocardiographic and pathoanatomical characteristics of pathological non-compaction, as a distinct cardiomyopathy. *Heart (British Cardiac Society).* 2001;86:666-671.

CHAPTER 16

Magnetic Resonance Imaging of the Heart

Jonathan Afilalo

QUESTIONS

DIRECTIONS: Choose the one best response to each question.

16-1. Tissue characterization with mapping or weighted imaging using assessments of T1, T2, or T2* relaxation is increasingly used in cardiovascular magnetic resonance (CMR).[1,2] Which of the following conditions *cannot* be identified by T2 or T2*-weighted imaging?

A. Myocardial edema in the setting of acute myocardial infarction (MI)
B. Myocardial edema in the setting of myocarditis
C. Myocardial hemorrhage
D. Iron-overload cardiomyopathy
E. None of the above

16-2. Although a relatively safe imaging modality, CMR does have the potential for serious and even lethal events. Which of the following statements regarding the safety of common metallic implants and electronic devices commonly found in cardiac patients is *false*?

A. Current coronary stents are safe and can be imaged immediately after implantation
B. Current prosthetic valves are safe and can be imaged immediately after implantation
C. Weakly ferromagnetic implants are safe and can be imaged immediately after implantation
D. Swan-Ganz catheters contain metal and are considered unsafe
E. Transdermal patches may need to be removed before the procedure

16-3. CMR is unique in that, with a single imaging modality, one can identify abnormalities of myocardial perfusion or wall motion with a relatively high spatial resolution and without ionizing radiation. Based on multimodality appropriate use criteria, in which of the following patients is stress CMR considered appropriate?

A. Patients presenting with chest pain at a high pretest probability of coronary artery disease (CAD)
B. Patients at an intermediate pretest probability of CAD with an uninterpretable ECG
C. Patients with an abnormal or uncertain exercise ECG
D. Patients with obstructive CAD of uncertain significance
E. All of the above

16-4. A 54-year-old obese woman was admitted to the emergency department complaining of worsening chest discomfort. After being diagnosed with an acute myocardial infarction, she underwent successful stenting of the left anterior descending artery. An echocardiogram was ordered to assess left ventricular function, but the image quality was suboptimal due to poor acoustic windows. A cardiac magnetic resonance exam was then ordered to provide an assessment of:

A. Myocardial salvage
B. Microvascular obstruction
C. The extent of late gadolinium enhancement (LGE) as a predictor of survival and adverse cardiac events
D. The presence of T2 hyperintensity in the affected territory as an indicator of infarct acuity
E. All of the above

16-5. A 65-year-old man with a 20-year history of poorly controlled diabetes presented to the emergency department complaining of acute dyspnea. After the initial tests, the diagnosis of acute decompensated heart failure (HF) was confirmed. In order to establish the underlying etiology and, importantly, to exclude chronic ischemic heart disease as a potentially reversible cause, a CMR was performed. An LGE image in a two-chamber long-axis orientation is illustrated in Figure 16-1. Which of the following statements regarding LGE is *false*?

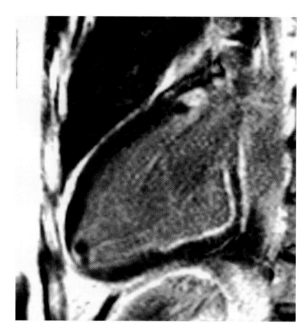

FIGURE 16-1 Late gadolinium-enhanced inversion recovery gradient echo image in a two-chamber long-axis orientation in a patient with systolic heart failure. Two areas of prior myocardial infarction are seen: a subendocardial infarct in the basal to midinferior wall and a small apical infarct with an associated apical thrombus.

A. The absence of LGE rules out the diagnosis of underlying CAD
B. Patients without obstructive CAD may have evidence of LGE
C. The presence and amount of LGE is prognostically important in the setting of CAD
D. CMR is considered an appropriate technique for the evaluation of patients with new-onset HF
E. Patients with nonischemic causes of HF may or may not have evidence of LGE

16-6. A 35-year-old man with no prior cardiac history was admitted to the emergency department with chest pain, troponin elevation, and no evidence of angiographically detectable stenoses within the epicardial coronary arteries. The patient underwent CMR, and an LGE image in a basal

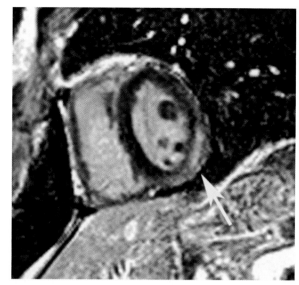

FIGURE 16-2 Late gadolinium-enhanced (LGE) inversion recovery gradient echo image in a basal short-axis orientation. LGE is noted in the midwall and subepicardium in the inferolateral wall (arrow).

short-axis orientation is shown in Figure 16-2. Which of the following is the most likely diagnosis?

A. Noncardiac chest pain
B. Hypertrophic cardiomyopathy (HCM)
C. Acute myocardial infarction
D. Viral myocarditis
E. Takotsubo or stress cardiomyopathy

16-7. A 57-year-old woman with no prior cardiac history was admitted to the emergency department complaining of a 6-month history of dyspnea. On physical examination, she had jugular venous distension, hepatomegaly, tense ascites, severe bilateral lower limb edema, and an S3 gallop. After an initial management she underwent CMR, and a four-chamber T1-weighted image as well as diastolic short-axis images from a real-time cine acquisition during free breathing are illustrated in Figure 16-3. Which of the following statements regarding the diagnosis is *false*?

A. Pericardial thickness of 4 mm or more is considered abnormal
B. Pericardial thickness may not be accurately quantified in the presence of an effusion
C. This disease can occur with normal pericardial thickness
D. The presence of extensive pericardial LGE may identify a subgroup of patients in whom the disease can revert with anti-inflammatory therapy
E. Pericardial LGE is synonymous with pericardial fibrosis

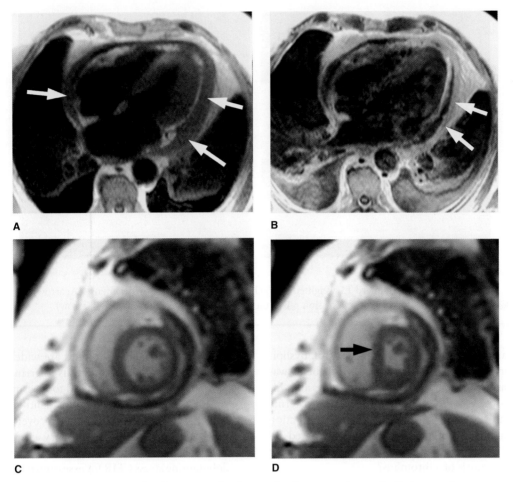

FIGURE 16-3 (A) Four-chamber T1-weighted spin echo demonstrating markedly increased pericardium (dark band, arrows). (B) Same image acquired after contrast showing pericardial enhancement (arrows). (C) and (D) Expiratory and inspiratory, respectively—diastolic short-axis frames from a real-time cine acquisition during free breathing. Note the marked septal flattening during inspiration (arrow) consistent with increased ventricular interdependence.

16-8. An 85-year-old woman with no prior cardiac history presented to the emergency department complaining of dizziness. The patient denied any other associated symptoms, and initial test results were within normal range. As part of the dizziness workup, a transthoracic echocardiogram was performed, which showed a large interatrial mass. For further characterization of the mass, the patient underwent CMR, and a T1-weighted image before and after the application of a fat suppression pulse is illustrated in Figure 16-4. Which of the following conditions is the most likely diagnosis?

A. Lymphoma
B. Rhabdomyosarcoma
C. Angiosarcoma
D. Lipoma
E. Myxosarcoma

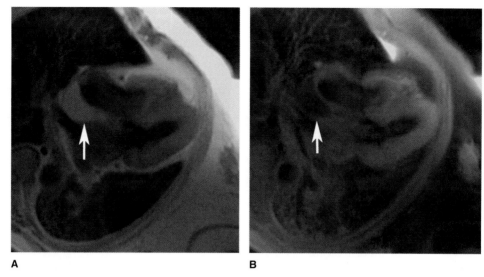

FIGURE 16-4 On standard T1-weighted spin echo images, the lesion is hyperintense (A; arrow). After the application of a fat suppression pulse, the signal from the lesion is nulled (B; arrow).

16-9. A 75-year-old man with a prior history of dyslipidemia, hypertension, and poorly controlled diabetes was referred to cardiology for a CMR exam, three days after his admission to the emergency department for retrosternal chest discomfort. A four-chamber long-axis orientation with different inversion times (TI) is illustrated in Figure 16-5. Which of the following feature does *not* support the diagnosis of a thrombus?

A. Homogenous appearance
B. Lack of mobility
C. Hyper- or iso-intense with short inversion time (TI) and hypointense with long TI
D. Location in the LV adjacent to areas of scar
E. None of the above

16-10. Although LGE techniques are widely used for identifying myocardial scar and thus inferring viability, dobutamine stress CMR is also used to measure LV myocardial contractile reserve and thus to identify myocardial segments that have the potential to recover systolic function after successful epicardial coronary arterial revascularization. Which of the following is *not* an advantage of using dobutamine stress CMR for assessing myocardial viability?

A. It can be administered to patients with reactive airways disease
B. It can be administered to patients with severe renal dysfunction
C. The prediction of improvements in regional wall motion or radial thickening is incremental above and beyond LGE
D. None of the above
E. All of the above

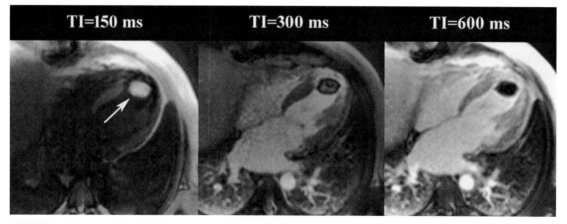

FIGURE 16-5 Four-chamber long-axis orientation with different inversion times (TI).

16-1. The answer is E. *(Hurst's The Heart, 14th Edition, Chap. 16)* High signal on T2-weighted imaging can demonstrate myocardial edema, such as in the setting of acute MI or myocarditis. T2*-weighted imaging is sensitive to iron in the heart and can identify iron overload cardiomyopathy and myocardial hemorrhage in the setting of acute MI.

16-2. The answer is C. *(Hurst's The Heart, 14th Edition, Chap. 16)* All current coronary stents and prosthetic valves are safe and can be imaged immediately after implantation. Many other cardiac or vascular implants are nonferromagnetic and can also be scanned at any time, or they are weakly ferromagnetic and a delay of 6 weeks before MRI is recommended to allow for endothelialization. Swan-Ganz catheters contain metal and are considered unsafe. Similarly, some medication patches (including transdermal patches) contain metallic foil and may need to be removed before the procedure.

16-3. The answer is E. *(Hurst's The Heart, 14th Edition, Chap. 16)* Based on multimodality appropriate use criteria, stress CMR is considered appropriate for patients at a high pretest probability of CAD or an intermediate pretest probability of CAD with an uninterpretable ECG or inability to exercise.[3] It is also appropriate for patients with an abnormal ECG who are intermediate to high risk as well as those with an abnormal or uncertain exercise ECG or those with obstructive CAD of uncertain significance noted on computed tomography (CT) or invasive coronary angiography.

16-4. The answer is E. *(Hurst's The Heart, 14th Edition, Chap. 16)* Today, perhaps the most widely used imaging method for identifying myocardial injury and fibrosis associated with myocardial infarction is through CMR-based assessments of LGE.[4] LGE has several important uses in the setting of patients with suspected CAD. These include identification of the extent of acute and remote MI, the prediction of recovery of myocardial contractility after successful coronary artery revascularization, characterization of prognosis, visualization of cardiac thrombus or microvascular obstruction and, when combined with T2 imaging methods, localization of the area of myocardial salvage and infarct acuity.

16-5. The answer is A. *(Hurst's The Heart, 14th Edition, Chap. 16)* The first step in the evaluation of the patient with new-onset HF is to establish the underlying etiology and, importantly, to exclude ischemic heart disease as a potentially reversible cause. CMR is considered an appropriate technique for the evaluation of patients with new-onset HF.[5] The presence of LGE in a coronary distribution can support the diagnosis of underlying CAD, but its absence does not rule it out because patients with extensive hibernating myocardium may not have LGE.[6] Patients with HF without obstructive CAD may not have evidence of LGE,[7] or they may have evidence of LGE, usually in a noninfarct pattern, but occasionally in an infarct pattern because of transient thrombotic occlusion of a nonobstructive artery, embolization, or spontaneous coronary dissection. The presence and amount of LGE are prognostically important.

16-6. The answer is D. *(Hurst's The Heart, 14th Edition, Chap. 16)* The pattern of LGE can be quite useful in differentiating causes of cardiomyopathies.[8] The finding of LGE in the midwall and subepicardium of the LV is seen in viral myocarditis and has been validated against histopathology.[8] The finding of "patchy" LGE in myocardial segments with marked hypertrophy, or in the septal insertion points, is suggestive of HCM. The finding of LGE in the subendocardium of the LV following a distinct coronary territory is characteristic of myocardial infarction. Takotsubo or stress cardiomyopathy is a clinical syndrome characterized by chest pain and ECG changes that mimic an acute myocardial infarction, in which there is generally no LGE.

16-7. The answer is E. *(Hurst's The Heart, 14th Edition, Chap. 16)* The hallmarks of constrictive pericarditis are increased pericardial thickness, pericardial inflammation, and ventricular interdependence. The pericardium can be visualized and measured in a number of sequences, although T1-weighted black-blood imaging is usually the standard,[9] where the pericardium appears as a hypointense linear structure surrounded by hyperintense fat layers (Figure 16-3A). Although normal pericardial thickness is less than 1 mm, on CMR, 1 to 3 mm is considered normal because of limitations in spatial resolution,[9] and a thickness of 4 mm or more is considered abnormal. Pericardial thickening may be focal or diffuse. It is important to realize that pericardial thickness may not be accurately quantified in the presence of an effusion (both are hypointense on black-blood imaging), that constriction can occur with normal pericardial thickness, and that increased thickness is not synonymous with constriction. The presence of extensive LGE, which may represent dense inflammation, identifies a subgroup of patients in whom constrictive pericarditis can revert with anti-inflammatory therapy.[10,11]

16-8. The answer is D. *(Hurst's The Heart, 14th Edition, Chap. 16)* High signal intensity on T1-weighted images, besides the presence of recent hemorrhage, can also be caused by fat. Together with signal reduction with fat suppression techniques, hyperintensity on T2-weighted imaging, a lack of first-pass perfusion, and an absence of LGE, CMR allows for the straightforward diagnosis of lipoma. Although less accurate, CMR can also help differentiate benign from malignant neoplasms (lymphoma, rhabdomyosarcomas, angiosarcomas, and myxosarcomas). Larger sizes, invasion of adjacent structure(s), the presence of pleural or pericardial effusions, prominent first-pass perfusion, or positive LGE are all features seen more commonly in malignancy.[12,13]

16-9. The answer is E. *(Hurst's The Heart, 14th Edition, Chap. 16)* The main strength of CMR in the evaluation of cardiac masses is probably the ability to differentiate between cardiac thrombi from tumors. Features supporting the diagnosis of thrombus include location in the LV adjacent to areas of scar or the left atrial appendage, homogenous appearance, lack of mobility, isointensity or hypointensity on T2-weighted imaging, and absence of perfusion or LGE. A thrombus is hyper- or iso-intense with short TI and hypointense with long TI.

16-10. The answer is D. *(Hurst's The Heart, 14th Edition, Chap. 16)* A particular advantage of low-dose dobutamine infusions for assessing myocardial viability is that they can be administered to patients with reactive airways disease as well as to those with renal dysfunction in whom the use of gadolinium may be contraindicated. In addition, there is some evidence that low-dose dobutamine stress CMR assessments of improvements in regional wall motion or radial thickening are complementary and may even be superior to the assessments of LGE, particularly in those individuals who have an intermediate nontransmural extent of LGE.[14]

References

1. Ferreira VM, Piechnik SK, Robson MD, Neubauer S, Karamitsos TD. Myocardial tissue characterization by magnetic resonance imaging: novel applications of T1 and T2 mapping. *J Thorac Imaging.* 2014;29(3).
2. Salerno M, Kramer CM. Advances in parametric mapping with CMR imaging. *JACC Cardiovasc Imaging.* 2013;6(7):806-822.
3. Wolk MJ, Bailey SR, Doherty JU, et al. ACCF/AHA/ASE/ASNC/HFSA/HRS/SCAI/SCCT/SCMR/STS 2013 multimodality appropriate use criteria for the detection and risk assessment of stable ischemic heart disease: a report of the American College of Cardiology Foundation Appropriate Use Criteria Task Force, American Heart Association, American Society of Echocardiography, American Society of Nuclear Cardiology, Heart Failure Society of America, Heart Rhythm Society, Society for Cardiovascular Angiography and Interventions, Society of Cardiovascular Computed Tomography, Society for Cardiovascular Magnetic Resonance, and Society of Thoracic Surgeons. *J Am Coll Cardiol.* 2014;63(4):380-406.
4. Rehwald WG. Myocardial magnetic resonance imaging contrast agent concentrations after reversible and irreversible ischemic injury. *Circulation.* 2002;105(2):224-229.

5. Patel MR, White RD, Abbara S, et al. 2013 ACCF/ACR/ASE/ASNC/SCCT/SCMR appropriate utilization of cardiovascular imaging in heart failure: A joint report of the American College of Radiology Appropriateness Criteria Committee and the American College of Cardiology Foundation Appropriate Use Criteria Task Force. *J Am Coll Cardiol.* 2013;61(21):2207-2231.

6. Soriano CJ, Ridocci F, Estornell J, Jimenez J, Martinez V, De Velasco JA. Noninvasive diagnosis of coronary artery disease in patients with heart failure and systolic dysfunction of uncertain etiology, using late gadolinium-enhanced cardiovascular magnetic resonance. *J Am Coll Cardiol.* 2005;45(5):743-748.

7. McCrohon JA, Moon JC, Prasad SK, et al. Differentiation of heart failure related to dilated cardiomyopathy and coronary artery disease using gadolinium-enhanced cardiovascular magnetic resonance. *Circulation.* 2003;108(1):54-59.

8. Mahrholdt H, Goedecke C, Wagner A, et al. Cardiovascular magnetic resonance assessment of human myocarditis: a comparison to histology and molecular pathology. *Circulation.* 2004;109(10):1250-1258.

9. Bogaert J, Francone M. Pericardial disease: value of CT and MR imaging. *Radiology.* 2013;267(2):340-356.

10. Feng D, Glockner J, Kim K, et al. Cardiac magnetic resonance imaging pericardial late gadolinium enhancement and elevated inflammatory markers can predict the reversibility of constrictive pericarditis after antiinflammatory medical therapy: a pilot study. *Circulation.* 2011;124(17):1830-1837.

11. Cremer PC, Tariq MU, Karwa A, et al. Quantitative assessment of pericardial delayed hyperenhancement predicts clinical improvement in patients with constrictive pericarditis treated with anti-inflammatory therapy. *Circ Cardiovasc Imaging.* 2015;8(5).

12. Patel R, Lim RP, Saric M, et al. Diagnostic performance of cardiac magnetic resonance imaging and echocardiography in evaluation of cardiac and paracardiac masses. *Am J Cardiol.* 2016;117(1):135-140.

13. Pazos-Lopez P, Pozo E, Siqueira ME, et al. Value of CMR for the differential diagnosis of cardiac masses. *JACC Cardiovasc Imaging.* 2014;7(9):896-905.

14. Wellnhofer E. Magnetic resonance low-dose dobutamine test is superior to scar quantification for the prediction of functional recovery. *Circulation.* 2004;109(18): 2172-2174.

CHAPTER 17
Computed Tomography of the Heart
Jonathan Afilalo

QUESTIONS

DIRECTIONS: Choose the one best response to each question.

17-1. Advancements in CT technology have made it possible to noninvasively image the beating heart. Which of the following statements regarding cardiac CT is *false*?

A. Cardiac CT can assess left and right ventricular remodeling
B. Cardiac CT can assess regional myocardial wall motion and thickening
C. Cardiac CT is comparable to first-pass radionuclide angiography for the calculation of post-MI LVEF
D. Cardiac CT can detect myocardial iron overload
E. Cardiac CT can detect intracardiac thrombus

17-2. A 35-year-old obese woman with a significant family history of premature coronary heart disease presented to the emergency department complaining of a 2-week history of intermittent chest pain. Initial ECG and biomarkers were within normal limits. After an equivocal stress test, she underwent cardiac CT. Which of the following statements about cardiac CT and coronary artery calcification (CAC) is *false*?

A. The severity of angiographic coronary artery stenosis is directly related to the total CAC
B. Cardiac CT can detect coronary atherosclerosis at its earliest stages
C. CAC is caused by atherosclerosis in the coronary arteries
D. CAC is not found in normal coronary arteries
E. There is a strong linear correlation between total coronary artery plaque area and the extent of CAC

17-3. A 55-year-old woman with a prior history of poorly controlled diabetes, hypertension, and dyslipidemia presented to the emergency department complaining of a retrosternal chest pain radiating to her left arm. In the absence of new ECG changes or cardiac biomarker elevation, she underwent cardiac CT. This patient was scanned with a dual-source CT, and the heart rate during the time of the scan was 105 beats/min. The rendered three-dimensional (3D) image of the heart as well as the maximum-intensity projection (MIP) image of the same patient are illustrated in Figure 17-1. Which of the following would *not* be useful for decreasing motion-related artifacts?

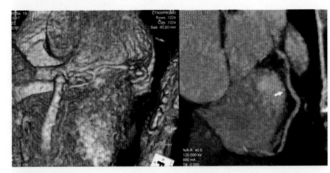

FIGURE 17-1 Left panel: Three-dimensional (3D) rendering image of a heart with significant motion artifact affecting the interpretation of the distal right coronary artery (RCA). Right panel: Maximum-intensity projection (MIP) image of the same patient showing significant transitional motion artifact in the proximal and mid RCA.

A. Image acquisition of less than 50 milliseconds
B. Use of oral and/or intravenous β-blockers prior to scanning
C. Use of sublingual tablets or spray of nitroglycerin
D. Breath-hold strategy during scanning
E. None of the above

17-4. A 64-year-old man with suspected acute coronary syndrome (ACS) was referred to cardiology for coronary CT angiography (CCTA). Which of the following statements about the diagnostic performance of the CCTA is *false*?

A. The diagnostic accuracy for ACS with CCTA is lower than stress echocardiography.

B. The diagnostic accuracy for ACS with CCTA is higher than stress nuclear imaging.

C. The high negative predictive value of CCTA is a valuable tool in the exclusion of obstructive CAD

D. CCTA is useful in the risk stratification of symptomatic CAD

E. CCTA is an accurate tool in the assessment of chest pain in patients with intermediate risk of CAD

17-5. A 78-year-old woman with multivessel coronary artery disease and prior PCI to the left anterior descending coronary artery (LAD) was referred to cardiology for coronary stent evaluation following an episode of severe central chest pain. A CCTA was performed, and it is shown in Figure 17-2. Which of the following factors can potentially *reduce* the diagnostic accuracy of CCTA for the noninvasive evaluation of in-stent restenosis?

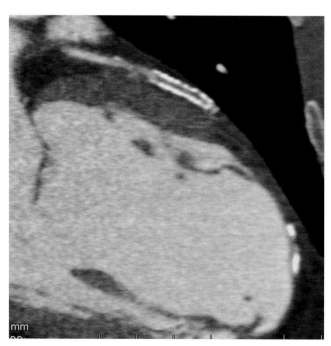

FIGURE 17-2 Evaluation of coronary stents. Occluded stent in the proximal left anterior descending (coronary artery).

A. Imaging artifacts
B. Stent location
C. Heart rate
D. Stent diameter
E. All of the above

17-6. A 37-year-old woman with no prior cardiac history was admitted to the emergency department complaining of atypical chest pain. After the initial ECG and biomarkers were within normal limits, she underwent coronary computed tomography angiography to exclude coronary artery disease. CCTA is illustrated in Figure 17-3. Which of the following statements about congenital anomalies of the coronary arteries is *false*?

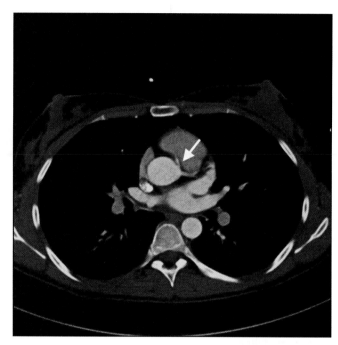

FIGURE 17-3 Anomalous right coronary artery. Note the right coronary artery (arrowhead) arising to the left of midline from the left sinus of Valsalva taking interarterial course.

A. Congenital anomalies of the coronary arteries are reported in 0.3% to 1% of the general population

B. Approximately 20% of coronary anomalies can be hemodynamically significant

C. An interarterial course is the coronary anomaly most commonly associated with sudden cardiac death

D. None of the above

E. All of the above

17-7. An 85-year-old woman with a prior history of poorly controlled type 2 diabetes, hypertension, dyslipidemia, rheumatoid arthritis, and multivessel coronary heart disease was admitted to the emergency department with severe symptomatic aortic stenosis. She underwent a contrast-enhanced CTA in advance of the transcatheter aortic valve replacement (TAVR). The left main coronary artery craniocaudal height is illustrated in Figure 17-4. Which of the following factors is predictive of an increased risk of coronary occlusion during TAVR?

A. Left main height of lesser than 12 mm

B. A shallow of Valsalva mean diameter (cusp to commissures) of < 30 mm

C. A sinus of Valsalva–to–annular ratio of less than 1.25

D. None of the above

E. All of the above

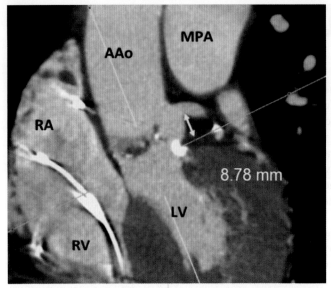

FIGURE 17-4 Left main coronary artery craniocaudal height measured perpendicular to the annular plane. The left main coronary artery height is 8.78 mm. AAo, ascending aorta; LV, left ventricle; MPA, main pulmonary artery; RA; right atrium; RV, right ventricle.

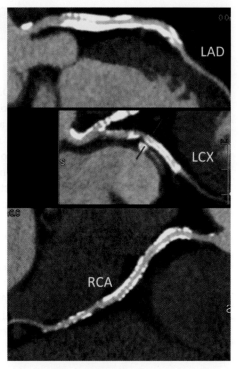

FIGURE 17-5 Conventional cardiac computed tomography angiography (CCTA) for evaluation of all three coronary artery vessels. LAD, left anterior descending (artery); LCX, left circumflex artery; and RCA, right coronary artery.

17-8. The main historical limitation of cardiac CT has been radiation exposure, which was previously reported to be two to four times the radiation dose of diagnostic invasive coronary angiography. Which of the following strategies has been shown to provide the greatest reduction in radiation dose during CCTA?

A. Using prospective ECG-gated or sequential CCTA image acquisition
B. Decreasing the tube voltage in nonobese patients
C. Adopting iterative reconstruction algorithms to allow for significant noise reduction
D. Using scan acquisition modes employing fast helical pitch technique
E. None of the above

17-9. A 75-year-old man with a prior history of dyslipidemia, hypertension, poorly controlled diabetes, multivessel CAD, and multivessel PCI was referred to cardiology for CCTA 3 days after his admission to the emergency department for retrosternal chest discomfort. A CCTA view of the 3 major epicardial vessels is illustrated in Figure 17-5. Which of the following statements regarding the prognostic value of CCTA is *false*?

A. The presence of any stenosis greater than 50% predicts an increased risk of cardiovascular events
B. CCTA is useful for establishing the diagnosis, but not the true extent, of CAD
C. Plaque morphology by CT confers incremental prognostic information beyond that provided by percent stenosis alone
D. CCTA measures of CAD severity and LVEF have independent prognostic value
E. None of the above

17-10. In patients undergoing repeat coronary artery bypass surgery (CABG), CTA scanning has several advantages. Which of the following does *not* support the use of CTA as a primary noninvasive imaging tool for the evaluation of patients prior to CABG?

A. CTA may guide the surgical approach by defining the position of the sternum relative to the underlying right ventricle and internal mammary artery bypass graft
B. CTA can assess the diameter and calcification of the aorta
C. CTA can assess the presence of coronary stenoses within the bypass graft
D. CTA can assess the presence of coronary stenoses within the native coronary arteries and anastomotic sites
E. None of the above

17-1. The answer is D. *(Hurst's The Heart, 14th Edition, Chap. 17)* While cardiac CT can provide some information about tissue characterization, it cannot reliably detect iron overload, and this is typically assessed by cardiac MR. Cardiac CT can assess left and right heart size as well as regional myocardial wall motion and thickening (options A and B).[1,2] Cardiac CT is comparable to first-pass radionuclide angiography for the calculation of left ventricular ejection fraction in patients with myocardial infarction (option C).[3] Cardiac CT could effectively detect intracardiac masses such as thrombi and tumors, particularly when these masses are nonmobile or calcified (option E).[4]

17-2. The answer is A. *(Hurst's The Heart, 14th Edition, Chap. 17)* The presence of CAC is clearly indicative of coronary atherosclerosis,[5,6] serving as a marker for CAD; but importantly, the severity of angiographic coronary artery stenosis is not directly related to the total CAC. CAC is thought to begin early in life, and CT can detect coronary atherosclerosis at its earliest stages. Although lack of calcification does not categorically exclude the presence of atherosclerotic plaque, calcification occurs exclusively in atherosclerotic arteries and is not found in normal coronary arteries. A strong linear correlation exists between total coronary artery plaque area and the extent of CAC.

17-3. The answer is E. *(Hurst's The Heart, 14th Edition, Chap. 17)* The coronary arteries move independently throughout the cardiac cycle, and even at relatively slower heart rates (< 70 beats/min), they exhibit significant translational motion of up to 60 mm/s for the RCA and 20 to 40 mm/s for the LAD and circumflex coronary arteries.[7,8] The velocity of coronary artery motion increases significantly with increasing heart rates. Image acquisition of less than 50 milliseconds is truly required to completely avoid cardiac motion artifacts.[7] Cardiac motion is minimized with the use of oral and/or intravenous β-blockers prior to scanning, thereby reducing the heart rate and prolonging the time during the cardiac cycle at which coronary artery velocity is low. Another crucial element for obtaining high-quality coronary images is to maximally dilate coronary vessels with nitroglycerin through the use of sublingual tablets or spray. Respiratory motion can be excluded by performing the scan during a breath-hold.

17-4. The answer is A. *(Hurst's The Heart, 14th Edition, Chap. 17)* Although there is still room for improvement in terms of image quality and elimination of artifacts, the diagnostic performance of the CCTA is now well established. Studies demonstrate higher diagnostic accuracy for ACS with CCTA than with other previously studied modalities, including exercise treadmill, stress nuclear imaging, and stress echocardiography. The high negative predictive value of CCTA makes 64-slice MDCT a valuable tool in the exclusion of obstructive CAD. Therefore, CCTA is useful in the risk stratification of symptomatic patients and can reduce the need for invasive diagnostic coronary angiography in patients without obstructive CAD. A recent scientific statement from the American Heart Association (AHA) on CCTA concluded that "CT coronary angiography is reasonable for the assessment of obstructive disease in symptomatic patients (class IIa, Level of Evidence: B)."[9] In particular, CCTA is an accurate tool in the assessment of chest pain in patients with intermediate risk of CAD or in patients with uninterpretable or equivocal stress tests.[10]

17-5. The answer is E. *(Hurst's The Heart, 14th Edition, Chap. 17)* Imaging artifacts caused by the metallic stent limit the overall visibility of the inner lumen of a deployed stent and can potentially reduce the diagnostic accuracy of CCTA for the noninvasive evaluation of in-stent restenosis. Stent location, heart rate, and stent diameter are also important determinants of accuracy and feasibility for CCTA in this setting.

17-6. The answer is D. *(Hurst's The Heart, 14th Edition, Chap. 17)* Anomalies of the coronary arteries are reported in 0.3% to 1% of the general population.[11] Approximately 20% of coronary anomalies can be hemodynamically significant and manifest as arrhythmias, syncope, MI, or sudden death.[12,13] An interarterial course between the pulmonary artery and aorta is the coronary anomaly most commonly associated with sudden cardiac death.[14]

17-7. The answer is E. *(Hurst's The Heart, 14th Edition, Chap. 17)* Cardiac CT is helpful in reducing the risk of coronary occlusion during TAVR. Coronary occlusion is said to occur in 0.66% of TAVR procedures and is associated with a poor clinical outcome. The mechanism of coronary occlusion relates to calcification on the native aortic valve leaflet being displaced up toward the coronary ostium. CT allows for accurate assessment of both the height of the coronaries and the size and capacity of the sinus of Valsalva.[15] Evidence suggests that a left main height of < 12 mm in conjunction with shallow of Valsalva mean diameter (cusp to commissures) of < 30 mm was associated with more than a fivefold increased risk of coronary occlusion. In addition, a sinus of Valsalva–to–annular ratio of less than 1.25 was also strongly predictive of an increased risk.

17-8. The answer is A. *(Hurst's The Heart, 14th Edition, Chap. 17)* The most significant, and routinely available, radiation reduction strategy (up to 79%) can be achieved through prospective ECG-gated or sequential CCTA image acquisition, which involves the use of axial scanning with the tube current on only during prespecified portions of the cardiac cycle, eliminating tube current (milliampere) during nonimaging portions of the cardiac cycle (ie, systole).[16,17] Additionally, radiation exposure can be further minimized by approximately 46% to 53% by decreasing the tube voltage in nonobese (body mass index < 30 kg/m^2) patients from 120 to 100 kVp.[18,19] More recently, new iterative reconstruction algorithms have been introduced and validated for use in cardiac CT to allow for significant noise reduction, enabling an uncoupling of tube current and image noise and thereby allowing for significant tube current and dose reduction.[20] Finally, new scan acquisition modes employing fast helical pitch technique afforded by dual source dual detector technology allow for rapid scan acquisition and significant dose reduction as a result.[21]

17-9. The answer is B. *(Hurst's The Heart, 14th Edition, Chap. 17)* CCTA yields independent prognostic information in addition to clinical risk factors in patients with suspected or known CAD.[22] In patients with chest pain, CCTA can identify obstructive lesions, such as proximal LAD stenosis, as well as the number of vessels with moderate to severe stenosis, which predict an increased risk for all-cause mortality.[23] The presence of any stenosis greater than 50% at CCTA has been associated with a 10-fold higher risk of cardiovascular events. In addition, the extent of CAD, reflected by the number of coronary segments involved, incrementally increased the risk of adverse outcomes.[24] Plaque morphology by CT confers incremental prognostic information beyond that provided by percent stenosis alone. CCTA measures of CAD severity and LVEF have independent prognostic value. Incorporation of CAD severity had incremental value for predicting all-cause death over routine clinical predictors and LVEF in patients with suspected obstructive CAD.[25]

17-10. The answer is E. *(Hurst's The Heart, 14th Edition, Chap. 17)* CTA may guide the surgical approach by defining the position of the sternum to the RV, establishing patency of existing grafts, and visualizing the aorta, thereby avoiding unnecessary trauma and bleeding.[26] CCTA may be clinically useful for the evaluation of coronary bypass grafts and coronary anatomy in symptomatic patients.[27,28] In the case of reoperation or revascularization, coronary CTA may provide critically important information on the status and anatomic location of the bypass grafts. The AHA Scientific Statement on CCTA states, "It might be reasonable in most cases to not only assess the patency of bypass graft but also the presence of coronary stenoses in the course of the bypass graft or at the anastomotic site as well as in the native coronary artery system (class IIb, Level of Evidence: C)."[9]

References

1. Roig E, Chomka EV, Castaner A, et al. Exercise ultrafast computed tomography for the detection of coronary artery disease. *J Am Coll Cardiol.* 1989;13(5):1073-1081.
2. Budoff MJ, Gillespie R, Georgiou D, et al. Comparison of exercise electron beam computed tomography and sestamibi in the evaluation of coronary artery disease. *Am J Cardiol.* 1998;81(6):682-687.
3. Gerber TC, Behrenbeck T, Allison T, Mullan BP, Rumberger JA, Gibbons RJ. Comparison of measurement of left ventricular ejection fraction by Tc-99m sestamibi first-pass angiography with electron beam computed tomography in patients with anterior wall acute myocardial infarction. *Am J Cardiol.* 1999;83(7):1022-1026.
4. Budoff MJ, Shittu A, Hacioglu Y, et al. Comparison of transesophageal echocardiography versus computed tomography for detection of left atrial appendage filling defect (thrombus). *Am J Cardiol.* 2014;113(1):173-177.

5. Rumberger JA, Simons DB, Fitzpatrick LA, Sheedy PF, Schwartz RS. Coronary artery calcium area by electron-beam computed tomography and coronary atherosclerotic plaque area. A histopathologic correlative study. *Circulation.* 1995;92(8):2157-2162.

6. Sangiorgi G, Rumberger JA, Severson A, et al. Arterial calcification and not lumen stenosis is highly correlated with atherosclerotic plaque burden in humans: a histologic study of 723 coronary artery segments using nondecalcifying methodology. *J Am Coll Cardiol.* 1998;31(1):126-133.

7. Lu B, Mao SS, Zhuang N, et al. Coronary artery motion during the cardiac cycle and optimal ECG triggering for coronary artery imaging. *Invest Radiol.* 2001;36(5):250-256.

8. Achenbach S, Ropers D, Holle J, Muschiol G, Daniel WG, Moshage W. In-plane coronary arterial motion velocity: measurement with electron-beam CT. *Radiology.* 2000;216(2):457-463.

9. Budoff MJ, Achenbach S, Blumenthal RS, et al. Assessment of coronary artery disease by cardiac computed tomography: a scientific statement from the American Heart Association Committee on Cardiovascular Imaging and Intervention, Council on Cardiovascular Radiology and Intervention, and Committee on Cardiac Imaging, Council on Clinical Cardiology. *Circulation.* 2006;114(16):1761-1791.

10. Taylor AJ, Cerqueira M, Hodgson JM, et al. ACCF/SCCT/ACR/AHA/ASE/ASNC/ NASCI/SCAI/SCMR 2010 appropriate use criteria for cardiac computed tomography. A report of the American College of Cardiology Foundation Appropriate Use Criteria Task Force, the Society of Cardiovascular Computed Tomography, the American College of Radiology, the American Heart Association, the American Society of Echocardiography, the American Society of Nuclear Cardiology, the North American Society for Cardiovascular Imaging, the Society for Cardiovascular Angiography and Interventions, and the Society for Cardiovascular Magnetic Resonance. *J Am Coll Cardiol.* 2010;56(22):1864-1894.

11. Angelini P, Velasco JA, Flamm S. Coronary anomalies: incidence, pathophysiology, and clinical relevance. *Circulation.* 2002;105(20):2449-2454.

12. Eckart RE, Scoville SL, Campbell CL, et al. Sudden death in young adults: a 25-year review of autopsies in military recruits. *Ann Intern Med.* 2004;141(11):829-834.

13. Budoff MJ, Ahmed V, Gul KM, Mao SS, Gopal A. Coronary anomalies by cardiac computed tomographic angiography. *Clin Cardiol.* 2006;29(11):489-493.

14. Taylor AJ, Rogan KM, Virmani R. Sudden cardiac death associated with isolated congenital coronary artery anomalies. *J Am Coll Cardiol.* 1992;20(3):640-647.

15. Ribeiro HB, Webb JG, Makkar RR, et al. Predictive factors, management, and clinical outcomes of coronary obstruction following transcatheter aortic valve implantation: insights from a large multicenter registry. *J Am Coll Cardiol.* 2013;62(17):1552-1562.

16. Gopal A, Mao SS, Karlsberg D, et al. Radiation reduction with prospective ECG triggering acquisition using 64-multidetector computed tomographic angiography. *Int J Cardiovasc Imaging.* 2009;25(4):405-416.

17. Pontone G, Andreini D, Bartorelli AL, et al. Diagnostic accuracy of coronary computed tomography angiography: a comparison between prospective and retrospective electrocardiogram triggering. *J Am Coll Cardiol.* 2009;54(4):346-355.

18. Hausleiter J, Meyer T, Hermann F, et al. Estimated radiation dose associated with cardiac CT angiography. *JAMA.* 2009;301(5):500-507.

19. Bischoff B, Hein F, Meyer T, et al. Impact of a reduced tube voltage on CT angiography and radiation dose: results of the PROTECTION I study. *JACC Cardiovasc Imaging.* 2009;2(8):940-946.

20. Leipsic J, Labounty TM, Heilbron B, et al. Estimated radiation dose reduction using adaptive statistical iterative reconstruction in coronary CT angiography: the ERASIR study. *AJR Am J Roentgenol.* 2010;195(3):655-660.

21. Achenbach S, Goroll T, Seltmann M, et al. Detection of coronary artery stenoses by low-dose, prospectively ECG-triggered, high-pitch spiral coronary CT angiography. *JACC Cardiovasc Imaging.* 2011;4(4):328-337.

22. Pundziute G, Schuijf JD, Jukema JW, et al. Prognostic value of multislice computed tomography coronary angiography in patients with known or suspected coronary artery disease. *J Am Coll Cardiol.* 2007;49(1):62-70.

23. Min JK, Shaw LJ, Devereux RB, et al. Prognostic value of multidetector coronary computed tomographic angiography for prediction of all-cause mortality. *J Am Coll Cardiol.* 2007;50(12):1161-1170.

24. Bamberg F, Sommer WH, Hoffmann V, et al. Meta-analysis and systematic review of the long-term predictive value of assessment of coronary atherosclerosis by contrast-enhanced coronary computed tomography angiography. *J Am Coll Cardiol.* 2011;57(24):2426-2436.

25. Chow BJ, Small G, Yam Y, et al. Incremental prognostic value of cardiac computed tomography in coronary artery disease using CONFIRM: COroNary computed tomography angiography evaluation for clinical outcomes: an InteRnational Multicenter registry. *Circ Cardiovasc Imaging.* 2011;4(5):463-472.

26. Cremer J, Teebken OE, Simon A, Hutzelmann A, Heller M, Haverich A. Thoracic computed tomography prior to redo coronary surgery. *Eur J Cardiothorac Surg.* 1998;13(6):650-654.

27. Meyer TS, Martinoff S, Hadamitzky M, et al. Improved noninvasive assessment of coronary artery bypass grafts with 64-slice computed tomographic angiography in an unselected patient population. *J Am Coll Cardiol.* 2007;49(9):946-950.

28. Weustink AC, Nieman K, Pugliese F, et al. Diagnostic accuracy of computed tomography angiography in patients after bypass grafting: comparison with invasive coronary angiography. *JACC Cardiovasc Imaging.* 2009;2(7):816-824.

CHAPTER 18

Nuclear Cardiology

Jonathan Afilalo

QUESTIONS

DIRECTIONS: Choose the one best response to each question.

18-1. The concept that CAD can be detected with radiopharmaceuticals used for SPECT-MPI is based on the ability to detect a relative reduction in myocardial perfusion in a region supplied by a significantly stenosed vessel when compared with a normal region during hyperemia. Which of the following factors beyond focal percent stenosis can affect the degree of hyperemia achievable in diseased vessels?

A. Myocardial mass distal to the stenosis
B. Endothelial dysfunction
C. Nonatherosclerotic microvascular disease
D. B and C
E. A, B, and C

18-2. A 55-year-old double-amputee man with a prior history of ischemic heart disease, migraine, dyslipidemia, and hypertension was admitted to the emergency department with central chest pain. His medications include bisoprolol, amlodipine, isosorbide dinitrate, aspirin, ramipril, rosuvastatin, and the over-the-counter Excedrin Migraine. Initial ECG and biomarkers were within normal limits. Three days after admission, the patient underwent stress nuclear SPECT-MPI for risk stratification. With regard to his medications, which of the following statements is *true*?

A. Bisoprolol should be discontinued for 12 hours before stress imaging
B. Amlodipine should be discontinued for 12 hours before stress imaging
C. Isosorbide dinitrate should be discontinued for 48 hours before stress imaging
D. Excedrin Migraine should be discontinued for 24 hours before stress imaging
E. All of the above

18-3. A frail 89-year-old woman with a prior history of asthma, multiple falls, peripheral vascular disease, and permanent atrial fibrillation was admitted to the hospital following an episode of retrosternal chest pain. Initial ECG and biomarkers were within normal limits. Three days after admission, the patient underwent stress nuclear SPECT-MPI. Which of the following types of stress testing is the preferred approach to stress nuclear SPECT-MPI for this patient?

A. Adenosine
B. Regadenoson
C. Dipyridamole
D. Dobutamine
E. Exercise

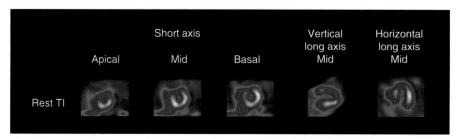

FIGURE 18-1 Rest thallium-201 (201Tl) single-photon emission computed tomography (SPECT) myocardial perfusion imaging (MPI) showing a large amount of resting ischemia in the left anterior descending. The stress SPECT-MPI study was canceled in this patient because of the unexpected perfusion defect.

18-4. A 75-year-old man with a prior history of myocardial infarction, dyslipidemia, and hypertension was admitted to the hospital following an episode of central chest pain. Initial ECG showed T-wave inversion in the anterior leads with negative biomarkers. Three days after admission, the patient underwent rest thallium-201 (201Tl) SPECT-MPI, which is illustrated in Figure 18-1. Which of the following is the optimal SPECT approach for the assessment of myocardial viability in this patient?

A. Rest ^{99m}Tc-sestamibi SPECT-MPI
B. Rest ^{99m}Tc-tetrofosmin SPECT-MPI
C. Rest/redistribution thallium-201 (Tl) SPECT-MPI
D. Stress SPECT-MPI
E. Any of the above

18-5. A 65-year-old woman with multiple risk factors for coronary artery disease presented to the emergency department with 2-day history of retrosternal chest discomfort at rest. The patient, whose images are shown in Figure 18-2, was referred for SPECT-MPI after an initial normal ECG and negative biomarkers. With regard to the use of SPECT-MPI in the evaluation of acute chest pain, which of the following statements is *false*?

A. A normal rest SPECT-MPI alone provides strong evidence of the absence of acute MI
B. There is a reduction in hospitalizations when rest SPECT-MPI is incorporated into an ED evaluation strategy of patients presenting with suspected ACS
C. Stress SPECT-MPI study is of no value in ruling out an ACS after a normal rest SPECT-MPI study
D. Stress SPECT-MPI study is safe in low-risk ED patients
E. A normal stress SPECT-MPI study is associated with a very low cardiac event rate

18-6. A 55-year-old man with a prior history of stage IV chronic kidney disease, hypertension, and dyslipidemia presented to the emergency department complaining of central chest pain. Initial ECG revealed an old LBBB, and the laboratory investigations showed negative biomarkers. Which of the following is the best imaging modality for this patient's risk assessment?

A. Vasodilator SPECT-MPI
B. Exercise stress SPECT-MPI
C. CMR imaging
D. CCTA
E. Any of the above

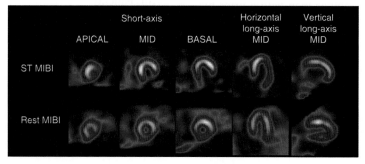

FIGURE 18-2 Adenosine stress/rest myocardial perfusion single-photon emission computed tomography images. Rest sestamibi (MIBI) demonstrated minimal (borderline) perfusion defect in the inferior wall. Stress imaging revealed evidence of severe and extensive ischemia in the inferior and inferolateral wall (41% of the left ventricle).

18-7. A 58-year-old morbidly obese woman with a prior history of poorly controlled type 2 diabetes, peripheral vascular disease, stage IV COPD, hypertension, dyslipidemia, and rheumatoid arthritis was admitted to the emergency department with severe retrosternal chest pain. There were no new changes on the initial ECG, and the labs revealed negative biomarkers. Which of the following is the best initial imaging modality for this patient's risk assessment?

A. Exercise stress ECG test
B. Exercise stress CMR imaging
C. Exercise stress nuclear MPI
D. Vasodilator stress nuclear MPI
E. Any of the above

18-8. Applications of nuclear MPI in stable ischemic heart disease are included in the recent ACCF/AHA clinical practice guidelines. Which of the following was assigned a class Ib level of evidence for exercise MPI?

A. Patients with an intermediate pretest risk who have an ECG for which the exercise response cannot be interpreted
B. Patients with an intermediate pretest risk who have an interpretable ECG
C. Patients with ongoing chest pain and uninterpretable ECG (as in old LBBB)
D. None of the above
E. All of the above

18-9. Several large randomized clinical trials have evaluated the application of CCTA to patients with suspected ACS in the ED in comparison to a standard of care approach. In which of the following settings of chest pain in the ED would SPECT-MPI be preferred over CCTA?

A. Elderly patients with known dense coronary calcification
B. Younger patients due to the radiation exposure with CCTA
C. Patients with documented allergy to gadolinium-based contrast agents
D. Patients with valvular heart disease
E. All of the above

18-10. The 2013 ACCF/AHA guideline for the management of heart failure summarized the recommendations for the use of imaging in heart failure patients. Based on this statement, in which of the following clinical applications may nuclear imaging *not* play a role?

A. Patients with ischemic cardiomyopathy who have had a significant change in their clinical status
B. Radionuclide ventriculography for the assessment of LVEF when device therapy is being considered
C. Patients who received treatment that may affect cardiac function
D. Patients with ischemic cardiomyopathy with EF < 35% who are not eligible for revascularization
E. Radionuclide ventriculography for the assessment of LVEF and LV volumes when echocardiography is inadequate

18-1. **The answer is E.** *(Hurst's The Heart, 14th Edition, Chap. 18)* Multiple factors beyond focal percent stenosis can also affect the degree of hyperemia achievable in diseased vessels. These include stenosis length, myocardial mass distal to the stenosis, plaque composition, diffuse atherosclerosis, nonatherosclerotic microvascular disease, and endothelial dysfunction.[1,2] In general, a significant reduction in maximal hyperemia is usually present when stenosis severity exceeds 70%.[3] However, when compared to assessment of fractional flow reserve (FFR), considered the gold standard, only 35% of vessels visually assessed as having 50% to 70% stenosis manifest a decrease in maximal hyperemia.[4]

18-2. **The answer is D.** *(Hurst's The Heart, 14th Edition, Chap. 18)* In general, for purposes of diagnosis or initial risk stratification, stress nuclear MPI is performed with the patient off anti-ischemic medications[5] because these medications may limit the development of ischemia during the stress test. When feasible, the use of beta-blockers or long-acting calcium channel blockers should be discontinued for 48 hours before stress imaging, and long-acting nitrates should be discontinued for 12 hours before stress imaging.[5] In general, discontinuation of compounds containing caffeine (Excedrin Migraine) for 24 hours prior to the use of adenosine or dipyridamole and 12 hours prior to the use of regadenoson is recommended.[5,6]

18-3. **The answer is B.** *(Hurst's The Heart, 14th Edition, Chap. 18)* For patients who cannot exercise (mobility impairment, severe peripheral vascular disease), pharmacologic stress testing is the preferred approach to stress.[7] The preferred pharmacologic stress agents for SPECT-MPI are coronary vasodilators: adenosine, regadenoson, or dipyridamole. Because of the potential adverse effect of severe bronchospasm, dipyridamole is contraindicated for asthmatics. Adenosine is considered contraindicated for patients with second- or third-degree AV block, sick sinus syndrome, or bronchospasm. Regadenoson has the potential to reduce the high frequency of uncomfortable systemic adverse effects and the risk of bronchospasm in asthmatics that are associated with adenosine and dipyridamole. A large phase IV study (999 patients) has reported the safety of regadenoson in patients with stable chronic obstructive pulmonary disease or asthma, but appropriate resuscitative measures should be available in case bronchospasm occurs.[6,8] An alternative to vasodilator stress is inotropic stress with dobutamine. With the increased use of regadenoson, which has fewer contraindications, dobutamine stress nuclear MPI has markedly decreased in many nuclear laboratories. Dobutamine stress results in a lower-rate pressure product than exercise and a lower peak coronary blood flow with vasodilator stress. Moreover, this patient has atrial fibrillation, and dobutamine may aggravate this arrhythmia.

18-4. **The answer is C.** *(Hurst's The Heart, 14th Edition, Chap. 18)* Although PET and MRI are considered superior for viability assessment, rest/redistribution 201Tl SPECT-MPI is the preferred SPECT approach for the assessment of myocardial viability.[9] Theoretically, the effectiveness of 201Tl SPECT-MPI for viability assessment could be improved by the administration of nitroglycerin prior to the rest injection. Importantly, 24-hour imaging may show additional redistribution compared to 4-hour imaging[10,11] because, in the setting of a critical coronary stenosis with reduced resting blood flow, the time to complete redistribution may be delayed. The stress SPECT-MPI study is not the optimal approach in this patient because of the unexpected perfusion defect at rest. Rest ^{99m}Tc-sestamibi and ^{99m}Tc-tetrofosmin can also be used to assess myocardial viability. However, they are not considered optimal because, unlike 201Tl, they reflect only myocardial perfusion and do not redistribute into the potassium pool. Furthermore, these agents underestimate viability in the presence of myocardial hibernation with resting hypoperfusion.

18-5. **The answer is C.** *(Hurst's The Heart, 14th Edition, Chap. 18)* Because of the very strong relationship between an acute MI and acute closure of a coronary artery, a normal rest MPI alone, without stress imaging, provides strong evidence of the absence of MI (option A). A 99% negative predictive value of rest SPECT-MPI alone for MI was reported in several studies beginning in the mid-1990s.[12] A prospective, randomized, controlled multicenter trial reported a reduction in hospitalizations when rest SPECT-MPI was incorporated into an ED evaluation strategy of patients presenting with suspected ACS (ERASE Trial) (option B).[13] When the radiopharmaceutical is injected after pain has subsided and the SPECT-MPI study is normal, stress SPECT-MPI studies are commonly used to further rule out an ACS because unstable angina might be associated with normal rest perfusion (Figure 18-2). This case illustrates this concept, that is, the value of stress testing when rest MPI is normal in the acute chest pain patient (option C). In fact, rest sestamibi (MIBI) demonstrated minimal (borderline) perfusion defect in the inferior wall, while stress imaging revealed evidence of severe and extensive ischemia in the inferior and inferolateral wall. Based on extensive literature documenting the safety of maximal exercise testing in low-risk ED with a normal ECG and normal serial enzymes (4 to 6 hours apart), a normal stress SPECT-MPI study was safe and associated with a very low cardiac event rate in several studies (options D and E).[14]

18-6. **The answer is A.** *(Hurst's The Heart, 14th Edition, Chap. 18)* Current guidelines support nuclear MPI in symptomatic patients with LBBB.[15] Vasodilator stress SPECT-MPI has been shown to be an excellent predictor of cardiac events in LBBB patients (option A).[16] Guidelines give a class I indication for the use of pharmacologic stress nuclear MPI in the patients with LBBB, regardless of the ability to exercise to an adequate workload (options A and B).[15] Nuclear MPI has a distinct advantage over the use of CMR imaging and CCTA for risk assessment of the CKD patient because there is no organ toxicity associated with the injection of the radionuclide tracers (options C and D). CMR with gadolinium contrast is contraindicated in these patients due to the risks of nephrogenic systemic fibrosis in renal failure patients. With CCTA, the nephrotoxicity of the iodinated contrast results in this study being contraindicated unless the patient is on dialysis. Even in the dialysis patient, the high CAC scores commonly found in the renal failure patient can reduce the diagnostic and prognostic value of the coronary CTA study.

18-7. **The answer is D.** *(Hurst's The Heart, 14th Edition, Chap. 18)* Patients may be categorized as unable to exercise if they are challenged with performing moderate household, yard, or recreational work.[17] In addition, patients with disabling comorbidities are also unable to exercise, and they include patients who are severely frail, markedly obese, with severe peripheral arterial disease, severe chronic obstructive pulmonary disease, or orthopedic limitations. These groups form a large proportion of patients who will be referred and have appropriate indications for nuclear MPI. In patients unable to exercise, guidelines support pharmacologic stress imaging as the initial test in symptomatic male and female patients with intermediate or high pretest likelihood of CAD.[5,18,19]

18-8. **The answer is A.** *(Hurst's The Heart, 14th Edition, Chap. 18)* The ACCF/AHA SIHD guideline assigned a class Ib level of evidence to exercise MPI for patients with an intermediate to high pretest risk who have an ECG for which the exercise response cannot be interpreted.[20] An exercise stress MPI in this same subset with an intermediate to high risk in the presence of an interpretable ECG was assigned a class IIa level of evidence. Exercise stress is not appropriate in the setting of ongoing chest pain, which may be the manifestation of a high-risk acute coronary syndrome.

18-9. **The answer is A.** *(Hurst's The Heart, 14th Edition, Chap. 18)* Coronary CTA is of value and generally preferred over SPECT-MPI in the ED setting. However, there are certain scenarios of chest pain in the ED in which SPECT-MPI would be preferred. These include patients with known dense coronary calcification (option A), often encountered in the elderly demographic, patients with prior stents causing artifacts within the stent lumen, and patients with contraindications to CCTA.[21-23] CCTA does expose the younger patient to radiation, although the dose with contemporary techniques is lower than that of SPECT-MPI. CCTA does require contrast administration, although this is iodinated contrast (not gadolinium-based contrast as is used for MRI).

18-10. The answer is D. *(Hurst's The Heart, 14th Edition, Chap. 18)* Based on the ACCF/AHA guideline for the management of heart failure, the clinical applications where imaging may play a role include:[24] (i) repeat measurement of LVEF in patients who have had a significant change in their clinical status, received treatment that may affect cardiac function, or are under consideration for device therapy (class I, level of evidence C); (ii) imaging to detect ischemia and viability in patients with de novo heart failure, known CAD, and no angina, unless the patient is not eligible for revascularization (class IIa, level of evidence C); (iii) viability assessment prior to revascularization in select situations is reasonable in the heart failure patient with CAD (class IIa, level of evidence B); and (iv) radionuclide ventriculography for the assessment of LVEF and LV volumes when echocardiography is inadequate (class IIa, level of evidence C).

References

1. Kern MJ, Samady H. Current concepts of integrated coronary physiology in the catheterization laboratory. *J Am Coll Cardiol.* 2010;55(3):173-185.

2. Park HB, Heo R, ó Hartaigh B, et al. Atherosclerotic plaque characteristics by CT angiography identify coronary lesions that cause ischemia: a direct comparison to fractional flow reserve. *JACC Cardiovasc Imaging.* 2015;8(1):1-10.

3. Ragosta M, Bishop AH, Lipson LC, et al. Comparison between angiography and fractional flow reserve versus single-photon emission computed tomographic myocardial perfusion imaging for determining lesion significance in patients with multivessel coronary disease. *Am J Cardiol.* 2007;99(7):896-902.

4. Tonino PA, Fearon WF, De Bruyne B, et al. Angiographic versus functional severity of coronary artery stenosis in the FAME study fractional flow reserve versus angiography in multivessel evaluation. *J Am Coll Cardiol.* 2010;55(25):2816-2821.

5. Klocke FJ, Baird MG, Lorell BH, et al. ACC/AHA/ASNC Guidelines for the clinical use of cardiac radionuclide imaging: A report of the American 1995 guidelines for the clinical use of radionuclide imaging. *Circulation.* 2003;108(11):1404-1418.

6. Henzlova MJ, Duvall WL, Einstein AJ, et al. Stress protocols and tracers. ASNC Imaging Guidelines for Nuclear Cardiology Procedures. 2009.

7. Verani MS, Mahmarian JJ, Hixson JB, et al. Diagnosis of coronary artery disease by controlled coronary vasodilation with adenosine and thallium-201 scintigraphy in patients unable to exercise. *Circulation.* 1990;82(1):80-87.

8. Prenner BM, Bukofzer S, Behm S, et al. A randomized, double-blind, placebo-controlled study assessing the safety and tolerability of regadenoson in subjects with asthma or chronic obstructive pulmonary disease. *J Nucl Cardiol.* 2012;19(4):681-692.

9. Pohost GM, Zir LM, Moore RH, et al. Differentiation of transiently ischemic from infarcted myocardium by serial imaging after a single dose of thallium-201. *Circulation.* 1977;55(2):294-302.

10. Kiat H, Friedman JD, Wang FP, et al. Frequency of late reversibility in stress-redistribution thallium-201 SPECT using an early reinjection protocol. *Am Heart J.* 1991;122(3 Pt 1):613-619.

11. Hayes SW, Berman DS, Germano G. Stress testing and imaging protocols. In: Germano G, Berman DS, eds. *Clinical Gated Cardiac SPECT.* Oxford, UK: Blackwell Publishing; 2006:47-68.

12. Amsterdam EA, Kirk JD, Bluemke DA, et al. Testing of low-risk patients presenting to the emergency department with chest pain: a scientific statement from the American Heart Association. *Circulation.* 2010;122(17):1756-1776.

13. Udelson JE, Beshansky JR, Ballin DS, et al. Myocardial perfusion imaging for evaluation and triage of patients with suspected acute cardiac ischemia: a randomized controlled trial. *JAMA.* 2002;288(21):2693-2700.

14. Duvall WL, Wijetunga MN, Klein TM, et al. Stress-only Tc-99m myocardial perfusion imaging in an emergency department chest pain unit. *J Emerg Med.* 2012;42(6):642-650.

15. Fihn SD, Blankenship JC, Alexander KP, et al. 2014 ACC/AHA/AATS/PCNA/SCAI/STS focused update of the guideline for the diagnosis and management of patients with stable ischemic heart disease: a report of the American College of Cardiology/American Heart Association Task Force on Practice Guidelines, and the American Association for Thoracic Surgery, Preventive Cardiovascular Nurses Association, Society for Cardiovascular Angiography and Interventions, and Society of Thoracic Surgeons. *J Thorac Cardiovasc Surg.* 2015;149(3):e5-e23.

16. Wagdy HM, Hodge D, Christian TF, et al. Prognostic value of vasodilator myocardial perfusion imaging in patients with left bundle-branch block. *Circulation.* 1998;97(16):1563-1570.

17. Fihn SD, Gardin JM, Abrams J, et al. 2012 ACCF/AHA/ACP/AATS/PCNA/SCAI/STS guideline for the diagnosis and management of patients with stable ischemic heart disease: a report of the American College of Cardiology Foundation/American Heart Association task force on practice guidelines, and the American College of Physicians, American Association for Thoracic Surgery, Preventive Cardiovascular Nurses Association, Society for Cardiovascular Angiography and Interventions, and Society of Thoracic Surgeons. *Circulation.* 2012;126(25):e354-e471.

18. Mieres JH, Shaw LJ, Arai A, et al. Role of noninvasive testing in the clinical evaluation of women with suspected coronary artery disease: Consensus statement from the Cardiac Imaging Committee, Council on Clinical Cardiology, and the Cardiovascular Imaging and Intervention Committee, Council on Cardiovascular Radiology and Intervention, American Heart Association. *Circulation*. 2005;111(5):682-696.

19. Hendel RC, Berman DS, Di Carli MF, et al. ACCF/ASNC/ACR/AHA/ASE/SCCT/SCMR/SNM 2009 appropriate use criteria for cardiac radionuclide imaging: a report of the American College of Cardiology Foundation Appropriate Use Criteria Task Force, the American Society of Nuclear Cardiology, the American College of Radiology, the American Heart Association, the American Society of Echocardiography, the Society of Cardiovascular Computed Tomography, the Society for Cardiovascular Magnetic Resonance, and the Society of Nuclear Medicine. *J Am Coll Cardiol*. 2009;53(23):2201-2229.

20. Fihn SD, Gardin JM, Abrams J, et al. 2012 ACCF/AHA/ACP/AATS/PCNA/SCAI/STS Guideline for the diagnosis and management of patients with stable ischemic heart disease: a report of the American College of Cardiology Foundation/American Heart Association Task Force on Practice Guidelines, and the American College of Physicians, American Association for Thoracic Surgery, Preventive Cardiovascular Nurses Association, Society for Cardiovascular Angiography and Interventions, and Society of Thoracic Surgeons. *J Am Coll Cardiol*. 2012;60(24):e44-e164.

21. Nabi F, Kassi M, Muhyieddeen K, et al. Optimizing evaluation of patients with low to intermediate risk acute chest pain: a randomized study comparing stress myocardial perfusion tomography incorporating stress-only imaging to cardiac computed tomography. *J Nucl Med*. 2016;57(3):378-384. doi: 10.2967/jnumed.115.166595. Epub 2015.

22. Hoffmann U, Truong QA, Schoenfeld DA, et al. Coronary CT angiography versus standard evaluation in acute chest pain. *N Engl J Med*. 2012;367(4):299-308.

23. Litt HI, Gatsonis C, Snyder B, et al. CT angiography for safe discharge of patients with possible acute coronary syndromes. *N Engl J Med*. 2012;366(15):1393-1403.

24. Yancy CW, Jessup M, Bozkurt B, et al. 2013 ACCF/AHA guideline for the management of heart failure: a report of the American College of Cardiology Foundation/American Heart Association Task Force on Practice Guidelines. *J Am Coll Cardiol*. 2013;62(16):e147-e239.

CHAPTER 19

Positron Emission Tomography in Heart Disease

Jonathan Afilalo

QUESTIONS

DIRECTIONS: Choose the one best response to each question.

19-1. Although the assessment of coronary flow and coronary flow reserve (CFR) is based on absolute rather than relative measures of myocardial perfusion, these measures may still appear reduced in the absence of obstructive epicardial coronary artery disease. Which of the following factors may lower stress perfusion to erroneously low ischemic levels?

A. Caffeine
B. Beta-blockers
C. Inadequate vasodilator stress
D. Small vessel disease
E. All of the above

19-2. The radioligand ^{18}F-FDG is the most important and most widely used for the noninvasive study of the myocardium substrate's metabolism with PET. In which of the following cells does ^{18}F-FDG *not* trace glucose utilization?

A. Mechanical heart valves
B. Skeletal muscle cells
C. Brain cells
D. Tumor cells
E. Inflammatory cells

19-3. Adequate patient preparation during the 24 hours before a ^{18}F-FDG PET scan is essential for reliable results due to the myocardium's ability to shift its energy needs among several fuel substrates, including free fatty acids, glucose, and lactate. Which of the following parameters does *not* affect the myocardium's selection of fuel substrates?

A. Concentrations of the substrates in the blood
B. The availability of adequate oxygenated coronary blood flow
C. Prior carbohydrate or fatty food intake
D. Hormonal influences
E. Neurological innervations

19-4. A 71-year-old woman with a prior history of multivessel PCI and whose images are shown in Figure 19-1 was referred for PET because of recent abnormal ECG and a 6-month history of exertional chest pain and dyspnea. Which of the following statements regarding the rest and stress PET images is *false*?

A. There is resting scar or hibernating myocardium in the distribution of the left circumflex
B. There is resting scar or hibernating myocardium in the distribution of the mid-LAD
C. There is a significant worsening of the defect after dipyridamole (stress)
D. There is a substantial mismatch with active FDG uptake in anterior, septal, and apical regions
E. The lateral LV has a predominantly transmural scar

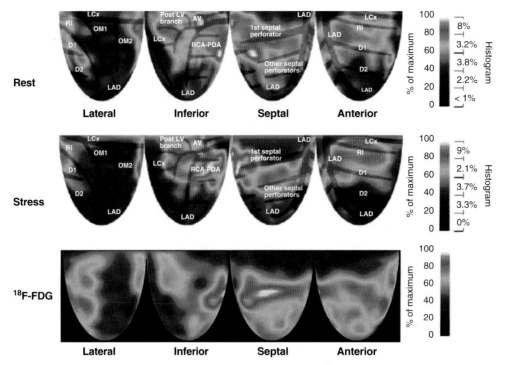

FIGURE 19-1. Relative rest and stress myocardial perfusion and ^{18}F-FDG images are color coded by the scale for relative myocardial uptake. For the rest stress relative perfusion images, the histogram on the right side of the color bar scale gives the relative activity as percent of maximum (100%) and percent of the left ventricle in each range of relative perfusion.

19-5. An 82-year-old hypertensive and diabetic man with prior history of multiple MIs was referred for viability PET to determine his treatment options (revascularization vs. medical treatment). Resting perfusion images are illustrated in Figure 19-2. Which of the following statements regarding rest/viability PET images is *false*?

A. There are apical perfusion defects
B. There are anterior perfusion defects
C. There are lateral perfusion defects
D. Most of the heart is no longer viable
E. None of the above

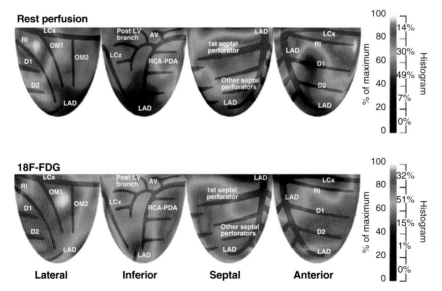

FIGURE 19-2. Relative rest perfusion and ^{18}F-FDG images are color coded by the scale for relative myocardial uptake. The histogram on the right side of the color scale gives the percent of the left ventricle in each range of relative uptake.

19-6. An 86-year-old woman was referred for PET scan after refusing a coronary angiography when she presented to the emergency department complaining of retrosternal chest pain after an emotionally stressful event. Initial ECG revealed ischemic-appearing ST changes with elevated biomarkers. Echocardiography showed apical akinesis and hyperdynamic function of the basal segments, with an EF of 28%. Which of the following statements about the stress and rest PET perfusion and ^{18}F-FDG findings of Takotsubo stress cardiomyopathy is *true*?

A. Stress perfusion activity is increased in the basal half of the LV
B. ^{18}F-FDG metabolic activity is decreased in the apical half of the LV
C. "Inverse flow metabolism mismatch" is a characteristic finding
D. B and C
E. A, B, and C

19-7. The assessment of myocardial viability is clinically used in patients with ischemic cardiomyopathy and severely impaired LV function in order to determine prognosis and guide therapeutic decision making. Which of the following clinical outcomes related to myocardial viability is *false*?

A. Revascularization of viable myocardium often leads to increases in LVEF
B. Revascularization of viable myocardium may lead to a reversal of LV remodeling
C. Revascularization of viable myocardium is associated with relief of heart failure symptoms
D. Postrevascularization improvements in physical activity are related to the amount of viable myocardium
E. Revascularization of nonviable myocardium never leads to functional or prognostic improvements in patient outcomes

19-8. A 67-year-old asymptomatic man whose images are shown in Figure 19-3 was referred for PET scan after an abnormal exercise stress test and coronary angiogram. The patient presented on the day of the examination after 16 hours of fasting. With regard to the PET perfusion and glucose metabolism images (Figure 19-3), which of the following statements is *false*?

A. Perfusion is severely reduced in the distal anterior wall
B. Perfusion is severely reduced in the apex
C. Perfusion is severely reduced in the mid lateral wall
D. ^{18}F-FDG activity is selectively increased in the region of the perfusion defect
E. ^{18}F-FDG uptake in normal myocardium is absent as a result of prolonged fasting.

19-9. A 37-year-old African-American woman whose images are shown in Figure 19-4 requested a second opinion and PET scan after series of nondiagnostic tests. She complained of a 2-month history of exertional dyspnea. Initial ECG showed a complete left bundle branch block. Echocardiography revealed a severely dilated left ventricle (LV) with an ejection fraction of 45%. Cardiac catheterization demonstrated dilatation of the LV, and the coronary arteries appeared normal. In which of the following conditions can the illustrated patterns of myocardial ^{18}F-FDG uptake occur?

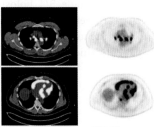

Fused PET/CT   PET images

FIGURE 19-4. Axial PET-only and PET/computed tomography (CT) images of the mediastinum (upper row) and the left ventricle (lower row). Multiple foci of intensely increased ^{18}F-FDG uptake are seen in the mediastinum (consistent with mediastinal lymph node involvement) and throughout the left and right ventricular myocardium.

A. Cardiac sarcoid
B. Tuberculous myocarditis
C. Epstein-Barr virus myocarditis
D. Chagas disease
E. All of the above

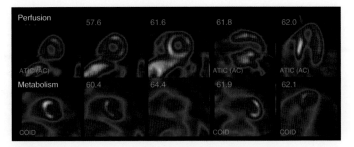

FIGURE 19-3. Positron emission tomography (PET) N-13 ammonia perfusion and glucose metabolism images.

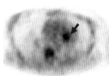 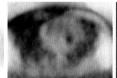 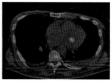

FIGURE 19-5. ^{18}F-FDG positron emission tomography (PET)/ computed tomography (CT) imaging of a case of suspected infective endocarditis. The increased ^{18}F-FDG activity (arrow) corresponds to an infected mitral valve. (Reproduced with permission from Kouijzer IJ, Vos FJ, Janssen MJ, et al. The value of ^{18}F-FDG PET/CT in diagnosing infectious endocarditis, *Eur J Nucl Med Mol Imaging.* 2013 Jul;40(7):1102-1107.)

19-10. The 42-year-old man whose images are shown in Figure 19-5 was referred for ^{18}F-FDG PET/CT imaging after an initial nondiagnostic transthoracic echocardiogram, which was followed by a negative transesophageal echocardiogram for vegetations. The patient had continuing fever, weight loss, and malaise. His cardiovascular examination revealed a grade 3/4 holosystolic murmur that had not been heard before. With regard to the use of ^{18}F-FDG PET/CT for the identification of infective endocarditis in this patient, which of the following statements is *false*?

A. Vegetations can be visualized with ^{18}F-FDG PET/CT

B. Vegetations are seen as small foci of increased ^{18}F-FDG activity in the region of the mitral valve

C. ^{18}F-FDG PET/CT is highly sensitive to rule out native valve endocarditis

D. ^{18}F-FDG PET/CT may contribute to the detection of downstream septic emboli

E. None of the above

ANSWERS

19-1. **The answer is E.** *(Hurst's The Heart, 14th Edition, Chap. 19)* Caffeine, beta-blockers, inadequate vasodilator stress, and diffuse or small-vessel disease may lower stress perfusion in cc/min/g to apparently low ischemic levels; therefore, concurrently measuring rest flow and CFR provides integrated diagnostic information for correct clinical interpretation from the coronary flow capacity map.

19-2. **The answer is A.** *(Hurst's The Heart, 14th Edition, Chap. 19)* As a glucose analog, ^{18}F-FDG tracks the initial transport of glucose from blood into cells and its phosphorylation to glucose-6-phosphate as the initial metabolic step of transformation of exogenously derived glucose. Because phosphorylated ^{18}F-FDG cannot be metabolized further, it is metabolically trapped in the cell, and it accumulates in tissue in proportion to rates of exogenous glucose utilization. However, the radiotracer ^{18}F-FDG is not cell specific for myocardium. It also traces glucose utilization in different organs, such as skeletal muscle and brain, as well as in tumors and inflammatory processes. While ^{18}F-FDG traces glucose utilization around prosthetic heart valves in cases of perivalvular infection, there is no utilization to trace within inert materials such as mechanical valve discs. Therefore, ^{18}F-FDG is clinically useful for imaging regional myocardial metabolism and for identifying inflammatory disease of the cardiovascular system

19-3. **The answer is E.** *(Hurst's The Heart, 14th Edition, Chap. 19)* The selection of fuel substrates depends on their concentrations in blood, prior carbohydrate or fatty food intake, availability of oxygenated coronary blood flow, and hormonal influences. Complicating factors include diabetes mellitus and elevated blood catecholamine concentrations, often present in heart failure patients. Neurological innervations do not play a direct role in myocardial fuel utilization.

19-4. **The answer is C.** *(Hurst's The Heart, 14th Edition, Chap. 19)* The rest and stress PET images showed a large, severe, lateral, apical, mid-anterior, and distal inferior resting scar or hibernating myocardium involving 60% to 70% of the left ventricle in the distribution of the left circumflex, mid-posterior descending, and mid-left anterior descending coronary arteries. After dipyridamole, the defect was minimally worse, indicating a fixed scar or viable, low-flow, hibernating myocardium. The viability ^{18}F-FDG images showed substantial mismatch with active FDG uptake in anterior, septal, and apical regions, indicating hibernating, viable, hypoperfused myocardium in mid to distal LAD and RCA distributions comprising approximately 30% of the LV. The lateral LV had a predominantly transmural scar comprising 25% of the LV with an additional 10% of the anterior, anterolateral wall, apex, and basal inferior wall being viable and hibernating in the distribution of a large first OM branch.

19-5. **The answer is D.** *(Hurst's The Heart, 14th Edition, Chap. 19)* Resting perfusion images showed large, severe, anterior, apical, lateral, and inferior perfusion defects involving 60% of the LV in the distribution of the mid LAD, mid LCX, and RCA coronary arteries. ^{18}F-FDG metabolic images showed myocardial uptake of ^{18}F-FDG, indicating viability of essentially the entire heart, with only a small distal inferior nontransmural scar comprising 3% of the LV taking up less ^{18}F-FDG.

19-6. **The answer is D.** *(Hurst's The Heart, 14th Edition, Chap. 19)* Transient apical ballooning, called Takotsubo (stress) cardiomyopathy, may mimic an acute coronary syndrome; it affects predominantly postmenopausal women and accounts for 1% to 2% of patients with troponin-positive acute coronary syndromes but with angiographically normal coronary vessels. It has been referred to as neurogenic myocardial stunning because it often follows a stressful event.[1] Wall motion is typically impaired in the apical portion of the LV, with concordantly reduced ^{18}F-FDG metabolic activity.[1,2] The typical finding of "inverse flow metabolism mismatch" refers to reduced apical ^{18}F-FDG metabolic activity in the presence of normal or near-normal apical perfusion.

19-7. **The answer is E.** *(Hurst's The Heart, 14th Edition, Chap. 19)* Patients with ischemic cardiomyopathy, severe LV dysfunction, and congestive heart failure symptoms will benefit most from the assessment of myocardial viability. Most studies have reported statistically significant postrevascularization increases in LVEF in patients with viability as compared to no or only minimal improvements in LVEF in patients without viable myocardium.[3] Revascularization of viable myocardium may lead to a reversal of LV remodeling[4] and relief of congestive heart failure symptoms.[5] Postrevascularization improvements in physical activity are related to the amount of viable myocardium with improved physical exercise during daily life prior to and 24 months after CABG.[6] It is important to emphasize that despite the presence of myocardial viability, even involving an adequate amount of the LV, revascularization may not always be followed by a functional improvement or reversed remodeling of the LV, and vice versa—revascularization may be associated with beneficial outcomes even in the absence of apparent viability.

19-8. **The answer is C.** *(Hurst's The Heart, 14th Edition, Chap. 19)* Perfusion is severely reduced in the distal anterior wall, the apex, and the distal inferior wall, suggestive of obstructive disease of the left anterior descending coronary artery. ^{18}F-FDG activity is selectively increased in the region of the perfusion defect, most likely consistent with myocardial viability; the perfusion metabolism mismatch corresponds in location to the distal left anterior descending coronary artery. ^{18}F-FDG uptake in normal myocardium is absent as a result of prolonged fasting. Among several approaches, prolonged fasting for 16 to 20 hours has been proven most effective in consistently suppressing ^{18}F-FDG uptake.[7-9] This is due to the shift of myocardium's substrate selection from glucose to free fatty acid, thereby reducing the accumulation of ^{18}F-FDG in normal myocardium.

19-9. **The answer is E.** *(Hurst's The Heart, 14th Edition, Chap. 19)* Multiple foci of intensely increased ^{18}F-FDG uptake are seen in the mediastinum (consistent with mediastinal lymph node involvement) and throughout the left and right ventricular myocardium (Figure 19-4), consistent with cardiac sarcoid associated with systemic sarcoid. This pattern of focally increased myocardial ^{18}F-FDG uptake is, however, not specific for cardiac sarcoid but also occurs in other types of granulomatous and nongranulomatous inflammatory processes of the myocardium as, for example, in tuberculous myocarditis,[10] Epstein-Barr virus myocarditis,[11] or Chagas disease.[12]

19-10. **The answer is C.** *(Hurst's The Heart, 14th Edition, Chap. 19)* There is now substantial evidence that ^{18}F-FDG PET/CT contributes to the identification of infective endocarditis, endovascular devices, and prosthetic vascular grafts, and, importantly, the detection of downstream septic emboli. Vegetations and abscesses of native and prosthetic valves can be visualized with ^{18}F-FDG PET/CT, though with a lower and clinically insufficient sensitivity (about 40%) and a specificity of about 70% to 100%.[13,14] They are typically seen as small foci of mildly to intensely increased ^{18}F-FDG activity in the region of the mitral or aortic valve (Fig. 19-5) and do not invariably correspond to findings on echocardiography. In one investigation in 30 patients with definite prosthetic valve infection, for example, findings by echocardiography and ^{18}F-FDG PET/CT agreed in only half of the patients; in nearly half of the remaining patients, focally increased ^{18}F-FDG uptake was seen in the valve area without corresponding vegetations on echocardiography, possibly because of an early stage of disease when echocardiography may still be negative.[14] Conversely, the absence of abnormal ^{18}F-FDG uptake effectively ruled out the presence of prosthetic valve infection in that study, so the authors proposed to include PET/CT as a major criterion for the diagnosis of infective endocarditis.[14]

References

1. Ibrahim T, Nekolla SG, Langwieser N, et al. Simultaneous positron emission tomography/magnetic resonance imaging identifies sustained regional abnormalities in cardiac metabolism and function in stress-induced transient midventricular ballooning syndrome: a variant of Takotsubo cardiomyopathy. *Circulation.* 2012;126:e324-e326.

2. Obunai K, Misra D, Van Tosh A, Bergmann SR. Metabolic evidence of myocardial stunning in takotsubo cardiomyopathy: a positron emission tomography study. *J Nucl. Cardiol.* 2005;12:742-744.

3. Schinkel AF, Bax JJ, Poldermans D, Elhendy A, Ferrari R, Rahimtoola SH. Hibernating myocardium: diagnosis and patient outcomes. *Curr Probl Cardiol.* 2007;32:375-410.

4. Carluccio E, Biagioli P, Alunni G, et al. Patients with hibernating myocardium show altered left ventricular volumes and shape, which revert after revascularization: evidence that dyssynergy might directly induce cardiac remodeling. *J Am Coll Cardiol.* 2006;47: 969-977.

5. Di Carli MF, Davidson M, Little R, et al. Value of metabolic imaging with positron emission tomography for evaluating prognosis in patients with coronary artery disease and left ventricular dysfunction. *Am J Cardiol.* 1994;73:527-533.

6. Di Carli MF, Asgarzadie F, Schelbert HR, et al. Quantitative relation between myocardial viability and improvement in heart failure symptoms after revascularization in patients with ischemic cardiomyopathy. *Circulation.* 1995;92:3436-3444.

7. Langah R, Spicer K, Gebregziabher M, Gordon L. Effectiveness of prolonged fasting [18]f-FDG PET-CT in the detection of cardiac sarcoidosis. *J Nucl Cardiol.* 2009;16:801-810.

8. Demeure F, Hanin FX, Bol A, et al. A randomized trial on the optimization of ^{18}F-FDG myocardial uptake suppression: implications for vulnerable coronary plaque imaging. *J Nucl Cardiol.* 2014;55:1629-1635.

9. Morooka M, Moroi M, Uno K, et al. Long fasting is effective in inhibiting physiological myocardial ^{18}F-FDG uptake and for evaluating active lesions of cardiac sarcoidosis. *EJNMMI Res.* 2014;4:1.

10. Sperry BW, Oldan JD, Hsich EM, Reynolds JP, Tamarappoo BK. Infectious myocarditis on FDG-PET imaging mimicking sarcoidosis. *J Nucl Cardiol.* 2015;22:840-844.

11. von Olshausen G, Hyafil F, Langwieser N, Laugwitz KL, Schwaiger M, Ibrahim T. Detection of acute inflammatory myocarditis in Epstein Barr virus infection using hybrid ^{18}F-fluoro-deoxyglucose-positron emission tomography/magnetic resonance imaging. *Circulation.* 2014;130:925-926.

12. Garg G, Cohen S, Neches R, Travin MI. Cardiac F-FDG uptake in chagas disease. *J Nucl Cardiol.* 2016 Apr;23(2):321-325.

13. Kouijzer IJ, Vos FJ, Janssen MJ, van Dijk AP, Oyen WJ, Bleeker-Rovers CP. The value of ^{18}F-FDG PET/CT in diagnosing infectious endocarditis. *Eur J Nucl Med Mol Imaging.* 2013;40:1102-1107.

14. Saby L, Laas O, Habib G, et al. Positron emission tomography/computed tomography for diagnosis of prosthetic valve endocarditis: increased valvular ^{18}F-fluorodeoxyglucose uptake as a novel major criterion. *J Am Coll Cardiol.* 2013;61:2374-2382.

CHAPTER 20

Cardiac Catheterization, Cardiac Angiography, and Coronary Blood Flow and Pressure Measurements

Jonathan Afilalo

DIRECTIONS: Choose the one best response to each question.

20-1. The radial artery approach is associated with reduced bleeding complications and increased patient satisfaction. Which of the following factors is not an additional reason to favor the right radial artery approach over the femoral artery approach?

A. Easy access
B. Direct cannulation of left internal mammary artery grafts in patients with prior coronary bypass
C. Most secure hemostasis in fully anticoagulated patients
D. Radial artery occlusion is generally well tolerated
E. Superficial location

20-2. A 68-year-old man with prior reactions to contrast media, history of type 2 diabetes, chronic kidney disease, and left ventricular systolic dysfunction presented to the emergency department with a 2-hour history of retrosternal chest pain. ECG on arrival showed ST-elevation in interior leads, and the patient was emergently taken to the cardiac catheterization laboratory for primary PCI. Which of the following radiographic contrast agents will be preferred in this case?

A. Iodixanol
B. Diatrizoate
C. Iothalamate
D. Metrizoate
E. Iopamidol

20-3. A 75-year-old woman with a prior history of uncontrolled type 2 diabetes and stage IV chronic kidney disease was admitted to the emergency department complaining of central chest pain and dyspnea. Initial ECG showed T-wave inversions in high lateral leads, and biomarkers were above the upper limit of normal. The patient was brought to the catheterization laboratory within 24 hours. Which of the following pharmacologic regimens has recently been demonstrated to perform better than volume loading with normal saline in reducing the risk for contrast-induced nephropathy (CIN)?

A. IV bolus of furosemide immediately before the procedure
B. Continuous IV furosemide infusion throughout the procedure
C. IV mannitol
D. Calcium channel blockers
E. None of the above

20-4. Intracoronary optical coherence tomography (OCT) is a catheter-based optical imaging modality that produces high-resolution cross-sectional images of the coronary wall. OCT has superior resolution as compared to intravascular ultrasound (IVUS) for all of the following features of the vulnerable plaque, *except*:

A. Plaque rupture
B. Thin-capped fibroatheroma
C. Macrophages within the fibrous caps
D. Plaque burden
E. Intracoronary thrombus

20-5. Myocardial blood flow has been assessed angiographically using the thrombolysis in myocardial infarction (TIMI) score for qualitative grading of coronary flow. Which of the following TIMI flow grades is *false*?

A. Flow equal to that in noninfarct arteries (TIMI-3)
B. Delayed or sluggish antegrade flow with complete filling of the distal coronary bed (TIMI-2)
C. Filling beyond the culprit lesion but faint antegrade flow with incomplete filling of the distal coronary bed (TIMI-1)
D. No flow beyond the occlusion (TIMI-0)
E. Flow faster than that in noninfarct arteries (TIMI-4)

20-6. Unlike fractional flow reserve (FFR), coronary flow reserve (CFR) is subject to variations in hemodynamics that may alter resting flow and limit maximal hyperemic flow. Which of the following clinical situations *cannot* affect CFR?

A. Tachycardia
B. Dyslipidemia
C. Diabetes
D. Age
E. Hypertension

20-7. An 85-year-old woman with a prior history of poorly controlled type 2 diabetes presented to the emergency department complaining of a 2-hour duration substernal chest pain and dyspnea. The initial ECG showed ST-elevation in the high lateral leads. The physical examination revealed a harsh, pansystolic murmur, loudest at the apex and radiating to the axilla. The patient was brought to the cardiac catheterization laboratory, and the left ventricular (LV) and left atrial (LA) pressure tracings are illustrated in Figure 20-1. In which of the following conditions may large *v* waves *not* be present?

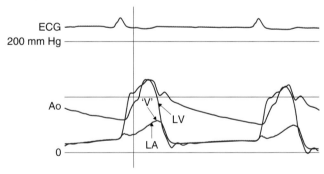

FIGURE 20-1 Left ventricular (LV) and left atrial (LA) pressures showing large V wave.

A. Mitral regurgitation
B. Postcardiac surgery
C. Infiltrative heart disease
D. Mitral stenosis
E. None of the above

20-8. Thermodilution and Fick techniques are the most commonly used methods to assess cardiac output in the cardiac catheterization laboratory. In which of the following clinical scenarios will the thermal dilution cardiac output be unreliable?

A. Severe tricuspid regurgitation
B. Severe pulmonary regurgitation
C. VSD with significant left-to-right shunt
D. Left ventricular heart failure with low output
E. All of the above

20-9. Valvular or vascular obstruction produces a pressure gradient across a stenosis or vascular conduit/chamber narrowing. Which of the following physiologic variables may *not* influence the pressure gradient?

A. Serial lesions
B. Shape of valve orifice
C. Length of valve orifice
D. Proximal chamber pressure
E. None of the above

20-10. In most patients, the pulmonary capillary wedge (PCW) is sufficient to assess LV filling pressure because it closely approximates LA pressure. In which of the following conditions may PCW pressure overestimate LA pressure?

A. Acute respiratory failure
B. Chronic obstructive lung disease with pulmonary hypertension
C. Pulmonary vein stenosis
D. LV failure with volume overload
E. All of the above

20-1. The answer is B. *(Hurst's The Heart, 14th Edition, Chap. 20)* The radial approach is favored for several additional reasons: (1) The radial artery is easily accessible and is not located near significant veins or nerves; (2) the superficial artery location permits rapid and secure compression band hemostasis; (3) the radial artery access provides the most secure hemostasis in fully anticoagulated patients; (4) because of the collateral flow to the hand through the ulnar artery, the rare case of radial artery occlusion is generally well tolerated; and (5) patient comfort is enhanced by the ability to sit up and walk immediately after the procedure. However, the right radial approach is not directly amenable to cannulation of the left internal mammary artery graft for patients with prior coronary bypass.

20-2. The answer is A. *(Hurst's The Heart, 14th Edition, Chap. 20)* The advantages of the nonionic, low-osmolar agents include less hemodynamic loading, less patient discomfort, less depression of myocardial function and blood pressure, and fewer anaphylactoid reactions. Currently, nonionic, low-osmolar agents are routine for nearly all patients, and they are especially helpful in patients with poor LV function, renal disease, diabetes, or prior reactions to contrast media. Iodixanol is a nonionic, iso-osmolar dimer that is particularly well tolerated and used selectively in patients with peripheral arterial procedures and prior contrast reactions. Diatrizoate, iothalamate, and metrizoate (options B, C, and D) are all high-osmolar ionic contrast agents, whereas iopamidol (option E) is a low-osmolar nonionic contrast agent.

20-3. The answer is E. *(Hurst's The Heart, 14th Edition, Chap. 20)* Dehydrated patients or those with diabetes or renal insufficiency are at risk for CIN. Advanced precautions to limit CIN include hydration, minimizing contrast delivered, and maintenance of large-volume urine flow (> 200 mL/h). These patients should be hydrated intravenously the night before the procedure. After the contrast study, intravenous fluids should be liberally continued unless intravascular volume overload is a problem. Furosemide, mannitol, and calcium channel blockers are not helpful in reducing CIN. No pharmacologic regimen has been demonstrated to perform better than volume loading with normal saline (options A, B, C, and D).

20-4. The answer is D. *(Hurst's The Heart, 14th Edition, Chap. 20)* Compared to IVUS, OCT has superior resolution to evaluate certain features of the vulnerable plaque, such as plaque rupture, intracoronary thrombus, thin-capped fibroatheroma, and macrophages within the fibrous caps. For stent placement, OCT can visualize stent malapposition and tissue protrusion after stenting and neointimal hyperplasia at late follow-up. OCT may replace IVUS for certain applications, such as assessing stent deployment. However, compared to IVUS, OCT has inferior depth of penetration and is therefore less suited to assess total plaque burden.

20-5. The answer is E. *(Hurst's The Heart, 14th Edition, Chap. 20)* TIMI flow grades 0 to 3 have become a standard description of angiographic coronary blood flow in clinical trials. There is no TIMI flow grade 4. In acute myocardial infarction trials, TIMI grade 3 flows have been associated with improved clinical outcomes. The four grades of flow are described as follows:[1]

1. Flow equal to that in noninfarct arteries (TIMI-3)
2. Distal flow in the artery less than in noninfarct arteries (TIMI-2)
3. Filling beyond the culprit lesion but no antegrade flow (TIMI-1)
4. No flow beyond the total occlusion (TIMI-0)

20-6. The answer is B. *(Hurst's The Heart, 14th Edition, Chap. 20)* Tachycardia increases basal flow; therefore, CFR is reduced by 10% for every 15 heartbeats.[2] Increasing mean arterial pressure reduces maximal vasodilatation, thus reducing hyperemia with less alteration in basal flow. CFR may be reduced in patients with essential hypertension or aortic stenosis, myocardial ischemia, and diabetes. The variability in CFR in nonobstructed arteries may also be due to age.[3] Dyslipidemia has no direct physiological effect on CFR.

20-7. **The answer is E.** *(Hurst's The Heart, 14th Edition, Chap. 20)* The *v* wave on an LA or PCW pressure tracing usually is associated with significant mitral regurgitation (Fig. 20.1). However, large *v* waves are neither highly sensitive nor specific for mitral regurgitation. Large *v* waves also may be present with mitral stenosis with or without mitral regurgitation or any condition in which the LA volume (eg, VSD or LA pressure relationship [the stiffness or compliance] is increased [such as in rheumatic heart disease, postcardiac surgery, and infiltrative heart diseases]).

20-8. **The answer is E.** *(Hurst's The Heart, 14th Edition, Chap. 20)* If severe tricuspid or pulmonary regurgitation or significant left-to-right shunting is present, the indicator (temperature loss) is attenuated, and the downslope of the temperature curve is prolonged, so the thermal dilution cardiac output will be unreliable. In general, when one uses thermal dilution, a true directional change in cardiac output is reflected by an observed change of ±10%. Thermodilution is also inaccurate in patients with low cardiac output.

20-9. **The answer is E.** *(Hurst's The Heart, 14th Edition, Chap. 20)* The pressure gradient is influenced by physiologic variables such as rate of blood flow (eg, cardiac output, coronary blood flow); resistance to flow; proximal chamber pressure and compliance; and anatomic variables, such as shape and length of valve orifice, tortuosities of the vessels (for arterial stenosis), or multiple or serial lesions (for both cardiac valves and arterial stenosis).

20-10. **The answer is D.** *(Hurst's The Heart, 14th Edition, Chap. 20)* PCW pressure closely approximates LA pressure. PCW pressure overestimates LA pressure in patients with acute respiratory failure, chronic obstructive lung disease with pulmonary hypertension, pulmonary vein stenosis, or LV failure with volume overload.

References

1. Gibson CM, Cannon CP, Daley WL, et al. TIMI frame count: a quantitative method of assessing coronary artery flow. *Circulation*. 1996;93:879-888.
2. McGinn AL, White CW, Wilson RF. Interstudy variability of coronary flow reserve: influence of heart rate, arterial pressure, and ventricular preload. *Circulation*. 1990;81:1319-1330.
3. Baumgart D, Haude M, Liu F, et al. Current concepts of coronary flow reserve for clinical decision making during cardiac catheterization. *Am Heart J*. 1998; 136:136-149.

CHAPTER 21

Coronary Intravascular Imaging

Jonathan Afilalo

QUESTIONS

DIRECTIONS: Choose the one best response to each question.

21-1. The echogenicity and texture of different tissue components may exhibit comparable acoustic properties. Which of the following items may *not* appear as an echolucent intraluminal image?

A. Thrombus
B. Coronary calcification
C. Atheroma with a high lipid content
D. Retained contrast
E. Air bubble

21-2. Most mechanical limitations of IVUS imaging are specific to the construct of each system. Which of the following parameters is a common cause of nonuniform rotation distortion (NURD) artifacts?

A. Tortuosity
B. Small guide lumen size
C. Slack in the catheter shaft
D. Tightened hemostatic valve
E. All of the above

21-3. Studies comparing optical coherence tomography (OCT) with IVUS suggest that time domain (TD)-OCT is safe and can be performed with success rates at least comparable to those of IVUS. Which of the following adverse effects are *not* empirically associated with the OCT procedure?

A. Chest discomfort
B. Tachycardia
C. ST-T changes on electrocardiography (ECG)
D. Decompensated heart failure
E. All of the above

21-4. Some image artifacts are common to both OCT and IVUS. Which of the following artifacts is specific to the new generation of Fourier-domain (FD-OCT) systems?

A. Foldover artifact
B. Sew-up artifact
C. Multiple reflection artifact
D. Saturation artifact
E. Attenuation artifact

21-5. Near-infrared spectroscopy (NIRS) is a new imaging modality able to detect necrotic core invasively. All of the following limitations of NIRS have considerably reduced its application in the clinical arena, *except*:

A. Inability to quantify plaque burden
B. Inability to assess plaque vulnerability
C. Inability to visualize lumen and outer vessel wall
D. Inability to detect neovascularization
E. Inability to detect microcalcification

21-6. Understanding of the structure of a normal coronary artery is essential to identify its pathologic conditions. Which of the following statements about coronary artery wall is *false*?

A. Normal coronary artery wall appears as a three-layer structure on IVUS
B. A trilayered appearance by IVUS suggests the presence of intimal thickening
C. Visualization of the perivascular structures is common with IVUS
D. Visualization of the perivascular structures is not possible with OCT
E. Normal coronary artery wall appears as a three-layer structure on OCT

21-7. The presence, depth, and circumferential distribution of calcification are important factors for selecting the type of interventional device and estimating the risk of vessel dissection and perforation during PCI. Which of the following statements about the detection of calcification is *false*?

A. IVUS can detect the leading edge of calcium as well as determining its thickness
B. IVUS is superior to fluoroscopy at detecting coronary calcification
C. OCT can depict calcification within plaques as well as quantifying calcium burden
D. OCT is superior to IVUS at estimating calcium component and extent
E. OCT can detect superficial microcalcifications

21-8. Pathologic studies have suggested a relationship between positive vessel remodeling and plaque vulnerability. Which of the following parameters is *not* characteristic of vessels with positive remodeling?

A. Paucity of smooth muscle cells
B. Thinner media
C. Thicker cap
D. Larger lipid cores
E. Increased inflammatory marker concentrations

21-9. Several IVUS studies have been performed to define predictors of restenosis after balloon angioplasty. Which of the following processes is the most important mechanism of long-term failures of nonstented coronary interventions?

A. Negative remodeling
B. Positive remodeling
C. Neointima hyperplasia
D. Neointima thickening
E. None of the above

21-10. Several studies have explored the accuracy of intravascular imaging at detecting hemodynamic significant stenosis. Which of the following parameters may *not* affect the hemodynamic implications of a stenotic lesion?

A. The IVUS minimum luminal cross-sectional area (MLA)
B. Length of the stenosis
C. Physiology of the microvascular bed
D. None of the above
E. All of the above

21-1. The answer is B. *(Hurst's The Heart, 14th Edition, Chap. 21)* The similar appearance of different materials represents an inherent limitation of all gray-scale IVUS systems. An echolucent intraluminal image, for instance, may represent thrombus, atheroma with a high lipid content, retained contrast, or an air bubble. Calcified structures are, conversely, very echobright.

21-2. The answer is E. *(Hurst's The Heart, 14th Edition, Chap. 21)* Common causes of NURD are tortuosity; severely stenotic segments; small guide lumen size; and guide catheters with sharp secondary curves, slack in the catheter shaft, or tightened hemostatic valve.

21-3. The answer is D. *(Hurst's The Heart, 14th Edition, Chap. 21)* The most frequent complication with TD-OCT using the occlusive OCT technique is transient chest discomfort, bradycardia or tachycardia, and ST-T changes on ECG, all of which tend to resolve immediately after the procedure.[1] Similar transient events were also seen during IVUS imaging procedures. Decompensated heart failure is not a reported complication of the OCT procedure.

21-4. The answer is A. *(Hurst's The Heart, 14th Edition, Chap. 21)* Foldover artifact is specific to the new generation of FD-OCT systems and is the consequence of the "phase wrapping" or "alias" along the Fourier transformation when structure signals are reflected beyond the field of view. This can occur at the site of bifurcations or in large vessels. Sew-up, multiple reflection, saturation, and attenuation artifacts are common to all intravascular imaging technologies.

21-5. The answer is B. *(Hurst's The Heart, 14th Edition, Chap. 21)* Extensive validation studies suggested that NIRS may be superior to IVUS in detecting lipid-rich plaques, but it has limited accuracy in characterizing their phenotype and detecting fibroatheroma (FA) and thin-cap fibroatheroma (TCFA).[2] Other significant limitations of NIRS that have considerably reduced its application in the clinical arena are its inability to quantify plaque burden, to visualize the lumen and outer vessel wall, and to assess plaque characteristics associated with increased vulnerability, such as plaque erosion, neovascularization, and microcalcification.

21-6. The answer is A. *(Hurst's The Heart, 14th Edition, Chap. 21)* A monolayer appearance is a common finding in normal coronary arteries, but a trilayered appearance by IVUS suggests the presence of intimal thickening.[3] The IVUS beam penetrates beyond the adventitial layer, allowing visualization of the perivascular structures, including the cardiac veins and the pericardium. In contrast, the normal coronary artery wall (< 1.5 mm thick) appears as a three-layer structure on OCT, but imaging beyond the adventitial layer is not possible.

21-7. The answer is A. *(Hurst's The Heart, 14th Edition, Chap. 21)* IVUS detects only the leading edge of calcium and cannot determine its thickness. Thus, calcification on IVUS is usually described based on its circumferential angle (arc), longitudinal length, and depth. IVUS has shown significantly higher sensitivity than fluoroscopy in the detection of coronary calcification.[4] OCT can depict calcification within plaques as well-delineated, low-backscattering heterogeneous regions. In addition to circumferential angulation, depth, and longitudinal length, OCT can quantify calcium burden. OCT allows more accurate estimation of the calcium component than IVUS, which significantly underestimates its extent.[5] Superficial microcalcifications can also be identified on OCT images as small calcific deposits separated from the lumen by a thin tissue layer.

21-8. The answer is C. *(Hurst's The Heart, 14th Edition, Chap. 21)* Vessels with positive remodeling showed increased inflammatory marker concentrations, larger lipid cores, a paucity of smooth muscle cells, and medial thinning.[6,7]

21-9. The answer is A. *(Hurst's The Heart, 14th Edition, Chap. 21)* One of the main contributions of intravascular imaging to this field was the realization that negative remodeling, not neointimal hyperplasia, was the most important mechanism of long-term failures of nonstented coronary interventions, namely restenosis. This was initially demonstrated in the peripheral vessels and later reported in the coronary circulation.[8] These studies revealed that more than 70% of lumen loss was attributable to the decrease in external elastic membrane (EEM) area; the neointima accounted for only 23% of the loss.

21-10. The answer is D. *(Hurst's The Heart, 14th Edition, Chap. 21)* The limited value of intravascular imaging in detecting flow-limiting lesions should be attributed to the fact that the hemodynamic implications of a stenosis depend not only on MLA but also on the length of the stenosis and the physiology of the microvascular bed, which cannot be assessed by imaging techniques.

References

1. Yamaguchi T, Terashima M, Akasaka T, et al. Safety and feasibility of an intravascular optical coherence tomography image wire system in the clinical setting. *Am J Cardiol.* 2008;101(5):562-567.
2. Kang SJ, Mintz GS, Pu J, et al. Combined IVUS and NIRS detection of fibroatheromas: histopathological validation in human coronary arteries. *JACC Cardiovasc Imaging.* 2015;8(2):184-194.
3. Davies MJ. Anatomic features in victims of sudden coronary death. Coronary artery pathology. *Circulation.* 1992;85(1 Suppl):I19-I24.
4. Mintz GS, Popma JJ, Pichard AD, et al. Patterns of calcification in coronary artery disease. A statistical analysis of intravascular ultrasound and coronary angiography in 1155 lesions. *Circulation.* 1995;91(7):1959-1965.
5. Kume T, Okura H, Kawamoto T, et al. Assessment of the coronary calcification by optical coherence tomography. *EuroIntervention.* 2011;6(6):768-772.
6. Pant R, Marok R, Klein LW. Pathophysiology of coronary vascular remodeling: relationship with traditional risk factors for coronary artery disease. *Cardiol Rev.* 2014;22(1):13-16.
7. Burke AP, Kolodgie FD, Farb A, Weber D, Virmani R. Morphological predictors of arterial remodeling in coronary atherosclerosis. *Circulation.* 2002;105(3):297-303.
8. Kimura T, Kaburagi S, Tamura T, et al. Remodeling of human coronary arteries undergoing coronary angioplasty or atherectomy. *Circulation.* 1997;96(2):475-483.

CHAPTER 22

Magnetic Resonance Imaging and Computed Tomography of the Vascular System

Jonathan Afilalo

QUESTIONS

DIRECTIONS: Choose the one best response to each question.

22-1. A rare, albeit serious, risk of contrast-enhanced magnetic resonance angiography (CE-MRA) is the association between gadolinium-based contrast agents and nephrogenic systemic fibrosis. In which of the following scenarios may the linear chelates of gadolinium be considered safe?

A. Chronic renal impairment with eGFR < 30 mL/m²
B. Acute renal impairment
C. Perioperative liver transplantation
D. Neonates
E. Severe heart failure

22-2. Before the advent of CE-MRA, nonenhanced magnetic resonance time of flight (TOF) imaging acquisitions were used to image the carotid arteries, demonstrating good agreement with digital subtraction angiography (DSA). Which of the following statements about the limitations of TOF imaging is *false*?

A. It is sensitive to turbulent flow
B. It tends to underestimate the severity of stenoses
C. It has long acquisition times
D. It increases the potential for motion artifacts
E. None of the above

22-3. A 67-year-old man with a prior history of uncontrolled hypertension presented to the emergency department complaining of an acute-onset excruciating and sharp retrosternal chest pain while watching a football game on television. Initial ECG revealed normal sinus rhythm with nonspecific ST changes in the lateral leads. Cardiac biomarkers were within normal limits, and a chest radiography showed moderate mediastinal widening. Which of the following imaging modalities has the highest sensitivity and specificity for detecting this condition?

A. MRI
B. Retrograde invasive aortography
C. Transthoracic echocardiography
D. Transesophageal echocardiography
E. They all have the same sensitivity and specificity for detecting this condition

22-4. Thoracic aortic aneurysms (TAAs) are typically discovered in asymptomatic patients, with symptoms occurring in the setting of either a complication of the disease (eg, a rupture or dissection) or when these complications are imminent. Which of the following statements about the recommendations for surgery is *false*?

A. Diameter of the ascending aorta > 50 mm is the threshold for degenerative aneurysm
B. Diameter of the ascending aorta > 50 mm is the threshold for aneurysm associated with bicuspid aortic valve
C. Diameter of the ascending aorta > 50 mm is the threshold for aneurysm associated with Marfan disease
D. Thresholds can be lowered in case of rapid expansion of TAA (> 5 mm/y)
E. Thresholds can be lowered in select connective tissue diseases (eg, Loeys-Dietz syndrome)

22-5. A 77-year-old man with a prior history of hypertension, type 2 diabetes, and a 150-pack-per-year tobacco smoking habit presented to his cardiologist for a health maintenance examination. He has been feeling generally well and has no particular complaints or concerns. On physical examination, there was an extensive palpable pulsatile abdominal mass. Which of the following represents the preferred imaging modality for preoperative evaluation of abdominal aortic aneurysms (AAA) before open or endovascular surgery?

A. CTA
B. Ultrasonography
C. TOF sequences MRI
D. CE-MRA
E. Digital subtraction angiography

22-6. A 55-year-old man with a prior history of poorly controlled type 2 diabetes, hypertension, and a 100-pack-per-year tobacco smoking habit, presented to the emergency department with a 6-month history of leg pain upon exertion. He noticed that he had bilateral calf pain (worse on the left) with walking and that it tended to go away when he stopped walking. Which of the following is the best initial investigation for this patient's complaint?

A. Ultrasound imaging
B. Ankle brachial pressure index
C. CTA
D. TOF imaging
E. CE-MRA

22-7. The diagnostic accuracy of CTA for the evaluation of peripheral vessels compares well with MRA and invasive angiography. Which of the following clinical settings does *not* represent one of the main clinical indications of CTA for imaging the lower extremities?

A. Evaluation of arterial and aneurysmal disease
B. Evaluation of patency and integrity of bypass grafts
C. Traumatic arterial injury
D. Acute ischemia
E. None of the above

22-8. Plaques that are at high risk for rupture represent a potential imaging target for identifying vulnerable patients likely to develop unstable manifestations of their atherosclerotic disease. Which of the following features is *not* a key characteristic of vulnerable plaques?

A. A fibrous cap with thickness between 65 µm and 85 µm
B. Few smooth muscle cells
C. Heavy infiltrate of inflammatory cells
D. Microcalcification
E. Large necrotic core

22-9. A key advantage of MRI of the vasculature is the soft-tissue contrast it provides, allowing detailed examination of the composition of individual atherosclerotic plaques. Which of the following features of atherosclerotic plaques *cannot* be directly assessed by MRI?

A. Intraplaque hemorrhage
B. Calcification
C. Luminal thrombosis
D. Angiogenesis
E. Fibrous cap

22-10. ^{18}F-fluoride is a PET tracer increasingly being used to measure the activity of calcific processes in the vasculature. Which of the following statements about ^{18}F-fluoride is *false*?

A. Preferentially binds regions of vascular microcalcification activity
B. The sensitivity of ^{18}F-fluoride/PET is superior to CT for detecting vascular microcalcification
C. Can identify patients with increased metabolic activity in their coronary arteries
D. Can prospectively identify the individual lesions responsible for coronary events
E. None of the above

22-1. The answer is E. *(Hurst's The Heart, 14th Edition, Chap. 22)* Different gadolinium contrast agents have been divided into low, medium, and high risk for causing nephrogenic systemic fibrosis[1] by the European Medicines Agency. High-risk agents include the linear chelates of gadolinium, and these are contraindicated in patients with an eGFR < 30 mL/m^2, acute renal impairment, and perioperative liver transplantation, as well as in neonates. Low-risk agents include newer cyclic preparations of gadolinium. These are considered safe in patients with an eGFR of more than 30 mL/m^2, and they can be used in patients with an eGFR below this threshold if the benefit of undergoing contrast MRI outweighs the risk. The volume of contrast agent used in this case should be minimized and repetition within 7 days avoided.[2] Gadolinium contrast agents are routinely used, and known to be safe, in the evaluation of patients with (often severe) forms of heart failure.

22-2. The answer is B. *(Hurst's The Heart, 14th Edition, Chap. 22)* TOF acquisitions are sensitive to turbulent flow, can overestimate stenoses, and have long acquisition times, increasing potential motion artifacts.[2] Although TOF MRA remains useful for patients with contraindications to MRI contrast, such as renal insufficiency, CE-MRA has become the technique of choice for imaging the carotid arteries.

22-3. The answer is A. *(Hurst's The Heart, 14th Edition, Chap. 22)* Of all the imaging techniques, MRI has the highest sensitivity and specificity for detecting aortic dissection (98%).[4] However, the use of MRI for the detection of aortic dissection is limited by its lack of availability in urgent situations and by the difficulty of monitoring and managing critically ill patients in the MRI scanner. Therefore, CTA is now considered the mainstay for the accurate and timely diagnosis of acute aortic syndromes.[5] Retrograde invasive aortography has an overall sensitivity of 88% and specificity of 94% for the detection of aortic dissection.[6,7] Transesophageal echocardiography, like CTA and MRA, has demonstrated high accuracy for the diagnosis of aortic dissection and is an alternative diagnostic technique.[8] Transthoracic echocardiography can, in most cases, visualize the aortic root and proximal ascending aorta, but it is not sufficiently comprehensive to rule out this diagnosis.

22-4. The answer is A. *(Hurst's The Heart, 14th Edition, Chap. 22)* When the diameter of the ascending aorta is > 55 mm for degenerative aneurysm (option A) and > 50 mm for aneurysm associated with bicuspid aortic valve (option B) or Marfan disease (option C), surgery is recommended.[9] These thresholds can be lowered in case of rapid expansion of TAA (> 5 mm/y) or in select connective tissue diseases (eg, Loeys–Dietz syndrome) (options D and E).

22-5. The answer is A. *(Hurst's The Heart, 14th Edition, Chap. 22)* Preoperative assessment of AAAs before open or endovascular repair should include determination of the maximum transverse diameter; the relation of the AAA to the renal arteries; the length, diameter, and angulation of the normal-caliber aorta below the renal arteries before the aneurysm (ie, the infrarenal neck); the presence of iliac or hypogastric aneurysms; and serious occlusive disease in the iliac or renal arteries. CTA represents the preferred imaging modality for preoperative evaluation of AAAs before open or endovascular surgery because it allows precise assessment of each of the aforementioned parameters. Ultrasonography remains the most cost-effective imaging technique for detection and follow-up of abdominal AAA expansion. MRI (TOF sequences, CE-MRA) represents an alternative to CTA for the preoperative evaluation of AAA, particularly in cases of renal insufficiency or advanced arterial calcification, although attention should be paid to the risk of developing nephrogenic systemic fibrosis following gadolinium administration in patients with the former. Digital subtraction angiography (DSA) has been largely replaced by the preceding imaging modalities.

22-6. The answer is B. *(Hurst's The Heart, 14th Edition, Chap. 22)* The most common initial investigation in patients presenting with suspected peripheral arterial disease is the ankle brachial pressure index. This is the ratio of the systolic blood pressure measured at the ankle to that measured at the brachial artery. An ankle brachial pressure index of 0.90 or less should then prompt further investigation to confirm a diagnosis of peripheral artery disease. This is commonly performed with either CTA or MRA.[10]

22-7. The answer is E. *(Hurst's The Heart, 14th Edition, Chap. 22)* The main clinical indications of CTA for imaging the lower extremities include the evaluation of arterial and aneurysmal disease, patency and integrity of bypass grafts, traumatic arterial injury, and acute ischemia.[11]

22-8. The answer is A. *(Hurst's The Heart, 14th Edition, Chap. 22)* Plaques that are at high risk for rupture usually have several key characteristics, consisting of a thin fibrous cap (< 65 μm) with few smooth muscle cells and a heavy infiltrate of inflammatory cells, principally macrophages, microcalcification, and a large necrotic core accounting for more than half of the volume of the plaque. Each of these characteristics therefore represents a potential imaging target for identifying high-risk plaques.

22-9. The answer is B. *(Hurst's The Heart, 14th Edition, Chap. 22)* MRI is useful in detecting intraplaque hemorrhage (option A), a process believed to play a key role in triggering plaque rupture and growth.[12] T2*-weighted sequences have been used to accurately image intraplaque hemorrhage in carotid atherosclerotic plaques.[13,14] Plaque hemorrhage and luminal thrombosis can also be detected on T1-weighted imaging as high-intensity plaques (option C).[15,16] Late gadolinium enhancement detects areas of interstitial edema, angiogenesis, and fibrosis (option D).[17] Late gadolinium enhancement can also improve the visualization of the atherosclerotic fibrous cap, allowing estimation of the carotid cap thickness and the size of its necrotic core (option E).[18] Given that calcification is hypointense on the various MRI sequences, plaque calcification is better assessed by CT and other modalities (option B).

22-10. The answer is D. *(Hurst's The Heart, 14th Edition, Chap. 22)* ^{18}F-fluoride[19-20] preferentially binds regions of vascular microcalcification activity.[21] These are beyond the resolution of CT, a technique that instead detects macroscopic calcium deposits. ^{18}F-fluoride can identify patients with increased metabolic activity in their coronary arteries, and it retrospectively appears to identify the individual lesions responsible for coronary events.[22]

References

1. Daftari Besheli L, Aran S, Shaqdan K, Kay J, Abujudeh H. Current status of nephrogenic systemic fibrosis. *Clin Radiol.* 2014;69:661-668.
2. Thomsen HS, Morcos SK, Almén T, et al. Nephrogenic systemic fibrosis and gadolinium-based contrast media: updated ESUR Contrast Medium Safety Committee guidelines. *Eur Radiol.* 2013;23:307-318.
3. Carriero A, Scarabino T, Magarelli N, et al. High-resolution magnetic resonance angiography of the internal carotid artery: 2D vs 3D TOF in stenotic disease. *Eur Radiol.* 1998;8:1370-1372.
4. Erbel R, Aboyans V, Boileau C, et al. 2014 ESC Guidelines on the diagnosis and treatment of aortic diseases: Document covering acute and chronic aortic diseases of the thoracic and abdominal aorta of the adult. The Task Force for the Diagnosis and Treatment of Aortic Diseases of the European Society of Cardiology (ESC). *Eur Heart J.* 2014;35:2873-2926.
5. LePage MA, Quint LE, Sonnad SS, Deeb GM, Williams DM. Aortic dissection: CT features that distinguish true lumen from false lumen. *AJR Am J Roentgenol.* 2001;177: 207-211.
6. Rizzo RJ, Aranki SF, Aklog L, et al. Rapid noninvasive diagnosis and surgical repair of acute ascending aortic dissection. Improved survival with less angiography. *J Thorac Cardiovasc Surg.* 1994;108:567-574–discussion 574-575.
7. Petasnick JP. Radiologic evaluation of aortic dissection. *Radiology.* 1991;180:297-305.
8. Shiga T, Wajima Z, Apfel CC, Inoue T, Ohe Y. Diagnostic accuracy of transesophageal echocardiography, helical computed tomography, and magnetic resonance imaging for suspected thoracic aortic dissection: systematic review and meta-analysis. *Arch Internal Med.* 2006;166:1350-1356.

9. Goldfinger JZ, Halperin JL, Marin ML, Stewart AS, Eagle KA, Fuster V. Thoracic aortic aneurysm and dissection. *J Am Coll Cardiol.* 2014;64:1725-1739.

10. Aboyans V, Criqui MH, Abraham P, et al. Measurement and interpretation of the ankle-brachial index: a scientific statement from the American Heart Association. *Circulation.* 2012;126:2890-2909.

11. Rubin GD, Leipsic J, Joseph Schoepf U, Fleischmann D, Napel S. CT angiography after 20 years: a transformation in cardiovascular disease characterization continues to advance. *Radiology.* 2014;271:633-652.

12. Kolodgie FD, Gold HK, Burke AP, et al. Intraplaque hemorrhage and progression of coronary atheroma. *N Engl J Med.* 2003;349:2316-2325.

13. Chu B, Kampschulte A, Ferguson MS, et al. Hemorrhage in the atherosclerotic carotid plaque: a high-resolution MRI study. *Stroke.* 2004;35:1079-1084.

14. Takaya N, Yuan C, Chu B, et al. Presence of intraplaque hemorrhage stimulates progression of carotid atherosclerotic plaques: a high-resolution magnetic resonance imaging study. *Circulation.* 2005;111:2768-2775.

15. Noguchi T, Yamada N, Higashi M, Goto Y, Naito H. High-intensity signals in carotid plaques on T1-weighted magnetic resonance imaging predict coronary events in patients with coronary artery disease. *J Am Coll Cardiol.* 2011;58:416-422.

16. Saam T, Hetterich H, Hoffmann V, et al. Meta-analysis and systematic review of the predictive value of carotid plaque hemorrhage on cerebrovascular events by magnetic resonance imaging. *J Am Coll Cardiol.* 2013;62:1081-1091.

17. Kerwin WS, O'Brien KD, Ferguson MS, Polissar N, Hatsukami TS, Yuan C. Inflammation in carotid atherosclerotic plaque: a dynamic contrast-enhanced MR imaging study. *Radiology.* 2006;241:459-468.

18. Cai J, Hatsukami TS, Ferguson MS, et al. In vivo quantitative measurement of intact fibrous cap and lipid-rich necrotic core size in atherosclerotic carotid plaque: comparison of high-resolution, contrast-enhanced magnetic resonance imaging and histology. *Circulation.* 2005;112:3437-3444.

19. Dweck MR, Chow MWL, Joshi NV, et al. Coronary arterial ^{18}F-sodium fluoride uptake. *J Am Coll Cardiol.* 2012;59:1539-1548.

20. Jenkins WSA, Vesey AT, Shah ASV, et al. Valvular (18)F-fluoride and (18)F fluorodeoxyglucose uptake predict disease progression and clinical outcome in patients with aortic stenosis. *J Am Coll Cardiol.* 2015;66:1200-1201.

21. Irkle A, Vesey AT, Lewis DY, et al. Identifying active vascular microcalcification by ^{18}F-sodium fluoride positron emission tomography. *Nat Commun.* 2015;6:1-11.

22. Joshi NV, Vesey AT, Williams MC, et al. ^{18}F-fluoride positron emission tomography for identification of ruptured and high-risk coronary atherosclerotic plaques: a prospective clinical trial. *Lancet.* 2014;383:705-713.

SECTION 4

Systemic Arterial Hypertension

CHAPTER 23

Epidemiology of Hypertension

Jacqueline Joza

QUESTIONS

DIRECTIONS: Choose the one best response to each question.

23-1. A 48-year-old man presents in follow-up to your outpatient clinic. He has no comorbidities apart from right knee osteoarthritis and obesity. His blood pressure on his initial visit with you was 136/86 mm Hg. After losing 5 lb, today's blood pressure is 132/80 mm Hg. This patient's blood pressure can be labeled:

A. White coat hypertension
B. Benign hypertension
C. Isolated systolic hypertension
D. Prehypertension
E. Pseudohypertension

23-2. Which of the following statements about prehypertension is *false*?

A. The lifetime risk of hypertension approaches 50%, warranting the importance of recognizing the concept of prehypertension to promote lifestyle changes to prevent the onset of hypertension
B. In persons without cardiovascular disease or cancer, the prevalence of prehypertension is 36%, and it is higher in men than in women
C. Prehypertension is associated with abnormalities of cardiac structure and function
D. Approximately 15% of BP-related deaths from coronary heart disease occur in individuals with BP in the prehypertensive range
E. Persons with prehypertension have a 43% higher risk of incident coronary heart disease than those with optimal blood pressure (< 120/80 mm Hg)

23-3. A 56-year-old woman is referred to you for workup of glaucoma. Despite her blood pressure being normal in your office, her home readings have all been above 135/85 mm Hg. Regarding this particular type of hypertension, which of the following is *true*?

A. It is present in approximately 5% of patients not receiving antihypertensive treatment
B. There is a twofold greater risk of future cardiovascular events in those with this type of hypertension as compared to normotensive persons
C. Home BP monitoring is the standard for diagnosing this type of hypertension
D. It is more common in younger persons
E. Persons with prehypertension are less likely to have this type of hypertension

23-4. A 65-year-old man is referred to you from his family physician for the management of hypertension. On history, he admits to snoring when sleeping and describes daytime fatigue. On exam, BP in both arms is 164/98, HR 86 O^2 sat 96% on RA. Normal heart sounds are present, and lungs are clear to auscultation. Which of the following statements is *false*?

A. The most common curable form of hypertension is sleep apnea
B. Treatment with a CPAP mask is most likely indicated
C. Both sleep apnea and hypertension are closely linked to obesity
D. Approximately 60% of sleep apnea patients are hypertensive
E. Approximately 25% of hypertensive patients have sleep apnea

23-5. There is a fundamental difference between the genesis of hypertension in younger and older patients. Which of the following does *not* represent a true difference?

A. In general, the systolic and diastolic BPs are increased in younger patients, whereas in people aged 60 years and older, the diastolic BP starts to fall, but there is a marked increase in systolic BP

B. Younger patients will have an increased peripheral resistance with a normal cardiac output, whereas older patients will have a selective increase of systolic BP as a result of increased arterial stiffness

C. In younger patients, the increased peripheral resistance is a result of active vasoconstriction that is mediated hormonally, particularly by the sympathetic nervous system and the renin-angiotensin system

D. The benefits of treatment in older patients with systolic pressures below 160 mm Hg remain unproven

E. There is some evidence for BP treatment of the very old (age 85 years or older) to improve mortality

23-6. You are going to counsel your 55-year-old female patient on her risk factors for hypertension. Which of the following statements is *false*?

A. The diastolic pressure will typically increase up to the age of 50, will plateau, and then will decrease throughout the remainder of the life span

B. Increasing body mass index correlates with an increased risk of hypertension

C. The incidence of hypertension is increased in those who smoke 15 or more cigarettes per day

D. There is a strong positive relation between sodium intake and blood pressure

E. Mexican Americans have prevalences that are similar to that of African Americans

23-7. The principal complications of hypertension include all of the following *except*:

A. Left ventricular hypertrophy
B. Peripheral arterial disease
C. Hypothyroidism
D. Stroke
E. Heart failure

23-8. A 58-year-old woman with a history of untreated hypertension presents to your office to discuss the results of her cardiac echocardiogram. Which of the following would be the least likely to be found on her echocardiogram report?

A. Diastolic dysfunction
B. Tricuspid valve regurgitation
C. Increased left atrial size
D. Systolic dysfunction
E. Left ventricular hypertrophy

23-9. Which of the following statements regarding stroke and hypertension is *incorrect*?

A. The linear relationship between stroke and hypertension is stronger for diastolic than for systolic pressure

B. BP typically rises acutely after a stroke, and it is postulated that this helps to maintain cerebral perfusion in the infarct's *penumbra* zone

C. Of all the risk factors for stroke, hypertension has the highest relative risk

D. Hypertension indirectly raises the risk of stroke through its role in atrial fibrillation and left atrial enlargement

E. Treatment of hypertension reduces stroke rates by approximately 35% to 45%

23-10. Your 65-year-old female patient presents to the office to discuss the results of her blood work. You have been treating her for hypertension over the last 10 years. Her creatinine has risen slightly, and you are concerned. Which of the following statements is *true*?

A. There is a twofold greater risk for end-stage renal disease with a systolic BP of > 140 mm Hg compared to a systolic BP of < 117 mm Hg

B. Chronic kidney disease causes remodeling of the arteries and increased stiffness

C. Hypertensive patients with mildly impaired renal function (estimated GFR < 60 mL/min) compared to normal renal function have an equivalent prevalence of target organ damage

D. Diastolic BP is a stronger risk factor for renal death than systolic BP

E. In a patient with chronic kidney disease, it is obvious whether the hypertension or the kidney disease came first

23-1. The answer is D. *(Hurst's The Heart, 14th Edition, Chap. 23).* The Joint National Committee on Prevention, Detection, Evaluation, and Treatment of High Blood Pressure (JNC) 7 classification for hypertension has defined normal BP as < 120 and < 80 mm Hg. What JNC-6 previously labeled as normal (120–129 mm Hg systolic BP or 80–84 mm Hg diastolic BP) and high normal (130–139 mm Hg systolic BP or 85–89 mm Hg diastolic BP) are now combined into a single group called *prehypertension* (option D), to increase the awareness of people with an intermediate level of risk that they may progress to definite hypertension. *White coat hypertension* (or *isolated office hypertension*) (option A) is diagnosed in patients not on any BP-lowering medications when the BP is elevated only persistently in the presence of a health care worker, particularly a physician. *Benign* hypertension, which alluded to less severe forms of hypertension, is a misnomer and is no longer used (option B). When the average systolic BP is at least 140 mm Hg or more and diastolic BP is < 90 mm Hg, the patient is classified as isolated systolic hypertensive (option C). The term *pseudohypertension* (option E) refers to a falsely elevated diastolic BP when in fact it is low. This condition represents wide pulse pressure isolated systolic hypertension in the elderly and often occurs with diabetes and diabetic kidney disease; it is associated with extensive calcification of many large arteries, including the brachial and elastic aorta.

23-2. The answer is A. *(Hurst's The Heart, 14th Edition, Chap. 23).* The lifetime risk of hypertension approaches 90%[1] (not 50%), which emphasizes the need to recognize prehypertension to help motivate physicians and patients alike to promote lifestyle modifications that will prevent or delay the transition to clinical hypertension. Data from the National Health and Nutrition Examination Survey (NHANES) 1999–2006 in persons without cardiovascular disease (CVD) or cancer shows a prevalence of prehypertension of 36.3%, higher in men than in women, and associated with adverse cardiometabolic risk factors[2] (option B). Prehypertension has recently been shown to be associated with abnormalities of cardiac structure and function, specifically increased left ventricular remodeling and impaired diastolic function[3] (option C). It is estimated that about 15% of BP–related deaths from coronary heart disease (CHD) occur in persons with BP in the prehypertensive range[4] (option D). A recent meta-analysis showed that, compared with optimal blood pressure (< 120/80 mm Hg), those with prehypertension had a 43% higher risk of incident CHD (hazard ratio [HR], 1.43; 95% confidence interval [CI], 1.26–1.63) a risk that was higher in Western subjects (relative risk [RR], 1.70; 95% CI, 1.49–1.94) than in Asian subjects (RR, 1.25; 95% CI, 1.12–1.38), with 24.1% of CHD attributable to prehypertension in Western subjects versus 8.4% in Asian subjects[5] (option E).

23-3. The answer is B. *(Hurst's The Heart, 14th Edition, Chap. 23).* The question refers to a patient with a diagnosis of *masked hypertension*, which is defined as a normal office BP (< 140/90 mm Hg) together with an elevated daytime BP (≥ 135/85 mm Hg). The Dallas Heart Study also showed a twofold greater risk of future cardiovascular events in those with masked hypertension compared to those who were normotensive.[6] Option A is false: masked hypertension is present in approximately 10% to 40% of patients not receiving antihypertensive treatment. Option C is false: Twenty-four-hour ambulatory BP monitoring is the standard for diagnosing masked hypertension; home BP monitoring can also be used, but it is not the standard. Masked hypertension is more common in older persons; those with mental stress; smokers; and those with metabolic syndrome, diabetes, chronic kidney disease, and obstructive sleep apnea (option D). Persons with prehypertension are *more* likely to have masked hypertension and can even develop target organ damage before transitioning to established sustained hypertension (option E).

23-4. The answer is A. *(Hurst's The Heart, 14th Edition, Chap. 23).* The most common curable form of hypertension is renal artery stenosis (not sleep apnea). Sleep apnea is emerging as one of the major causes of hypertension that is of epidemiologic significance. Support for a causal association between sleep-disordered breathing and hypertension includes physiological mechanisms involving vascular dysfunction secondary to altered sympathovagal balance and insulin resistance (option B). Both sleep apnea and hypertension are common, and unsurprisingly there are many people with both conditions. Furthermore, both are closely linked to obesity (particularly central obesity, as seen in the metabolic syndrome), so there is a cluster of related syndromes: hypertension, sleep apnea, diabetes, and the metabolic syndrome (option C). Option D: Approximately 60% of sleep apnea patients are hypertensive[7], and, conversely, approximately 25% of hypertensive patients have sleep apnea[8,9] (option E).

23-5. **The answer is E.** *(Hurst's The Heart, 14th Edition, Chap. 23).* There is evidence that in the very old (age 85 years or older), mortality may be *higher* in those with the lowest blood pressures.[10] The benefit or harm of treating this patient population is currently being evaluated. In younger patients, whatever the underlying etiology of the hypertension (with a few exceptions), both systolic and diastolic BPs are raised, whereas in people aged 60 years and older, the diastolic BP starts to fall, but there is a marked increase of systolic BP (option A). The underlying hemodynamics are also different: in younger patients, the characteristic changes are an increased peripheral resistance with a normal cardiac output, whereas in older patients, the reason for the selective increase of systolic BP is increased arterial stiffness[11] (option B). In younger patients, the increased peripheral resistance is a result of active vasoconstriction that is mediated hormonally, particularly by the sympathetic nervous system and the renin-angiotensin system. In older patients with systolic hypertension, hormonal mediation is less important, and the changes are mostly mechanical (eg, loss of elastin fibers in the media of the arterial wall[11] (option C). In younger patients, it is clearly established that starting drug treatment when the pressure exceeds 140/90 mm Hg is beneficial. This may also be true in older patients, but the clinical trials that have investigated the benefits of treatment have almost all used an initial systolic BP of 160 mm Hg or greater as an entry criterion and have not lowered the pressure to below 140 or 150 mm Hg[12] (option D).

23-6. **The answer is E.** *(Hurst's The Heart, 14th Edition, Chap. 23).* African Americans have among the highest prevalences of hypertension compared to other major ethnic groups, and Mexican Americans have prevalences that are similar to that of whites. Age is the factor most strongly associated with hypertension. Systolic BP rises monotonically with age, whereas diastolic BP increases to about age 50, plateaus, and then decreases throughout the remainder of the life span (option A). More than 42% of those with a body mass index of 30 kg/m^2 or greater have hypertension, compared to 28% in those who are overweight (body mass index 25 to less than 30 kg/m^2)[13,14] (option B). Cigarette smoking has an acute effect on increasing blood pressure, primarily through stimulation of the sympathetic nervous system, with adverse effects on arterial stiffness and wave reflection (option C). Dietary sodium is implicated by many genetic, epidemiological, migrational, and intervention studies to contribute to increasing BP in the population, and higher salt intake is likely to contribute to coronary vascular disease mainly through its effects on BP but also independently by increasing arterial stiffness and albuminuria[15] (option D). The INTERSALT study involved 10,079 persons and found a strong positive relation between sodium intake and BP, with an increase of 6 g/d in salt intake estimated to elevate systolic BP 9 mm Hg over 30 years.[16]

23-7. **The answer is C.** *(Hurst's The Heart, 14th Edition, Chap. 23).* The principal complications of hypertension include coronary heart disease, left ventricular hypertrophy (option A), peripheral arterial disease (option B), stroke (option D), heart failure (option E), and chronic kidney disease. The 36-year follow-up data from the Framingham Heart Study show that while the relative impact of hypertension is greatest for stroke and heart failure (RRs, 2.6–4.0), because the overall incidence of CHD is greater than that for stroke or heart failure, the absolute impact of hypertension on CHD is greatest, even though the RR is lower (2.0–2.2).[17]

23-8. **The answer is B.** *(Hurst's The Heart, 14th Edition, Chap. 23)* There is no direct association between tricuspid regurgitation and systemic hypertension (option A). Approximately half of the patients who present with classic signs and symptoms of heart failure appear to have a normal ejection fraction of more than 50% on echocardiography, termed "diastolic dysfunction," diastolic heart failure," or "heart failure with preserved ejection fraction." Diastolic heart failure is thought to be responsible for as many as 74% of cases of heart failure in hypertensive patients.[18] Left ventricular hypertrophy (option E) and systolic dysfunction and heart failure (option D) are known complications of hypertension. Increased left atrial size (option C) associated with left ventricular hypertrophy can result with systemic hypertension.

23-9. **The answer is A.** *(Hurst's The Heart, 14th Edition, Chap. 23)* As with coronary events, there is a strong log-linear relationship between both systolic and diastolic pressure and stroke, although the relationship is steeper for strokes than for CHD events and much stronger for systolic than diastolic pressure.[19] BP typically rises acutely after a stroke, and it is postulated that this helps to maintain cerebral perfusion in the infarct's *penumbra* zone (option B).[20] This forms the rationale for avoiding excessive reduction of BP immediately after a stroke. Of all the risk factors for stroke, hypertension has the highest relative risk (4.0 at 40 to 50 years, falling to 2.0 at ages 70 to 80 years), and the highest population attributable risk (40% at ages 40 to 50 years and 30% at ages 70 to 80 years) (option C). Hypertension also indirectly raises the risk of stroke through its role as an important risk factor for atrial fibrillation and left atrial enlargement, which both relate directly to stroke risk (option D). Treatment of hypertension reduces stroke rates by 35% to 44%; this has been shown in both younger patients with systolic and diastolic hypertension and in older patients with isolated systolic hypertension (option E).

23-10. **The answer is B.** *(Hurst's The Heart, 14th Edition, Chap. 23)* There are two main effects of CKD on the arteries: (1) increased prevalence of atherosclerosis and (2) remodeling of the arteries and increased stiffness, which has been related to increased mortality. The Multiple Risk Factor Intervention Trial showed systolic BP of > 140 mm Hg to be associated with a five- to sixfold (not twofold) greater risk for end-stage renal disease (ESRD) compared to systolic BP of less than 117 mm Hg (option A). Hypertensive patients with mildly impaired renal function (estimated GFR < 60 mL/min) have an increased prevalence of target organ damage, such as left ventricular hypertrophy, increased carotid intima-media thickness, and microalbuminuria (option C). In a large pooled cohort study of more than 500,000 individuals from the Asia-Pacific region followed for a median of 6.8 years, systolic BP was the strongest risk factor for renal death, with each standard deviation increase in systolic BP (19 mm Hg) associated with a more than 80% higher risk (HR, 1.84; 95% CI, 1.60–2.12)[21] (option D). Although chronic kidney disease is certainly a major cause of hypertension, it is often difficult to decide whether the hypertension or the kidney disease came first because a vicious cycle can develop where one condition exacerbates the other (option E).

References

1. Vasan RS, Beiser A, Seshadri S, et al. Residual lifetime risk for developing hypertension in middle-aged women and men: the Framingham Heart Study. *JAMA.* 2002;287(8):1003-1010.
2. Gupta AK, McGlone M, Greenway FL, Johnson WD. Prehypertension in disease-free adults: a marker for an adverse cardiometabolic risk profile. *Hypertens Res.* 2010;33:905-910.
3. Santos AB, Gupta DK, Bello NA, et al. Prehypertension is associated with abnormalities of cardiac structure and function in the Atherosclerosis Risk in Communities Study. *Am J Hypertens.* 2015;pii:hpv156.
4. Miura K, Daviglus ML, Dyer AR, et al. Relationship of blood pressure to 25-year mortality due to coronary heart disease, cardiovascular diseases, and all causes in young adult men: the Chicago Heart Association Detection Project in Industry. *Arch Intern Med.* 2001;161(12):1501-1508.
5. Huang Y, Cai X, Liu C, et al. Prehypertension and the risk of coronary heart disease in Asian and Western populations: a meta-analysis. *J Am Heart Assoc.* 2015;4:pii:e001519.

6. Tientcheu D, Ayers C, Das SR, et al. Target organ complications and cardiovascular events associated with masked hypertension and white-coat hypertension: analysis from the Dallas Heart Study. *J Am Coll Cardiol.* 2015;66(20):2159-2169.

7. Fletcher EC, DeBehnke RD, Lovoi MS, et al. Undiagnosed sleep apnea in patients with essential hypertension. *Ann Intern Med.* 1985;103(2):190-195.

8. Nieto FJ, Young TB, Lind BK, et al. Association of sleep-disordered breathing, sleep apnea, and hypertension in a large community-based study. Sleep Heart Health Study. *JAMA.* 2000;283(14):1829-1836.

9. Haas DC, Foster GL, Nieto FJ, et al. Age-dependent associations between sleep-disordered breathing and hypertension: importance of discriminating between systolic/diastolic hypertension and isolated systolic hypertension in the Sleep Heart Health Study. *Circulation.* 2005;111(5):614-621.

10. Mattila K, Haavisto M, Rajala S, et al. Blood pressure and five year survival in the very old. *BMJ.* 1988;296(6626):887-889.

11. Nichols WW, O'Rourke MF. *McDonald's Blood Flow in Arteries.* 5th ed. London, UK: Hodder Arnold; 2005.

12. Bulpitt CJ. Controlling hypertension in the elderly. *QJM.* 2000;93(4):203-205.

13. Chobanian AV, Bakris GL, Black HR, et al. The seventh report of the Joint National Committee on Prevention, Detection, Evaluation, and Treatment of High Blood Pressure: the JNC 7 report. *JAMA.* 2003;289(19):2560-2572.

14. Wang Y, Qang QJ. The prevalence of prehypertension and hypertension among US adults according to the new Joint National Committee guidelines. *Arch Intern Med.* 2004;164:2126-2134.

15. He FJ, MacGregor GA. A comprehensive review on salt and health and current experience of worldwide salt reduction programmes. *J Hum Hypertens.* 2009;23:363-384.

16. Elliott P, Stamler J, Nichols R, et al. Intersalt revisited: further analyses of 24 hour sodium excretion and blood pressure within and across populations. Intersalt Cooperative Research Group. *BMJ.* 1996;312:1249-1253.

17. Kannel WB, Wilson PWF. Chapter B81. Cardiovascular risk factors and hypertension. In: Izzo JL, Black HR, eds., *Hypertension Primer.* 3rd ed. Dallas, TX: American Heart Association; 2003.

18. Vasan RS, Benjamin EJ, Levy D. Prevalence, clinical features and prognosis of diastolic heart failure: an epidemiologic perspective. *J Am Coll Cardiol.* 1995;26(7):1565-1574.

19. Nielsen WB, Lindenstrom E, Vestbo J, et al. Is diastolic hypertension an independent risk factor for stroke in the presence of normal systolic blood pressure in the middle-aged and elderly? *Am J Hypertens.* 1997;10(6):634-639.

20. Staessen JA, Wang JG, Thijs L. Cardiovascular prevention and blood pressure reduction: a quantitative overview updated until 1 March 2003. *J Hypertens.* 2003;21(6):1055-1076.

21. O'Seaghdha CM, Perkovic V, Lam TH, et al. Asia Pacific Cohort Studies Collaboration. Blood pressure is a major risk factor for renal death: an analysis of 560 352 participants from the Asia-Pacific region. *Hypertension.* 2009;54:509-515.

CHAPTER 24

Pathophysiology of Hypertension

Ravi Karra

QUESTIONS

DIRECTIONS: Choose the one best response to each question.

24-1. A 52-year-old man presents to your office for prevention of cardiovascular disease. His examination is notable for a blood pressure (BP) of 153/98 mm Hg. He wants to know about factors that would predispose him to hypertension. Which of the following is *not* associated with hypertension?

A. Excess sodium intake
B. Excess potassium intake
C. Obesity
D. Sedentary lifestyle
E. A and D

24-2. A 23-year-old man is involved in a car accident and is bleeding into his abdomen. Which of the following systems *do not* regulate blood pressure (BP) acutely?

A. Arterial baroreceptors
B. Chemoreceptors
C. Central nervous system (CNS)
D. Renin-angiotensin-aldosterone system (RAAS)
E. Increase in vasodilation

24-3. Which of the following alters pressure-natriuresis in chronic hypertension?

A. Increased tubular resorption
B. Decreased antinatriuretic hormones
C. Decreased activity of the sympathetic nervous system (SNS)
D. A and C
E. None of the above

24-4. Which of the following is *not true* of the two-kidney, one-clip Goldblatt model of hypertension?

A. The clipped kidney is at greater risk for nephron loss than the untouched kidney
B. The clipped kidney produces more renin than the untouched kidney
C. Blood flow through the untouched kidney may be increased compared to the flow before clipping of the contralateral kidney
D. Removal of clipping will restore blood pressure to normal levels, even after the untouched kidney becomes dysfunctional
E. None of the above

24-5. Which of the following are *true* regarding salt-sensitive hypertension?

A. Loss of functional nephrons contributes to salt-sensitive hypertension
B. High levels of Ang II or mineralocorticoids contribute to salt-sensitive hypertension by increasing renal tubular resorption
C. A and B
D. Increased sensitivity of the RAAS is associated with salt-sensitive hypertension
E. None of the above

24-6. A 45-year-old air traffic controller presents to your office for evaluation of hypertension. Which of the following is *not true* about how the SNS contributes to hypertension?

A. Activation of the renal sympathetic nerves causes increases in renin secretion and sodium resorption
B. Radiofrequency renal denervation is an effective way to treat refractory hypertension
C. Epidemiologic studies have suggested a relationship between chronic stress and hypertension
D. Obesity results in increased renal sympathetic activity
E. Renal sympathetic activity is regulated by various regions of the brain

24-7. A 58-year-old man with hypertension presents to your office to establish care. His blood pressure is well controlled with lisinopril. Which of the following is *true* about renin-angiotensin-aldosterone system (RAAS) blockade and hypertension?

A. Blood pressure is very salt-sensitive in the setting of RAAS blockade
B. Angiotensin II (Ang II) elevation promotes sodium and water retention
C. ACE inhibitors can reduce GFR by inhibition of the constrictor effect of Ang II on efferent arterioles
D. RAAS blockade can prevent glomerular injury when the nephrons are hyperfiltering
E. All of the above are true

24-8. A 55-year-old man is being treated with bevacizumab for his lung cancer. He is seeing you for management of his hypertension. Which of the following is *not true* about hypertension associated with VEGF inhibitors?

A. VEGF-inhibitor-induced hypertension is likely to result from decreased NO
B. VEGF inhibition is likely to result from increased endothelin-1
C. VEGF-induced hypertension is solely to be mediated by its effects on the vasculature and is less likely to involve a direct effect on the kidney
D. All of the above are false
E. All of the above are true

24-9. A 53-year-old woman presents with hypertension. Her serum laboratory tests are notable for hypokalemia and metabolic alkalosis. Examination is notable for the absence of acne, adiposity, or hair loss. Which is the next best diagnostic test?

A. Dexamethasone suppression test
B. Plasma renin and aldosterone
C. Serum metanephrines
D. Genetic testing
E. None of the above

24-10. A 35-year-old obese woman presents to you for evaluation of hypertension. She wants to know whether her hypertension would resolve if she were to lose weight. Which of the following is *true* about obesity and hypertension?

A. Central adiposity is more strongly associated with hypertension than subcutaneous fat
B. Obesity results in increased activity of the SNS
C. Obesity results in activation of the RAAS
D. Obesity results in physical compression of the kidneys
E. All of the above are true

24-1. **The answer is B.** *(Hurst's The Heart, 14th Edition, Chap. 24)* Although primary hypertension is heterogeneous, some of the main causes of high BP are known. For example, overweight and obesity may account for 65% to 75% of the risk for primary hypertension (option C). Sedentary lifestyle, excess intake of alcohol or salt, and low potassium intake are also known to increase BP in some patients (options A, B, D, and E).[1]

24-2. **The answer is E.** *(Hurst's The Heart, 14th Edition, Chap. 24)* With rapid blood loss, three important neural control systems begin to function powerfully within seconds: (1) the arterial baroreceptors, which detect changes in BP and send appropriate autonomic reflex signals back to the heart and blood vessels to return the BP toward normal (option A); (2) the chemoreceptors, which detect changes in oxygen or carbon dioxide in the blood and initiate autonomic feedback responses that influence BP (option B); and (3) the central nervous system (CNS) (option C), which responds within a few seconds to ischemia of the vasomotor centers in the medulla, especially when BP falls below about 50 mm Hg. Within a few minutes or hours after a BP disturbance, additional controls react, including (1) a shift of fluid from the interstitial spaces into the blood in response to decreased BP (or a shift of fluid out of the blood into the interstitial spaces in response to increased BP); (2) the RAAS, which is activated when BP falls too low and suppressed when BP increases above normal (option D); and (3) multiple vasodilator systems that are suppressed when BP decreases and stimulated when BP increases above normal (option E).

24-3. **The answer is D.** *(Hurst's The Heart, 14th Edition, Chap. 24)* In all types of human or experimental hypertension studied thus far, there is a shift of pressure natriuresis that appears to sustain the hypertension. In some cases, abnormal pressure natriuresis is caused by intrarenal disturbances that alter renal hemodynamics or increased tubular reabsorption (option A). In other cases, altered kidney function is caused by extrarenal disturbances, such as increased SNS activity or excessive formation of antinatriuretic hormones that reduce the kidney's ability to excrete sodium and water and eventually increase BP (options B and C). Consequently, effective treatment of patients with hypertension requires interventions that reset pressure natriuresis toward normal BP either by directly increasing renal excretory capability (eg, with diuretics), or by reducing antinatriuretic influences (eg, with RAAS blockers) on the kidneys.

24-4. **The answer is D.** *(Hurst's The Heart, 14th Edition, Chap. 24)* In the two-kidney, one-clip Goldblatt model of hypertension, the clipped kidney has reduced blood flow, while the untouched kidney has normal or increased blood flow (option C). This differential in blood flow results in high levels of renin being made by the clipped kidney but almost no renin from the untouched kidney (option B).[1] Over time, the untouched kidney will develop injury from the increased blood flow, leading to nephron loss (option A). Once damage has occurred to the untouched kidney, reversal of clipping will no longer be able to completely reverse hypertension (option D).

24-5. **The answer is C.** *(Hurst's The Heart, 14th Edition, Chap. 24)* After the loss of entire nephrons, the surviving nephrons must excrete greater amounts of sodium and water to maintain balance. This is achieved by increasing GFR and decreasing reabsorption in the remaining nephrons, resulting in increased sodium chloride delivery to the macula densa and suppression of renin release (option A). This, in turn, impairs the kidney's ability to further decrease renin secretion during high sodium intake, and BP becomes salt sensitive. Factors that increase renal tubular sodium reabsorption, such as excessive levels of mineralocorticoids or Ang II, can also cause hypertension (option B). Reduced sensitivity of the RAAS contributes to salt-sensitive hypertension (option D).

24-6. **The answer is B.** (*Hurst's The Heart, 14th Edition, Chap. 24*) It is widely believed that chronic stress may lead to long-term increases in blood pressure. Support for this concept comes largely from a few epidemiologic studies showing that air traffic controllers, lower socio-economic groups, and other groups who are believed to lead more stressful lives also have increased prevalence of hypertension (option C).[2] Even mild increases in renal sympathetic activity stimulate renin secretion and sodium reabsorption in multiple segments of the nephron, including the proximal tubule, the loop of Henle, and distal segments (option A). Obese persons have elevated SNS activity in various tissues, including the kidneys and skeletal muscle, as assessed by microneurography, tissue catecholamine spillover, and other methods (option D). The preganglionic neurons that synapse with the renal sympathetic postganglionic fibers are located in the lower thoracic and upper lumbar segments of the spinal cord and receive multiple inputs from various regions of the brain, including the brainstem, forebrain, and cerebral cortex (option E). Whether renal denervation will prove to be an effective therapy for patients who are resistant to the usual pharmacological treatments remains to be determined (option B).

24-7. **The answer is E.** (*Hurst's The Heart, 14th Edition, Chap. 24*) Ang II causes salt and water retention by increasing renal sodium reabsorption through the stimulation of aldosterone secretion, by direct effects on epithelial transport, and by hemodynamic effects (option B). Blockade of the RAAS, with Ang II–receptor blockers (ARBs) or angiotensin-converting enzyme (ACE) inhibitors, increases renal excretory capability so that sodium balance can be maintained at reduced BP. However, blockade of the RAAS also makes BP salt sensitive (option A). The impairment of GFR after RAAS blockade is caused, in part, by inhibition of the constrictor effects of Ang II on efferent arterioles as well as reduced BP (option C). RAAS blockade is often beneficial when nephrons are hyperfiltering, especially if Ang II is not appropriately suppressed (option D). For example, in diabetes mellitus and certain forms of hypertension associated with glomerulosclerosis and nephron loss, Ang II blockade decreases BP, efferent arteriolar resistance, and glomerular hydrostatic pressure, and it attenuates glomerular hyperfiltration.[3]

24-8. **The answer is C.** (*Hurst's The Heart, 14th Edition, Chap. 24*) VEGF and VEGF receptors are highly expressed in the kidney. VEGF is expressed in glomerular podocytes, and VEGF receptors are present on endothelial, mesangial, and peritubular capillary cells. Signaling between endothelial cells and podocytes is thought to be important for maintenance of the filtration function of the glomerulus, and inhibitors of VEGF signaling have been shown to alter glomerular structure and function (option C). Because the endothelium is a major target for VEGF actions, it is likely that decreases in the production of endothelium-derived relaxing factors such as NO and PGs or enhanced production of vasoconstricting factors such as thromboxane and ET-1 play a role in the hypertensive response to drugs that block the VEGF pathway (options A and B).[4]

24-9. **The answer is B.** (*Hurst's The Heart, 14th Edition, Chap. 24*) This patient is most likely to have Conn syndrome or primary aldosteronism. Conn syndrome is manifest by expansion of extracellular fluid volume, hypertension, suppression of renin secretion, hypokalemia, and metabolic alkalosis. Therefore, testing of renin and aldosterone levels can be useful to establish a diagnosis (option B). A dexamethasone suppression test can be useful to differentiate ACTH-dependent and ACTH-independent Cushing syndrome (option A). Serum metanephrines can be useful for diagnosing pheochromocytoma (option C). Genetic testing is unlikely to be of high yield at this stage of diagnostics (option D).

24-10. **The answer is E.** (*Hurst's The Heart, 14th Edition, Chap. 24*) Adipose tissue distribution is important to the risk for obesity-related hypertension. Most population studies that have investigated the relationship between obesity and BP have measured BMI rather than visceral or retroperitoneal fat, which appear to be better predictors of increased BP than subcutaneous fat (option A).[5] Additionally, three mechanisms appear to be especially important in increasing sodium reabsorption and impairing renal-pressure natriuresis in obesity hypertension: (1) increased SNS activity (option B), (2) activation of the RAAS (option C), and (3) physical compression of the kidneys by fat accumulation within and around the kidneys and by increased abdominal pressure (option D).

References

1. Hall JE, Granger JP, do Carmo JM, et al. Hypertension: physiology and pathophysiology. *Compr Physiol.* 2012;2(4):2393-2442.
2. Kaplan NM. *Clinical Hypertension.* 8th ed. Philadelphia, PA: Lippincott Williams & Wilkins; 2002.
3. Hall JE, Brands MW, Henegar JR. Angiotensin II and long-term arterial pressure regulation: the overriding dominance of the kidney. *J Am Soc Nephrol.* 1999;10 Suppl 12:S258-S265.
4. Facemire CS, Nixon AB, Griffiths R, Hurwitz H, Coffman TM. Vascular endothelial growth factor receptor 2 controls blood pressure by regulating nitric oxide synthase expression. *Hypertension.* 2009;54(3):652-658.
5. Tchernof A, Despres JP. Pathophysiology of human visceral obesity: an update. *Physiol Rev.* 2013;93(1):359-404.

CHAPTER 25

Diagnosis and Treatment of Hypertension

Patrick R. Lawler

QUESTIONS

DIRECTIONS: Choose the one best response to each question.

25-1. Which of the following statements about hypertension is *false*?

A. Hypertension is a public health problem worldwide
B. Treating hypertension with antihypertensive drugs is effective for the long-term prevention of cardiovascular disease
C. Normal (optimal) pressure is classified as blood pressure < 120/80 mm Hg
D. Blood pressure measurements outside the office or clinic are always identical to office or clinic pressure measurement
E. The prevalence of hypertension is increasing in relation to increased overweight

25-2. During a routine checkup, a 55-year-old male factory worker's recorded blood pressure is 150/90 mm Hg. What is the goal for the initial evaluation of hypertensive patients?

A. Estimate the average blood pressure
B. Consider the overall cardiovascular risk status
C. Determine the presence or absence of target organ pathology
D. Educate the patient on long-term cardiovascular risk reduction
E. All of the above

25-3. Which of the following is considered *correct* blood pressure measurement in the clinic?

A. Using the same cuff size for all patients
B. Taking blood pressures in both arms, in the seated and standing positions

C. Taking the blood pressure in one arm with the patient standing
D. Taking the blood pressure in one arm with the patient seated
E. Using the brachial artery pressure as a substitute for central aortic pressure

25-4. A 36-year-old woman patient has a blood pressure of 140/90 mm Hg in the clinic. An out-of-office ambulatory blood pressure monitor is requested for the next 24 hours. Which of the following is *not* an advantage of this monitoring device?

A. It predicts the risk of morbid events better than clinic blood pressure
B. It can diagnose white coat hypertension
C. It can diagnose masked hypertension
D. It eliminates the need for medical history and physical examination in determining cardiovascular disease risk
E. It can measure systolic and diastolic pressures while the patient sleeps

25-5. After initial assessment in clinic followed by a 24-hour ambulatory pressure monitoring, a 50-year-old male banker is diagnosed with hypertension. Which of the following is *not* an appropriate course of action?

A. Recommendation of the DASH diet
B. Recommendation of an exercise routine
C. Recommendation of smoking cessation and scheduled follow-up in 1 year
D. Prescription of antihypertensive medications
E. Performance of laboratory biochemical testing and imaging to define cardiovascular risk

25-6. Which of the following diuretics used as an antihypertensive drug does *not* cause hypokalemia as a side effect?

A. Spironolactone
B. Thiazides
C. Loop-active diuretics
D. All of the above
E. None of the above

25-7. A 62-year-old female office worker is evaluated for hypertension. She currently takes a beta-receptor blocker for angina, but due to inadequate blood pressure control, a second-line agent is being selected to achieve optimal blood pressure control. Which antihypertensive drug class is *not* appropriate to prescribe?

A. Thiazide diuretic
B. Non-dihydropyridine calcium channel blocker
C. Angiotensin converting enzyme (ACE) inhibitor
D. Angiotensin receptor blocker (ARB)
E. Alpha-receptor blocker

25-8. Which of the following statements about hypertension management is *correct*?

A. Beta-blockers may cause hypoglycemic unawareness
B. The coexistence of diabetes and hypertension increases the risk of future cardiovascular disease compared to hypertension alone
C. The incidence of new hypertension is very low in cancer patients undergoing chemotherapy treatment with vascular endothelial growth factor (VEGF) inhibitors such as bevacizumab
D. Once a stroke has occurred, antihypertensive drug therapy cannot help prevent additional cerebrovascular pathology and disease
E. The prevalence and severity of hypertension are uniform across different ethnic groups

25-9. A 65-year-old man presents to the emergency room with blood pressure of 220/120 mm Hg, altered mental status, and seizures. This hypertensive emergency could be caused by which of the following?

A. Poor adherence to antihypertensive medication
B. Use of NSAIDs
C. Alcohol or substance abuse
D. Underlying pheochromocytoma
E. All of the above

25-10. A 42-year-old woman in her second trimester of gestation requires antihypertensive therapy for her chronic hypertension. Which of the following is *not* safe to prescribe to her?

A. ACEI
B. Methyldopa
C. Labetalol
D. Nifedipine
E. All of the above

25-1. The answer is D. *(Hurst's The Heart, 14th Edition, Chap. 25)* By current guidelines, normal (optimal) pressure is classified as blood pressure < 120/80 mm Hg (option C). Hypertension is highly prevalent in adult populations throughout the world and is increasing in relation to increased overweight and reduced daily exercise (option E), and it is a growning cause of fatal and nonfatal cardiovascular and renal disease worldwide (option A).[1,2] The benefits of treating hypertension have been firmly established.[3,4]

The introduction of 24-hour ambulatory blood pressure monitoring and systematic home blood pressure monitoring has brought to light the fact that blood pressure measured outside the office or clinic may differ substantially from office or clinic pressure (option D). The importance of out-of-office blood pressures for accurate prognosis is now supported by several national and international guidelines.[5-8]

25-2. The answer is E. *(Hurst's The Heart, 14th Edition, Chap. 25)* Most hypertensive patients are initially identified during office or clinic visits when seen for checkups or nonemergent symptoms. Initial evaluation and classification of these patients is crucial because hypertension is mostly a silent disorder, and patients are often asymptomatic for long periods of time. The goals for the initial evaluation of hypertensive patients include: estimating the average blood pressure (option A), considering the overall cardiovascular risk status (option B), determining the presence or absence of target organ pathology (option C), and beginning the process of education that will lead the patient to recognize and collaborate in long-term risk reduction (option D). It is also an opportune moment to assess the patient for identifiable (secondary) hypertension. Therefore, all of the above are correct (option E).

25-3. The answer is B. *(Hurst's The Heart, 14th Edition, Chap. 25)* Blood pressure measurement in the clinic requires careful and consistent practice.[9] Choosing an appropriate cuff size is essential for accurate pressure readings; therefore, larger adult cuffs are mandatory for most large or obese patients (option A). In general, a cuff that is too large will underestimate blood pressure. During measurement, the patient should be seated comfortably, and pressures should be taken in both arms due to possible variability. Blood pressures can also be measured in the standing position (option B) to assess for orthostatic hypotension, particularly in the elderly and in those with dizziness.[10] Brachial artery pressures may fail to reflect central aortic pressures (option E), the latter of which is measured directly by invasive catheterization.

25-4. The answer is D. *(Hurst's The Heart, 14th Edition, Chap. 25)* Ambulatory blood pressure measurement is a noninvasive, fully automated technique in which multiple blood pressure measurements are recorded over an extended period (typically 24 hours). It can thus measure blood pressure when a patient is awake during the day, as well as when the patient is sleeping during the night (option E). Studies suggest that the average level of ambulatory blood pressure predicts risk of morbid events better than clinic blood pressure (option A).[11] Ambulatory blood pressure monitoring is valuable for determining whether the patient's usual pressure, in "real life," is either higher or lower than the clinic pressure, thereby enabling the diagnosis of both white coat (option B) and masked hypertension (option C). Nevertheless, a careful and well-focused medical history and physical examination are the foundation for the initial appraisal of a hypertensive patient and his or her risk for cardiovascular disease, and these cannot be substituted by the use of this device (option D).

25-5. The answer is C. *(Hurst's The Heart, 14th Edition, Chap. 25)* After the initial assessment of hypertensive patients, appropriate follow-up reassessment is crucial. Studies have shown that increased cardiovascular event rates were related to failure to intensify treatment, delays of more than 1.4 months for intensification, and delays in follow-up of more than 2.7 months after intensification.[12] In general, the higher the blood pressure, the greater the need for shorter intervals between revisits. Therefore, while smoking cessation is important for cardiovascular prevention, 1 year is too long an interval for follow-up (option C). There is general agreement that in the absence of clues to identifiable hypertension, efficient use and appropriate selection of laboratory resources can be confined to those needed to define cardiovascular risk, to target organ pathology, and to establish a baseline for treatment (option E). Subsequently, appropriate treatment should focus on lifestyle improvement such as adherence to an adequate diet (option A) and increased exercise (option B), as well as prescription of antihypertensive drugs (option D).

25-6. The answer is A. (*Hurst's The Heart, 14th Edition, Chap. 25*) Thiazides have been the mainstay of antihypertensive drug treatment since the 1960s as single agents or in effective two-drug combinations. The most frequent adverse reaction to these drugs is hypokalemia, due to their effect on potassium excretion by the kidneys (option B). Loop-active diuretics are preferred over thiazides when renal function is impaired or in the presence of congestive heart failure, but they share similar adverse reactions, including hypokalemia (option C). Potassium-sparing diuretics, on the other hand, reduce potassium excretion by the kidneys and therefore do not cause hypokalemia (option A). They are valuable for treating primary aldosteronism or thiazide-related hypokalemia.

25-7. The answer is B. (*Hurst's The Heart, 14th Edition, Chap. 25*) The effectiveness of beta-receptor blockers for the prevention of cardiovascular disease in the absence of coronary artery disease is uncertain.[13,14] However, the role of beta-blockers in the management of coronary heart disease, especially angina, remains well accepted.[15] Alpha-blockers may be combined with a beta-blocker for persons with highly variable blood pressure associated with tachycardia (option E). Likewise, ACEIs (option C) and ARBs (option D) can be safely used with beta-receptor blockers as antihypertensive drugs in the context of coronary heart disease. Non-dihydropyridine calcium channel blocker, on the other hand, inhibits cardiac AV conduction and should not be combined with beta-receptor blockers because of the risk of bradycardia (option B).

25-8. The answer is B. (*Hurst's The Heart, 14th Edition, Chap. 25*) The prevalence and severity of hypertension are not entirely uniform in comparing populations with different ethnic status, with increased prevalence in non-Hispanic (black) groups.[16] In addition, the treatment rates and drug responses vary across groups (option E). Beta-blockers may mask the symptoms of hypoglycemia ("hypoglycemic unawareness"), while diuretics and ACEIs have no discernable effect (option A).[17] In addition, the coexistence of diabetes and hypertension confers a two- to threefold greater risk of future cardiovascular disease compared to hypertension alone (option B).[18,19] Antihypertensive drug therapy continues to be important even after a stroke has occurred, as studies have shown that the combination of an ACEI and diuretic is effective for preventing the occurrence of a second stroke (option D).[20] Finally, the occurrence of cancer in hypertensive patients is all too frequent, and the incidence of new hypertension or worsening of previous hypertension in cancer patients may result from chemotherapy with the VEGF inhibitors, varying from 20% to 70% (option C).[21]

25-9. The answer is E. (*Hurst's The Heart, 14th Edition, Chap. 25*) A hypertensive emergency is defined by a rapid increase in blood pressure linked to an immediate threat to target organs.[22,23] Although there is no blood pressure threshold for the diagnosis of hypertensive emergencies, most end-organ damage is noted with systolic blood pressures exceeding 220 mm Hg or diastolic blood pressures exceeding 120 mm Hg. The condition is usually related to a rapid increase in pressure from already high levels in established hypertension, perhaps related to poor adherence to antihypertensive medications. However, abrupt increases in pressure with threat to target organs may appear without prior warning as in some patients with pheochromocytoma or some forms of renal disease (eg, scleroderma renal crisis). The medical history should include queries about the use of nonsteroidal anti-inflammatory drugs (NSAIDs), alcohol, and substance use.

25-10. The answer is A. (*Hurst's The Heart, 14th Edition, Chap. 25*) The goals and strategy for treating hypertension in pregnancy differ from the usual pattern for nonpregnant women.[24]

For women with treated hypertension before pregnancy, pressure should be kept in the range of 120–160/80–105 mm Hg. However, the range of drug classes suitable for treating hypertension in pregnancy is a restricted one, excluding the renin system blockers such as ACEIs (option A) because of the risk of fetal damage.[25,26] Recommended drugs are methyldopa (option B), labetalol (option C), and nifedipine (option D) because these have acceptable evidence of safety in pregnancy.

References

1. Lewington S, Clarke R, Qizilbash N, Peto R, Collins R. Prospective studies collaboration. Age-specific relevance of usual blood pressure to vascular mortality: a meta-analysis of individual data for one million adults in 61 prospective studies. *Lancet.* 2002;360(9349):1903-1913.

2. Hypertension: uncontrolled and conquering the world. *Lancet.* 2007;370:539.

3. Staessen JA, Wang JG, Thijs L. Cardiovascular protection and blood pressure reduction: a meta-analysis. *Lancet.* 2001;358:1305-1315.

4. Hebert PR, Moser M, Mayer J, Hennekens CH. Recent evidence on drug therapy of mild to moderate hypertension and decreased risk of coronary heart disease. *Arch Intern Med.* 1993;153:578-581.

5. Piper MA, Evans CV, Burda BU, Margolis KL, O'Connor E, Whitlock EP. Diagnostic and predictive accuracy of blood pressure screening methods with consideration of rescreening intervals: an updated systematic review for the U.S. Preventive Services Task Force. *Ann Intern Med.* 2014;162:192-204.

6. Parati G, Stergiou G, O'Brien E, et al. European Society of Hypertension practice guidelines for ambulatory blood pressure monitoring. *J Hypertens.* 2014;32(7):1359-1366.

7. Mayor S. Hypertension diagnosis should be based on ambulatory blood pressure monitoring, NICE recommends. *BMJ.* 2011;343:d5421.

8. Pickering TG, White WB. ASH position paper: home and ambulatory blood pressure monitoring. When and how to use self (home) and ambulatory blood pressure monitoring. *J Clin Hypertens (Greenwich).* 2008;10(11):850-855.

9. Pickering TG, Hall JE, Appel LJ, et al. Recommendations for blood pressure measurement in humans and experimental animals: Part 1: blood pressure measurement in humans: a statement for professionals from the Subcommittee of Professional and Public Education of the American Heart Association Council on High Blood Pressure Research. *Hypertension.* 2005;45(1):142-161.

10. Benvenuto LJ, Krakoff LR. Morbidity and mortality of orthostatic hypotension: implications for management of cardiovascular disease. *Am J Hypertens.* 2011;24:135-144.

11. Dolan E, Stanton A, Thijs L, et al. Superiority of ambulatory over clinic blood pressure measurement in predicting mortality: the Dublin outcome study. *Hypertension.* 2005;46(1):156-161.

12. Xu W, Goldberg SI, Shubina M, Turchin A. Optimal systolic blood pressure target, time to intensification, and time to follow-up in treatment of hypertension: population based retrospective cohort study. *BMJ.* 2015;350:h158.

13. Lindholm LH, Carlberg B, Samuelsson O. Should beta blockers remain first choice in the treatment of primary hypertension? A meta-analysis. *Lancet.* 2005;366(9496):1545-1553.

14. Devereux RB, Dahlof B, Kjeldsen SE, et al. Effects of losartan or atenolol in hypertensive patients without clinically evident vascular disease: A substudy of the LIFE randomized trial. *Ann Intern Med.* 2003;136:169-177.

15. Rosendorff C, Lackland DT, Allison M, et al. Treatment of hypertension in patients with coronary artery disease: a scientific statement from the American Heart Association, American College of Cardiology, and American Society of Hypertension. *Hypertension.* 2015;9(6):453-498.

16. Cutler JA, Sorlie PD, Wolz M, Thom T, Fields LE, Roccella EJ. Trends in hypertension prevalence, awareness, treatment, and control rates in United States adults between 1988-1994 and 1999-2004. *Hypertension.* 2008;52(5):818-827.

17. Gress TW, Nieto J, Shahar E, Wofford MR, Brancati FL. Hypertension and antihypertensive therapy as risk factors for type 2 diabetes mellitus: Atherosclerosis Risk in Communities Study. *N Engl J Med.* 2000;342:905-912.

18. Stamler J, Vaccaro O, Neaton JD, Wentworth D. Diabetes, other risk factors, and 12-yr cardiovascular mortality for men screened in the Multiple Risk Factor Intervention Trial. *Diabetes Care.* 1993;16(2):434-444.

19. Almdal T, Scharling H, Jensen JS, Vestergaard H. The independent effect of type 2 diabetes mellitus on ischemic heart disease, stroke, and death: a population-based study of 13,000 men and women with 20 years of follow-up. *Arch Intern Med.* 2004;164(13):1422-1426.

20. PROGRESS Collaborative. Group. Randomised trial of a perindopril-based blood pressure lowering regimen among 6105 individuals with previous stroke or transient ischemic attack. *Lancet.* 2001;358:1033-1041.

21. Maitland ML, Bakris GL, Black HR, et al. Initial assessment, surveillance, and management of blood pressure in patients receiving vascular endothelial growth factor signaling pathway inhibitors. *J Natl Cancer Inst.* 2010;102(9):596-604.

22. Phillips RA, Greenblatt J, Krakoff LR. Hypertensive emergencies: diagnosis and management. *Prog Cardiovasc Dis.* 2002;45:33-48.

23. Zampaglione B, Pascale C, Marchiso M, Cavallo-Perin P. Hypertensive urgencies and emergencies: prevalence and clinical presentation. *Hypertension.* 1996;27:144-147.

24. American College of Obstetricians and Gynecologists, Task Force on Hypertension in Pregnancy. Hypertension in pregnancy. Report of the American College of Obstetricians and Gynecologists' Task Force on Hypertension in Pregnancy. *Obstet Gynecol.* 2013;122(5):1122-1131.

25. Hanssens M, Keirse MJ, Vankelecom F, Van Assche FA. Fetal and neonatal effects of treatment with angiotensin-converting enzyme inhibitors in pregnancy. *Obstet Gynecol.* 1991;78:128-135.

26. Hunseler C, Paneitz A, Friedrich D, et al. Angiotensin II receptor blocker induced fetopathy: 7 cases. *Klin Padiatr.* 2011;223(1):10-14.

SECTION 5

Metabolic Disorders and Cardiovascular Disease

CHAPTER 26

The Metabolic Syndrome

Mark J. Eisenberg

QUESTIONS

DIRECTIONS: Choose the one best response to each question.

26-1. Which of the following is *not* considered a component of the metabolic syndrome (MetS)?

A. Central adiposity
B. Insulin resistance
C. High serum low-density lipoprotein (LDL) cholesterol
D. High serum triglycerides
E. Hypertension

26-2. Which of the following statements concerning the MetS is *not true*?

A. Insulin resistance and central adiposity are required for a diagnosis of MetS
B. Three of the five criteria are always required for a diagnosis of MetS
C. Between 20% and 35% of the worldwide adult population have MetS
D. Atherosclerotic risk rises in association with the severity of MetS
E. Residual risk describes the remaining increased risk for atherosclerosis after the treatment of a specific risk factor

26-3. Which of the following is *not* a mechanism by which physical activity affects metabolism?

A. Activation of brown fat
B. Improvement in insulin sensitivity
C. Modulation of endothelial and adipose tissue function
D. Gene activation
E. All of the above are mechanisms by which physical activity affects metabolism

26-4. Which of the following concerning sleep is *true*?

A. Six hours of sleep per night is sufficient for the average adult
B. Reduced sleep is associated with hypertension
C. Sleep quality has no known effects on metabolism
D. Shift workers do not differ from the general population in rates of obesity
E. Adults sleep more on average today than 50 years ago

26-5. Which environmental factors could affect the prevalence of MetS?

A. Modern agricultural practices
B. Exposure to endocrine-disrupting chemicals
C. Industrial production of sugars
D. Antidepressant and antibiotic use
E. All of the above

26-6. Which of the following is considered the common starting pathway for the development of MetS?

A. Genetic predisposition
B. Insulin resistance
C. Systemic inflammation
D. Accumulation of fat in adipose or nonadipose tissue
E. Hypertension

26-7. The presence of which of the following would *not* raise a suspicion of MetS?

A. Alzheimer's disease
B. Polycystic ovary syndrome
C. Obstructive sleep apnea
D. Gestational diabetes
E. Family history of hypertension

26-8. What is the approximate annual risk of developing type 2 diabetes in a patient with obesity and MetS?

A. 2.5%
B. 5%
C. 7.5%
D. 10%
E. 12.5%

26-9. What is the most important factor when selecting a dietary intervention for a patient with MetS?

A. Minimization of refined carbohydrates
B. Avoidance of processed foods
C. Consumption of lean meats
D. Consumption of large amounts of vegetables and fruits
E. Ability to maintain the dietary intervention long-term

26-10. Which of the following procedures is associated with the least improvement in type 2 diabetes?

A. Roux-en-Y gastric bypass (RYGB)
B. Sleeve gastrectomy (SG)
C. Laparoscopic gastric banding (LGB)
D. Biliopancreatic diversion with duodenal switch
E. Biliopancreatic diversion without duodenal switch

26-1. The answer is C. *(Hurst's The Heart, 14th Edition, Chap. 26)* The metabolic syndrome is a theoretical construct from the clustering of interrelated processes to better represent complex pathophysiology for actionable and effective clinical decision making. Specifically, the rationale and practical utility of MetS is to facilitate early diagnosis, risk stratification, and management of cardiometabolic risk factors. This topic is relevant, but it also remains controversial because many aspects remain unproven. Nevertheless, the core principle is that the value of MetS is related to the impact of residual risk (total risk minus the aggregate of known specific risk factors) on cardiovascular disease (CVD). Currently, the diagnosis of MetS is based on a set of commonly measured metabolic markers: abdominal girth (option A), hyperglycemia (option B), hypertriglyceridemia (option D), hypertension (option E), and low high-density lipoprotein (HDL) levels. However, debate still exists over the relative weighting of each of these measures in a predictive model for morbidity and mortality risk. Low-density lipoprotein levels are not among the diagnostic criteria (option C).

26-2. The answer is A. *(Hurst's The Heart, 14th Edition, Chap. 26)* While the diagnostic criteria for MetS vary by organization, either insulin resistance or central adiposity (but not both) are generally required for a diagnosis of MetS (option A). The exception is the criteria of the American Heart Association/National Heart, Lung, and Blood Institute, which do not make a specific requirement for either. By all definitions, three of five criteria (abdominal girth, hyperglycemia, hypertriglyceridemia, hypertension, and low HDL levels) are required for a diagnosis of MetS (option B). Depending on the specific criteria used, approximately 20% to 35% of various reported worldwide adult populations have MetS (option C). Overall, atherosclerotic risk rises in association with the severity of MetS (option D).[1,2] The practical decisions of diagnosis and clinical intervention should take into consideration the continuum of risk imposed by MetS. The term *residual risk* complements the concept of the MetS. Specifically, residual risk describes the remaining increased potential for atherosclerotic CVD, after the treatment of a specific risk factor, such as using cholesterol-lowering agents with dyslipidemia (option E).[3] Factors that contribute to residual risk include lifestyle factors, such as eating patterns and nutrient content, endocrine-disrupting compounds (EDCs), physical activity, sleep hygiene, and others.

26-3. The answer is E. *(Hurst's The Heart, 14th Edition, Chap. 26)* Physical activity has multiple effects on metabolism, including the activation of brown fat (option A), improvement in insulin sensitivity (option B), and modulation of endothelial function and adipose tissue function (option C).[4,5] Shifts in internal energy use among highly active people may also contribute to more efficient carbohydrate processing and reduced insulin resistance.[6] Additionally, gene activation following physical activity can influence insulin resistance and mitochondrial function (option D).[7] Interventional studies consistently demonstrate a great reduction in the prevalence and severity of MetS among highly active subjects.[1] Most notably, trials that incorporate increased physical activity demonstrate a 29% to 58% reduction in the incidence of type 2 diabetes among at-risk subjects.[8]

26-4. The answer is B. *(Hurst's The Heart, 14th Edition, Chap. 26)* Many studies demonstrate that a reduced amount of sleep, generally 6 hours or less per night (option A), is associated with increased insulin resistance, hypertension (option B), and obesity.[9] One large study demonstrated that reduced time of slow-wave sleep was specifically associated with increased waist circumference.[10] Quality of sleep can also affect metabolism (option C). Shift workers with frequent changes in circadian patterns have higher rates of obesity and type 2 diabetes compared to the general population (option D). Insulin resistance also worsens in the presence of obstructive sleep apnea. Current trends over the past 50 years demonstrate a 1.5- to 2-hour reduction in time spent sleeping each night, which may further contribute to the rising prevalence of MetS (option E).[11]

26-5. **The answer is E.** (*Hurst's The Heart, 14th Edition, Chap. 26*) The potential adverse metabolic effects of modern agricultural techniques (option A), food processing, and the resultant food chain in the United States with respect to nutrient content and endocrine disruptors are only just becoming clear, but they are still not without controversy. For example, the use of corn for animal feed rather than grass for beef production or seeds for poultry yields a higher n-6 fatty acid content, which may have proinflammatory effects.[12] A number of man-made industrial chemicals have properties that can interrupt normal hormone signaling either through molecular mimicry of natural hormones, blockade of hormone activity, or by affecting hormonal synthesis, transport, binding, or catabolism (option B). Animal models and population exposure studies identify specific endocrine-disrupting chemicals, such as pesticides, plasticizers, preservatives, and artificial sweeteners, among other chemicals that hinder glucose metabolism and cause insulin resistance.[13-16] However, the degree to which endocrine-disrupting chemicals (EDCs) contribute to the high prevalence of MetS is unclear. The high content of fructose within industrially produced sugars (option C), such as sucrose and high-fructose corn syrup, makes this inefficiently metabolized monosaccharide highly available. Multiple longitudinal and cross-sectional studies demonstrate a strong association among high fructose intake and the development of obesity, MetS, and/or vascular disease.[17-20] The rising use of certain antidepressant and other psychotropic medications (option D) that affect metabolic control within the hypothalamus leads to insulin resistance and weight gain. Even the widespread use of antibiotics may influence metabolism through the alteration of intestinal microbiota (option D).[21] The average American adult is given one to two prescriptions for antibiotics annually, which has been associated with the development of obesity.[21] Macrolides confer the greatest risk, perhaps reflecting a greater effect on intestinal microbiota.[21,22]

26-6. **The answer is D.** (*Hurst's The Heart, 14th Edition, Chap. 26*) It is useful to view a common starting pathway for the MetS as the accumulation of fat in adipose or nonadipose tissue (option D), which increases systemic inflammation (option C) and insulin resistance (option B). Pancreatic β-cell dysfunction ensues via degeneration or transformation to inactive cells.[23] Impaired insulin signaling leads to further accumulation of fat mass.[24] Reduced release and reduced activity of glucagon-like peptide-1 (GLP-1) by L-cells of the distal ileum worsens insulin resistance and drives further increases in adipose tissue.[25] Nutrient sensing within the paraventricular nucleus of the hypothalamus becomes impaired, and resistance to leptin develops within the arcuate nucleus.[26] Adiponectin production within adipose tissue is also diminished, which further promotes insulin resistance.[27] Insulin resistance reduces endothelial and adipose lipoprotein lipase activity, yielding small, dense LDL particles that enter the circulation and are highly atherogenic.[28] Circulating free fatty acids further drive insulin resistance through oxidative stress and accumulation of intracellular derivatives such as ceramides.[29] Visceral fat stores increase, leading to hepatosteatosis and fat accumulation within the pancreas, promoting insulin resistance and β-cell dysfunction.[30,31] Within the vascular endothelium, insulin resistance also impairs nitric oxide (NO) synthase activity, which diminishes NO production, affecting vasodilation and leading to the development of essential hypertension (option E).[32] Low circulating adiponectin and resistance to leptin induce increased expression of endothelin-1, further driving vasoconstriction and promoting hypertension.[32] High levels of circulating lipid particles naturally oxidize and are taken up by macrophages that become activated.[33] Free fatty acids also bind toll-like receptor 4 on macrophage cell surfaces.[34] Both processes trigger the release of inflammatory cytokines such as tumor necrosis factor-α (TNFα), interleukin (IL)-1, and IL-6. These cytokines promote the degradation of insulin receptor substrate-1, a downstream mediator of insulin activity, further driving insulin resistance.[33] Very few genes have been identified that specifically confer a risk of MetS (option A).[35] However, epigenetic phenomena secondary to behavioral and environmental factors do have great potential to influence the development of obesity and MetS.

26-7. **The answer is A.** (*Hurst's The Heart, 14th Edition, Chap. 26*) The high prevalence of MetS should trigger aggressive case finding in a large portion of the general population.[36] Signs of obesity, weight gain, hypertension, hyperlipidemia, and hyperglycemia can be early markers of MetS. People with a family history of type 2 diabetes, hypertension (option E), and CVD should also be evaluated for MetS. Additionally, the presence of other conditions associated with insulin resistance, such as polycystic ovary syndrome (option B), hepatosteatosis, obstructive sleep apnea (option C), or gestational diabetes (option D), should raise suspicion for MetS. Diagnosing a person with MetS emphasizes the decision to intervene.

26-8. **The answer is B.** *(Hurst's The Heart, 14th Edition, Chap. 26)* The annual risk of type 2 diabetes (T2D) is approximately 2.5% when stratified by fasting glucose (option A).[37] In people with obesity and MetS, the annual risk of T2D is nearly 5% (option B), although annual regression of hyperglycemia is about 10%, emphasizing the need for intensive lifestyle changes as part of a preventive care paradigm.[37] By virtue of its syndromic nature, this preventive care approach to people at high risk for MetS should follow the same treatment strategies for MetS. The intensity of intervention should parallel the severity of each MetS component.[36] A striking theme among the major clinical trials investigating individual criteria of MetS is that early, intensive intervention is best at reducing adverse outcomes, especially with the intention of atherosclerotic risk reduction.[8,38-42]

26-9. **The answer is E.** *(Hurst's The Heart, 14th Edition, Chap. 26)* In early MetS, when the severity of component risks is mild, lifestyle interventions should be implemented that minimize refined carbohydrates (option A), avoid processed foods (option B), favor meats that are lean (option C), and contain large amounts of fruits, vegetables, and fish (option D). Debate continues over the ideal diet, but beneficial dietary pattern examples include the Mediterranean diet, the New Nordic diet, the Dietary Approaches to Stop Hypertension (DASH) diet, and the Ornish diet. The use of very low carbohydrate diets, such as the Atkins diet, can also be considered. The most important consideration for dietary intervention is the person's ability to maintain this new lifestyle over the long term (option E).[43]

26-10. **The answer is C.** *(Hurst's The Heart, 14th Edition, Chap. 26)* Approved bariatric surgical procedures include the RYGB (option A), SG (option B), biliopancreatic diversion with or without duodenal switch (BPD) (options D and E), and LGB (option C). Surgically induced changes in the gastrointestinal tract affect energy physiology, insulin resistance, hypertension, hyperlipidemia, and other weight-related complications.[44] Additionally, many of the factors contributing to MetS improve, and the risk of cardiovascular events and mortality is reduced.[45] In people undergoing RYGB, SG, or BPD, insulin resistance improves in the immediate postoperative period, signifying the predominance of improved energy regulatory hormone signaling well before weight loss occurs.[46] Following LGB, insulin resistance declines in association with weight loss.[46] The significant improvement and possible resolution of T2D is also substantially higher following RYGB, SG, and BPD, when compared to LGB.[47-49] These observations suggest that the metabolic benefits of RYGB, SG, and BPD may confer additional improvement to people with MetS.

References

1. Singh GM, Danaei G, Farzadfar F, et al. The age-specific quantitative effects of metabolic risk factors on cardiovascular diseases and diabetes: a pooled analysis. *PLoS One.* 2013;8(7):e65174.
2. Einhorn D, Reaven GM, Cobin RH, et al. American College of Endocrinology position statement on the insulin resistance syndrome. *Endocr Pract.* 2003;9(3):237-252.
3. Fruchart JC, Davignon J, Hermans MP, et al. Residual macrovascular risk in 2013: what have we learned? *Cardiovasc Diabetol.* 2014;13:26.
4. Sepa-Kishi DM, Ceddia RB. Exercise-mediated effects on white and brown adipose tissue plasticity and metabolism. *Exerc Sport Sci Rev.* 2016;44(1):37-44.
5. Zaccardi F, O'Donovan G, Webb DR, et al. Cardiorespiratory fitness and risk of type 2 diabetes mellitus: a 23-year cohort study and a meta-analysis of prospective studies. *Atherosclerosis.* 2015;243(1):131-137.
6. Pontzer H, Raichlen DA, Wood BM, Mabulla AZ, Racette SB, Marlowe FW. Hunter-gatherer energetics and human obesity. *PLoS One.* 2012;7(7):e40503.
7. Hargreaves M. Exercise and gene expression. *Prog Mol Biol Transl Sci.* 2015;135:457-469.
8. The Diabetes Prevention Program (DPP): description of lifestyle intervention. *Diabetes Care.* 2002; 25(12):2165-2171.
9. Patel SR, Hu FB. Short sleep duration and weight gain: a systematic review. *Obesity (Silver Spring).* 2008; 16(3):643-653.

10. Rao MN, Blackwell T, Redline S, Stefanick ML, Ancoli-Israel S, Stone KL. Association between sleep architecture and measures of body composition. *Sleep.* 2009;32(4):483-490.

11. Unhealthy sleep-related behaviors–12 States, 2009. *MMWR Morb Mortal Wkly Rep.* 2011;60(8):233-238.

12. Wang Y, Lehane C, Ghebremeskel K, Crawford MA. Modern organic and broiler chickens sold for human consumption provide more energy from fat than protein. *Public Health Nutr.* 2010;13(3):400-408.

13. Baillie-Hamilton PF. Chemical toxins: a hypothesis to explain the global obesity epidemic. *J Altern Complement Med.* 2002;8(2):185-192.

14. Valvi D, Mendez MA, Martinez D, et al. Prenatal concentrations of polychlorinated biphenyls, DDE, and DDT and overweight in children: a prospective birth cohort study. *Environ Health Perspect.* 2012;120(3):451-457.

15. Verhulst SL, Nelen V, Hond ED, et al. Intrauterine exposure to environmental pollutants and body mass index during the first 3 years of life. *Environ Health Perspect.* 2009;117(1):122-126.

16. Suez J, Korem T, Zeevi D, et al. Artificial sweeteners induce glucose intolerance by altering the gut microbiota. *Nature.* 2014;514(7521):181-186.

17. Maersk M, Belza A, Stodkilde-Jorgensen H, et al. Sucrose-sweetened beverages increase fat storage in the liver, muscle, and visceral fat depot: a 6-mo randomized intervention study. *Am J Clin Nutr.* 2012;95(2):283-289

18. Aeberli I, Gerber PA, Hochuli M, et al. Low to moderate sugar-sweetened beverage consumption impairs glucose and lipid metabolism and promotes inflammation in healthy young men: a randomized controlled trial. *Am J Clin Nutr.* 2011;94(2):479-485.

19. Aeberli I, Hochuli M, Gerber PA, et al. Moderate amounts of fructose consumption impair insulin sensitivity in healthy young men: a randomized controlled trial. *Diabetes Care.* 2013;36(1):150-156.

20. Stanhope KL, Medici V, Bremer AA, et al. A dose-response study of consuming high-fructose corn syrup-sweetened beverages on lipid/lipoprotein risk factors for cardiovascular disease in young adults. *Am J Clin Nutr.* 2015;101(6):1144-1154.

21. Schwartz BS, Pollak J, Bailey-Davis L, et al. Antibiotic use and childhood body mass index trajectory. *Int J Obes (Lond).* 2016;40(4):615-621.

22. Morotomi N, Fukuda K, Nakano M, et al. Evaluation of intestinal microbiotas of healthy Japanese adults and effect of antibiotics using the 16S ribosomal RNA gene based clone library method. *Biol Pharm Bull.* 2011;34(7):1011-1020.

23. Malin SK, Finnegan S, Fealy CE, Filion J, Rocco MB, Kirwan JP. Beta-cell dysfunction is associated with metabolic syndrome severity in adults. *Metab Syndr Relat Disord.* 2014;12(2):79-85.

24. Ali AT, Ferris WF, Naran NH, Crowther NJ. Insulin resistance in the control of body fat distribution: a new hypothesis. *Horm Metab Res.* 2011;43(2):77-80.

25. Habegger KM, Al-Massadi O, Heppner KM, et al. Duodenal nutrient exclusion improves metabolic syndrome and stimulates villus hyperplasia. *Gut.* 2014;63(8):1238-1246.

26. Munzberg H, Bjornholm M, Bates SH, Myers MG, Jr. Leptin receptor action and mechanisms of leptin resistance. *Cell Mol Life Sci.* 2005;62(6):642-652.

27. Deng Y, Scherer PE. Adipokines as novel biomarkers and regulators of the metabolic syndrome. *Ann N Y Acad Sci.* 2010;1212:E1-E19.

28. Cho Y, Lee SG, Jee SH, Kim JH. Hypertriglyceridemia is a major factor associated with elevated levels of small dense LDL cholesterol in patients with metabolic syndrome. *Ann Lab Med.* 2015;35(6):586-594.

29. Randle PJ, Garland PB, Hales CN, Newsholme EA. The glucose fatty-acid cycle. Its role in insulin sensitivity and the metabolic disturbances of diabetes mellitus. *Lancet.* 1963;1(7285):785-789.

30. Targher G. Non-alcoholic fatty liver disease as a determinant of cardiovascular disease. *Atherosclerosis.* 2007;190(1):18-19; author reply 20-11.

31. Wong VW, Wong GL, Yeung DK, et al. Fatty pancreas, insulin resistance, and beta-cell function: a population study using fat-water magnetic resonance imaging. *Am J Gastroenterol.* 2014;109(4):589-597.

32. Potenza MA, Marasciulo FL, Chieppa DM, et al. Insulin resistance in spontaneously hypertensive rats is associated with endothelial dysfunction characterized by imbalance between NO and ET-1 production. *Am J Physiol Heart Circ Physiol.* 2005;289(2):H813-H822.

33. Martins AR, Nachbar RT, Gorjao R, et al. Mechanisms underlying skeletal muscle insulin resistance induced by fatty acids: importance of the mitochondrial function. *Lipids Health Dis.* 2012;11:30.

34. Eguchi K, Manabe I. Toll-like receptor, lipotoxicity and chronic inflammation: the pathological link between obesity and cardiometabolic disease. *J Atheroscler Thromb.* 2014;21(7):629-639.

35. Kvaloy K, Holmen J, Hveem K, Holmen TL. Genetic effects on longitudinal changes from healthy to adverse weight and metabolic status—The HUNT Study. *PLoS One.* 2015;10(10):e0139632.

36. Sperling LS, Mechanick JI, Neeland IJ, et al. The CardioMetabolic Health Alliance: working toward a new care model for the metabolic syndrome. *J Am Coll Cardiol.* 2015;66(9):1050-1067.

37. DeFina LF, Vega GL, Leonard D, Grundy SM. Fasting glucose, obesity, and metabolic syndrome as predictors of type 2 diabetes: the Cooper Center Longitudinal Study. *J Investig Med.* 2012;60(8):1164-1168.

38. Wing RR, Bolin P, Brancati FL, et al. Cardiovascular effects of intensive lifestyle intervention in type 2 diabetes. *N Engl J Med.* 2013;369(2):145-154.

39. Gerstein HC, Miller ME, Byington RP, et al. Effects of intensive glucose lowering in type 2 diabetes. *N Engl J Med.* 2008;358(24):2545-2559.

40. Ridker PM, Danielson E, Fonseca FA, et al. Rosuvastatin to prevent vascular events in men and women with elevated C-reactive protein. *N Engl J Med.* 2008;359(21):2195-2207.

41. Sleight P. The HOPE Study (Heart Outcomes Prevention Evaluation). *J Renin Angiotensin Aldosterone Syst.* 2000;1(1):18-20.

42. King P, Peacock I, Donnelly R. The UK prospective diabetes study (UKPDS): clinical and therapeutic implications for type 2 diabetes. *Br J Clin Pharmacol.* 1999;48(5):643-648.

43. Dansinger ML, Gleason JA, Griffith JL, Selker HP, Schaefer EJ. Comparison of the Atkins, Ornish, Weight Watchers, and Zone diets for weight loss and heart disease risk reduction: a randomized trial. *JAMA.* 2005;293(1):43-53.

44. Rubino F, Kaplan LM, Schauer PR, Cummings DE. The Diabetes Surgery Summit consensus conference: recommendations for the evaluation and use of gastrointestinal surgery to treat type 2 diabetes mellitus. *Ann Surg.* 2010;251(3):399-405.

45. Sjostrom L, Narbro K, Sjostrom CD, et al. Effects of bariatric surgery on mortality in Swedish obese subjects. *N Engl J Med.* 2007;357(8):741-752.

46. Buchwald H, Estok R, Fahrbach K, et al. Weight and type 2 diabetes after bariatric surgery: systematic review and meta-analysis. *Am J Med.* 2009;122(3):248-256 e245.

47. Mingrone G, Panunzi S, De Gaetano A, et al. Bariatric surgery versus conventional medical therapy for type 2 diabetes. *N Engl J Med.* 2012;366(17):1577-1585.

48. Schauer PR, Kashyap SR, Wolski K, et al. Bariatric surgery versus intensive medical therapy in obese patients with diabetes. *N Engl J Med.* 2012;366(17):1567-1576.

49. Ikramuddin S, Korner J, Lee WJ, et al. Roux-en-Y gastric bypass vs intensive medical management for the control of type 2 diabetes, hypertension, and hyperlipidemia: the Diabetes Surgery Study randomized clinical trial. *JAMA.* 2013;309(21):2240-2249.

CHAPTER 27

Obesity and Cardiovascular Disease

Mark J. Eisenberg

QUESTIONS

DIRECTIONS: Choose the one best response to each question.

27-1. What approximate proportion of the adult population worldwide is overweight or obese?

A. 20%
B. 30%
C. 40%
D. 50%
E. 60%

27-2. What proportion of a person's risk for obesity is attributable to genetic factors?

A. < 10%
B. 10% to 20%
C. 30% to 40%
D. 50% to 60%
E. > 60%

27-3. Which of the following does *not* occur in response to weight loss?

A. Increased secretion of ghrelin
B. Increased secretion of leptin, cholecystokinin, glucagon-like peptide-1, amylin, and peptide YY
C. Decreased resting energy expenditure
D. Increased hunger
E. Increased calorie-dense food preferences

27-4. What proportion of body weight must be lost to achieve predictable therapeutic benefits for obstructive sleep apnea?

A. 2.5%
B. 5%
C. 7.5%
D. 10%
E. 12.5%

27-5. Which of the following is *not true* concerning body mass index (BMI)?

A. National Institutes of Health obesity-defined BMI is divided into three classes: obese class I (BMI 30–34.9), obese class II (BMI 35–39.9), and obese class III (BMI ≥ 40)
B. Cutoff values for classifying individuals as underweight, normal, overweight, or obese vary by population
C. BMI will overestimate adiposity in athletes with high muscle mass
D. BMI is a significant independent predictor of cardiovascular disease (CVD)
E. In patients with congestive heart failure, overweight and obesity are protective against mortality

27-6. Which of the following statements concerning the clinical component of the diagnosis of obesity is *not true*?

A. Individuals who meet the anthropometric criterion for overweight or obesity should undergo a clinical evaluation for weight-related complications
B. In many cases, information gathered in the initial examination is sufficient for the diagnosis of certain weight-related complications
C. The goal of weight-loss therapy is to treat and prevent weight-related complications
D. Even metabolically healthy obese patients should be treated aggressively to reduce risk for coronary heart disease
E. BMI does not indicate the impact of excess adiposity on the health of individual patients

27-7. Which of the following is *not true* about the effects of weight loss on CVD risk factors?

A. Weight loss is the most effective therapeutic approach for treating and preventing the progression of cardio-metabolic disease

B. If weight loss is not sustained over time, its beneficial effect on type 2 diabetes incidence is lost

C. Weight loss is an effective approach for reducing blood pressure

D. Weight loss decreases triglycerides and LDL, while increasing HDL

E. Weight loss has beneficial effects on LDL subclasses characterized by reductions in small, dense LDL particle concentrations and an increase in medium and large LDL particles

27-8. Which of the following is *not* appropriate for staging cardiometabolic risk in insulin resistant patients?

A. American College of Cardiology/American Heart Association Omnibus risk estimator

B. Framingham Coronary Heart Disease Risk Score

C. Reynolds Risk Score

D. Cardiometabolic Disease Staging System

E. American Heart Association/National Heart, Lung, and Blood Institute diagnostic criteria for metabolic syndrome (MetS)

27-9. Which of the following weight-loss medications is approved for the treatment of obese adolescents?

A. Orlistat

B. Lorcaserin

C. Phentermine/topiramate

D. Naltrexone/bupropion

E. None of the above

27-10. In which of the following patient group(s) could bariatric surgery be considered?

A. BMI of 35 kg/m^2 or more

B. BMI of 35 kg/m^2 or more with at least one associated comorbidity

C. BMI of 40 kg/m^2 or more

D. Both B and C

E. A, B, and C

ANSWERS

27-1. The answer is C. *(Hurst's The Heart, 14th Edition, Chap. 27)* Prevalence rates of obesity have increased sharply worldwide over the past 30 years.[1] Worldwide, the proportion of adults with a BMI of 25 kg/m[2] or greater increased between 1980 and 2013 from 28.8% to 36.9% in men, and from 29.8% to 38.0% in women.[2] Prevalence has increased substantially in children and adolescents in developed countries, to the point where 23.8% of boys and 22.6% of girls were overweight or obese in 2013.[2] In the United States, data from the National Health and Nutrition Examination Survey (NHANES) show that roughly two out of three US adults are overweight or obese, more than one-third are obese, and 17% of children are obese.[3,4] This has created a global health crisis with a profound impact on morbidity, mortality, and health care costs largely attributable to weight-related complications.

27-2. The answer is D. *(Hurst's The Heart, 14th Edition, Chap. 27)* Like many other chronic diseases, genetic factors constitute a substantial component of disease risk[5] that can explain 50% to 60% of individual variation in body weight in monozygotic/dizygotic twin studies. Monogenic forms of the disease are rare, such as in families with leptin or leptin receptor mutations or deletion of the *SNORD116* gene cluster in patients with Prader–Willi syndrome. Susceptibility to obesity in most people results from the inheritance of multiple genes, with each allele conferring a very small relative risk for the disease. Genomewide association studies have identified more than 100 susceptibility loci for obesity.[6] Particularly strong association signals have been detected for the fat mass- and obesity-associated gene (*FTO*) and the melanocortin-4 receptor (*MC4R*) gene, but even these variants confer odds for obesity of less than 1.7.[7,8] The multiple susceptibility genes interact with each other and with the environment, behavior, and biological factors to produce individual variation in the risks of obesity. The development of excess adiposity is a complex process; however, those individuals who inherit larger subsets of obesity susceptibility genes will tend to be more overweight in any given environment.[9,10] Progressive weight gain is not a lifestyle choice and cannot be viewed in terms of a simple thermodynamic equation of greater energy in than energy out. Rather, gene-environment interactions generate a human biological and behavioral interface unique to each person that not only determines body weight but also explains individual variation in the net effect on body weight for any given amount of food intake or physical activity.

27-3. The answer is B. *(Hurst's The Heart, 14th Edition, Chap. 27)* Homeostatic dysregulation in the hypothalamus adversely affects appetite and satiety as they respond to peripheral hormones that register fuel storage and availability. With obesity, these mechanisms drive an increase in appetite, producing a positive energy balance, which generates and maintains a higher body weight.[11,12] Following a weight-loss intervention, secretion of ghrelin from the stomach is increased above baseline both before and after meals (option A). Ghrelin stimulates neuropeptide Y (NPY) and Agouti-related peptide neurons in the arcuate nucleus of the hypothalamus, causing the release of NPY, which activates orexigenic neural pathways, leading to an increase in appetite (option D). At the same time, hormones from the gastrointestinal tract and pancreas (eg, leptin, cholecystokinin, glucagon-like peptide-1, amylin, and peptide YY) are reduced below baseline levels (option B).[12] These latter hormones circulate to the hypothalamus and stimulate proopiomelanocortin-expressing neurons in the arcuate nucleus to produce α-melanocyte-stimulating hormone (MSH). The α-MSH binds upstream MC4R receptors to activate anorexigenic neural pathways, resulting in suppression of appetite. The fall in these satiety-producing hormones has an additional effect to stimulate appetite. Furthermore, in response to weight loss, resting energy expenditure rates are decreased (option C), and the energy that muscles use for any given amount of work is also decreased (ie, increased muscle energy efficiency). These energetic changes also promote weight regain.[13] Finally, psychological food preferences become oriented to foods of greater caloric density with high fat and sugar content (option E).

27-4. **The answer is D.** *(Hurst's The Heart, 14th Edition, Chap. 27)* Obesity markedly augments the risk of obstructive sleep apnea, which interrupts normal sleep with periods of hypoxia. This establishes a vicious cycle whereby progressive weight gain exacerbates sleep apnea and sleep apnea promotes further weight gain.[14,15] Obstructive sleep apnea adversely affects psychological health, causing fatigue and depression, affects metabolic health by predisposing to MetS and type 2 diabetes, and affects cardiovascular health as an independent risk factor for refractory hypertension, stroke, and CVD.[16-20] The therapeutic options for obstructive sleep apnea include continuous positive airway pressure therapy and weight loss.[21,22] The severity of sleep apnea is quantified by the apnea–hypopnea index (AHI), which reflects the average number of apneic/hypopneic episodes per hour during a polysomnography study.[23] Weight loss, whether achieved by lifestyle therapy[22] or obesity medications,[22] can dramatically improve both AHI scores and symptomatology; however, therapeutic benefits are most predictably achieved with at least 10% weight loss.[21,22]

27-5. **The answer is D.** *(Hurst's The Heart, 14th Edition, Chap. 27)* The criteria established by the World Health Organization in 1998[24] defines that BMI values 18.5 to 24.9 kg/m^2 are indicative of lean individuals, BMIs 25 to 29.9 kg/m^2 overweight, and BMIs of 30 kg/m^2 or more represent obesity categorized as obese class I (BMI 30–34.9), obese class II (BMI 35–39.9), or obese class III (BMI ≥ 40) (option A). These criteria were soon thereafter adopted by the National Institutes of Health.[25] However, in South Asian, East Asian, and Southeast Asian populations, health is adversely affected at lower levels of BMIs, and alternate criteria have been advocated, with BMIs of 18.5 to 22.9 kg/m^2 indicative of normal weight, 23 to 24.9 kg/m^2 overweight, and 25 or more kg/m^2 obese (option B).[26] BMI is an anthropometric measure that interrelates the height and weight of individuals, and, therefore, is only an indirect measure of adiposity of total body fat mass. BMI incorporates lean mass, fat mass, bone mass, and fluid status, all of which can vary independently from fat mass. BMI will overestimate adiposity in athletes with high muscle mass (option C) and in patients with edema and will underestimate adiposity in elderly patients with sarcopenia. For this reason, patients with elevated BMI measurements must be clinically evaluated to confirm excess adiposity. It is important to consider that the association between BMI and CVD is largely explained by its association with other risk factors, such that independent risk conferred by BMI is usually minimized in multivariate analyses (option D). For example, when adjusted for waist circumference or the presence of MetS, BMI is no longer a significant independent risk factor for CVD or becomes a much weaker predictor.[27-31] Regarding congestive heart failure (CHF), the presence of overweight or obesity may be protective against mortality, referred to as the *obesity paradox* (option E). Elevations in BMI are associated with increased risk of developing CHF in part by predisposing to hypertension, type 2 diabetes, sleep apnea, and CVD. However, once patients present with CHF, the presence of overweight and/or obesity has been observed to be protective regarding risks of future CVD mortality and hospitalizations when compared with lean individuals.[32-34] Better outcomes in overweight or obese subjects may reflect reverse causality resulting from processes that both lower body weight and increase mortality (eg, cardiac cachexia and cigarettes).

27-6. **The answer is D.** *(Hurst's The Heart, 14th Edition, Chap. 27)* Body mass index status as lean, overweight, or obese does not substantially affect coronary heart disease risk in metabolically healthy patients (those with no other MetS traits), so aggressive weight-loss treatment would not be expected to reduce the risk for coronary heart disease in these patients (option D). Metabolically healthy obese individuals exhibit relatively low rates of future type 2 diabetes, cardiovascular events, and mortality.[27,35-38] BMI does not indicate the impact of excess adiposity on the health of individual patients (option E).[39] Therefore, individuals who meet the anthropometric criterion for overweight or obesity must then undergo a clinical evaluation for the presence or absence of weight-related complications (option A).[39,40] The presence and severity of complications or relevant risk factors will indicate the need for more aggressive therapy to improve the health of individual patients. The identification of complications does not involve an extensive or extraordinary degree of testing but can be ascertained in the course of an initial patient evaluation consisting of medical history, review of systems, physical examination, and laboratory studies. In many cases, the information gathered in the initial examination is sufficient for the diagnosis of certain weight-related complications (option B). For other complications, the initial information augments the degree of suspicion, and additional testing consistent with standards of care is then needed to confirm the diagnosis and to stage the severity of the complication. The goals of weight-loss therapy are to improve the health of patients with obesity by treating and preventing weight-related complications (option C).

27-7. **The answer is B.** (*Hurst's The Heart, 14th Edition, Chap. 27*) Weight loss is perhaps the most effective therapeutic approach for treating and preventing the progression of cardiometabolic disease (option A) via improvements in the core physiological processes that confer risk of future type 2 diabetes (T2D) and CVD events. Three major randomized clinical trials, the Diabetes Prevention Program,[41] the Finnish Diabetes Study,[42] and the Da Qing Study,[43] all demonstrated the impressive efficacy of lifestyle/behavioral therapy to prevent T2D. With observational follow-up after termination of the Diabetes Prevention Program study, there was still a significant reduction in the cumulative incidence of T2D in the lifestyle treatment group at 10 years, despite the fact that BMI levels had equalized among the three treatment arms (option B).[41] Hypertension is an established consequence of overweight and obesity. It is therefore not surprising that one of the associated benefits of weight reduction is lowering blood pressure (option C). A meta-analysis suggests that blood pressure decreases by 1.2/1.0 mm Hg for every kilogram of weight lost. Weight loss of 5% to 10% has been shown to amplify the benefits of changes in macronutrient composition, resulting in a 20% decrease in triglycerides, a 15% reduction in LDL cholesterol, and an 8% to 10% increase in HDL cholesterol (option D). However, greater degrees of weight loss can achieve progressive improvements in dyslipidemia. Meta-analyses have reported that for every kilogram of weight loss, triglyceride levels decrease about 1.9% or 1.5 mg/dL.[44] Furthermore, there are beneficial effects of weight loss on LDL subclasses characterized by reductions in small, dense LDL particle concentrations and an increase in medium and large LDL particles, coupled to a mean increase in LDL particle size and reductions in total LDL particle concentration (option E).[44,45]

27-8. **The answer is E.** (*Hurst's The Heart, 14th Edition, Chap. 27*) Estimates of cardiometabolic disease risk can be used to identify patients at greatest risk for future type 2 diabetes (T2D) and CVD in order to target more aggressive weight-loss therapy to those individuals who will receive the greatest benefit. The clinician should evaluate patients for MetS and prediabetes, because this effectively identifies individuals at high risk for future T2D and CVD. However, MetS and prediabetes have high specificity but low sensitivity for identifying patients with insulin resistance and cardiometabolic disease,[37,46] and these entities alone will not identify significant proportions of at-risk patients (option E). Various indices using information from history and physical examination, such as the American College of Cardiology (ACC)/American Heart Association (AHA) Omnibus risk estimator (option A),[47] Framingham Coronary Heart Disease Risk Score (option B),[48] the Reynolds Risk Score (option C),[49] or commercial products that use clinical laboratory assays, can be used to stage risk in insulin-resistant patients whether or not they meet diagnostic criteria for MetS or prediabetes. Another approach to cardiometabolic disease risk stratification for the patient with obesity is the Cardiometabolic Disease Staging system (CMDS) (option D).[27,28] CMDS defines five stages of risk that are based on established physiological and epidemiological observations to quantitatively stratify the risk of both T2D and CVD.

27-9. **The answer is A.** (*Hurst's The Heart, 14th Edition, Chap. 27*) Orlistat (option A) is the only approved long-term drug for obese adolescents aged at least 12 years, while all others (options B, C, and D) are only approved for adult patients. Since 2012, there have been four new weight-loss medications approved for the chronic treatment of obesity by the FDA.[50,41,51,52] These medications are in addition to orlistat (120 mg), approved in 1999, which was the only preexisting medication for long-term pharmacotherapy and the only one currently permitted in Europe and many other countries. The newer medications include lorcaserin, phentermine/topiramate extended-release (ER), naltrexone ER/bupropion ER, and high-dose liraglutide (3 mg). The availability of these new medications has greatly expanded treatment options for patients with obesity and has led to more robust approaches to patient management.[40] All these medications are approved in the United States as adjuncts to lifestyle modification in overweight patients with BMIs of 27 to 29.9 kg/m^2 having at least one weight-related comorbidity (generally taken to be diabetes, hypertension, or dyslipidemia), or obese patients (BMI ≥ 30 kg/m^2) whether or not comorbidities are present.

27-10. The answer is D. *(Hurst's The Heart, 14th Edition, Chap. 27)* Bariatric surgery is the most effective method for treating class II and III obesity[53,54] and can be considered in patients with (1) BMIs of 35 kg/m^2 or more and associated comorbidities (option B) or (2) BMIs of 40 kg/m^2 whether or not accompanied by comorbidities, particularly after failure of lifestyle modification and medical therapies (option C). Bariatric surgery can provide substantial weight loss (15% to more than 40%), but this varies by procedure.[54] The most commonly performed procedures are Roux-en-Y gastric bypass (RYGB), adjustable gastric banding, sleeve gastrectomy, and biliopancreatic diversion with or without duodenal switch. Many patients achieve long-term weight loss; however, it is not uncommon for patients to gradually regain weight over time.[55] Sustained weight loss also depends on ongoing lifestyle therapy, patient reeducation in terms of active lifestyle changes, and long-term medical follow-up.

References

1. Finucane MM, Stevens GA, Cowan MJ, et al. National, regional, and global trends in body-mass index since 1980: systematic analysis of health examination surveys and epidemiological studies with 960 country-years and 9.1 million participants. *Lancet.* 2011;377(9765):557-567.
2. Ng M, Fleming T, Robinson M, et al. Global, regional, and national prevalence of overweight and obesity in children and adults during 1980-2013: a systemic analysis for the Global Burden of Disease Study 2013. *Lancet.* 2014;384(9945):766-781.
3. Ogden CL, Carroll MD, Kit BK, et al. Prevalence of childhood and adult obesity in the United States, 2011-2012. *JAMA.* 2014;311(8):806-814.
4. Ogden CL, Carroll MD, Fryar CD, et al. Prevalence of obesity among adults and youth: United States 2011-2014. *NCHS Data Brief.* 2015;219:1-8.
5. Farooqi IS, O'Rahilly S. Genetic factors in human obesity. *Obes Rev.* 2007;8(Suppl 1): 37-40.
6. Haqq S, Ganna A, van der Laan SW, et al. Gene-based meta-analysis of genome wide association studies implicates new loci involved in obesity. *Hum Mol Genet.* 2015;24(23):6849-6860.
7. Frayling TM, Timpson NJ, Weedon MN, et al. A common variant in the FTO gene is associated with body mass index and predisposes to childhood and adult obesity. *Science.* 2007;316(5826):889-894.
8. Loos RJF, Lindgren CM, Li S, et al. Common variants near MC4R are associated with fat mass, weight and risk of obesity. *Nat Genet.* 2008;40(6):768-775.
9. Qi Q, Chu AY, Kang JH, et al. Sugar-sweetened beverages and genetic risk of obesity. *N Engl J Med.* 2012;367:1387-1396.
10. Willer CJ, Speliotes EK, Loos RJF, et al. Six new loci associated with body mass index highlight neuronal influence on body weight regulation. *Nat Genet.* 2009;41(1):25-34.
11. Sumithran P, Proietto J. The defence of body weight: a physiological basis for weight regain after weight loss. *Clin Sci (Lond).* 2013;124:231-241.
12. Maclean PS, Bergouignan A, Cornier MA, et al. Biology's response to dieting: the impetus for weight regain. *Am J Physiol Regul Integr Comp Physiol.* 2011;301:R581-R600.
13. Leibel RL, Rosenbaum M, Hirsch J. Changes in energy expenditure resulting from altered body weight. *N Engl J Med.* 1995;332:621-628.
14. Xiao Q, Arem H, Moore SC, et al. A large prospective investigation of sleep duration, weight change, and obesity in the NIH-AART Diet and Health Study cohort. *Am J Epidemiol.* 2013;178:1600-1610.
15. Young T, Skatrud J, Peppard PE. Risk factors for obstructive sleep apnea in adults. *JAMA.* 2004;291(16):2013-2016.
16. Young T, Peppard PE, Gottlieb DJ. Epidemiology of obstructive sleep apnea: a population health perspective. *Am J Respir Crit Care Med.* 2002;165(9):1217-1239.
17. Coughlin SR, Mawdsley L, Mugarza JA, Calverley PM, Wilding JP. Obstructive sleep apnoea is independently associated with an increased prevalence of metabolic syndrome. *Eur Heart J.* 2004;25(9):735-741.
18. Loke YK, Brown JW, Kwok CS, Niruban A, Myint PK. Association of obstructive sleep apnea with risk of serious cardiovascular events: a systematic review and meta-analysis. *Circ Cardiovasc Qual Outcomes.* 2012;5(5):720-728.
19. Wolk R, Shamsuzzaman AS, Somers VK. Obesity, sleep apnea, and hypertension. *Hypertension.* 2003;42(6):1067-1074.

20. Marcus JA, Pothineni A, Marcus CZ, et al. The role of obesity and obstructive sleep apnea in the pathogenesis and treatment of resistant hypertension. *Curr Hypertens Rep.* 2014;16:410.

21. Foster GD, Borradaile KE, Sanders MH, et al; Sleep AHEAD Research Group of Look AHEAD Research Group. A randomized study on the effect of weight loss on obstructive sleep apnea among obese patients with type 2 diabetes: the Sleep AHEAD study. *Arch Intern Med.* 2009;169(17):1619-1626.

22. Winslow DH, Bowden CH, DiDonato KP, McCullough PA. A randomized, double-blind, placebo-controlled study of an oral, extended-release formulation of phentermine/topiramate for the treatment of obstructive sleep apnea in obese adults. *Sleep.* 2012;35(11):1529-1539.

23. Araghi MH, Chen YF, Jagielski A, et al. Effectiveness of lifestyle interventions on obstructive sleep apnea (OSA): systematic review and meta-analysis. *Sleep.* 2013;36(10): 1553-1562.

24. World Health Organization (WHO). Report of a WHO consultation on obesity. Obesity: preventing and managing the global epidemic. Geneva, Switzerland: WHO; 1998. National Heart, Lung, and Blood Institute. Clinical Guidelines on the Identification, Evaluation, and Treatment of Overweight and Obesity in Adults: The Evidence Report. Bethesda, MD: National Institutes of Health; 1998. Accessed at www .nhlbi.nih.gov/guidelines/obesity/ob_gdlns.pdf. Available at: http://whqlibdoc.who.int/hq/1998/WHO_ NUT_NCD_98.1_ (p1-158).pdf.

25. National Heart, Lung, and Blood Institute. *Clinical Guidelines on the Identification, Evaluation, and Treatment of Overweight and Obesity in Adults: The Evidence Report.* Bethesda, MD: National Institutes of Health; 1998. Accessed at www.nhlbi .nih.gov/guidelines/obesity/ob_gdlns.pdf.

26. World Health Organization Expert Consultation. Appropriate body-mass index for Asian populations and its implications for policy and intervention strategies. *Lancet.* 2004;363:157-163.

27. Guo F, Moellering DR, Garvey WT. The progression of cardiometabolic disease: validation of a new cardiometabolic disease staging system applicable to obesity. *Obesity (Silver Spring).* 2014;22:110-118.

28. Ridker PM, Buring JE, Rifai N, Cook NR. Development and validation of improved algorithms for the assessment of global cardiovascular risk in women: the Reynolds Risk Score. *JAMA.* 2007;297(6):611-619.

29. Yusuf S, Hawken S, Ounpuu S, et al. Obesity and the risk of myocardial infarction in 27,000 participants from 52 countries: a case-control study. *Lancet.* 2005;366(9497): 1640-1649.

30. Meigs JB, Wilson PW, Fox CS, et al. Body mass index, metabolic syndrome, and risk of type 2 diabetes or cardiovascular disease. *J Clin Endocrinol Metab.* 2006;91(8): 2906-2912.

31. Kip KE, Marroquin OC, Kelley DE, et al. Clinical importance of obesity versus the metabolic syndrome in cardiovascular risk in women: a report from the Women's Ischemia Syndrome Evaluation (WISE) study. *Circulation.* 2004;109(6):706-713.

32. Sharma A, Lavie CJ, Borer JS, et al. Meta-analysis of the relation of body mass index to all-cause and cardiovascular mortality and hospitalization in patients with chronic heart failure. *Am J Cardiol.* 2015;115(10):1428-1434.

33. Khalid U, Ather S, Bavishi C, et al. Pre-morbid body mass index and mortality after incident heart failure: the ARIC Study. *J Am Coll Cardiol.* 2014;64(25):2743-2749.

34. Oreopoulos A, Padwal R, Kalantar-Zadeh K, et al. Body mass index and mortality in heart failure: a meta-analysis. *Am Heart J.* 2008;156(1):13-22.

35. Krauss RM, Blanche PJ, Rawlings RS, Fernstrom HS, Williams PT. Separate effects of reduced carbohydrate intake and weight loss on atherogenic dyslipidemia. *Am J Clin Nutr.* 2006; 83(5):1025-1031.

36. Stefan N, Kantartzis K, Machann J, et al. Identification and characterization of metabolically benign obesity in humans. *Arch Intern Med.* 2008;168:1609-1616.

37. Wildman RP, Muntner P, Reynolds K, et al. The obese without cardiometabolic risk factor clustering and the normal weight with cardiometabolic risk factor clustering: prevalence and correlates of 2 phenotypes among the US population (NHANES 1999-2004). *Arch Intern Med.* 2008;168(15):1617-1624.

38. Meigs JB, Wilson PW, Fox CS, et al. Body mass index, metabolic syndrome, and risk of type 2 diabetes or cardiovascular disease. *J Clin Endocrinol Metab.* 2006;91:2906-2912.

39. Garvey WT, Garber AJ, Mechanick JI, et al; on behalf of the AACE Obesity Scientific Committee. American Association of Clinical Endocrinologists and American College of Endocrinology position statement on the 2014 advanced framework for a new diagnosis of obesity as a chronic disease. *Endocr Pract.* 2014;20(9):977-989.

40. Garvey WT. New tools for weight-loss therapy enable a more robust medical model for obesity treatment: rationale for a complications-centric approach. *Endocr Pract.* 2013;19(5):864-874.

41. Diabetes Prevention Program Research Group, Knowler WC, Fowler SE, Hamman RF, et al. 10-year follow-up of diabetes incidence and weight loss in the Diabetes Prevention Program Outcomes Study. *Lancet.* 2009;374:1677-1686.

42. Lindström J, Ilanne-Parikka P, Peltonen M, et al; Finnish Diabetes Prevention Study Group. Sustained reduction in the incidence of type 2 diabetes by lifestyle intervention: follow-up of the Finnish Diabetes Prevention Study. *Lancet.* 2006;368:1673-1679.

43. Pan XR, Li GW, Hu YH, et al. Effects of diet and exercise in preventing NIDDM in people with impaired glucose tolerance. The Da Qing IGT and Diabetes Study. *Diabetes Care.* 1997;20:537-544.

44. Nordmann AJ, Nordmann A, Briel M, et al. Effects of low-carbohydrate vs low-fat diets on weight loss and cardiovascular risk factors: a meta-analysis of randomized controlled trials. *JAMA Intern Med.* 2006;166(3):285-293. Erratum in: *JAMA Intern Med.* 2006;166(8):932.

45. Varady KA, Bhutani S, Klempel MC, Kroeger CM. Comparison of effects of diet versus exercise weight loss regimens on LDL and HDL particle size in obese adults. *Lipids Health Dis.* 2011;10:119.

46. Yusuf S, Hawken S, Ounpuu S, et al. Obesity and the risk of myocardial infarction in 27,000 participants from 52 countries: a case-control study. *Lancet.* 2005;366:1640-1649.

47. Liao Y, Kwon S, Shaughnessy S, et al. Critical evaluation of adult treatment panel III criteria in identifying insulin resistance with dyslipidemia. *Diabetes Care.* 2004;27:978-983.

48. Lloyd-Jones DM, Leip EP, Larson MG, et al. Prediction of lifetime risk for cardiovascular disease by risk factor burden at 50 years of age. *Circulation.* 2006;113(6):791-798.

49. Kannel WB, McGee D, Gordon T. A general cardiovascular risk profile: the Framingham Study. *Am J Cardiol.* 1976;38(1):46-51.

50. Cefalu WT, Bray GA, Home PD, et al. Advances in the science, treatment, and prevention of the disease of obesity: reflections from a Diabetes Care editors' expert forum. *Diabetes Care.* 2015;38(8):1567-1582.

51. Apovian CM, Garvey WT, Ryan DH. Challenging obesity: Patient, provider, and expert perspectives on the roles of available and emerging nonsurgical therapies. *Obesity.* 2015;23 Suppl 2:S1-S26.

52. Fujioka K. Current and emerging medications for overweight or obesity in people with comorbidities. *Diabetes Obes Metab.* 2015;17(11):1021-1032.

53. Carnethon MR, De Chavez PJ, Biggs ML, et al. Association of weight status with mortality in adults with incident diabetes. *JAMA.* 2012;308(6):581-590.

54. Adams TD, Davidson LE, Litwin SE, et al. Health benefits of gastric bypass surgery after 6 years. *JAMA.* 2012;308:1122-1131.

55. Sjostrom L, Lindroos AK, Peltonen M, et al. Lifestyle, diabetes, and cardiovascular risk factors 10 years after bariatric surgery. *N Engl J Med.* 2004;351:2683-2693.

CHAPTER 28

Diabetes and Cardiovascular Disease

Mark J. Eisenberg

QUESTIONS

DIRECTIONS: Choose the one best response to each question.

28-1. A 41-year-old woman with a history of atrial fibrillation presents to your office. Which of the following is *incorrect*?

A. A normal glycated hemoglobin should be < 6.0%, while a glycated hemoglobin of 6.0% to 6.5% is considered prediabetes
B. A glycated hemoglobin level of 6.5% or higher on two separate occasions indicates diabetes
C. Prediabetes can be diagnosed by a fasting plasma glucose of 100 mg/dL or more (impaired fasting glucose), a postglucose load of 140 to 199 mg/dL (impaired glucose tolerance), or both
D. Diabetes can be diagnosed by a fasting plasma glucose > 126 mg/dL or a 2-hour postprandial glucose of > 200 mg/dL during an oral glucose tolerance test involving a glucose solution containing the equivalent of 75 grams of glucose dissolved in water
E. Diabetes can be diagnosed in the patient who has a random plasma glucose of > 200 mg/dL with classic symptoms of hyperglycemia

28-2. An obese 17-year-old woman now present with her second pregnancy. Which of the following is *incorrect*?

A. Patients who are overweight or obese with a body mass index (BMI) of > 25 kg/m^2 or in the case of Asian Americans of 23 kg/m^2 or higher should be screened for diabetes
B. Children and adolescents who are overweight or obese should be screened for diabetes

C. With regard to gestational diabetes, patients with risk factors should be tested in the first prenatal visit. At 28 weeks' of gestation, pregnant women who are not previously known to have diabetes should be tested for gestational diabetes
D. Women with a history of gestational diabetes are considered to have prediabetes and should receive lifestyle interventions for the prevention of diabetes
E. All are correct

28-3. Which of the following is *incorrect*?

A. In 1985, an estimated 30 million people worldwide had diabetes
B. It is expected that there will be 350 million people worldwide with diabetes by 2025
C. In the United States in 2012, the unadjusted prevalence of diabetes was 19.3% (95% confidence interval [CI], 7.8%–11.1%)
D. Within the diabetes population, 25.2% (95% CI, 21.1%–29.8%) were undiagnosed
E. All are correct

28-4. A 70-year-old man with a history of diabetes, coronary artery disease (CAD), and hypertension has now developed diabetic nephropathy. Which of the following should *not* be used when treating this patient?

A. Control of hypertension with an angiotensin converting enzyme (ACE) inhibitor or angiotensin receptor blocker (ARB)
B. Glycemic control
C. Sodium restriction
D. Adjustment of protein intake
E. Renal arteriography if systolic blood pressure is > 170 mm Hg despite treatment with two antihypertensive agents

28-5. Which of the following statements is *not true* regarding type 2 diabetes mellitus and coronary heart disease?

A. Coronary heart disease (CHD) is strongly associated with type 2 diabetes mellitus and is the leading cause of death regardless of the duration of disease

B. There is a two- to fourfold increase in the relative risk ratio of cardiovascular disease in type 2 diabetes patients compared to the general population. This increase is particularly disproportionate in diabetic women when compared with diabetic men

C. The protection that premenopausal women have against CHD is not seen if they suffer from diabetes

D. The degree of hyperglycemia and the duration of hyperglycemia are strong risk factors for the development of microvascular but not macrovascular complications

E. Even impaired glucose tolerance increases cardiovascular risk, although there is minimal hyperglycemia

28-6. Which of the following statements is *not true* regarding insulin resistance?

A. The insulin resistance syndrome is a composite of dyslipidemia, hypertension, hypercoagulability, and microalbuminuria

B. Insulin resistance is the predominant defect in > 90% of type 2 diabetes patients and the major pathologic mechanism for the susceptibility to premature cardiovascular disease

C. Hyperinsulinemia is an independent risk factor when adjusted for lipid profile, hypertension, and family history

D. Studies of multiple ethnic groups show increased carotid intima-medial thickness (a reliable marker for coronary disease) in subjects with insulin resistance

E. Because insulin resistance precedes clinically diagnosed type 2 diabetes by 10 to 15 years in as many as 90% of patients, this extensive period of atherogenic exposure may account for the higher rates of cardiovascular disease in type 2 diabetics

28-7. One of your patients who has a history of diabetes and multivessel percutaneous coronary intervention (PCI) has a glycated hemoglobin of 7.0%. With respect to intensive (< 7.0% glycated hemoglobin) versus usual care strategies for the treatment of diabetes, meta-analyses of clinical trial results indicate which of the following?

A. For cardiovascular death, there is no difference between the intensive (< 7.0% glycated hemoglobin) and usual care strategies

B. In long-term studies that combine UKPDS, ACCORD, and VADT, myocardial infarction (MI) was reduced by about approximately 15% over the long term

C. Apart from a modest reduction in MI rates, there is no significant benefit of a more intensive lowering of glycated hemoglobin with regard to cardiovascular macrovascular end points

D. One meta-analysis of 27,000 participants with 2370 major cardiovascular events, including hospitalization or death from heart failure, showed no important differences between the more intensive arm compared to the less intensive arm

E. All of the above are true

28-8. Which of the following statements is *not true* about the treatment of diabetic patients with statins?

A. For patients with diabetes and known cardiovascular disease, high-intensity statin therapy is recommended according to the American College of Cardiology/American Heart Association (ACC/AHA) guidelines of 2013

B. For patients with diabetes under the age of 40 with one additional cardiovascular risk factor or those age 40 to 75 without any cardiovascular risk factors, moderate to high-intensity statins are recommended

C. Much of the evidence for the treatment of diabetics with statins comes from subgroup analyses from large randomized trials of lipid-lowering therapies in which diabetic patients represented < 10% of all the patients enrolled

D. In the trials of statin therapy with hyperlipidemia, the relative benefit appears to be increased among diabetic patients compared with nondiabetic patients

E. In a pooled analysis from the TNT (Treating to New Targets) and IDEAL (Incremental Decrease in Clinical Endpoints Through Aggressive Lipid Lowering) trials, patients with prediabetes treated with high-intensity compared to low-intensity statins were more likely to develop new onset diabetes over 5 years

28-9. A 45-year-old man with diabetes and palpitations presents to your clinic. Which of the following statements regarding antiplatelet therapy in patients with diabetes is *false*?

A. For men over age 50 and women over age 60 with at least one additional major cardiovascular risk factor, it is recommended that aspirin therapy at 81 mg daily be instituted as a primary prevention strategy for type 1 and type 2 diabetic patients

B. For men over age 50 and women over age 60 with at least one additional major cardiovascular risk factor, clopidogrel can be considered as an alternative to aspirin as a primary prevention strategy for type 1 and type 2 diabetic patients

C. For patients who are under age 50 for men and 60 for women with no additional major risk factors, aspirin therapy is not recommended

D. For diabetic patients with acute coronary syndromes, the evidence suggests that there is no heterogeneity in the response to newer antiplatelet agents and strategies based on diabetes status

E. Clopidogrel is associated with a lower bleeding risk than are prasugrel and ticagrelor

28-10. An asymptomatic 65-year-old man with diabetes is referred to you for screening. With respect to screening for coronary artery disease (CAD) in patients with diabetes, which of the following statements is *true*?

A. Exercise testing in diabetic patients is more likely to be accurate when combined with echocardiography or radionuclide imaging

B. Diabetic patients are less likely to have an appropriate blood pressure and heart rate response to exercise and less likely to experience any pain corresponding to ST-segment changes caused in part by autonomic dysfunction

C. The AHA recommends that the finding of subclinical CAD should prompt clinicians to initiate more aggressive preventive measures

D. The DIAD study has shown that the prevalence of silent ischemia in the diabetic population is not insignificant, but the annual cardiac event rate is < 1% overall at 4.8 years of follow-up, and routine screening for inducible coronary ischemia did not reduce cardiovascular events

E. All of the above are correct

28-1. **The answer is A.** *(Hurst's The Heart, 14th Edition, Chap. 28)* The universally recognized criteria for the diagnosis of prediabetes and diabetes are as follows: (1) a normal glycated hemoglobin should be < 5.7%, (2) a glycated hemoglobin of 5.7% to 6.4% is considered prediabetes, and (3) a level of 6.5% or higher on two separate occasions indicates diabetes (option B).[1] Prediabetes can be diagnosed by a fasting plasma glucose of 100 mg/dL or more (impaired fasting glucose), a postglucose load of 140 to 199 mg/dL (impaired glucose tolerance), or both (option C). Other recognized criteria include a fasting plasma glucose > 126 mg/dL or a 2-hour postprandial glucose of > 200 mg/dL during an oral glucose tolerance test involving a glucose solution containing the equivalent of 75 grams of glucose dissolved in water (option D). Diabetes can also be diagnosed in the patient who has a random plasma glucose of > 200 mg/dL with classic symptoms of hyperglycemia (option E).

28-2. **The answer is E.** *(Hurst's The Heart, 14th Edition, Chap. 28)* New recommendations identify patients who are at increased risk for diabetes and who require testing. These include patients who were overweight or obese with a body mass index (BMI) of > 25 kg/m^2 or in the case of Asian Americans of 23 kg/m^2 or higher (option A). Recommendations for screening for diabetes have now expanded to screening of children and adolescents who are overweight or obese (option B). With regard to gestational diabetes, patients are tested in the first prenatal visit with risk factors. At 28 weeks' of gestation, there is a test for gestational diabetes in pregnant women who are not previously known to have diabetes (option C). It is recommended that women with a history of gestational diabetes are considered to have prediabetes and should receive lifestyle interventions for the prevention of diabetes (option D).

28-3. **The answer is C.** *(Hurst's The Heart, 14th Edition, Chap. 28)* The number of people with diabetes has increased alarmingly since 1985, and the rate of new cases is escalating. In 1985, an estimated 30 million people worldwide had diabetes (option A), and this figure is expected to rise to almost 350 million by 2025 (option B).[2] In the United States in 2012, the unadjusted prevalence of diabetes was 12.3% (95% confidence interval [CI], 10.8%–14.1%) (option C). Within the diabetes population, 25.2% (95% CI, 21.1%–29.8%) were undiagnosed (option D).[3]

28-4. **The answer is E.** *(Hurst's The Heart, 14th Edition, Chap. 28)* There is insufficient evidence to recommend angiotensin-converting enzyme (ACE) inhibitors in normotensive patients without microalbuminuria. Nonetheless, physicians should still recommend screening on at least a yearly basis, because the risk-to-benefit ratio of diagnosing microalbuminuria justifies treatment with an ACE inhibitor, if not for renal disease alone, then for reducing the incidence of myocardial infarction (MI) (option A). Clinical trials evaluating angiotensin receptor blockers (ARBs), including losartan and irbesartan, have demonstrated a significant renal protective effect in the diabetic patient with nephropathy (option A). There were no differences between the ARB and usual care groups with regard to cardiovascular outcomes.[4] An optimal approach toward diabetic nephropathy combines control of hypertension, preferably with an ACE inhibitor or ARB, glycemic control (option B), sodium restriction (option C), and adjustment of protein intake (option D). If increasing macroalbuminuria occurs or if renal insufficiency is progressive despite these measures, the patient should be referred to a nephrologist. It is strongly recommended that renal arteriography be avoided (option E). Dietary protein restriction in patients who have progressive renal insufficiency will reduce the accumulation of nitrogen-containing waste products and can have a beneficial influence on the progression of renal insufficiency.

28-5. **The answer is D.** *(Hurst's The Heart, 14th Edition, Chap. 28)* Coronary heart disease (CHD) is strongly associated with type 2 diabetes mellitus and is the leading cause of death regardless of the duration of disease (option A). There is a two- to fourfold increase in the relative risk ratio of cardiovascular disease in type 2 diabetes patients compared to the general population. This increase is particularly disproportionate in diabetic women when compared with diabetic men (option B). The protection that premenopausal women have against CHD is not seen if they suffer from diabetes (option C). The degree of hyperglycemia and the duration of hyperglycemia are strong risk factors for the development of *both* microvascular and macrovascular complications (option D). Even impaired glucose tolerance increases cardiovascular risk, although there is minimal hyperglycemia (option E).[5]

28-6. **The answer is A.** *(Hurst's The Heart, 14th Edition, Chap. 28)* The insulin resistance syndrome is a composite of dyslipidemia, hypertension, and hypercoagulability (option A).[6] The syndrome composite does not require microalbuminuria. It is only now being recognized that insulin resistance is the predominant defect in more than 90% of type 2 diabetes patients and the major pathologic mechanism for the susceptibility to premature cardiovascular disease (option B). Insulin resistance and hyperinsulinemia accelerate the development of atherosclerosis. Hyperinsulinemia is an independent risk factor when adjusted for lipid profile, hypertension, and family history (option C). Studies of multiple ethnic groups show increased carotid intima-medial thickness (a reliable marker for coronary disease) in subjects with insulin resistance (option D). Impaired glucose tolerance can increase the risk of heart disease. Because insulin resistance precedes clinically diagnosed type 2 diabetes by 10 to 15 years in as many as 90% of patients, this extensive period of atherogenic exposure may account for the higher rates of cardiovascular disease in type 2 diabetics (option E).[7,8]

28-7. **The answer is E.** *(Hurst's The Heart, 14th Edition, Chap. 28)* Evidence from updated meta-analyses indicates that, for cardiovascular death, there is no difference between the intensive (< 7.0% glycated hemoglobin) and usual care strategies (option A).[9] In long-term studies that combine UKPDS, ACCORD, and VADT, myocardial infarction (MI) was reduced by about 15% over the long term (option B). Apart from this modest reduction in MI rates, there was no significant benefit of a more intensive lowering of glycated hemoglobin with regard to cardiovascular macrovascular end points (option C). One meta-analysis of 27,000 participants with 2370 major cardiovascular events, including hospitalization or death from heart failure, showed no important differences between the more intensive arm compared to the less intensive arm (option D).[10]

28-8. **The answer is D.** *(Hurst's The Heart, 14th Edition, Chap. 28)* Hydroxymethylglutaryl coenzyme A (HMG-CoA) reductase inhibitors—statins—are the frontline therapy in lowering LDL cholesterol levels in type 2 diabetes patients without having an adverse effect on glycemic control. Important evidence from large randomized trials of lipid-lowering therapies is based on subgroup analyses in which diabetic patients represented < 10% of all the patients enrolled (option C); however, more recently studies have been done exclusively in diabetic patients. In the Cholesterol and Recurrent Events (CARE) Trial, which compared pravastatin with a placebo in secondary prevention, the baseline mean LDL concentration in diabetic patients was 136 mg/dL. LDL was reduced 27% in the group receiving pravastatin, which translated into a 25% reduction in coronary events over 5 years compared with the control group.[11] The Heart Protection Study (HPS), with a subgroup of 5963 diabetic patients, showed a 28% reduction in total coronary heart disease (CHD), including nonfatal myocardial infarction and CHD death, nonfatal and fatal strokes, coronary and noncoronary revascularizations, and major vascular events (total CHD, total stroke, or revascularizations) with simvastatin therapy.[12] *In the trials of statin therapy with hyperlipidemia, the relative benefit appears to be similar between diabetic patients and nondiabetic patients* (option D).

Secondary prevention: For patients with diabetes and known cardiovascular disease, high-intensity statin therapy is recommended according to the American College of Cardiology/American Heart Association (ACC/AHA) guidelines of 2013 (option A).[13] Primary prevention: For patients with diabetes under age 40 with one additional cardiovascular risk factor or those age 40 to 75 without any cardiovascular risk factors, moderate to high-intensity statins are recommended (option B). In a pooled analysis from the TNT

(Treating to New Targets) and IDEAL (Incremental Decrease in Clinical Endpoints Through Aggressive Lipid Lowering) trials, patients with prediabetes treated with high-intensity compared to low-intensity statins were more likely to develop new onset diabetes over 5 years (HR 1.20, 95% CI; 1.04–1.37) (option E).[14]

28-9. The answer is B. *(Hurst's The Heart, 14th Edition, Chap. 28)* For men over age 50 and women over age 60 with at least one additional major cardiovascular risk factor, aspirin therapy at 81 mg daily is recommended as a primary prevention statin strategy for type 1 and type 2 diabetic patients (option A). *Clopidogrel is not recommended for primary prevention among diabetic patients among patients who can take aspirin* (option B). However, for men under age 50 and women under age 60 with no additional major risk factors, aspirin therapy is not recommended (option C).[1] The use of antiplatelet therapy is the mainstay of management of acute coronary syndromes in diabetic patients. With the advent of newer antiplatelet drugs, there have been recommendations for greater use of prasugrel and ticagrelor. The evidence suggests that there is no heterogeneity in the response to newer agents and strategies based on diabetes status (option D).[15-20] The optimal strategy and regimen in diabetic patients is still elusive and remains the question of ongoing trials focused on limiting the thrombotic burden and not increasing the risk of major bleeding. Clopidogrel is associated with a lower bleeding risk than are prasugrel and ticagrelor (option E).

28-10. The answer is E. *(Hurst's The Heart, 14th Edition, Chap. 28)* The significant increase in major microvascular and macrovascular complications makes it important to begin screening for diabetes at an age younger than 45 years.[21] It has become necessary to implement aggressive screening strategies to be able to identify populations at the highest risk of developing diabetes.[22] Current measures of cardiovascular surveillance for coronary artery disease (CAD) in asymptomatic diabetic patients focus on routine stress testing in accordance with the American College of Cardiology/American Heart Association (ACC/AHA) guidelines. Exercise testing in diabetic patients is more likely to be accurate when combined with echocardiography or radionuclide imaging (option A).[23] Diabetic patients are less likely to have an appropriate blood pressure and heart rate response to exercise and less likely to experience any pain corresponding to ST-segment changes caused in part by autonomic dysfunction (option B). The AHA recommends that the finding of subclinical CAD should prompt clinicians to initiate more aggressive preventive measures (option C). The DIAD study has shown that the prevalence of silent ischemia in the diabetic population is not insignificant, but the annual cardiac event rate is < 1% overall at 4.8 years of follow-up, and routine screening for inducible coronary ischemia did not reduce cardiovascular events (option D).[24]

References

1. American Diabetes Association. Standards of Medical Care in Diabetes—2016. *Diabetes Care* 2016;39(Suppl 1).
2. World Health Organization. *Diabetes Fact Sheet 236.* 2016.
3. Menke A, Casagrande S, Geiss L, Cowie CC. Prevalence of and trends in diabetes among adults in the United States, 1988-2012. *JAMA.* 2015;314(10):1021-1029.
4. Brenner BM, Cooper ME, de Zeeuw D, et al. Effects of losartan on renal and cardiovascular outcomes in patients with type 2 diabetes and nephropathy. *N Engl J Med.* 2001;345:861-869.
5. Li C, Ford ES, Zhao G, Mokdad AH. Prevalence of pre-diabetes and its association with clustering of cardiometabolic risk factors and hyperinsulinemia among U.S. adolescents: National Health and Nutrition Examination Survey 2005-2006. *Diabetes Care.* 2009;32(2):342-347.
6. Bansilal S, Farkouh ME, Fuster V. Role of insulin resistance and hyperglycemia in the development of atherosclerosis. *Am J Cardiol.* 2007;99(4A):6B-14B.
7. Hanley AJ, Williams K, Stern MP, Haffner SM. Homeostasis model assessment of insulin resistance in relation to the incidence of cardiovascular disease: the San Antonio Heart Study. *Diabetes Care.* 2002;25(7):1177-1184.
8. Forst T, Lubben G, Hohberg C, et al. Influence of glucose control and improvement of insulin resistance on microvascular blood flow and endothelial function in patients with diabetes mellitus type 2. *Microcirculation.* 2005;12:543-550.

9. Kähler P, Grevstad B, Almdal T, et al. Targeting intensive versus conventional glycaemic control for type 1 diabetes mellitus: a systematic review with meta-analyses and trial sequential analyses of randomised clinical trials. *BMJ Open*. 2014;4(8).

10. Turnbull FM, Abraira C, Anderson RJ, et al; Control Group. Intensive glucose control and macrovascular outcomes in type 2 diabetes. *Diabetologia*. 2009;52(11):2288-2298.

11. Goldberg RB, Mellies MJ, Sacks FM, et al. Cardiovascular events and their reduction with pravastatin in diabetic and glucose-intolerant myocardial infarction survivors with average cholesterol levels: subgroup analyses in the cholesterol and recurrent events (CARE) trial: the CARE investigators. *Circulation*. 1998;98(23):2513-2519.

12. Collins R, Armitage J, Parish S, et al; Heart Protection Study Collaborative Group. Effects of cholesterol-lowering with simvastatin on stroke and other major vascular events in 20,536 people with cerebrovascular disease or other high-risk conditions. *Lancet*. 2004;363(9411):757-767.

13. Stone NJ, Robinson JG, Lichtenstein AH, et al; American College of Cardiology/American Heart Association Task Force on Practice Guidelines. 2013 ACC/AHA guideline on the treatment of blood cholesterol to reduce atherosclerotic cardiovascular risk in adults: a report of the American College of Cardiology/American Heart Association Task Force on Practice Guidelines. *J Am Coll Cardiol*. 2014; 63(25 Pt B):2889-2934.

14. Kohli P, Waters DD, Nemr R, et al. Risk of new-onset diabetes and cardiovascular risk reduction from high-dose statin therapy in pre-diabetics and non-pre-diabetics: an analysis from TNT and IDEAL. *J Am Coll Cardiol*. 2015;65(4):402-404.

15. CURRENT-OASIS 7 Investigators, Mehta SR, Bassand JP, et al. Dose comparisons of clopidogrel and aspirin in acute coronary syndromes. *N Engl J Med*. 2010;363:930-942.

16. James S, Angiolillo DJ, Cornel JH, et al. Ticagrelor versus clopidogrel in patients with acute coronary syndromes and diabetes: a substudy from the PLATelet inhibition and patient Outcomes (PLATO) trial. *Eur Heart J*. 2010;31:3006-3016.

17. Ferreiro JL, Ueno M, Tello-Montoliu A, et al. Effects of cangrelor in coronary artery disease patients with and without diabetes mellitus: an in vitro pharmacodynamics investigation. *J Thromb Thrombolysis*. 2013;35:155-164.68.

18. Angiolillo DJ, Capranzano P, Ferreiro JL, et al. Impact of adjunctive cilostazol therapy on platelet function profiles in patients with and without diabetes mellitus on aspirin and clopidogrel therapy. *Thromb Haemost*. 2011;106:253-262.

19. Angiolillo DJ, Badimon JJ, Saucedo JF, et al. A pharmacodynamic comparison of prasugrel versus high-dose clopidogrel in patients with type 2 diabetes mellitus and coronary artery disease: Results of the OPTIMUS-3 trial. *Eur Heart J*. 2011;32:838-846.

20. Wiviott SD, Braunwald E, Angiolillo DJ, et al; TRITON-TIMI 38 Investigators. Greater clinical benefit of more intensive oral antiplatelet therapy with prasugrel in patients with diabetes mellitus in the trial to assess improvement in therapeutic outcomes by optimizing platelet inhibition with prasugrel-Thrombolysis in Myocardial Infarction 38. *Circulation*. 2008;118(16):1626-1636.

21. Gillies CL, Lambert PC, Abrams KR, et al. Different strategies for screening and prevention of type 2 diabetes in adults: cost effectiveness analysis. *BMJ*. 2008;336(7654):1180-1185.

22. Jansson SP, Andersson DK, Svärdsudd K. Mortality and cardiovascular disease outcomes among 740 patients with new-onset type 2 diabetes detected by screening or clinically diagnosed in general practice. *Diabetes Med*. 2016;33(3):324-331.

23. Hage FG, Lusa L, Dondi M, Giubbini R, Iskandrian AE; IAEA Diabetes Investigators. Exercise stress tests for detecting myocardial ischemia in asymptomatic patients with diabetes mellitus. *Am J Cardiol*. 2013;112(1):14-20.

24. Bansal S, Wackers FJ, Inzucchi SE, et al; DIAD Study Investigators. Five-year outcomes in high-risk participants in the Detection of Ischemia in Asymptomatic Diabetics (DIAD) study: a post hoc analysis. *Diabetes Care*. 2011;34(1):204-209.

CHAPTER 29

Hyperlipidemia

Mark J. Eisenberg

DIRECTIONS: Choose the one best response to each question.

29-1. Lipoproteins contain which of the following?

A. Neutral lipid
B. Nonesterified cholesterol
C. Phospholipid
D. Proteins
E. All of the above

29-2. A 40-year-old man with a history of hyperlipidemia has an inferior MI. Multiple members of his family have had coronary events in their early 40s. Which of the following types of studies do *not* provide evidence to support the idea that an elevated plasma LDL is a major risk factor for atherosclerotic cardiovascular disease (ASCVD)?

A. Animal studies
B. Genetic forms of elevated LDL
C. Epidemiological associations
D. Randomized controlled trials
E. All of the above support the idea

29-3. Which of the following steps in the progression of atherosclerosis is *incorrect*?

A. Accumulation of large numbers of foam cells gives rise to fatty streaks
B. Some foam cells die and release their cholesterol esters into the interstitium, and over time the core of extracellular lipid expands
C. Osteoclasts from the medium begin to produce fibrous connective tissue
D. This tissue forms a covering of the fatty streak; here the lesion is called a fibrous plaque (fibroatheroma)
E. Continuous filtration of LDL into the arterial wall leads to several steps to plaque progression

29-4. Which of the following is *not true* about familial hypercholesterolemia (FH)?

A. Heterozygous FH occurs in about one in 500 persons; homozygous FH occurs in only one in a million persons
B. Patients with heterozygous FH commonly develop premature ASCVD, most often between the ages of 30 and 60 years, and estimates are that it accounts for at least 2% of premature myocardial infarctions (MIs). Homozygous FH leads to very premature disease, often in the teens or earlier
C. A clinical feature of FH is the presence of cholesterol deposition in tendons (xanthomas) of the hands, elbows, knees, and feet, especially the Achilles tendon
D. Deposition of cholesterol in the skin about the eyes is called xanthelasma
E. In individuals with hypercholesterolemia, the presence of xanthelasmas is pathognomonic of FH

29-5. One of your patients is morbidly obese and consults you with respect to the advisability of bariatric surgery. Which of the following is *not true* about obesity?

A. Excess body weight can be defined as *overweight* (body mass index [BMI] 25 to 30 kg/m^2) and *obesity* (BMI > 30 kg/m^2)
B. More than one-third (34.9% or 78.6 million) of US adults are obese
C. More than 15% of American children and teens are clinically obese
D. Non-Hispanic blacks have the highest age-adjusted rates of obesity (47.8%) followed by Hispanics (42.5%), non-Hispanic whites (32.6%), and non-Hispanic Asians (10.8%)
E. Obesity is higher among middle-aged adults (ages 40 to 59 years; 39.5%) than among younger adults (ages 20 to 39 years; 30.3%) or older adults (≥ age 60 years; 35.4%)

29-6. A patient is referred to you with the possible diagnosis of metabolic syndrome. Which of the following is *not true* about the criteria used for the clinical definition of the metabolic syndrome?

A. Increased blood pressure is one of the criteria
B. Dyslipidemia (increased triglycerides and lowered HDL-C) is one of the criteria
C. Increased fasting glucose is one of the criteria
D. Abdominal obesity (increased waist circumference) is one of the criteria
E. Any three of five abnormal findings constitute a diagnosis of the metabolic syndrome, and a single set of cut points are used for all components

29-7. One of your patients has suffered from multiple MIs yet is statin-intolerant. You are considering starting the patient on a PCSK9 inhibitor. Which of the following is *not true* about PCSK9 inhibitors?

A. PCSK9 inhibitors bind PCSK9 from the circulation and thereby prevent the action of PCSK9 to promote the degradation of LDL receptors
B. As a result of PCSK9 inhibition, fewer LDLRs are expressed by the liver, and serum LDL-C levels are reduced
C. US Food and Drug Administration (FDA)–approved PCSK9 inhibitors are evolocumab and alirocumab
D. These drugs must be given systemically once or twice a month, and they cause marked incremental reductions of LDL-C even when given with statins
E. To date, they appear to be safe and have not been reported to cause myopathy

29-8. Which of the following is *true* about cholesteryl ester transfer protein (CETP) inhibitors?

A. CETP inhibitors inhibit CETP, 353 which transfers cholesterol ester from HDL-C to VLDL or LDL. As a result, HDL-C levels are increased, whereas VLDL-C and LDL-C are decreased
B. Three randomized controlled trials with CETP inhibitors have failed to show an ASCVD risk reduction
C. Torcetrapib gave an increase in total mortality, and the trial was discontinued
D. Trials with two other CETP inhibitors, dalcetrapib and evacetrapib, were discontinued before completion because of futility
E. All are true

29-9. A 73-year-old woman who was recently started on a statin comes to you complaining of muscle pain. According to the 2014 National Lipid Association Statin Muscle Safety Task Force, which of the following terms is *incorrect* with respect to statin-associated adverse muscle events?

A. Myalgia: A symptom of muscle discomfort, including muscle aches, soreness, stiffness, tenderness, or cramps with or soon after exercise, with a normal creatine kinase (CK) level. Myalgia symptoms can be described as flu-like symptoms
B. Myopathy: Muscle weakness (not due to pain), with or without an elevation in CK level
C. Myositis: Muscle inflammation
D. Myonecrosis: Elevation in muscle enzymes compared with either baseline CK levels (while not on statin therapy) or the upper limit of normal that has been adjusted for age, race, and sex: Mild: 3- to 5-fold elevation in CK above baseline; moderate: 5- to 10-fold elevation in CK above baseline; severe: 10-fold or greater elevation in CK above baseline or an absolute level of 10,000 U/L or more
E. Clinical rhabdomyolysis: Myonecrosis with myoglobinuria or acute renal failure (an increase in serum creatinine of least 0.5 mg/dL [44 µM/L])

29-10. A patient in your practice cannot tolerate high-dose statin therapy. Which of the following statements is *not true* regarding alternatives for patients who are statin intolerant?

A. Efforts should be doubled to start and maintain lifestyle modification, which can lower cholesterol levels by 10% to 15%
B. Both bile acid resins and ezetimibe can lower LDL-C by 25% to 35%
C. Ezetimibe plus a moderate-intensity statin will reduce cholesterol levels as much as high-intensity statins
D. Fibrates and niacin are alternative add-on drugs for patients with hypertriglyceridemia
E. In patients with severe hypercholesterolemia, PCSK9 inhibitors may be an option for patients who are statin intolerant, especially in those with ASCVD or very high LDL-C levels

29-1. **The answer is E.** *(Hurst's The Heart, 14th Edition, Chap. 29)* The basic structure of all lipoproteins is similar. They contain a core of neutral lipid (triglyceride and cholesterol ester) (option A) that is surrounded by a polar coat containing nonesterified cholesterol (option B), phospholipid (option C), and proteins (called apolipoproteins) (option D). The major categories of lipoproteins consist of low-density lipoprotein (LDL), very-low-density lipoprotein (VLDL), high-density lipoprotein (HDL), and chylomicrons. These lipoproteins vary in size and density. Because lipoproteins can be separated by electrophoresis, they also have been named according to their migration relative to serum proteins. LDL is called beta lipoprotein, VLDL is pre-beta lipoprotein, and HDL is alpha lipoprotein.

29-2. **The answer is E.** *(Hurst's The Heart, 14th Edition, Chap. 29)* An elevated plasma LDL is designated a major risk factor for ASCVD. Several lines of evidence support a strong association: animal studies (option A), genetic forms of elevated LDL (option B), epidemiological associations (option C), and randomized controlled trials (RCTs) of LDL-lowering therapies (option D).

29-3. **The answer is C.** *(Hurst's The Heart, 14th Edition, Chap. 29).* Steps in the progression of atherosclerosis have been studied in detail. Accumulation of large numbers of foam cells gives rise to fatty streaks (option A). Some foam cells die and release their cholesterol esters into the interstitium, and over time the core of extracellular lipid expands (option B). Later, smooth muscle cells *(not osteoclasts)* from the medium begin to produce fibrous connective tissue (option C). This tissue forms a covering for the fatty streak; here the lesion is called a fibrous plaque (fibroatheroma) (option D). Continuous filtration of LDL into the arterial wall leads to several steps to plaque progression (option E); after many years, atheromas degenerate into complicated lesions, become unstable, and are prone to rupture. When rupture occurs, plaque material discharges into the lumen of the artery, producing thrombosis and cardiovascular events. At any stage of this process, LDL-lowering therapy reduces plaque progression and decreases the likelihood of plaque rupture and acute ASCVD events.

29-4. **The answer is E.** *(Hurst's The Heart, 14th Edition, Chap. 29).* Classic estimates were that heterozygous FH occurs in about one in 500 persons; homozygous FH occurs only one in a million persons (option A). In some populations, the prevalence of both forms can be higher. Patients with heterozygous FH commonly develop premature ASCVD, most often between the ages of 30 and 60 years, and estimates are that it accounts for at least 2% of premature MIs. Homozygous FH leads to very premature disease, often in the teens or earlier (option B). Another clinical feature of FH is the presence of cholesterol deposition in tendons (xanthomas) of the hands, elbows, knees, and feet, especially the Achilles tendon (option C). Deposition of cholesterol in the skin about the eyes is called xanthelasma (option D); in individuals with hypercholesterolemia, this finding suggests but is not pathognomonic of FH (option E). The same is true for corneal arcus.

29-5. **The answer is A.** *(Hurst's The Heart, 14th Edition, Chap. 29).* Obesity in the general population is associated with an increased risk of ASCVD and other disorders. Among the latter are hypertensive cardiovascular disease, type 2 diabetes, fatty liver disease, gallstone disease, obstructive sleep apnea, and certain forms of cancer (colon, breast, and endometrial). Excess body weight can be defined as *overweight* (BMI 25 to 29 kg/m^2) *(not BMI 25-30 kg/m^2)* and *obesity* (BMI ≥ 30 kg/m^2) *(not BMI > 30 kg/m^2)* (option A). According to the Centers for Disease Control and Prevention (CDC), more than one-third (34.9% or 78.6 million) of US adults are obese (option B). In addition, more than one-third of American adults (35.7%) and 17% (12.5 million) of American children and teens are clinically obese (option C). The CDC notes that non-Hispanic blacks have the highest age-adjusted rates of obesity (47.8%), followed by Hispanics (42.5%), non-Hispanic whites (32.6%), and non-Hispanic Asians (10.8%) (option D). Moreover, obesity is higher among middle-aged adults (ages 40 to 59 years; 39.5%) than among younger adults (ages 20 to 39 years; 30.3%) or older adults (≥ age 60 years; 35.4%) (option E).

29-6. **The answer is E.** *(Hurst's The Heart, 14th Edition, Chap. 29).* A clinical diagnosis of the metabolic syndrome can be made in accord with a clinical definition.[1] The risk factors of this definition include increased blood pressure (option A), dyslipidemia (increased triglycerides and lowered HDL-C) (option B), increased fasting glucose (option C), and abdominal obesity (increased waist circumference) (option D). This diagnosis harmonized previous recommendations from the International Diabetes Federation and the American Heart Association/ National Heart, Lung, and Blood Institute. Any three of five abnormal findings constitute a diagnosis of the metabolic syndrome. A single set of cut points is used for all components *except waist circumference, for which different national or regional thresholds for waist increased circumference were recommended* (option E).

29-7. **The answer is B.** *(Hurst's The Heart, 14th Edition, Chap. 29).* Monoclonal antibody inhibitors of PCSK9 are a new class of LDL-lowering drugs. They bind PCSK9 from the circulation and thereby prevent the action of PCSK9 to promote the degradation of LDL receptors (option A).[2,3] As a result, more *(not fewer)* LDLRs are expressed by the liver, and serum LDL-C levels are reduced (option B).[4,5] US Food and Drug Administration (FDA)–approved PCSK9 inhibitors are evolocumab[4,5] and alirocumab (option C).[6] Another agent (bococizumab) is under investigation. These drugs must be given systemically once or twice a month. They cause marked incremental reductions of LDL-C even when given with statins (option D). To date, they appear to be safe and have not been reported to cause myopathy (option E). Interim reports from randomized controlled trials (RCTs) indicate that they enhance risk reduction in high-risk patients treated with statins.[7,8] Meta-analysis of several smaller trials further suggests ASCVD benefit.[9]

29-8. **The answer is E.** *(Hurst's The Heart, 14th Edition, Chap. 29).* CETP inhibitors inhibit CETP.[10] The protein transfers cholesterol ester from HDL-C to very-low-density or low-density lipoproteins (VLDL or LDL). As a result, HDL-C levels are increased, whereas VLDL-C and LDL-C are decreased (option A). This exchange theoretically could be beneficial by raising HDL-C, the so-called good cholesterol. However, to date three randomized controlled trials (RCTs) with CETP inhibitors have failed to show an ASCVD risk reduction (option B). One inhibitor, torcetrapib, gave an increase in total mortality, and the trial was discontinued (option C).[11] Trials with two other CETP inhibitors, dalcetrapib and evacetrapib, were discontinued before completion because of futility (option D).[12]

29-9. **The answer is D.** *(Hurst's The Heart, 14th Edition, Chap. 29).* Although the main concern with statins is the risk of rhabdomyolysis, this is a rare occurrence that affects 0.1% of patients.[13,14] Terminology relating to statin-associated adverse muscle events is variable and has changed over time. According to the 2014 National Lipid Association Statin Muscle Safety Task Force:[13] Myalgia: A symptom of muscle discomfort, including muscle aches, soreness, stiffness, tenderness, or cramps with or soon after exercise, with a normal creatine kinase (CK) level. Myalgia symptoms can be described as flu-like symptoms (option A). Myopathy: Muscle weakness (not due to pain), with or without an elevation in CK level (option B). Myositis: Muscle inflammation (option C). Myonecrosis: Elevation in muscle enzymes compared with either baseline CK levels (while not on statin therapy) or the upper limit of normal that has been adjusted for age, race, and sex: *Mild: 3- to 10-fold elevation in CK above baseline; Moderate: 10- to 50-fold elevation in CK above baseline; Severe: 50-fold or greater elevation in CK above baseline or an absolute level of 10,000 U/L or more* (option D). Clinical rhabdomyolysis: Myonecrosis with myoglobinuria or acute renal failure (an increase in serum creatinine of least 0.5 mg/dL [44 μM/L]) (option E).

29-10. **The answer is B.** *(Hurst's The Heart, 14th Edition, Chap. 29).* Statins are first-line cholesterol-lowering therapy, but if they are not tolerated, other ways to achieve cholesterol goals can be considered. Efforts should be doubled to start and maintain lifestyle modification, which can lower cholesterol levels by 10% to 15% (option A).[15] Both bile acid resins and ezetimibe can lower LDL-C by 15% to 25% *(not 25% to 35%)* (option B). Ezetimibe plus a moderate-intensity statin will reduce cholesterol levels as much as high-intensity statins (option C). Fibrates and niacin are alternative add-on drugs for patients with hypertriglyceridemia (option D). Finally, in patients with severe hypercholesterolemia, PCSK9 inhibitors may be an option for patients who are statin intolerant, especially in those with ASCVD or very high LDL-C levels (option E).

References

1. Alberti KG, Eckel RH, Grundy SM, et al. Harmonizing the metabolic syndrome: a joint interim statement of the International Diabetes Federation Task Force on Epidemiology and Prevention; National Heart, Lung, and Blood Institute; American Heart Association; World Heart Federation; International Atherosclerosis Society; and International Association for the Study of Obesity. *Circulation.* 2009;120(16):1640-1645.

2. Kwon HJ, Lagace TA, McNutt MC, Horton JD, Deisenhofer J. Molecular basis for LDL receptor recognition by PCSK9. *Proc Natl Acad Sci U S A.* 2008;105(6):1820-1825.

3. Horton JD, Cohen JC, Hobbs HH. PCSK9: a convertase that coordinates LDL catabolism. *J Lipid Res.* 2009;50(Suppl):S172-S177.

4. Roth EM, McKenney JM, Hanotin C, Asset G, Stein EA. Atorvastatin with or without an antibody to PCSK9 in primary hypercholesterolemia. *N Engl J Med.* 2012;367(20):1891-1900.

5. Blom DJ, Hala T, Bolognese M, et al. A 52-week placebo-controlled trial of evolocumab in hyperlipidemia. *N Engl J Med.* 2014;370(19):1809-1819.

6. Kereiakes DJ, Robinson JG, Cannon CP, et al. Efficacy and safety of the proprotein convertase subtilisin/kexin type 9 inhibitor alirocumab among high cardiovascular risk patients on maximally tolerated statin therapy: The ODYSSEY COMBO I study. *Am Heart J.* 2015;169(6):906-915 e913.

7. Robinson JG, Farnier M, Krempf M, et al. Efficacy and safety of alirocumab in reducing lipids and cardiovascular events. *N Engl J Med.* 2015;372(16):1489-1499.

8. Sabatine MS, Giugliano RP, Wiviott SD, et al. Efficacy and safety of evolocumab in reducing lipids and cardiovascular events. *N Engl J Med.* 2015;372(16):1500-1509.

9. Navarese EP, Kolodziejczak M, Schulze V, et al. Effects of proprotein convertase subtilisin/kexin type 9 antibodies in adults with hypercholesterolemia: a systematic review and meta-analysis. *Ann Intern Med.* 2015;163(1):40-51.

10. Tall AR. CETP inhibitors to increase HDL cholesterol levels. *N Engl J Med.* 2007;356(13):1364-1366.

11. Barter PJ, Caulfield M, Eriksson M, et al. Effects of torcetrapib in patients at high risk for coronary events. *N Engl J Med.* 2007;357(21):2109-2122.

12. Schwartz GG, Olsson AG, Abt M, et al. Effects of dalcetrapib in patients with a recent acute coronary syndrome. *N Engl J Med.* 2012;367(22):2089-2099.

13. Rosenson RS, Baker SK, Jacobson TA, Kopecky SL, Parker BA, The National Lipid Association's Muscle Safety Expert Panel. An assessment by the Statin Muscle Safety Task Force: 2014 update. *J Clin Lipidol.* 2014;8(3 Suppl):S58-S71.

14. Stroes ES, Thompson PD, Corsini A, et al. Statin-associated muscle symptoms: impact on statin therapy–European Atherosclerosis Society Consensus Panel Statement on Assessment, Aetiology and Management. *Eur Heart J.* 2015;36(17):1012-1022.

15. National Cholesterol. Education Program Expert Panel on Detection, Evaluation, Treatment of High Blood Cholesterol in Adults (Adults Treatment Panel III). Third Report of the National Cholesterol Education Program (NCEP) Expert Panel on Detection, Evaluation, and Treatment of High Blood Cholesterol in Adults (Adult Treatment Panel III) final report. *Circulation.* 2002;106(25):3143-3421.

SECTION 6

Cigarette Smoking and Cardiovascular Disease

CHAPTER 30

Epidemiology of Smoking and Pathophysiology of Cardiovascular Damage

Mark J. Eisenberg

QUESTIONS

DIRECTIONS: Choose the one best response to each question.

30-1. At its peak in the 1960s, what proportion of the United States population consumed cigarettes?

A. 35%
B. 45%
C. 55%
D. 65%
E. 75%

30-2. What proportion of the world's 1 billion smokers are male?

A. 50%
B. 60%
C. 70%
D. 80%
E. 90%

30-3. Which of the following statements concerning smoking prevalence and trends in the United States is *false*?

A. The prevalence of smoking among adults in the US decreased by 25% between 1998 and 2013
B. Smoking among US high school students decreased by > 50% between 1997 and 2013
C. A larger proportion of adults 20 to 49 years of age smoke compared to adults age 50 and older
D. Hispanic men are almost twice as likely to smoke as Hispanic women
E. All of the above are true

30-4. By approximately how many years does smoking throughout adulthood reduce life expectancy?

A. 2 years
B. 5 years
C. 7 years
D. 10 years
E. 12 years

30-5. Which of the following statements concerning smoking and cardiovascular disease is *false*?

A. Smoking increases the risk of peripheral arterial disease and abdominal aortic aneurysm by fivefold
B. Smoking increases the risk of ischemic heart disease and stroke by threefold
C. There is a linear and independent relationship between smoking duration and intensity and increasing arterial stiffness
D. Only three constituents of cigarette smoking have been shown to play a role in the initiation and progression of cardiovascular disease: nicotine, carbon monoxide, and reactive oxygen species
E. Cigarette smoking disrupts cardiovascular homeostasis, leading to hemodynamic changes, endothelial dysfunction, inflammation, thrombosis and plaque progression, and abnormalities in lipid and glucose metabolism

30-6. Which of the following statements concerning the effects of cigarette smoking is *false*?

A. Nicotine consumption results in acute, but not chronic, increases in heart rate up to 7 to 10 beats per minute, and elevation in systolic blood pressure up to 5 to 10 mm Hg

B. A combination of nicotine-induced increased oxygen demands and carbon monoxide-associated reduced oxygen availability may lower the threshold for angina onset in smokers

C. The primary mechanism by which smoking leads to vascular and endothelial dysfunction is thought to be suppression of endothelial nitric oxide synthase (eNOS) expression and subsequent decreased bio-availability of NO caused by oxidant chemicals from cigarette smoke

D. Cigarette smoking promotes a prothrombotic state through alterations in platelet activity as well as antithrombotic and prothrombotic factors, including fibrinolytic factors and platelet-mediated pathways

E. Chronic vascular inflammation mediated by cigarette smoking may play an important role in the progression of atherosclerosis

30-7. Smokers are how much more likely to have diabetes than individuals who have never smoked?

A. 0% (incidence of diabetes is not affected by smoking)
B. 25%
C. 45%
D. 65%
E. 100%

30-8. Which of the following statements concerning electronic cigarettes (e-cigarettes) is *false*?

A. There are currently no results from appropriately powered randomized controlled trials examining e-cigarettes for smoking cessation

B. Studies looking at the long-term safety of e-cigarettes are lacking

C. Population-based studies suggest e-cigarette use is associated with 28% lower odds of quitting compared to nonusers

D. The use of e-cigarettes by youth is increasing

E. E-cigarettes are marketed for therapeutic purposes in the United States

30-9. Which of the following statements concerning smoking cessation in cardiovascular patients is *false*?

A. Smokers with myocardial infarction are more likely to quit than similar patients undergoing percutaneous coronary intervention (PCI) who did not present with myocardial infarction

B. Patients with cardiovascular disease who continue to smoke have nearly double the risk of death, myocardial infarction, or stroke compared to patients who quit

C. Patients who quit smoking after PCI have fewer anginal episodes within the first year than patients who continue to smoke

D. Only one in three smokers hospitalized with acute coronary syndrome (ACS) remains abstinent following discharge

E. Varenicline does not increase abstinence following ACS

30-10. What public health intervention has had the largest impact on cigarette consumption?

A. Taxation of tobacco
B. Restrictions on tobacco advertisements
C. Policies to reduce exposure to secondhand smoke
D. Graphic warnings on cigarette packs
E. Public quitlines

ANSWERS

30-1. The answer is B. *(Hurst's The Heart, 14th Edition, Chap. 30)* Although the Surgeon General's report in 1957 concluded that cigarette smoking is associated with an increased risk of lung cancer, it was not until publication of the landmark 1964 Surgeon General's report that the adverse relationship between cigarette smoking and cardiovascular disease was seriously recognized. The Surgeon General's report concluded that cigarette smoking is strongly associated with myocardial infarction and coronary heart disease deaths, and it laid the foundation for tobacco control.[1] Unfortunately, health care providers, professional societies, civic bodies, and governments have also played negative or timid roles, largely attributed to the smoking industry's exploitation of the natural skepticism and probabilistic nature inherent in scientific evidence, serious conflicts of interest, and lack of a strong public will. Smoking has claimed more than 20 million lives with premature deaths in the United States alone since the publication of the 1964 report. The annual per capita cigarette consumption in the United States was at its peak in the early 1960s, with a prevalence smoking of about 45% of the population in 1965 (option B). Through concerted efforts over more than half a century, the cigarette consumption in the United States has declined to half of its peak prevalence rates—to about 18% in 2012.[2] Multiple factors, including an improved understanding of the adverse effects of secondhand smoke, policy measures such as a ban on broadcast advertising, increased public awareness, and the increase in cigarette taxes have contributed to this epidemiological transition. Despite years of progress, cigarette smoking remains the leading cause of preventable cardiovascular morbidity and mortality across the globe.

30-2. The answer is D. *(Hurst's The Heart, 14th Edition, Chap. 30)* Globally, about 1 billion individuals smoke. The majority (about 800 million) are males (80%, option D). Although the prevalence of smoking has declined over the past few decades, the total number of smokers has increased globally owing to population growth. The worldwide prevalence of smoking is highly variable by country and region, suggesting a heavy influence of socioeconomic and cultural currents as well as national policies. In 2012, the prevalence of smoking among adults was 49% in eastern Europe, 45% in China, 36% in Japan, 28% in western Europe, 23% in India, and about 18% in Australia, the United States, and Canada.[3] When considering differences by age groups, the highest prevalence of smoking worldwide in 2012 was seen in males aged 44 to 49 (41% prevalence) and females aged 50 to 54 (8.7% prevalence). There is a disproportionately high burden of smoking among males compared to females in countries such as China and India. This is also reflected in the recent estimates of deaths attributable to smoking in China; of the nearly 1 million deaths in 2010, 840,000 were among males in contrast to 130,000 among females.[4] A high burden of smoking among adolescents and young adults (more than 150 million smokers were 25 years or younger) remains a major concern and challenge.[3] During 2012, the prevalence of smoking among 20- to 24-year-old males was above 50% in eastern Europe, Russia, and Indonesia, 41% in China, 37% in Japan, 28% in Latin America, 24% in Pakistan, 21% in Australia, 19% in Canada and the United States, and 13% in India.

30-3. The answer is E. *(Hurst's The Heart, 14th Edition, Chap. 30)* According to the Behavioral Risk Factor Surveillance System (BRFSS) survey, the prevalence of smoking among US adults has declined by 25%, with only 17.9% smokers in 2013 as compared to 24.1% smokers in 1998 (option A).[5] A larger change in smoking prevalence has been seen among US high school students: 15.7% in 2013 compared to 36.4% in 1997 (option B). There are important differences in the smoking prevalence by states and regions in the United States. Similarly, US population-based survey data (National Health and Nutrition Examination Survey [NHANES]) for 2011–2012 showed a much higher smoking prevalence among people 20 to 49 years of age (23.1%) compared to those 50 years of age and older (16.3%) (option C).[5] There is significant heterogeneity in smoking prevalence by race/ethnicity and gender. The smoking rate among Hispanic men (16%) is almost two times higher than it is among Hispanic women (8.3%) (option D).

30-4. The answer is D. *(Hurst's The Heart, 14th Edition, Chap. 30)* A loss of about a decade of life expectancy is estimated because of smoking throughout adulthood among both men and women in various countries, including the United Kingdom, the United States, Japan, and India (option D).[6] Importantly, people who have smoked cigarettes since early adulthood but stopped at 30, 40, or 50 years of age gain back 10, 9, and 6 years of life expectancy, respectively.[6] About 5 to 6 million yearly deaths worldwide and about 0.5 million in the United States are attributable to cigarette smoking each year. This estimate is projected to increase to more than 10 million in a few decades.[6,7] In 1990, smoking was the third-ranked risk factor after childhood malnutrition and indoor pollution from biofuels for loss of disability-adjusted life years (ie, sum of years of life lost and years lived with disability [DALY]). With improvements in nutrition and clean fuel availability, in 2010, it has become the second most common contributor to loss of DALYs (6.3%; 95% confidence interval, 6.2 to 7.7).[8] Smoking is the highest contributor to loss of DALYs in males worldwide and in both males and females in many developing countries. The US societal costs of cigarette smoking per year are around $289 billion; this includes about $151 billion in lost productivity caused by premature deaths and remaining as direct health care costs.[5]

30-5. The answer is B. *(Hurst's The Heart, 14th Edition, Chap. 30)* Smoking has been associated with increased and accelerated atherosclerosis and acute plaque rupture and all cardiovascular end points, including myocardial infarction, stroke, and peripheral arterial disease.[9] While smoking causes incremental and independent risk with other risk factors such as hypertension and diabetes on coronary and cerebral vasculature, its prominent role in peripheral vasculature and small-vessel disease has been appreciated: fivefold increased risk of peripheral arterial disease and abdominal aortic aneurysm (option A) compared to a 1.5- to 2-fold increased risk of ischemic heart disease and stroke (option B).[10] A linear and independent relationship of smoking duration and intensity has been reported, with an increase in arterial stiffness measured using brachial-ankle pulse wave velocity (option C).[11] Cigarette smoke is a mixture of more than 5000 toxic chemicals[12] and 1015 to 1017 free radicals.[13,14] It is conventionally divided into two chemically different phases: a tar phase and a gas phase.[15] The tar or particulate phase is material that is trapped when the smoke steam is passed through the glass-fiber (cigarette) filter. The cigarette filter retains 99.9% of all particles larger than 0.1 μm. Nicotine is a major chemical component of the particulate phase of cigarette smoke.[16] The gas (or vapor) phase consists of the material that passes through the cigarette filter.[16] The common chemical components of the gas phase include carbon monoxide (CO), acetaldehyde, formaldehyde, acrolein, nitrogen oxides, and carbon dioxide. Both phases are high in reactive oxygen species (ROS).[17] Despite the presence of many constituents in both phases, only three constituents (nicotine, CO, and ROS) have been shown to play a role in the initiation and progression of cardiovascular disease (option D).[18] The net effect of various endogenous chemicals from cigarette smoke, such as oxidative free radicals and nicotine, together with inflammatory molecules and endogenous-produced ROS released by activated inflammatory cells, is disruption of cardiovascular homeostasis, leading to hemodynamic changes, endothelial dysfunction, inflammation, thrombosis and plaque progression, and abnormalities in lipid and glucose metabolism (option E).[14]

30-6. The answer is A. *(Hurst's The Heart, 14th Edition, Chap. 30)* Via sympathetic stimulation, nicotine leads to an increase in cardiac contractility, acute and chronic increase in heart rate up to 7 to 10 beats per minute,[19] and elevation in systolic blood pressure up to 5 to 10 mm Hg from baseline (option A).[18] Carbon monoxide (CO) is another component of cigarette smoke that has been implicated in cigarette smoke-induced hemodynamic changes. By binding to hemoglobin, CO reduces the oxygen-carrying capacity of hemoglobin, resulting in relative hypoxemia and subsequent dilation of coronary arteries.[20] A combination of nicotine-induced increased oxygen demands on one side and CO-associated reduced oxygen availability on the other side may lower the threshold for angina onset in smokers (option B).[21] Cigarette smoking-induced endothelial dysfunction is an important factor in coronary hemodynamic disturbances and the progression of atherosclerosis. The primary mechanism by which smoking leads to vascular and endothelial dysfunction is thought to be suppression of eNOS expression and subsequent decreased bioavailability of

NO caused by oxidant chemicals from cigarette smoke (option C).[22] Cigarette smoking has also been shown to promote a prothrombotic state through several mechanisms. These mechanisms include alterations in platelet activity as well as alterations in antithrombotic and prothrombotic factors, including fibrinolytic factors and platelet-mediated pathways (option D).[15,23] Chronic vascular inflammation mediated by cigarette smoking may play an important role in the progression of atherosclerosis (option E).[24] The exact molecular-pathogenic mechanisms by which smoking induces vascular inflammation are not completely established. Nonetheless, the role of several proinflammatory cytokines as well as activation and interaction between leukocytes and endothelial cells is well recognized in this process.

30-7. **The answer is E.** (*Hurst's The Heart, 14th Edition, Chap. 30*) Cigarette smoking increases the risk of development of diabetes mellitus type 2.[25] A dose-response relationship has been found between the smoking and the incidence of diabetes mellitus in both men and women.[26] Data from the Cancer Prevention Study have shown that there is a 45% higher diabetes rate among smokers than among men who had never smoked (option C). Higher levels of HbA1C have been found in smokers with diabetes than in nonsmokers with diabetes. Smoking also increases requirements for insulin and causes insulin resistance in nondiabetics.[27] Studies have also shown an increased risk of microvascular complications of diabetes such as diabetic neuropathy and faster progression of renal disease.[28] There has been a debate about whether possible weight gain associated with quitting smoking is associated with increased risk, too.[29] Although confounding in observational studies makes it difficult to test this relationship further, the increased risk of weight gain after cessation ameliorates with the duration of smoking cessation.[29] The pathogenesis of smoking and glucose metabolism is not well understood, but nicotine appears to have a central role in this process.[14,30] Nicotine stimulates catecholamine release from the adrenal medulla and sympathetic nervous system, which may lead to insulin resistance. It also increases the release of corticosteroids, which are known hyperglycemic hormones.[18]

30-8. **The answer is E.** (*Hurst's The Heart, 14th Edition, Chap. 30*) Invented in the early 2000s by a Chinese pharmaceutical company and patented in 2004, e-cigarettes deliver a nicotine-containing vapor when a solution of nicotine with humectant solution (glycerol or propylene glycol) and flavoring is heated by a battery-powered atomizer. Currently, there are no appropriately powered randomized controlled trials with e-cigarettes to examine their efficacy in smoking cessation (option A).[31] Also, studies looking at the long-term safety of e-cigarettes are lacking (option B). When using population-based studies of smoking cessation in the absence of good randomized controlled trials, e-cigarette users are associated with 28% lower relative odds of quitting compared to nonusers (option C).[32] There are growing concerns about their use due to the absence of studies showing either safety or efficacy. For instance, among high school students, the use of e-cigarettes tripled in 2014 to 2 million (13.4%) from 0.67 million (4.5%) in 2013 (option D).[33] Because of a lack of evidence supporting the safety or efficacy of e-cigarettes at this time, e-cigarette companies cannot advertise them as an alternative for smoking cessation or for therapeutic purposes in the United States (option E).

30-9. **The answer is E.** (*Hurst's The Heart, 14th Edition, Chap. 30*) In a retrospective analysis of over 2000 patients who underwent percutaneous coronary intervention (PCI) from 1999 to 2009 at Olmsted County, Minnesota, smoking cessation rates at 6 to 12 months were around 50% and did not change over a decade.[34] The odds of cessation were 2.6 times higher among those who had presented with myocardial infarction (option A) and three times among those who participated in cardiac rehabilitation, and cessation was associated with better prognosis.[34] Similarly, a cessation rate of about 60% was seen in Synergy between PCI with Taxus and Cardiac Surgery (SYNTAX) trial participants, and those who continued to smoke had a 1.8 times higher risk of death, myocardial infarction, or stroke compared to those who had quit (option B).[35] Smokers have worse outcomes than nonsmokers after PCI, and those who quit smoking after PCI had fewer anginal episodes at 1-year follow-up than those who continued (option C).[36] It is a big challenge and a big opportunity for us that less than one in three of the current smokers hospitalized with acute coronary syndrome (ACS) remains abstinent following discharge (option D). In a recent study of patients presenting with ACS, varenicline was associated with an abstinence rate of 47.3% versus 32.5% in the placebo group at 6 months (option E).[37]

30-10. The answer is A. *(Hurst's The Heart, 14th Edition, Chap. 30)* The most common and successful step that has been used to reduce tobacco consumption is excise taxes (option A). About a 20% decrease in cigarette consumption has been reported with a 50% increase in inflation-adjusted tobacco price.[38] Tobacco taxes have proven to be more effective among younger adults, and among poor or less educated groups.[6] However, a rapid growth in income and purchasing power parity in developing countries, and the availability of low-priced alternatives such as "bidis," is a challenge. The lower excise tax in the low-income countries makes cigarettes cheaper than in developed countries. Additionally, organized smuggling of cigarettes after excise taxes are raised remains another challenge that will require stricter tax administration.[6] Profits from tobacco manufacturing exceeded 50 billion US dollars in 2012,[39] and beyond the industry's lobbying effort for keeping a check on excise taxes, the major portal for more than half a century has been the influence and use of mass media. Although a complete or partial ban on tobacco advertisements remains a strong tool to reduce smoking rates, comprehensive bans may be needed to prevent the tobacco industry from using advertising media (option B).[6] Legislative developments to protect people from secondhand smoke (option C), research to continue to study the influence of various interventions to reduce smoking rates, and understanding the counterforces, such as smoking industry activities and human behavior, will be important. Other interventions, such as graphic warnings on cigarette packs (option D) and public quitlines (option E), have been used to reduce tobacco consumption.

References

1. Filion KB, Luepker RV. Cigarette smoking and cardiovascular disease: Lessons from framingham. *Global Heart.* 2013;8:35-41.

2. General S. *The health Consequences of Smoking—50 Years of Progress: A Report of the Surgeon General.* US Department of Health and Human Services. 2014.

3. Ng M, Freeman MK, Fleming TD, et al. Smoking prevalence and cigarette consumption in 187 countries, 1980-2012. *JAMA.* 2014;311:183-192.

4. Chen Z, Peto R, Zhou M, Iona A, et al, for the China Kadoorie Biobank (CKB) Collaborative Group. Contrasting male and female trends in tobacco-attributed mortality in China: evidence from successive nationwide prospective cohort studies. *Lancet.* 2015;386:1447-1456.

5. Mozaffarian D, Benjamin EJ, Go AS, et al, on behalf of the American Heart Association Statistics Committee and Stroke Statistics Subcommittee. Heart disease and stroke statistics—2015 update: a report from the American Heart Association. *Circulation.* 2015;131:e29-e322.

6. Jha P, Peto R. Global effects of smoking, of quitting, and of taxing tobacco. *N Engl J Med.* 2014;370:60-68.

7. Proctor RN. The cigarette catastrophe continues. *Lancet.* 2015;385:938-939.

8. Lim SS, Vos T, Flaxman AD, et al. A comparative risk assessment of burden of disease and injury attributable to 67 risk factors and risk factor clusters in 21 regions, 1990-2010: a systematic analysis for the global burden of disease study 2010. *Lancet.* 2012;380:2224-2260.

9. Pan A, Wang Y, Talaei M, Hu FB. Relation of smoking with total mortality and cardiovascular events among patients with diabetes mellitus: A meta-analysis and systematic review. *Circulation.* 2015;132:1795-1804.

10. Pujades-Rodriguez M, George J, Shah AD, et al. Heterogeneous associations between smoking and a wide range of initial presentations of cardiovascular disease in 1,937,360 people in England: lifetime risks and implications for risk prediction. *Int J Epidemiol.* 2015;44:129-141.

11. Tomiyama H, Hashimoto H, Tanaka H, et al. Continuous smoking and progression of arterial stiffening: a prospective study. *J Am Coll Cardiol.* 2010;55:1979-1987.

12. Borgerding M, Klus H. Analysis of complex mixtures—cigarette smoke. *Exp Toxicol Pathol.* 2005;57(Suppl 1): 43-73.

13. Rafacho BP, Azevedo PS, Polegato BF, et al. Tobacco smoke induces ventricular remodeling associated with an increase in NADPH oxidase activity. *Cell Physiol Biochem.* 2011;27:305-312.

14. Kitami M, Ali MK. Tobacco, metabolic and inflammatory pathways, and CVD risk. *Global Heart.* 2012;7:121-128.

15. Ambrose JA, Barua RS. The pathophysiology of cigarette smoking and cardiovascular disease: an update. *J Am Coll Cardiol.* 2004;43:1731-1737.

16. Pryor WA, Stone K, Zang LY, Bermúdez E. Fractionation of aqueous cigarette tar extracts: fractions that contain the tar radical cause DNA damage. *Chem Res Toxicol.* 1998;11:441-448.

17. Ichiki T. Collaboration between smokers and tobacco in endothelial dysfunction. *Cardiovasc Res.* 2011;90:395-396.

18. Benowitz NL. Cigarette smoking and cardiovascular disease: pathophysiology and implications for treatment. *Prog Cardiovasc Dis.* 2003;46:91-111.

19. Benowitz NL, Kuyt F, Jacob P. Influence of nicotine on cardiovascular and hormonal effects of cigarette smoking. *Clin Pharmacol Ther.* 1984;36:74-81.

20. Czernin J, Waldherr C. Cigarette smoking and coronary blood flow. *Prog Cardiovasc Dis.* 2003;45:395-404.

21. Yamada S, Zhang XQ, Kadono T, et al. Direct toxic effects of aqueous extract of cigarette smoke on cardiac myocytes at clinically relevant concentrations. *Toxicol Appl Pharmacol.* 2009;236:71-77.

22. Barua RS, Ambrose JA, Srivastava S, DeVoe MC, Eales-Reynolds LJ. Reactive oxygen species are involved in smoking-induced dysfunction of nitric oxide biosynthesis and upregulation of endothelial nitric oxide synthase: an in vitro demonstration in human coronary artery endothelial cells. *Circulation.* 2003;107:2342-2347.

23. Salahuddin S, Prabhakaran D, Roy A. Pathophysiological mechanisms of tobacco-related CVD. *Global Heart.* 2012;7:113-120.

24. Hasnis E, Bar-Shai M, Burbea Z, Reznick AZ. Cigarette smoke-induced NF-kappaB activation in human lymphocytes: the effect of low and high exposure to gas phase of cigarette smoke. *J Physiol Pharmacol.* 2007;58 Suppl 5:263-274.

25. Eliasson B. Cigarette smoking and diabetes. *Prog Cardiovasc Dis.* 2003;45:405-413.

26. Will JC, Galuska DA, Ford ES, Mokdad A, Calle EE. Cigarette smoking and diabetes mellitus: evidence of a positive association from a large prospective cohort study. *Int J Epidemiol.* 2001;30:540-546.

27. Zhu Y, Zhang M, Hou X, et al. Cigarette smoking increases risk for incident metabolic syndrome in Chinese men–Shanghai diabetes study. *Biomed Environl Sci.* 2011;24:475-482.

28. Chuahirun T, Khanna A, Kimball K, Wesson DE. Cigarette smoking and increased urine albumin excretion are interrelated predictors of nephropathy progression in type 2 diabetes. *Am J Kid Dis* 2003;41:13-21.

29. Pan A, Wang Y, Talaei M, Hu FB, Wu T. Relation of active, passive, and quitting smoking with incident type 2 diabetes: a systematic review and meta-analysis. *Lancet Diabetes Endocrinol.* 2015;3:958-967.

30. Axelsson T, Jansson PA, Smith U, Eliasson B. Nicotine infusion acutely impairs insulin sensitivity in type 2 diabetic patients but not in healthy subjects. *J Intern Med.* 2001;249:539-544.

31. Franck C, Budlovsky T, Windle SB, Filion KB, Eisenberg MJ. Electronic cigarettes in North America: history, use, and implications for smoking cessation. *Circulation.* 2014;129:1945-1952.

32. Kalkhoran S, Glantz SA. E-cigarettes and smoking cessation in real-world and clinical settings: a systematic review and meta-analysis. *Lancet Respir Med.* 2016;4:116-128.

33. Arrazola RA, Singh T, Corey CG, et al. Tobacco use among middle and high school students—United States, 2011–2014. *MMWR Morb Mortal Wkly Rep.* 2015;64(14):381-385.

34. Sochor O, Lennon RJ, Rodriguez-Escudero JP, et al. Trends and predictors of smoking cessation after percutaneous coronary intervention (from Olmsted County, Minnesota, 1999 to 2010). *Am J Cardiol.* 2015;115:405-410.

35. Zhang YJ, Iqbal J, van Klaveren D, et al. Smoking is associated with adverse clinical outcomes in patients undergoing revascularization with PCI or CABG: the SYNTAX trial at 5-year follow-up. *J Am Coll Cardiol.* 2015;65:1107-1115.

36. Jang JS, Buchanan DM, Gosch KL, et al. Association of smoking status with health-related outcomes after percutaneous coronary intervention. *Circ Cardiovasc Interv.* 2015;8.

37. Eisenberg MJ, Windle SB, Roy N, et al, EVITA Investigators. Varenicline for smoking cessation in hospitalized patients with acute coronary syndrome. *Circulation.* 2016;133:21-30.

38. International Agency for Research on Cancer. *Effectiveness of Tax and Price Policies for Tobacco Control.* Lyon, France: IARC; 2011.

39. Eriksen M, Mackay J, Ross H. *The Tobacco Atlas.* 4th ed. Atlanta, GA, and New York, NY: American Cancer Society and World Lung Foundation; 2012.

CHAPTER 31

Preventing and Mitigating Smoking-Related Heart Disease

Mark J. Eisenberg

QUESTIONS

DIRECTIONS: Choose the one best response to each question.

31-1. What percentage of smokers interested in quitting are reported to have received tobacco cessation medication during outpatient physician office visits?

A. 69%
B. 50%
C. 21%
D. 8%
E. 75%

31-2. Which of the following statements about the cardiovascular benefits of smoking cessation is *false*?

A. In one year following smoking cessation, half the excess risk of a myocardial infarction is gone
B. Smoking cessation before the age of 30 years eliminates nearly all the risk of death from smoking-related disease
C. The risk of cardiac events drops approximately one month after quitting smoking
D. Those who quit when they are older gain years of life compared to those who continue to smoke
E. The risk of myocardial infarction and other cardiac events drops 15% to 20% by a month after implementing comprehensive smoke-free laws to protect people from secondhand smoke

31-3. Which of the following statements is *not* included within the US Public Health Service "5As" model for smoking cessation intervention and screening for tobacco use?

A. *Advocate* for patients who wish to quit smoking
B. *Advise* tobacco users to quit

C. *Arrange* for follow-up to monitor progress
D. *Assist* patients interested in quitting with counseling and/or pharmacotherapy
E. *Assess* patient interest in and willingness to quit

31-4. A 52-year-old female smoker presents to your clinic and expresses her desire to quit smoking. Which of the following treatment options should *not* be recommended to your patient as a first-line therapy for smoking cessation?

A. Nicotine patch
B. Electronic cigarette
C. Varenicline
D. Bupropion
E. Nicotine inhaler

31-5. A 43-year-old male smoker expresses his desire to quit smoking. He says he has previously tried to quit cold turkey but was unable to abstain from smoking in the long run. What is the maximum recommended duration of nicotine replacement therapy (NRT) use?

A. 8 weeks
B. 10 weeks
C. 12 weeks
D. 24 weeks
E. 52 weeks

31-6. Which of the following interventions has *not* been associated with long-term smoking cessation compared with sham interventions?

A. Motivational interviewing
B. Printed self-help materials
C. Acupuncture
D. Telephone counseling
E. Mobile phone-based interventions

31-7. A smoker with two previous quit attempts is interested in combining NRT with a second form of pharmacotherapy. Which of the following statements about combination therapy is *correct*?

A. Treatment with a combination of long-acting and short-acting NRT is not associated with increased smoking cessation when compared to a single type of NRT

B. Varenicline combined with NRT is associated with higher tobacco abstinence at 12 weeks and 6 months compared to varenicline alone

C. Participants receiving combination therapy do not report more anxiety and depressive symptoms

D. Combination of bupropion and NRT treatment is associated with a significant difference in smoking cessation compared to NRT alone

E. There is no evidence that combination therapy is effective for smoking cessation

31-8. A 30-year-old man who self-identifies as a social smoker (5 or fewer cigarettes per day) presents to your clinic for an unrelated clinical concern. He is unbothered by his smoking, which he does *not* feel compelled to reduce due to his already low number of cigarettes smoked per day. Which of the following statements about the health effects of smoking reduction is *true*?

A. The dose-response relationship between smoking and cardiovascular disease is highly linear

B. Smoking reduction has not been associated with improved levels of biomarkers associated with cardiovascular disease in some studies

C. Smoking as few as five cigarettes a day is associated with a higher risk of death from ischemic heart disease

D. Cigarette smoking at low levels is not associated with an increased risk of cardiovascular disease

E. Complete cessation should not be encouraged in all patients

31-9. The World Health Organization's Framework Convention on Tobacco Control (FCTC) emphasizes the importance of promoting public health through the implementation of policies, including which of the following?

A. Smoke-free environments to protect people from secondhand smoke and to provide an environment that helps people stop smoking

B. Elimination of tobacco advertising and promotion

C. Increased taxes to reduce demand for cigarettes

D. Education of the public on the risks of smoking, such as with large graphic warning labels on tobacco products

E. All of the above

31-10. A 21-year-old smoker is interested in finding alternatives to cigarette smoking and asks about using electronic cigarettes (e-cigarettes) to help him quit smoking. Which of the following statements about e-cigarettes is *false*?

A. E-cigarettes are relatively new products, so their long-term health effects are unknown

B. As of January 2016, e-cigarettes were regulated by the FDA

C. As currently being used in the real world, e-cigarettes are associated with significantly less quitting than NRT or no cessation aids

D. E-cigarettes should not be recommended as effective smoking cessation aids until there is evidence that they assist in smoking cessation

E. Use of e-cigarettes by patients may signal readiness to quit cigarettes, and thus clinicians should be prepared to support patients in their quit attempts

31-1. **The answer is D.** *(Hurst's The Heart, 14th Edition, Chap. 31)* Even though 69% of smokers are interested in quitting (option A) and over half report having made a quit attempt in the past year (option B),[1] only 21% of adult current tobacco users received tobacco cessation counseling (option C) and 8% received tobacco cessation medication during outpatient visits (option D).[2] Screening for interest in tobacco cessation is particularly important because physician advice to quit smoking is associated with increased smoking cessation compared to no advice to quit or usual care, with higher cessation seen with more intensive advice compared to minimal advice.[3] It is important that screening be incorporated into all clinical encounters, including those with cardiologists and other specialists, not only to identify and assist patients who are ready to stop smoking, but also to encourage those who are not yet ready to move toward making the decision to quit.

31-2. **The answer is C.** *(Hurst's The Heart, 14th Edition, Chap. 31)* In addition to contributing to the long-term development of atherosclerosis, smoking (and secondhand smoke exposure) has immediate effects (within minutes) on endothelial function[4,5] and platelet activation[6] and so can trigger a cardiac event. The risk of cardiac events begins to drop immediately after quitting and declines rapidly (option C). The heart rate drops 20 minutes after quitting, and in a year, half the excess risk of a myocardial infarction is gone (option A). The risk of myocardial infarction and other cardiac events drops 15% to 20% by a month after implementing comprehensive smoke-free laws to protect people from secondhand smoke (option E).[7,8] Smoking cessation before the age of 30 years eliminates nearly all of the risk of death from smoking-related disease (option B), and even those who quit when they are older gain years of life compared to those who continue to smoke (option D).[4] This fact highlights both the importance of encouraging smokers to quit early and the importance of encouraging all smokers to quit, no matter how old they are.

31-3. **The answer is A.** *(Hurst's The Heart, 14th Edition, Chap. 31)* The US Public Health Service recommends the 5As model for smoking cessation intervention, in which providers (1) *ask* patients about tobacco use to identify current users, (2) *advise* tobacco users to quit (option B), (3) *assess* patient interest in and willingness to quit (option E), (4) *assist* patients interested in quitting with counseling and/or pharmacotherapy (option D), and (5) *arrange* for follow-up to monitor progress (option C). Although current smokers report high rates of being asked about tobacco use (88%), fewer report being advised to quit (66%), and even fewer report being asked if they wanted to quit (43%).[9] If smokers are not properly identified, those interested in cessation cannot be connected with resources that can help them with their quit attempt. Therefore, screening should be incorporated into all outpatient and hospital encounters.

31-4. **The answer is B.** *(Hurst's The Heart, 14th Edition, Chap. 31)* Various prescription and nonprescription medications approved by the US Food and Drug Administration (FDA) are available to help patients in their attempt to quit, provided patients do not have contraindications to their use.[10] Nicotine replacement therapy, which provides patients with nicotine to manage cravings and nicotine withdrawal symptoms, comes in a variety of forms. Types of NRT include patches (option A), lozenges, inhalers (option E), and nasal sprays. FDA-approved medications include NRT, varenicline (option C), and bupropion (option D). They are all first-line treatments for smoking cessation, and the choice of agent should take into consideration patient preferences, medical comorbidities, and potential drug-drug interactions.

31-5. **The answer is D.** *(Hurst's The Heart, 14th Edition, Chap. 31)* With respect to treatment duration, a randomized clinical trial of different durations of nicotine patch treatment (8, 24, or 52 weeks) found higher rates of smoking abstinence at 24 weeks in those still using nicotine patches, but no significant difference was seen at 52 weeks.[11] This result suggests that, while nicotine patch treatment can continue longer than 8 to 10 weeks (options A and B), evidence does not support extending treatment past 24 weeks (option D). For the timing of treatment initiation, there is some evidence that starting nicotine patches prior to a patient's quit day is associated with increased smoking cessation compared to starting after the quit day. However, no difference was seen with nicotine gum or lozenges.[12] Thus, it is not necessary to wait until the quit date to initiate treatment with nicotine patches. It is important to note that, while clinical trials have demonstrated the efficacy of NRT when used as part of an organized cessation effort, unsupervised NRT bought over the counter is associated with significantly less quitting than the use of no smoking cessation aids (odds ratio [OR] 0.68, confidence interval [CI] 0.49–0.94).[13] Thus, patients using NRT should be followed and encouraged to maintain their quit attempt. Such combinations of counseling and NRT can be accomplished through telephone quitlines, which also provide certain types of NRT to eligible callers.

31-6. **The answer is C.** *(Hurst's The Heart, 14th Edition, Chap. 31)* Counseling delivered by telephone (option D), either through telephone quitlines or other sources, is associated with smoking cessation,[14] as are some mobile phone-based interventions (option E),[15] printed self-help materials (option B),[16] and interactive, tailored Internet-based interventions.[17] Motivational interviewing, which consists of counseling to improve one's motivation for and interest in behavioral change, has also been associated with increased smoking cessation compared to brief advice or usual care.[18] In people using pharmacotherapy for smoking cessation, the addition of behavioral support through in-person or telephone contact is also associated with increased smoking cessation compared to control groups.[19] Assistance via telephone is available from state telephone quitlines toll-free at 1-800-QUIT-NOW (1-800-784-8669). Support through text messaging can also be found through the National Cancer Institute's Smokefree TXT program, which is available at smokefree.gov/smokefreetxt, or by texting the word QUIT to 47848 from a mobile phone. Acupuncture, acupressure, or laser therapy has not been associated with long-term smoking cessation compared with sham interventions.[20]

31-7. **The answer is B.** *(Hurst's The Heart, 14th Edition, Chap. 31)* Treatment with a combination of long-acting and short-acting NRT is associated with increased smoking cessation compared to a single type of NRT (option A).[12] A randomized controlled trial found that varenicline combined with NRT was associated with higher tobacco abstinence at 12 weeks and 6 months compared to varenicline alone (option B).[21] Another randomized controlled trial found that treatment with both varenicline and bupropion for 12 weeks was associated with significantly greater smoking cessation than treatment with varenicline alone at 12 weeks (OR 1.49, 95% CI 1.05–2.12) and 26 weeks (OR 1.52, 95% CI 1.04–2.22)—but not at 52 weeks (OR, 1.32, 95% CI 0.91–1.91).[22] Participants receiving combination therapy, however, reported more anxiety and depressive symptoms (option C). Combination bupropion and NRT treatment is not associated with a significant difference in smoking cessation compared to NRT alone (option D).[23] While combining different forms of NRT is a recommended, effective strategy for smoking cessation, combination of NRT with bupropion has not proven to be effective, and while combination varenicline and NRT has shown some promise of efficacy at 6 months, further studies on long-term efficacy and safety are needed.

31-8. **The answer is C.** *(Hurst's The Heart, 14th Edition, Chap. 31)* Cigarette smoking, even at low levels, is associated with an increased risk of cardiovascular disease.[24-26] The dose-response relationship between smoking and cardiovascular disease is highly nonlinear, with more rapid increases in risk at low levels of exposure and flattening of the curve at higher levels of exposure.[24] In fact, smoking as few as five cigarettes a day is associated with a higher risk of death from ischemic heart disease.[26] Smoking a few cigarettes a day should not be promoted as a long-term use pattern, and complete cessation should be encouraged in all patients. Smoking reduction has been associated with improved levels of biomarkers associated with cardiovascular disease in some studies,[27,28] but not in others.[29] It is not clear whether improvements in these biomarkers also result in improvements in the risk of smoking-related disease.

31-9. **The answer is E.** *(Hurst's The Heart, 14th Edition, Chap. 31)* There is great variability in the prevalence of cigarette smoking worldwide. The World Health Organization's Framework Convention on Tobacco Control (FCTC), the first global public health treaty, adopted in 2003 and implemented in 2005, emphasizes the importance of promoting public health through the implementation of policies, including smoke-free environments to protect people from secondhand smoke and to provide an environment that helps people stop smoking; elimination of tobacco advertising and promotion; increased taxes to reduce the demand for cigarettes; and education on the risks of smoking, such as with large graphic warning labels on tobacco products.[30] Although the FCTC has accelerated the implementation of smoke-free laws[31] and strong health warning labels,[32] only about half of nations report 100% smoke-free restaurants and even fewer smoke-free private workplaces.[33] As of 2016, the United States was one of the few countries that had not ratified the FCTC, and the United States lags behind the rest of the world in several areas, notably strong graphic warning labels on tobacco products, restrictions on advertising and promotion, and tobacco taxation. More comprehensive smoking laws are needed worldwide to ensure the maximum health benefits conferred to both smokers and nonsmokers by such tobacco control legislation.

31-10. **The answer is B.** *(Hurst's The Heart, 14th Edition, Chap. 31)* As of January 2016, e-cigarettes were not regulated by the FDA. E-cigarettes, a type of electronic nicotine delivery system, are battery-powered devices that heat a solution of humectants such as propylene glycol or glycerol, generally with nicotine and/or flavorings, to form an aerosol that is inhaled by the user. E-cigarettes are relatively new products, so their long-term health effects are unknown (option A). Although many smokers report using e-cigarettes to quit smoking, randomized controlled trials on their efficacy for smoking cessation have been limited, and their results have been equivocal.[34,35] As currently being used in the real world, e-cigarettes are associated with significantly less quitting than NRT or no cessation aids (option C).[36] Data from three studies[37-39] suggest that specific e-cigarette use patterns (daily use of high nicotine delivery devices, which represents the minority of users in these studies) may be associated with increased quitting; as e-cigarette product types and use patterns continue to evolve, this association should continue to be studied. Nevertheless, e-cigarettes should not be recommended as effective smoking cessation aids until there is evidence that, as promoted and used, they assist in smoking cessation (option D).[36,40] A policy statement by the American Heart Association in 2014 encourages the inclusion of e-cigarette use in tobacco screening questions.[41] Use of e-cigarettes by patients may signal readiness to quit cigarettes, and thus clinicians should be prepared to support patients in their quit attempts and to discuss evidence-based practices for smoking cessation, including counseling, NRT, or stop-smoking pharmacotherapy, with these patients (option E).[40]

References

1. Quitting smoking among adults—United States, 2001-2010. *MMWR Morb Mortal Wkly Rep.* 2011;60(44):1513-1519.
2. Jamal A, Dube SR, Malarcher AM, Shaw L, Engstrom MC. Tobacco use screening and counseling during physician office visits among adults—National Ambulatory Medical Care Survey and National Health Interview Survey, United States, 2005-2009. *MMWR Suppl.* 2012;61:38-45.
3. Stead LF, Buitrago D, Preciado N, Sanchez G, Hartmann-Boyce J, Lancaster T. Physician advice for smoking cessation. *Cochrane Database Syst Rev.* 2013;5:Cd000165.
4. Pinnamaneni K, Sievers RE, Sharma R, et al. Brief exposure to secondhand smoke reversibly impairs endothelial vasodilatory function. *Nicotine Tob Res.* 2014;16(5):584-590.
5. Heiss C, Amabile N, Lee AC, et al. Brief secondhand smoke exposure depresses endothelial progenitor cells activity and endothelial function: sustained vascular injury and blunted nitric oxide production. *J Am Coll Cardiol.* 2008;51(18):1760-1771.
6. US Department of Health and Human Services. *How Tobacco Smoke Causes Disease: The Biology and Behavioral Basis for Smoking-Attributable Disease: A Report of the Surgeon General.* Atlanta, GA: Centers for Disease Control and Prevention; 2010:2.
7. Tan CE, Glantz SA. Association between smoke-free legislation and hospitalizations for cardiac, cerebrovascular, and respiratory diseases: a meta-analysis. *Circulation.* 2012;126(18):2177-2183.
8. US Department of Health and Human Services. *The Health Consequences of Smoking—50 Years of Progress. A Report of the Surgeon General.* Rockville, MD: US Department of Health and Human Services. Public Health Service; 2014.
9. King BA, Dube SR, Babb SD, McAfee TA. Patient-reported recall of smoking cessation interventions from a health professional. *Prev Med.* 2013;57(5):715-717.
10. Fiore MC, Jaén CR, Baker TB, et al. *Clinical Practice Guideline.* Rockville, MD: US Department of Health and Human Services. Public Health Service; 2008:101-103.
11. Schnoll RA, Goelz PM, Veluz-Wilkins A, et al. Long-term nicotine replacement therapy: a randomized clinical trial. *JAMA Intern Med.* 2015;175(4):504-511.

12. Stead LF, Perera R, Bullen C, et al. Nicotine replacement therapy for smoking cessation. *Cochrane Database Syst Rev.* 2012;11:Cd000146.

13. Kotz D, Brown J, West R. Prospective cohort study of the effectiveness of smoking cessation treatments used in the "real world." *Mayo Clin Proc.* 2014;89(10):1360-1367.

14. Stead LF, Hartmann-Boyce J, Perera R, Lancaster T. Telephone counselling for smoking cessation. *Cochrane Database Syst Rev.* 2013;8:Cd002850.

15. Whittaker R, McRobbie H, Bullen C, Borland R, Rodgers A, Gu Y. Mobile phone-based interventions for smoking cessation. *Cochrane Database Syst Rev.* 2012;11:Cd006611.

16. Hartmann-Boyce J, Lancaster T, Stead LF. Print-based self-help interventions for smoking cessation. *Cochrane Database Syst Rev.* 2014;6:Cd001118.

17. Civljak M, Stead LF, Hartmann-Boyce J, Sheikh A, Car J. Internet-based interventions for smoking cessation. *Cochrane Database Syst Rev.* 2013;7:Cd007078.

18. Lindson-Hawley N, Thompson TP, Begh R. Motivational interviewing for smoking cessation. *Cochrane Database Syst Rev.* 2015;3:Cd006936.

19. Stead LF, Koilpillai P, Lancaster T. Additional behavioural support as an adjunct to pharmacotherapy for smoking cessation. *Cochrane Database Syst Rev.* 2015;10:Cd009670.

20. White AR, Rampes H, Liu JP, Stead LF, Campbell J. Acupuncture and related interventions for smoking cessation. *Cochrane Database Syst Rev.* 2014;1:Cd000009.

21. Koegelenberg CF, Noor F, Bateman ED, et al. Efficacy of varenicline combined with nicotine replacement therapy vs varenicline alone for smoking cessation: a randomized clinical trial. *JAMA.* 2014;312(2):155-161.

22. Ebbert JO, Hatsukami DK, Croghan IT, et al. Combination varenicline and bupropion SR for tobacco-dependence treatment in cigarette smokers: a randomized trial. *JAMA.* 2014;311(2):155-163.

23. Hughes JR, Stead LF, Hartmann-Boyce J, Cahill K, Lancaster T. Antidepressants for smoking cessation. *Cochrane Database Syst Rev.* 2014;1:Cd000031.

24. Pope CA, 3rd, Burnett RT, Krewski D, et al. Cardiovascular mortality and exposure to airborne fine particulate matter and cigarette smoke: shape of the exposure-response relationship. *Circulation.* 2009;120(11):941-948.

25. Schane RE, Ling PM, Glantz SA. Health effects of light and intermittent smoking: a review. *Circulation.* 2010;121(13):1518-1522.

26. Bjartveit K, Tverdal A. Health consequences of smoking 1-4 cigarettes per day. *Tob Control.* 2005;14(5):315-320.

27. Eliasson B, Hjalmarson A, Kruse E, Landfeldt B, Westin A. Effect of smoking reduction and cessation on cardiovascular risk factors. *Nicotine Tob Res.* 2001;3(3):249-255.

28. Hatsukami DK, Kotlyar M, Allen S, et al. Effects of cigarette reduction on cardiovascular risk factors and subjective measures. *Chest.* 2005;128(4):2528-2537.

29. Joseph AM, Hecht SS, Murphy SE, et al. Smoking reduction fails to improve clinical and biological markers of cardiac disease: a randomized controlled trial. *Nicotine Tob Res.* 2008;10(3):471-481.

30. World Health Organization. WHO Framework Convention on Tobacco Control. Geneva: *World Health Organization;* 2003: http://apps.who.int/iris/bit-stream/10665/42811/1/9241591013.pdf. Accessed April 18, 2016.

31. Uang R, Hiilamo H, Glantz SA. Accelerated adoption of smoke-free laws after ratification of the World Health Organization Framework Convention on Tobacco Control. *Am J Public Health.* 2016;106(1):166-171.

32. Sanders-Jackson AN, Song AV, Hiilamo H, Glantz SA. Effect of the Framework Convention on Tobacco Control and voluntary industry health warning labels on passage of mandated cigarette warning labels from 1965 to 2012: transition probability and event history analyses. *Am J Public Health.* 2013;103(11):2041-2047.

33. World Health Organization. 2012 *Global Progress Report on Implementation of the WHO Framework Convention on Tobacco Control.* Geneva, Switzerland: World Health Organization; 2012.

34. Bullen C, Howe C, Laugesen M, McRobbie H, Parag V, Williman J, Walker N. Electronic cigarettes for smoking cessation: a randomized controlled trial. *Lancet.* 2013;382(9905):1629-1637.

35. Caponnetto P, Campagna D, Cibella F, Morjaria JB, Caruso M, Russo C, et al. Efficiency and safety of an electronic cigarette (ECLAT) as tobacco cigarettes substitute: a prospective 12-month randomized control design study. *PloS One.* 2013;8(6):e66317.

36. Kalkhoran S, Glantz SA. E-cigarettes and smoking cessation in real world and clinical settings: a systematic review and meta-analysis. *Lancet Resp Med.* 2016;4(2)116-128.

37. Hitchman SC, Brose LS, Brown J, Robson D, McNeill A. Associations between e-cigarette type, frequency of use, and quitting smoking: findings from a longitudinal online panel survey in Great Britain. *Nicotine Tob Res.* 2015;17(10):1187-1194.

38. Biener L, Hargraves JL. A longitudinal study of electronic cigarette use among a population-based sample of adult smokers: association with smoking cessation and motivation to quit. *Nicotine Tob Res.* 2015;17(2):127-133.

39. Zhuang YL, Cummins SE, Y Sun J, Zhu SH. Long-term e-cigarette use and smoking cessation: a longitudinal study with US population. *Tob Control.* 2016;25(Suppl 1):i90-i95.

40. Grana R, Benowitz N, Glantz SA. E-cigarettes: a scientific review. *Circulation.* 2014;129(19):1972-1986.

41. Bhatnagar A, Whitsel LP, Ribisl KM, et al. Electronic cigarettes: a policy statement from the American Heart Association. *Circulation.* 2014;130(16):1418-1436.

SECTION 7

Atherosclerosis and Coronary Heart Disease

CHAPTER 32

Atherothrombosis: Disease Burden, Activity, and Vulnerability

Mark J. Eisenberg

QUESTIONS

DIRECTIONS: Choose the one best response to each question.

32-1. Which of the following statements is *not true*?

A. Causal and modifiable risk factors for atherosclerotic cardiovascular disease are well known but account for < 50% of heart attacks in both sexes

B. Individual susceptibility to conventional risk factors varies greatly, and therefore their predictive value is limited

C. Most first heart attacks occur among people with average or only slightly elevated risk factor levels

D. Better detection of at-risk individuals may be achieved by visualizing the diseased arterial wall rather than just assessing risk factors

E. All of the statements are true

32-2. Which of the following statements is *not true*?

A. Atherosclerosis is a chronic, lipid-driven inflammatory disease of the arterial wall leading to multifocal plaque development

B. Atherosclerosis predominates at sites characterized by high and nonoscillatory endothelial shear stress

C. The speed of disease progression varies greatly, but it usually takes decades to develop the advanced atherosclerotic lesions responsible for clinical disease

D. Plaques are very heterogeneous in size and composition, even plaques located next to each other

E. Most plaques remain asymptomatic, some become obstructive, and a few, if any, become vulnerable

32-3. Which of the following statements is *not true*?

A. Approximately 50% of symptomatic coronary thrombi are caused by plaque rupture

B. Plaque rupture with mural thrombosis is also a common cause of episodic but asymptomatic progression to severe stenosis

C. Of the coronary thrombi not caused by plaque rupture, most are caused by plaque erosion

D. Plaque rupture is a more frequent cause of coronary thrombosis in men than in women

E. All of the statements are true

32-4. Which of the following are characteristics of vulnerable plaques of the erosion-prone type?

A. A plaque that contains a large and soft lipid-rich necrotic core

B. A necrotic core covered by a thin and inflamed fibrous cap

C. Big plaque size and expansive positive remodeling mitigating luminal obstruction

D. Neovascularization (angiogenesis), plaque hemorrhage, and adventitial inflammation

E. None of the above

32-5. Which of the following statements is *not true* regarding the fibrous cap in a fibroatheroma?

A. The fibrocellular part of the plaque located between the necrotic core and the lumen is called the fibrous cap
B. Assessed by microscopic examination postmortem, ruptured caps are typically < 65 μm thick
C. In thin-cap fibroatheroma (TCFA), the necrotic core occupies > 50% of plaque area
D. Thin fibrous caps are usually heavily inflamed, particularly those that have ruptured
E. Apoptosis is common at the site of fibrous cap rupture

32-6. The coronary heart disease (CHD) risk equivalent concept includes all of the following *except*:

A. Symptomatic disease in noncoronary arteries
B. Carotid stenosis of > 50%
C. Ankle-brachial blood pressure index < 0.8
D. Abdominal aortic aneurysm
E. Asymptomatic carotid bruit

32-7. Which of the following statements is *not true*?

A. The total amount of CAC (usually expressed as the *Agatston score*) is a strong predictor of coronary events and provides prognostic information beyond that provided by traditional risk factor scoring
B. Contrast-enhanced CT angiography visualizes not only the lumen but also the arterial wall
C. Intravascular ultrasound (IVUS) can detect and localize plaque as well as quantitate plaque burden, but it requires selective catheterization and motorized pullback in the arteries of interest
D. Serial examinations of well-defined coronary segments have been used to monitor the speed of plaque progression (or regression) over time in patients with established CHD
E. Most acute coronary events originate from angiographically obstructive plaques

32-8. Which of the following is *not* a common characteristic of the TCFA?

A. Large necrotic core
B. Inflamed fibrous cap
C. Uniform pattern of calcification
D. Expansive remodeling
E. Neovascularization

32-9. Which of the following statements is *not true* of coronary CT angiography?

A. Coronary CT may visualize the lumen and detect obstructive and nonobstructive plaques
B. Coronary CT may quantify calcified and noncalcified plaque burden
C. Coronary CT may provide additional prognostic information by the detection of higher-risk plaques characterized by large plaque volume
D. Coronary CT may provide additional prognostic information by the detection of higher-risk plaques characterized by high CT attenuation
E. Coronary CT may provide additional prognostic information by the detection of higher-risk plaques characterized by the napkin-ring sign and expansive remodeling

32-10. Which of the following catheter-based technologies may have potential for the assessment of coronary atherosclerosis and vulnerable plaques?

A. Conventional grayscale IVUS and virtual histology IVUS
B. Coherence tomography and angioscopy
C. Near-infrared spectroscopy
D. Intracoronary magnetic resonance imaging and thermography
E. All of the above

32-1. The answer is A. (*Hurst's The Heart, 14th Edition, Chap. 32*) Causal and modifiable risk factors for atherosclerotic cardiovascular disease are well known (eg, smoking, dyslipidemia, high blood pressure, diabetes) and account for most (*not less than 50%*) of heart attacks in both sexes (option A).[1] However, for unknown reasons, the individual susceptibility to these risk factors varies greatly, and consequently, their predictive value is limited (option B).[2,3] Most first heart attacks occur among people with average or only slightly elevated risk factor levels (option C).[4-6] Recurrent events still occur despite lowering of these levels,[7,8] indicating that we need both better detection and better treatment of those who are destined for a heart attack. Better detection of at-risk individuals may be achieved by visualizing the diseased arterial wall rather than just assessing risk factors (option D).

32-2. The answer is B. (*Hurst's The Heart, 14th Edition, Chap. 32*) Atherosclerosis is a chronic, lipid-driven inflammatory disease of the arterial wall leading to multifocal plaque development (option A),[9-11] predominantly at sites characterized by low and oscillatory (*not high and nonoscillatory*) endothelial shear stress (bifurcations, inner wall of curvatures) and pre-existing intimal thickenings (option B).[12,13] The speed of disease progression varies greatly, but it usually takes decades to develop the advanced atherosclerotic lesions responsible for clinical disease (option C). Plaques are very heterogeneous in size and composition, even plaques located next to each other and exposed for the same systemic risk factors (option D). Most plaques remain asymptomatic (subclinical disease), some become obstructive (stable angina), and a few, if any, become vulnerable and lead to atherothrombotic events such as a fatal heart attack or a disabling stroke (option E).

32-3. The answer is A. (*Hurst's The Heart, 14th Edition, Chap. 32*) The great majority of symptomatic coronary thrombi (~75%) (*not approximately 50%*) are caused by *plaque rupture* (option A).[11] Plaque rupture with mural thrombosis (with or without plaque hemorrhage) is also a common cause of episodic but asymptomatic progression to severe stenosis (option B).[14,15] The remaining thrombi are caused by less well-defined mechanisms, of which so-called *plaque erosion* is the most common type (option C).[11] Plaque rupture is a more frequent cause of coronary thrombosis in men (~80%) than in women (~60%) but, except for sex and menopause, no other risk factors have consistently been connected with a particular mechanism of thrombosis (option D).[11] By inference, there are two major types of vulnerable plaques, rupture-prone and erosion-prone, that are presumed to look like the corresponding thrombosed plaques, just without rupture and thrombosis.[16]

32-4. The answer is E. (*Hurst's The Heart, 14th Edition, Chap. 32*) All of the listed characteristics are properties of rupture-prone rather than erosion-prone plaques (option E). Vulnerable plaques of the erosion-prone type are heterogeneous and defined only by their fate (thrombosis, mostly mural).[11,16] The surface endothelium is missing, but whether it vanished before or after thrombosis remains unknown. No distinct morphologic features have been identified, but in general, eroded plaques with thrombosis are scarcely calcified, rarely associated with expansive remodeling, and only sparsely inflamed.[11,16] So, irrespective of plaque type, it is a misconception that vulnerable plaques are heavily inflamed. In contrast with the erosion-prone plaque, the prototype of a presumed rupture-prone plaque contains a large and soft lipid-rich necrotic core covered by a thin and inflamed fibrous cap.[16,17] Associated features include big plaque size, expansive positive remodeling mitigating luminal obstruction (mild stenosis by angiography), neovascularization (angiogenesis), plaque hemorrhage, adventitial inflammation, and a *spotty* pattern of calcifications. Although the macrophage density in ruptured caps is high,[16,17] whole-plaque macrophage density rarely exceeds a small percent because ruptured caps are tiny.

32-5. The answer is C. (*Hurst's The Heart, 14th Edition, Chap. 32*) The fibrocellular part of the plaque located between the necrotic core and the lumen is called the *fibrous cap* (option A).

It is extremely thin in coronary plaque rupture.[16,17] Assessed by microscopic examination postmortem, ruptured caps were usually < 65 μm thick (option B).[18] Assessed by optical coherence tomography in vivo, the mean thickness was only 49 μm.[19] If the fibrous cap is thin, the plaque is called a *thin-cap fibroatheroma* (TCFA).[18,20] In TCFA, the necrotic core occupies approximately 23% of plaque area *(not more than 50%)* (option C).[20] Thin fibrous caps are usually heavily inflamed (macrophage density ~14%), particularly those that have ruptured (macrophage density ~26%) (option D),[20] but because they are thin, their ability to accommodate macrophages is limited. Apoptosis is common at the site of fibrous cap rupture, usually confined to macrophages because the vascular SMCs already have vanished when rupture occurs.[20,21] With their ability to synthesize extracellular matrix, including collagen, SMC apoptosis is associated with impaired healing and repair, increasing the risk of plaque rupture.

32-6. **The answer is C.** *(Hurst's The Heart, 14th Edition, Chap. 32)* Atherosclerosis is a generalized, multifocal arterial disease. However, compared with other arteries, the coronary arteries are in general the most susceptible to atherosclerosis and its thrombotic complications.[22,23] Therefore, if atherosclerosis is present in noncoronary arteries, the coronary arteries will usually also be diseased, irrespective of symptoms.[24] The CHD risk equivalent concept introduced in the previous prevention guidelines included symptomatic disease in noncoronary arteries (option A), carotid stenosis of > 50% (option B), ankle-brachial blood pressure index < 0.9 *(not 0.8)* (option C), and abdominal aortic aneurysm (option D).[25] Asymptomatic carotid bruit is also associated with high CHD risk (option E).[26,27]

32-7. **The answer is E.** *(Hurst's The Heart, 14th Edition, Chap. 32)* The number and severity of stenoses determined by coronary angiography are signs of atherosclerosis with diagnostic, therapeutic, and prognostic implications.[28-30] However, most acute coronary events originate from angiographically nonobstructive *(not obstructive)* plaques (option E), probably because they are much more numerous.[17,16,31-34] An irregular lumen and/or filling defects indicating plaque disruption and/or thrombosis are associated with worse outcomes.[35] In contrast to coronary *luminography*, CAC detected by computed tomography (CT) imaging reveals the diseased arterial wall directly and correlates strongly with plaque burden.[36,37] The total amount of CAC (usually expressed as the *Agatston score*) is a strong predictor of coronary events and provides prognostic information beyond that provided by traditional risk factor scoring (option A).[38] Contrast-enhanced CT angiography visualizes not only the lumen but also the arterial wall (option B). Because the strong relationship between the CAC score and coronary events is mediated predominantly by coexisting noncalcified or less calcified vulnerable plaques, total or noncalcified plaque burden detected by CT angiography may prove to be an even better marker of risk than the CAC score.[39,40] Intravascular ultrasound (IVUS) can detect and localize plaque as well as quantitate plaque burden, but it requires selective catheterization and motorized pullback in the arteries of interest (option C). Serial examinations of well-defined coronary segments have been used to monitor the speed of plaque progression (or regression) over time in patients with established CHD (option D).[41]

32-8. **The answer is C.** *(Hurst's The Heart, 14th Edition, Chap. 32)* The TCFA has a distinct microstructure, including a large necrotic core (option A) covered by a thin and inflamed fibrous cap (option B), and other characteristic plaque features are common, such as a large, expansive remodeling (option D), neovascularization (angiogenesis) (option E), and a spotty *(not uniform)* pattern of calcification (option C).[16,17]

32-9. **The answer is D.** *(Hurst's The Heart, 14th Edition, Chap. 32)* Coronary CT angiography may not only visualize the lumen and detect obstructive and nonobstructive plaques (option A), it may also quantify calcified and noncalcified plaque burden (option B). Furthermore, coronary CT angiography may also provide additional prognostic information by the detection of higher-risk plaques characterized by large plaque volume (option C), low *(not high)* CT attenuation (option D), napkin-ring sign, expansive remodeling (option E), and spotty calcification.[42,43]

32-10. The answer is E. (*Hurst's The Heart, 14th Edition, Chap. 32*) Many catheter-based technologies have been developed or are under development for the assessment of coronary atherosclerosis and vulnerable plaques, including conventional grayscale IVUS, virtual histology IVUS (option A) and other ultrasound-based tissue characterization modalities, optical coherence tomography, angioscopy (option B), near-infrared spectroscopy (option C), intracoronary magnetic resonance imaging, thermography (option D), and vascular profiling.[44-47] Because vulnerable coronary plaques of the rupture-prone type (TCFA) are relatively large, not numerous, and often cluster proximally in the major coronary arteries, their detection in patients undergoing percutaneous coronary interventions might be feasible.[48]

References

1. Yusuf S, Hawken S, Ounpuu S, et al; INTERHEART Study Investigators. Effect of potentially modifiable risk factors associated with myocardial infarction in 52 countries (the INTERHEART study): case-control study. *Lancet*. 2004;364:937-952.
2. Ware JH. The limitations of risk factors as prognostic tools. *N Engl J Med*. 2006;355: 2615-2617.
3. Wald NJ, Morris JK, Rish S. The efficacy of combining several risk factors as a screening test. *J Med Screen*. 2005;12:197-201.
4. Mortensen MB, Falk E. Real-life evaluation of European and American high-risk strategies for primary prevention of cardiovascular disease in patients with first myocardial infarction. *BMJ Open*. 2014;4:e005991
5. Lauer MS. Primary prevention of atherosclerotic cardiovascular disease: the high public burden of low individual risk. *JAMA*. 2007;297:1376-1378.
6. Kulenovic I, Mortensen MB, Bertelsen J, et al. Statin use prior to first myocardial infarction in contemporary patients: Inefficient and not gender equitable. *Prev Med*. 2016;83:63-69.
7. Libby P. The forgotten majority: unfinished business in cardiovascular risk reduction. *J Am Coll Cardiol*. 2005;46:1225-1228.
8. Sampson UK, Fazio S, Linton MF. Residual cardiovascular risk despite optimal LDL cholesterol reduction with statins: the evidence, etiology, and therapeutic challenges. *Curr Atheroscler Rep*. 2012;14:1-10.
9. Libby P, Hansson GK. Inflammation and immunity in diseases of the arterial tree: players and layers. *Circ Res*. 2015;116:307-311.
10. Hansson GK. Inflammation, atherosclerosis, and coronary artery disease. *N Engl J Med*. 2005;352:1685-1695.
11. Falk E, Nakano M, Bentzon JF, Finn AV, Virmani R. Update on acute coronary syndromes: the pathologists' view. *Eur Heart J*. 2013;34:719-728.
12. Stary HC, Blankenhorn DH, Chandler AB, et al. A definition of the intima of human arteries and of its atherosclerosis-prone regions. A report from the Committee on Vascular Lesions of the Council on Arteriosclerosis, American Heart Association. *Circulation*. 1992;85:391-405.
13. Wentzel JJ, Chatzizisis YS, Gijsen FJ, Giannoglou GD, Feldman CL, Stone PH. Endothelial shear stress in the evolution of coronary atherosclerotic plaque and vascular remodelling: current understanding and remaining questions. *Cardiovasc Res*. 2012;96:234-243.
14. Mann J, Davies MJ. Mechanisms of progression in native coronary artery disease: role of healed plaque disruption. *Heart*. 1999;82:265-268.
15. Burke AP, Kolodgie FD, Farb A, et al. Healed plaque ruptures and sudden coronary death: evidence that subclinical rupture has a role in plaque progression. *Circulation*. 2001;103:934-940.
16. Bentzon JF, Otsuka F, Virmani R, Falk E. Mechanisms of plaque formation and rupture. *Circ Res*. 2014;114:1852-1866.
17. Falk E, Shah PK, Fuster V. Coronary plaque disruption. *Circulation*. 1995;92:657-667.
18. Virmani R, Kolodgie FD, Burke AP, et al. Lessons from sudden coronary death: a comprehensive morphological classification scheme for atherosclerotic lesions. *Arterioscler Thromb Vasc Biol*. 2000;20:1262-1275.
19. Kubo T, Imanishi T, Takarada S, et al. Assessment of culprit lesion morphology in acute myocardial infarction: ability of optical coherence tomography compared with intravascular ultrasound and coronary angioscopy. *J Am Coll Cardiol*. 2007;50: 933-939.
20. Kolodgie FD, Burke AP, Farb A, et al. The thin-cap fibroatheroma: a type of vulnerable plaque: the major precursor lesion to acute coronary syndromes. *Curr Opin Cardiol*. 2001;16:285-292.
21. Kolodgie FD, Narula J, Burke AP, et al. Localization of apoptotic macrophages at the site of plaque rupture in sudden coronary death. *Am J Pathol*. 2000;157:1259-1268.
22. Dalager S, Paaske WP, Kristensen IB, et al. Artery-related differences in atherosclerosis expression: implications for atherogenesis and dynamics in intima-media thickness. *Stroke*. 2007;38:2698-2705.
23. Dalager S, Falk E, Kristensen IB, et al. Plaque in superficial femoral arteries indicates generalized atherosclerosis and vulnerability to coronary death: an autopsy study. *J Vasc Surg*. 2008;47:296-302.
24. Gallino A, Aboyans V, Diehm C, et al; European Society of Cardiology Working Group on Peripheral Circulation. Non-coronary atherosclerosis. *Eur Heart J*. 2014;35:1112-1119.

25. National Cholesterol Education Program (NCEP) Expert Panel on Detection, Evaluation, and Treatment of High Blood Cholesterol in Adults (Adult Treatment Panel III). Third Report of the National Cholesterol Education Program (NCEP) Expert Panel on Detection, Evaluation, and Treatment of High Blood Cholesterol in Adults (Adult Treatment Panel III) final report. *Circulation*. 2002;106:3143-3421.

26. Lackland DT, Elkind MS, D'Agostino R Sr, et al. Inclusion of stroke in cardiovascular risk prediction instruments: a statement for healthcare professionals from the American Heart Association/American Stroke Association. *Stroke*. 2012;43:1998-2027.

27. Pickett CA, Jackson JL, Hemann BA, et al. Carotid bruits as a prognostic indicator of cardiovascular death and myocardial infarction: a meta-analysis. *Lancet*. 2008;371:1587-1594.

28. Min JK, Shaw LJ, Devereux RB, et al. Prognostic value of multidetector coronary computed tomographic angiography for prediction of all-cause mortality. *J Am Coll Cardiol*. 2007;50:1161-1170.

29. Mancini GBJ, Bates ER, Maron DJ, et al; on behalf of the COURAGE Trial Investigators and Coordinators. Quantitative results of baseline angiography and percutaneous coronary intervention in the COURAGE Trial. *Circ Cardiovasc Qual Outcomes*. 2009;2:320-327.

30. Gulati M, Cooper-DeHoff RM, McClure C, et al. Adverse cardiovascular outcomes in women with non-obstructive coronary artery disease: a report from the Women's Ischemia Syndrome Evaluation Study and the St James Women Take Heart Project. *Arch Intern Med*. 2009;169:843-850.

31. Kern MJ, Meier B. Evaluation of the culprit plaque and the physiological significance of coronary atherosclerotic narrowings. *Circulation*. 2001;103:3142-3149.

32. Boden WE, O'Rourke RA, Teo KK, et al. Optimal medical therapy with or without PCI for stable coronary disease. *N Engl J Med*. 2007;356:1503-1516.

33. BARI 2D Study Group; Frye RL, August P, Brooks MM, et al. A randomized trial of therapies for type 2 diabetes and coronary artery disease. *N Engl J Med*. 2009;360:2503-2515.

34. Stone GW, Maehara A, Lansky AJ, et al; PROSPECT Investigators. A prospective natural-history study of coronary atherosclerosis. *N Engl J Med*. 2011;364:226-235.

35. Goldstein JA, Demetriou D, Grines CL, et al. Multiple complex coronary plaques in patients with acute myocardial infarction. *N Engl J Med*. 2000;343:915-922.

36. Sangiorgi G, Rumberger JA, Severson A, et al. Arterial calcification and not lumen stenosis is highly correlated with atherosclerotic plaque burden in humans: a histologic study of 723 coronary artery segments using nondecalcifying methodology. *J Am Coll Cardiol*. 1998;31:126-133.

37. Tota-Maharaj R, Al-Mallah MH, Nasir K, et al. Improving the relationship between coronary artery calcium score and coronary plaque burden: addition of regional measures of coronary artery calcium distribution. *Atherosclerosis*. 2015;238:126-131.

38. Blaha MJ, Silverman MG, Budoff MJ. Is there a role for coronary artery calcium scoring for management of asymptomatic patients at risk for coronary artery disease? Clinical risk scores are not sufficient to define primary prevention treatment strategies among asymptomatic patients. *Circ Cardiovasc Imaging*. 2014;7:398-408.

39. Motoyama S, Sarai M, Harigaya H, et al. Computed tomographic angiography characteristics of atherosclerotic plaques subsequently resulting in acute coronary syndrome. *J Am Coll Cardiol*. 2009;54:49-57.

40. Choi EK, Choi SI, Rivera JJ, et al. Coronary computed tomography angiography as a screening tool for the detection of occult coronary artery disease in asymptomatic individuals. *J Am Coll Cardiol*. 2008;52:357-365.

41. Nicholls SJ, Tuzcu EM, Sipahi I, et al. Intravascular ultrasound in cardiovascular medicine. *Circulation*. 2006;114:e55-e59.

42. Maurovich-Horvat P, Ferencik M, Voros S, et al. Comprehensive plaque assessment by coronary CT angiography. *Nat Rev Cardiol*. 2014;11:390-402.

43. Thomsen C, Abdulla J. Characteristics of high-risk coronary plaques identified by computed tomographic angiography and associated prognosis: a systematic review and meta-analysis. *Eur Heart J Cardiovasc Imaging*. 2016;17(2):120-129.

44. Tomey MI, Narula J, Kovacic JC. Advances in the understanding of plaque composition and treatment options: year in review. *J Am Coll Cardiol*. 2014;63:1604-1616.

45. Toutouzas K, Benetos G, Karanasos A, et al. Vulnerable plaque imaging: updates on new pathobiological mechanisms. *Eur Heart J*. 2015;36:3147-3154.

46. Garcia-Garcia HM, Jang IK, Serruys PW, et al. Imaging plaques to predict and better manage patients with acute coronary events. *Circ Res*. 2014;114:1904-1917.

47. Stone PH, Coskun AU. Conceptual new biomechanical approaches to identify coronary plaques at risk of disruption. *JACC Cardiovasc Imaging*. 2015;8:1167-1169.

48. Waxman S, Ishibashi F, Muller JE. Detection and treatment of vulnerable plaques and vulnerable patients: novel approaches to prevention of coronary events. *Circulation*. 2006;114:2390-2411.

CHAPTER 33

Coronary Thrombosis: Local and Systemic Factors

Patrick R. Lawler

QUESTIONS

DIRECTIONS: Choose the one best response to each question.

33-1. Initial atherosclerotic lesions result from the accumulation of inflammatory cells and lipids in which part or layer of the arterial wall?

A. Arterial lumen
B. Intima
C. Media
D. Adventitia
E. All of the above

33-2. Which of the following factors contributes to the attenuation of the proatherogenic state and lesion progression?

A. Vascular cell adhesion molecule-1 (VCAM-1)
B. Matrix metalloproteinases (MMPs)
C. Elevated high-density lipoprotein (HDL)
D. Lipids at injury site
E. Interferon (IFN)-gamma

33-3. Which of the following statements about the coagulation cascade is *correct*?

A. Injury to vessel wall exposes subendothelial proteins such as collagen and von Willebrand factor (vWF) that can potently activate platelets
B. Activated factor Xa is responsible for cleaving fibrinogen to fibrin, which forms a stable hemostatic plug over the injury site
C. Vitamin K is crucial for *de novo* synthesis of four clotting factors, including prothrombin
D. Platelets play an important role in coagulation via their ability to upregulate DNA replication following binding of tissue factor to their surface receptor
E. Upon stimulation, intracellular calcium blocks platelet degranulation, thereby inhibiting platelet activation

33-4. Which of the following is an intrinsic mechanism developed to control coagulation reactions?

A. Hemodilution of coagulation factors
B. Proteolytic feedback by thrombin
C. Protein C
D. Fibrinolysis
E. All of the above

33-5. A 55-year-old female flight attendant with a history of hypertension and atrial fibrillation recently underwent coronary angioplasty, transient ischemic attack, and stenting in the setting of a troponin-positive acute coronary syndrome. Which antithrombotic therapy is recommended for this patient?

A. Aspirin and prasugrel
B. Aspirin and warfarin
C. Aspirin and clopidogrel and warfarin
D. Clopidogrel and warfarin
E. Warfarin alone

33-6. The P2Y and P2X receptors play an important role in platelet activation and thrombus formation. Which of the following statements about these receptors is *false*?

A. $P2Y_1$ is responsible for platelet shape change and calcium mobilization
B. $P2X_1$ is an ADP-gated calcium channel receptor involved in platelet shape change
C. $P2Y_{12}$ is responsible for the platelet aggregation response to ADP
D. $P2Y_1$ is responsible for TXA_2 generation
E. cAMP is an important signaling molecule downstream of $P2Y_{12}$ activation

33-7. Which of the following statements about atherosclerotic plaque neovascularization is *correct*?

A. Vasa vasorum in the intima spreads into the adventitia, where it prompts neovascularization and plaque growth
B. Neovascularization is responsible for stabilizing and strengthening atherosclerotic plaques
C. Promotion of plaque neovascularization is a potential therapeutic strategy to prevent plaque disruption
D. Leaky vasa vasorum in the intima results in macrophage infiltration and plaque destabilization
E. All of the above

33-8. The innate and acquired immune systems are important modulators of inflammation and atherosclerosis. Which of the following associations is *false*?

A. Monocytes and Ly6C/GR-1
B. Dendritic cells and CD4
C. Platelets and CD40L
D. T cells and CD8
E. Mast cell and histamine

33-9. A 60-year-old man is rushed to the emergency room after sustaining a myocardial infarction (MI) during strenuous exercise. What is the *most likely* explanation for this patient's coronary thrombosis?

A. An atherosclerotic plaque rupture led to exposure of subendothelial matrix elements and resulted in a persistent thrombotic occlusion and MI
B. The ruptured plaque had a very small atheromatous core, which increased plaque thrombogenicity and risk of MI
C. A residual mural thrombus resulted in a decreased shear rate, which facilitated the activation and deposition of platelets on the lesion
D. Lack of macrophages in the atherosclerotic plaque led to activation of MMPs that resulted in plaque disruption and thrombus formation
E. None of the above

33-10. A mother brings her 4-year-old daughter to the emergency room with a severe nosebleed. After careful examination and proper testing, she is diagnosed with von Willebrand disease, characterized by a missing or defective vWF. Given what is known about blood clotting, what step in the coagulation cascade is dysregulated in this disease?

A. Proteolytic cleavage of prothrombin to thrombin
B. Platelet degranulation
C. Binding of TF to factor VII
D. Platelet adhesion to injury site
E. Binding of ADP to $P2Y_1$ receptor

33-1. The answer is B. *(Hurst's The Heart, 14th Edition, Chap. 33)* Atherosclerosis is a systemic disease involving the intima of large and medium-sized arteries that is characterized by intimal thickening caused by the accumulation of cells and lipids (option B).[1] However, secondary changes may occur in the underlying media (option C) and adventitia (option D), particularly in advanced disease stages. The early atherosclerotic lesions might progress without compromising the lumen because of compensatory vascular enlargement (Glagovian remodeling) (option A).[2] Importantly, the culprit lesions leading to acute coronary syndromes are usually mildly stenotic and therefore barely detected by angiography.[3] These high-risk, rupture-prone lesions usually have a large lipid core, a thin fibrous cap, and a high density of inflammatory cells.

33-2. The answer is C. *(Hurst's The Heart, 14th Edition, Chap. 33)* Inflammation is an important process that affects plaque progression, vulnerability, and subsequent thrombus formation. Inflammatory cells (monocyte/macrophages, T cells, and mast cells) present in the core and shoulder of atherosclerotic lesions release inflammatory cytokines and MMPs that affect each step of atherosclerosis from lesion formation, to progression, to disruption and ACS (option B). The circulating monocytes are recruited within the subendothelial space in response to the synthesis and exposure of adhesive proteins triggered by the early accumulation of lipids (option D). The internalized monocytes release inflammatory mediators, such as netrin-1 and VCAM-1, that are responsible for their retention in the lesions (option A). Mast cells are proinflammatory through the release of histamine, leukotrienes, interleukin (IL)-6, and interferon (IFN)-gamma (option E). Attenuation of the proatherogenic state occurs through HDL-raising and may facilitate the efflux of the wall macrophages (option C).

33-3. The answer is A. *(Hurst's The Heart, 14th Edition, Chap. 33)* The coagulation cascade constitutes a series of molecules that interact with each other in a controlled manner to produce a rapid and amplified response to vessel wall injury. In the case of an atherosclerotic lesion, plaque rupture facilitates the interaction of the inner plaque components with the circulating blood.[4] At the site of vascular lesion, circulating von Willebrand factor (vWF) binds to the exposed collagen that subsequently binds to the glycoprotein (GP) Ib/IX receptor on the platelet membrane (option A). Tissue factor (TF), another plaque component, exhibits a potent activating effect on platelets and coagulation. Platelet activation triggers intracellular signaling via second messengers, such as calcium, that induce shape change and secretion of their granular contents (option E). While platelets are nucleated cells that are devoid of genomic DNA, they contain messenger RNA and have the ability to synthesize proteins following activation (option D). Some clotting factors, namely factors VII, IX, X, and prothrombin, require vitamin K to undergo a posttranslational modification necessary for their ability to bind cell membrane surfaces. Without vitamin K, these factors can be synthesized but will not participate in proper clotting reactions (option C). Finally, clotting factors must be enzymatically cleaved in order to become active. Activated factor Xa is responsible for cleaving prothrombin to thrombin, which can then cleave fibrinogen to fibrin to form the hemostatic plug over the injury site (option B).

33-4. The answer is E. *(Hurst's The Heart, 14th Edition, Chap. 33)* Several mechanisms exist to control and limit coagulation reactions and maintain hemostasis. Coagulation is normally restricted to the site of injury by hemodilution of clotting elements, thereby limiting the size of the platelet plug and washing away coagulation factors as blood flows (option A). Although thrombin plays a pivotal role in maintaining the complex balance of initial prothrombotic reparative events, it also controls the subsequent anticoagulant and fibrinolytic pathways through proteolytic feedback mechanisms (option B). Thrombin has a specific receptor in endothelial cell surfaces, thrombomodulin, which triggers a physiologic anticoagulation system. Thrombin generated at the site of injury binds to thrombomodulin, and the complex serves as a receptor for the vitamin K-dependent protein C, which is activated and released from the endothelial cell surface. Activated protein C then inactivates factors Va and VIIIa and limits thrombin effects (option C). Fibrinolysis, the enzymatic breakdown of the fibrin clots, involves catalytic activation of zymogens, positive and negative feedback control, and inhibitor blockade (option D). Blood clotting is blocked at the level of the prothrombinase complex by the physiologic anticoagulant-activated protein C. Activated protein C cleaves factor Va, rendering it functionally inactive, thereby blocking thrombin formation.

33-5. **The answer is C.** *(Hurst's The Heart, 14th Edition, Chap. 33)* Patients presenting with troponin-positive acute coronary syndromes should be considered for treatment with dual antiplatelet therapy to reduce the risk of ischemic complications, irrespective of whether an intracoronary artery stent was used in the management of the patient. Patients treated with intracoronary stenting particularly should receive dual antiplatelet therapy to reduce the risk of stent thrombosis (option A). In addition, oral anticoagulants such as warfarin or NOACs are considered as part of "triple therapy" when an indication for antithrombotic therapy is present (eg, atrial fibrillation, venous thromboembolic disease) (option B). Although such triple therapy increases bleeding risk, this is the current standard of care, although several ongoing clinical trials are examining alternative regimens (options C, D, and E).

33-6. **The answer is A.** *(Hurst's The Heart, 14th Edition, Chap. 33)* Great interest in the platelet ADP receptors (P2Y, P2X) has recently been generated because of available pharmacologic inhibitors. The $P2Y_1$ receptor is responsible for inositol trisphosphate formation through the activation of phospholipase C, leading to transient increase in the concentration of intracellular calcium, platelet shape change, and weak transient platelet aggregation (option A).[5,6] Pharmacologic data have also revealed an essential role for the $P2Y_1$ receptor in the initiation of platelet ADP-induced activation, TXA_2 generation, and platelet activation in response to other agonists (option D). The $P2Y_{12}$ receptor is responsible for completion of the platelet aggregation response to ADP (option C), and it has several important downstream signaling molecules, including cAMP (option E). Pharmacologic approaches have shown a role for the $P2Y_{12}$ receptor in dense granule secretion, fibrinogen-receptor activation, P-selectin expression, and thrombus formation. Although not activated by ADP, platelets possess a third purinergic receptor ($P2X_1$), which is a fast adenosine triphosphate (ATP)-gated calcium channel receptor mainly involved in platelet shape change.

33-7. **The answer is D.** *(Hurst's The Heart, 14th Edition, Chap. 33)* Recent evidence has highlighted the importance of lesion neovascularization in plaque destabilization and plaque growth.[7-9] Preexisting vasa vasorum in the adventitia is thought to spread into the intima, prompting intimal neovascularization (option A).[8] Leaky vasa vasorum with the subsequent red blood cell extravasation is thought to be a major source of macrophage infiltration, and it increases the vulnerability of the atherosclerotic lesions (option D). A recent study using optical coherence tomography has associated vasa vasorum increase with fibrous plaque volume and intraplaque neovessels with plaque vulnerability (option B).[10] Inhibition of plaque neovascularization could thus be seen as a potential new therapeutic intervention to prevent plaque disruption (option C).

33-8. **The answer is B.** *(Hurst's The Heart, 14th Edition, Chap. 33)* Monocytes, dendritic cells, and mast cells are the major players in innate immunity (Figure 33-1). Mast cells are inflammatory by releasing histamine, leukotrienes, interleukin (IL)-6, and interferon (IFN)-gamma (option E). Dendritic cells are responsible for antigen presentation via human leukocyte antigen (HLA) molecules CD80/86 and CD40 (option B). Monocytes are divided into two major types according to their expression of CD14 and CD16, and can be further classified by their expression of the proinflammatory molecule Ly6C/GR-1 (option A). Platelets also play an important role in the inflammatory environment by secreting various vasoactive chemokines and cytokines such as CD40L (option C). Finally, T cells of the acquired immunity are either $CD4^+$ or $CD8^+$ and likewise play a crucial role in the destabilization of atherosclerotic lesions (option D).

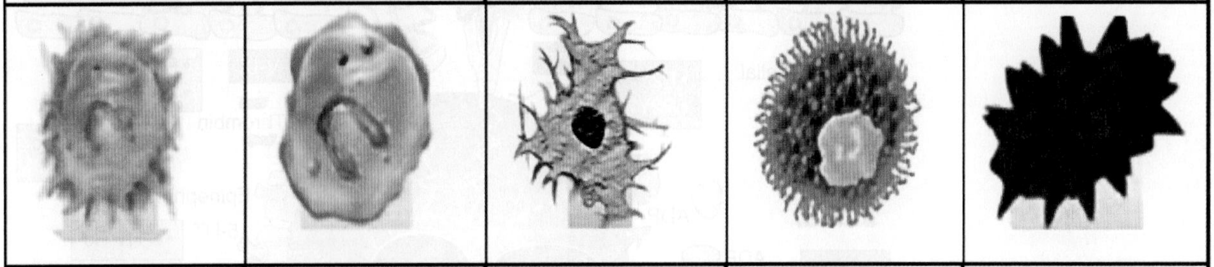

Monocytes		Dendritic cells	Mast cells	Activated platelets
Ly6C/GR-1 positive TLRs Proteases Redox species TNF IL-1 Cytokines	Ly6C/GR-1 negative TGF-β CD36 SR-A CD163 VEGF	HLA molecules CD80/86 CD40	Histamine Leukotrienes Chymase IL-6 Interferon	CD40L RANTES MRP-8/14 PDGF TGF-β
Pro-inflammatory	Anti-inflammatory?	Antigen presentation	Inflammatory	Hemostasis

FIGURE 33-1 Major cell players involved in innate immunity.

33-9. **The answer is A.** (*Hurst's The Heart, 14th Edition, Chap. 33*) The mechanisms of platelet deposition and thrombus formation after vascular damage are modulated by the type of injury, the local geometry, and local hemodynamic conditions.[11,12] Tissue factor (TF) readily available in the atherosclerotic intimal space exposed by endothelial loss contributes to the high thrombogenicity of atherosclerotic plaques.[13,14] As such, when injury to the vessel wall is mild, the thrombogenic stimulus is relatively limited, and the resulting thrombotic occlusion is transient, as occurs in UA. On the other hand, deep vessel injury secondary to plaque rupture or ulceration results in exposure of collagen, TF, and other elements of the vessel matrix, leading to relatively persistent thrombotic occlusion and MI (option A). Studies show that the atheromatous core is up to sixfold more active than the other plaque substrates in triggering thrombosis.[11] Therefore, ruptured plaques with a large atheromatous core are at high risk of leading to ACS (option B). Macrophages are suggested to play a key role in inducing plaque rupture by secreting proteases capable of destroying the ECM that provides physical strength to the fibrous cap. Recently, it has been shown that macrophage-mediated matrix degradation by MMPs can induce plaque rupture (option D). Additionally, because platelet deposition increases with increasing degrees of vessel stenosis, residual mural thrombus encroaching into the vessel lumen may result in an increased shear rate, which facilitates the activation and deposition of platelets on the lesion (option C).

33-10. **The answer is D.** (*Hurst's The Heart, 14th Edition, Chap. 33*) Von Willebrand factor (vWF) is an important clotting factor present in blood plasma, endothelium, and subendothelial connective tissue. Its primary function is binding to other proteins and stimulating platelet adhesion to wound sites (option D). At the site of vascular lesions, circulating vWF binds to the exposed collagen that subsequently binds to the glycoprotein (GP) Ib/IX receptor on the platelet membrane. Under pathological conditions and in response to changes in shear stress, vWF can be secreted from the storage organelles in platelets or endothelial cells, reinforcing the activation process. vWF is not an enzyme, and thus it has no catalytic activity or effect on the conversion of prothrombin to thrombin (option A). Platelet activation by various agonists, such as ADP, leads to the mobilization of calcium and subsequent release of its granular content (option B). Likewise, vWF is not responsible for TF binding to factor VII, which happens physiologically or pathologically following exposure of TF during injury (option C). vWF is also not required for the binding of the ADP agonist to its receptor, $P2Y_1$ (option E). Figure 33-2 highlights the mechanisms involved in platelet adhesion, activation, and aggregation.

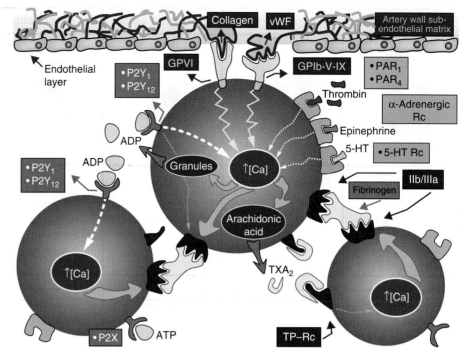

FIGURE 33-2 Mechanisms and agonists involved in platelet adhesion, activation, and aggregation. (Reproduced with permission from Ibanez B, Vilahur G, Badimon J. Pharmacology of thienopyridines: rationale for dual pathway inhibition, *Eur Heart J Suppl.* 2006;8(Suppl G):G3-G9.)

References

1. Santos-Gallego CG, Picatoste B, Badimón JJ. Pathophysiology of acute coronary syndrome. Biologic aspects of vulnerable plaque. *Curr Atheroscler Rep.* 2014;16(4):401.

2. Glagov S, Weisenberg E, Zarins CK, Stankunavicius R, Kolettis GJ. Compensatory enlargement of human atherosclerotic coronary arteries. *N Engl J Med.* 1987;316:1371-1375.

3. Libby P, Hansson GK. Inflammation and immunity in disease of the arterial tree: players and layers. *Circ Res.* 2015;116(2):307-311.

4. Angiolillo DJ, Ferreiro JL Antiplatelet and anticoagulant therapy for atherothrombotic disease: the role of current and emerging agents. *Am J Cardiovasc Drugs.* 2013;13(4): 233-250.

5. Jacobson KA, Gao ZG, Paoletta S, et al. John Daly Lecture: Structure-guided drug design for adenosine and P2Y receptors. *Comput Struct Biotechnol J.* 2014;13:286-298.

6. Tang XF, Fan JY, Meng J et al. Impact of new oral or intravenous P2Y$_{12}$ inhibitors and clopidogrel on major ischemic and bleeding events in patients with coronary artery disease: a meta-analysis of randomized trials. *Atherosclerosis.* 2014;233(2):568-578.

7. Moreno PR, Purushothaman KR, Fuster V, et al. Plaque neovascularization is increased in ruptured atherosclerotic lesions of human aorta: implications for plaque vulnerability. *Circulation.* 2004;110:2032-2038.

8. Virmani R, Kolodgie FD, Burke AP, et al. Atherosclerotic plaque progression and vulnerability to rupture: angiogenesis as a source of intraplaque hemorrhage. *Arterioscler Thromb Vasc Biol.* 2005;25:2054-2061.

9. Fuster V, Moreno PR, Fayad ZA, et al. Atherothrombosis and high-risk plaque: part I: evolving concepts. *J Am Coll Cardiol.* 2005;46:937-954.

10. Taruya A, Tanaka A, Nishiguchi T, et al. Vasa vasorum restructuring in human atherosclerotic plaque vulnerability: a clinical optical coherence tomography study. *J Am Coll Cardiol.* 2015;65:2469-2477.

11. Badimon L, Badimon JJ, Turitto VT, Vallabhajosula S, Fuster V. Platelet thrombus formation on collagen type I. A model of deep vessel injury. Influence of blood rheology, von Willebrand factor, and blood coagulation. *Circulation.* 1988;78:1431-1442.

12. Badimon L, Badimon JJ, Galvez A, Chesebro JH, Fuster V. Influence of arterial damage and wall shear rate on platelet deposition. Ex vivo study in a swine model. *Arteriosclerosis.* 1986;6:312-320.

13. Badimon L, Badimon JJ. Mechanisms of arterial thrombosis in nonparallel streamlines: platelet thrombi grow on the apex of stenotic severely injured vessel wall. Experimental study in the pig model. *J Clin Invest.* 1989;84:1134-1144.

14. Fernandez-Ortiz A, Badimon JJ, Falk E, et al. Characterization of the relative thrombogenicity of atherosclerotic plaque components: implications for consequences of plaque rupture. *J Am Coll Cardiol.* 1994;23:1562-1569.

CHAPTER 34

Coronary Blood Flow and Myocardial Ischemia

Patrick R. Lawler

QUESTIONS

DIRECTIONS: Choose the one best response to each question.

34-1. Which of the following statements about myocardial ischemia is *true*?

A. Elective revascularization trials driven by ischemia on diagnostic testing has not yet been shown to reduce myocardial infarction despite relief of angina

B. Revascularization of routinely identified coronary stenoses can improve mortality

C. Revascularization is more effective than medical treatment in preventing myocardial infarction and coronary death in stable CAD

D. Immediate percutaneous coronary intervention (PCI) in acute coronary syndrome (ACS) fails to reduce the risk of subsequent myocardial infarction

E. All of the above

34-2. A 66-year-old man undergoes exercise testing with myocardial perfusion imaging. What effect will dipyridamole administration have on this patient in the presence of a 95% diameter stenosis in a coronary artery?

A. It will cause progressive coronary narrowing, reducing coronary flow reserve (CFR) but not resting flow

B. A fall in coronary perfusion pressure due to a steal phenemenon and associated subendocardial ischemia

C. Coronary control mechanisms will be activated and will prevent the invocation of maximal vasodilatory capacity

D. Vasodilator-mediated increased coronary flow will cause a rise in coronary perfusion pressure to the epicardium

E. None of the above are correct

34-3. In a fluid dynamic model of stenosis and diffuse narrowing, what is the relationship between arterial radius and coronary flow?

A. Coronary flow is directly proportional to arterial radius

B. Coronary flow is inversely proportional to arterial radius

C. Coronary flow is proportional to the arterial radius divided by four

D. Coronary flow is proportional to the arterial radius raised to the fourth power

E. Coronary flow is independent of arterial radius

34-4. Which of the following statements about coronary blood flow in women is *correct*?

A. Women have larger coronary arteries and higher myocardial perfusion

B. Women have low endothelial shear, which reduces "leaky" endothelial cell junctions

C. Women have high endothelial shear that promotes atheroma formation

D. Women can have high endothelial shear that inhibits low-density lipoprotein transport

E. Women upregulate endothelial NADPH oxidase, thereby increasing oxidative stress

34-5. Which of the following accurately describes the difference in blood flow through a nonstenotic artery compared with a stenotic artery?

A. A stenosis imposes an area of low wall pressure

B. Flow velocity is greater through a nonstenotic section of an artery

C. A section of nonstenosis is an area of high endothelial shear

D. High endothelial shear stress is atherogenic

E. The viscous pressure loss across a stenosis is linearly proportional to flow squared

34-6. Which of the following is *true* about myocardial steal and its mechanisms?

A. Intramyocardial steal refers to blood flow being withdrawn from the subendocardium by the subepicardium

B. As flow increases through a stenosis, the pressure gradient increases, and distal coronary pressure falls

C. Pharmacological vasodilators increase epicardial flow, thereby decreasing the pressure gradient across the stenosis

D. It manifests as stress-induced ST elevations on ECG and angina with reduced average transmural perfusion

E. All of the above

34-7. Which of the following mechanisms regulating coronary blood flow is *incorrect*?

A. Metabolic demand is the primary controller of coronary blood flow

B. Both sympathetic and parasympathetic neurons enervate the coronary arteries

C. Increased coronary blood flow increases endothelial shear and results in vasodilation

D. A sudden rise in coronary pressure results in a sustained increase in coronary blood flow

E. All of the above are incorrect

34-1. The answer is A. *(Hurst's The Heart, 14th Edition, Chap. 34)* Immediate PCI in ACS reduces the risk of recurrent myocardial infarction (option D). However, elective revascularization trials driven by "ischemia" on diagnostic testing has not yet been shown to reduce myocardial infarction or cardiovascular deaths despite relief of angina (option A; not option B). In addition, the failure of randomized revascularization trials to reduce myocardial infarction or coronary deaths compared to medical treatment alone in "stable CAD" has been demonstrated in the Clinical Outcomes Utilizing Revascularization and Aggressive Drug Evaluation (COURAGE) trial[1] (option C).

34-2. The answer is B. *(Hurst's The Heart, 14th Edition, Chap. 34)* Experimentally and clinically, maximal hyperemic flow for determining CFR is achieved pharmacologically by arteriolar vasodilating drugs such dipyridamole, adenosine, and regadenoson. Progressive coronary narrowing reduces CFR with little change in resting flow until an approximately 80% to 90% diameter stenosis. At these levels of severe stenosis, resting blood flow falls (option A), but some residual CFR capacity remains upon pharmacologic vasodilator stimulus. Stenosis severe enough to reduce resting perfusion does not elicit all remaining reserve vasodilator capacity because of a self-regulating mechanism that protects subendocardial perfusion. At such severe stenosis reducing resting perfusion, any increase in vasodilator-mediated increased coronary flow causes a proportionately greater fall in coronary perfusion pressure, thereby reducing subendocardial perfusion more than subepicardial perfusion, and causing subendocardial (option D is incorrect) ischemia, angina, and ST depression on ECG. When exercise or pharmacologic vasodilation forces greater vasodilation than stable resting conditions, this protective control is overridden (option C), with ensuing subendocardial ischemia (option B).

34-3. The answer is D. *(Hurst's The Heart, 14th Edition, Chap. 34)* The relationship between arterial radius and coronary flow is depicted in Figure 34-1. Coronary flow is a function of the arterial radius raised to the fourth power (option D).

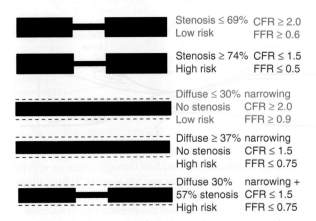

Stenosis ≤ 69%   CFR ≥ 2.0
Low risk   FFR ≥ 0.6

Stenosis ≥ 74%   CFR ≤ 1.5
High risk   FFR ≤ 0.5

Diffuse ≤ 30% narrowing
No stenosis   CFR ≥ 2.0
Low risk   FFR ≥ 0.9

Diffuse ≥ 37% narrowing
No stenosis   CFR ≤ 1.5
High risk   FFR ≤ 0.75

Diffuse 30%   narrowing +
57% stenosis CFR ≤ 1.5
High risk   FFR ≤ 0.75

FIGURE 34-1 Computer models of stenosis and calculated coronary flow reserve (CFR) and fractional flow reserve (FFR) based on fluid dynamic analysis of the entire branching coronary artery tree with and without stenosis or diffuse narrowing. (Reproduced with permission from Gould KL, Johnson NP, Kaul S, et al. Patient selection for elective revascularization to reduce myocardial infarction and mortality: New lessons from randomized trials, coronary physiology, and statistics, *Circ Cardiovasc Imaging* 2015 May;8(5). pii: e003099.)

34-4. The answer is D. *(Hurst's The Heart, 14th Edition, Chap. 34)* CAD in women is characterized by atypical chest pain, diffuse epicardial coronary atherosclerosis, microvascular dysfunction, inaccurate diagnostic tests, delayed or late ACS associated with high mortality, and differential responses to medical treatment or invasive procedures in women compared to men. Coronary arteries in women are smaller than in men (option A), but myocardial perfusion is higher in women. Accordingly, average endothelial shear is higher in women. High endothelial shear stress inhibits low-density lipoprotein transport (option D) by reducing "leaky" endothelial cell junctions (option B); inhibiting inflammation, platelet activation, and thrombosis; retarding oxidative processes; promoting mild stable uniform remodeling; and inhibiting focal atheroma (option C), focal stenosis, and plaque instability. These beneficial effects are mediated by high shear that upregulates endothelial nitric oxide (NO), NO synthase (eNOS) gene expression, eNOS phosphorylation, and manganese superoxide dismutase (Mn-SOD) expression and downregulates endothelial NADPH oxidase, thereby decreasing superoxide ion and oxidative stress (option E).

34-5. The answer is A. *(Hurst's The Heart, 14th Edition, Chap. 34)* Figure 34-2 shows the fluid dynamic equations relating stenosis dimensions, coronary blood flow, pressure gradient, flow profiles, exit vortex shedding, and endothelial shear stress. A normal nonstenotic artery is defined by low flow velocity (option B), high pressure and low shear (option C). Meanwhile, a stenotic artery is defined by high flow velocity, low pressure, and high shear (option A). The quadratic equation has a viscous pressure loss linearly proportional to flow (option E) and an exit separation loss proportional to flow squared. Both viscous and separation pressure losses are related to the arterial radius raised to the fourth power. Consequently, small changes in arterial diameter that are not visible or quantifiable on angiogram may have major effects on coronary flow or CFR, incurring high or low risk. High endothelial shear stress has antiatherogenic effects, whereas low shear stress is atherogenic (option D), with implications for the different manifestations of CAD in women versus men.

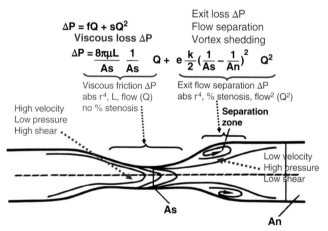

FIGURE 34-2 Schema of blood flow through a stenosis with fluid dynamic equation characterizing stenosis severity. Abbreviations: μ, blood viscosity; ΔP, pressure gradient across the stenosis; An, cross-sectional area of the normal nonstenotic artery; As, cross-sectional lumen area of the stenosis; k, constant; L, stenosis length; ΔP, pressure gradient; Q, flow; fQ, friction coefficient of flow; sQ, separation coefficient of flow squared.

34-6. The answer is B. *(Hurst's The Heart, 14th Edition, Chap. 34)* Intramyocardial steal, also called subendocardial-subepicardial steal, manifests as stress-induced ST depression on ECG and usually angina with reduced average transmural perfusion in cc/min/g to the ischemic threshold of 0.9 cc/min/g (option D). As flow increases through a stenosis, the pressure gradient increases, and distal coronary pressure falls (option B), thereby impairing subendocardial perfusion more than the subepicardium. This subepicardial to subendocardial perfusion gradient is called intramyocardial steal because of the superficial appearance of perfusion being "stolen away" from the subendocardium by the subepicardium (option A). As epicardial perfusion pressure and flow fall because of stenosis, the subendocardium vasodilates maximally as a result of ATP release from red blood cells that prevents ischemia up to a limit. At that level of epicardial perfusion pressure and flow, the subepicardium sees higher pressure and flow, thereby not vasodilating maximally. With added pharmacologic vasodilator stress, the epicardial flow increases, the pressure gradient across the stenosis increases (option C), and perfusion pressure falls, thereby making the subendocardium ischemic.

34-7. **The answer is D.** *(Hurst's The Heart, 14th Edition, Chap. 34)* Of the many factors affecting coronary blood flow, the primary controller is metabolic demand (option A) that nearly instantaneously regulates regional coronary flow, even in small separate myocardial regions independently. Myocardial oxygen demand regulates coronary blood flow via ATP release from oxygenated red blood cells at low myocardial pO_2. Coronary arterial smooth muscle inherently responds to changes in arterial pressure even with adequate arterial oxygenation and in the absence of myocardium or neural connections. A sudden rise in coronary pressure that initially increases coronary blood flow incurs coronary artery vasoconstriction that reduces flow back toward baseline (option E). Both sympathetic and parasympathetic neural networks enervate the coronary arteries (option B). The direct neural effect of parasympathetic stimulation is coronary vasodilation that would increase coronary blood, while the direct neural effect of beta-sympathetic blockade causes coronary vasoconstriction. As a component of its complex molecular biology, arteriolar vasodilation with increased coronary blood flow also increases endothelial shear stress that normally triggers epicardial coronary artery vasodilation mediated by NO (option C). However, with endothelial dysfunction, shear-induced epicardial vasodilation is lost, or vasoconstriction occurs.

References

1. Boden WE, O'Rourke RA, Teo, KK, et al. Optimal medical therapy with or without PCI for stable coronary disease. *The N Engl J Med.* 2007;356:1503-1516.
2. Gould KL, Johnson NP, Kaul S, et al. Patient selection for elective revascularization to reduce myocardial infarction and mortality: new lessons from randomized trials, coronary physiology, and statistics. *Circ Cardiovasc Imaging.* 2015;8:e003099.

CHAPTER 35

Nonobstructive Atherosclerotic and Nonatherosclerotic Coronary Heart Disease

Patrick R. Lawler

QUESTIONS

DIRECTIONS: Choose the one best response to each question.

35-1. Which of the following statements about normal coronary physiology and function is *correct*?

A. Conductance and flow in the coronary microcirculation are governed by Poiseuille's law
B. Resistance in the conductive vessels of the precapillary coronary tree is primarily responsive to metabolic stimuli
C. Epicardial vessels represent the predominant resistance within the coronary flow circuit
D. All of the above
E. None of the above

35-2. A 45-year-old woman presents to clinic with chest pain and shortness of breath. She had revascularization performed in the past, but her latest angiography results did not demonstrate residual obstructive epicardial coronary stenoses. Which of the following is *correct* about nonobstructive coronary artery disease (CAD)?

A. Nonobstructive CAD is diagnosed much more often in men than in women
B. Results from noninvasive stress testing will likely be normal
C. The patient likely has preserved LV systolic function
D. All of the above are correct
E. None of the above are correct

35-3. A 45-year-old female patient is evaluated for the presence of coronary microvascular dysfunction (CMD). Which of the following measurement techniques and expected outcomes is *not* correct?

A. Administration of adenosine results in smooth muscle relaxation
B. Regadenoson is associated with a reduced risk of bradycardia and bronchoconstriction compared with adenosine
C. Invasive Doppler flow wire can measure coronary blood flow velocity and pressures
D. Acetylcholine has direct effects on smooth muscle relaxation and vasodilation
E. Adenosine has both endothelium-dependent and endothelium-independent effects on smooth muscle cells

35-4. A 65-year-old man complains of new onset dyspnea and presyncopal episodes. He previously underwent heart transplantation six years ago for idiopathic dilated cardiomyopathy. Following a stress test and coronary CT, the patient is diagnosed with cardiac allograft vasculopathy (CAV) with diffuse narrowing of the coronary arteries. Which of the following is expected to be of limited efficacy in this patient without focal stenosis?

A. Repeat heart transplantation
B. Statin
C. Percutaneous coronary intervention (PCI)
D. Calcium channel blocker
E. ACE inhibitors

35-5. Which of the following statements about vasculitides that manifest with coronary arteritis is *correct*?

A. Kawasaki disease affects medium arteries and can result in coronary artery aneurysms

B. Takayasu's arteritis is an autoimmune process affecting the vasa vasorum of large vessels

C. ANCA-associated vasculitides can manifest with myocardial scarring

D. Giant cell arteritis (GCA) may present initially with coronary manifestations

E. All of the above

35-6. A 43-year-old man presents to the emergency room with anginal symptoms. Coronary angiography demonstrates patent coronary arteries, however, a tunneled (bridging) LAD artery is present. Which of the following could account for this patient's symptoms?

A. The tunneled artery is surrounded by epicardial fat, which compresses the lumen and limits blood flow

B. Compression of the tunneled artery occurs during diastole because myocardial blood flow occurs predominantly during systole

C. The tunneled artery runs deep in the myocardium, creating a greater myocardial bridge and accounting for greater compression of the vessel lumen

D. Greater myocardial demand results in increased blood flow during diastole because systole is limited by the increase in heart rate

E. None of the above; a tunneled artery cannot account for this patient's symptoms

35-7. A 43 year old man presents to clinic with exertional dyspnea and is is found to be in clinical heart failure. Angiography revealed a fistula between the LAD and the pulmonary artery. What is the *most* appropriate treatment for this patient?

A. Interventional (transcatheter) closure of the fistula

B. Beta-blocking agent

C. ACE inhibitor

D. Observation and continued follow-up

E. Answers B and C

35-8. Which of the following statements about the pathophysiology of aneurysms is *correct*?

A. The most common cause of aneurysms is dilatation secondary to vessel trauma

B. Dilatation involves the entire vessel wall (intima, media, and adventitia)

C. Aneurysms are often symptomatic and are discovered following patients' complaints

D. A "giant" aneurysm is defined as one having a dilatation diameter > 10 mm

E. All of the above are correct

35-9. A 36-year-old woman presents to the emergency room with chest pains, which started 5 days after delivering her child. A coronary angiography revealed a retrograde dissection of the LAD. Which of the following is *true* regarding this patient's condition?

A. Retrograde dissections should be treated surgically to prevent ischemic complications

B. Pregnancy is unrelated to the coronary dissection

C. Dissections always occur secondary to a triggering event, such as blunt force trauma

D. Coronary dissections are not associated with ischemic ECG changes

E. Retrograde dissections can be treated conservatively without further investigation

35-10. Which of the following characteristics appropriately defines epicardial coronary spasms?

A. Symptoms of angina pectoris occurring at rest

B. ST-segment changes on ECG

C. Minor elevations in serum C-reactive protein

D. Younger age and female predominance

E. All of the above are correct

35-1. The answer is A. *(Hurst's The Heart, 14th Edition, Chap. 35)* Vessels branch and decrease in size, from prearterioles to arterioles to capillaries. Myocardial blood flow is regulated mostly in the coronary microcirculation, where only small changes in arteriolar diameter can result in large changes in conductance and flow as predicted by Poiseuille's law (option A). Despite a historical focus on the epicardial coronary macrovessels, the microvessels represent the predominant resistance within the coronary flow circuit (option C), and they are innumerable in comparison to the epicardial vessels seen during invasive coronary angiography. The precapillary coronary tree consists of conductive, prearteriolar, and arteriolar vessels. Resistance in these vessel components is primarily responsive to flow, pressure, and metabolic stimuli, respectively (option B) (Figure 35-1).

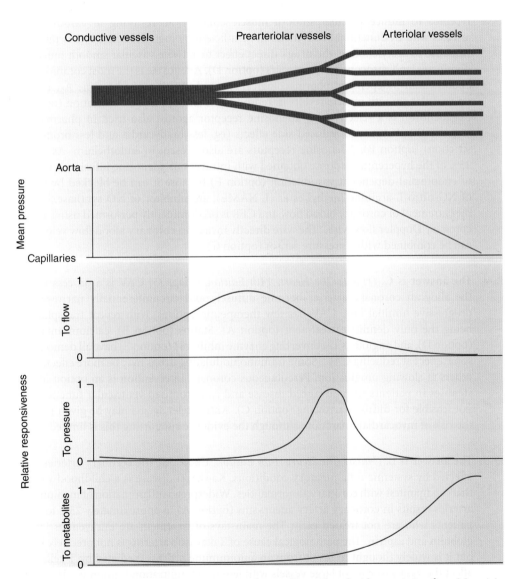

FIGURE 35-1 Components of the coronary circulation. (Reproduced with permission from Maseri A. *Ischemic Heart Disease*. New York: Churchill Livingstone; 1995.)

35-2. The answer is C. *(Hurst's The Heart, 14th Edition, Chap. 35)* A nontrivial proportion of patients with anginal symptoms and ischemia on stress testing (option B) have been noted to have an absence of fixed epicardial coronary arterial stenosis on coronary angiography.[1] The condition of angina with normal angiography, more accurately termed nonobstructive CAD, is being increasingly observed and is significantly more prevalent among women than men (option A).[2] In addition to those without fixed obstructive coronary stenosis, contemporary data suggest that 20% to 30% of patients with angina remain symptomatic despite technically successful revascularization and resolution of fixed epicardial coronary stenosis. In large international registries of patients referred for coronary angiography, the prevalence of nonobstructive CAD in women with angina symptoms may be as high as 65%.[3] Even in the presence of preserved LV systolic function (option C), patients with nonobstructive CAD are at elevated long-term risk when compared to healthy cohorts.

35-3. **The answer is D.** (*Hurst's The Heart, 14th Edition, Chap. 35*) To evaluate for the presence of CMD, several provocative agents are dependent on functional endothelium, whereas others act directly on vascular smooth muscle and are considered endothelium-independent. The most commonly used pharmacological agent for endothelium-dependent testing is acetylcholine. In normal coronary arteries, acetylcholine releases nitric oxide (NO) from endothelium, overriding its direct effects at the vascular smooth muscle muscarinic receptor to induce vascular smooth muscle contraction, resulting in vasodilation. In arteries with dysfunctional endothelium, insufficient biologically active NO is released in response to acetylcholine, the drug's direct effect to activate vascular smooth muscle predominates, and vasoconstriction occurs (option D). Adenosine is the most commonly used endothelium-independent pharmacological agent. Activation of adenosine A_{2A} receptors on vascular smooth muscle results in reproducible smooth muscle relaxation (option A). Regadenoson is a selective A_{2A} adenosine receptor agonist also used in pharmacologic stress testing because of reduced side effects (eg, less bradycardia and less bronchoconstriction) (option B). Adenosine receptors are also present in endothelium. As much as 25% of the hyperemic response obtained with intravenous adenosine infusion is the result of endothelial-dependent vasodilation (option E) because it can be blocked by infusion of NG-nitro-L-arginine methyl ester (L-NAME), an inhibitor of NO synthase.[4] Invasive measurement of coronary blood flow and CFR is predominantly performed using an intracoronary Doppler flow wire.[5] The wire directly measures coronary blood flow velocity and can be combined with a pressure sensor (option C).

35-4. **The answer is C.** (*Hurst's The Heart, 14th Edition, Chap. 35*) CAV is a process whereby the allograft coronary arteries become diffusely and circumferentially narrowed with progressive luminal loss. CAV has few therapeutic options, with repeat transplantation being the only definitive treatment (option A). Statins (option B), calcium antagonists (option D), and angiotensin-converting enzyme inhibitors (option E) have all demonstrated some effect at reducing CAV.[6] Some immunomodulating drugs may be more effective than others at slowing progression. Percutaneous coronary intervention is an option for focal stenoses in patients with advanced disease and compromised ventricular function but is not feasible for diffuse narrowing (option C). Antiplatelet agents may be given to reduce the risk of myocardial infarction, although the evidence supporting this is limited.

35-5. **The answer is E.** (*Hurst's The Heart, 14th Edition, Chap. 35*) The coronary arteries can be affected by systemic inflammatory conditions. Kawasaki disease is a childhood vasculitis that can manifest with coronary abnormalities. Widespread inflammation of medium-sized arteries results in coronary artery aneurysms (option A) in approximately 25% to 30% of patients who are not treated early. The mainstays of treatment are intravenous immune globulin and aspirin. The pathological cause of Takayasu's arteritis is not precisely known, but it is widely thought to result from an autoimmune process mediated by T cells and to affect the vasa vasorum of large vessels with leukocyte infiltration (option B). The ANCA-associated diseases most commonly affect the kidneys, lungs, eyes, nerves, and skin, and cardiac involvement may not be considered part of the typical presentation. However, up to half of patients may have cardiac abnormalities, and cardiac MRI often demonstrates myocardial scarring (option C).[7,8] Giant cell arteritis is a vasculitis predominantly of older patients. Infiltration of the intima with giant cells can result in granuloma formation and thickening of the internal elastic lamina. In rare cases, GCA may present initially with coronary manifestations (option D).

35-6. The answer is C. *(Hurst's The Heart, 14th Edition, Chap. 35)* Occasionally, coronary artery segments of varying lengths may travel within the myocardium and reappear on the epicardium more distally in the arterial course. This is sometimes referred to as a *tunneled artery*, but the clinical phenomenon is most often referred to as the description of the overlying muscle, a *myocardial bridge*. On pathological specimens, the coronary artery is surrounded, not by epicardial fat, but by myocardium (option A). The degree of bridging and compression of the vessel lumen is variable, possibly relating to the varying depth of the tunneled segment within myocardium, with thicker myocardial bridges being potentially more symptomatic (Figure 35-2) (option C). Conceptually, the compression of a tunneled artery should be limited mostly to myocardial systole because coronary blood flow occurs predominantly during diastole. However, many bridges also restrict expansion of the coronary artery in diastole (option B). Additionally, augmentation of coronary blood flow required to meet increasing demands, such as exercise, is often accompanied by an increase in flow during systole because diastole is progressively limited by the increase in heart rate (option D). Thus ischemia, myocardial infarction, arrhythmias, and sudden death have all been attributed to myocardial bridging (option E).

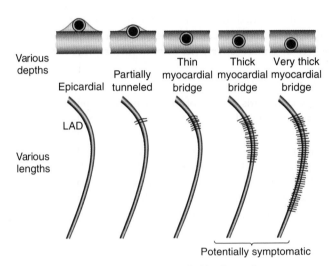

FIGURE 35-2 Diagram of myocardial bridging showing morphologic variations in tunneling (length of tunneled segment, depth of tunneled segment). (Reproduced with permission from Pepine CJ. *Acute Myocardial Infarction.* Philadelphia: FA Davis; 1989.)

35-7. The answer is A. *(Hurst's The Heart, 14th Edition, Chap. 35)* An abnormal communication between an epicardial coronary artery and a cardiac chamber, major vessel (vena cava, subpulmonary veins, pulmonary artery), or other vascular structure (mediastinal vessels, coronary sinus) is known as a coronary artery fistula. Fistulas that connect the left circulation to left-sided chambers may not result in clinical disease and may be incidentally found on angiography. Fistulas between the left and right circulation result in a shunt of blood flow, which may be clinically relevant, depending on the volume of flow. Fistulas predispose to endocarditis and may present with continuous murmur, myocardial ischemia/angina, acute myocardial infarction, sudden death, coronary steal, congestive heart failure, arrhythmias, or coronary aneurysm formation.[9] If patients present with heart failure or ischemia symptoms, the traditional evaluation often includes coronary angiography, which is the most reliable method of detecting coronary fistulas. Patients with incidentally found, asymptomatic, left-to-left fistulas can be managed conservatively (eg, with beta-blockers) and will often remain stable and symptom-free for long periods of time. Interventional occlusion or surgical repair (option A) is indicated for patients with symptoms attributable to the fistula or heart failure/cardiac remodeling caused by shunting of blood.

35-8. The answer is B. *(Hurst's The Heart, 14th Edition, Chap. 35)* An aneurysm of the coronary artery is a pathological dilation of the entire vessel wall: intima, media, and adventitia (option B). "Giant" aneurysms are often defined as those with diameters more than four times the normal diameter (option D), but dilations of 20, 30, and 40 mm are not uncommon. Aneurysms are present in about 1% of people at autopsy; the most common (up to 50% of cases) etiology is dilation secondary to vessel damage from atherosclerosis (option A). The malformation can be congenital or acquired secondary to atherosclerosis, trauma (external or iatrogenic), or inflammatory illnesses. Aneurysms are typically asymptomatic (option C) and are sometimes incidentally found on CT, angiography or, rarely, on echocardiography.

35-9. **The answer is E.** *(Hurst's The Heart, 14th Edition, Chap. 35)* Dissection refers to the separation of arterial wall layers and can occur spontaneously or as a secondary event (option C). Depending on the nature and severity of the dissection, the false lumen can compress or occlude the true lumen, resulting in ischemia, infarction, or death. Spontaneous or primary dissections are less common than secondary and are most commonly reported in young women, often associated with pregnancy (option B). Vessels can dissect in antegrade (toward the distal vessel) or retrograde (toward the vessel origin) patterns. The signs and symptoms of dissection are similar to ACS resulting from atherosclerotic disease: chest pain, ischemic ECG changes (option D), and elevated cardiac biomarkers. Antegrade dissections are often treated with stenting to prevent further propagation of the dissection and ischemic complications. Because of the direction of blood flow, retrograde dissections can often be treated conservatively (ie, without further intervention) (option E).

35-10. **The answer is E.** *(Hurst's The Heart, 14th Edition, Chap. 35)* The syndrome of coronary spasm includes symptoms typical of angina pectoris, but occurring at rest (option A) and typically associated with transient elevation of the ST segments. The clinical findings (symptoms and ECG changes) associated with coronary spasm may occur without ST-segment elevation, and in fact they are often associated with ST-segment depression and/or T-wave changes (option B) and may also at times result from small-vessel or regional coronary dysfunction. Minor elevations of serum C-reactive protein (option C) suggest chronic low-grade inflammation may be involved in the pathogenesis of coronary spasm.[10] Finally, coronary spasm is more common in younger patients and women (option D) than angina pectoris occurring because of obstructive atherosclerosis. So all of the above are correct (option E).

References

1. Likoff W, Segal BL, Kasparian H. Paradox of normal selective coronary arteriograms in patients considered to have unmistakable coronary heart disease. *N Engl J Med.* 1967;276(19):1063-1066.
2. Pepine CJ. Multiple causes for ischemia without obstructive coronary artery disease: not a short list. *Circulation.* 2015;131(12):1044-1046.
3. Sedlak TL, Lee M, Izadnegahdar M, Merz CN, Gao M, Humphries KH. Sex differences in clinical outcomes in patients with stable angina and no obstructive coronary artery disease. *Am Heart J.* 2013;166(1):38-44.
4. Buus NH, Bottcher M, Hermansen F, Sander M, Nielsen TT, Mulvany MJ. Influence of nitric oxide synthase and adrenergic inhibition on adenosine-induced myocardial hyperemia. *Circulation.* 2001;104(19):2305-2310.
5. Pries AR, Habazettl H, Ambrosio G, et al. A review of methods for assessment of coronary microvascular disease in both clinical and experimental settings. *Cardiovasc Res.* 2008;80(2):165-174.
6. Vecchiati A, Tellatin S, Angelini A, Iliceto S, Tona F. Coronary microvasculopathy in heart transplantation: consequences and therapeutic implications. *World J Transplant.* 2014;4(2):93-101.
7. Mavrogeni S, Karabela G, Gialafos E, et al. Cardiac involvement in ANCA (+) and ANCA (−) Churg–Strauss syndrome evaluated by cardiovascular magnetic resonance. *Inflamm Allergy Drug Targets.* 2013;12(5):322-327.
8. Hazebroek MR, Kemna MJ, Schalla S, et al. Prevalence and prognostic relevance of cardiac involvement in ANCA-associated vasculitis: eosinophilic granulomatosis with polyangiitis and granulomatosis with polyangiitis. *Int J Cardiol.* 2015;199:170-179.
9. Mangukia CV. Coronary artery fistula. *Ann Thorac Surg.* 2012;93(6):2084-2092.
10. Hung MJ, Cherng WJ, Cheng CW, Li LF. Comparison of serum levels of inflammatory markers in patients with coronary vasospasm without significant fixed coronary artery disease versus patients with stable angina pectoris and acute coronary syndromes with significant fixed coronary artery disease. *Am J Cardiol.* 2006;97(10):1429-1434.

CHAPTER 36

Definitions of Acute Coronary Syndromes

Mark J. Eisenberg

QUESTIONS

DIRECTIONS: Choose the one best response to each question.

36-1. Coronary artery disease (CAD) accounts for what proportion of all global deaths?

A. 20%
B. 30%
C. 40%
D. 50%
E. 60%

36-2. In 2011, the costs associated with myocardial infarction (MI) and coronary heart disease (CHD) in the United States were $11 billion and $10 billion, respectively. These costs are projected to do what by 2030?

A. Decrease by 100%
B. Decrease by 50%
C. Stay approximately the same
D. Increase by 50%
E. Increase by 100%

36-3. Which of the following concerning acute coronary syndrome (ACS) is *false*?

A. ACS is usually, but not always, caused by atherosclerotic plaque rupture, fissuring, erosion, or a combination with superimposed intracoronary thrombosis
B. ACS encompasses unstable angina (UA), ST-segment elevation MI (STEMI), and acute non–ST-segment elevation MI (NSTEMI)
C. ACS without myocardial necrosis is defined as UA
D. Myocardial necrosis is a necessary, but not sufficient, component of either STEMI or NSTEMI
E. Classification of ACS as STEMI, NSTEMI, or UA is determined within the initial hours of presentation

36-4. Initial triage of patients suspected of having acute coronary ischemia should include consideration which of the following possible alternative conditions?

A. Myocarditis/myopericarditis
B. Pulmonary embolism
C. Gastroesophageal reflux
D. Sepsis
E. Any of the above

36-5. Which of the following concerning UA is *false*?

A. UA is usually secondary to abrupt reduction in myocardial perfusion as a result of nonocclusive coronary thrombosis
B. UA and NSTEMI have distinct clinical presentations and pathogenesis
C. The incidence of UA has decreased over the last several decades
D. The diagnosis of UA relies primarily on clinical history
E. Patients with UA may present with either rest or minimal exertion angina lasting at least 20 minutes, new-onset severe angina, or crescendo angina

36-6. The risk of all-cause mortality, new or recurrent MI, or severe recurrent ischemia requiring urgent revascularization within 14 days in individuals with the highest Thrombolysis in Myocardial Infarction (TIMI) risk scores is:

A. 25%
B. 40%
C. 55%
D. 70%
E. 85%

36-7. Historically, myoglobin, creatine kinase, and the cardiac-specific CK-MB isoform have served as serum biomarkers indicating myocardial injury or necrosis. What is the most significant limitation of these biomarkers for the diagnostic evaluation of patients with presumed cardiac chest pain?

A. Cost of the test
B. Delay in release into the peripheral blood after onset of injury
C. Lack of cardiac specificity
D. Difficulty of use
E. Instability in vitro

36-8. Which of the following concerning biomarkers of cardiac injury is *false*?

A. Both troponin I and troponin T are only found in cardiac tissue
B. Troponin elevation occurs only in the context of ACS
C. Cardiac troponins demonstrate a graded, dose-dependent association with increasing cardiovascular risk
D. Changes in cardiac troponins confer an independent and stronger impact on subsequent risk than clinical symptoms or ECG signs
E. American College of Cardiology/American Heart Association guidelines recommend against the routine measurement of CK-MB for the diagnosis of MI

36-9. Which of the following is *not* one of the criteria that must be present in the proper clinical setting leading to evidence of myocardial necrosis, according to the World Heart Federation's Universal Definition of Myocardial Infarction?

A. Detection of the rise or fall of troponin or CK-MB with at least one value above the 99th percentile of the upper reference limit (URL), in addition to evidence of myocardial ischemia by one of the following: (1) Symptoms of ischemia; (2) ECG changes indicative of new ischemia (new ST/T-wave changes or new left bundle branch block [LBBB]); (3) Development of new pathologic Q waves on ECG; (4) Imaging evidence of new loss of viable myocardium or new regional wall motion abnormality

B. Sudden or unexpected cardiac death, involving cardiac arrest, often preceded by symptoms of coronary ischemia and accompanied by new ST-segment elevation or new LBBB, with or without evidence of fresh intracoronary thrombus or an expected rise in serum biomarkers

C. For patients with normal baseline biomarker levels undergoing PCI, a periprocedural increase of cardiac biomarkers above the 99th percentile URL is deemed abnormal. An increase of a biomarker greater than five times the 99th percentile URL is defined as a PCI-related MI

D. For patients undergoing coronary artery bypass graft (CABG) with normal baseline biomarker levels, increases greater than five times the 99th percentile URL accompanied by either new pathologic Q waves or new LBBB, angiographically documented graft or native artery occlusion, or new imaging evidence of loss of viable myocardium are labeled as CABG-related MIs

E. Pathologic evidence of MI

36-10. The global task force that introduced the Universal Definition of Myocardial Infarction also added a clinical classification of MI encompassing most of the common etiologies leading to myocardial necrosis. A patient with a history of recent MI who presents with ST-segment elevation and positive troponin is found to have an occlusive stent thrombosis upon emergent angiography. This would be classified as what type of MI?

A. Type 1
B. Type 2
C. Type 4a
D. Type 4b
E. Type 5

ANSWERS

36-1. The answer is B. *(Hurst's The Heart, 14th Edition, Chap. 36)* Coronary artery disease accounts for 30% of all global deaths, representing the single most common cause of adult mortality and equivalent to the combined number of deaths caused by nutritional deficiencies, infectious diseases, and maternal/perinatal complications.[1,2] Recent growth in the global burden of cardiovascular disease (CVD) is primarily attributable to the rising incidence across low- and middle-income countries.[3] Among European member states of the World Health Organization (WHO), for example, CVD death rates for men and women were highest in the Russian Federation and Uzbekistan, respectively, whereas risk was lowest in France and Israel.[4] Conversely, in the United States, over 15 million Americans, or 6.2% of the adult population, have CHD, with an MI occurring once every 43 seconds.[5]

36-2. The answer is E. *(Hurst's The Heart, 14th Edition, Chap. 36)* Health care resource utilization for CHD is significant; over 1.1 million hospital discharges in 2010 listed MI or UA as a primary or secondary diagnosis.[5] Health care expenditures are also substantial; costs for MI and CHD were approximately $11 billion and $10 billion, respectively, in 2011.[6] These diagnoses constitute two of the most expensive discharge diagnoses and are expected to increase by 100% by 2030. Despite these sobering statistics, important strides in the diagnosis, prevention, and management of CHD have occurred over the past 50 years. In the United States, for example, several population-based studies have shown a reduction in both the incidence and the case fatality rate associated with MI.[7,8] These favorable trends have been attributed to greater utilization of evidence-based therapies and improvements in the control and burden of risk factors.[9] Concordant changes in the epidemiology of ACS have occurred over the past 10 years as a result of changing demographics and updated definitions of MI.

36-3. The answer is E. *(Hurst's The Heart, 14th Edition, Chap. 36)* The term *acute coronary syndrome (ACS)* is a unifying construct representing a pathophysiologic and clinical spectrum culminating in acute myocardial ischemia. This is usually, but not always, caused by atherosclerotic plaque rupture, fissuring, erosion, or a combination with superimposed intracoronary thrombosis and is associated with an increased risk of myonecrosis and cardiac death (option A).[10] ACS encompasses UA and ST-segment elevation MI (STEMI) or acute non–ST-segment elevation MI (NSTEMI) (option B). Distinguishing these presentations is predicated on the presence or absence of myocyte necrosis coupled with the electrocardiographic tracing at the time of symptoms. ACS without myocardial necrosis is defined as UA (option C), whereas myocardial necrosis is a necessary, but not sufficient, component of either STEMI or NSTEMI (option D). The diagnosis of ACS relies on integrating clinical information from the patient history with the initial ECG and laboratory results. In the initial hours after presentation, distinguishing between STEMI, NSTEMI, and UA may be difficult because biomarkers of myonecrosis can initially be normal (option E). However, as a result of the life-threatening nature of ACS, it is prudent to have a low threshold in suspecting this diagnosis, and therefore, diagnostic sensitivity is usually favored over specificity.

36-4. The answer is E. *(Hurst's The Heart, 14th Edition, Chap. 36)* Initial triage of patients suspected of having acute coronary ischemia should identify patients as having (1) ACS; (2) a non-ACS cardiovascular condition such as myocarditis/myopericarditis (option A), stress-related cardiomyopathy, aortic dissection, or pulmonary embolism (option B); (3) a noncardiac cause of chest pain such as gastroesophageal reflux (option C); or (4) a noncardiac condition that is yet undefined, such as sepsis (option D).[11] ACS patients with new ST-segment elevation on the presenting electrocardiogram (ECG) are labeled as having STEMI and should be considered for immediate reperfusion therapy by thrombolytics or percutaneous coronary intervention; those without ST-segment elevation but with evidence of myonecrosis are deemed to have an NSTEMI; and those without any evidence of myonecrosis are diagnosed with UA.

36-5. **The answer is B.** *(Hurst's The Heart, 14th Edition, Chap. 36)* UA is usually secondary to abrupt reduction in myocardial perfusion as a result of nonocclusive coronary thrombosis (option A). In this event, however, the nonocclusive thrombus that developed on a disrupted atherosclerotic plaque does not result in biochemical evidence of myocardial necrosis. Accordingly, UA and NSTEMI can be viewed as very closely related clinical conditions with similar presentations and pathogenesis but variable clinical severity (option B). Nevertheless, given the increased reliance on highly sensitive biomarkers of myocyte necrosis, the incidence of troponin-negative ACS or UA is decreasing (option C).[12] This shift in ACS epidemiology was illustrated in a report from the US Nationwide Inpatient Sample, which demonstrated an 87% decline in the prevalence of UA between 1998 and 2001 but an increase in NSTEMI.[13] As a result of the lack of objective criteria used to define this condition, UA must be diagnosed from the clinical history (option D) and is thus the most subjective of the ACS diagnoses. There are three principal clinical presentations of UA (option E): (1) rest angina or angina with minimal exertion usually lasting at least 20 minutes; (2) new-onset severe angina (Canadian Cardiovascular Society grade III or higher); and (3) crescendo angina, defined as previously diagnosed angina that has become distinctly more frequent, precipitated by less severe degrees of exertion, or more severe.[14,15] Despite a clear and consistent definition for UA, the subjective nature of these criteria may compromise diagnostic accuracy, thereby leading to misclassification. In one report, for example, 20% of patients diagnosed with UA and referred for coronary angiography did not have any angiographically apparent obstructive epicardial CAD.[16]

36-6. **The answer is B.** *(Hurst's The Heart, 14th Edition, Chap. 36)* Once CAD has been established as the likely cause of chest pain, it is necessary to estimate, or stratify, risk for adverse events using qualitative or quantitative methods. The tempo and severity of chest pain, the extent of electrical abnormality, and the magnitude of serum biomarker elevation all portend a higher risk for adverse events. Among these, biomarker evidence of myocyte necrosis is the strongest and most consistent correlate of risk. Quantitative risk scores provide an alternative and more precise approach to risk stratification. Perhaps the most widely used is the integer-based TIMI risk score, which allots a single point for each of the following in patients with chest pain: age > 65 years; aspirin use within 7 days prior to presentation; ST deviation > 0.5 mm; severe angina; at least three risk factors for CAD; raised cardiac biomarker; and known coronary stenosis.[17] The short-term risk of all-cause mortality, new or recurrent MI, or severe recurrent ischemia requiring urgent revascularization within 14 days varied from 1.4% for patients with very low scores (0–1) to 40% for those with the highest scores (option B).

36-7. **The answer is C.** *(Hurst's The Heart, 14th Edition, Chap. 36)* Serum biomarkers indicating myocardial injury or necrosis are critical elements in the diagnostic evaluation of a patient with presumed cardiac chest pain and are essential to distinguishing between UA and overt infarction. Ideally, such biomarkers would be specific to cardiac muscle, would be absent from nonmyocardial tissue, would be released quickly into the peripheral blood after onset of injury, and would reflect the magnitude of necrosis. Moreover, the marker should be easy to use, quick and inexpensive to measure, and stable in vitro. Historically, myoglobin, creatine kinase, and the cardiac-specific CK-MB isoform have served this purpose in the diagnosis of MI. The main limitation of these markers is the lack of cardiac specificity (option C) because each may also be variably released from skeletal muscle and other tissues, such as the tongue, small intestine, uterus, and prostate. As a result, earlier definitions of MI did not require the presence of these cardiac biomarkers for diagnosis but rather considered their elevation along with clinical symptoms and electrical signs of myocardial ischemia.[18]

36-8. **The answer is B.** *(Hurst's The Heart, 14th Edition, Chap. 36)* Troponin I (TnI) and troponin T (TnT) are found only in myocardial tissue (option A), therefore elevated levels of either marker reflect myocyte injury. The advantages to cardiac troponin (cTn) testing (TnI or TnT) notwithstanding, as with any diagnostic test, gains in sensitivity occur at the expense of specificity. Several studies have shown that troponin elevations may occur in non–acute coronary syndrome clinical settings (option B), such as heart failure, renal dysfunction, and pulmonary embolism. Troponin may even be detected in apparently healthy community-dwelling adults, as shown in the Dallas Heart Study.[19] In that report, investigators found the following clinical conditions independently associated with detectable levels of cardiac troponin: left ventricular hypertrophy, diabetes mellitus, chronic kidney disease, and heart failure. As a result, the diagnosis of type 1 MI requires not only the presence of elevated cardiac troponin, but also a clinical context supporting an ischemic etiology. From a prognostic perspective, cTns demonstrate a graded, dose-dependent association with increasing cardiovascular risk (option C). Antman et al[20] illustrated this relationship in a post hoc analysis of a randomized trial evaluating various pharmacologic approaches in patients with ACS, demonstrating that unadjusted mortality rates at 42 days increased from 1.0% to 7.5% among those with the lowest versus highest levels of cTn. In addition, changes in cTn confer an independent and stronger impact on subsequent risk than clinical symptoms, ECG signs, or other biomarkers (option D).[21] Given these benefits of assessing and formulating clinical decisions based on detecting cTn, the Universal Definition of MI considers this biomarker preferentially over CK-MB. In addition, American College of Cardiology/American Heart Association guidelines no longer consider the routine measurement of CK-MB as necessary for the diagnosis of MI, and they provide a class III recommendation against routine use of this test (option E).[11]

36-9. **The answer is B.** (*Hurst's The Heart, 14th Edition, Chap. 36*) In 2007, the World Heart Federation, in concert with major European and American cardiovascular societies, convened a global task force to introduce the Universal Definition of MI. The result was a clinicopathologic classification of MI that considers five different MI types, each representing a distinct clinical and pathologic entity culminating in myocyte necrosis. The Universal Definition has been updated twice, with the most recent iteration published in 2012.[22] The new accepted universal criteria for diagnosing an acute MI state that one of five criteria must be present in the proper clinical setting leading to evidence of myocardial necrosis. Options A, B, D, and E are four of these criteria. Option C is incorrect; for a diagnosis of MI to be made in the event of sudden or unexpected cardiac death, involving cardiac arrest, often preceded by symptoms of coronary ischemia and accompanied by new ST-segment elevation or new LBBB, evidence of fresh intracoronary thrombus must be detected by angiography or autopsy when death occurred before blood was obtained or an expected rise in serum biomarkers could occur.

36-10. **The answer is D.** (*Hurst's The Heart, 14th Edition, Chap. 36*) In addition to revising the criteria for MI diagnosis, the global task force added a clinical classification of MI encompassing most of the common etiologies leading to myocardial necrosis. Each etiology of MI differs with respect to short- and long-term mortality rates. Type 1 MI (option A) occurs as a result of a primary coronary event such as plaque erosion and/or rupture, fissuring, or dissection. Type 2 MI (option B) occurs secondary to ischemia from either increased oxygen demand or decreased supply, for example, coronary artery spasm, embolism, anemia, arrhythmias, hypertension, or hypotension. Type 3 MI occurs in the setting of sudden cardiac death, including cardiac arrest, that may be preceded by ischemic symptoms, accompanied by new ST-segment elevation, new LBBB, or evidence of fresh thrombus by coronary arteriography or autopsy. Death could occur before blood samples are obtained or before cardiac biomarkers appear in the blood. Type 4 MI is associated with PCI and is further classified as Type 4a or 4b. Type 4a MI (option C) is associated with PCI. Type 4b MI (option D) is associated with stent thrombosis as documented by angiography or at autopsy. Type 5 MI (option E) is associated with CABG.

References

1. Bansilal S, Castellano JM, Fuster V. Global burden of CVD: focus on secondary prevention of cardiovascular disease. *Int J Cardiol*. 2015;201(Suppl 1):S1-S7.

2. Lopez AD, Mathers CD, Ezzati M, Jamison DT, Murray CJ, eds. *Global Burden of Disease and Risk Factors*. New York: Oxford University Press and The World Bank; 2006.

3. World Health Organization, United Nations Programme on HIV/AIDS. *Prevention of Cardiovascular Disease.* Geneva, Switzerland: World Health Organization; 2007.

4. Nichols M, Townsend N, Scarborough P, Rayner M. Cardiovascular disease in Europe: epidemiological update. *Eur Heart J.* 2013;34:3028-3034.

5. Mozaffarian D, Benjamin EJ, Go AS, et al. Heart disease and stroke statistics–2015 update: a report from the American Heart Association. *Circulation.* 2015;131:e29-322.

6. Pfuntner A, Weir L, Steiner C. *Costs for Hospital Stays in the United States, 2011.* HCUP Statistical Brief #168. Rockville, MD: US Agency for Healthcare Research and Quality; 2013.

7. Rogers WJ, Frederick PD, Stoehr E, et al. Trends in presenting characteristics and hospital mortality among patients with ST elevation and non-ST elevation myocardial infarction in the National Registry of Myocardial Infarction from 1990 to 2006. *Am Heart J.* 2008;156:1026-1034.

8. Yeh RW, Sidney S, Chandra M, Sorel M, Selby JV, Go AS. Population trends in the incidence and outcomes of acute myocardial infarction. *N Engl J Med.* 2010;362:2155-2165.

9. Ford ES, Ajani UA, Croft JB, et al. Explaining the decrease in U.S. deaths from coronary disease, 1980-2000. *N Engl J Med.* 2007;356:2388-2398.

10. Fuster V, Moreno PR, Fayad ZA, Corti R, Badimon JJ. Atherothrombosis and high-risk plaque: part I: evolving concepts. *J Am Coll Cardiol.* 2005;46:937-954.

11. Amsterdam EA, Wenger NK, Brindis RG, et al. 2014 AHA/ACC guideline for the management of patients with non-ST-elevation acute coronary syndromes: a report of the American College of Cardiology/American Heart Association Task Force on Practice Guidelines. *J Am Coll Cardiol.* 2014;64:e139-228.

12. Braunwald E, Morrow DA. Unstable angina: is it time for a requiem? *Circulation.* 2013;127:2452-2457.

13. Bertoni AG, Bonds DE, Thom T, Chen GJ, Goff DC Jr. Acute coronary syndrome national statistics: challenges in definitions. *Am Heart J.* 2005;149:1055-1061.

14. Braunwald E. Unstable angina. A classification. *Circulation.* 1989;80:410-414.

15. Campeau L. Letter: grading of angina pectoris. *Circulation.* 1976;54:522-523.

16. Goldberg A, Yalonetsky S, Kopeliovich M, Azzam Z, Markiewicz W. Appropriateness of diagnosis of unstable angina pectoris in patients referred for coronary arteriography. *Exp Clin Cardiol.* 2008;13:133-137.

17. Antman EM, Cohen M, Bernink PJ, et al. The TIMI risk score for unstable angina/non-ST elevation MI: a method for prognostication and therapeutic decision making. *JAMA.* 2000;284:835-842.

18. World Health Organization: Working Group on the Establishment of Ischemic Heart Disease Registers: Report of the Fifth Working Group, Copenhagen. In Report No. Eur 8201 (5). Geneva, Switzerland: World Health Organization; 1971.

19. Wallace TW, Abdullah SM, Drazner MH, et al. Prevalence and determinants of troponin T elevation in the general population. *Circulation.* 2006;113:1958-1965.

20. Antman EM, Tanasijevic MJ, Thompson B, et al. Cardiac-specific troponin I levels to predict the risk of mortality in patients with acute coronary syndromes. *N Engl J Med.* 1996;335:1342-1349.

21. Apple FS, Smith SW, Pearce LA, Murakami MM. Delta changes for optimizing clinical specificity and 60-day risk of adverse events in patients presenting with symptoms suggestive of acute coronary syndrome utilizing the ADVIA Centaur TnI-Ultra assay. *Clin Biochem.* 2012;45:711-713.

22. Thygesen K, Alpert JS, Jaffe AS, et al. Third universal definition of myocardial infarction. *Eur Heart J.* 2012;33:2551-2567.

CHAPTER 37

Pathology of Myocardial Infarction and Sudden Death

Patrick R. Lawler

DIRECTIONS: Choose the one best response to each question.

37-1. Which of the following statements about myocardial energy metabolism is *correct*?

A. Under normal aerobic conditions, most cardiac energy is derived from glycolysis

B. Decreased adenosine triphosphate (ATP) production due to ischemia results in decreased cytosolic Na$^+$ and cell swelling

C. Myocardial ischemia primarily affects mitochondrial metabolism and oxidative phosphorylation

D. Reversibly injured myocytes are characterized by cell membrane breaks and amorphous densities in the mitochondria

E. Only one-third of the ATP used by the heart goes to contractile shortening

37-2. A 63-year-old man presents to the emergency department with onset of chest pain while washing his car. He has a history of angina and MI due to culprit LAD disease. Which of the following could be a contributor to smaller infarct size?

A. The absence of coronary collateral vessels

B. The extended duration of coronary occlusion

C. The earlier occlusion of the same coronary artery

D. Ventricular remodeling

E. None of the above

37-3. A 67-year-old man has an acute myocardial infarction (MI) with occlusion of the LAD. He receives thrombolysis and coronary artery revascularization by PCI, but in the following months, he develops left ventricular systolic dysfunction. Which of the following is *not correct* about the mechanisms of reperfusion injury?

A. Reperfusion-mediated infiltration of neutrophils into the ischemic region causes inflammation

B. Reperfusion results in decreased intracellular Ca^{2+}, ATP depletion, and cell death

C. Rapid restoration of physiologic pH contributes to reperfusion injury

D. Reperfusion generates oxidative stress that extends the myocardial injury

E. Decreased nitric oxide allows for neutrophil accumulation and reduced coronary blood flow during reperfusion

37-4. Which of the following is *not* a feature of myocardial hibernation?

A. Decreased calcium responsiveness

B. Upregulation of nitric oxide synthase, COX-2, and heat shock protein

C. Decreased number of sarcomeres

D. Upregulation of myosin, titin, and actinin

E. Chronic ischemia with contractile dysfunction

37-5. A 45-year-old woman is recovering in the hospital from a myocardial infarct with ST-segment elevation. Which of the following is *correct* about plaque morphology?

A. The majority of thrombi leading to acute MI are caused by plaque erosion

B. Plaque erosions are more common in men than in women

C. Most plaques occur in the proximal portion of the coronary arteries

D. Most thrombi in plaque rupture are organizing (> 1 day)

E. All of the above are correct

37-6. Which of the following depicts the *correct* pathologic progression of nonreperfused myocardial infarcts?

A. Wavy fibers, neutrophil infiltration, coagulation necrosis, fibroblast activity

B. Fibroblast activity, granulation tissue, neutrophil infiltration, coagulation necrosis

C. Wavy fibers, coagulation necrosis, hypereosinophilic myocyte, neutrophil infiltration

D. Fibroblast activity, wavy fibers, neutrophil infiltration, coagulation necrosis

E. None of the above

37-7. A 59-year-old man presents with chest pain that precipitated while he was mowing the lawn. He did not seek medical attention until 4 hours after the onset of symptoms. Which of the following is *correct* about reperfusion following acute MI?

A. Myocardium is not salvageable 4 hours after the onset of chest pain

B. In perfused infarcts, neutrophils are concentrated at the margins

C. The rate of healing by fibroblasts is greater in nonreperfused infarcts

D. Reperfused infarcts have areas of necrosis at the center mixed with noninfarcted myocardium

E. Reperfusion within 6 hours of the onset of chest pain is likely to result in significant myocardial salvage

37-8. Which of the following is *incorrect* about myocardial remodeling following MI?

A. Myocardial infarction induces a systemic inflammatory response

B. Transition to M2 macrophages causes expansion of the infarcted area

C. M1 macrophages set up the proinflammatory environment following an infarct

D. Prolonged M1 macrophage activation results in expansion of the injured ventricular wall

E. All of the above are incorrect

37-9. A 64-year-old woman developed an aneurysm following an MI caused by occlusion of the LAD. Which of the following is *correct* about aneurysms?

A. Patients receiving reperfusion therapy have a higher incidence of aneurysms

B. Female gender is an independent determinant of aneurysm formation after infarction

C. The wall of a true aneurysm consists of fibrous pericardium

D. Subendocardial infarcts are the most likely to result in true aneurysms

E. All of the above are correct

37-10. Which of the following is *not correct* regarding complications of MI?

A. Right ventricular wall rupture is much more common than left ventricle rupture

B. Anticoagulation should be discontinued or used with caution in the presence of significant (≥ 1 cm) pericardial effusion after MI

C. Cardiogenic shock is caused by decreased systemic cardiac output with adequate intravascular volume

D. Ventricular arrhythmias are associated with decreased survival post-MI

E. Right ventricular cardiogenic shock is associated with younger age

37-1. The answer is C. (*Hurst's The Heart, 14th Edition, Chap. 37*) The normal function of the heart muscle is supported by high rates of myocardial blood flow, oxygen consumption, and combustion of fat and carbohydrates (glucose and lactate). Under normal aerobic conditions, cardiac energy is derived from fatty acids, supplying 60% to 90% of the energy for ATP synthesis (option A). The rest (10% to 40%) comes from the oxidation of pyruvate formed from glycolysis and lactate oxidation. Almost all of the ATP formed comes from oxidative phosphorylation in the mitochondria; only a small amount of ATP (< 2%) is produced by glycolysis. Approximately two-thirds of the ATP used by the heart goes to contractile shortening (option E), and the remaining third is used by sarcoplasmic reticulum Ca^{2+} ATPase and other ion pumps. Myocardial ischemia primarily affects mitochondrial metabolism, resulting in a decrease in ATP formation by shutting off oxidative phosphorylation (option C). Decreased ATP inhibits Na^+/K^+-ATPase, increasing intracellular Na^+ and Cl, leading to cell swelling (option B). Reversibly injured myocytes are edematous and swollen from the osmotic overload. Irreversibly injured myocytes contain shrunken nuclei with marked chromatin margination. The two hallmarks of irreversible injury are cell membrane breaks and the mitochondrial presence of small osmiophilic amorphous densities (option D).

37-2. The answer is C. (*Hurst's The Heart, 14th Edition, Chap. 37*) Myocardial ischemia occurs when oxygen and nutrient supply do not meet myocardial demand, and necrosis or infarction occurs when ischemia is severe and prolonged. The extent of coronary collateral flow is one of the principal determinants of infarct size. Indeed, at autopsy, it is common to see chronic total coronary occlusion and an absence of MI in the distribution of that artery. The absence of myocardial ischemia following coronary artery occlusion is associated with the presence of well-developed collateral vessels (option A). Reimer and Jennings showed that if a canine coronary artery was occluded for 15 minutes, for 40 minutes, for 3 hours, or permanently for 4 days, myocardial necrosis progressed as a "wave front phenomenon."[1,2] The extent of myocardial necrosis therefore depended on the duration of coronary occlusion (option B). Other than the presence of collateral circulation, factors that influence infarct size include preconditioning (option C), which may greatly reduce infarct size, and reperfusion. Transmural infarcts may increase in size for weeks after the initial event, and the degree of this expansion is associated with a decrease in the survival rate. The processes involved in postinfarction ventricular dilatation are known as ventricular remodeling. In general, the transmural extent of necrosis is a major determinant of infarct expansion (remodeling) based on large infarct size and the persistence of the occlusion (option D).

37-3. The answer is B. (*Hurst's The Heart, 14th Edition, Chap. 37*) The process of restoring blood flow to ischemic myocardium has shown utility in limiting cell death in the presence of severe ischemia. Reperfusion, however, has paradoxical effects on myocardium that can result in adverse reactions, termed reperfusion injury. During reperfusion, the myocardium is subject to abrupt biochemical and metabolic changes governed by several mediators that interact with each other in complex ways. Reperfusion markedly enhances the infiltration of neutrophils into the ischemic region and amplifies the inflammatory response (option A). At the time of myocardial reperfusion, there is an abrupt increase in intracellular Ca^{2+} known as the calcium paradox (option B). This intracellular Ca^{2+} causes opening of the mitochondrial permeability transition pore (PTP), which uncouples oxidative phosphorylation, resulting in ATP depletion and cell death. In addition, studies have shown that reperfusion of ischemic myocardium generates reactive oxygen species (oxygen paradox). This oxidative stress results in the extension of the myocardial injury beyond that induced by ischemia alone (option D). A key mechanism involves the reduction of the bioavailability of the nitric oxide, which normally inhibits neutrophil accumulation, inactivates superoxide radicals, and improves coronary blood flow (option E). Further contributing to reperfusion injury is the rapid restoration of physiologic pH (option C) that occurs after washout of lactic acid and the activation of the sodium-hydrogen exchanger and the sodium-bicarbonate symporter. The final consequence of reperfusion injury is left ventricular (LV) systolic dysfunction leading to increased morbidity and mortality.

37-4. **The answer is D.** *(Hurst's The Heart, 14th Edition, Chap. 37)* In the early 1980s, Rahimtoola et al.[3] found significant improvement in left ventricular function after coronary revascularization in a subset of patients with depressed ventricular performance. They postulated that the mechanism of poor myocardial contractility was chronic ischemia (option E), which could be improved by revascularization. The premise behind this rationale was dependent on the surviving myocardium being in a functional, albeit depressed, state, suggesting that the myocardium may adapt to chronic ischemia by decreasing its contractility but preserving viability. Chronically hibernating myocardium demonstrates changes in adrenergic control and calcium responsiveness (option A). Substances that are upregulated in chronic hibernating myocardium include heat shock protein, hypoxia-inducible factor, inducible nitric oxide synthase, cyclooxygenase-2, and monocyte chemotactic protein (option B). Morphologically, hibernating myocytes show a loss of contractile elements, the sarcomeres (option C), with increased glycogen. There is a disorderly increase in cytoskeletal desmin, tubulin, and vinculin, with a decrease in contractile proteins myosin, titin, and actinin (option D).

37-5. **The answer is C.** *(Hurst's The Heart, 14th Edition, Chap. 37)* The vast majority of MIs occur in patients with coronary atherosclerosis, with > 90% associated with superimposed luminal thrombi. Arbustini et al.[4] found coronary thrombi in 98% of patients dying with clinically documented acute MI, and of those thrombi, 75% were caused by plaque rupture and 25% by plaque erosion (option A). There are gender differences in the causation of coronary thrombi leading to acute MI: Arbustini et al.[4] showed that 37% of thrombi in women were erosion compared with only 18% in men (option B). The thrombus age also varies; the majority of acute thrombi (< 1 day) have been observed in plaque rupture, whereas the majority of thrombi in plaque erosion are organizing (> 1 day)[5] (option D). The majority of thin cap fibroatheromas, acute and healed ruptures, and lesions with fibroatheromas occur predominantly in the proximal portion of the three major coronary arteries (option C), and about 50% arise in the midportion of these arteries.

37-6. **The answer is A.** *(Hurst's The Heart, 14th Edition, Chap. 37)* The earliest morphologic characteristic of MI that can be discerned and observed between 12 and 24 hours after the onset of chest pain is the hypereosinophilic myocyte. It has been suggested in experimentally induced infarction that the appearance of "wavy fibers" (1) may be the earliest change and is thought to be the result of stretching of the ischemic noncontractile fibers by the adjoining viable contracting myocytes. Neutrophil infiltration (2) is present by 24 hours at the border areas. As the infarct progresses between 24 and 48 hours, coagulation necrosis (3) is established with various degrees of nuclear pyknosis, early karyorrhexis, and karyolysis. At 3 to 5 days, the central portion of the infarct shows loss of myocyte nuclei and striations. The influx of inflammatory cells, including mast cells, induces a cascade of chemokines, which suppress further inflammation and result in scar tissue.[6] Macrophages and fibroblasts (4) begin to appear in the border areas. By 1 week, neutrophils decline, and granulation tissue is established with neocapillary invasion and lymphocytic and plasma cell infiltration. By the second week, fibroblasts are prominent, and there is continued removal of the necrotic myocytes as the fibroblasts are actively producing collagen and angiogenesis occurs in the area of healing. Option A is therefore correct.

37-7. **The answer is E.** *(Hurst's The Heart, 14th Edition, Chap. 37)* If reperfusion occurs within 4 to 6 hours after the onset of chest pain or electrocardiographic (ECG) changes, there is myocardial salvage (option A), and the infarct is likely to be subendocardial without transmural extension (option E). Within a few hours of reperfusion, neutrophils are evident within the area of necrosis, but they are usually sparse. In contrast to nonreperfused infarcts, neutrophils do not show concentration at the margins (option B). However, reperfused infarcts often demonstrate areas of necrosis at the periphery with interdigitation with noninfarcted myocardium (option D). Macrophages begin to appear by day 2 or 3, and stromal cells show enlarged nuclei and nucleoli by days 3 and 4. Neutrophil debris, which may be concentrated at the border areas in cases of incomplete reperfusion, is seen by

3 to 5 days. Fibroblasts appear by days 3 to 5, with an accelerated rate of healing compared with nonreperfused infarcts (option C).

37-8. The answer is B. (*Hurst's The Heart, 14th Edition, Chap. 37*) Myocardial remodeling is defined as changes in size, shape, and function of the heart occurring secondary to molecular, cellular, and interstitial events after MI. Left ventricular remodeling begins within the first few hours after an infarct and continues to progress, and the infarcted myocardium undergoes rapid turnover during the first 1 to 2 weeks after MI. MI generates a systemic inflammatory response (option A), with activation of the complement cascade, transforming growth factor-β, and chemokines and free radical generation. During the healing phase, infiltrating monocytes differentiate into macrophages, which, along with mast cells, accumulate in the healing scar, inducing fibroblast proliferation. Classically activated M1 macrophages are the first line of defense that influences the subsequent phase of the healing process by M2 macrophages. The prolonged presence of M1 macrophages extends the proinflammatory environment (option C) and causes expansion of the infarcted area (option B). A delayed transition to M2 macrophages thus hampers the formation of scar tissue, predisposing to heart failure development as a result of expansion of the injured ventricular wall (negative remodeling) (option D). Improved healing may be attained by modulating macrophage polarization toward the M2 phenotype, thus promoting the resolution of inflammation and improved infarct healing.

37-9. The answer is B. (*Hurst's The Heart, 14th Edition, Chap. 37*) Single-vessel disease, absence of previous angina, total LAD occlusion, and female gender (option B) are independent predictors of left ventricular aneurysm formation after anterior infarction. Patients receiving reperfusion therapy and exhibiting a patent infarct-related artery have a lower incidence of aneurysm formation (option A). A large acute transmural myocardial infarction that has undergone expansion is the most likely infarct to result in a true aneurysm (option D). Morphologically, the wall of a true aneurysm develops after MI, and it consists of fibrous tissue (option C) with or without interspersed myocytes. In contrast, the wall of a false aneurysm is formed by fibrous pericardium (not from the left ventricular MI and healing).

37-10. The answer is A. (*Hurst's The Heart, 14th Edition, Chap. 37*) The complications of MI may manifest immediately or they may appear late, and they depend on the location and extent of infarction. The acute complications consist of arrhythmias and sudden death, cardiogenic shock, infarct extension, fibrinous pericarditis, cardiac rupture, and mural thrombus and embolization. Ventricular arrhythmias are important markers of electrical instability and are associated with decreased survival in the acute post-MI phase. Left ventricular wall rupture is much more common than right ventricle rupture (option A). Although reperfusion therapy has reduced the incidence of cardiac rupture, late thrombolytic therapy may increase the risk of cardiac rupture. Heart failure after MI ranges from pulmonary congestion to profound organ hypoperfusion or cardiogenic shock. Cardiogenic shock is caused by decreased systemic cardiac output in the presence of adequate intravascular volume (option C). Right ventricular cardiogenic shock after acute infarction is associated with younger age, a lower prevalence of previous infarctions, fewer anterior infarct locations, and less multivessel disease (option E). Pericardial effusion after MI usually takes several months to reabsorb. Anticoagulation should be discontinued in the presence of a significant (≥ 1 cm) or enlarging pericardial effusion (option B).

References

1. Reimer KA, Jennings RB. The "wavefront phenomenon" of myocardial ischemic cell death. II. Transmural progression of necrosis within the framework of ischemic bed size (myocardium at risk) and collateral flow. *Lab Invest.* 1979;40:633-664.
2. Reimer KA, Jennings RB, Tatum AH. Pathobiology of acute myocardial ischemia: metabolic, functional and ultrastructural studies. *Am J Cardiol.* 1983;52:72A-81A.
3. Rahimtoola SH, Grunkemeier GL, Teply JF, et al. Changes in coronary bypass surgery leading to improved survival. *JAMA.* 1981;246:1912-1916.

4. Arbustini E, Dal Bello B, Morbini P, et al. Plaque erosion is a major substrate for coronary thrombosis in acute myocardial infarction. *Heart.* 1999;82:269-272.

5. Kramer MC, Rittersma SZ, de Winter RJ, et al. Relationship of thrombus healing to underlying plaque morphology in sudden coronary death. *J Am Coll Cardiol.* 2010;55:122-132.

6. Frangogiannis NG. Chemokines in the ischemic myocardium: from inflammation to fibrosis. *Inflamm Res.* 2004;53:585-595.

CHAPTER 38

Molecular and Cellular Mechanisms of Myocardial Ischemia/Reperfusion Injury

Ravi Karra

QUESTIONS

DIRECTIONS: Choose the one best response to each question.

38-1. Which of the following is *not* a determinant of infarct size?

A. Time to reperfusion
B. The presence of collaterals
C. Blood pressure
D. Temperature
E. Ischemia/reperfusion injury

38-2. Which of the following does *not* contribute to myocyte necrosis after reperfusion?

A. Sarcolemma disruption and calcium overload
B. ATP depletion and reversal of the Na^+/Ca^{2+} exchanger, resulting in increased intracellular calcium
C. The no-reflow phenomenon
D. Tissue edema
E. Autophagy

38-3. Which of the following is *true* about intracellular Ca^{2+} during ischemia-reperfusion injury?

A. The Na^+/Ca^{2+} exchanger extrudes Ca^{2+} from the cytoplasm
B. Calpains are activated by increases in Ca^{2+}
C. The RyR2 does not contribute to increased intracellular Ca^{2+}
D. Sarcolemma membranes remain intact
E. Calpains are only active at low pH

38-4. Which of the following is *correct* regarding mitochondrial function during reperfusion?

A. Mitochondrial calcium decreases
B. The mitochondrial permeability transition pore (MPTP) is open during acidosis
C. Cyclophilin D closes the MPTP
D. Restoration of DNA synthesis occurs immediately following reperfusion
E. Succinate levels increase during ischemia and scavenge reactive oxygen species (ROS) following reperfusion

38-5. Which of the following is *not true* regarding coronary circulation during reperfusion injury?

A. Interstitial edema occurs in part because of a dysfunctional endothelial barrier
B. Edema peaks at 120 minutes and again at 7 days
C. The release of vasodilators from the culprit lesion dilates the microvasculature
D. Cellular aggregates from the culprit lesion impair flow in the microcirculation
E. Hemorrhage of the microcirculation is associated with an adverse prognosis

38-6. Which of the following is *true* of ischemic preconditioning (IPC)?

A. Repeated episodes of ischemia increase reperfusion injury
B. Ischemic preconditioning results in a cardioprotective phase 7 days after preconditioning
C. Ischemic preconditioning results in the release of protective autacoids
D. Ischemic preconditioning is thought to increase calcium load
E. The presence of angina before an MI is associated with larger injuries following MI

38-7. Which of the following is *true* about ischemic postconditioning?

A. In preclinical models, intermittent reperfusion reduces infarct size
B. Ischemic postconditioning is unlikely to involve the same mechanisms as preconditioning
C. Early clinical studies demonstrate a benefit of ischemic postconditioning on improving outcomes following myocardial infarction in humans
D. Ischemic postconditioning increases myocardial edema
E. Ischemic postconditioning increases infiltration by polymorphonuclear monocytes

38-8. Which of the following is *not correct* regarding remote ischemic conditioning (RIC)?

A. RIC is likely mediated by bloodborne factors
B. RIC requires an intact neural pathway to be effective
C. The mechanism of RIC is likely to involve the RISK and SAFE pathways
D. RIC results in the release of autacoids
E. Treatment with SDF-1 can increase infarct size by mimicking RIC

38-9. Which of the following pharmacologic options may reduce ischemia-reperfusion injury?

A. Cyclosporine A
B. Adenosine
C. Hypothermia
D. Metoprolol
E. Antioxidants

38-10. When does myocardial edema peak after reperfusion following acute myocardial infarction?

A. Immediately after reperfusion
B. 7 days post reperfusion
C. 3 days post reperfusion
D. A and B
E. B and C

38-1. **The answer is C.** *(Hurst's The Heart, 14th Edition, Chap. 38)* Shorter time to reperfusion and an increased number of collaterals are associated with smaller infarct sizes (options A and B). Lower temperatures and larger ischemia/reperfusion injury are associated with larger infarct sizes (options D and E). Blood pressure by itself is not directly associated with infarct size (option C).

38-2. **The answer is E.** *(Hurst's The Heart, 14th Edition, Chap. 38)* Calcium overload that results from disruption of the sarcolemma and reversal of the Na^+/Ca^{2+} exchanger contribute to reperfusion injury (options A and B).[1] Impairment of the microcirculation via the no-reflow phenomenon or by compression through tissue edema can exacerbate reperfusion injury (options C and D).[2,3] Autophagy is not known to contribute to reperfusion injury (option E).

38-3. **The answer is B.** *(Hurst's The Heart, 14th Edition, Chap. 38)* Altered Ca^{2+} handling is one of the most prominent and relevant aspects of cardiomyocyte reperfusion. Reperfusion causes further Ca^{2+} influx through the Na^+/Ca^{2+} exchanger in response to Na^+ overload (option A). An important consequence of increased Ca^{2+} is activation of the Ca^{2+}-dependent proteases calpains. Calpains translocate to the sarcolemma during ischemia in response to Ca^{2+} overload but are activated only during reperfusion when intracellular pH is normalized because they are inhibited by low pH (options B and E).[4] When the Ca^{2+} capacity of the sarcoplasmic reticulum (SR) is exceeded, Ca^{2+} is released back into the cytosol through the ryanodine receptor channel (RyR2) (option C). Excessive contractile activation may cause hypercontracture, resulting in disruption of cardiomyocyte architecture that can cause sarcolemma rupture and cell death (option D).

38-4. **The answer is D.** *(Hurst's The Heart, 14th Edition, Chap. 38)* Restoration of the mitochondrial membrane potential favors mitochondrial Ca^{2+} uptake through the Ca^{2+} uniporter and Ca^{2+} overload (option A).[5] Mitochondrial permeability transition is caused by the opening of the MPTP. During ischemia, the MPTP does not open because of the inhibiting effect of intracellular acidosis (option B). Cyclophilin D modulates the sensitivity of MPTP to Ca^{2+} (option C).[6] Reperfusion results in immediate restoration of respiration, proton gradient across the inner mitochondrial membrane, and ATP synthesis (option D). Reactive oxygen species levels increase following reperfusion, in part, because of oxidation of the excess succinate that builds up during ischemia (option E).[7,8]

38-5. **The answer is C.** *(Hurst's The Heart, 14th Edition, Chap. 38)* Interstitial edema develops as a consequence of increased interstitial osmolarity from increased ion and catabolite concentrations and a dysfunction of the endothelial barrier during myocardial ischemia (option A). Edema development during reperfusion follows a bimodal pattern, where an initial maximum of water content after 120 minutes is associated with the beginning of leukocyte infiltration and a secondary peak after 7 days is associated with enhanced collagen deposition (option B).[9,10] The release of vasoconstrictor substances such as thromboxane, serotonin, and endothelin from the culprit lesion into the microcirculation, in conjunction with the impairment of endothelial function by ischemia/reperfusion per se or by tumor necrosis factor-α (TNF-α), can contribute to enhanced vasoconstrictor responsiveness of the microcirculation during myocardial ischemia/reperfusion (option C).[11-13] Cellular aggregates are either released from the epicardial atherosclerotic culprit lesion and dislodged into the microcirculation or are formed in the coronary microcirculation, resulting in impaired flow (option D). No-reflow and hemorrhage carry an adverse prognosis (option E).[14,15]

38-6. **The answer is C.** *(Hurst's The Heart, 14th Edition, Chap. 38)* Repeated episodes of ischemia decrease reperfusion injury (option A).[16,17] IPC has been shown to induce two distinct windows of cardioprotection. The first, usually referred to as classic preconditioning, occurs immediately after the IPC stimulus and lasts 2 to 3 hours, followed by a disappearance of the effect. This is followed by a second window of protection, or delayed effect, appearing 12 to 24 hours later and lasting 48 to 72 hours (option B).[18,19]The sublethal cycles of short bursts of ischemia and reperfusion, which make up the IPC stimulus, produce a number of endogenous biological factors (i.e., autacoids) from the myocyte, including adenosine, bradykinin, endothelin, acetylcholine, and opioids, which can bind to their respective receptors on the plasma membrane. This will direct the appropriate cardioprotective communication pathway that will convey the protective signal to the mitochondria (option C). Although the end effectors of cardioprotection in classical and delayed IPC remain unclear, it has been suggested that preservation of mitochondrial function with less calcium overload, attenuated ROS production, and MPTP inhibition all contribute to the protective effect (option D).[20-22] The presence of angina before an MI is associated with smaller injuries following MI (option E).[23]

38-7. **The answer is A.** *(Hurst's The Heart, 14th Edition, Chap. 38)* Ischemic postconditioning (IPost) confers myriad protective effects, including the preservation of endothelial function, reduced levels of myocardial edema, reduced levels of oxidative stress, and reduced neutrophil accumulation (options A, D, and E).[24] IPost has been shown to reduce myocardial infarction size in rodents, rabbits, pigs, and other species including humans, although the cardioprotective effects of IPost do not appear to be as robust as with ischemic preconditioning.[25,26] Mechanistically, IPost appears to share many of the same signaling mechanisms recruited at the time of reperfusion by ischemic preconditioning (option B).[25,27] While animal data are promising, early phase clinical studies have yielded mixed results (option C).[28]

38-8. **The answer is E.** *(Hurst's The Heart, 14th Edition, Chap. 38)* Remote ischemic conditioning is the phenomenon whereby the application of one or more brief cycles of nonlethal ischemia and reperfusion to an organ or tissue protect the heart against a lethal episode of acute reperfusion injury. Blood taken from a rabbit that has been preconditioned reduces MI size when transfused into a naïve rabbit, suggesting that RIC occurs via bloodborne factors (option A). The generation of this cardioprotective factor has been shown to be dependent on an intact neural pathway.[29] The exact factor remains unknown, but SDF-1 is a candidate (option E).[25] RIC involves the release of autacoid and depends on an intact neural system (options B and D). The mechanism of RIC is likely to involve the RISK and SAFE pathways (option C).[30]

38-9. **The answer is D.** *(Hurst's The Heart, 14th Edition, Chap. 38)* The history of pharmacologic cardioprotection has been hugely disappointing, with adenosine, antioxidants, magnesium, calcium channel blockers, anti-inflammatory agents, erythropoietin, and atorvastatin all failing to reduce myocardial infarction size or to improve clinical outcomes (options A, B, C, and E).[24,31] Initial clinical trials using early metoprolol in patients with acute myocardial infarction have suggested a reduction in infarct size (option D).[32] Large clinical studies are under way.

38-10. **The answer is D.** *(Hurst's The Heart, 14th Edition, Chap. 38)* Edema development during reperfusion follows a bimodal pattern, where an initial maximum of water content after 120 minutes is associated with a beginning leukocyte infiltration, and a secondary peak after 7 days is associated with enhanced collagen deposition (options A, B, and C).[9,10,32] It has been proposed that edema during reperfusion reflects the area at risk on cardiac magnetic resonance (CMR), but such a bimodal pattern raises questions about the use of T2-weighted edema measurement for AAR delineation.[33]

References

1. Piper HM, Garcia-Dorado D, Ovize M. A fresh look at reperfusion injury. *Cardiovasc Res.* 1998;38(2):291-300.
2. Garcia-Dorado D, Andres-Villarreal M, Ruiz-Meana M, Inserte J, Barba I. Myocardial edema: a translational view. *J Mol Cell Cardiol.* 2012;52(5):931-939.
3. Kloner RA, Ganote CE, Jennings RB. The "no-reflow" phenomenon after temporary coronary occlusion in the dog. *J Clin Invest.* 1974;54(6):1496-1508.
4. Inserte J, Hernando V, Garcia-Dorado D. Contribution of calpains to myocardial ischaemia/reperfusion injury. *Cardiovasc Res.* 2012;96(1):23-31.
5. Tisdale MJ. Biology of cachexia. *J Natl Cancer Inst.* 1997;89(23):1763-1773.
6. Baines CP, Kaiser RA, Purcell NH, et al. Loss of cyclophilin D reveals a critical role for mitochondrial permeability transition in cell death. *Nature.* 2005;434(7033):658-662.
7. Chouchani ET, Pell VR, Gaude E, et al. Ischaemic accumulation of succinate controls reperfusion injury through mitochondrial ROS. *Nature.* 2014;515(7527):431-435.
8. Valls-Lacalle L, Barba I, Miro-Casas E, et al. Succinate dehydrogenase inhibition with malonate during reperfusion reduces infarct size by preventing mitochondrial permeability transition. *Cardiovasc Res.* 2016;109(3):374-384.
9. Fernandez-Jimenez R, Sanchez-Gonzalez J, Aguero J, et al. Myocardial edema after ischemia/reperfusion is not stable and follows a bimodal pattern: imaging and histological tissue characterization. *J Am Coll Cardiol.* 2015;65(4):315-323.
10. Fernandez-Jimenez R, Garcia-Prieto J, Sanchez-Gonzalez J, et al. Pathophysiology underlying the bimodal edema phenomenon after myocardial ischemia/reperfusion. *J Am Coll Cardiol.* 2015;66(7):816-828.
11. Kleinbongard P, Bose D, Baars T, et al. Vasoconstrictor potential of coronary aspirate from patients undergoing stenting of saphenous vein aortocoronary bypass grafts and its pharmacological attenuation. *Circ Res.* 2011;108(3):344-352.
12. Kleinbongard P, Baars T, Mohlenkamp S, et al. Aspirate from human stented native coronary arteries vs. saphenous vein grafts: more endothelin but less particulate debris. *Am J Physiol Heart Circ Physiol.* 2013;305(8):H1222-H1229.
13. Ku DD. Coronary vascular reactivity after acute myocardial ischemia. *Science.* 1982;218(4572):576-578.
14. Niccoli G, Scalone G, Lerman A, Crea F. Coronary microvascular obstruction in acute myocardial infarction. *Eur Heart J.* 2016;37(13):1024-1033.
15. Betgem RP, de Waard GA, Nijveldt R, et al. Intramyocardial haemorrhage after acute myocardial infarction. *Nat Rev Cardiol.* 2015;12(3):156-167.
16. Murry CE, Jennings RB, Reimer KA. Preconditioning with ischemia: a delay of lethal cell injury in ischemic myocardium. *Circulation.* 1986;74(5):1124-1136.
17. Reimer KA, Murry CE, Yamasawa I, Hill ML, Jennings RB. Four brief periods of myocardial ischemia cause no cumulative ATP loss or necrosis. *Am J Physiol.* 1986;251(6 Pt 2):H1306-J1315.
18. Marber MS, Latchman DS, Walker JM, Yellon DM. Cardiac stress protein elevation 24 hours after brief ischemia or heat stress is associated with resistance to myocardial infarction. *Circulation.* 1993;88(3):1264-1272.
19. Kuzuya T, Hoshida S, Yamashita N, et al. Delayed effects of sublethal ischemia on the acquisition of tolerance to ischemia. *Circ Res.* 1993;72(6):1293-1299.
20. Yellon DM, Downey JM. Preconditioning the myocardium: from cellular physiology to clinical cardiology. *Physiol Rev.* 2003;83(4):1113-1151.
21. Ong SB, Dongworth RK, Cabrera-Fuentes HA, Hausenloy DJ. Role of the MPTP in conditioning the heart—translatability and mechanism. *Br J Pharmacol.* 2015;172(8):2074-2084.
22. Hausenloy DJ. Cardioprotection techniques: preconditioning, postconditioning and remote conditioning (basic science). *Curr Pharm Des.* 2013;19(25):4544-4563.
23. Eitel I, and Thiele H. Cardioprotection by pre-infarct angina: training the heart to enhance myocardial salvage. *Eur Heart J Cardiovasc Imaging.* 2013;14(11):1115-1116.
24. Zhao ZQ, Corvera JS, Halkos ME, et al. Inhibition of myocardial injury by ischemic postconditioning during reperfusion: comparison with ischemic preconditioning. *Am J Physiol Heart Circ Physiol.* 2003;285(2):H579-H588.
25. Heusch G. Molecular basis of cardioprotection: signal transduction in ischemic pre-, post-, and remote conditioning. *Circ Res.* 2015;116(4):674-699.
26. Tsang A, Hausenloy DJ, Yellon DM. Myocardial postconditioning: reperfusion injury revisited. *Am J Physiol Heart Circ Physiol.* 2005;289(1):H2-H7.
27. Bulluck H, Hausenloy DJ. Ischaemic conditioning: are we there yet? *Heart.* 2015;101(13):1067-1077.
28. Hahn JY, Song YB, Kim EK, et al. Ischemic postconditioning during primary percutaneous coronary intervention: the effects of postconditioning on myocardial reperfusion in patients with ST-segment elevation myocardial infarction (POST) randomized trial. *Circulation.* 2013;128(17):1889-1896.

29. Steensrud T, Li J, Dai X, et al. Pretreatment with the nitric oxide donor SNAP or nerve transection blocks humoral preconditioning by remote limb ischemia or intra-arterial adenosine. *Am J Physiol Heart Circ Physiol.* 2010;299(5):H1598-H1603.

30. Skyschally A, Gent S, Amanakis G, et al. Across-species transfer of protection by remote ischemic preconditioning with species-specific myocardial signal transduction by reperfusion injury salvage kinase and survival activating factor enhancement pathways. *Circ Res.* 2015;117(3):279-288.

31. Kloner RA, Forman MB, Gibbons RJ, et al. Impact of time to therapy and reperfusion modality on the efficacy of adenosine in acute myocardial infarction: the AMISTAD-2 trial. *Eur Heart J.* 2006;27(20):2400-2405.

32. Ibanez B, Prat-Gonzalez S, Speidl WS, et al. Early metoprolol administration before coronary reperfusion results in increased myocardial salvage: analysis of ischemic myocardium at risk using cardiac magnetic resonance. *Circulation.* 2007;115(23):2909-2916.

33. Heusch P, Nensa F, Heusch G. Is MRI really the gold standard for the quantification of salvage from myocardial infarction? *Circ Res.* 2015;117(3):222-224.

CHAPTER 39

Evaluation and Management of Non–ST-Segment Elevation Myocardial Infarction

Patrick R. Lawler

DIRECTIONS: Choose the one best response to each question.

39-1. Which of the following factors is associated with a low likelihood that chest pain is caused by myocardial ischemia attributable to obstructive coronary artery disease (CAD)?

A. Known coronary disease (particularly recent PCI)
B. Typical angina reproducing prior documented angina
C. Hemodynamic or ECG changes during pain
D. Dynamic ST-segment elevation or depression of ≥1 mm
E. T waves flat or inverted < 1 mm

39-2. A 55-year-old woman with a history of hypertension and obstructive sleep apnea presents with two days of an intermittent "squeezing" sensation in her chest. The last episode was approximately six hours ago. Which of the following is *true* about the use of the electrocardiogram to diagnose an acute coronary syndrome?

A. Persistent 0.5 mm ST segment depression is strongly suggestive of an acute coronary syndrome
B. T-wave inversions do not localize well the territory of myocardial ischemia
C. The presence of ST depressions confers a higher risk of 30-day mortality
D. The presence of isolated T-wave inversions confers a worse prognosis compared with ST depression
E. None of the above are true

39-3. A 52-year-old woman presents with an episode of substernal chest pressure. An initial conservative ("ischemia-guided") strategy is selected, and she undergoes stress testing. Which of the following findings would be consistent with a low-risk result, supporting ongoing medical management without coronary angiography with the intent to perform percutaneous coronary intervention (PCI)?

A. Duke treadmill score of 6
B. Echocardiographic wall motion abnormality (involving > 2 segments) developing at a heart rate of 120 beats per minute
C. Lung uptake on thallium scanning
D. Large stress-induced perfusion defect
E. Exercise-related left ventricular ejection fraction < 35%

39-4. A 76-year-old man, an active smoker, with a history of diabetes and hypertension, presents with accelerating angina over the past week that is now present at rest. In addition to his age and the presence of ≥3 risk factors for CAD, all of the following would also put this patient at higher risk, according to the TIMI Risk Score, *except*:

A. Known coronary artery stenosis ≥50%
B. Aspirin use within the past 7 days
C. ≥2 episodes of angina within the past 24 hours
D. ST changes ≥1 mm on ECG
E. Positive cardiac biomarkers

39-5. Which of the following is *not true* about ticagrelor?

A. Ventricular pauses are a known side effect of ticagrelor that usually develop early after treatment initiation, tend to decrease in frequency over time, are rarely symptomatic, and are not usually associated with clinically significant bradycardia

B. Dyspnea tends to occur early after starting the drug in 10% to 15% of treated patients, is not associated with evidence of heart failure, and usually lasts less than a week.

C. Dyspnea and ventricular pauses are thought to be mediated by interference with adenosine reuptake in erythrocytes

D. Ticagrelor is a twice daily, reversible ADP antagonist, and hence its antiplatelet effects are no longer present within 12 hours of discontinuation

E. Ticagrelor is preferred over clopidogrel in the management of patients with acute coronary syndromes when possible

39-6. In selecting a parenteral anticoagulant to treat patients with unstable angina/NSTEMI, which of the following is *true* about the evidence base supporting the use of fondaparinux compared with enoxaparin?

A. In clinical trials, fondaparinux has been shown to reduce the composite risk of death, MI, or refractory ischemia when compared with enoxaparin

B. No meaningful differences in bleeding risk have been observed with fondaparinux over enoxaparin

C. The risk of catheter-related thrombotic complications is higher in patients referred for percutaneous coronary artery intervention who were initially treated with enoxaparin versus fondaparinux

D. A criticism of the OASIS 5 trial that compared fondaparinux with enoxaparin was that patients with renal failure were allowed into the trial, and the hazard was driven by this group

E. Fondaparinux has received a class I recommendation for use in patients with unstable angina/NSTEMI by the ACCF/AHA

39-7. A 39-year-old woman presents to the emergency room with chest pain and marked ST segment changes. She continues to complain of crushing chest pain that began abruptly 2 hours ago. Her brother has a history of aortic dissection at a young age. She is referred for urgent coronary angiography, which is shown in Figure 39-1. Based on the angiographic findings and the patient's clinical picture, which of the following is the most likely diagnosis?

A. Acute plaque rupture (type I) myocardial infarction in the setting of atherosclerotic CAD

B. Coronary artery embolization

C. Coronary artery dissection

D. Aortic dissection with extension into the coronary arteries

E. Takayasu arteritis

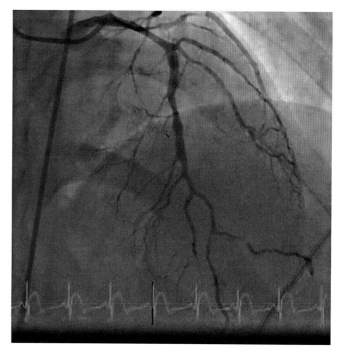

FIGURE 39-1 Coronary angiogram for the patient described in question 39-7.

39-8. A 52-year-old female cigarette smoker presents with chest pain and ST segment elevations in leads V4 to V6 on a 12-lead ECG, which abruptly resolve accompanied by the resolution of chest pain with a dose of sublingual nitroglycerin in the emergency room. She undergoes coronary angiography, which demonstrates only a 60% stenosis in the circumflex artery. A diagnosis of variant angina is made. All of the following are potentially beneficial treatments *except*:

A. Nifedipine

B. Amlodipine

C. Atorvastatin

D. Isosorbide mononitrate

E. Metoprolol

39-9. A 65-year-old woman presents with two days of chest pain and progressive dyspnea. She has anterolateral ST elevations, and her troponin is 5 times the upper limit for normal. She undergoes coronary angiography and ventriculography, which is shown in Figure 39-2. Which of the following statements is *true* about the underlying diagnosis?

A. The incidence is rare, approximately 1 in 1000 patients presenting with ACS

B. Emotional stress in the presence of symmetric T-wave inversion in most leads is diagnostic for the condition

C. At angiography, most patients with this condition will not have obstructive CAD

D. Inotropes in this patient are likely to improve hemodynamics

E. The condition is more common in women

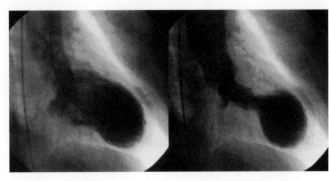

FIGURE 39-2 Left ventriculogram for the patient described in question 39-9. (Reproduced with permission from Abe Y, Kondo M, Matsuoka R, et al. Assessment of clinical features in transient left ventricular apical ballooning, *J Am Coll Cardiol*. 2003 Mar 5; 41(5):737-742.)

39-10. A 67-year-old man presents to the emergency department with chest pain and is diagnosed with NSTEMI. According to the 2014 ACCF/AHA guidelines, all of the following represent class III recommendations *except*:

A. Ibuprofen for early pericarditis
B. Nitroglycerin for pain relief in a patient with recent sildenafil use
C. Immediate release nifidipine in the absence of a beta-blocker
D. Intravenous metoprolol if the oral route is unavailable
E. Withholding oxygen therapy to when SpO$_2$ is < 90%

39-1. The answer is E. *(Hurst's The Heart, 14th Edition, Chap. 39)* T wave flattening or low-level inversion (< 1 mm) is associated with a lower likelihood of obstructive CAD as the basis for chest symptoms, whereas more marked symmetric T-wave inversion in multiple precordial leads is highly suggestive of CAD. A number of factors increase or decrease the likelihood of CAD (Table 39-1; answers A through D are incorrect).

TABLE 39-1 **Likelihood that Chest Symptoms Are Caused by Myocardial Ischemia Attributable to Obstructive Coronary Artery Disease**

High likelihood
Known coronary disease (particularly recent PCI)
Typical angina reproducing prior documented angina
Hemodynamic or ECG changes during pain
Dynamic ST-segment elevation or depression of ≥1 mm
Marked symmetric T-wave inversion in multiple precordial leads
Elevated cardiac enzymes in a rising and falling pattern
Intermediate likelihood
Absence of high-likelihood features and any of the following:
Typical angina in a patient without prior documented angina
Atypical anginal symptoms in diabetics or in nondiabetics with two or more other risk factors
Male gender
Age older than 70 y
Extracardiac vascular disease
ST depression 0.5-1.0 mm or T-wave inversion of ≥1 mm
Low-level troponin elevation that is "flat" and does not rise or fall
Low likelihood
Absence of high- or intermediate-likelihood features but may have:
Chest discomfort reproduced by palpation
T waves flat or inverted < 1 mm
Normal ECG

39-2. The answer is C. *(Hurst's The Heart, 14th Edition, Chap. 39)* Even minor ST depression is associated with a markedly increased mortality rate. Among 9461 patients enrolled in the PURSUIT (Platelet Glycoprotein IIb/IIIa in Unstable Angina: Receptor Suppression Using Integrilin Therapy) study, mortality at 30 days was 5.1% in patients with ST-segment depression versus 2.1% among those without ST-segment depression.[1]

Transient ST-segment depression of at least 0.5 mm that appears during chest discomfort and disappears after relief provides objective evidence of transient myocardial ischemia. When it is a constant finding with or without chest pain, it is less specific (option A is incorrect). A common but nonspecific ECG pattern in patients with UA/NSTEMI consists of persistent negative T waves over the involved area (option B is incorrect). Deeply negative T waves across the precordial (anterior) leads suggest a proximal, severe, left anterior descending coronary artery stenosis as the culprit lesion and are considered a marker of high risk. However, patients with isolated T-wave inversion have a more favorable prognosis than do those with ST-segment depression (option D is incorrect).[2]

39-3. The answer is A. *(Hurst's The Heart, 14th Edition, Chap. 39)* Stress testing is commonly used for risk stratification in patients with UA/NSTEMI who are managed with an initial conservative ("ischemia-guided") strategy. The Duke treadmill score (DTS) is used to objectify risk during exercise stress testing. The score is calculated as: DTS = Exercise time (minutes) – (5 × ST deviation in mm) – (4 × angina index). The angina index is scored as: 0 points if no angina occurs, 1 point if nonlimiting angina occurs, and 2 points if angina occurs that limits exercise. Scores are considered low (> 5), intermediate (between 4 and –11), and high (< –11). The other answer choices confer a high risk (Table 39-2; options B through E are incorrect). Stress tests should be symptom limited rather than submaximal, and a stress ECG without adjunctive imaging is appropriate unless baseline

TABLE 39-2 American College of Cardiology/American Heart Association Noninvasive Risk Stratification

High risk (> 3% annual mortality rate)
1. Severe resting LV dysfunction (LVEF < 0.35)
2. High-risk treadmill (score ≤ 11)
3. Severe exercise LV dysfunction (exercise LVEF < 0.35)
4. Stress-induced large perfusion defect (particularly if anterior)
5. Stress-induced multiple perfusion defects of moderate size
6. Large, fixed perfusion defect with LV dilatation or increased lung uptake
7. Stress-induced moderate perfusion defect with LV dilatation or increased lung uptake (thallium-201)
8. Echocardiographic wall motion abnormality (involving > 2 segments) developing at a low dose of dobutamine (≤ 10 mg/kg/min) or at a low heart rate (≤120 bpm)
9. Stress echocardiographic evidence of extensive ischemia

Intermediate risk (1%-3% annual mortality rate)
1. Mild to moderate resting LV dysfunction (LVEF 0.35-0.49)
2. Intermediate-risk treadmill score (score –11 to +5)
3. Stress-induced moderate perfusion defect without LV dilatation or increased lung intake
4. Limited stress echocardiographic ischemia with a wall motion abnormality only at higher doses of dobutamine involving ≤ 2 segments.

Low risk (< 1% annual mortality rate)
1. Low-risk treadmill (score ≥ +5)
2. Normal or small myocardial perfusion defect at rest or with stress
3. Normal stress echocardiographic wall motion or no change of limited resting wall motion abnormalities during stress

ECG abnormalities would preclude adequate interpretation. Those with high-risk findings should undergo coronary arteriography; those with negative or low-risk results can be treated medically. Low-risk patients who complete a stay in a chest pain unit without objective evidence of myocardial ischemia can safely undergo stress testing for diagnosis and prognostic purposes either immediately or, when possible, within 48 hours as an outpatient. In patients who cannot exercise, pharmacologic testing with dipyridamole, adenosine, regadenoson, or dobutamine can be used to provide the stress, and sestamibi imaging or echocardiography can be used as a method of assessment.

39-4. **The answer is D.** (*Hurst's The Heart, 14th Edition, Chap. 39*) The TIMI Risk Score for unstable angina/NSTEMI errs in the risk stratification of patients presenting with suspected acute coronary syndromes. The score allocates points for all of the above risk factors, except for ST changes ≥ 0.5 mm (not 1 mm) on ECG (options A, B, C, and E are incorrect). Patients with unstable angina/NSTEMI at low risk based on TIMI Risk Scores 0 or 1 (or GRACE Risk Score of < 109) can be managed by an "ischemia-guided" strategy.

39-5. **The answer is D.** (*Hurst's The Heart, 14th Edition, Chap. 39*) Although reversible, ticagrelor still has residual antiplatelet effects for up to 5 days among individuals on chronic therapy, and it should be withheld for at least 5 days if possible prior to nonemergent surgery. Ticagrelor has several known, usually self-limited, side effects, which likely arise from its interference with adenosine uptake (options A through C are incorrect). In the PLATO trial,[3] at the end of the 12-month follow-up period, the primary end point (CV death, MI, and stroke) was reduced from 11.7% in the clopidogrel arm to 9.8% in the ticagrelor arm (HR, 0.84; 95% CI, 0.77–0.92; P < .001). In addition to significant reductions in MI alone, there was also a significant 21% relative risk reduction in vascular mortality and a 22% reduction in total mortality (5.9% vs 4.5%; P < .001).

39-6. **The answer is B.** (*Hurst's The Heart, 14th Edition, Chap. 39*) Fondaparinux receives a class I recommendation in the most recent AHA/ACC NSTEMI guidelines. In the OASIS 5 trial, which enrolled > 20,000 patients with UA/NSTEMI, 2.5 mg/d of fondaparinux versus 1 mg/kg twice a day of enoxaparin yielded similar rates of the primary end point of death, MI, or refractory ischemia at 9 days (5.8% vs 5.7%; option A is incorrect). However, major bleeding events were reduced by 48% with fondaparinux, and mortality trended lower in the fondaparinux group at 30 days (2.9% vs 3.5%; *P* = .02) and at 180 days (5.8% vs 6.5%; *P* = .05); all but three of the 64 excess deaths with enoxaparin were associated with major or minor bleeding (option B is incorrect). However, several caveats to the OASIS 5 trial merit mention. First, patients were allowed entry with a creatinine up to 3.0 mg/dL. Major bleeding risk was particularly high among patients treated with weight-adjusted enoxaparin who had a creatinine clearance below 30 mL/min (9.9% rate of major bleeding; option D is incorrect). Second, UFH was administered after randomization in a larger proportion of enoxaparin-treated patients, a practice that is thought to increase bleeding risks. Third, the long half-life of fondaparinux may create logistical problems in centers that perform early cardiac catheterization. Finally, among patients undergoing cardiac catheterization, an excess in catheter-related thrombotic complications was observed, a finding that has also been observed in other trials using fondaparinux (option C is incorrect). Finally, it should be noted that, as of the time of writing, fondaparinux has not been approved by the United States Food and Drug Administration for use in patients with acute coronary syndromes, although it received a class I recommendation from the ACCF/AHA Guidelines and is used off-label.

39-7. **The answer is C.** *(Hurst's The Heart, 14th Edition, Chap. 39)* Figure 39-1 demonstrates the coronary angiogram of a patient with spontaneous coronary artery dissection (SCAD); diffuse irregularity of the left anterior descending artery is noted, along with extension into side branches, including the diagonal artery. SCAD is an increasingly recognized cause of ACS, particularly in women age 30 to 50 years. The pathophysiology of SCAD is unknown; many cases occur in situations such as uncontrolled hypertension, in the puerperium, in those with fibromuscular dysplasia, or as a complication of disorders of collagen integrity, such as Marfan syndrome. The diagnosis of SCAD should be entertained when younger (usually female) patients present with symptoms and signs of acute coronary ischemia in the absence of other risk factors. Diagnostic studies for those with SCAD should be similar to those without the diagnosis; the presence of a coronary dissection plane may be challenging to recognize at the time of coronary angiography, so a high level of suspicion for the presence of the diagnosis should be maintained during such procedures. Standard treatment for SCAD is not established. For many, conservative management may be quite effective, particularly if flow is present in the coronary artery at the time of diagnostic coronary angiography; spontaneous healing of the dissection may be seen at the time of follow-up angiography. Revascularization, by PCI or CABG, is potentially indicated in the presence of an occlusion of a coronary vessel. Given the high prevalence of unrecognized fibromuscular dysplasia in affected patients, some recommend screening for the presence of intracranial aneurysm in those affected by SCAD.

39-8. **The answer is E.** *(Hurst's The Heart, 14th Edition, Chap. 39)* Variant angina, also called Prinzmetal's angina, is characterized by transient marked ST-segment elevation in the absence of plaque rupture and is thought to be caused by coronary spasm, which is usually focal and often at the site of a coronary artery stenosis. It is thought that coronary spasm is a result of abnormalities in endothelial function and nitric oxide activity at sites of coronary spasm.

Patients with variant angina are often difficult to treat because attacks are unpredictable and often occur without an obvious precipitating factor. NTG relieves variant angina attacks within minutes and should be used promptly; long-acting nitrates are initially effective in preventing variant angina attacks (option D is incorrect). CCBs are very effective in preventing attacks of variant angina (options A and B are incorrect); higher CCB doses are often required. For example, long-acting nifedipine (90 mg/d), diltiazem (360 mg/d), verapamil (480 mg/d), and amlodipine (20 mg/d) are commonly used. Statin therapy is indicated (option C is incorrect), given beneficial effects on endothelial function and the common presence of atherosclerosis underlying focal spasm. There is no documented role for beta-blockers.

39-9. **The answer is E.** *(Hurst's The Heart, 14th Edition, Chap. 39)* Figure 39-2 demonstrates the characteristic left ventriculogram of a patient with stress cardiomyopathy. Widely recognized as an ACS "mimic," stress cardiomyopathy (also known as "apical ballooning" syndrome or takotsubo cardiomyopathy as a result of the resemblance of the dysfunctional LV to a Japanese octopus pot trap) is found in 1.7% to 2.2% of patients presenting with ACS, and the vast majority (> 90%) are women (option E is correct). Stress cardiomyopathy most often follows an acute emotional stress, such as the death of a loved one, and it may be indistinguishable from a high-risk ACS, with typical angina, rise and fall of troponin, and onset of heart failure symptoms. Characteristic ECG changes of stress cardiomyopathy include the development of symmetric T-wave inversion in most leads; however, such changes are not specific enough to stress cardiomyopathy to avoid diagnostic coronary angiography (option B is incorrect). At angiography, nonobstructed coronary arteries are the rule (option C is incorrect), along with characteristic myocardial dysfunction of the LV apex, with compensatory basal hyperkinesis. Management of patients with stress cardiomyopathy is typically supportive; patients most often recover rapidly after presentation, though shock at presentation is not uncommon. The use of vasodilating inotropic agents or intra-aortic balloon counterpulsation in those with shock may actually worsen hemodynamics because such treatment may precipitate LV outflow tract obstruction in the context of basal hyperkinesis (option D is incorrect). β-Blockers and ACE inhibitors or ARBs are often used during convalescent periods, but their value in stress cardiomyopathy is unknown.

39-10. **The answer is E.** *(Hurst's The Heart, 14th Edition, Chap. 39)* A number of pharmacologic strategies are proposed in patients with unstable angina/NSTEMI, as outlined in Table 39-3 (options A through D are incorrect).

TABLE 39-3 American College of Cardiology/American Heart Association Guideline Recommendations for Early Care of Patients with Suspected Acute Coronary Syndrome Treatment Recommendation Level of Evidence

Treatment		Recommendation	Level of Evidence
Oxygen	Administer supplemental oxygen only with oxygen saturation < 90%, respiratory distress, or other high-risk features for hypoxemia	I	C
Nitrates	Administer sublingual nitroglycerin every 5 minutes × 3 for continuing ischemic pain and then assess need for IV nitroglycerin	I	C
	Administer IV nitroglycerin for persistent ischemia, HF, or hypertension	I	B
	Nitrates are contraindicated with recent use of a phosphodiesterase inhibitor	III:Harm	B
Analgesic therapy	IV morphine sulfate may be reasonable for continued ischemic chest pain despite maximally tolerated anti-ischemic medications	IIb	B
	NSAIDs (except aspirin) should not be initiated and should be discontinued during hospitalization	III:Harm	B
β-Adrenergic blockers	Initiate oral β-blockers within the first 24 hours in the absence of HF, low-output state, risk for cardiogenic shock, or other contraindications to β-blockade	I	A
	Use of sustained-release metoprolol succinate, carvedilol, or bisoprolol is recommended for β-blocker therapy with concomitant NSTE-ACS, stabilized HF, and reduced systolic function	I	C
	Reevaluate to determine subsequent eligibility in patients with initial contraindications to β-blockers	I	C
	It is reasonable to continue β-blocker therapy in patients with normal LV function with NSTE-ACS	IIa	C
	IV β-blockers are potentially harmful when risk factors for shock are present	III:Harm	B
Calcium channel blockers	Administer initial therapy with nondihydropyridine calcium channel blockers with recurrent ischemia and contraindications to β-blockers in the absence of LV dysfunction, increased risk for cardiogenic shock, PR interval > 0.24 seconds, or second- or third-degree atrioventricular block without a pacemaker	I	B
	Administer oral nondihydropyridine calcium antagonists with recurrent ischemia after use of β-blocker and nitrates in the absence of contraindications	I	C
	Calcium channel blockers are recommended for ischemic symptoms when β-blockers are not successful, are contraindicated, or cause unacceptable side effects	I	C
	Long-acting calcium channel blockers and nitrates are recommended for patients with coronary artery spasm	I	C
	Immediate-release nifedipine is contraindicated in the absence of a β-blocker	III:Harm	B
Cholesterol management	Initiate or continue high-intensity statin therapy in patients with no contraindications	I	A
	Obtain a fasting lipid profile, preferably within 24 hours	IIa	C

Abbreviations: HF, heart failure; IV, intravenous; NSAIDs, nonsteroidal anti-inflammatory drugs; NSTE-ACS, non–ST-segment elevation acute coronary syndrome.

Reproduced with permission from Amsterdam EA, Wenger NK, Brindis RG, et al. 2014 AHA/ACC Guideline for the Management of Patients with Non-ST-Elevation Acute Coronary Syndromes: a report of the American College of Cardiology/American Heart Association Task Force on Practice Guidelines, *J Am Coll Cardiol.* 2014 Dec 23;64(24):e139-e228.

References

1. Boersma E, Pieper KS, Steyerberg EW, et al. Predictors of outcome in patients with acute coronary syndromes without persistent ST-segment elevation. Results from an international trial of 9461 patients. The PURSUIT investigators. *Circulation.* 2000;101(22):2557-2567.

2. Mueller C, Neumann FJ, Perach W, Perruchoud AP, Buettner HJ. Prognostic value of the admission electrocardiogram in patients with unstable angina/non–ST-segment elevation myocardial infarction treated with very early revascularization. *Am J Med.* 2004;117(3):145-150.

3. Wallentin L, Becker RC, Budaj A, et al. Ticagrelor versus clopidogrel in patients with acute coronary syndromes. *N Engl J Med.* 2009;361(11):1045-1057.

CHAPTER 40

ST-Segment Elevation Myocardial Infarction

Patrick R. Lawler

QUESTIONS

DIRECTIONS: Choose the one best response to each question.

40-1. All of the following electrocardiographic findings can potentially support the diagnosis of a myocardial infarction in the presence of a known old left bundle branch block *except*:

A. Precordial R-wave regression
B. ST-segment elevation ≥ 1 mm concordant with the QRS complex
C. ST-segment elevation ≥ 5 mm discordant with the QRS
D. ST-segment depression ≥ 1 mm in leads V_1, V_2, or V_3
E. T-wave inversions in the anterior precordial leads

40-2. A 55-year-old man with a history of coronary artery disease is brought to the emergency room with chest pain by his wife. His ECG demonstrates ST-segment elevation. Which of the following is *true* about his initial management?

A. If he presents to a non–PCI-capable hospital, lytic therapy should be administered promptly, in the absence of contraindications, and the patient should emergently be transferred to a PCI-capable hospital for "facilitated PCI"
B. If the patient presents to a PCI-capable hospital, the desired first medical contact (FMC)-to-device time is < 120 minutes
C. If the patient presents to a non–PCI-capable hospital, and the anticipated FMC-to-device time, including transfer to a PCI-capable hospital, is < 120 minutes, then the patient should be transferred for primary PCI without receiving fibrinolysis
D. When PCI is unavailable, a fibrinolytic should be administered within 90 minutes
E. Patients treated successfully with fibrinolysis do not require follow-up angiography

40-3. All of the following are reasons to preferentially transfer a patient with STEMI for primary PCI rather than administer fibrinolytic therapy *except*:

A. Diagnosis of plaque rupture myocardial infarction in doubt
B. Cardiogenic shock
C. Suspected aortic dissection
D. History of ischemic stroke 6 months prior
E. Anticipated FMC-to-device time of 90 minutes, including transfer

40-4. Which of the following is *true* about the administration of fibrinolytic therapy for patients with STEMI?

A. Reperfusion therapy is reasonable for patients with STEMI and symptom onset within the prior 12 to 24 hours who have clinical and/or ECG evidence of ongoing ischemia. Primary PCI is the preferred strategy in this population
B. Fibrinolysis and primary PCI are associated with equivalent vessel patency rates
C. While there is no mortality benefit associated with primary PCI over fibrinolysis, the lower risk of stroke makes primary PCI the preferred reperfusion strategy in most cases
D. Fibrinolysis should generally be considered up to 6 hours following symptoms onset
E. There are no circumstances under which fibrinolysis should be administered for patients with ST depressions

40-5. A 56-year-old woman presents with crushing chest pain for 30 minutes. Which of the following 12-lead ECG changes would suggest involvement of the left main coronary artery?

A. ST-segment elevation in lead V_1 in the setting of inferior myocardial infarction
B. ST-segment elevation in leads I, aVL, V_5, and V_6
C. Peaking following by a loss of anterior R waves
D. Failure of T waves to invert within 48 hours following the administration of fibrinolysis
E. ST elevation in lead aVR greater than or equal to the extent of ST-segment elevation in lead V_1

40-6. A 67-year-old man is admitted with an anterior STEMI, and he undergoes successful reperfusion with primary PCI. His left ventricular ejection fraction is 35%. All of the following represent potential angiotensin-converting enzyme (ACE) inhibitor regimens to begin ideally within the first 24 hours for this patient *except*:

A. Captopril 6.25 to 12.5 mg 3 times/d to start; titrate to 25 to 50 mg 3 times/d as tolerated
B. Lisinopril 2.5 to 5 mg/d to start; titrate to 10 mg/d or higher as tolerated
C. Ramipril 2.5 mg twice daily to start; titrate to 5 mg twice daily as tolerated
D. Trandolapril test dose 0.5 mg; titrate up to 4 mg daily as tolerated
E. Enalaprilat 1 mg/dose IV over a two-hour period, followed by oral enalopril

40-7. Which of the following is *true* about the epidemiology of cardiogenic shock complicating myocardial infarction?

A. No therapy has meaningfully improved the mortality rate from cardiogenic shock
B. The incidence of cardiogenic shock as a result of severe LV dysfunction complicating MI has decreased over time
C. No trials have successfully demonstrated improvement in outcomes in patients with cardiogenic shock
D. Mortality from cardiogenic shock now is approximately 25%
E. None of the above statements are true

40-8. A 52-year-old man presents with myocardial infarction and undergoes placement of a pulmonary artery catheter, which demonstrated a cardiac index of 2.6 L/min/m^2 and a pulmonary capillary wedge pressure of 22 mm Hg. Which of the following Forrester classifications applies to this patient?

A. Class I
B. Class II
C. Class III
D. Class IV
E. Class V

40-9. A 78-year-old woman presents with chest pain and ST elevation in leads II, III, and aVF. She has ST-segment elevation in lead V4R. Within several minutes of assessment, she becomes progressive hypotensive. The cardiac catheterization team is en route to the hospital. All of the following principles apply to therapy for patients with STEMI and RV infarction and ischemic dysfunction *except*:

A. Nitroglycerine is beneficial to relieve symptoms of chest pain and to decrease endogenous catecholamine release
B. Atrioventricular synchrony should be achieved, and bradycardia should be corrected
C. RV preload should be optimized, which usually requires initial volume challenge in patients with hemodynamic instability provided the jugular venous pressure is normal or low
D. RV afterload should be optimized, which usually requires therapy for concomitant LV dysfunction
E. Inotropic support should be used for hemodynamic instability not responsive to volume challenge

40-10. Which of the following is *true* of patients with acute mitral regurgitation (MR) in the setting of myocardial infarction?

A. The onset of MR due to papillary muscle is usually 14 days following myocardial infarction
B. Acute MR will be detectable at the bedside by the presence of a new-onset, loud, apical systolic murmur
C. When papillary muscle rupture occurs, the posteromedial papillary muscle is more often involved than the anterolateral muscle
D. Echocardiography is often insufficient to make the diagnosis
E. IABP and blood pressure control are used to treat patients acutely and to allow the myocardium to heal; surgery is rarely required

ANSWERS

40-1. The answer is E. *(Hurst's The Heart, 14th Edition, Chap. 40)* New-onset (or not known to be old) LBBB in the setting of chest pain is typically considered and treated as an STEMI. Conversely, the diagnosis of STEMI in the setting of old LBBB can be difficult. Findings suggesting STEMI include (1) a pathologic Q wave in leads I, aVL, V_5, or V_6 (two leads); (2) precordial R-wave regression (option A is incorrect); (3) late notching of the S wave in V_1 to V_4; and (4) deviation of the ST segment in the same direction as that of the major QRS deflection.

An analysis of ECG data from the Global Use of Strategies to Open Occluded Coronary Arteries (GUSTO) I study identified three criteria for diagnosing myocardial infarction in the presence of the LBBB: (1) ST-segment elevation ≥ 1 mm concordant with the QRS complex; (2) ST-segment depression ≥ 1 mm in leads V_1, V_2, or V_3; and (3) ST-segment elevation ≥ 5 mm discordant with the QRS (options B through D are incorrect).[1] Such findings are often referred to as the Sgarbossa criteria.

40-2. The answer is C. *(Hurst's The Heart, 14th Edition, Chap. 40)* Primary PCI is superior to fibrinolytic therapy, and when available should be pursued. Patients who present with STEMI to a non–PCI-capable hospital should receive prompt (< 30 minutes; option D is incorrect) fibrinolytic therapy in the absence of contraindications. Such patients should then usually be transferred to a PCI-capable hospital, where follow-up angiography between 3 and 24 hours later (not sooner; option A is incorrect) can be undertaken. If there is evidence of failed thrombolytic therapy (shock, recurrent chest pain, failure of ST segments to decrease by > 50%), then the patient should be transferred more urgently for PCI. On the other hand, for patients who present with STEMI to a PCI-capable hospital, the desired FMC-to-device (eg, coronary stent) time is < 90 minutes (option B is incorrect).

40-3. The answer is D. *(Hurst's The Heart, 14th Edition, Chap. 40)* Patients who present with STEMI to a non–PCI-capable hospital can be managed with fibrinolysis or early transfer to a PCI-capable hospital. If the anticipated FMC-to-device time is anticipated to be < 120 minutes, then transfer should be undertaken (option E is incorrect). Patients presenting with an uncertain diagnosis, such as those with suspected coronary artery dissection, aortic dissection (option C is incorrect), or pericarditis, should be considered for transfer for primary PCI. Additionally, patients with contraindications to fibrinolysis, including ischemic stroke within 3 months (option D is incorrect), should be transferred, as well as those with cardiogenic shock (option B is incorrect).

40-4. The answer is A. *(Hurst's The Heart, 14th Edition, Chap. 40)* While the efficacy of reperfusion declines over time, patients with evidence of ongoing ischemia (ie, chest pain or ongoing ECG changes suggestive of ischemia) can be considered for reperfusion, although in this population the efficacy is anticipated to be lower, and primary PCI is preferred over fibrinolysis. Approximately 95% of patients who are treated with primary PCI obtain complete reperfusion versus 50% to 60% of patients who are treated with fibrinolytics (option B is incorrect). Primary PCI is also associated with a lower risk of stroke than treatment with fibrinolysis, and diagnostic angiography quickly defines coronary anatomy, LV function, and mechanical complications. In meta-analyses, primary PCI is associated with a lower mortality rate (7% vs 9%; $P = .0002$), less reinfarction (3% vs 7%; $P = .0001$), and fewer strokes (1% vs 2%; $P = .0004$) at 30 days when compared with fibrinolysis (option C is incorrect).[2]

Fibrinolysis should be considered up to 12 hours following symptoms onset (option D is incorrect). Fibrinolytic therapy should not be administered to patients with ST depression, except when a true posterior (inferobasal) MI is suspected or when associated with ST elevation in lead aVR (option E is incorrect).

40-5. The answer is E. *(Hurst's The Heart, 14th Edition, Chap. 40)* ST-segment elevation in lead aVR is an ominous sign and is more frequent in patients with left main artery occlusion than in patients with left anterior descending coronary artery or right coronary artery occlusion. In a study of STEMI patients, ST-segment elevation in lead aVR that was greater than or equal to the extent of ST-segment elevation in lead V_1 had 81% accuracy for diagnosing left main occlusion.[3] Generally, ST-elevation myocardial infarction is defined by new ST elevation at the J point in at least two contiguous leads of 2 mm (0.2 mV) in men or 1.5 mm (0.15 mV) in women in leads V_2 to V_3 and/or of 1 mm (0.1 mV) in other contiguous chest leads or the limb leads. ST-segment elevation in lead V_1 in the setting of inferior myocardial infarction suggests RV involvement (option A is incorrect). Because no leads on the standard 12-lead ECG directly represent the posterior myocardium, isolated infarction of this area may be difficult to diagnose but is typically manifested by ST-segment depression in V_1 to V_3, a mirror image of anterior myocardial infarct. ST-elevation in leads I, aVL, V_5, and V_6 suggests lateral wall infarction (option B is incorrect). While the R wave may initially increase in height but then soon decrease, this finding is not specific for left main coronary artery disease (option C is incorrect). Failure of the T wave to invert within 24 to 48 hours suggests early postinfarction regional pericarditis (option D is incorrect).

40-6. **The answer is E.** (*Hurst's The Heart, 14th Edition, Chap. 40*) In the Cooperative New Scandinavian Enalapril Survival Study-2 (CONSENSUS-2) trial, intravenous enalaprilat was administered within 24 hours of presentation followed by oral enalapril. In CONSENSUS-2, mortality was nonsignificantly increased in the treatment group. Conversely, a number of trials demonstrated a benefit with other ACE inhibitor regimens in patients with myocardial infarction, including the Survival and Ventricular Enlargement (SAVE) and Captopril and Thrombolysis Study (CATS) trials of captopril (option A is incorrect), the Gruppo Italiano per lo Studio della Sopravvivenza nell'infarto Miocardico (GISSI-3) trial of lisinopril (option B is incorrect), the Acute Infarction Ramipril Efficacy (AIRE) trial (option C is incorrect), and the Trandolapril Cardiac Evaluation (TRACE) trial (option D is incorrect).

40-7. **The answer is E.** (*Hurst's The Heart, 14th Edition, Chap. 40*) Cardiogenic shock as a result of severe LV dysfunction occurs in approximately 7% of patients with myocardial infarction; it previously had a mortality rate of approximately 80% before the widespread implementation of early revascularization (option A is incorrect). There was a trend toward increased in-hospital survival in the mid- to late 1990s, which correlated with the increased application of reperfusion technologies. The SHOCK II (Should We Emergently Revascularize Occluded Coronaries for Cardiogenic Shock II) trial demonstrated the benefit of early revascularization in patients with MI and cardiogenic shock (option C is incorrect). In most recent studies, the mortality from cardiogenic shock remains approximately 50% (option D is incorrect).

40-8. **The answer is B.** (*Hurst's The Heart, 14th Edition, Chap. 40*) Forrester described the treatment of patients on the basis of hemodynamic subsets related to pulmonary artery wedge pressure and cardiac output (Table 40-1). The basic goals of this approach include adjustment of the intravascular volume status to bring the pulmonary artery capillary wedge pressure from 18 to 20 mm Hg and optimization of cardiac output with inotropic and/or vasodilating agents. Severely hypotensive patients can be temporarily aided by intra-aortic balloon pumping or possibly by a ventricular assist device. However, the benefits from these mechanical treatments are often temporary, and there may be a significant risk of complications.

TABLE 40-1 Forrester Classification of Myocardial Infarction

	Cardiac Index (L/min/m^2)	Pulmonary Capillary Wedge Pressure (mm Hg)
Class I	> 2.2	< 18
Class II	> 2.2	> 18
Class III	< 2.2	< 18
Class IV	< 2.2	> 18

40-9. **The answer is A.** *(Hurst's The Heart, 14th Edition, Chap. 40)* Patients with right ventricular myocardial infarction should not receive therapies that could deplete preload, such as nitroglycerine. Patients with right ventricular infarction (RVI) present with a mix of left ventricular and right ventricular injury, and the overall balance between the extent of RV and LV dysfunction is a major determinant of long-term outcome. Most patients with RVI and significant hemodynamic compromise have evidence of extensive biventricular infarction and cardiogenic shock. Treatment of RVI initially involves volume loading with normal saline to achieve a pulmonary artery wedge pressure of 18 to 20 mm Hg. In some patients, this alone is sufficient to improve cardiac output and systemic pressure. However, some patients will not respond to fluid loading alone. This may be a result of marked RV enlargement within a relatively noncompliant pericardium, which may result in functional LV compression because of ventricular interaction. In addition to volume loading, the use of dobutamine improves cardiac index. Patients requiring temporary pacing for heart block may also benefit from arteriovenous sequential pacing rather than lone ventricular pacing.

40-10. **The answer is C.** *(Hurst's The Heart, 14th Edition, Chap. 40)* Severe MR caused by papillary muscle rupture is responsible for approximately 5% of deaths in AMI patients. Rupture may be complete or partial, and it usually involves the posteromedial papillary muscle because its blood supply is derived only from the posterior descending artery, whereas the anterolateral papillary muscle has a dual blood supply from both the left anterior descending and the circumflex coronary arteries. Most patients have relatively small areas of infarction with poor collaterals, and up to half of the patients may have single-vessel disease. The clinical presentation of papillary muscle rupture is the acute onset of pulmonary edema, usually within 2 to 7 days after inferior myocardial infarction (option A is incorrect). The characteristics of the murmur vary; as a result of a rapid increase of pressure in the left atrium, no murmur may be audible (option B is incorrect). Thus a high degree of suspicion, especially in patients with inferior wall infarction, is necessary for diagnosis. Two-dimensional echocardiographic examination demonstrates the partially or completely severed papillary muscle head and a flail segment of the mitral valve (option D is incorrect). LV function is hyperdynamic as a result of the severe regurgitation into the low-impedance left atrium; this finding alone, in a patient with severe congestive heart failure, should suggest the diagnosis. The cornerstones of successful therapy are prompt diagnosis and emergency surgery (option E is incorrect). Emergent placement of an IABP and blood pressure control may be beneficial. The current approach of emergency surgery accrues an overall operative mortality of 0% to 21%, but this appears to be decreasing, and the late results of this approach can be excellent.

References

1. Sgarbossa EB, Pinski SL, Barbagelata A, et al. Electrocardiographic diagnosis of evolving acute myocardial infarction in the presence of left bundle-branch block. GUSTO-1 (Global Utilization of Streptokinase and Tissue Plasminogen Activator for Occluded Coronary Arteries) Investigators. *N Engl J Med.* 1996;334: 481-487.
2. Keeley EC, Boura JA, Grines CL. Primary angioplasty versus intravenous thrombolytic therapy for acute myocardial infarction: a quantitative review of 23 randomised trials. *Lancet.* 2003;361:13-20.
3. Yamaji H, Iwasaki K, Kusachi S, et al. Prediction of acute left main coronary artery obstruction by 12-lead electrocardiography. ST segment elevation in lead aVR with less ST segment elevation in lead V(1). *J Am Coll Cardiol.* 2001;38:1348-1354.

CHAPTER 41

Antiplatelet and Anticoagulant Therapy in Acute Coronary Syndromes

Patrick R. Lawler

QUESTIONS

DIRECTIONS: Choose the one best response to each question.

41-1. A 45-year-old man undergoes coronary stent implantation for stable ischemic heart disease. He is prescribed clopidogrel and aspirin. Which of the following is *true* about his antithrombotic regimen?

A. The dose of aspirin should be between 75 and 100 mg per day
B. Higher doses of aspirin could be more effective at preventing ischemic events, but at the expense of a higher risk of bleeding
C. Clinical trials support a higher dose (ie, 300 to 325 mg daily) of aspirin in patients with ischemic heart disease
D. When used with newer-generation oral P2Y$_{12}$ receptor inhibitors (prasugrel and ticagrelor), no preference to aspirin dosing is given
E. None of the above

41-2. All of the following are actions of thromboxane A$_2$ (TXA$_2$) *except*:

A. Induces platelet aggregation
B. Potent vasoconstrictor
C. Regulation of renal blood flow
D. Induces proliferation of vascular smooth-muscle cells
E. Proatherogenic

41-3. Which of the following is *true* about clopidogrel?

A. Clopidogrel is approved only in patients receiving percutaneous coronary intervention (PCI) for myocardial infarction
B. All patients with ST-elevation myocardial infarction (STEMI) should receive a loading dose of 600 mg of clopidogrel
C. Renal dose adjustment in the loading and mantainance dose should be undertaken when the estimated glomerular filtration rate (eGFR) is < 30 mL/min per 1.73 m^2
D. In patients scheduled for nonemergent coronary artery bypass graft (CABG) surgery, clopidogrel should be held for 5 days if it is safe to do so clinically
E. Clopidogrel is a bioactive immediately medication

41-4. Which of the following is *true* about intravenous antiplatelet agents?

A. Cangrelor is an intravenous adenosine diphosphate (ADP) analog
B. Cangrelor requires conversion into a bioactive metabolite in the liver
C. Cangrelor's use is experimental only.
D. Parenteral glycoprotein IIb/IIIa inhibitors (such as abciximab, eptifibatide, and tirofiban) have demonstrated an evidence-based reduction in major adverse cardiac events in patients undergoing percutaneous coronary intervention
E. Thrombocytopenia is uncommon with glycoprotein IIb/IIIa inhibitors

41-5. According to the American College of Cardiology Foundation/American Heart Association guidelines for the use of thrombolytics in the management of ST-segment elevation myocardial infarction, all of the following are true *except*:

A. In the absence of contraindications, fibrinolytic therapy should be administered to patients with STEMI at non–PCI-capable hospitals when the anticipated first medical contact (FMC)-to-device time at a PCI-capable hospital exceeds 90 minutes because of unavoidable delays

B. When fibrinolytic therapy is indicated or chosen as the primary reperfusion strategy, it should be administered within 30 minutes of hospital arrival

C. In the absence of contraindications and when PCI is not available, fibrinolytic therapy is reasonable for patients with STEMI if there is clinical and/or ECG evidence of ongoing ischemia within 12 to 24 hours of symptom onset and a large area of myocardium at risk or hemodynamic instability

D. Fibrinolytic therapy should not be administered to patients with ST depression except when a true posterior (inferobasal) MI is suspected or when it is associated with ST elevation in lead aVR

E. Fibrin-specific fibrinolytic agents (tenecteplase, reteplase, alteplase) are preferred over streptokinase if available

41-6. All of the following are *true* about aspirin pharmacokinetics *except*:

A. Peak plasma levels occur 30 to 40 minutes after ingestion

B. Aspirin absorption in the upper gastrointestinal tract occurs within 60 minutes

C. Enteric coating of aspirin has negligible effects on absorption pharmacokinetics

D. COX-mediated TXA_2 synthesis is prevented for the entire life span of the platelet

E. COX-1 and COX-2 are not similarly blocked by equivalent doses of aspirin

41-7. The following are absolute contraindications to fibrinolytic therapy *except*:

A. Structural intracranial disease

B. Previous intracranial hemorrhage

C. Previous ischemic stroke

D. Active bleeding or bleeding diathesis

E. Recent brain or spinal surgery or recent head trauma with fracture or brain injury

41-8. All of the following anticoagulants act by interrupting factor Xa *except*:

A. Enoxaparin

B. Fondaparinux

C. Unfractionated heparin

D. Rivaroxaban

E. Bivalirudin

41-9. According to the American College of Cardiology Foundation/American Heart Association guidelines for the use of anticoagulants in the management of ST-segment elevation myocardial infarction, all of the following are true *except*:

A. Patients with STEMI undergoing reperfusion with fibrinolytic therapy should receive enoxaparin administered according to age, weight, and creatinine clearance, given as an intravenous bolus, followed in 15 minutes by subcutaneous injection for the duration of the index hospitalization, up to 8 days or until revascularization

B. The recommended dosing for enoxaparin for age < 75 years is 30-mg IV bolus followed by 1 mg/kg SC every 12 h (maximum of 100 mg for the first 2 SC doses) and for age > 75 years is no IV bolus, 0.7 mg/kg SC every 12 h (maximum of 7 mg for the first 2 SC doses)

C. For patients with STEMI undergoing PCI after receiving fibrinolytic therapy with enoxaparin, if the last dose of enoxaparin was given < 8 h before PCI, is recommended no additional anticoagulant therapy. If the last dose of enoxaparin was given 8 to 12 h before PCI, is recommended a 0.3mg/kg bolus of IV enoxaparin at the time of PCI

D. For patients receiving alteplase, tenecteplase, or reteplase for fibrinolysis, weight-based IV bolus and infusion of UFH adjusted to obtain aPTT of 1.5 to 2.0 times control are recommended for 48 h or until revascularization. IV bolus of 60 U/kg (maximum 4000 U) followed by an infusion of 12 U/kg/h (maximum 1000 U) initially, adjusted to maintain aPTT at 1.5 to 2.0 times control (approximately 50 to 70 s) for 48 h or until revascularization

E. All of the above are consistent with recommendations in the guidelines

41-1. **The answer is A.** (*Hurst's The Heart, 14th Edition, Chap. 41*) While some pharmacodynamic studies have suggested high-dose aspirin (eg, 325 mg) may be associated with enhanced antithrombotic effects as a result of COX-1–independent mechanisms, these pharmacodynamic observations do not appear to translate into improved clinical outcomes, and when given in combination with clopidogrel, the maintenance dose of aspirin should generally be lowered to 75 to 100 mg. This is based on a post hoc analysis of data from the CURE[1] (Clopidogrel in Unstable Angina to Prevent Recurrent Events) study in which similar efficacy but less major bleeding was seen in the low-dose (< 100 mg) aspirin group (option B is incorrect). Furthermore, a large-scale prospective randomized study to compare high- versus low-dose aspirin, the CURRENT/OASIS-7 (Clopidogrel Optimal Loading Dose Usage to Reduce Recurrent Events—Organization to Assess Strategies in Ischemic Syndromes)[2] trial did not show a benefit to higher dose (300 to 325 mg) versus lower dose (75 to 100 mg) daily aspirin (option C is incorrect). Finally, the introduction into clinical practice of newer-generation oral P2Y$_{12}$ receptor inhibitors (prasugrel and ticagrelor) that are characterized by greater potency than clopidogrel and are used in combination with aspirin has also led to questions about the optimal dose of aspirin in these patients. Although aspirin dosing did not affect the safety and efficacy profile of patients treated with prasugrel in the TRITON (Trial to Assess Improvement in Therapeutic Outcomes by Optimizing Platelet Inhibition with Prasugrel) study, a higher dose of aspirin ($\geq$ 300 mg) was associated with reduced efficacy, albeit with no differences in bleeding, in patients treated with ticagrelor in the PLATO (Platelet Inhibition and Outcomes) trial[3] (option D is incorrect).

41-2. **The answer is C.** (*Hurst's The Heart, 14th Edition, Chap. 41*) The cyclooxygenase (COX) isozymes catalyze the conversion of arachidonic acid to prostaglandin H$_2$, an unstable intermediate that is the substrate for multiple downstream isomerases that lead to the generation of several prostanoids, including TXA$_2$ and prostacyclin (PGI$_2$). Thromboxane A$_2$ plays roles in platelet aggregation, vasoconstriction, the proliferation of vascular smooth-muscle cells, and the acceleration of atherosclerosis (options A, B, D, and E are incorrect). Conversely, prostacyclin plays a role in regulating renal blood flow, and it functions as a platelet inhibitor and a vasodilator. Only COX-1 is expressed in mature platelets. Importantly, TXA$_2$ (an amplifier of platelet activation and a vasoconstrictor) is derived largely from COX-1 (mostly from platelets), and its biosynthesis is highly sensitive to inhibition by aspirin, whereas vascular PGI$_2$ (a platelet inhibitor and a vasodilator) is derived predominantly from COX-2 and is less susceptible to inhibition by low doses of aspirin. Therefore, low-dose aspirin ultimately preferentially blocks platelet formation of TXA$_2$, diminishing platelet aggregation mediated by thromboxane (TP) receptor pathways.

41-3. **The answer is D.** (*Hurst's The Heart, 14th Edition, Chap. 41*) In patients taking a thienopyridine in whom CABG is planned and can be delayed, it is recommended that the drug be discontinued to allow for dissipation of the antiplatelet effect. The period of withdrawal should be at least 5 days in patients receiving clopidogrel. Clopidogrel is approved for the treatment and prevention of secondary atherothrombotic events across the spectrum of patients with ACS, irrespective of the treatment strategy (invasive or noninvasive; option A is incorrect). This recommendation is independent of whether patients are revascularized or not (ie, medical management) and irrespective of strategy for those undergoing PCI (ie, similar for bare metal stent [BMS], drug-eluting stent [DES], or balloon angioplasty). Clopidogrel is also the only oral P2Y$_{12}$ receptor inhibitor approved for patients with stable CAD undergoing PCI. The recommended loading dose of clopidogrel is 300 to 600 mg. However, in the setting of PCI, a 600-mg loading dose is most commonly used. A 300-mg loading dose of clopidogrel, in addition to aspirin, should also be given in patients under age 75 with STEMI treated with fibrinolytic therapy; patients 75 or older treated with fibrinolytic therapy should be treated with clopidogrel 75 mg (without a loading dose; option B is incorrect). After loading dose administration, a maintenance dose of 75 mg daily should be initiated. No dosage adjustment is necessary for patients with renal impairment, including patients with end-stage renal disease (option D is incorrect). Clopidogrel is an inactive prodrug that requires oxidation by the CYP system to generate an active metabolite (option E is incorrect).

41-4. **The answer is D.** (*Hurst's The Heart, 14th Edition, Chap. 41*) Glycoprotein IIb/IIIa inhibitors (GPIs) have been shown to reduce major adverse cardiac events (death, MI, and urgent revascularization) by 35% to 50% in patients undergoing PCI. However, their broad use has been limited because they are associated with an increased risk of bleeding complications. Moreover, their use has declined in recent years because of treatment alternatives, such as bivalirudin, associated with a more favorable safety profile (ie, less bleeding) as well as the introduction of potent $P2Y_{12}$ receptor inhibitors. Cangrelor is an intravenous adenosine triphosphate (ATP) analog (option A is incorrect). Due to structural modifications, cangrelor has high affinity for the $P2Y_{12}$ receptor and a higher resistance to ectonucleotidases, does not require hepatic conversion, and is directly active (option B is incorrect). Cangrelor was approved by the FDA in 2015 as an adjunct to PCI for reducing the risk of periprocedural MI, repeat coronary revascularization, and stent thrombosis in patients who have not been treated with a $P2Y_{12}$ platelet receptor inhibitor and are not being given a GPI (option C is incorrect).

Acute coronary syndrome trials tended to report higher incidence of thrombocytopenia among patients treated with abciximab compared with PCI trials (option E is incorrect). Some of this risk may by mediated by the need for longer heparin infusions and an increased risk of heparin-induced thrombocytopenia (HIT). Eptifibatide or tirofiban does not appear to increase mild or severe thrombocytopenia compared with placebo. Severe and profound (< 20,000) thrombocytopenia is more commonly associated with abciximab use and requires immediate cessation of therapy. Pseudothrombocytopenia secondary to platelet clumping and HIT needs to be ruled out. The platelet count returns to normal within 48 to 72 hours in most cases.

41-5. **The answer is A.** (*Hurst's The Heart, 14th Edition, Chap. 41*) In the absence of contraindications, fibrinolytic therapy should be administered to patients with STEMI at non–PCI-capable hospitals when the anticipated FMC-to-device time at a PCI-capable hospital exceeds 120 minutes because of unavoidable delays. The remainder of the statements provided are correct (options B through E are incorrect).

41-6. **The answer is C.** (*Hurst's The Heart, 14th Edition, Chap. 41*) Enteric-coated aspirin delays absorption, with peak plasma levels at 3 to 4 hours, as opposed to 30 to 40 minutes for non-enteric coated (option A is incorrect). Aspirin is rapidly absorbed in the upper gastrointestinal tract and is associated with measurable platelet inhibition within 60 minutes (option B is incorrect). Because the blockade of COX-1 induced by aspirin is irreversible, COX-mediated TXA_2 synthesis is prevented for the entire life span of the platelet (about 7 to 10 days; option D is incorrect). Therefore, even low doses of aspirin can produce long-lasting platelet inhibition. Higher doses of aspirin are needed to inhibit COX-2 than to inhibit COX-1 (option E is incorrect). These differences explain why very high doses of aspirin are needed to achieve anti-inflammatory and analgesic effects, whereas low doses of aspirin lead to antiplatelet effects.

41-7. **The answer is C.** (*Hurst's The Heart, 14th Edition, Chap. 41*) Ischemic stroke within the past 3 months is an absolute contraindication to fibrinolytic therapy; ischemic stroke > 3 months prior is a relative contraindication only. The remainder of the options provided are absolute contraindications to fibrinolytic therapy (options A, B, D, and E are incorrect). In addition to ischemic stroke > 3 months prior, other relative contraindications include: systolic blood pressure > 180 or diastolic blood pressure > 110 mm Hg, recent bleeding (nonintracranial), recent surgery, recent invasive procedure, anticoagulation (eg, vitamin K therapy), traumatic or prolonged cardiopulmonary resuscitation, pericarditis or pericardial fluid, and diabetic retinopathy, among others.

41-8. **The answer is E.** (*Hurst's The Heart, 14th Edition, Chap. 41*) Anticoagulants act by antagonizing or synergizing various factors along the clotting cascade (Figure 41-1).

Coagulation cascade and site of action of various anticoagulants

Exposed tissue factor from vascular injury binds to circulating activated factor VII to form the extrinsic tenase complex. This complex is a potent activator of factors IX and X.

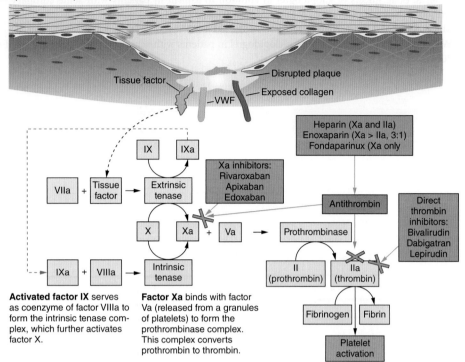

Activated factor IX serves as coenzyme of factor VIIIa to form the intrinsic tenase complex, which further activates factor X.

Factor Xa binds with factor Va (released from a granules of platelets) to form the prothrombinase complex. This complex converts prothrombin to thrombin.

Thrombin is a powerful stimulant of platelet activator (via PAR 1), further propagating the platelet plug. It also converts soluble fibrinogen to insoluble fibrin, leading to clot formation, and it activates factor XIII, leading to cross-linking of fibrin and further stabilization of the clot.

FIGURE 41-1 Coagulation cascade and site of action of various anticoagulants. Exposed tissue factor from vascular injury binds to circulating activated factor VII to form the extrinsic tenase complex. This complex is a potent activator of factors IX and X. Activated factor IX serves as a coenzyme of factor VIIIa to form the intrinsic tenase complex, which further activates factor X. Factor Xa binds with factor Va (released from a granules of platelets) to form the prothrombinase complex. This complex converts prothrombin to thrombin. Thrombin is a powerful stimulant of platelet activator, further propagating the platelet plug. It also converts soluble fibrinogen to insoluble fibrin, leading to clot formation, and it activates factor XIII, leading to cross-linking of fibrin and further stabilization of the clot.
(Reprinted with permission from Singh D, Gupta K, Vacek JL. Anticoagulation and antiplatelet therapy in acute coronary syndromes, *Cleve Clin J Med*. 2014 Feb;81(2):103-114. Copyright © 2014 Cleveland Clinic. All rights reserved.)

Exposed tissue factor from vascular injury binds to circulating activated factor VII to form the extrinsic tenase complex. This complex is a potent activator of factors IX and X. Activated factor IX serves as a coenzyme of factor VIIIa to form the intrinsic tenase complex, which further activates factor X. Factor Xa binds with factor Va (released from granules of platelets) to form the prothrombinase complex. This complex converts prothrombin to thrombin. Thrombin is a powerful stimulant of platelet activator, further propagating the platelet plug. It also converts soluble fibrinogen to insoluble fibrin, leading to clot formation, and it activates factor XIII, leading to cross-linking of fibrin and further stabilization of the clot. Factor Xa is antagonized either directly (rivaroxaban, apixaban, or edoxaban; option D is incorrect) or indirectly by agents that synergize antithrombin (unfractionated heparin, enoxaparin, and fondaparinux; options A through C are incorrect). Conversely, direct thrombin inhibitors, including bivalirudin, dabigatran, and lepirudin act to block thrombin (factor IIa) directly.

41-9. **The answer is E.** *(Hurst's The Heart, 14th Edition, Chap. 41)* All of the options above are consistent with American College of Cardiology Foundation/American Heart Association recommendations as of 2017 (options A through D are incorrect).

271

References

1. Yusuf S, et al. Effects of Clopidogrel in addition to aspirin in patients with acute coronary syndromes without ST-segment elevation. *N Engl J Med*. 2001;345(7):494-502.
2. Metha SR, et al. *Lancet*. 2010 Oct 9;376(9748):1233-1243.
3. Wallentin L, et al. Ticagrelor versus clopidogrel in patients with acute coronary syndromes. *N Engl J Med*. 2009;361(11):1045-1057.

CHAPTER 42

Percutaneous Coronary Interventions in Acute Myocardial Infarction and Acute Coronary Syndromes

Patrick R. Lawler

QUESTIONS

DIRECTIONS: Choose the one best response to each question.

42-1. Which of the following is *not* an advantage of primary percutaneous coronary intervention (PCI) over fibrinolytic therapy for ST-segment elevation myocardial infarction (STEMI)?

A. Primary PCI is associated with a reduced incidence of intracranial hemorrhage
B. Primary PCI is superior in reducing short-term mortality
C. Primary PCI has a lower overall risk of major bleeding
D. Primary PCI is associated with fewer nonfatal reinfarctions
E. All of the above are correct

42-2. A 58-year-old man begins to experience chest pain that radiates to his left arm while jogging. He initially dismisses the symptoms and is admitted to the emergency department 6 hours later with an anterior myocardial infarction (MI) confirmed by ECG. Which of the following may be associated with smaller infarct size?

A. TIMI grade 1 flow in the infarct artery
B. Remote ischemic conditioning
C. Anterior MI location
D. Reperfusion with PCI at 6 hours
E. None of the above

42-3. A 64-year-old woman with long-standing hypertension is admitted to the hospital with an anterior myocardial infaction. She is promptly reperfused by primary PCI, including stenting of the left anterior descending coronary artery. Which of the following are associated with reduced infarct size?

A. Baseline TIMI grade 3 flow
B. Total ischemia time < 3 hours
C. Nonanterior MI location
D. Remote ischemic conditioning
E. All of the above

42-4. A 54-year-old woman presents with an anterior STEMI. Which of the following is *not true* about ticagrelor administration in this patient?

A. Ticagrelor is an oral P2Y$_{12}$ inihbitor
B. Ticagrelor is not inferior to clopidogrel in the treatment of patients with STEMI
C. The rates of stent thrombosis are similar with ticagrelor and clopidogrel
D. Crushed oral ticagrelor can increase the time to onset of platelet inhibition
E. Dyspnea is a frequent reason for switching from ticagrelor to clopidogrel

42-5. A 48-year-old man presents with an anterior MI and is found to have complete occlusion of the left anterior descending (LAD) artery, as well as an 80% stenosis in the mid-right coronary artery. He is hemodynamically stable and chest pain free following PCI of the LAD. Which of the following is *correct* about the treatment of multivessel disease?

A. PCI of the infarct artery only has better clinical outcomes than multivessel PCI
B. Primary angioplasty of stenosed vessels with normal blood flow is associated with worse survival
C. Multivessel PCI is associated with increased cardiac mortality
D. Mutivessel PCI in the setting of MI is associated with decreased major adverse cardiovascular events
E. All of the above

42-6. Which of the following is *incorrect* regarding adjunctive thrombectomy methods?

A. Adjunctive aspiration thrombectomy enhances angiographic blush scores and ST-segment resolution

B. Routine thrombectomy before or after stent implantation enhances outcomes for all thrombi sizes

C. There is no benefit to the routine use of rheolytic thrombectomy with primary PCI for STEMI

D. It is reasonable to consider adjunctive thrombectomy in all patients with angiographically large thrombus burden before primary PCI

E. None of the above are incorrect

42-7. Which of the following constitutes a *correct* sequence of events following the arrival of a STEMI patient to the hospital?

A. 12-lead ECG, heparin and $P2Y_{12}$ inhibitor administration, transfer to catheterization lab, revascularization with DES, aspirin treatment indefinitely

B. 12-lead ECG, discontinue anticoagulation, transfer to catheterization lab, routine thrombectomy and PCI, aspirin treatment indefinitely

C. Remote ischemic conditioning, 12-lead ECG, transfer to catheterization lab, revascularization with DES, aspirin treatment indefinitely

D. 12-lead ECG, transfer to catheterization lab, revascularization with DES, heparin and $P2Y_{12}$ administration

E. None of the above are correct

42-8. A 44-year-old man presents to the hospital with ongoing acute chest pain and ST depressions on ECG. He has elevated troponin and a history of coronary artery disease. Which treatment is most appropriate for this patient?

A. "Cool off" the acute thrombotic lesion with antiplatelet and anticoagulant agents for a few days

B. Coronary angiography performed the next working day

C. Immediate Coronary angiography

D. Noninvasive stress testing when troponin is down-trending

E. None of the above

42-9. A 53-year-old woman is admitted with acute chest pain and ECG signs of non–ST-segment elevation MI. Revascularization the following morning is planned. Which of the following adjunctive pharmacological strategies is *incorrect*?

A. Pre-PCI treatment with clopidogrel

B. Aspirin loading dose of 300 to 325 mg

C. Subcutaneous injection of low-molecular-weight heparin

D. Pre-PCI treatment with prasugrel

E. All of the above

42-10. A 70-year-old man is brought to the emergency department with acute chest pain, ST-segment depressions on ECG, and sinus bradycardia. Which adjunctive therapy is *not* appropriate in this patient?

A. IV nitroglycerin

B. Beta-blockers

C. Statin

D. Oxygen therapy

E. Dual antiplatelet therapy

42-1. The answer is C. *(Hurst's The Heart, 14th Edition, Chap. 42)* Over the past 40 years, improvements in the design and development of highly effective antithrombotic and anti-platelet therapy have made PCI a widely used revascularization strategy. This technique gained particular success as it became apparent that a severe residual stenosis persisted in most patients after successful fibrinolysis treatment. A meta-analysis of 23 randomized trials incorporating 7739 patients compared primary PCI with fibrinolytic therapy for STEMI.[1] Primary PCI was superior to fibrinolytic therapy in reducing short-term mortality (option B), nonfatal reinfarction (option D), stroke, and the composite end point of death, nonfatal reinfarction, and stroke. These results were maintained at long-term follow-up and were independent of the type of thrombolytic agent used (streptokinase vs fibrin-specific thrombolytics) and whether patients were directly admitted or transferred emergently for primary PCI. The incidence of intracranial hemorrhage was significantly less with primary PCI (option A), although the overall risk of major bleeding (mostly related to access site bleeding) was not lower with primary PCI (option C).

42-2. The answer is B. *(Hurst's The Heart, 14th Edition, Chap. 42)* Once consensus was reached that primary PCI is the superior reperfusion modality, attention turned to limiting infarction size. The last decade has seen many pharmacologic and mechanical strategies to limit infarct size, which are summarized in Table 42-1. Achieving TIMI grade 3 flow has a major impact on short- and long-term mortality. Indeed, there appears to be an inverse relationship between the ability to achieve TIMI grade 3 flow and short-term mortality with either reperfusion strategy (option A). Infarctions involving the LAD artery tend to be larger than left circumflex or right coronary artery infarcts (option C). Symptom onset to balloon time was critically important at up to 3 hours of symptom duration. After 3 hours, MI size did not appear to vary with prolonged times to reperfusion (option D). Experimental models suggest that remote ischemic conditioning, such as transient intermittent limb ischemia, may reduce myocardial infarct size in ischemia-reperfusion models (option B); studies are ongoing.

TABLE 42-1 **Infarct Size Reduction.**

Proven
1. Baseline TIMI grade 3 flow
2. Total ischemia time < 3 hours
3. Nonanterior MI location
4. Remote ischemic conditioning
Potentially useful in anterior STEMI
1. IV metoprolol
2. SSA O$_2$
3. IV adenosine (high dose, early treatment)
4. Hypothermia
Ongoing trials
1. LV unloading
2. Steroids
3. Colchicine

Methods or factors associated with small final infarction size are tabulated. Remote ischemic conditioning is the only therapy to appear to decrease MI size and provide lasting clinical benefit.

Abbreviations: IV, intravenous; LV, left ventricular; MI, myocardial infarction; SSA O$_2$, hyperoxemic oxygen therapy; STEMI, ST-segment elevation myocardial infarction; TIMI, thrombolysis in myocardial infarction.

42-3. The answer is E. *(Hurst's The Heart, 14th Edition, Chap. 42)* In addition to proven approaches to reducing infarct size (options A–D), several experimental approaches are currently under development, such as methods to decrease reperfusion injury.[2] Reperfusion injury refers to damage to the myocardial tissue caused when blood supply returns to the tissues after a period of ischemia. In this situation, the restoration of flow results in inflammation and oxidative stress damage. Adenosine can potentially reduce reperfusion injury by suppressing free radical formation and by preventing neutrophil activation. Intracoronary administration of supersaturated oxygen with an arterial oxygen partial pressure of 760 to 1000 mm Hg has been tested in two clinical trials.[3,4] Patients with anterior MI who were treated with less than 6 hours of symptom duration or a 90-minute selective intracoronary infusion of supersaturated oxygen after PCI had a reduction in infarct size. In addition, many experimental studies have documented the effectiveness of systemic hypothermia, initiated before reperfusion, in reducing infarct size. More recently, two small trials have pooled results and demonstrated a reduction of infarct size and a decrease in heart failure for anterior MI. Finally, IV metoprolol has been shown to reduce infarct size in patients with anterior MI presenting < 6 hours after symptom onset, although currently due to the findings from the COMMIT-CCS2 trial, its routine use in STEMI is not recommended.

42-4. **The answer is A.** (*Hurst's The Heart, 14th Edition, Chap. 42*) Ticagrelor is a rapid oral $P2Y_{12}$ inhibitor (option A). Oral ticagrelor has been compared to clopidogrel in the PLATO (Platelet Inhibition and Patient Outcomes) trial. A total of 18,624 patients with AMI and ACS PCI were randomized to clopidogrel 300 mg or ticagrelor 90 mg loading dose and subsequent therapy of 90 mg twice a day. A total of 7008 patients (37%) were undergoing STEMI intervention. The ticagrelor group had a lower event rate (9.8% vs 11.7%; $P < .0001$; option B). Stent thrombosis was decreased from 3.8% to 2.9% ($P = .01$; option C). An even more rapid onset of platelet inhibition can be achieved by crushing the ticagrelor tablet for oral administration (option D). Time to maximal plasma concentration decreased from 4 to 2 hours, and substantial platelet inhibition occurred within 1 hour of oral administration. Dyspnea is a potential complication of ticagrelor, potentially due to its effects on adenosine reuptake, but this side effect is usually self-limited (option E).

42-5. **The answer is D.** (*Hurst's The Heart, 14th Edition, Chap. 42*) In initial trials of primary PCTA, plaque dissection and intraluminal thrombosis were difficult to treat with balloon angioplasty and heparin alone. Reocclusion of the infarct-related artery occurred in 5% to 15% of cases and worsened survival. In this context, treating non-culprit stenoses with normal blood flow was considered harmful, and thus the practice of primary angioplasty evolved with treatment of the infarct artery only. However, as antithrombotic, antiplatelet, and coronary stenting improved, the issue of complete revascularization was again raised. Three recently performed well-done randomized trials[6-8] demonstrated that the primary end point of death, recurrent MI, or refractory angina was lower in the multivessel PCI group (option A). Cardiac mortality was also lower (option C). They also showed that major adverse cardiovascular events (MACEs) were lower in patients assigned to multivessel PCI (option D) and that on a background of high usage of $P2Y_{12}$ inhibitors, multivessel PCI is safe and is associated with improved clinical outcomes compared with culprit-only revascularization.

42-6. **The answer is B.** (*Hurst's The Heart, 14th Edition, Chap. 42*) Primary PCI is effective in restoring normal epicardial coronary flow (TIMI grade 3 flow) in more than 90% of patients with STEMI, but more than half of these patients will have suboptimal flow at the tissue level, as evidenced by poor angiographic blush scores or lack of complete ECG ST-segment resolution. The AIMI (rheolytic thrombectomy) study investigators demonstrated that there is no indication for the routine use of rheolytic thrombectomy with primary PCI for STEMI (option C). However, patients with large thrombus burden often have distal macroembolization, and studies have shown that macroembolization is harmful and leads to impaired myocardial reperfusion and worse clinical outcomes. Therefore, it may be reasonable to consider adjunctive thrombectomy in patients with angiographically large thrombus burden before primary PCI (option D). In another trial involving 1071 patients with STEMI, adjunctive aspiration resulted in enhanced rates of normal angiographic myocardial perfusion (blush) and ST-segment resolution (option A). However, the initial enthusiasm for routine use of aspiration thrombectomy has been dramatically tempered by findings that rates of mortality, TVR, recurrent MI, and stent thrombosis were the same for thrombectomy and primary PCI patients. Only stroke was different and higher in the thrombectomy patients. Thus, routine thrombectomy does not enhance outcomes and should be reserved for large thrombus burden before or after stent implantation (option B).

42-7. **The answer is A.** *(Hurst's The Heart, 14th Edition, Chap. 42)* Regardless of mode of presentation, rapid performance and competent analysis of the 12-lead ECG are the first steps. Skilled reading either on site or by transmission is essential so that "false activations" can be limited. Once a firm diagnosis of STEMI is made, activation of the STEMI team and transport to the catheterization lab are essential. A heparin bolus and a $P2Y_{12}$ inhibitor should be rapidly administered. If logistically feasible, consideration should be given to remote ischemic conditioning while en route to the catheterization lab. Once the infarct artery is identified, intracoronary abciximab may be considered if not already administered. Routine thrombectomy is not useful, but if extensive clot burden exists, it will prevent extensive macroembolization. The use of DESs should be routine. Proper sizing and proper stent opposition are essential to prevent stent thrombosis, and intravascular ultrasound-guided implantation should be strongly considered. After the procedure, anticoagulation is discontinued unless there are other reasons to resume it. All patients without contraindications should be treated with aspirin indefinitely following PCI. The correct sequence of events is therefore described in option A.

42-8. **The answer is C.** *(Hurst's The Heart, 14th Edition, Chap. 42)* Most patients with non–ST-segment elevation (NSTE)-ACS in the United States undergo cardiac catheterization. The evidence for invasive management is based on several randomized trials that showed improvement in MACE, improved symptoms, improved quality of life, and reduction in readmission. The benefits were greater in patients with higher risk (ie, elevated biomarker, ST-segment changes, higher TIMI or GRACE risk scores).[9] The timing of catheterization has been evaluated in randomized and observational trials. Initially, it was thought that it may be beneficial to "cool off" an ulcerated thrombotic lesion with antiplatelet and anticoagulant agents for a few days (option A). However studies found that earlier intervention is better, particularly in higher-risk patients (option C). Early catheterization was also associated with a reduction in death or large MI at 30 days (option B), and studies consistently favor early invasive strategies over conservative strategies in high-risk patients (option D). In this patient, the presence of ongoing chest pain and the absence of contraindications call for immediate angiography.

42-9. **The answer is D.** *(Hurst's The Heart, 14th Edition, Chap. 42)* The primary goal of pharmacotherapy for NSTE-ACS is to alleviate ischemia using antiplatelets, antithrombotics, and adjunctive therapies to reduce myocardial oxygen demand. Pharmacotherapy in NSTE-ACS is crucial for management because a substantial portion of patients will not immediately undergo coronary angiography and/or revascularization. Evidence-based guidelines universally advocate that patients with NSTE-ACS should routinely and indefinitely receive low-dose (75 to 100 mg) non–enteric-coated aspirin, after an initial loading dose of 300 to 325 mg (option B). Aspirin is routinely given to all patients with CAD, and it is assumed to equally benefit those undergoing and not undergoing an invasive management strategy.[10,11] The administration of clopidogrel prior to PCI is known to improve outcomes (option A). A study revealed that patients who received pre-PCI treatment with clopidogrel had reduced cardiovascular death, MI, and stent thrombosis when compared with placebo.[12] This can be explained by clopidogrel's slow onset, which is circumvented by early administration. In another trial, pretreatment with prasugrel did not decrease ischemic complications when compared with administration at the time of PCI and was associated with a higher risk for major bleeding.[13] Prasugrel has a very fast onset, thereby rendering pretreatment unnecessary; clinical trials therefore examined its efficacy by administering it at the time of coronary angiography (option D). Finally, anticoagulation is recommended for all NSTE-ACS patients undergoing PCI at the time of diagnosis (class I practice guideline).[11] This is typically administered as an IV infusion of UFH or a subcutaneous injection of low-molecular-weight heparin, or in some countries as subcutaneous fondaparinux (option C).

42-10. The answer is B. (*Hurst's The Heart, 14th Edition, Chap. 42*) In addition to antiplatelets and antithrombotics, adjunctive therapy with oxygen (options D and E are incorrect) is empirically administered in all patients, and especially for patients with oxygen saturation < 90%. If patients are experiencing ischemic chest discomfort, sublingual or IV nitroglycerin can be used (option A is incorrect). Oral beta-blockade should be initiated within 24 hours to reduce heart rate, contractility, and blood pressure, as long as patients are not experiencing heart failure or low output, are at increased risk of cardiogenic shock, or have other contraindications to beta-blockade such as bradycardia or wheezing (option B is correct).[14] Nondihydropyridine calcium channel blockers can be administered to reduce myocardial oxygen demand if beta-blockers are contraindicated, but they would not be indicated here due to bradycardia. Lastly, high-intensity statin therapy (option C is incorrect) should be administered as soon as possible in patients presenting with NSTE-ACS because it has been associated with reduced rates of recurrent MI, coronary heart disease mortality, need for revascularization, and stroke.[15]

References

1. Keeley EC, Boura JA, Grines CL. Primary angioplasty vs. intravenous thrombolytic therapy for acute myocardial infarction, a quantitative review of 23 randomized trials. *Lancet*. 2003;361:13-20.

2. Hausenloy DJ, Yellon DM. Targeting myocardial reperfusion injury—the search continues. *N Engl J Med*. 2015;373:1073-1075.

3. O'Neill WW, Martin JL, Dixon SR, et al. Acute myocardial infarction with hyperoxemic therapy (AMIHOT): a prospective, randomized trial of intracoronary hyperoxemic reperfusion after percutaneous coronary intervention. *J Am Coll Cardiol*. 2007;50:397-405.

4. Stone GW, Martin JL, de Boer MJ, et al. Effect of supersaturated oxygen delivery on infarct size after percutaneous coronary intervention in acute myocardial infarction. *Circ Cardiovasc Interv*. 2009;2:366-375.

5. Stadius ML, Davis K, Maynard C, Ritchie JL, Kennedy JW. Risk stratification for 1 year survival based on characteristics identified in the early hours of acute myocardial infarction. The Western Washington Intracoronary Streptokinase Trial. *Circulation*. 1986;74:703-711.

6. Wald DS, Morris JK, Wald NJ, et al. Randomized trial of preventive angioplasty in myocardial infarction. *N Engl J Med*. 2013;369:1115-1123.

7. Gershlick AH, Khan JN, Kelly DJ, et al. Randomized trial of complete versus lesion- only revascularization in patients undergoing primary percutaneous coronary intervention for STEMI and multivessel disease: the CvLPRIT trial. *J Am Coll Cardiol*. 2015;65:963-972.

8. Engstrøm T, Kelbæk H, Helqvist S, et al. Complete revascularisation versus treatment of the culprit lesion only in patients with ST-segment elevation myocardial infarction and multivessel disease (DANAMI-3—PRIMULTI): an open-label, randomised controlled trial. *Lancet*. 2015;386:665-671.

9. Hansen KW, Sorensen R, Madsen M, et al. Effectiveness of an early versus a conservative invasive treatment strategy in acute coronary syndromes: a nationwide cohort study. *Ann Intern Med*. 2015;163:737-742.

10. Kolh P, Windecker S, Alfonso F, et al. 2014 ESC/EACTS guidelines on myocardial revascularization: The Task Force on Myocardial Revascularization of the European Society of Cardiology (ESC) and the European Association for Cardio-Thoracic Surgery (EACTS) developed with the special contribution of the European Association of Percutaneous Cardiovascular Interventions (EAPCI). *Eur J Cardiothorac Surg*. 2014;46(4):517-592.

11. Levine GN, Bates ER, Blankenship JC, et al. 2011 ACCF/AHA/SCAI guideline for percutaneous coronary intervention. A report of the American College of Cardiology Foundation/American Heart Association Task Force on Practice Guidelines and the Society for Cardiovascular Angiography and Interventions. *J Am Coll Cardiol*. 2011;58(24):e44-e122.

12. Mehta SR, Yusuf S, Peters RJG, et al. Effects of pretreatment with clopidogrel and aspirin followed by long-term therapy in patients undergoing percutaneous coronary intervention: the PCI-CURE study. *Lancet*. 2001;358(9281):527-533.

13. Montalescot G, Bolognese L, Dudek D, et al. Pretreatment with prasugrel in non-ST- segment elevation acute coronary syndromes. *N Engl J Med*. 2013;369(11):999-1010.

14. Amsterdam EA, Wenger NK, Brindis RG, et al. 2014 AHA/ACC guideline for the management of patients with non-ST-elevation acute coronary syndromes: a report of the American College of Cardiology/American Heart Association Task Force on Practice Guidelines. *J Am Coll Cardiol*. 2014;64(24): e139-e228.

15. Cannon CP, Braunwald E, McCabe CH, et al. Intensive versus moderate lipid lowering with statins after acute coronary syndromes. *N Engl J Med*. 2004;350(15):1495-1504.

CHAPTER 43

The Evaluation and Management of Stable Ischemic Heart Disease

Patrick R. Lawler

QUESTIONS

DIRECTIONS: Choose the one best response to each question.

43-1. A 65-year-old man with a history of obstructive coronary artery disease (CAD) is evaluated in your clinic. He complains that he develops chest pain walking approximately one city block and climbing one flight of stairs. Which of the following Canadian Cardiovascular Society (CCS) angina classes best describes the patient's symptoms?

A. CCS I
B. CCS II
C. CCS III
D. CCS IV
E. None of the above are correct

43-2. All of the following are criteria for defining vulnerable plaque *except*:

A. Active inflammation (eg, monocyte, macrophage, ± T-cell infiltration)
B. Thin cap with large lipid core
C. Endothelial denudation with superficial platelet aggregation
D. Fissured plaque
E. Luminal stenosis > 60%

43-3. A 64-year-old woman presents to your clinic with progressive exertional chest pressure over the past several months. All of the following are advantages of stress echocardiography over stress myocardial perfusion imaging *except*:

A. Higher specificity
B. Versatility; more extensive evaluation of cardiac anatomy and function

C. Greater convenience/efficacy/availability
D. Lower cost
E. Higher sensitivity, especially for single-vessel coronary disease involving the left circumflex artery

43-4. A 54-year-old woman is evaluated for chest pain and dyspnea with noninvasive testing. Which of the following is *not* considered a high-risk finding?

A. Severe resting LV dysfunction (LVEF < 35%) not readily explained by noncoronary causes
B. Resting perfusion abnormalities ≥ 10% of the myocardium in patients without prior history or evidence of MI
C. Stress ECG findings including ≥ 2 mm of ST-segment depression at low workload or persisting into recovery, exercise-induced ST-segment elevation, or exercise-induced VT/VF
D. Severe stress-induced LV dysfunction (peak exercise LVEF < 45% or drop in LVEF with stress ≥ 10%)
E. Stress-induced perfusion abnormalities encumbering 5% to 9.9% of the myocardium or stress segmental scores (in multiple segments) indicating one vascular territory with abnormalities but without LV dilation

43-5. A 56-year-old man undergoes coronary angiography and is found to have a 70% left main coronary artery (LMCA) stenosis. Which of the following factors would suggest similar efficacy between coronary stenting and coronary artery bypass surgery?

A. Comorbid diabetes mellitus
B. Additional lesions involving the right coronary artery
C. Left main stenosis involving calcified plaque at the bifurcation of the LAD and LCx arteries
D. Reduced ejection fraction
E. SYNTAX score of 20

43-6. All of the following are key angiographic features important for calculating the SYNTAX score *except*:

A. Right, left, or codominant coronary circulation
B. Number of atherosclerotic lesions
C. Number of artery segments involved per atherosclerotic lesion
D. Trifurcation lesion: number of vessel segments diseased
E. All of the above

43-7. Which of the following is *not true* about coronary calcium scoring?

A. Calcification observed on cardiac CT correlates inversely with the overall extent of CAD
B. The coronary artery calcification score is a quantitative measure of overall vascular calcium burden
C. Coronary calcium does not correlate with the degree of luminal obstruction
D. The overall burden may predict future coronary heart disease events
E. Serial screening of patients for progression of CAC is not recommended

43-8. Which of the following are core components of a cardiac rehabilitation/secondary prevention program?

A. Nutritional counseling
B. Blood pressure management
C. Tobacco cessation
D. Lipid management
E. All of the above

43-9. Which of the following is *incorrect* about patients with human immunodeficiency virus (HIV) and cardiac disease?

A. Highly active antiretroviral therapy (HAART) is considered a risk factor for CAD
B. Compared to HIV-negative patients, the prevalence of noncalcified coronary plaques is approximately threefold higher in HIV-positive patients on HAART therapy
C. The risk of incident MI is increased approximately fourfold among those with HIV
D. Lipodystrophy is unlikely to mediate the relationship between HIV and CAD
E. In selected HIV patients at elevated risk for cardiovascular disease, protease inhibitors may be inappropriate

43-10. A 70-year-old man with hypertension is seen in your clinic. Which of the following is *not true* about blood pressure control and the risk of cardiac events?

A. In patients with stable ischemic heart disease, hypertension is a risk factor for recurrent MI
B. In patients with diabetes, uncontrolled hypertension is a strong predictor of premature death, cardiovascular morbidity, and progressive nephropathy
C. Compared to a standard treatment goal SBP < 140 mm Hg, patients treated to intensive blood pressure targets (SBP < 120 mm Hg) have a lower risk for the combination of MI, other ACSs, stroke, HF, and death from cardiovascular causes
D. Blood pressure control in the elderly need not be as rigorous as in younger patients
E. Blood pressure control is an important preventive strategy for incident heart failure

43-1. The answer is C. *(Hurst's The Heart, 14th Edition, Chap. 43)* Canadian Cardiovascular Society (CCS) angina classification is described in Table 43-1. This patient's symptoms are most consistent with class III (option C).

TABLE 43-1 The Canadian Cardiovascular Society Angina Scale

I	II	III	IV
Ordinary physical activity does not cause angina including: Walking and climbing stairs	Slight limitation of ordinary activity including: Walking stairs rapidly Walking uphill Stair climbing after meals	Marked limitation of ordinary physical activity.	Inability to perform any physical activity without discomfort.
Angina occurs: Only with strenuous, rapid, or prolonged exertion at work or recreation	*Angina occurs:* A few hours after awakening Walking > 2 city blocks (level ground) Walking 1 flight of ordinary stairs at a normal pace	*Angina occurs:* Walking ≤ 1 city block (level ground) Climbing one flight of stairs under normal conditions and at a normal pace	*Angina occurs:* With minimal activity May be present at rest

Data from Campeau L. The Canadian Cardiovascular Society grading of stable angina pectoris after a quarter of a century of use, *Can J Cardiol.* 2002 Sep;18(9):941-944.

43-2. The answer is E. *(Hurst's The Heart, 14th Edition, Chap. 43)* Major criteria for the defining vulnerable plaque include options A through D.[1] Additionally, luminal stenosis > 90% is also a major criterion. Minor criteria include: superficial calcified nodule, glistening yellow appearance (pathologic diagnosis), intraplaque hemorrhage, outward remodeling, and endothelial dysfunction.

43-3. The answer is E. *(Hurst's The Heart, 14th Edition, Chap. 43)* Advantages of echocardiography (options A through D) are outlined. Conversely, advantages of stress myocardial perfusion imaging include: higher technical success rate; higher sensitivity, especially for single-vessel coronary disease involving the left circumflex artery (option E); better accuracy for evaluating possible ischemia when multiple resting left ventricular wall motion abnormalities are present; and more extensive published database, especially in the evaluation of the prognosis.[2]

43-4. The answer is E. *(Hurst's The Heart, 14th Edition, Chap. 43)* High-risk findings on noninvasive testing include options A through D, as well as: stress-induced perfusion abnormalities encumbering ≥ 10% myocardium or stress segmental scores indicating multiple vascular territories with abnormalities; stress-induced LV dilation; inducible wall motion abnormality (involving > 2 segments or 2 coronary beds); wall motion abnormality developing at a low dose of dobutamine (≤ 10 mg/kg/min) or at a low heart rate (< 1 20 beats/min); coronary artery calcium score > 400 Agatston units; and multivessel obstructive CAD (≥ 70% stenosis) or left main stenosis (≥ 50% stenosis) on coronary CT angiography (Table 43-2). Other features are considered low risk, or moderate risk, such as stress-induced perfusion abnormalities encumbering 5% to 9.9% of the myocardium or stress segmental scores (in multiple segments) indicating one vascular territory with abnormalities but without LV dilation (option E).

TABLE 43-2 Noninvasive Risk Stratification of Coronary Artery Disease

High risk (> 3% annual death or MI)

1. Severe resting LV dysfunction (LVEF < 35%) not readily explained by noncoronary causes
2. Resting perfusion abnormalities ≥ 10% of the myocardium in patients without prior history or evidence of MI
3. Stress ECG findings including ≥ 2 mm of ST-segment depression at low workload or persisting into recovery, exercise-included ST-segment elevation, or exercise-induced VT/VF
4. Severe stress-induced LV dysfunction (peak exercise LVEF < 45% or drop in LVEF with stress ≥ 10%)
5. Stress-induced perfusion abnormalities encumbering ≥ 10% myocardium or stress segmental scores indicating multiple vascular territories with abnormalities
6. Stress-induced LV dilation
7. Inducible wall motion abnormality (involving > 2 segments or 2 coronary beds)
8. Wall motion abnormality developing at low dose of dobutamine (≤ 10 mg/kg/min) or at a low heart rate (< 120 beats/min)
9. CAC score > 400 Agatston units
10. Multivessel obstructive CAD (≥ 70% stenosis) or left main stenosis (≥ 50% stenosis) on CCTA

Intermediate risk (1% to 3% annual death or MI)

1. Mild/moderate resting LV dysfunction (LVEF 35% to 49%) not readily explained by noncoronary causes
2. Resting perfusion abnormalities in 5% to 9.9% of the myocardium in patients without a history or prior evidence of MI
3. ≥ 1 mm of ST-segment depression occurring with exertional symptoms
4. Stress-induced perfusion abnormalities encumbering 5% to 9.9% of the myocardium or stress segmental scores (in multiple segments) indicating 1 vascular territory with abnormalities but without LV dilation
5. Small wall motion abnormality involving 1 to 2 segments and only 1 coronary bed
6. CAC score 100 to 399 Agatston units
7. One vessel CAD with ≥ 70% stenosis or moderate CAD stenosis (50% to 69% stenosis) in ≥ 2 arteries on CCTA

Low risk (< 1% annual death or MI)

1. Low-risk treadmill score (score ≥ 5) or no new ST segment changes or exercise-induced chest pain symptoms; when achieving maximal levels of exercise
2. Normal or small myocardial perfusion defect at rest or with stress encumbering < 5% of the myocardium*
3. Normal stress or no change of limited resting wall motion abnormalities during stress
4. CAC score < 100 Agaston units
5. No coronary stenosis > 50% on CCTA

Abbreviations: CAC, coronary artery calcium; CAD, coronary artery disease; CCTA, coronary computed tomography angiography; EEG, electrocardiogram; LV, left ventricular; LVEF, left ventricular ejection fraction; MI, myocardial infarction; VF, ventricular fibrillation; VT, ventricular tachycardia.
Reproduced with permission from Fihn SD, Gardin JM, Abrams J, et al. 2012 ACCF/AHA/ACP/AATS/ PCNA/ SCAI/STS Guidelines for the diagnosis and management of patients with stable ischemic heart disease: a report of the American College of Cardiology Foundation/American Heart Association Task Force on Practice Guidelines, and the American College of Physicians, American Association of Thoracic Surgery, Preventative Cardiovascular Nurses Association, Society of Cardiovascular Angiography and Interventions, and Society of Thoracic Surgeons, *J Am Coll Cardiol.* 2012 Dec 18;60(24):e44-e164.

43-5. The answer is E. *(Hurst's The Heart, 14th Edition, Chap. 43)* A number of factors are associated with benefit from coronary artery bypass over coronary stenting (options A through D). However, in individuals without such factors, and who have favorable anatomy (option E), disease involving the LMCA can be managed with coronary artery stenting or bypass with similar efficacy (Figure 43-1). Among the strengths of the SYNTAX trial was the use of a numerical score for the objective evaluation of coronary disease severity and the likelihood of revascularization success. The SYNTAX score is generated by summarizing various qualitative plaque features and stenosis locations, and it serves as an objective measure of coronary disease severity that can be used to stratify anticipated patient outcomes (see syntaxscore.com).[3] Patients with high (≥ 33) and intermediate (23–32) SYNTAX scores had lower rates of MACCEs with surgery compared with PCI out to 5 years (high SYNTAX score: 26.8% surgery versus 44.0% PCI; *P* < .0001; intermediate SYNTAX score: 25.8% surgery vs 36.0% PCI). Event rates were similar for patients with low SYNTAX scores (≤ 22). The trial also established that PCI is noninferior to bypass surgery for the treatment of left main CAD (31.0% MACCE rate in the CABG surgery group versus 36.9% in the PCI group; *P* = .12).

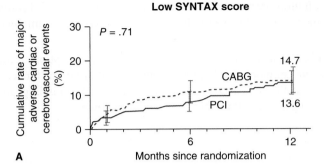

Low SYNTAX score

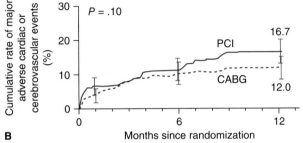

Intermediate SYNTAX score

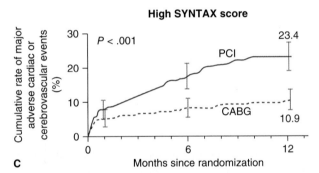

High SYNTAX score

FIGURE 43-1 SYNTAX score and benefit of revascularization strategy. The rates of major adverse cardiac or cerebrovascular events 12 months following therapy are reported for patients with low (A), intermediate (B), or high (C) SYNTAX score. The bars indicate 1.5 standard errors. Note the improved outcomes among patients with high SYNTAX scores who underwent revascularization. CABG, coronary artery bypass graft; PCI, percutaneous coronary intervention. (Reproduced with permission from Serruys PW, Morice MC, Kappetein AP, et al. Percutaneous coronary intervention versus coronary-artery bypass grafting for severe coronary artery disease, *N Engl J Med*. 2009 Mar 5;360(10):961-972.)

43-6. **The answer is E.** (*Hurst's The Heart, 14th Edition, Chap. 43*) The SYNTAX score can support decision making about the optimal strategy for revascularization of left main stenosis. Angiographic features that contribute to the score include options A through D, as well as: total occlusion (number of segments involved, age of total occlusion, presence of a blunt stump, presence of bridging collateral, antegrade versus retrograde filling of the first segment beyond the occlusion, side branch involvement); bifurcation lesion: angulation between the distal main vessel and the side branch < 70°; the presence of an aorto-ostial atherosclerotic lesion; the presence of severe vessel tortuosity at the lesion site; atherosclerotic lesion length > 20 mm; the presence of heavily calcified plaque; the presence of thrombus; and the presence of diffuse or small-vessel disease.

43-7. **The answer is A.** (*Hurst's The Heart, 14th Edition, Chap. 43*) Coronary artery calcification observed on cardiac CT correlates positively with the presence of established atherosclerosis (option A). The coronary artery calcification score is a quantitative measure of overall vascular calcium burden (option B). The presence of calcium in the vessel wall does not correlate with the degree of luminal obstruction (option C), although the overall burden may predict future coronary heart disease events (option D). Serial coronary artery calcification scoring to assess the rate of disease progression is not recommended (option E).

43-8. **The answer is E.** *(Hurst's The Heart, 14th Edition, Chap. 43)* Options A through D represent important, core components of optimal management programs for secondary prevention in those with established CAD. In addition, psychosocial counseling, physical activity, and exercise training are important and beneficial components.

43-9. **The answer is D.** *(Hurst's The Heart, 14th Edition, Chap. 43)* Patients infected with the HIV appear to be at increased risk for a wide range of inflammatory vascular diseases, including CAD. This may occur as a manifestation of HIV itself; low CD4$^+$ T-cell count has been associated with the presence of coronary artery stenotic lesions > 50% of the luminal diameter. Alternatively, CAD in HIV-infected persons could occur as a result of HAART use (option A). Compared to HIV-negative patients, the prevalence of non-calcified coronary plaques is approximately threefold higher in HIV-positive patients on HAART therapy (option B), which may account for parallel findings in similar patients suggesting that the risk of incident MI is increased approximately fourfold (option C). The mechanistic link between HAART and CAD remains speculative, but it may involve cross-reactivity between protease inhibitors and lipid metabolism–regulating proteins that results in dyslipidemia, insulin resistance, central adiposity, and lipodystrophy (option D). In selected HIV patients at elevated risk for cardiovascular disease, protease inhibitors may be inappropriate; under these circumstances, consultation with an infectious disease specialist to determine optimal HIV therapy is advised, as is the early institution of aggressive risk factor control (eg, statin therapy).

43-10. **The answer is D.** *(Hurst's The Heart, 14th Edition, Chap. 43)* Many observational studies have demonstrated a positive, continuous, and graded relationship between systemic blood pressure and cardiovascular disease risk. In patients with stable ischemic heart disease, hypertension is a risk factor for recurrent MI (option A), an observation that is likely a consequence of the associated endothelial dysfunction and the adverse effects of persistently elevated afterload on myocardial function and oxygen demand. In patients with diabetes, uncontrolled hypertension is a strong predictor of premature death, cardiovascular morbidity, and progressive nephropathy (option B). The Systolic Blood Pressure Intervention Trial (SPRINT) tested whether the conventional systolic blood pressure (SBP) goal of 140 mm Hg is sufficient to reduce cardiovascular events in nondiabetic, nonstroke patients at increased cardiovascular risk. Compared to a standard treatment goal SBP < 140 mm Hg, patients randomized to intensive therapy (SBP < 120 mm Hg) had lower risk for the composite end point of MI, other ACSs, stroke, HF, and death from cardiovascular causes at 1 year (HR, 0.75; 95% CI, 0.64–0.89; $P < .001$; option C). Directionally similar findings were observed for all-cause mortality, although the beneficial effects of intensive therapy were associated with an attendant increase in the number of medications prescribed, systemic hypotension, syncope, electrolyte abnormalities, and acute kidney injury. Studies have affirmed the benefit of treating hypertension in the elderly, although debate continues about the optimal targets and thresholds (option D). Blood pressure control is an important preventive strategy for incident heart failure (option E).

References

1. Naghavi M, Libby P, Falk E, et al. From vulnerable plaque to vulnerable patient. A call for new definitions and risk assessment strategies: part I. *Circulation*. 2003;108:1664-1672.
2. Gibbons RJ, et al. ACC/AHA/ACP-ASIM guidelines for the management of patients with chronic stable angina: a report of the American College of Cardiology/American Heart Association Task Force on Practice Guidelines (Committee on Management of Patients With Chronic Stable Angina). *J Am Coll Cardiol*. 1999;33(7):2092-2197.
3. Capodanno D, Capranzano P, Di Salvo ME, et al. Usefulness of SYNTAX score to select patients with left main coronary artery disease to be treated with coronary artery bypass graft. *JACC Cardiovasc Interv*. 2009;2:731-738.

CHAPTER 44

Coronary Artery Bypass Grafting and Percutaneous Interventions in Stable Ischemic Heart Disease

Patrick R. Lawler

QUESTIONS

DIRECTIONS: Choose the one best response to each question.

44-1. Which of the following findings on noninvasive testing should prompt referral of a patient for coronary angiography?

A. Exercise treadmill, > 2 mm of ST depression
B. Failure to increase systolic pressure to > 120 mm Hg or a sustained decrease of > 10 mm Hg during exercise
C. Resting perfusion abnormalities > 10% of the myocardium
D. Stress-induced left ventricular dilatation
E. All of the above

Questions 44-2, 44-3, and 44-4 relate to the following vignette:

A 55-year-old man with hypertension, dyslipidemia, and type II diabetes mellitus treated with subcutaneous insulin undergoes coronary angiography following a high-risk stress test with hypotensive blood pressure response. He is found to have proximal left anterior descending coronary artery (LAD) stenosis of 85%, as well as a 70% lesion in the mid-right coronary artery.

44-2. Which of the factors in this patient's history would favor referral for surgical revascularization?

A. A history of diabetes
B. The presence of two or more preexisting risk factors
C. Young age
D. SYNTAX score of 20
E. None of the above

44-3. In this patient, what benefits would be expected from surgical revascularization with coronary artery bypass grafting (CABG) versus percutaneous coronary intervention (PCI)?

A. Reduction in the composite end point of death, nonfatal myocardial infarction, and nonfatal stroke
B. Reduced all-cause mortality risk compared to PCI at 5 years
C. Reduction in the need for repeat revascularization
D. All of the above
E. None of the above

44-4. If this patient were to undergo surgical revascularization, which of the following would be true about the risk of stroke?

A. CABG and PCI are associated with similar risks of stroke
B. Higher stroke risk in patients undergoing CABG is evident only at 1 year follow-up
C. Previous stroke is a risk factor for CABG-related stroke in this population
D. Chronic renal failure is not related to long-term stroke risk in this population
E. The risk of stroke over longitudinal follow-up is five-fold higher in patients undergoing CABG compared with PCI in this population

Questions 44-5 and 44-6 relate to the following vignette:

A 76-year-old man with angina is found to have multivessel coronary artery disease (MV CAD) involving his proximal left anterior descending coronary artery (95%) as well as in an obtuse marginal branch from the left circumflex coronary artery (80%), and distal right coronary artery (75%). An echocardiogram demonstrates no valvular disease, but the left ventricular ejection fraction is 30%.

44-5. Which strategy represents the optimal approach to this patient's management?

A. Optimal medical therapy
B. CABG
C. Multivessel PCI
D. Durable left ventricular device consideration
E. Noninvasive ischemia testing to guide revascularization decisions

44-6. What is the optimal modality of viability testing to inform the decision to undertake surgical revascularization in this patient?

A. Single-photon emission computed tomography (SPECT)
B. Dobutamine stress echocardiography (DSE)
C. Thallium scan
D. Evidence of Q-waves on ECG
E. There is no certain, evidence-based role for viability testing in this setting

Questions 44-7, 44-8, and 44-9 relate to the following vignette:

A 55-year-old man without diabetes presents with typical angina symptoms and no prior history of coronary artery disease. Noninvasive stress testing is positive, and he is referred for coronary angiography, which demonstrates an 80% proximal LAD stenosis as well as a 90% mid-vessel stenosis in a dominant right coronary artery.

44-7. If there is uncertainty as to the hemodynamic significance of this patient's coronary stenoses, which of the following can be undertaken during the catheterization procedure to support a role for revascularization:

A. Fractional flow reserve (FFR) measurement
B. Optical coherence tomography (OCT)
C. Intravascular ultrasound (IVUS)
D. Noninvasive FFR by coronary CT
E. None of the above

44-8. In reviewing this patient's coronary angiogram, which of the following are important elements to ascertain when assessing the anatomic complexity of underlying coronary artery disease?

A. Number of lesions
B. Bifurcation types and angulation
C. Aorto-ostial lesions
D. Severe tortuosity
E. All of the above

44-9. Which of the following statements is true regarding a hybrid approach (percutaneous coronary intervention and surgical revascularization) to revascularization?

A. A hybrid approach is used commonly in all patients without diabetes mellitus where center of expertise is present
B. Insufficient data exist to strongly recommend hybrid revascularization
C. Hybrid approach is strongly preferred in this patient
D. PCI would be preferred in this patient
E. None of the above

44-10. In patients with ischemia identified on noninvasive stress testing, which of the following is true?

A. The role of PCI in the absence of uncontrolled symptoms is uncertain in such patients
B. PCI should be undertaken in all patients with documented ischemia and anatomically amenable disease
C. Optimal medical therapy (OMT) is usually ineffective at controlling angina symptoms
D. PCI is associated with improved mortality in patients with stable coronary artery disease
E. None of the above

44-1. The answer is E. (*Hurst's The Heart, 14th Edition, Chap. 44*) Patients referred for diagnostic noninvasive stress testing should be considered for coronary angiography in the presence of high-risk findings. A number of such factors are suggested (Table 44-1; options A through D are incorrect).

TABLE 44-1 Criteria for Referring Patients to Coronary Angiography

Exercise Treadmill
  Exercise treadmill, > 2 mm of ST depression;
  Exercise-induced ST-segment elevation;
  Exercise-induced ventricular tachycardia/ventricular fibrillation; and
  Failure to increase systolic pressure to > 120 mm Hg or a sustained decrease of > 10 mm Hg during exercise
Myocardial Perfusion Imaging
  Severe left ventricular dysfunction, not readily explained;
  Resting perfusion abnormalities > 10% of the myocardium;
  Severe stress-induced left ventricular dysfunction;
  Stress-induced perfusion abnormalities involving > 10% of the myocardium or stress and mental scores indicating multiple territories at risk;
  Stress-induced left ventricular dilatation; and
  Increased lung uptake.
Stress Echocardiography
  Inducible wall motion abnormalities involving > 2 segments or 2 coronary beds
Coronary Computed Tomography
  Multivessel obstructive coronary disease or left main stenosis

Modified with permission from Mancini GB, Gosselin G, Chow B, et al. Canadian Cardiovascular Society. Canadian Cardiovascular Society guidelines for the diagnosis and management of stable ischemic heart disease, *Can J Cardiol.* 2014 Aug;30(8):837-849.

44-2. The answer is A. (*Hurst's The Heart, 14th Edition, Chap. 44*) Patients with diabetes mellitus have consistently been found to have more favorable outcomes with surgical revascularization than with percutaneous revascularization (Figure 44-1).[1] This is true even among contemporary trials employing the use of drug-eluting stents. Other clinical variables (options B through E) in this patient would not have an obvious influence on preference for one modality of revascularization over another.

44-3. The answer is D. (*Hurst's The Heart, 14th Edition, Chap. 44*) The FREEDOM trial was designed to address the optimal coronary revascularization strategy in patients with diabetes and multivessel CAD in the absence of left main disease, prior CABG, prior stenting within 6 months, and current ST-segment elevation myocardial infarction.[2] In FREEDOM, the overall 5-year Kaplan-Meyer estimates of the primary composite end point of death, nonfatal myocardial infarction, and nonfatal stroke indicated a 26.6% event rate in the first-generation DES group compared to 18.7% in the CABG group (*P* < .005; option A alone is incorrect). Indeed, in FREEDOM, CABG was associated with a significantly reduced all-cause mortality risk compared to PCI at 5 years, and the mortality curves continued to diverge in favor of CABG throughout follow-up (option B alone is incorrect). The results of FREEDOM and subsequent meta-analyses lead to a Class I recommendation in the 2014 ACC/AHA guidelines stating that CABG was associated with improved survival in diabetics with multivessel CAD. This was upgraded from a Class II recommendation in 2012. CABG remains the revascularization treatment of choice for diabetic patients with multivessel disease. This is particularly true if a left internal mammary artery (LIMA) graft to the left anterior descending artery was performed. In general, the need for repeat revisualization is reduced with coronary artery bypass surgery versus PCI (option C alone is incorrect).

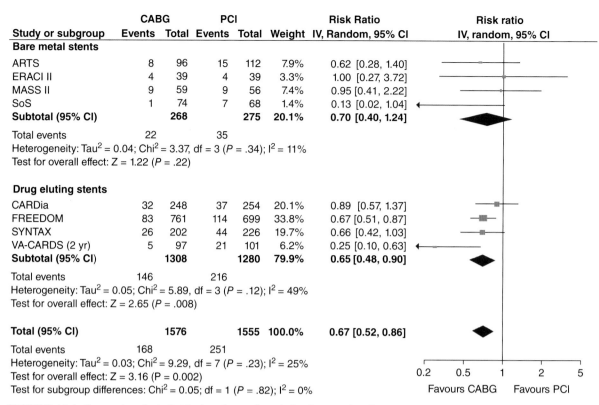

Study or subgroup	CABG Events	Total	PCI Events	Total	Weight	Risk Ratio IV, Random, 95% CI	Risk ratio IV, random, 95% CI
Bare metal stents							
ARTS	8	96	15	112	7.9%	0.62 [0.28, 1.40]	
ERACI II	4	39	4	39	3.3%	1.00 [0.27, 3.72]	
MASS II	9	59	9	56	7.4%	0.95 [0.41, 2.22]	
SoS	1	74	7	68	1.4%	0.13 [0.02, 1.04]	
Subtotal (95% CI)		**268**		**275**	**20.1%**	**0.70 [0.40, 1.24]**	
Total events	22		35				

Heterogeneity: Tau^2 = 0.04; Chi^2 = 3.37, df = 3 (P = .34); I^2 = 11%
Test for overall effect: Z = 1.22 (P = .22)

Study or subgroup	CABG Events	Total	PCI Events	Total	Weight	Risk Ratio IV, Random, 95% CI	Risk ratio IV, random, 95% CI
Drug eluting stents							
CARDia	32	248	37	254	20.1%	0.89 [0.57, 1.37]	
FREEDOM	83	761	114	699	33.8%	0.67 [0.51, 0.87]	
SYNTAX	26	202	44	226	19.7%	0.66 [0.42, 1.03]	
VA-CARDS (2 yr)	5	97	21	101	6.2%	0.25 [0.10, 0.63]	
Subtotal (95% CI)		**1308**		**1280**	**79.9%**	**0.65 [0.48, 0.90]**	
Total events	146		216				

Heterogeneity: Tau^2 = 0.05; Chi^2 = 5.89, df = 3 (P = .12); I^2 = 49%
Test for overall effect: Z = 2.65 (P = .008)

	CABG	Total	PCI	Total	Weight	Risk Ratio	
Total (95% CI)		**1576**		**1555**	**100.0%**	**0.67 [0.52, 0.86]**	
Total events	168		251				

Heterogeneity: Tau^2 = 0.03; Chi^2 = 9.29, df = 7 (P = .23); I^2 = 25%
Test for overall effect: Z = 3.16 (P = 0.002)
Test for subgroup differences: Chi^2 = 0.05; df = 1 (P = .82); I^2 = 0%

Favours CABG Favours PCI

FIGURE 44-1 Forest plots for individual studies and pooled risk ratios for all-cause mortality in randomized controlled trials comparing patients with diabetes and multivessel coronary artery disease who underwent coronary artery bypass grafting (CABG) versus percutaneous coronary intervention (PCI) after 5 years or the longest follow-up. CI, confidence interval. (Reproduced with permission from Verma S, Farkouh ME, Yanagawa B, et al. Comparison of coronary artery bypass surgery and percutaneous coronary intervention in patients with diabetes: a meta-analysis of randomised controlled trials, *Lancet Diabetes Endocrinol* 2013 Dec;1(4):317-328.)

44-4. The answer is C. *(Hurst's The Heart, 14th Edition, Chap. 44)* For patients with diabetes undergoing CABG in the FREEDOM trial, there was an excess of early stroke compared to PCI (option A is incorrect). The difference accrued mostly over the first 30 days after follow-up (option B is incorrect). In an analysis from the FREEDOM CABG cohort, predictors of early stroke included a prior history of stroke, the use of warfarin, and whether CABG was performed outside North America. In long-term follow-up, the strongest predictor of stroke was the presence of chronic renal insufficiency (option D is incorrect). Over 5 years of follow-up, CABG was still associated with a significantly higher stroke rate compared to PCI (5.2% vs 2.4%; *P* = .03; option E is incorrect).

44-5. The answer is B. *(Hurst's The Heart, 14th Edition, Chap. 44)* In the Surgical Treatment for Ischemic Heart Failure (STICH) study, patients with ischemic cardiomyopathy and an ejection fraction of 35% or less were randomly assigned to CABG versus OMT alone and followed for 9.8 years.[3] Although there was no significant difference between OMT alone and OMT plus CABG with respect to the primary end point (death from any cause), there were more cardiovascular deaths in the OMT group (297 deaths, 49.3%) compared to the CABG group (247 deaths, 40.5%; hazard ratio, 0.79; 95% CI, 0.66–0.93; *P* = .006; option A is incorrect). A 2009 meta-analysis has suggested that CABG is the preferred mode of revascularization in patients with left ventricular dysfunction (option C is incorrect),[4] although this analysis was largely limited to patients in the bare metal stent era. The patient does not currently have indications for durable LVAD consideration (option D is incorrect). Noninvasive, ischemia-guided revascularization decisions in patients with left ventricular systolic dysfunction have not been shown to improve outcomes (option E is incorrect).

44-6. **The answer is E.** *(Hurst's The Heart, 14th Edition, Chap. 44)* In a substudy of the STICH trial, among the 1212 patients enrolled in the overall randomized trial, 601 underwent viability assessment with SPECT or DSE.[5] Of these 601, 298 were randomly assigned to receive OMT plus CABG and 303 to receive OMT alone. There was no significant mortality interaction between viability status and treatment assignment ($P = 0.53$), suggesting that viability assessment did not identify patients with a differential survival benefit from CABG + OMT versus OMT alone. In all patients, while there was an unadjusted association between the presence of viable myocardium and mortality, this was no longer significant after adjusting for potential confounders. Thus, the role of viability testing across modalities (options A through D) remains uncertain in this population.

44-7. **The answer is A.** *(Hurst's The Heart, 14th Edition, Chap. 44)* The fractional flow reserve (FFR) is a lesion-specific index of stenosis severity defined as the ratio of maximum flow in the presence of stenosis to normal maximum flow. In practice, FFR is estimated as the ratio of coronary artery pressure distal to a lesion of interest to aortic pressure, averaged over the entire cardiac cycle, with variation in microvascular resistance minimized by pharmacologic induction of maximal hyperemia. FFR is useful to reclassify the functional severity of angiographically indeterminate coronary lesions and to define the utility of PCI. Evidence to date suggests that when a lesion is functionally significant, as defined by an FFR ≤ 0.80, revascularization may be beneficial. For example, in the FAME study, which randomized 1005 patients with multivessel CAD to PCI guided by angiography alone or angiography plus FFR, a strategy of FFR guidance was associated with a reduced rate of death, nonfatal myocardial infarction, and repeat revascularization at 1 year (13.2% vs 18.3%; $P = .02$) as well as a reduced usage of stents per patient (1.9 ± 1.3 vs 2.7 ± 1.2; $P < .001$).[6] In the FAME 2 trial, which randomized 888 patients with at least one functionally significant stenosis to PCI plus medical therapy or medical therapy alone, PCI conferred a significant reduction in death, nonfatal myocardial infarction, and urgent revascularization at 2 years.[7] Figure 44-2 depicts the overall decision making regarding revascularization in patients with stable ischemic heart disease, including the role of FFR.

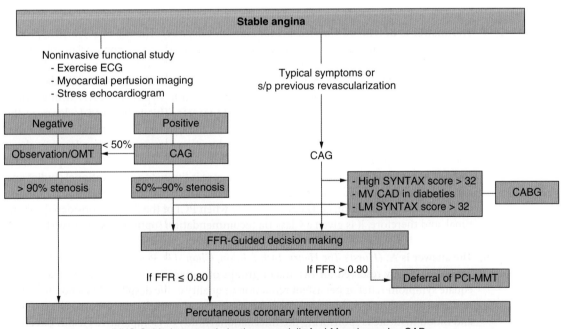

FIGURE 44-2 Proposed algorithm for assignment to revascularization in stable ischemic heart disease. CABG, coronary artery bypass grafting; CAG, coronary angiography; ECG, electrocardiogram; FFR, fractional flow reserve; IVUS, intravascular ultrasound; LM, left main; OMT, optimal medical therapy; MV CAD, multivessel coronary artery disease; PCI, percutaneous coronary intervention; SYNTAX, Synergy Between Percutaneous Coronary Intervention With Taxus and Cardiac Surgery.

TABLE 44-2 The SYNTAX Score Algorithm

1. Dominance
2. Number of lesions
3. Segments involved per lesion, with lesion characteristics
4. Total occlusions with subtotal occlusions:
   a. Number of segments
   b. Age of total occlusions
   c. Blunt stumps
   d. Bridging collaterals
   e. First segment beyond occlusion visible by antegrade or retrograde filling
   f. Side branch involvement
5. Trifurcation, number of segments diseased
6. Bifurcation type and angulation
7. Aorto-ostial lesion
8. Severe tortuosity
9. Lesion length
10. Heavy calcification
11. Thrombus
12. Diffuse disease, with number of segments

Adapted with permission from Sianos G, Morel MA, Kappetein AP, et al. The SYNTAX Score: an angiographic tool grading the complexity of coronary artery disease, *EuroIntervention*. 2005 Aug;1(2):219-227.

44-8. **The answer is E.** *(Hurst's The Heart, 14th Edition, Chap. 44)* The extent and complexity of CAD are important parameters informing triage to percutaneous coronary intervention (PCI) versus CABG in patients with stable multivessel CAD. The SYNTAX Score (SS), developed for use in the multicenter Synergy Between Percutaneous Coronary Intervention With Taxus and Cardiac Surgery (SYNTAX) trial provides a semiquantitative angiographic measure of disease complexity that is useful for this purpose. For a given patient, the SS represents a sum of scores for every lesion with > 50% diameter stenosis in vessels with a diameter > 1.5 mm. Elements of this score are listed in Table 44-2 (including options A through D; option E is correct).

44-9. **The answer is B.** *(Hurst's The Heart, 14th Edition, Chap. 44)* The use of a hybrid approach to coronary revascularization is gaining popularity and may be an appropriate alternative for a carefully selected subset of patients with limited CAD involving the proximal or mid LAD and at least one other non-LAD coronary artery. In hybrid coronary revascularization (HCR), a minimally invasive surgical approach is used to bypass the LAD with a LIMA graft in combination with stenting of non-LAD targets. This is believed to leverage the advantages of surgical arterial revascularization of the LAD and substitution of advanced stent technology for saphenous vein grafts for the other targets. HCR is offered in about one third of hospitals in the United States but represents less than 1% of CABG procedures (option A is incorrect). The current body of evidence is limited to observational studies and a small pilot randomized trial (option B is correct). The current ACC/AHA guidelines on coronary revascularization consider HCR only when PCI of the LAD is considered suboptimal, and therefore, it is given a Class IIa recommendation (option C is incorrect).

44-10. **The answer is A.** *(Hurst's The Heart, 14th Edition, Chap. 44)* Percutaneous coronary intervention is largely reserved for two major groups of patients, namely those who have inadequate symptom relief or persistent reduction in quality of life despite OMT and those with noninvasive testing indicating risk for ischemic events. Currently, the National Heart, Lung, and Blood Institute is sponsoring the International Study of Comparative Health Effectiveness with Medical and Invasive Approaches (ISCHEMIA) trial to evaluate the benefit of PCI in patients with high-risk features on noninvasive testing compared to OMT alone. In a prior pivotal randomized trial (COURAGE), 2287 patients with objective evidence of myocardial ischemia and significant coronary artery disease were randomized to undergo PCI with OMT or OMT alone. The primary outcome (death from any cause and nonfatal myocardial infarction during a follow-up period of median 4.6 years) did not differ during the two groups at follow-up (hazard ratio for the PCI group, 1.05; 95% confidence interval [CI], 0.87–1.27; P = 0.62). Similarly, there were no significant differences in the composite of death, myocardial infarction, and stroke ($P = 0.62$); hospitalization for acute coronary syndrome ($P = 0.56$); or myocardial infarction ($P = 0.33$). The ISCHEMIA trial will critically inform this ongoing question in the contemporary treatment era, but at the present time the role of routine PCI in the absence of symptoms refractory to OMT is uncertain.

References

1. Verma S, Farkouh ME, Yanagawa B, et al. Comparison of coronary artery bypass surgery and percutaneous coronary intervention in patients with diabetes: a meta-analysis of randomised controlled trials. *Lancet Diabetes Endocrinol*. 2013;1(4):317-328.
2. Farkouh ME, Domanski M, Sleeper LA, et al. Strategies for multivessel revascularization in patients with diabetes. *N Engl J Med*. 2012;367:2375-2384.
3. Velazquez EJ, Lee KL, Jones RH, et al. Coronary-artery bypass surgery in patients with ischemic cardiomyopathy. *N Engl J Med*. 2016;374(16):1511-1520.
4. Hlatky MA, Boothroyd DB, Bravata DM, et al. Coronary artery bypass surgery compared with percutaneous coronary interventions for multivessel disease: a collaborative analysis of individual patient data from ten randomised trials. *Lancet*. 2009;373(9670):1190-1197.
5. Bonow RO, Maurer G, Lee KL, et al. Myocardial viability and survival in ischemic left ventricular dysfunction. *N Engl J Med*. 2011;364(17):1617-1625.
6. Tonino PA, De Bruyne B, Pijls NH, et al. Fractional flow reserve versus angiography for guiding percutaneous coronary intervention. *N Engl J Med*. 2009;360:213-224.
7. De Bruyne B, Fearon WF, Pijls NH, et al. Fractional flow reserve-guided PCI for stable coronary artery disease. *N Engl J Med*. 2014;371:1208-1217.

CHAPTER 45

Rehabilitation of the Patient with Coronary Heart Disease

Patrick R. Lawler

QUESTIONS

DIRECTIONS: Choose the one best response to each question.

45-1. Which of the following is *not* a benefit of cardiac rehabilitation (CR)?

A. Improved heart rate recovery
B. Decreased levels of high-density lipoprotein (HDL) cholesterol
C. Dose-dependent reduction in mortality
D. Improved left ventricular (LV) function
E. Decreased depression symptoms

45-2. A 54-year-old man recovering from a cardiovascular event is referred to you for medical evaluation prior to initiating CR. Which of the following is a contraindication to enrollment in a CR program?

A. Hypertension
B. Coronary artery bypass graft (CABG) surgery
C. Myocardial infarction (MI)
D. Unstable angina
E. All of the above

45-3. A 59-year-old man with long-standing hypertension is admitted to the ER with a myocardial infarction (MI). Following revascularization with coronary stenting, he improves clinically. Which of the following signs suggests that the patient is ready for a gradual mobilization program and CR?

A. No signs of decompensated heart failure
B. New or recurrent chest pain in the past hour
C. Steadily increasing troponin levels
D. A recent change in cardiac rhythm
E. None of the above

45-4. During a treadmill exercise stress test, a 60-year-old male patient becomes tired and asks to stop the test. Which of the following signs and symptoms is *not* considered an absolute test termination criterion?

A. Cyanosis
B. Dyspnea
C. Ataxia
D. Severe chest pain
E. Dizziness

45-5. Following medical evaluation, a 60-year-old male patient is determined to be in the class C risk category for exercise training. Which of the following statements about his exercise capacity is *true*?

A. His exercise capacity is approximately 10 METs
B. His oxygen uptake during exercise is < 21 mL O_2 uptake/kg/min
C. His maximum HR during exercise (HR_{max}) is 140 beats per minute
D. He is unlikely to develop angina at a workload < 6 METs
E. None of the above

45-6. A 65-year-old woman with stable angina is evaluated for an exercise training program. Which of the following is a *correct* method for determining appropriate exercise intensity?

A. Exercise intensity is determined by the patient's oxygen consumption at rest
B. Exercise intensity is equal to the maximum heart rate achieved during the exercise test
C. Exercise intensity is estimated as the heart rate equal to 220 minus the age in years
D. Exercise intensity is extrapolated from a plot of the heart rate versus oxygen consumption
E. All of the above

45-7. Which of the following is *not* a physiologic effect of smoking on the cardiovascular system?

A. Cell migration to the intima
B. Increased fibrinogen levels
C. Decreased platelet adhesion to the endothelium
D. Smooth muscle proliferation
E. None of the above

45-8. A 57-year-old hypertensive male patient is evaluated following myocardial infarction. Which of the following findings would suggest that this patient has secondary hypertension?

A. Uncontrolled hypertension despite three medications
B. Nocturnal dipping of blood pressure on 24-hour ambulatory monitoring
C. Minimal alcohol consumption
D. Low salt sensitivity
E. All of the above

45-9. Following a psychological evaluation of a 48-year-old woman recovering from a myocardial infarction, you observe that she feels anxious about her cardiovascular health and upcoming CR. Which of the following is *not* a physiologic response to anxiety?

A. Platelet and macrophage cell activation
B. Increased levels of blood lipids
C. Increased heart rate
D. Decreased myocardial oxygen demand
E. Increased blood pressure

45-10. Which of the following is the most common reason for the underutilization of CR programs?

A. Lack of physician referral
B. Higher socioeconomic status
C. Patient age < 65 years old
D. Male gender
E. None of the above

ANSWERS

45-1. **The answer is B.** *(Hurst's The Heart, 14th Edition, Chap. 45)* Clinical trials have demonstrated many clinical benefits of exercise-based CR.[1] A number of mechanistic effects seem to contribute to this clinical benefit. For example, exercise has anti-inflammatory effects by *increasing* HDL cholesterol levels (option B). Heart rate recovery is an indicator of cardiovascular (CV) health, and impaired heart rate recovery predicts mortality. In a study of patients with abnormal heart rate recovery prior to starting CR, the exercise program resulted in a 41% improvement in heart rate recovery (option A).[2] Following MI, exercise training has proven benefits on LV function and remodeling (option D), and the effects were greatest when the exercise training was started 1 week after MI and lasted longer than 12 weeks.[3] It has been estimated that 20% to 45% of patients demonstrate depression following MI.[4] Improved fitness was associated with decreased depressive symptoms and decreased mortality (option E).[5] Furthermore, the relationship between the number of CR sessions completed in older patients and improved outcomes found a dose-dependent reduction in mortality and recurrent MI (option C).

45-2. **The answer is D.** *(Hurst's The Heart, 14th Edition, Chap. 45)* To establish a safe and effective program of comprehensive CV disease risk reduction and rehabilitation, each patient should undergo a careful medical evaluation and exercise test before participating in an outpatient CR/SP program. CR was initially implemented to reduce hospitalizations after MI (option C), but given the benefits for CV health, the concept was expanded to include patients with several conditions. This includes patients undergoing cardiac surgery and coronary interventions (option B), and those with a high cardiovascular risk, namely hypertensives (option A). Nevertheless, there are absolute contraindications to CR, including all conditions where physical exercise carries a significant risk of adverse effect, such as unstable angina (option D). The indications and contraindications for CR are summarized in Table 45-1.

TABLE 45-1 Clinical Indications and Contraindications for Inpatient and Outpatient Cardiac Rehabilitation.

Indications
- Medically stable after myocardial infarction
- Stable angina
- Coronary artery bypass graft surgery
- Percutaneous transluminal coronary angioplasty or other transcatheter procedure
- Compensated congestive heart failure
- Cardiomyopathy
- Heart or other organ transplantation
- Other cardiac surgery including valvular and pacemaker insertion (including implantable-cardioverter defibrillator)
- Peripheral arterial-vascular disease
- High-risk cardiovascular disease ineligible for surgical intervention
- Sudden cardiac death syndrome
- End-stage renal disease
- At risk for coronary artery disease, with diagnosis of diabetes mellitus, hyperlipidemia, hypertension, etc.
- Other patients who may benefit from structured exercise and/or patient education (based on physician referral and consensus of the rehabilitation team)

(Continued)

TABLE 45-1 Clinical Indications and Contraindications for Inpatient and Outpatient Cardiac Rehabilitation. (*Continued*)

Contraindications
- Unstable angina
- Resting systolic blood pressure > 200 mm Hg or diastolic > 110 mm Hg
- Orthostatic blood pressure decrease of > 20 mm Hg with symptoms
- Critical aortic stenosis (peak systolic pressure gradient of > 50 mm Hg with an aortic valve orifice area of < 0.75 cm^2 in an average-size adult)
- Acute systemic illness or fever
- Uncontrolled atrial or ventricular arrhythmias
- Uncontrolled sinus tachycardia (> 120 bpm)
- Uncompensated congestive heart failure
- Third-degree heart block (without pacemaker)
- Active pericarditis or myocarditis
- Recent embolism
- Thrombophlebitis
- Resting ST-segment displacement (> 2 mm)
- Uncontrolled diabetes (resting blood glucose > 300 mg/dL [17 mmol/L] or > 250 mg/dL [14 mmol/L]) with ketones present
- Orthopedic problems prohibiting exercise
- Other metabolic conditions such as acute thyroiditis, hypokalemia or hyperkalemia, hypovolemia, etc.

45-3. **The answer is A.** (*Hurst's The Heart, 14th Edition, Chap. 45*) Phase I of CR traditionally begins in the hospital and lasts for the duration of hospitalization. This phase emphasizes a gradual, progressive approach to exercise and an education program that helps the patient understand the disease process, the rehabilitation process, and initial preventive efforts to slow the progression of disease. Simple breathing and leg exercises are commenced with a program of gradual mobilization. The emphasis at this stage is to counteract the negative effects of deconditioning after a cardiac event. A patient is considered appropriate for daily ambulation/mobilization if he or she meets four criteria: there is no new or recurrent chest pain during the previous 8 hours (option B), neither troponin nor creatine phosphokinase (CPK) is increasing (option C), there are no signs of decompensated heart failure (option A), and there is no significant change in ECG or rhythm in the previous 8 hours (option D).

45-4. **The answer is B.** (*Hurst's The Heart, 14th Edition, Chap. 45*) Exercise stress testing in CR is performed to measure the ischemic threshold, assess for arrhythmias, assess exercise tolerance, evaluate hemodynamic response (blood pressure, heart rate), and observe for signs and symptoms of ischemia. The test is traditionally carried out using a treadmill or a cycle ergometer with monitoring of ECG, heart rate, and blood pressure. The RPE Scale and the individual's description of his or her levels of angina and dyspnea (option B) are also assessed. The exercise test usually lasts for 8 to 12 minutes and is terminated when the patient develops symptoms, such as chest pain (option D), or when he or she achieves a physiologic end point, such as 85% of maximal predicted heart rate. The subject's general appearance during the exercise test is also of value and should be carefully observed during the exercise test. Signs of poor perfusion, such as cyanosis (option A) or pallor, and increasing nervous system symptoms, such as ataxia (option C), dizziness (option E), and vertigo, serve as absolute test termination criteria.

45-5. **The answer is B.** (*Hurst's The Heart, 14th Edition, Chap. 45*) The exercise goals of a CR program are developed based on an individual's baseline ability and limitations. Risk stratification is performed with each patient before the initiation of an exercise program. The guidelines published by the AHA use four categories (A, B, C, and D) according to clinical characteristics. Class C individuals are at moderate or high risk of cardiac complications during exercise due to one of the following: a history of multiple MIs or cardiac arrest, New York Heart Association class III or IV angina, exercise capacity of less than 6 METs (option A), and significant angina or ischemia at a workload < 6 METs (option D). One MET is defined as 3.5 mL O_2 uptake/kg/min, therefore this patient has an oxygen uptake capacity of < 21 mL O_2 uptake/kg/min during exercise (option B). His maximum HR can be estimated as 220 minus his age in years, therefore his HR_{max} is equal to 160 beats per minute (option C).

45-6. **The answer is D.** (*Hurst's The Heart, 14th Edition, Chap. 45*) The intensity for exercise training can be calculated from the exercise test (option A), and for cardiac patients, the heart rate is the most common method used. There are three methods of using the heart rate, and these include the direct method, the percentage of HR_{max}, and the heart rate reserve.[6] In the direct method, the heart rate is plotted against oxygen consumption, and the appropriate exercise intensity is extrapolated (option D). The percentage of HR_{max} method uses 65% to 75% of the heart rate achieved during the exercise test, which approximates from 40% to 60% of an individual's maximal oxygen consumption (VO_2 max) (option B). In the heart rate reserve method, the resting heart rate is subtracted from the maximal heart rate (estimated as 220 minus the age in years) to give the heart rate reserve. If an exercise prescription of 60% to 80% of maximal oxygen consumption is required, then 60% and 80% values of the heart rate reserve are calculated, and the resting heart rate is added to each value to give the training heart rate values (option C).

45-7. **The answer is C.** (*Hurst's The Heart, 14th Edition, Chap. 45*) Cigarette smoking, a major risk factor for the development of CHD, remains a leading cause of preventable death worldwide. The causal relationship between smoking and CV disease is well established. The effects of smoking on the CV system include stimulation of smooth muscle proliferation (option D) and cell migration to intima (option A), increase in platelet adhesion to the endothelium (option C), and an increase in fibrinogen levels (increased clotting) (option B). Smoking cessation will reduce the subsequent risk of mortality by up to 9%.[7] Observational studies in post-MI patients suggest that this may be reflected as a halving of long-term mortality.[8]

45-8. **The answer is A.** (*Hurst's The Heart, 14th Edition, Chap. 45*) Evidence exists regarding the importance of hypertension as a risk factor for CV disease and the importance of lifestyle measures and appropriate medication to treat and control hypertension. Ambulatory blood pressure monitoring can confirm the diagnosis of hypertension. A change in lifestyle behaviors may have important effects on BP control. Excessive alcohol consumption (option C) is associated with hypertension, and reduction or cessation of alcohol consumption has been shown to improve blood pressure and to reduce need for medication. Most people with hypertension are salt-sensitive (option D), and reductions in dietary salt are effective. There is a direct link between increasing body weight and blood pressure levels, particularly if fat distribution is central. Stress has a major effect on blood pressure, and recognizing and eliminating this factor may have important effects. Secondary causes of hypertension may be diagnosed if one of the following is noted: blood pressure of ≥ 180/110 mm Hg, uncontrolled hypertension despite three medications (option A), or nondipping of blood pressure during 24-hour ambulatory blood pressure monitoring (option B).

45-9. **The answer is D.** (*Hurst's The Heart, 14th Edition, Chap. 45*) Psychosocial factors may affect the occurrence and recurrence of CHD and may affect rehabilitation. Anxiety and depression are prevalent in both cardiac patients and their families and are associated with increased morbidity and mortality. Although they may be normal responses after a cardiac event and a natural part of recovery after any life-threatening or stressful event, in excess, they may seriously impede rehabilitation. Anxiety can affect both short- and long-term recovery after a cardiac event. It may relate more to how an individual responds to his or her condition than to its severity. Anxiety may trigger a variety of physiologic responses such as increased levels of circulating lipids (option B), platelet and macrophage cell activation (option A), and increased heart rate (option C), blood pressure (option E), and myocardial oxygen demand (option D), all of which have have implications for the development of atherosclerosis, ischemia, MI, and sudden death.

45-10. The answer is A. *(Hurst's The Heart, 14th Edition, Chap. 45)* The most common barrier to CR is a lack of physician referral (option A). Despite national guidelines in the United States designating CR as a Class IA recommendation, Menezes et al.[9] report that up to 80% are not referred. In particular, women (option D), those of lower socioeconomic status (option B), and patients over age 65 (option C) have lower rates of referral.[10] The EuroAspire survey analyzed records and interviews of 9000 patients and reported that only one-third of patients with CHD received any form of CR.[11] Even among those referred to CR, the dropout rate is high among post-MI patients. Importantly, once referred to CR, the reasons for nonattendance were more likely due to personal factors, such as perceptions of heart disease and family influence, versus physical issues.

References

1. Lawler PR, Filion KB, Eisenberg MJ. Efficacy of exercise-based cardiac rehabilitation post-myocardial infarction: a systemic review and meta-analysis of randomized controlled trials. *Am Heart J.* 2011;162:571.
2. Jolly MA, Brennan DM, Cho L. Impact of exercise on heart rate recovery. *Circulation.* 2011;124:1520-1526.
3. Haykowsky M, Scott J, Esch B, et al. A meta-analysis of the effects of exercise training on left ventricular remodeling following myocardial infarction: start early and go longer for greatest exercise benefits on remodeling. *Trials.* 2011;12:92.
4. Wenger N. Current status of cardiac rehabilitation. *J Am Coll Cardiol.* 2008;51:1619-1631.
5. Milani RV, Lavie CJ. Impact of cardiac rehabilitation on depression and its associated mortality. *Am J Med.* 2007;120:799-806.
6. Fletcher G, Ades P, Kligfield P, et al. Exercise standards for testing and training: a scientific statement on behalf of the American Heart Association Exercise, Cardiac Rehabilitation, and Prevention Committee of the Council on Clinical Cardiology, Council on Nutrition, Physical Activity and Metabolism, Council on Cardiovascular and Stroke Nursing, and Council on Epidemiology and Prevention. *Circulation.* 2013;128:873-934.
7. Camm A, Luscher T, Serruys P. *The ESC Textbook of Cardiovascular Medicine.* Oxford, United Kingdom: Blackwell Publishing; 2015.
8. McIntyre D. *Lifestyle Management: Smoking in Coronary Heart Disease Prevention, a Handbook for the Healthcare Team.* Edinburgh, United Kingdom: Churchill Livingstone; 1996.
9. Menezes AR, Lavie CJ, Milani RV, et al. Cardiac rehabilitation in the United States. *Prog Cardiovasc Dis.* 2014;56(5):522-529.
10. Leon AS, Franklin BA, Costa F, et al. Cardiac rehabilitation and secondary prevention of coronary heart disease: an American Heart Association scientific statement from the Council on Clinical Cardiology (Subcommittee on Exercise, Cardiac Rehabilitation, and Prevention) and the Council on Nutrition, Physical Activity, and Metabolism (Subcommittee on Physical Activity), in collaboration with the American Association of Cardiovascular and Pulmonary Rehabilitation. *Circulation.* 2005;111:369-376.
11. EUROASPIRE III: a survey on the lifestyle, risk factors and use of cardioprotective drug therapies in coronary patients from 22 European countries. *Eur J Cardiovasc Prev Rehabil.* 2009;16(2):121-137.

SECTION 8

Valvular Heart Disease

CHAPTER 46

Acute Rheumatic Fever

Jonathan Afilalo

QUESTIONS

DIRECTIONS: Choose the one best response to each question.

46-1. Acute rheumatic fever (ARF) is a multisystem autoimmune response to untreated or partially treated group A *Streptococcus* (GAS) pharyngitis. Which of the following statements about ARF is *false*?

A. First attacks are rare in the very young
B. The peak incidence of ARF occurs in those age 5 to 15 years
C. ARF is rare in adults older than age 35
D. ARF is equally common in males and females
E. No association with ethnic origin has been found

46-2. The incidence of ARF began to decline in developed countries toward the end of the 19th century, and by the second half of the 20th century, ARF had become rare in most affluent populations. Which of the following factors contributed *least* to this decline?

A. More hygienic living conditions
B. Less crowded living conditions
C. Better nutrition
D. Improved access to medical care
E. The advent of antibiotics

46-3. A 31-year-old man with a prior history of rheumatism in every joint at the age of 15 presented to the emergency department complaining of pain in the left hip and right knee. His physical examination revealed a systolic murmur, loudest at the apex and radiating to the axilla. Which of the following statements about the antibodies that contribute to this rheumatic valvulitis is *false*?

A. They target the N-acetyl-β-D-glucosamine–dominant epitope of the GAS carbohydrate

B. They recognize sequences in α-helical proteins (eg, myosin and tropomyosin)
C. They are neutralized by appropriate antibiotic therapy
D. Their serum levels fall significantly after surgical removal of inflamed valves
E. None of the above

46-4. A 29-year-old healthy woman with a past medical history of ARF as a child is seen in the clinic because her 12-year-old daughter has recently been diagnosed with ARF. She is concerned that ARF may be running in her family and that her 2-year-old son may thus be at increased risk of having ARF. Which of the following genetic factors has been associated with the development of ARF?

A. Human leukocyte antigen (HLA) Class II alleles
B. Polymorphisms of transforming growth factor-β1
C. Immunoglobulin genes
D. Certain B-cell alloantigens
E. All of the above

46-5. The long-term clinical consequence of ARF is related to permanent cardiac damage. Which of the following patients is most likely to have permanent cardiac damage from ARF?

A. 15-year-old boy with pleuritic chest pain and diffuse concave-shaped ST-elevation on ECG
B. 25-year-old man with acute heart failure with an EF of 25% and recurrent tachyarrhythmias
C. 27-year-old man with joint pain and a pansystolic murmur loudest at the apex and radiating to the axilla
D. 19-year-old woman with central pleuritic chest pain, positive troponins, and raised inflammatory markers
E. All of the above

46-6. ARF usually has an acute febrile onset and presents with variable combinations of major and minor manifestations. In which of the following presentations is the evidence of a preceding GAS infection *not* needed to diagnose ARF?

A. 12-year-old girl with involuntary, purposeless, rapid, and abrupt movements associated with muscular weakness and emotional lability

B. 13-year-old boy with polyarthritis, temperature of 38.5°C, and ESR of 60 mm in the first hour

C. 9-year-old girl with polyarthritis, temperature of 39.5°C, and ESR of 120 mm in the first hour

D. 12-year-old boy with pleuritic chest pain, arthralgia, fever, and ESR of 72 mm in the first hour

E. None of the above

46-7. A 10-year-old girl was brought by her mother to the emergency department complaining of personality changes, with inappropriate behavior, restlessness, and outbursts of anger or crying. During the physical examination, the patient was asked to squeeze the examiner's hand. This resulted in repetitive irregular squeezes. Which of the following statements about the patient's condition is *false*?

A. It must be associated with other manifestations of ARF in order to confirm the diagnosis

B. It may be the sole expression of the ARF

C. It is a neurologic disorder

D. It occurs in up to 30% of cases of ARF

E. The abnormal movements disappear during sleep

46-8. An 11-year-old girl was brought to the emergency department by her parents complaining of pains in the right hip and left knee. On physical examination, there was a pink rash on the patient's trunk. She had a temperature of 39.5°C, and the ESR was 120 mm in the first hour. Which of the following statements about this rash is *false*?

A. It is itchy and evanescent in nature

B. It affects the trunk predominantly

C. It may be fleeting and disappear within hours

D. It may be brought out by a warm bath or shower

E. It is found in only 4% to 15% of cases

46-9. A 12-year-old boy was brought by his parents to the emergency department complaining of a rash over the bony surfaces of his elbows, wrists, and knees. Three to 4 weeks ago, the patient presented to the same hospital with pleuritic chest pain, arthralgia, fever, and ESR of 72 mm in the first hour. The physical examination revealed some nodules over the bony surfaces of his elbows, wrists, and knees. Which of the following statements about these nodules is *false*?

A. They generally appear later in the course of the disease after several weeks of illness

B. They are seen most commonly in patients with carditis

C. They are firm and painful

D. The overlying skin is not usually inflamed

E. They occur in less than 10% of cases of ARF

46-10. There is no definitive laboratory test for ARF, with the diagnosis based on a combination of clinical manifestations and laboratory evidence of previous streptococcal infection. Which of the following laboratory findings *cannot* be used as evidence of a preceding strep infection?

A. Increased or rising antistreptolysin O titer

B. Increased or rising of other streptococcal antibodies

C. A positive throat swab culture

D. Rapid antigen test for group A β-hemolytic streptococci

E. None of the above

46-1. **The answer is C.** (*Hurst's The Heart, 14th Edition, Chap. 46*) Acute rheumatic fever is equally common in males and females, but RHD is more common in females in almost all populations.[1,2] First attacks are rare in the very young (option A); only 5% of first episodes arise in children younger than age 5, and the disease is almost unheard of in those younger than age 2 (option A). The peak incidence of ARF occurs in those age 5 to 15 (option B), with a decline thereafter such that cases are rare in adults older than age 35 (option C).[3] No association with sex or ethnic origin has been found (options D and E).

46-2. **The answer is E.** (*Hurst's The Heart, 14th Edition, Chap. 46*) This decline is attributed to more hygienic and less crowded living conditions, better nutrition, improved access to medical care, and, to a lesser extent, the advent of antibiotics in the 1950s. The decline in the prevalence of RHD in wealthy countries has followed a similar pattern, albeit with a delay compared to ARF incidence, which is explained by the chronic nature of RHD.

46-3. **The answer is C.** (*Hurst's The Heart, 14th Edition, Chap. 46*) The antibodies that contribute to rheumatic valvulitis target the N-acetyl-β-D-glucosamine–dominant epitope of the GAS carbohydrate,[4] but they also recognize sequences in α-helical proteins (eg, myosin and tropomyosin).[5] These antibodies are elevated in patients with valvular involvement in ARF, significantly reduce after the surgical removal of inflamed valves, and correlate with poor prognosis.[6] At this stage, antibiotics are ineffective and do not reduce the level of circulating antibodies.

46-4. **The answer is E.** (*Hurst's The Heart, 14th Edition, Chap. 46*) Host factors have been considered to be important ever since familial clustering was reported last century. Associations between disease and HLA Cass II alleles have been identified, but the alleles associated with susceptibility or protection differ depending on the population investigated.[7] High concentrations of circulating mannose-binding lectin and polymorphisms of transforming growth factor-β1 and immunoglobulin genes also are associated with ARF.[8-10] Certain B-cell alloantigens are expressed to a greater level in patients with ARF or RHD than controls, with family members having intermediate expression, suggesting that these antigens are markers of inherited susceptibility.

46-5. **The answer is C.** (*Hurst's The Heart, 14th Edition, Chap. 46*) Although rheumatic carditis involves the pericardium, myocardium, and endocardium, fibrinous pericarditis (options A and D) and interstitial myocardial involvement (options B and D) typically resolve without residual damage, whereas verrucous valvulitis (option C) is usually associated with lasting damage. Notably, the pathologic changes also indicate that, unlike in the more common lymphocytic form of myocarditis, heart muscle cells are spared in rheumatic carditis.[11]

46-6. **The answer is A.** (*Hurst's The Heart, 14th Edition, Chap. 46*) The diagnosis of ARF is made when the patient develops two major manifestations, or one major manifestation and at least two minor manifestations; in addition, evidence of a preceding infection with GAS must be demonstrated using streptococcal serology. The exceptions are patients who present with chorea (option A) or indolent carditis because these manifestations may only become apparent months after the inciting streptococcal infection, so additional manifestations may not be present and streptococcal serology testing may be normal.[12]

46-7. **The answer is A.** (*Hurst's The Heart, 14th Edition, Chap. 46*) Mild chorea may best be demonstrated by asking the patient to squeeze the examiner's hand. This results in repetitive irregular squeezes labeled as the milking sign. Emotional lability manifests in personality changes, with inappropriate behavior, restlessness, and outbursts of anger or crying.[13] Sydenham chorea may be associated with other manifestations of ARF but may also be the sole expression of the disease (options A and B). It is a neurologic disorder characterized by involuntary, purposeless, rapid, and abrupt movements associated with muscular weakness and emotional lability (option C). Chorea occurs in up to 30% of cases of ARF (option D). The abnormal movements disappear during sleep (option E).

46-8. **The answer is A.** *(Hurst's The Heart, 14th Edition, Chap. 46)* Erythema marginatum is a nonitchy (option A), evanescent rash that is pink or slightly red and that affects the trunk predominantly (option B). The rash extends centrifugally, and the skin in the center returns toward normal. The rash may be fleeting and may disappear within hours (option C). It may be brought out by a warm bath or shower (option D). It is reported to be found in only 4% to 15% of cases and may be difficult to detect in dark-skinned patients (option E).

46-9. **The answer is C.** *(Hurst's The Heart, 14th Edition, Chap. 46)* These nodules generally appear later in the course of the disease after several weeks of illness and are seen most commonly in patients with carditis. They are firm and painless; the overlying skin is not inflamed and may vary in size from a few millimeters to several centimeters. They are most commonly located over bony surfaces or tendons such as elbows, wrists, knees, occiput, and spinous processes of the vertebrae. These occur in less than 10% of cases of ARF.

46-10. **The answer is E.** *(Hurst's The Heart, 14th Edition, Chap. 46)* Evidence of preceding streptococcal infection may be demonstrated by increased or rising antistreptolysin O titer, other streptococcal antibodies, a positive throat swab culture, or a rapid antigen test for group A β-hemolytic streptococci.

References

1. Lawrence JG, Carapetis JR, Griffiths K, Edwards K, Condon JR. Acute rheumatic fever and rheumatic heart disease: incidence and progression in the Northern Territory of Australia, 1997 to 2010. *Circulation.* 2013;128:492-501.
2. Rothenbuhler M, O'Sullivan CJ, Stortecky S, et al. Active surveillance for rheumatic heart disease in endemic regions: a systematic review and meta-analysis of prevalence among children and adolescents. *Lancet Glob Health.* 2014;2:e717-e726.
3. Carapetis JR, McDonald M, Wilson NJ. Acute rheumatic fever. *Lancet.* 2005;366:155-168.
4. Goldstein I, Rebeyrotte P, Parlebas J, Halpern B. Isolation from heart valves of glycopeptides which share immunological properties with *Streptococcus haemolyticus* group A polysaccharides. *Nature.* 1968;219: 866-868.
5. Galvin JE, Hemric ME, Ward K, Cunningham MW. Cytotoxic mAb from rheumatic carditis recognizes heart valves and laminin. *J Clin Invest.* 2000;106:217-224.
6. Ellis NM, Kurahara DK, Vohra H, et al. Priming the immune system for heart disease: a perspective on group A streptococci. *J Infect Dis.* 2010;202:1059-1067.
7. Bessen DE, Carapetis JR, Beall B, et al. Contrasting molecular epidemiology of group A streptococci causing tropical and nontropical infections of the skin and throat. *J Infect Dis.* 2000;182:1109-1116.
8. Berdeli A, Celik HA, Ozyurek R, Aydin HH. Involvement of immunoglobulin FcgammaRIIA and FcgammaRIIIB gene polymorphisms in susceptibility to rheumatic fever. *Clin Biochem.* 2004;37:925-929.
9. Chou HT, Chen CH, Tsai CH, Tsai FJ. Association between transforming growth factor-beta1 gene C-509T and T869C polymorphisms and rheumatic heart disease. *Am Heart J.* 2004;148:181-186.
10. Schafranski MD, Stier A, Nisihara R, Messias-Reason IJ. Significantly increased levels of mannose-binding lectin (MBL) in rheumatic heart disease: a beneficial role for MBL deficiency. *Clin Exp Immunol.* 2004;138:521-525.
11. Tandon R, Sharma M, Chandrashekhar Y, Kotb M, Yacoub MH, Narula J. Revisiting the pathogenesis of rheumatic fever and carditis. *Nat Rev Cardiol.* 2013;10:171-177.
12. Taranta A, Stollerman GH. The relationship of Sydenham's chorea to infection with group A streptococci. *Am J Med.* 1956;20:170-175.
13. Cilliers AM. Rheumatic fever and its management. *Br Med J.* 2006;333:1153A-1156A.

CHAPTER 47

Aortic Valve Disease

Jonathan Afilalo

QUESTIONS

DIRECTIONS: Choose the one best response to each question.

47-1. A 65-year-old man was referred for cardiac consultation following a 2-year history of dyspnea on minimal exertion. He had a coronary angiography in the past that revealed normal coronaries. His physical examination revealed a 3/6 systolic ejection systolic murmur across the precordium. An echo was obtained showing left ventricular dysfunction with an EF of 38%, a calcified aortic valve with a mean gradient of 29 mm Hg, and AVA (aortic valve area) of 0.9 cm^2. Which of the following is the best next step in the management of this patient?

A. SAVR after coronary angiography
B. Left and right cardiac catheterization
C. Exercise treadmill testing
D. TAVR
E. Dobutamine stress echocardiography (DSE)

47-2. A 67-year-old man with a prior medical history of hypertension and atrial fibrillation was referred for cardiac consultation following a 2-year history of chest discomfort on minimal exertion. His physical examination revealed a late peaking 3/6 ejection systolic murmur with a soft and single S2. An echo was obtained showing left ventricular hypertrophy with an EF of 62%, moderate right ventricular dysfunction, moderate mitral regurgitation, a calcified aortic valve with a mean gradient of 29 mm Hg, and AVA of 0.7 cm^2. Which of the following parameters may *not* be a contributor to paradoxical low-flow, low-gradient severe aortic stenosis?

A. Hypertensive heart disease
B. Atrial fibrillation
C. Right ventricular dysfunction
D. Occult aortic regurgitation
E. Mitral regurgitation

47-3. A 52-year-old man with no prior medical history was referred for cardiac consultation following a 1-year history of chest pain and dyspnea on exertion. Palpation of the carotid arteries demonstrated a pulse low in volume and delayed in upstroke. His remaining physical examination revealed a late-peaking 3/6 systolic ejection murmur with a soft and single S2. An echo was obtained showing left ventricular hypertrophy with an EF of 62%, a calcified bicuspid aortic valve with a mean gradient of 44 mm Hg, and AVA of 0.7 cm^2. Which of the following is the best next step in the management of this patient?

A. SAVR after coronary angiography
B. Stress cardiac magnetic resonance
C. Exercise treadmill testing
D. TAVR
E. DSE

47-4. A 65-year-old man was referred for cardiac consultation following a 2-year history of dyspnea on exertion. He had a coronary angiography in the past that revealed normal coronaries. Palpation of the carotid arteries demonstrated a pulse low in volume and delayed in upstroke. His remaining physical examination revealed a late-peaking 3/6 systolic ejection murmur with a soft and single S2. An echo was obtained showing left ventricular hypertrophy with an EF of 64%, a calcified aortic valve with a mean gradient of 28 mm Hg, and AVA of 1.5 cm^2. Which of the following is the best management approach for this patient?

A. SAVR after coronary angiography
B. Left and right cardiac catheterization
C. Exercise treadmill testing
D. TAVR
E. Observe

47-5. An 89-year-old woman with a prior history of CABG, hypertension, type 2 diabetes, stage III CKD, COPD, and peripheral artery disease presented to the clinic for routine follow-up. The patient appeared frail but denied any cardiovascular symptoms. Her physical examination revealed parvus tardus carotid pulse and a late-peaking 3/6 systolic ejection murmur with a single S2. An echo was obtained showing left ventricular dysfunction with an EF of 44%, a calcified aortic valve with a mean gradient of 48 mm Hg, and AVA of 0.8 cm². Which of the following is the best management approach for this patient?

A. SAVR after coronary angiography
B. Left and right cardiac catheterization
C. Exercise treadmill testing
D. TAVR
E. Observe

47-6. A 29-year-old man with no known cardiovascular history presented to the emergency department complaining of acute dyspnea. On arrival, the patient appeared pale with cool distal extremities, peripheral cyanosis, and tachycardia. The physical examination revealed a relatively unsustained left ventricular impulse that was neither hyperdynamic nor significantly displaced to the left, a short and soft diastolic murmur, pulmonary rales, and an elevated JVP. A wide pulse pressure was *not* seen during the examination. An echo was obtained showing a premature mitral valve closure and fluttering of the mitral valve leaflets, most effectively demonstrated using M-mode echocardiography. Continuous-wave Doppler of the regurgitant jet demonstrated a markedly shortened pressure half-time. Which of the following is the best next step in the management of this patient?

A. Aortic balloon counterpulsation
B. Beta-blocker infusion
C. Atrial pacing
D. SAVR
E. TAVR

47-7. Holodiastolic reversal of flow within the descending aorta detected by pulsed-wave Doppler is an abnormal finding typically consistent with at least moderate (present in the proximal descending aorta) or severe (present in the abdominal aorta) AR. In which of the following scenarios can holodiastolic retrograde aortic flow *not* be seen in the absence of AR?

A. Ruptured sinus of Valsalva aneurysm
B. Left-to-right shunt across a patent ductus arteriosus
C. Upper extremity arterio-venous fistula
D. Aortic dissection with diastolic flow into the false lumen
E. None of the above

47-8. A 66-year-old woman with a prior history of type 2 diabetes, depression, and childhood asthma was referred by her GP to the cardiology clinic because of a 2-year history of progressive dyspnea on exertion. Physical examination revealed a holodiastolic murmur best heard along the left sternal border and a 2/4 diastolic rumble noted at the apex. In addition, there was a sharp carotid upstroke followed by a rapid decline. An echocardiogram was obtained demonstrating severe aortic regurgitation, a left ventricular ejection fraction of 52%, and left ventricular end systolic dimension of 49 mm. Which of the following is the best next step in the management of this patient?

A. Nitroprusside infusion
B. Initiation of an angiotensin-converting enzyme inhibitor
C. Angiotensin-converting enzyme inhibitor and follow-up
D. TAVR
E. SAVR

47-9. A 71-year-old man with a prior history of diet-controlled type 2 diabetes and COPD was referred by his GP to the cardiology clinic because of a heart murmur. He was a very active gentleman without any cardiovascular symptoms. Physical examination revealed a diastolic blowing sound best heard along the left sternal border with the patient sitting up and leaning forward and an exaggerated carotid upstroke. In addition, the apical beat was easily visible and palpable, and it was oriented downward and to the left. An echocardiogram was obtained demonstrating severe aortic regurgitation, a left ventricular ejection fraction of 65%, and left ventricular end systolic dimension of 67 mm. Which of the following is the best next step in the management of this patient?

A. Initiation of nifedipine
B. Exercise treadmill testing
C. SAVR
D. Exercise echocardiography
E. Follow-up

47-10. A 61-year-old man with no known cardiovascular history was referred by his GP to the cardiology clinic because of a heart murmur. He was active and asymptomatic. Physical examination revealed a holodiastolic murmur best heard along the left sternal border. In addition, there was a sharp carotid upstroke followed by a rapid decline. An echocardiogram was obtained demonstrating severe aortic regurgitation, a left ventricular ejection fraction of 45%, and left ventricular end systolic dimension of 37 mm. Which of the following is the best next step in the management of this patient?

A. Initiation of a vasodilator
B. Exercise treadmill testing
C. Follow-up
D. Exercise echocardiography
E. SAVR

47-1. **The answer is E.** *(Hurst's The Heart, 14th Edition, Chap. 47)* There is a discrepancy between gradient and valve area calculation, and this needs to be sorted out before making any decision with regard to the interventions (options A and D are thus not correct). This patient may have low-flow/low-gradient severe AS with reduced EF. AS severity may be difficult to assess under resting conditions in low LVEF patients,[1-5] and DSE (option E) can help clarify the issue by allowing reassessment of the AVA at a higher flow. With normalized flow, a patient with true severe AS increases the mean transaortic gradient in tandem with valve flow so that AVA remains nearly constant. A patient with pseudo-severe AS, a condition where low flow causes an overestimation of AS severity, increases valve flow with little increase in gradient, resulting in increased AVA. Options B and C would not be useful in resolving the discrepancy between gradient and valve area calculation in this case.

47-2. **The answer is D.** *(Hurst's The Heart, 14th Edition, Chap. 47)* Multiple explanations for low forward flow in the setting of normal EF have been proposed.[6-8] It is generally held that this group has small LV volumes (concentric remodeling), so a normal EF of a small end-diastolic volume produces a small stroke volume and hence a low gradient. Hypertension (option A) has been shown to reduce the transaortic gradients in experimental models and patients, primarily because of changes in transvalvular flow rates and not directly as a result of changes in arterial compliance.[6,7] Right ventricular dysfunction (option C), atrial fibrillation (option B), and mitral regurgitation (option E) are independently associated with low-flow, low-gradient AS.[8] Aortic regurgitation (option D) is associated with higher transaortic flow rates and, consequently, should not cause low-flow, low-gradient AS. Option D is therefore the correct answer.

47-3. **The answer is A.** *(Hurst's The Heart, 14th Edition, Chap. 47)* All evidence (clinical, physical exam findings, aortic gradient, and AVA) points to severe symptomatic AS in a patient with high-flow and normal EF, so SAVR is indicated (option A). No further tests are needed (options B, C, and E). SAVR remains the standard of care in low-risk patients, especially in individuals with a congenital bicuspid aortic valve. (Insufficient data are currently available for the routine use of TAVR (option D) in bicuspid aortic valve patients.)

47-4. **The answer is B.** *(Hurst's The Heart, 14th Edition, Chap. 47)* There are discrepancies between clinical, physical exam, and echocardiographic findings; and this needs to be sorted out before making any decision with regard to the interventions (options A and D are thus not correct). Invasive hemodynamic measurement is the best next step for such situations when there is discordance in clinical presentation and noninvasive data regarding AS severity (option B). In such cases direct measurement of aortic valve gradient (g) and cardiac output (CO) is indicated. These data are entered into the Gorlin equation: $AVA = CO/44.3\sqrt{g}$, where cardiac output is expressed as flow per systole. Careful attention must be paid to proper pressure and cardiac output measurement.[9] Options C and E would be inappropriate for these reasons.

47-5. **The answer is D.** *(Hurst's The Heart, 14th Edition, Chap. 47)* In the truly asymptomatic AS patient, the risk of sudden death is small, probably less than 1% per year.[10,11] However, AVR is recommended for very rare asymptomatic patients who have developed LV dysfunction and for the patient with severe AS undergoing another cardiac operation where it would be unwise to fail to correct severe AS during surgery.[12,13] Because this is a high-risk patient (elderly, frail, multiple comorbidities and history of a prior CABG), TAVR (instead of SAVR) would be the best option in this case (options A and D). This patient has some indications for AVR, and therefore options B, C, and E would be inappropriate.

47-6. **The answer is D.** *(Hurst's The Heart, 14th Edition, Chap. 47)* This is a case of acute AR. Vasodilator therapy with sodium nitroprusside may stabilize the patient during transport to the operating department. Aortic balloon counterpulsation (option A) is contraindicated because it worsens AR. Beta-blockers (option B) should be avoided in acute AR because they prolong diastole and may worsen AR. Atrial pacing (option C) to increase heart rate might be of theoretical benefit[14]; however, this does not have an established role in clinical practice. Several studies have demonstrated that emergency aortic valve replacement (SAVR, and thus option D) can be performed with low operative mortality and good long-term results in acute AR. The data with TAVR are currently lacking (option E).

47-7. **The answer is E.** *(Hurst's The Heart, 14th Edition, Chap. 47)* In the absence of AR, holo-diastolic retrograde aortic flow can be seen most commonly in hypertensive patients with reduced aortic compliance[15] but also in other conditions such as a left-to-right shunt across a patent ductus arteriosus (option B), upper extremity arterio-venous fistula (option C), a ruptured sinus of Valsalva (option A), or aortic dissection with diastolic flow into the false lumen (option D). It is thus important to assess diastolic flow reversal in the context of these possible confounders. The correct answer is therefore option E.

47-8. **The answer is E.** *(Hurst's The Heart, 14th Edition, Chap. 47)* As with all valve disease, the onset of symptoms represents a negative demarcation in the natural history of the disease, and symptom onset is a clear indication of surgical intervention (options A, B, and C are thus not correct).[16] In most cases, SAVR is standard therapy (option E). Because TAVR (option D) relies on native valve calcification to hold the TAVR in place, TAVR is not widely used in treating AR, although newer valve designs may overcome this problem. The correct answer is therefore option E.

47-9. **The answer is C.** *(Hurst's The Heart, 14th Edition, Chap. 47)* As with all valve disease, the onset of symptoms represents a negative demarcation in the natural history of the disease, and symptom onset is a clear indication of surgical intervention.[16] However, some patients develop LV dysfunction without having or noticing symptom onset. To avoid persistent postoperative LV dysfunction, AVR should occur before the LV end-diastolic dimension increases from 50 to 55 mm (option C is thus the correct answer).[17,18] Although adding stress imaging is of uncertain value (option D), if exercise imaging is performed, attention should be focused on LV ejection fraction at exercise. However the utility of imaging LV function during exercise remains controversial (option D). Because afterload is often excessive in AR, there have been attempts to lower afterload using ACE inhibitors, direct vasodilators, or dihyropyridine calcium channel blockers (option A) in the hope of forestalling the need for AVR. These efforts have met with confusing and contradictory results, such that no clear recommendation can be made about their usage.[19-21] Options B and E are not correct for the reasons explained above.

47-10. **The answer is E.** *(Hurst's The Heart, 14th Edition, Chap. 47)* As with all valve disease, the onset of symptoms represents a negative demarcation in the natural history of the disease, and symptom onset is a clear indication of surgical intervention.[16] However, some patients develop LV dysfunction without having or noticing symptom onset. To avoid persistent postoperative LV dysfunction, AVR should occur before EF declines to 50% to 55% (option E is thus the correct answer) or before LV end-diastolic dimension increases from 50 to 55 mm.[17,18] Although adding stress imaging is of uncertain value (option D), if exercise imaging is performed, attention should be focused on LV ejection fraction at exercise. However, the utility of imaging LV function during exercise remains controversial (option B and D). Because afterload is often excessive in AR, there have been attempts to lower afterload using ACE inhibitors, direct vasodilators (option A), or dihyropyridine calcium channel blockers in the hope of forestalling the need for AVR. These efforts have met with confusing and contradictory results, such that no clear recommendation can be made about their usage.[19-21] Options B and C are not correct for the reasons explained above.

References

1. Clavel MA, Berthelot-Richer M, Le Ven F, et al. Impact of classic and paradoxical low flow on survival after aortic valve replacement for severeaortic stenosis. *J Am Coll Cardiol.* 2015;65(7):645-653.

2. deFilippi CR, Willett DL, Brickner ME, et al. Usefulness of dobutamine echocardiography in distinguishing severe from nonsevere valvular aortic stenosis in patients with depressed left ventricular function and low transvalvular gradients. *Am J Cardiol.* 1995;75(2):191-194.

3. Nishimura RA, Grantham JA, Connolly HM, Schaff HV, Higano ST, Holmes DR Jr. Low-output, low-gradient aortic stenosis in patients with depressed left ventricular systolic function: the clinical utility of the dobutamine challenge in the catheterization laboratory. *Circulation.* 2002;106(7):809-813.

4. Monin JL, Monchi M, Gest V, Duval-Moulin AM, Dubois-Rande JL, Gueret P. Aortic stenosis with severe left ventricular dysfunction and low transvalvular pressure gradients: risk stratification by low-dose dobutamine echocardiography. *J Am Coll Cardiol.* 2001;37(8):2101-2107.

5. Clavel MA, Fuchs C, Burwash IG, et al. Predictors of outcomes in low-flow, low-gradient aortic stenosis: Results of the multicenter TOPAS study. circulation. 2008;118(14 suppl):S234-S242.

6. Dayan V, Vignolo G, Magne J, Clavel MA, Mohty D, Pibarot P. Outcome and impact of aortic valve replacement in patients with preserved LVEF and low-gradient aortic stenosis. *J Am Coll Cardiol.* 2015;66(23):2594-2603.

7. Kadem L, Dumesnil JG, Rieu R, Durand L-G, Garcia D, Pibarot P. Impact of systemic hypertension on the assessment of aortic stenosis. *Heart.* 2005;91(3):354-361.

8. Leong DP, Pizzale S, Haroun MJ, et al. Factors associated with low flow in aortic valve stenosis. *J Am Soc Echocardiogr.* Feb 2016;29(2):158-165.

9. Carabello BA. Advances in hemodynamic assessment of stenotic cardiac valves (editorial review). *J Am Coll Cardiol.* 1987;10(4):912-919.

10. Rosenhek R, Zilberszac R, Schemper M, et al. Natural history of very severe aortic stenosis. *Circulation.* 2010;121(1):151-156.

11. Pellikka PA, Sarano ME, Nishimura RA, et al. Outcome of 622 adults with asymptomatic, hemodynamically significant aortic stenosis during prolonged follow-up. *Circulation.* 2005;111:3290-3295.

12. Nishimura RA, Otto CM, Bonow RO, et al. 2014 AHA/ACC guideline for the management of patients with valvular heart disease. Executive summary: A report of the American College of Cardiology/American Heart Association task force on practice guidelines. *J Am Coll Cardiol.* 2014;63(22):2438-2488.

13. Vahanian A, Alfieri O, Andreotti F, et al. Guidelines on the management of valvular heart disease (version 2012): the joint task force on the management of valvular heart disease of the European Society of Cardiology (ESC) and the European Association for Cardio-Thoracic Surgery (EACTS). *Eur J Cardiothorac Surg.* 2012;42(4):S1-S44.

14. Firth BG, Dehmer GJ, Nicod P, Willerson JT, Hillis LD. Effect of increasing heart rate in patients with aortic regurgitation. Effect of incremental atrial pacing on scintigraphic, hemodynamic and thermodilution measurements. *Am J Cardiol.* 1982;49(8): 1860-1867.

15. Hashimoto J, Ito S. Aortic stiffness determines diastolic blood flow reversal in the descending thoracic aorta: Potential implication for retrograde embolic stroke in hypertension. *Hypertension.* 2013;62(3):542-549.

16. Klodas E, Enriquez-Sarano M, Tajik AJ, Mullany CJ, Bailey KR, Seward JB. Optimizing timing of surgical correction in patients with severe aortic regurgitation: role of symptoms. *J Am Coll Cardiol.* 1997;30:746-752.

17. Henry WL, Bonow RO, Rosing DR, Epstein SE. Observations on the optimum time for operative intervention for aortic regurgitation. II. Serial echocardiographic evaluation of asymptomatic patients. *Circulation.* 1980;61(3):484-492.

18. Chaliki HP, Mohty D, Avierinos JF, et al. Outcomes after aortic valve replacement in patients with severe aortic regurgitation and markedly reduced left ventricular function. *Circulation.* 2002;106:2687-2693.

19. Scognamiglio R, Rahimtoola Sh, Faoli G, et al. Nifedipine in asymptomatic patients with severe aortic regurgitation and normal left ventricular function. *N Engl J Med.* 1994;331:689-694.

20. Evangelista A, Tornos P, Samola A, et al. Long-term vasodilator therapy in patients with severe aortic regurgitation. *N Engl J Med.* 2005;353:1342-1349.

21. Greenberg B, Massie B, Bristow JD, et al. Long-term vasodilator therapy of chronic aortic insufficiency. A randomized double-blinded, placebo-controlled clinical trial. *Circulation.* 1988;78(1):92-103.

CHAPTER 48

Degenerative Mitral Valve Disease

Jonathan Afilalo

QUESTIONS

DIRECTIONS: Choose the one best response to each question.

48-1. A 45-year-old woman with a prior history of diet-controlled type 2 diabetes and chronic obstructive pulmonary disease (COPD) was referred by her GP to the cardiology clinic because of a heart murmur. She was very active and without any cardiovascular symptoms. Physical examination revealed a soft late-systolic murmur best heard at the apex and radiating to the axilla. An echocardiogram was obtained demonstrating mild prolapse and leaflet thickening with normal coaptation. Left ventricular function and dimensions are normal (ejection fraction 65%). Which of the following is the best next step in the management of this patient?

A. Vasodilator therapy
B. Beta-blocker therapy
C. Elective mitral valve repair
D. Elective mitral valve replacement
E. Observe with echocardiographic annual follow-up

48-2. Mortality after mitral valve repair in patients with degenerative disease correlates with age, with an average risk of 1% for patients below 65 years, 2% for those aged 65 to 80 years, and 4% for octogenarians. Which of the following is *not* an independent predictor of postoperative survival?

A. Severe symptoms (NYHA class III or IV)
B. LV dysfunction
C. A regurgitant orifice area ≥ 40 mm^2
D. A large color Doppler jet appearance
E. The presence of long-standing atrial fibrillation

48-3. A 55-year-old woman with no prior cardiac history was referred by her GP to the cardiology clinic because of a heart murmur. She admitted to living a sedentary lifestyle, and she denied overt cardiovascular symptoms. Physical examination revealed a mid-to-late systolic murmur best heard at the apex and radiating to the axilla. An echocardiogram was obtained, clearly demonstrating moderate to severe mitral valve prolapse and regurgitation without flail segments. Left ventricular function and dimensions were normal (ejection fraction 62%). Which of the following is the best next step in the management of this patient?

A. Exercise Doppler echocardiography
B. Cardiac CT
C. Cardiac magnetic resonance
D. Nuclear perfusion scan
E. Cardiac catheterization

48-4. A 69-year-old man with a prior history of type 2 diabetes and dyslipidemia was referred by his GP to the cardiology clinic because of a heart murmur. He was a very active person without any cardiovascular symptoms. Physical examination revealed a holosystolic murmur best heard at the apex and radiating to the axilla. An echocardiogram was obtained demonstrating severe prolapse with loss of coaptation, LVEF of 63%, and LVESD of 38 mm. According to the ACC/AHA guidelines, which of the following statements does *not* justify prompt correction of MR in general?

A. Severe MR is not a benign condition
B. Surgical correction in patients with severe MR is unavoidable
C. Patients with severe MR may or may not develop symptoms
D. Mitral valve prolapse is almost always a repairable disease in reference centers
E. The risk of operative mortality in mitral valve repair surgery is, on average, only 10%

48-5. A 59-year-old woman with a prior history of depression and childhood asthma was referred by her GP to the cardiology clinic because of a new onset atrial fibrillation. During the visit, the patient denied any cardiovascular symptoms. Physical examination revealed a holosystolic murmur best heard at the apex and radiating to the axilla. The ECG showed atrial fibrillation with a controlled ventricular response. An echocardiogram was obtained demonstrating severe mitral valve prolapse with loss of coaptation, LVEF of 66%, and LVESD of 36 mm. Which of the following is the best next step in the management of this patient?

A. Vasodilator therapy
B. Exercise Doppler echocardiography
C. Elective mitral valve repair
D. Elective mitral valve replacement
E. Observe with echocardiographic annual follow-up

48-6. Tricuspid regurgitation does *not* always regress after correction of left-sided valve disease, and reoperations for residual or recurrent tricuspid regurgitation are associated with a higher mortality risk even in experienced centers (up to 15%). Which of the following factors may be used as a guide in deciding on concomitant tricuspid valve repair in patients undergoing mitral valve repair?

A. Degree of TR
B. Annular dimensions
C. Leaflet coaptation or mismatch between leaflet and annulus
D. Presence of atrial fibrillation
E. All of the above

48-7. A 71-year-old woman with a prior history of type 2 diabetes, COPD, and dyslipidemia was referred by her GP to the cardiology clinic because of a heart murmur. She reported otherwise feeling fit and well. Physical examination revealed a holosystolic murmur best heard at the apex and radiating to the axilla. An echocardiogram was obtained demonstrating severe mitral valve prolapse with loss of coaptation, LVEF of 62%, LVESD of 38 mm, and SPAP of 62 mm Hg. Which of the following is the best next step in the management of this patient?

A. Beta-blocker therapy
B. Exercise Doppler echocardiography
C. Elective mitral valve repair
D. Elective mitral valve replacement
E. Observe with echocardiographic annual follow-up

48-8. Severe mitral valve regurgitation in the setting of degenerative mitral valve disease is a mechanical problem, with the only definitive solution being mechanical (ie, mitral valve repair or replacement). Which of the following factors may be a reason to favor mitral valve replacement over repair?

A. Lower perioperative risk
B. Improved preservation of left ventricular function
C. Improved event-free survival in the majority of patients
D. Greater freedom from prosthetic valve–related complications
E. Greater certitude to correct complex lesions with extensive distortion of multiple scallops

48-9. A 58-year-old man with a history of mitral valve prolapse and mild mitral regurgitation, was referred by his GP to the cardiology clinic because of a 6-month history of exertional dyspnea. Physical examination revealed a pansystolic murmur best heard at the apex and radiating to the axilla. An echocardiogram was obtained demonstrating severe prolapse with a coaptation gap, LVEF of 62%, and LVESD of 38 mm. Which of the following is the best next step in the management of this patient?

A. Immediate admission for management of acute severe MR
B. Exercise Doppler echocardiography
C. Elective mitral valve repair
D. Elective mitral valve replacement
E. Observe with echocardiographic annual follow-up

48-10. An ejection fraction ≤ 60% or a left ventricular end-systolic dimension ≥ 40 mm, though useful at indicating the onset of LV dysfunction, are imprecise and reflect changes in the LV after the negative impact of MR has already been realized. Which of the following new markers indicating an adverse myocardial response to MR has the potential to determine the optimum timing of surgery in the very near future?

A. High brain natriuretic peptide (BNP) levels
B. A lower percentage of age- or sex-predicted metabolic equivalents
C. Lower heart rate recovery after exercise
D. Left atrial dimensions
E. All of the above

48-1. **The answer is E.** *(Hurst's The Heart, 14th Edition, Chap. 48)* Currently there is no indication to intervene (options C and D) in less than severe primary mitral regurgitation, except in symptomatic patients where there is a high suspicion that MR grade may be underestimated. The use of beta-blockers (option B) or vasodilators (option A) to treat mitral valve prolapse in normotensive subjects is not recommended. The correct answer is therefore to observe with echocardiographic annual follow-up (option E).

48-2. **The answer is D.** *(Hurst's The Heart, 14th Edition, Chap. 48)* Some of the identified independent predictors of postoperative survival include severe symptoms (NYHA class III or IV—option A is thus true and therefore incorrect), LV dysfunction (EF < 60% or LVESD > 40 mm—option B is thus incorrect), a regurgitant orifice area $\geq$ 40 mm^2 (option C is thus incorrect), left atrial dimensions (left atrial index $\geq$ 60 mL/m^2 or LA > 55 mm), or the presence of pulmonary hypertension or long-standing atrial fibrillation (option E is thus incorrect). The size of the color Doppler jet is subject to many technical parameters, and it is not reliably predictive of outcomes after repair. The correct answer is therefore D.

48-3. **The answer is A.** *(Hurst's The Heart, 14th Edition, Chap. 48)* Again, currently there is no indication to intervene in less than severe mitral regurgitation, except in symptomatic patients where there is a high suspicion that MR grade may be underestimated. In such patients, exercise testing is useful to clarify the decision making (option A is thus the correct answer).[1] In fact, exercise Doppler echocardiography can be used in asymptomatic patients with moderate to severe primary MR with preserved LV ejection fraction for immediate risk stratification and to guide the timing of mitral valve surgery, especially for those in whom the risk-to-benefit ratio of surgical intervention is uncertain or borderline.[2] Computed tomography (option B), cardiac magnetic resonance (option C), and nuclear perfusion scan (option D) techniques have been compared to echocardiography for MR assessment, but they are not routinely recommended unless there are critical considerations about chamber remodeling or viability.[3,4] Although TEE is more accurate than TTE in locating the site and severity of structural abnormalities and quantifying the severity of MR, TEE during an initial diagnostic evaluation is only indicated in patients with inconclusive or technically difficult TTE examinations. Once the mainstay of evaluation, invasive hemodynamic evaluation (option E) is now reserved for cases in which the diagnosis of the severity and impact of mitral regurgitation is uncertain.

48-4. **The answer is E.** *(Hurst's The Heart, 14th Edition, Chap. 48)* Prompt correction of asymptomatic mitral regurgitation with preserved left ventricular function (class IIa), in other words before the development of traditional triggers, is based on several axioms: (1) severe MR is not a benign condition (option A is thus incorrect),[5] and if left uncorrected it carries a significant rate of excess mortality associated with increased rates of heart failure and atrial fibrillation[6]; (2) surgical correction in patients with severe MR is unavoidable (option B is thus incorrect); (3) patients with severe MR or ventricular dysfunction may or may not develop classical symptoms (option C is thus incorrect); and (4) mitral valve prolapse is a repairable disease in reference centers (option D is thus incorrect) with excellent operative outcomes (mortality and stroke rates < 1%; not 10% as stated in option E, which is therefore the correct answer) and durability.[7-9]

48-5. **The answer is C.** *(Hurst's The Heart, 14th Edition, Chap. 48)* According to the 2014 ACC/AHA new classification of the severity of valve lesions, this patient is at stage C1 of degenerative mitral valve disease, and the presence of the new onset of atrial fibrillation[12] is considered a class IIa trigger for mitral surgery in asymptomatic patients with preserved left ventricular function (options B and E are not the best next step in the management of this patient, who needs her valve to be fixed).[13] Severe mitral valve regurgitation in the setting of degenerative mitral valve disease is a mechanical problem with only a mechanical solution (option A is thus not correct); at this time the only definitive treatment is mitral valve repair (option C is thus the correct answer). All prolapsing valves are repairable, and mitral valve replacement should not be an option if appropriate referral patterns are followed (option D is thus not correct).[14]

48-6. **The answer is E.** *(Hurst's The Heart, 14th Edition, Chap. 48)* The final decision should be guided not only by the degree of regurgitation (≥ moderate) (option A is thus incorrect) but also by annular dimensions (≥ 40 mm when measured by echocardiography in the apical 4-chamber view) (option B is also thus incorrect); leaflet coaptation or mismatch between leaflet and annulus on direct inspection (option C is thus incorrect); and the presence of atrial fibrillation (option D is thus incorrect), pulmonary hypertension, right ventricular dysfunction, and/or left ventricular dysfunction. The correct answer is therefore option E.

48-7. **The answer is C.** *(Hurst's The Heart, 14th Edition, Chap. 48)* According to the 2014 ACC/AHA new classification of the severity of valve lesions, this patient is at stage C1 of degenerative mitral valve disease, and the presence of pulmonary hypertension[12] is also considered a class IIa trigger for mitral surgery in asymptomatic patients with preserved left ventricular function (options B and E are not the best next step in the management of this patient, who needs her valve to be fixed).[13] Again, severe mitral valve regurgitation in the setting of degenerative mitral valve disease is a mechanical problem (option A is thus not correct) with only a mechanical solution; at this time the only definitive treatment is mitral valve repair (option C is thus the correct answer). All prolapsing valves are repairable, and mitral valve replacement should not be an option if appropriate referral patterns are followed (option D is thus not correct).[14]

48-8. **The answer is E.** *(Hurst's The Heart, 14th Edition, Chap. 48)* Mitral valve repair is favored over replacement for several reasons, including a lower perioperative risk (option A is thus not correct), improved preservation of left ventricular function (option B is thus not correct), improved event-free survival in most patients (option C is thus not correct), and greater freedom from prosthetic valve–related complications (option D is thus not correct) such as thromboembolism, anticoagulant-related hemorrhage, and endocarditis.[15-17,19] However, in a minority of cases, anatomical factors pertaining to the extent of valvular disruption (eg, perforation) and operator-related factors pertaining to local experience and expertise make replacement more appropriate than repair (option E is thus the correct answer).

48-9. **The answer is C.** *(Hurst's The Heart, 14th Edition, Chap. 48)* This patient is symptomatic but stable and therefore does not require immediate admission for the management of acute severe MR (option A). The standard class I indications for mitral valve surgery are the onset of symptoms or of left ventricular dysfunction.[19,20] Although guidelines currently contemplate mitral valve replacement (option D) as an acceptable option, mitral valve repair is the preferred option in patients with mitral valve prolapse (option C is therefore the correct answer).[14] Options B and E are not the best next step in the management of this patient, who needs her valve to be fixed.

48-10. **The answer is E.** *(Hurst's The Heart, 14th Edition, Chap. 48)* In this context, new potential triggers for surgical intervention in asymptomatic patients might include high BNP levels (option A is thus correct),[21] a lower percentage of age- or sex-predicted metabolic equivalents (option B is thus correct), or lower heart rate recovery after exercise (option C is thus correct),[1] the left ventricular ejection index,[22,23] and left atrial dimensions (option D is thus correct).[24,25] The correct answer is therefore option E.

References

1. Naji P, Griffin BP, Asfahan F, et al. Predictors of long-term outcomes in patients with significant myxomatous mitral regurgitation undergoing exercise echocardiography. *Circulation.* 2014;129:1310-1319.

2. Magne J, Mahjoub H, Dulgheru R, et al. Left ventricular contractile reserve in asymptomatic primary mitral regurgitation. *Eur Heart J.* 2014;35:1608-1616.

3. Cawley PJ, Hamilton-Craig C, Owens DS, et al. Prospective comparison of valve regurgitation quantitation by cardiac magnetic resonance imaging and transthoracic echocardiography. *Circ Cardiovasc Imaging.* 2013;6:48-57.

4. Uretsky S, Gillam L, Lang R, et al. Discordance between echocardiography and MRI in the assessment of mitral regurgitation severity: a prospective multicenter trial. *J Am Coll Cardiol.* 2015;65:1078-1088.

5. Grigioni F, Tribouilloy C, Avierinos JF, et al. Outcomes in mitral regurgitation due to flail leaflets: a multicenter European study. *JACC Cardiovasc Imaging.* 2008;1:133-141.

6. Suri RM, Schaff HV, Enriquez-Sarano M. Mitral valve repair in asymptomatic patients with severe mitral regurgitation: pushing past the tipping point. *Semin Thorac Cardiovasc Surg.* 2014;26:95-101.

7. Goldstone AB, Patrick WL, Cohen JE, et al. Early surgical intervention or watchful waiting for the management of asymptomatic mitral regurgitation: a systematic review and meta-analysis. *Ann Cardiothorac Surg.* 2015;4:220-229.

8. Suri RM, Vanoverschelde JL, Grigioni F, et al. Association between early surgical intervention vs watchful waiting and outcomes for mitral regurgitation due to flail mitral valve leaflets. *JAMA.* 2013;310:609-616.

9. Yazdchi F, Koch CG, Mihaljevic T, et al. Increasing disadvantage of "watchful waiting" for repairing degenerative mitral valve disease. *Ann Thorac Surg.* 2015;99:1992-2000.

10. Adams DH, Anyanwu AC. Valve disease: asymptomatic mitral regurgitation. Does surgery save lives? *Nat Rev Cardiol.* 2009;6:330-332.

11. Iung B, Vahanian A. Valvular disease: Implications of the new AHA/ACC valvular disease guidelines. *Nat Rev Cardiol.* 2014;11:317-318.

12. Kang DH, Park SJ, Sun BJ, et al. Early surgery versus conventional treatment for asymptomatic severe mitral regurgitation: a propensity analysis. *J Am Coll Cardiol.* 2014;63:2398-2407.

13. Rosenhek R. Watchful waiting for severe mitral regurgitation. *Semin Thorac Cardiovasc Surg.* 2011;23:203-208.

14. Castillo JG, Anyanwu AC, El-Eshmawi A, et al. All anterior and bileaflet mitral valve prolapses are repairable in the modern era of reconstructive surgery. *Eur J Cardiothorac Surg.* 2014;45:139-145; discussion 145.

15. Russo A, Grigioni F, Avierinos JF, et al. Thromboembolic complications after surgical correction of mitral regurgitation incidence, predictors, and clinical implications. *J Am Coll Cardiol.* 2008;51:1203-1211.

16. Shuhaiber J, Anderson RJ. Meta-analysis of clinical outcomes following surgical mitral valve repair or replacement. *Eur J Cardiothorac Surg.* 2007;31:267-275.

17. Dreyfus GD, Corbi PJ, Chan KM, et al. Secondary tricuspid regurgitation or dilatation: which should be the criteria for surgical repair? *Ann Thorac Surg.* 2005;79:127-132.

18. Nishimura RA, Otto CM, Bonow RO, et al. 2014 AHA/ACC guideline for the management of patients with valvular heart disease: executive summary. A report of the American College of Cardiology/American Heart Association task force on practice guidelines. *J Am Coll Cardiol.* 2014;63:2438-2488.

19. Jeganathan R, Armstrong S, Al-Alao B, et al. The risk and outcomes of reoperative tricuspid valve surgery. *Ann Thorac Surg.* 2013;95:119-124.

20. Vahanian A, Alfieri O, Andreotti F, et al. Guidelines on the management of valvular heart disease (version 2012). *Eur Heart J.* 2012;33:2451-2496.

21. Pizarro R, Bazzino OO, Oberti PF, et al. Prospective validation of the prognostic usefulness of brain natriuretic peptide in asymptomatic patients with chronic severe mitral regurgitation. *J Am Coll Cardiol.* 2009;54:1099-1106.

22. Magne J, Szymanski C, Fournier A, et al. Clinical and prognostic impact of a new left ventricular ejection index in primary mitral regurgitation because of mitral valve prolapse. *Circ Cardiovasc Imaging.* 2015;8:e003036.

23. Delling FN. Left ventricular ejection index as a marker of early myocardial dysfunction in primary mitral regurgitation: novel or old in disguise? *Circ Cardiovasc Imaging.* 2015;8:e003995.

24. Athanasopoulos LV, McGurk S, Khalpey Z, et al. Usefulness of preoperative cardiac dimensions to predict success of reverse cardiac remodeling in patients undergoing repair for mitral valve prolapse. *Am J Cardiol.* 2014;113:1006-1010.

25. Zito C, Manganaro R, Khandheria B, et al. Usefulness of left atrial reservoir size and left ventricular untwisting rate for predicting outcome in primary mitral regurgitation. *Am J Cardiol.* 2015;116:1237-1244.

CHAPTER 49

Ischemic Mitral Regurgitation

Jonathan Afilalo

QUESTIONS

DIRECTIONS: Choose the one best response to each question.

49-1. A 61-year-old man with a prior history of diet-controlled type 2 diabetes, ischemic heart disease, and COPD was referred for cardiology consultation for a heart murmur. He was a very active man without any cardiovascular symptoms. His physical examination revealed a 2/6 holosystolic murmur loudest at the apex. An echo was obtained showing normal valve leaflets, chords, and annulus; small central MR jet area of 15% LA on Doppler; and mildly dilated LV size with fixed regional wall motion abnormalities. According to the ACC/AHA stages for ischemic MR (IMR), at which of the following stages would this patient be?

A. Stage A
B. Stage B
C. Stage C1
D. Stage C2
E. Stage D

49-2. IMR is an independent predictor of cardiovascular mortality and HF following MI. Which of the following statements about IMR is *false*?

A. The magnitude of risk is proportional to the severity of MR
B. The estimated 1-year mortality for patients with severe IMR ranges from 15% to 40%
C. For patients with moderate IMR undergoing coronary artery bypass surgery, concomitant mitral valve replacement should always be performed
D. Adverse outcomes are associated with a smaller calculated effective regurgitant orifice (ERO) in IMR when compared to primary MR
E. None of the above

49-3. The MitraClip is a transcatheter mitral device for use in high-risk or inoperable patients with severe MR and suitable anatomic criteria. Which of the following characteristics is *not* part of the desirable anatomic criteria for percutaneous edge-to-edge repair of MR using this type of device?

A. Coaptation length ≥ 2 mm
B. Short posterior leaflet
C. Flail width < 15 mm
D. MV orifice area > 4 cm^2
E. MV leaflet length > 1 cm

49-4. IMR is a dynamic lesion, and MR severity can vary over time and during exercise. Which of the following statements about IMR during exercise is *false*?

A. The severity of IMR at rest predictably determines the severity of IMR during exercise
B. Exercise-induced increase in IMR provides additional prognostic information over resting evaluation
C. Exercise echocardiography may be used to further evaluate patients with exertional dyspnea out of proportion to the degree of resting IMR
D. An increase in EROA of ≥ 13 mm^2 during exercise is associated with increased mortality
E. An increase in EROA of ≥ 13 mm^2 during exercise is associated with increased HF hospitalizations

49-5. A 68-year-old man with a prior history of myocardial infarction with PCI to the LAD was referred for cardiology consultation for decreased exercise tolerance. His physical examination revealed a displaced apex beat downward and to the left and a holosystolic murmur loudest at the apex and radiating to the axilla. An echo was obtained showing regional wall motion abnormalities with reduced LV systolic function, LV dilation with severe tethering of mitral leaflets, and a large wall-impinging jet pattern with an estimated regurgitant volume of 40 mL. Defining severe

MR requires the careful integration of multiple echocardiographic parameters. Which of the following echo findings is *not* an indicator of severe MR?

A. Peak mitral valve E-wave velocity < 1.2 m/s
B. A dense triangular continuous-wave Doppler profile
C. Systolic flow reversal in the pulmonary veins
D. Vena contracta width ≥ 0.7 cm
E. MR regurgitant jet area/left atrial area ratio ≥ 40%

49-6. A 75-year-old woman with a prior history of ischemic heart failure was referred for cardiology consultation for a heart murmur. During the visit the patient denied any cardiovascular symptoms. Her physical exam revealed a displaced apex beat downward and to the left and a holosystolic murmur loudest at the apex and radiating to the axilla. An echo was obtained showing LV dilation and systolic dysfunction due to primary myocardial disease, annular dilation with severe loss of central coaptation of the mitral leaflets, and an estimated regurgitant fraction of 55%. In addition, there was systolic flow reversal in the pulmonary veins. According to the ACC/AHA Stages for IMR, at which of the following stages would this patient be?

A. Stage A
B. Stage B1
C. Stage B2
D. Stage C
E. Stage D

49-7. A 65-year-old woman with a prior history of myocardial infarction and multivessel PCI was referred for cardiology consultation for a 3-month history of progressive exertional dyspnea despite optimal guideline-directed medical therapy. Her physical examination revealed an irregularly irregular pulse, a displaced apex beat downward and to the left, an elevated JVP, and a holosystolic murmur loudest at the apex and radiating to the axilla. An ECG was obtained and revealed atrial fibrillation (AF). An echo was also obtained showing regional wall motion abnormalities with reduced LV systolic function and LV dilation with severe tethering of mitral leaflets, and an estimated regurgitant volume of 50 mL. A dense, triangular continuous-wave Doppler profile was also noted. Which of the following statements about this patient's AF is *false*?

A. AF is present in up to 20% of patients undergoing MV surgery
B. AF may be a marker of disease progression in IMR
C. AF may be a marker of worse prognosis in IMR
D. Surgical approaches for AF can be considered in patients undergoing MV surgery
E. The duration of preoperative AF is a risk factor for recurrence after the MAZE procedure

49-8. Although a variety of percutaneous therapies for MR have been developed, the MitraClip system has emerged clinically as the most tolerated and effective approach to date. Which of the following statements about MitraClip is *false*?

A. It may be used in high-risk or inoperable patients with severe MR and suitable anatomic criteria
B. It is currently approved for use in symptomatic patients with primary (degenerative) MR who are at prohibitive risk for surgery
C. It is currently approved for the treatment of IMR in the United States
D. It has already received a class IIb recommendation from the European Society of Cardiology for secondary MR
E. Approximately two-thirds of the MitraClip procedures have been performed in patients with secondary MR worldwide

49-9. A 67-year-old man with a prior history of ischemic heart failure was referred for cardiology consultation for a 2-month history of dyspnea on minimal exertion despite optimal guideline-directed medical therapy for HF. During the visit, the patient had a fast radial pulse with a reduced pulse pressure, the apex beat was displaced downward and to the left, JVP was elevated, and there was a holosystolic murmur loudest at the apex and radiating to the axilla. In addition, an S3 gallop was present. An echo was obtained showing LV dilation and systolic dysfunction, annular dilation with severe loss of central coaptation of the mitral leaflets, a vena contracta width of 0.8 cm, and an estimated regurgitant fraction of 70%. After careful review, the patient's cardiologist decided to refer the patient for surgery as per the ACC/AHA guidelines (class of recommendation: IIb; level of evidence: B).[1] In the setting of severe IMR, which of the following statements about the role of MV repair versus MV replacement (MVR) is *false*?

A. Repair may be safer with lower perioperative mortality and morbidity
B. There is a lower rate of recurrent MR with MV repair than with MV replacement
C. No differences in survival have been reported between the two strategies
D. No differences exist between the two strategies in the incidence of major adverse cardiac and cerebrovascular events
E. More adverse events related to HF and cardiovascular readmissions occur for MR repair

49-10. Many observational studies have identified echocardiographic predictors of recurrent MR following MV annuloplasty. In the randomized trial of repair versus replacement, which of the following factors was significantly associated with recurrent moderate or severe MR in patients following repair for severe IMR?

A. LV end-diastolic diameter > 65 mm
B. Coaptation depth > 1 cm
C. Systolic sphericity index > 0.7
D. Basal aneurysms and dyskinesis
E. All of the above

49-1. The answer is A. *(Hurst's The Heart, 14th Edition, Chap. 49)* The clinical presentation and the echo findings are consistent with stage A, which includes asymptomatic patients at risk of MR, as is the case for this patient (option A). Stages B (option B), C (options C and D), and D (option E) typically include patients with progressive MR, asymptomatic patients with severe disease, and symptomatic subjects with severe MR, respectively. Options B through E are therefore not correct. Stages of secondary MR with associated valve anatomy, valve hemodynamics, cardiac findings, and symptoms are presented in Table 49-1.[1]

TABLE 49-1 Stages of Secondary Mitral Regurgitation with Associated Valve Anatomy, Valve Hemodynamics, Cardiac Findings, and Symptoms

Grade	Definition	Valve Anatomy	Valve Hemodynamics*	Associated Cardiac Findings	Symptoms
A	At risk of MR	• Normal valve leaflets, chords, and annulus in a patient with coronary disease or cardiomyopathy	• No MR jet or small central jet area < 20% LA on Doppler • Small vena contracta < 0.30 cm	• Normal or mildly dilated LV size with fixed (infarction) or inducible (ischemia) regional wall motion abnormalities • Primary myocardial disease with LV dilation and systolic dysfunction	• Symptoms due to coronary ischemia or HF may be present that respond to revascularization and appropriate medical therapy
B	Progressive MR	• Regional wall motion abnormalities with mild tethering of mitral leaflet • Annular dilation with mild loss of central coaptation of the mitral leaflets	• ERO < 0.20 cm²† • Regurgitant volume < 30 mL • Regurgitant fraction < 50%	• Regional wall motion abnormalities with reduced LV systolic function • LV dilation and systolic dysfunction due to primary myocardial disease	• Symptoms due to coronary ischemia or HF may be present that respond to revascularization and appropriate medical therapy
C	Asymptomatic severe MR	• Regional wall motion abnormalities and/or LV dilation with severe tethering of mitral leaflet • Annular dilation with severe loss of central coaptation of the mitral leaflets	• ERO ≥ 0.20 cm²† • Regurgitant volume ≥ 30 mL • Regurgitant fraction ≥ 50%	• Regional wall motion abnormalities with reduced LV systolic function • LV dilation and systolic dysfunction due to primary myocardial disease	• Symptoms due to coronary ischemia or HF may be present that respond to revascularization and appropriate medical therapy
D	Symptomatic severe MR	• Regional wall motion abnormalities and/or LV dilation with severe tethering of mitral leaflet • Annular dilation with severe loss of central coaptation of the mitral leaflets	• ERO ≥ 0.20 cm²† • Regurgitant volume ≥ 30 mL • Regurgitant fraction ≥ 50%	• Regional wall motion abnormalities with reduced LV systolic function • LV dilation and systolic dysfunction due to primary myocardial disease	• HF symptoms due to MR persist even after revascularization and optimization of medical therapy • Decreased exercise tolerance • Exertional dyspnea

Reproduced with permission from Nishimura RA, Otto CM, Bonow RO, et al. 2014 AHA/ACC guideline for the management of patients with valvular heart disease: Executive summary. A report of the American College of Cardiology/American Heart Association Task Force on Practice Guidelines. *J Am Coll Cardiol*. 2014 Jun 10;63(22):2438-2488.

*Several valve hemodynamic criteria are provided for the assessment of MR severity, but not all criteria for each category will be present in each patient. Categorization of MR severity as mild, moderate, or severe depends on data quality and integration of these parameters in conjunction with other clinical evidence.

†The measurement of the proximal isovelocity surface area by 2D TTE in patients with secondary MR underestimates the true ERO due to the crescentic shape of the proximal convergence.

49-2. The answer is C. *(Hurst's The Heart, 14th Edition, Chap. 49)* The magnitude of risk is proportional to the severity of MR (option A is thus incorrect).[2,3] Although even mild MR is associated with increased mortality, prognosis is particularly poor for patients with severe IMR, with 1-year mortality estimates ranging from 15% to 40% (option B is thus incorrect).[4] Adverse outcomes are associated with a smaller calculated effective regurgitant orifice (ERO) of > 0.2 cm^2 in IMR compared to primary MR (option D is thus incorrect).[1] The role and expected benefits of concomitant mitral valve replacements remain controversial in moderate secondary mitral valve lesions such as IMR.

49-3. The answer is B. *(Hurst's The Heart, 14th Edition, Chap. 49)* The desirable anatomic criteria for percutaneous edge-to-edge repair of MR using MitraClip may include coaptation length ≥ 2 mm (option A), flail width < 15 mm (option C), MV orifice area > 4 cm^2 (option D), and MV leaflet length > 1 cm (option E). A short posterior leaflet is actually among the undesirable criteria for MitraClip. The correct answer is therefore option B. The favorable and unfavorable anatomic criteria are presented in Table 49-2.[5]

TABLE 49-2 **Favorable and Unfavorable Anatomic Criteria for Percutaneous Edge-to-Edge Repair of MR**

Anatomical MV and LV Characteristics for Percutaneous Edge-to-Edge Repair of MR	
Desirable Criteria	Undesirable Criteria
• Moderate to severe MR (≥ grade 3)	• Commissural lesion
• Pathology in the A2-P2 zone	• Short posterior leaflet
• Coaptation length ≥ 2 mm	• Severe asymmetric tethering
• Flail gap < 10 mm	• Calcification in the grasping area
• Flail width < 15 mm	• Severe annular calcification
• MV orifice area > 4 cm^2	• MV cleft
• MV leaflet length > 1 cm	• Severe annular dilation
	• Severe LV remodeling
	• Large (> 50%) inter-commissural extension of regurgitant jet
	• Severe myxomatous degeneration with multi-scallop prolapse

Reproduced with permission from De Bonis M, Al-Attar N, Antunes M, et al. Surgical and interventional management of mitral valve regurgitation: a position statement from the European Society of Cardiology Working Groups on Cardiovascular Surgery and Valvular Heart Disease, *Eur Heart J.* 2016 Jan 7;37(2):133-139.

49-4. The answer is A. *(Hurst's The Heart, 14th Edition, Chap. 49)* The severity of IMR at rest does not necessarily reflect nor predict the severity of MR during exercise (option A is thus false, and therefore the correct answer). Exercise-induced increase in IMR provides additional prognostic information over resting evaluation and identifies patients at higher risk of adverse clinical outcomes (option B is thus incorrect).[6] For example, an increase in EROA of ≥13 mm^2 during exercise is associated with increased mortality and HF hospitalizations (options D and E are thus incorrect).[7] Exercise echocardiography has been proposed to evaluate patients with exertional dyspnea out of proportion to the degree of resting IMR (option C is thus incorrect) and LV dysfunction, patients with IMR and unexplained acute pulmonary edema, and patients with moderate IMR at rest who are due to undergo surgical revascularization with CABG.[6,8]

49-5. The answer is A. *(Hurst's The Heart, 14th Edition, Chap. 49)* Indicators of severe MR should be integrated[12] and include a peak mitral valve E-wave velocity > 1.2 m/s (not E-wave velocity < 1.2 m/s as stated in option A, which is thus the correct answer), a dense triangular continuous-wave Doppler profile (option B is thus incorrect), vena contracta width ≥ 0.7 cm (option D is thus incorrect), MR regurgitant jet area/left atrial area ratio ≥ 40% (option E is thus incorrect), and systolic flow reversal in the pulmonary veins (option C is thus incorrect).[10]

49-6. The answer is D. *(Hurst's The Heart, 14th Edition, Chap. 49)* The clinical presentation and the echo findings are consistent with stage C, which includes asymptomatic patients with severe MR as is the case for this patient (option D). Stages A (option A), B (options B and C), and D (option E) typically include patients at risk of MR, patients with progressive MR, and symptomatic patients with severe MR, respectively. Options A, B, C, and E are therefore not correct. Stages of secondary MR with associated valve anatomy, valve hemodynamics, cardiac findings, and symptoms are presented in Table 49-1.[1]

49-7. The answer is A. *(Hurst's The Heart, 14th Edition, Chap. 49)* Atrial fibrillation (AF) is commonly associated with MR, and it is present in up to 50% of patients undergoing MV surgery (option A is thus false, and therefore is the correct answer).[11] LA chamber enlargement as a consequence of increased pressure and volume load to the LA from MR is implicated in the genesis of AF.[12] AF may be a marker of disease progression (option B is thus incorrect) and worse prognosis in IMR (option C is thus incorrect). Surgical approaches for AF with or without left atrial appendage ligation can be considered in patients undergoing MV surgery (option D is thus incorrect). Risk factors for the return of AF after the MAZE procedure include duration of preoperative AF, left atrial size, and reduced LV function (option E is thus incorrect).[13]

49-8. The answer is C. *(Hurst's The Heart, 14th Edition, Chap. 49)* The MitraClip is a transcatheter mitral device for use in high-risk or inoperable patients with severe MR and suitable anatomic criteria (option A is true and thus incorrect). It is currently approved by the US Food and Drug Administration for use in symptomatic patients with primary (degenerative) MR who are at prohibitive risk for surgery (option B is thus incorrect); it is not approved for the treatment of IMR in the United States (option C is thus false, and therefore is the correct answer), but is under investigation for this indication through the Clinical Outcomes Assessment of MitraClip Percutaneous Therapy for Extremely High-Surgical-Risk Patients (COAPT) trial.[10] In contrast, the MitraClip system has already received a class IIb recommendation from the European Society of Cardiology for secondary MR (option D is thus incorrect). Worldwide, it is estimated that approximately two-thirds of the MitraClip procedures have been performed in patients with secondary MR (option E is thus incorrect).

49-9. The answer is B. *(Hurst's The Heart, 14th Edition, Chap. 49)* In the setting of severe IMR, debate has focused on the role of MV repair versus MV replacement (MVR). Repair has been considered safer with lower perioperative mortality and morbidity (option A is thus incorrect), though generally associated with a higher rate of recurrent MR compared with replacement (option B is thus false, and therefore is the correct answer). A randomized multicenter trial assigned 251 patients with severe IMR to undergo either MV repair (*n* = 126) or chordal-sparing MVR (*n* = 125) and did not demonstrate any significant difference in LV end-systolic volume indexed to body surface area at 1 and 2 years (primary end point). No differences in survival (option C is thus incorrect) or the incidence of major adverse cardiac and cerebrovascular events (option D is thus incorrect) were found. The rate of recurrence of moderate or severe MR was significantly higher in the repair compared to the replacement group (32.6% vs 2.3% at 1 year, *P* < .001; and 58.8% versus 3.8% at 2 years, *P* < .001), resulting in more adverse events related to HF and cardiovascular readmissions (option E is thus incorrect).[14,4]

49-10. The answer is D. *(Hurst's The Heart, 14th Edition, Chap. 49)* Many observational studies have identified echocardiographic predictors of recurrent MR following MV annuloplasty, including an LV end-diastolic diameter > 65 mm (option A), coaptation depth > 1 cm (option B), and systolic sphericity index > 0.7 (option C).[5] These options (A, B, and C) would be correct in the setting of MV annuloplasty, but this question is about the factors associated with recurrent moderate or severe MR in patients following repair for severe IMR. In the randomized trial of repair versus replacement, only basal aneurysms and dyskinesis were significantly associated with recurrent moderate or severe MR in patients following repair for severe IMR (option D is thus the correct answer).[15] It is important to note that none of the prediction models for recurrent MR have been externally validated.

The durability of repair is also influenced by the natural history of underlying ventricular dilation over time; progressive dilation will undermine the integrity of MV repair.

References

1. Nishimura RA, Otto CM, Bonow RO, et al. 2014 AHA/ACC guideline for the management of patients with valvular heart disease: Executive summary. A report of the American College of Cardiology/American Heart Association Task Force on Practice Guidelines. *J Am Coll Cardiol.* 2014;63:2438-2488.

2. Bursi F, Enriquez-Sarano M, Nkomo VT, et al. Heart failure and death after myocardial infarction in the community: the emerging role of mitral regurgitation. *Circulation.* 2005;111:295-301.

3. Hillis GS, Moller JE, Pellikka PA, Bell MR, Casaclang-Verzosa GC, Oh JK. Prognostic significance of echocardiographically defined mitral regurgitation early after acute myocardial infarction. *Am Heart J.* 2005;150:1268-1275.

4. Goldstein D, Moskowitz AJ, Gelijns AC, et al. Two-year outcomes of surgical treatment of severe ischemic mitral regurgitation. *N Engl J Med.* 2016;374:344-353.

5. De Bonis M, Al-Attar N, Antunes M, et al. Surgical and interventional management of mitral valve regurgitation: a position statement from the European Society of Cardiology Working Groups on Cardiovascular Surgery and Valvular Heart Disease. *Eur Heart J.* 2016;37:133-139.

6. Lancellotti P, Pierard LA. Chronic ischaemic mitral regurgitation: exercise testing reveals its dynamic component. *Eur Heart J.* 2005;26:1816-1817.

7. Lancellotti P, Gerard PL, Pierard LA. Long-term outcome of patients with heart failure and dynamic functional mitral regurgitation. *Eur Heart J.* 2005;26:1528-1532.

8. Picano E, Pibarot P, Lancellotti P, Monin JL, Bonow RO. The emerging role of exercise testing and stress echocardiography in valvular heart disease. *J Am Coll Cardiol.* 2009;54:2251-2260.

9. Grayburn PA, Carabello B, Hung J, et al. Defining "severe" secondary mitral regurgitation: emphasizing an integrated approach. *J Am Coll Cardiol.* 2014;64:2792-2801.

10. Writing C, Kron IL, Acker MA, et al. The American Association for Thoracic Surgery Consensus Guidelines: ischemic mitral valve regurgitation. *J Thorac Cardiovasc Surg.* 2016;151:940-956.

11. Gillinov AM. Ablation of atrial fibrillation with mitral valve surgery. *Curr Opin Cardiol.* 2005;20:107-114.

12. Kim JB, Lee SH, Jung SH, et al. The influence of postoperative mitral valve function on the late recurrence of atrial fibrillation after the maze procedure combined with mitral valvuloplasty. *J Thorac Cardiovasc Surg.* 2010;139:1170-1176.

13. Gillinov AM, Sirak J, Blackstone EH, et al. The Cox maze procedure in mitral valve disease: predictors of recurrent atrial fibrillation. *J Thorac Cardiovasc Surg.* 2005;130:1653-1660.

14. Acker MA, Parides MK, Perrault LP, et al. Mitral-valve repair versus replacement for severe ischemic mitral regurgitation. *N Engl J Med.* 2014;370:23-32.

15. Kron IL, Hung J, Overbey JR, et al. Predicting recurrent mitral regurgitation after mitral valve repair for severe ischemic mitral regurgitation. *J Thorac Cardiovasc Surg.* 2015;149:752-761 e1.

CHAPTER 50

Mitral Stenosis

Jonathan Afilalo

QUESTIONS

DIRECTIONS: Choose the one best response to each question.

50-1. Rheumatic heart disease (RHD) remains prevalent in developing countries. Which of the following statements about RHD in developing countries is *false*?

A. The prevalence ranges from 1 to 2 per 1000 school children
B. Ten percent of patients with RHD have isolated MS
C. Only 10% of patients with isolated MS report a past history of rheumatic fever
D. Symptoms occur after at least 4 decades from the initial attack of ARF
E. All of the above

50-2. A 52-year-old woman with a prior history of type 2 diabetes, depression, and SLE presented to her family physician for a routine visit. The patient denied any symptoms such as exertional dyspnea, chest pain, or palpitations. Physical examination revealed a loud first heart sound and a middiastolic rumble. A transthoracic echocardiogram was performed and showed rheumatic valve changes with commissural fusion and diastolic doming of the mitral valve leaflets, a planimetered MVA of 1.8 cm², and a diastolic pressure half-time of 145 ms. The patient was in normal sinus rhythm and had a valve morphology that was suitable for BMV. According to the ACC/AHA Stages for MS, at which of the following stages would this patient be?

A. Stage A
B. Stage B
C. Stage C1
D. Stage C2
E. Stage D

50-3. A 56-year-old woman with no prior medical history was referred for cardiac consultation following a 6-month history of exertional dyspnea. Physical examination revealed a loud P2 and a middiastolic rumble. A transthoracic echocardiogram was performed that showed rheumatic valve changes with commissural fusion and diastolic doming of the mitral valve leaflets, a planimetered MVA of 0.9 cm², a diastolic pressure half-time of 230 ms, and a PASP of 69 mm Hg. In addition, there was right ventricular dilatation and dysfunction. Which of the following statements about this patient's pulmonary hypertension is *false*?

A. Secondary vasoconstriction in the pulmonary bed may play a role in its development
B. The specific cause of the observed pulmonary vasoconstriction is well established
C. It is almost always reversed by relief of MS
D. It can be improved by the administration of sildenafil
E. The nitric oxide pathway may be involved in the mechanism of pulmonary vasoconstriction

50-4. A 19-year-old man with a prior history of acute rheumatic fever presented to the emergency department complaining of dyspnea on minimal exertion, orthopnea, and paroxysmal nocturnal dyspnea. Physical examination revealed a loud first heart sound and a low-pitched diastolic rumble best heard at the apex. The initial investigations, including a chest x-ray, were consistent with the diagnosis of pulmonary edema. A transthoracic echocardiogram was performed and showed rheumatic valve changes with commissural fusion and diastolic doming of the mitral valve leaflets, and an MVA of 1.2 cm² with a PASP of 62 mm Hg. Which of the following statements about this patient is *false*?

A. Juvenile MS is the most likely diagnosis
B. The likely diagnosis may constitute up to a quarter of rheumatic MS cases in developing countries
C. Boys are more commonly affected
D. Atrial fibrillation is uncommon
E. MV calcification and LA thrombi are common findings

50-5. A 28-year-old primigravid woman at 31 weeks' gestation was admitted to the hospital because of NYHA class II heart failure symptoms. Physical examination revealed a loud first heart sound and a middiastolic rumble. An initial ECG revealed AF with fast ventricular response. A transthoracic echocardiogram was performed; it showed rheumatic valve changes with commissural fusion and diastolic doming of the mitral valve leaflets, and a diastolic pressure half-time of 138 ms. The patient had a valve morphology that was suitable for BMV. Which of the following will *not* be appropriate as an initial next best step?

A. Diuretics
B. Restriction of physical activity
C. Metoprolol
D. Digoxin
E. BMV

50-6. A 55-year-old woman with a prior history of acute rheumatic fever at age 15 presented to the emergency department complaining of exertional dyspnea and intermittent palpitations. Physical examination revealed a loud first heart sound and a middiastolic rumble. In addition, there was an irregularly irregular pulse. Atrial fibrillation was confirmed on the initial ECG. A transthoracic echocardiogram was performed and revealed rheumatic valve changes with commissural fusion and diastolic doming of the mitral valve leaflets, and an MVA of 1.1 cm². In addition there were extensive calcifications and severe subvalvular disease. Which of the following would be the surgical treatment of choice for this patient?

A. Closed mitral valvotomy (CMV)
B. Open mitral valvotomy (OMV)
C. Mitral valve replacement (MVR)
D. BMV
E. All of the above

50-7. A 49-year-old woman with no prior medical history presented to her cardiologist complaining of a reduced exercise tolerance. Physical examination revealed a loud first heart sound and a middiastolic rumble. A transthoracic echocardiogram was performed and showed rheumatic valve changes with commissural fusion and diastolic doming of the mitral valve leaflets, a planimetered MVA of 1.1 cm², a diastolic pressure half-time of 210 ms, and a PASP of 49 mm Hg. The patient was in normal sinus rhythm and had a valve morphology that was suitable for BMV. According to the ACC/AHA Stages for MS, at which of the following stages would this patient be?

A. Stage A
B. Stage B
C. Stage C1
D. Stage C2
E. Stage D

50-8. Relief of MS by surgery may be done either by CMV, OMV, or MVR. Which of the following is a class 2b indication for MVR?

A. Severely symptomatic MS (MVA < 1.5 cm²; NYHA class III/IV) who are not high risk for surgery and who are not candidates for BMV
B. Severe symptomatic MS (MVA < 1.5 cm²; NYHA class III/IV) who are not high risk for surgery and who have failed previous BMV
C. Severe MS (MVA ≤ 1.5 cm²) with recurrent embolic events despite adequate anticoagulation
D. Severe MS (MVA < 1.5 cm²) undergoing aortic valve surgery
E. Severe MS (MVA < 1.5 cm²) undergoing CABG

50-9. A 62-year-old woman with no prior medical history was referred for cardiac consultation following a 6-month history of exertional dyspnea and intermittent palpitations. Physical examination revealed an irregularly irregular pulse, a loud P2 and a middiastolic rumble. In addition, the assessment of the jugular venous pressure revealed absent "a" wave and "x" descent. The initial ECG confirmed AF. A transthoracic echocardiogram was performed, and it showed rheumatic valve changes with commissural fusion and diastolic doming of the mitral valve leaflets, a planimetered MVA of 0.7 cm², a diastolic pressure half-time of 240 ms, and a PASP of 79 mm Hg. In addition, there was right ventricular dilatation and dysfunction. Which of the following statements about this patient's AF is *false*?

A. The prevalence in MS patients is approximately 40%
B. Age and the severity of MS are the most important determinants for the development of AF
C. LA enlargement is the cause of AF rather than the result of AF
D. AF in MS may also be secondary to rheumatic scarring and histologic changes in the LA
E. Relief of mitral obstruction may or may not prevent AF

50-10. The echocardiogram is the modality of choice in the assessment of MS. In terms of the assessment of the valve area, which of the following echo modalities has the closest agreement with invasive Gorlin-derived MVA?

A. Direct 2D planimetry
B. Direct 3D planimetry
C. Continuity equation method
D. Pressure half-time technique
E. Proximal isovelocity surface area (PISA) method

50-1. The answer is E. (*Hurst's The Heart, 14th Edition, Chap. 50*) Using echocardiographic screening, the prevalence of RHD ranges from 20 to 30 per 1000 school children (option A is thus not correct).[1,2] This leads to a large pool of rheumatic MS. Forty percent of patients with RHD have isolated MS (option B is thus not correct) but only 60% of these patients report a past history of rheumatic fever (option C is also not correct).[2,3] In developing countries, the disease may progress much more rapidly, leading to symptoms by the age of 20 (juvenile MS), often within five years of the initial attack of RF (option D is thus not correct).[4] All the above statements are false, and therefore, the best option is E.

50-2. The answer is B. (*Hurst's The Heart, 14th Edition, Chap. 50*) The clinical presentation and the echo findings are consistent with stage B, which includes patients with progressive MS (not severe). Stages A, C, and D typically include patient at risk of MS, asymptomatic patients but with severe disease, and symptomatic subjects with severe MS, respectively. Therefore, options A, C, D, and E are not correct. The stages and severity of MS are presented in Table 50-1.[5]

TABLE 50-1 Stages and Severity of Mitral Stenosis

Stage	Definition	Valve Anatomy	Valve Hemodynamics	Hemodynamic Consequences	Symptoms
A	At risk of MS	Mild diastolic valve doming	Normal transmitral flow velocity	None	None
B	Progressive MS	1. Rheumatic valve changes with commissural fusion and diastolic doming of the mitral valve leaflets 2. Planimetered MVA > 1.5 cm^2	1. Increased transmitral flow velocities 2. MVA > 1.5 cm^2 3. Diastolic pressure half-time < 150 ms	1. Mild-to-moderate LA enlargement 2. Normal pulmonary pressure at rest	None
C	Asymptomatic severe MS	1. Rheumatic valve changes with commissural fusion and diastolic doming of the mitral valve leaflets 2. Planimetered MVA ≤ 1.5 cm^2 (MVA ≤ 1.0 cm^2 with very severe MS)	1. MVA ≤ 1.5 cm^2 (MVA ≤ 1.0 cm^2 with very severe MS) 2. Diastolic pressure half-time ≥ 150 ms (diastolic pressure half-time ≥ 220 ms with very severe MS)	1. Severe LA enlargement 2. Elevated PASP > 30 mm Hg	None
D	Symptomatic severe MS	1. Rheumatic valve changes with commissural fusion and diastolic doming of the mitral valve leaflets 2. Planimetered MVA ≤ 1.5 cm^2	1. MVA ≤ 1.5 cm^2 (MVA ≤ 1.0 cm^2 with very severe MS) 2. Diastolic pressure half-time ≥ 150 ms (diastolic pressure half-time ≥ 220 ms with very severe MS)	1. Severe LA enlargement 2. Elevated PASP > 30 mm Hg	1. Reduced exercise tolerance 2. Exertional dyspnea

MVA, Mitral valve area.
(Data from Nishimura RA, Otto CM, Bonow RO, et al. 2014 AHA/ACC guideline for the management of patients with valvular heart disease: A report of the American College of Cardiology/American Heart Association Task Force on Practice Guidelines, *J Am Coll Cardiol.* 2014 Jun 10;63(22):2438-2488.)

50-3. The answer is B. (*Hurst's The Heart, 14th Edition, Chap. 50*) The force needed to overcome the increased LA pressure and to drive blood past the stenotic mitral valve is generated by the right ventricle (RV), such that right ventricular pressure and pulmonary pressure become elevated. As MS becomes severe, secondary vasoconstriction in the pulmonary bed causes a further increase in pulmonary artery pressure (option A is thus incorrect), and pulmonary hypertension may become extreme. The exact cause of pulmonary vasoconstriction in MS is unknown (option B is thus false and is the correct answer). It is known that pulmonary hypertension is usually reversed by relief of MS (option C is thus incorrect)[6] and also that it can at times be improved by the administration of phosphodiesterase inhibitors such as sildenafil (option D is thus incorrect)[7] or by nitric oxide inhalation.[8] These data suggest that the nitric oxide pathway is in some way involved in the mechanism of pulmonary vasoconstriction and pulmonary hypertension in MS (option E is thus incorrect). Occasionally, patients have structural changes in the pulmonary bed, leading to a disproportionate pulmonary hypertension that is not completely resolved with relief of MS.

50-4. **The answer is E.** (Hurst's The Heart, 14th Edition, Chap. 50) This patient suffers from rheumatic mitral stenosis, which when presenting below 20 years is termed juvenile MS as in this case (option A is thus incorrect).[4] This condition is uncommon in developed countries, but it may constitute up to a quarter of cases of all rheumatic MS in developing countries (option B is thus incorrect).[4] Unlike in adults, boys are more commonly affected (option C is thus incorrect).[4] Heart failure/pulmonary edema is a frequent finding, while atrial fibrillation is uncommon (option D is thus incorrect). Severe pulmonary hypertension is common. Although MV calcification and LA thrombi are absent (option E is false and is thus the correct answer), the valve morphology is associated with severe subvalvular disease and thickened leaflets.

50-5. **The answer is E.** (Hurst's The Heart, 14th Edition, Chap. 50) Diuretics can usually be used safely to control mild symptoms; thus they should be administered as part of the initial management (option A). Overaggressive use of diuretics can lead to placental hypoperfusion. Therapy is targeted to reduce heart rate and prolong diastolic filling period. This includes restrictions on physical activity (option B) and the use of beta-blockers (those with selective beta-1 activity is preferred). Metoprolol is preferred over atenolol because it has a lower incidence of intrauterine growth retardation (option C).[5] In patients with atrial fibrillation, digoxin can be safely used (option D). Pregnant patients with severe MS (MVA ≤ 1.5 cm^2) and mild symptoms are best managed medically (options A, B, C, and D are thus true), while those who continue to manifest severe symptoms (NYHA class III-IV) despite medical therapy should undergo BMV if the valve is suitable (option E).[5]

50-6. **The answer is C.** (Hurst's The Heart, 14th Edition, Chap. 50) Relief of MS by surgery may be done either by CMV (option A), OMV (option B), or MVR. CMV, via the transatrial or transventricular route, is still practiced successfully in many developing countries. However, the results of BMV are superior to CMV with lower morbidity. When extensive calcification and severe subvalvular disease make BMV/OMV unfeasible (option D), as in this case, MVR is the surgical treatment of choice (option C).

50-7. **The answer is E.** (Hurst's The Heart, 14th Edition, Chap. 50) The clinical presentation and the echo findings are consistent with stage D, which includes symptomatic patients with severe MS (option E). Stages A, B, and C typically include patient at risk of MS, patient with progressive MS, and asymptomatic patients but with severe disease, respectively. Therefore, options A, B, C, and D are not correct. The stages and severity of MS are presented in Table 50-1.[5]

50-8. **The answer is C.** (Hurst's The Heart, 14th Edition, Chap. 50) The indications for MVR are as follows:[5] (1) Severely symptomatic patients (NYHA class III/IV) with severe MS (MVA < 1.5 cm^2) who are not high risk for surgery and who are not candidates for, or have failed, previous BMV (options A and B, respectively) are class 1 indications, not class 2b; (2) severe MS (MVA < 1.5 cm^2) patients undergoing other cardiac surgery (eg, aortic valve surgery, CABG), which are options D and E respectively, are class 2a indications; and (3) mitral valve surgery and LAA excision may be considered for patients with severe MS (MVA ≤ 1.5 cm^2, stages C and D) with recurrent embolic events despite adequate anticoagulation (option C); these are class 2b indications, and therefore C is the correct answer.

50-9. **The answer is C.** (Hurst's The Heart, 14th Edition, Chap. 50) Atrial fibrillation is the most common complication of MS, developing in approximately 40% of patients (option A is thus incorrect).[9] Age and the severity of MS are the most important determinants for the development of AF (option B is thus incorrect).[10] AF is related to LA enlargement, the latter often a result rather than the cause of AF (option C is thus false and is therefore the correct answer for this question).[11] Although it is often hoped that relief of MS will result in restoration of sinus rhythm, AF in MS is due not only to increased LA size but also to rheumatic scarring and histologic changes in the LA.[12] Thus relief of mitral obstruction may[13] or may not prevent AF[14] or allow for a return to sinus rhythm (option E is thus incorrect).

50-10. The answer is B. (*Hurst's The Heart, 14th Edition, Chap. 50*) Valve area can be estimated by direct planimetry (either 2D or 3D), by the continuity equation, by the pressure half-time technique (dividing an empirical constant of 220 by the mitral inflow pressure half-time), and by the PISA method. In some cases these measures are concordant, but in others, all measures must be taken into account and clinical judgment used to decide on MS severity. Planimetry by three-dimensional echocardiography (option B) has better reproducibility than two-dimensional echocardiography (option A) and has the closest agreement with invasive Gorlin-derived MVA.[15] Options C, D, and E are not correct for the above-mentioned reasons.

References

1. Saxena A, Ramakrishnan S, Roy A, et al. Prevalence and outcome of subclinical rheumatic heart disease in India: the RHEUMATIC (Rheumatic Heart Echo Utilisation and Monitoring Actuarial Trends in Indian Children) study. *Heart*. 2011;97:2018-2022.
2. Marijon E, Ou P, Celermajer DS, et al. Prevalence of rheumatic heart disease detected by echocardiographic screening. *N Engl J Med*. 2007;35:470-476.
3. Rowe JC, Bland EF, Sprague HB, et al. The course of mitral stenosis without surgery: ten- and twenty-year perspectives. *Ann Intern Med*. 1960;52:741-749.
4. Roy SB, Bhatia ML, Lazaro EJ, et al. Juvenile mitral stenosis in India. *Lancet*. 1963;2:1193-1195.
5. Nishimura RA, Otto CM, Bonow RO, et al. 2014 AHA/ACC guideline for the management of patients with valvular heart disease: A report of the American College of Cardiology/American Heart Association Task Force on Practice Guidelines. *J Am Coll Cardiol*. 2014;63:2438-2488.
6. Dalen JE, Matloff JM, Evans GL, et al. Early reduction of pulmonary vascular resistance after mitral-valve replacement. *N Engl J Med*. 1967;277(8):387-394.
7. Trachte AL, Lobato EB, Urdaneta F, et al. Oral sildenafil reduces pulmonary hypertension after cardiac surgery. *Ann Thorac Surg*. 2005;79(1):194-197.
8. Mahoney PD, Loh E, Bllitz LR, et al. Hemodynamic effects of inhaled nitric oxide in women with mitral stenosis and pulmonary hypertension. *Am J Cardiol*. 2001;87(2):188-192.
9. Selzer A, Cohn KE. Natural history of mitral stenosis: a review. *Circulation*. 1972;45:878-890.
10. Probst P, Goldschlager N, Selzer A. Left atrial size and atrial fibrillation in mitral stenosis. Factors influencing their relationship. *Circulation*. 1973;48:1282-1287.
11. Sanfilippo AJ, Abascal VM, Sheehan M, et al. Atrial enlargement as a consequence of atrial fibrillation. A prospective echocardiographic study. *Circulation*. 1990;82:792-797.
12. Alessandri N, Tufano F, Petrassi M, et al. Atrial fibrillation in pure rheumatic mitral valvular disease is expression of an atrial histological change. *Eur Rev Med Pharmacol Sci*. 2009;13(6):431-442.
13. Eid Fawzy M, Shoukri M, Al Sergani H, et al. Favorable effect of balloon mitral valvuloplasty on the incidence of atrial fibrillation in patients with severe mitral stenosis. *Catheter Cardiovasc Interv*. 2006;68(4):536-541.
14. Krasuski RA, Assar MD, Wang A, et al. Usefulness of percutaneous balloon mitral commissurotomy in preventing the development of atrial fibrillation in patients with mitral stenosis. *Am J Cardiol*. 2004;93(7):936-939.
15. Zamorano J, Cordeiro P, Sugeng L, et al. Real-time three-dimensional echocardiography for rheumatic mitral valve stenosis evaluation: an accurate and novel approach. *J Am Coll Cardiol*. 2004;43:2091-2096.

CHAPTER 51

Tricuspid and Pulmonary Valve Disease

Jonathan Afilalo

QUESTIONS

DIRECTIONS: Choose the one best response to each question.

51-1. A 15-year-old boy with a prior medical history of childhood murmur presented to the emergency department after a series of presyncopal episodes. The physical examination revealed a systolic ejection click, a loud systolic murmur peaking in late systole as well as a soft P2. Initial ECG and chest radiography showed evidence of right heart chamber enlargement. An echocardiogram was obtained and showed doming and restricted opening of the pulmonary valve. In addition, spectral and color-flow Doppler revealed high-velocity turbulent flow in the main pulmonary artery consistent with pulmonary stenosis. The patient underwent cardiac catheterization, which revealed an RV–to–pulmonary artery peak-to-peak gradient of 37 mm Hg. Which of the following would be the best step in the management of this patient?

A. Medical therapy with follow-up
B. Surgical valvotomy
C. Percutaneous balloon valvotomy
D. Bioprosthetic valve replacement
E. Mechanical valve replacement

51-2. In which of the following settings is surgical correction of tricuspid valve regurgitation (TR) most commonly performed?

A. Isolated procedure for primary TR
B. Isolated procedure for secondary TR
C. Concomitant procedure during mitral valve surgery
D. Concomitant procedure during aortic valve surgery
E. Concomitant procedure during coronary artery bypass grafting

51-3. A 19-year-old man with no known medical history presented to the emergency department complaining of flushing, diarrhea, and dyspnea. The cardiovascular examination revealed a 2/6 decrescendo diastolic murmur at the left upper sternal border, along with an RV heave and an elevated JVP. An echocardiogram demonstrated thickened barely mobile pulmonary valve cusps, with severe pulmonary regurgitation; subcostal imaging incidentally reveals a hepatic mass. Which of the following is the most likely diagnosis?

A. Infective endocarditis
B. Viral gastroenteritis
C. Congenital pulmonary insufficiency
D. Rheumatic heart disease
E. Carcinoid disease

51-4. An asymptomatic 47-year-old man with a remote history of rheumatic fever as a child is found to have a diastolic murmur during a routine physical examination; the murmur is best heard at the left lower sternal border and increases on inspiration. He is referred for an echocardiogram, which shows a thickened, distorted tricuspid valve with moderate tricuspid stenosis and mild-to-moderate tricuspid regurgitation. Which of the following statements regarding rheumatic tricuspid valve disease is *false*?

A. Rheumatic involvement of the tricuspid valve is more common than the aortic valve
B. Tricuspid stenosis and regurgitation are often seen in combination
C. A Kussmaul sign may be appreciated on examination
D. Valve repair with balloon valvotomy or annuloplasty is preferred in cases where the valve is not severely distorted
E. When valve replacement is needed, a bioprosthesis is preferred over a mechanical prosthesis

51-5. A 25-year-old woman with no significant past medical history was referred to the cardiology clinic complaining of a 6-month history of exertional chest discomfort. The physical examination revealed a systolic murmur peaking in late systole and best heard over the pulmonary area, and a well-preserved but delayed P2. Initial ECG and chest radiography showed evidence of right heart chamber enlargement. An echocardiography was obtained and showed normal pulmonary valve cusps, midsystolic cusp closure, a prominent presystolic a-wave, and a normal main pulmonary artery diameter. In addition, spectral and color-flow Doppler revealed a late-peaking, high-velocity flow with turbulence in the right ventricular outflow tract. Which of the following is the most likely diagnosis?

A. Pulmonary valve stenosis
B. Infundibular pulmonary stenosis
C. Pulmonary regurgitation
D. Idiopathic pulmonary artery dilatation
E. Pulmonary valve endocarditis

51-6. A 19-year-old woman is followed in cardiology clinic for pulmonary valve stenosis, but she has missed her last appointments because she "felt fine." She now notes progressive exertional dyspnea and can no longer play sports with her friends. Four years ago, the physical examination revealed a systolic ejection click, a preserved but delayed P2, and a 2/6 systolic murmur peaking in early-to-mid systole that was best heard over the pulmonary area. Given the clinical suspicion of worsening pulmonary valve stenosis, which of the following physical examination findings would *not* be expected at this time?

A. Murmur has gotten louder
B. Murmur peaks later in systole
C. Systolic ejection click is more prominent in inspiration
D. P2 has gotten softer
E. All of the above

51-7. A 67-year-old man with a remote history of pulmonary emboli complains of increased abdominal girth. A physical examination revealed elevated JVP, systolic RV heave, a 3/6 pansystolic murmur best heard at the left lower sternal border, and ascites. An echo showed right ventricular dilation, tricuspid annular dilation with loss of central coaptation of the tricuspid leaflets, and a vena contracta width of 0.8 cm. The findings were consistent with severe functional tricuspid regurgitation, and loop diuretic therapy is prescribed. Which of the following statements about tricuspid regurgitation (TR) is *false*?

A. If treated medically, this patient will have a mortality of 26% at 5 years
B. Cardiac MRI may be considered for the assessment of RV size and function
C. Aldosterone antagonists may be of additive benefit, especially in the setting of hepatic congestion
D. Pulmonary vasodilators may be helpful
E. None of the above

51-8. A 55-year-old woman with a prior history of myxomatous mitral valve disease, having been lost to follow-up, presented to the emergency department complaining of dyspnea on minimal exertion and leg swelling. Physical examination revealed a 4/6 systolic murmur best heard at the apex, along with an elevated JVP, pitting leg edema, and mild ascites. An echo was obtained showing biventricular dilation and systolic dysfunction, severe mitral regurgitation, and moderate functional tricuspid regurgitation. The tricuspid leaflets were tethered, but the annular diameter was within normal limits. Which of the following would be the best recommendation according to current guidelines?

A. Mitral valve surgery only
B. Mitral valve surgery with tricuspid valve replacement
C. Mitral valve surgery with tricuspid annuloplasty
D. Medical therapy with aggressive diuresis
E. Isolated tricuspid annuloplasty

51-9. The recommendation to offer surgical correction of the mitral and tricuspid valve lesions is discussed with the patient in Question 8. She asks about the success rate of the additional tricuspid valve procedure being recommended. Which of the following best approximates the probability that this patient will be free from significant tricuspid regurgitation 5 to 10 years post-annuloplasty?

A. 20%
B. 40%
C. 60%
D. 85%
E. 95%

51-10. Because tricuspid regurgitation is a dynamic lesion, tricuspid regurgitation may be graded as moderate or severe on preoperative transthoracic echocardiography under normal loading conditions, but it may appear only mild on intraoperative transesophageal echocardiography under general anesthesia. Other than tricuspid regurgitation severity under normal loading conditions, which of the following parameters should be taken into account when deciding about the need for concomitant tricuspid annuloplasty at the time of mitral valve repair?

A. Annular dimensions
B. Leaflet malcoaptation or leaflet-annulus mismatch on direct inspection
C. The presence of pulmonary hypertension
D. The presence of atrial fibrillation
E. All of the above

ANSWERS

51-1. **The answer is C.** *(Hurst's The Heart, 14th Edition, Chap. 51)* According to the American College of Cardiology/American Heart Association Guidelines for the Management of Patients with Valvular Heart Disease,[1] balloon valvotomy is recommended in adolescent and young adult patients with pulmonic stenosis who have exertional dyspnea, angina, syncope, or presyncope and an RV-to-pulmonary artery peak-to-peak gradient greater than 30 mm Hg at catheterization (Class I and Level of Evidence: C). Moderately severe and severe pulmonary valve stenosis is currently treated by percutaneous balloon valvotomy (option C). Surgical valvotomy or replacement is rarely needed (options B, D, E). There is no effective medical therapy for this structural condition (option A).

51-2. **The answer is C.** *(Hurst's The Heart, 14th Edition, Chap. 51)* Surgical correction of tricuspid valve disease is most commonly performed at the time of mitral valve surgery (option C).[2] Significant TR is less frequently observed in patients with aortic valve or ischemic heart disease, and therefore tricuspid valve surgery is less often needed at the time of these surgeries (options D, E). Furthermore, the majority of patients with TR, whether primary or secondary, are effectively managed medically with diuretics, such that tricuspid valve surgery is not often performed as an isolated procedure, unless it is refractory to medical therapy (options A, B).

51-3. **The answer is E.** *(Hurst's The Heart, 14th Edition, Chap. 51)* The patient is presenting with cutaneous (flushing) and gastrointestinal (diarrhea) symptoms that are typical of the carcinoid syndrome. The pathognomonic echocardiographic appearance of markedly thickened retracted leaflets is more common on the tricuspid valve but is also observed on the pulmonary valve, as in this case. The gold standard treatment for carcinoid heart disease is usually tricuspid valve replacement and pulmonary valve replacement with patch enlargement of the right ventricular outflow tract. Endocarditis does not have this echocardiographic appearance and is not suspected in the absence of fever (option A). Viral gastroenteritis is not associated with these cardiac findings (option B) whereas congenital pulmonary insufficiency is not associated with these noncardiac findings (option C). Rheumatic involvement of the pulmonary valve may manifest as thickening and restriction at the commissural level, and it would typically be associated with the involvement of other valves without the cutaneous and gastrointestinal symptoms (option D).

51-4. **The answer is A.** *(Hurst's The Heart, 14th Edition, Chap. 51)* Rheumatic involvement of the tricuspid valve is far less common than with the mitral and the aortic valves (option A), reported in between 10% and 20% of patients. Rheumatic tricuspid valve disease is often predominantly functional, but it is occasionally characterized by leaflet involvement with thickened, fibrosed, and shortened leaflets, and commissural fusion. The resulting clinical syndrome is one of mixed stenosis and regurgitation (option B). Inspiratory increase in jugular venous pressure is common and simulates the Kussmaul sign in constrictive pericarditis (option C). However, the jugular venous pulse with rheumatic tricuspid valve stenosis and regurgitation fails to show rapid "y" descent. Treatment of rheumatic tricuspid valve disease consists of balloon valvotomomy for predominant stenosis, valve repair with annuloplasty (option D), or valve replacement with a low-profile bioprosthetic valve for severely distorted valves (option E).

51-5. **The answer is B.** *(Hurst's The Heart, 14th Edition, Chap. 51)* Although the valve cusps are normal in infundibular stenosis, a characteristic midsystolic cusp closure (caused by dynamic subvalvular obstruction) and prominent presystolic a-wave are often diagnostic clues, along with high-velocity turbulent flow in the right ventricular outflow tract. The pulmonary valve morphology shows doming and restricted opening in the presence of pulmonary valve stenosis, with high-velocity turbulent flow in the main pulmonary artery (option A). The pulmonary artery and branches are dilated in pulmonary hypertension, idiopathic pulmonary artery dilatation, and severe pulmonary regurgitation (options C and D). In cases of pulmonary valve endocarditis, a mobile vegetation may be observed (option E).

51-6. The answer is C. *(Hurst's The Heart, 14th Edition, Chap. 51)* With progressive pulmonary valve stenosis severity, the murmur gets louder, longer, and peaks later in systole (options A and B). The ejection click is often more prominent in expiration (option C). This seemingly paradoxical behavior of the pulmonary ejection click is explained by an inspiratory increase in right ventricular end-diastolic pressure, which opens the valve in late diastole and hence the absence of systolic ejection clicks during the inspiratory phase. The pulmonary component of the second heart sound (P2) becomes softer (option D), and in very severe cases, the murmur spills past the aortic component, and the pulmonary component is inaudible.

51-7. The answer is E. *(Hurst's The Heart, 14th Edition, Chap. 51)* Several large studies have reported on the adverse effects of longstanding tricuspid regurgitation.[3-5] If treated medically, moderate to severe tricuspid regurgitation carries a mortality of 26% at 5 years (option A). In addition to echocardiography, cardiac MRI can provide complementary information about the severity of tricuspid regurgitation and its impact on RV dilation and dysfunction (option B). The mainstay of medical management for functional tricuspid regurgitation includes loop diuretics and aldosterone antagonists to decrease volume overload in patients with peripheral edema and ascites (option C).[1] Specific pulmonary vasodilators may be helpful to reduce right ventricular afterload in patients with reversible pulmonary hypertension evaluated with cardiac catheterization (option D).

51-8. The answer is C. *(Hurst's The Heart, 14th Edition, Chap. 51)* According to the American College of Cardiology/American Heart Association Guidelines for the Management of Patients with Valvular Heart Disease,[1] tricuspid valve repair can be beneficial for patients with mild, moderate, or greater functional tricuspid regurgitation at the time of left-sided valve surgery, with either (1) tricuspid annular dilatation or (2) prior evidence of right heart failure (Class IIa and Level of Evidence: B). This patient has evidence of right heart failure, and therefore should be considered for tricuspid annuloplasty (option C), which would also be a consideration if she had evidence of annular dilatation.[6] Tricuspid valve replacement (option B) is not indicated for the repair of moderate functional regurgitation because it introduces the additional risks of thromboembolic and hemorrhagic complications inherent with mechanical prostheses, or the risk of structural valve degeneration requiring reoperation inherent with bioprostheses.[7] Isolated tricuspid valve surgery (option E) is not appropriate because this patient has severe symptomatic mitral regurgitation that requires correction. Medical therapy is not a curative option for this patient (option D).

51-9. The answer is D. *(Hurst's The Heart, 14th Edition, Chap. 51)* Data from the surgical literature suggest that 85% of patients having a ring annuloplasty for functional tricuspid regurgitation will be free from moderate or severe tricuspid regurgitation from 5 to 10 years after surgery (option D).[8] Risk factors for recurrent moderate or severe tricuspid regurgitation include: higher preoperative regurgitation grade, poor left ventricular function, permanent pacemaker, and repair type other than ring annuloplasty.[9]

51-10. The answer is E. *(Hurst's The Heart, 14th Edition, Chap. 51)* In this context, the final decision should be guided not only by the degree of regurgitation but also by annular enlargement (diameter > 7 cm from the anteroseptal to anteroposterior commissures when measured by direct inspection, or > 40 mm from the 4-chamber view when measured by echo), leaflet malcoaptation, and the presence of atrial fibrillation, pulmonary hypertension, right ventricular dysfunction, or left ventricular dysfunction.

References

1. Nishimura RA, Otto CM, Bonow RO, et al. 2014 AHA/ACC guideline for the management of patients with valvular heart disease: executive summary. A report of the American College of Cardiology/American Heart Association Task Force on Practice Guidelines. *J Am Coll Cardiol.* 2014;63:2438-2488.

2. Chikwe J, Itagaki S, Anyanwu A, Adams DH. Impact of concomitant tricuspid annuloplasty on tricuspid regurgitation, right ventricular function, and pulmonary artery hypertension after repair of mitral valve prolapse. *J Am Coll Cardiol.* 2015;65:1931-1938.

3. Nath J, Foster E, Heidenreich PA. Impact of tricuspid regurgitation on long-term survival. *J Am Coll Cardiol.* 2004;43:405-409.

4. Neuhold S, Huelsmann M, Pernicka E, et al. Impact of tricuspid regurgitation on survival in patients with chronic heart failure: unexpected findings of a long-term observational study. *Eur Heart J.* 2013;34:844-852.

5. Lee JW, Song JM, Park JP, Lee JW, Kang DH, Song JK. Long-term prognosis of isolated significant tricuspid regurgitation. *Circ J.* 2010;74:375-380.

6. Goldstone AB, Howard JL, Cohen JE, MacArthur JW Jr., Atluri P, Kirkpatrick JN, Woo YJ. Natural history of coexistent tricuspid regurgitation in patients with degenerative mitral valve disease: implications for future guidelines. *J Thorac Cardiovasc Surg.* 2014;148:2802-2809.

7. Buzzatti N, Iaci G, Taramasso M, et al. Long-term outcomes of tricuspid valve replacement after previous left-side heart surgery. *Eur J Cardiothorac Surg.* 2014;46:713-719; discussion 719.

8. Chen Y, Seto WK, Ho LM, et al. Relation of tricuspid regurgitation to liver stiffness measured by transient elastography in patients with left-sided cardiac valve disease. *Am J Cardiol.* 2016;117:640-646.

9. McCarthy PM et al. Tricuspid valve repair: durability and risk factors for failure. *J Thorac Cardiovasc Surg.* 2004;127(3):674-685.

CHAPTER 52
Prosthetic Heart Valves
Jonathan Afilalo

QUESTIONS

DIRECTIONS: Choose the one best response to each question.

52-1. A 62-year-old man with a prior history of infective endocarditis and a porcine aortic bioprosthesis that was implanted 12 weeks ago attended the cardiology clinic for a routine visit. At the clinic, a complete evaluation was unremarkable, including anticoagulation adherence, clinical questioning, physical examination, 12-lead ECG, and transthoracic echocardiography for the assessment of ventricular and prosthetic valve function. Which of the following actions would be the most appropriate at this time?

A. Discharge the patient from the clinic
B. Discharge the patient from the clinic with family physician follow-up
C. Discharge the patient from the clinic and advise him to get in touch if symptoms occur
D. Follow the patient for another year, and if he is stable, discharge him with family physician follow-up
E. None of the above

52-2. Having undergone an echocardiogram before and shortly after his aortic valve replacement surgery, the patient described in Question 52-1 would like to know when the next echocardiogram will be scheduled. Which of the following statements about the use of transthoracic echocardiography after the bioprosthetic valve replacement is *false*?

A. Should be performed annually after the 10th postoperative year
B. Should be performed annually after the fifth postoperative year

C. Should be performed annually after the second or third postoperative year in patients who are at higher risk of accelerated valve dysfunction
D. Should be performed sooner if new symptoms occur
E. All of the above

52-3. A 60-year-old man with a past medical history of a mechanical mitral valve replacement presents to the cardiology clinic and would like to have an expert opinion regarding antibiotic prophylaxis before dental procedures. Which of the following would be the best recommendation regarding antibiotic prophylaxis?

A. 2 g of amoxicillin before any dental procedure
B. 2 g of ampicillin before any dental procedure
C. 600 mg of clindamycin before any dental procedure
D. Antibiotic prophylaxis is no longer recommended
E. Antibiotic prophylaxis only if there is manipulation of gingival or periapical tissue, or perforation of oral mucosa

52-4. You receive a phone call from a urologist for a consultation regarding a 55-year-old man with a past medical history of a bioprosthetic aortic valve replacement. The patient is scheduled to undergo a cystoscopy as part of his investigation for bladder cancer. Which of the following would be the best recommendation regarding antibiotic prophylaxis?

A. 2 g of amoxicillin before the urological procedure
B. 2 g of ampicillin before the urological procedure
C. 600 mg of clindamycin before the urological procedure
D. Antibiotic prophylaxis is no longer recommended
E. Cancel the cystoscopy and advise alternate noninvasive diagnostic testing

52-5. A 79-year-old man with a prior history of arterial hypertension, dyslipidemia, and stage IV chronic kidney disease presented to the emergency department complaining of worsening dyspnea and decreasing exercise tolerance. The patient underwent bioprosthetic aortic valve replacement 8 years earlier for aortic stenosis. The physical examination revealed reduced carotid upstroke bilaterally and a 5/6 systolic ejection murmur across the precordium. A transthoracic echocardiogram was obtained and revealed severe prosthetic valve stenosis. Which of the following may potentially explain the echocardiographic findings?

A. Bioprosthetic valve degeneration
B. Bioprosthetic valve thrombosis
C. Endocarditis with a large burden of vegetation
D. Pannus
E. All of the above

52-6. A 65-year-old woman with a prior history of arterial hypertension, coronary heart disease, and depression is referred for a routine echocardiogram 4 weeks after having undergone an aortic valve replacement with a 21-mm bioprosthesis. The echocardiogram revealed normal left ventricular function with a mean transprosthetic gradient of 68 mm Hg, and a calculated indexed effective orifice area was 0.61 cm^2/m^2. The mobility of prosthetic leaflets was normal, and there were no findings to suggest prosthetic pannus or thrombus. Patient-prosthesis mismatch was suspected. Which of the following may *not* be a clinical consequence of this diagnosis?

A. Decreased cardiac index
B. Reduced functional improvement
C. Higher risk of stroke in the first 30 days
D. Less left ventricular mass regression
E. More adverse events in long-term follow-up

52-7. A 37-year-old obese man with a history of mechanical mitral valve replacement for congenital mitral valve disease presented to the emergency department complaining of dyspnea. Upon further questioning, the patient also reported a prior history of four embolic strokes with no residual neurologic deficit, all of which were related to poor medication adherence. The physical examination revealed 4/6 systolic ejection murmur across the precordium. A transthoracic echocardiography was obtained and revealed prosthetic valve thrombosis. Which of the following is the strongest independent predictor of nonadherence to an anticoagulation regimen?

A. Age less than 55 years
B. Age older than 55 years
C. Living in a rural geographic area
D. Living in an urban geographic area
E. Pregnancy in the first trimester

52-8. A 42-year-old woman has a history of bioprosthetic mitral valve replacement 12 years ago for myxomatous mitral valve disease (bioprosthesis implanted because of childbearing at the time). She comes to the emergency department complaining of a 2-day history of dyspnea, orthopnea, and paroxysmal nocturnal dyspnea. The physical examination revealed bilateral crackles and a pansystolic murmur heard across the precordium. An urgent transthoracic echocardiography was obtained, and it revealed diffuse thickening and reduced mobility of the bioprosthesis. Which of the following is the most likely diagnosis and the most common bioprosthetic valve-related complication leading to reoperation?

A. Paravalvular leak
B. Structural valve degeneration
C. Endocarditis
D. Pannus formation
E. Thrombus formation

52-9. The patient described in Question 52-8 asks whether she should have chosen a mechanical prosthesis at the time of her index surgery (and accepted the risks associated with anticoagulation and childbearing). In counseling her, which of the following statements is *true* regarding the expected long-term risk of reoperation after a mitral valve replacement surgery?

A. The risk is higher with aortic valve replacement than with mitral valve replacement
B. The risk is higher with younger patients
C. The risk is higher with mechanical prostheses than with bioprostheses
D. There is a higher short-term risk with mechanical prostheses but no difference in long-term risk
E. The risk is negligible short- and long-term with newer-generation prosthetic valves

52-10. After initial medical management and discussions with the patient and the heart team, the decision was made to offer reoperative valve replacement to the patient described in Question 52-9. Which of the following may be helpful in preparation for the redo procedure?

A. Transesophageal echocardiography
B. Cardiac catheterization
C. Noncontrast chest CT
D. Prior operative reports
E. All of the above

ANSWERS

52-1. The answer is E. *(Hurst's The Heart, 14th Edition, Chap. 52)* At 6 to 12 weeks after surgery, a complete evaluation including clinical history and examination, 12-lead ECG, and transthoracic echocardiography should be performed to assess functional status, blood pressure and rhythm, ventricular function, prosthetic valve function, gradients, and any paravalvular regurgitation, and anticoagulation adherence should be reviewed. Consensus guidelines recommend annual and symptom-triggered follow-up by a cardiologist for life, with the aim of detecting prosthesis dysfunction and the progression of other valvular heart disease. Follow-up solely by a family physician or as needed is not sufficient (options A, B, C, D).

52-2. The answer is A. *(Hurst's The Heart, 14th Edition, Chap. 52)* Transthoracic echocardiography should be performed annually after the fifth year postoperatively in patients with bioprosthetic valves; earlier in young patients who are at higher risk of accelerated valve dysfunction; and in any patient with a prosthetic valve if any new symptoms occur or there is clinical suspicion of complications based on clinical examination.

52-3. The answer is E. *(Hurst's The Heart, 14th Edition, Chap. 52)* The risk of infectious endocarditis is significantly higher in patients with prosthetic heart valves, but there is insufficient evidence available (1) to define the threshold for and type of prophylaxis required to minimize this risk and (2) to define the incremental risk posed to by adverse outcomes related to antibiotic use, including anaphylaxis and antibiotic resistance.[1,2] Current consensus guidelines recommend antibiotic prophylaxis prior to dental procedures that involve manipulation of gingiva or apical tissue, or breach of the oral mucosa.

52-4. The answer is D. *(Hurst's The Heart, 14th Edition, Chap. 52)* Routine antibiotic prophylaxis is not recommended for patients with prosthetic valves who undergo genitourinary procedures, gastroscopy, colonoscopy, bronchoscopy, transesophageal echocardiography, vaginal or caesarian delivery, or skin or soft-tissue procedures, unless the patient has an active infection or is immunocompromised.[1,2]

52-5. The answer is E. *(Hurst's The Heart, 14th Edition, Chap. 52)* The causes of prosthetic valve stenosis include bioprosthetic valve dysfunction, valve thrombosis, endocarditis with large burden of vegetation, and ingrowth of fibrous tissue (pannus).[3]

52-6. The answer is C. *(Hurst's The Heart, 14th Edition, Chap. 52)* Patient-prosthesis mismatch has been associated with decreased cardiac index, reduced functional improvement, less left ventricular mass regression, worse survival, and more adverse events in long-term follow-up. However, there are several confounding variables associated with a smaller indexed effective orifice area and with worse postoperative outcomes, including advanced age, female gender, and obesity; it is unclear to what extent these confounding variables contribute to the worse outcomes observed in patients with patient-prosthesis mismatch.[4] Stroke is not typically associated with patient-prosthesis mismatch because this is an insidious hemodynamic issue.

52-7. The answer is A. *(Hurst's The Heart, 14th Edition, Chap. 52)* The reasons for anticoagulation nonadherence may include comorbidities and associated side effects, patient preference, socioeconomic barriers, and childbearing. Pregnancy in the first trimester is a contraindication to warfarin therapy. In an analysis of Medicaid patients, age less than 55 years was one of the strongest independent predictors of nonadherence to an anticoagulation regimen.[5] This study also identified inadequate housing and care support, mental illness, and substance abuse as significant barriers to patient adherence with anticoagulation.

52-8. The answer is B. *(Hurst's The Heart, 14th Edition, Chap. 52)* Bioprosthetic structural valve degeneration is defined as any change in function of an operated valve resulting from an intrinsic abnormality of the valve that causes stenosis or regurgitation. Structural valve degeneration is the most common valve-related complication in bioprosthetic valves.[6] It occurs more rapidly in younger patients than in older patients, and earlier in the mitral position compared to the aortic position. Paravalvular leak is common but generally mild, and it infrequently leads to reoperation (option A). Endocarditis is not likely in this case due to the absence of constitutional symptoms or oscillatory mass seen on echo (option C). Pannus and thrombus formation are not suggested by the echo findings (options D and E).

52-9. The answer is B. *(Hurst's The Heart, 14th Edition, Chap. 52)* The risk of reoperation to replace a mechanical or bioprosthetic valve is similar over the first few years (option D), but the risk of having to replace a bioprosthesis after 8 to 12 years is higher (option C) as a result of an increasing incidence of structural valve dysfunction, which is the most common indication for reoperation on bioprostheses.[7-12] Structural valve dysfunction occurs more rapidly in younger patients than in older patients (option B), and earlier in the mitral position compared to the aortic position (option A). Although newer-generation valves have enhanced durability, structural valve dysfunction remains a nonnegligible risk (option E).

52-10. The answer is E. *(Hurst's The Heart, 14th Edition, Chap. 52)* Investigation of the patient requiring reoperative valve replacement should include transesophageal echocardiography to assess native and prosthetic valve function, to evaluate the presence and extent of endocarditis, thrombus, and pannus, and to determine cardiac function, including the presence of pulmonary hypertension and right ventricular dysfunction.[13,14] Cardiac catheterization should be performed to document native coronary artery anatomy, the presence and patency of coronary bypass grafts, and hemodynamics, including pulmonary artery pressures, cardiac output, and transvalvular gradients. Noncontrast chest CT is helpful to plan sternal reentry, which may be complicated by inadvertent division of structures adherent to the sternum, including the right ventricle, pulmonary artery, aorta, innominate vein, and patent bypass grafts. Prior operative reports are useful to confirm the size and type of previous prosthesis, location of bypass grafts, and technical challenges encountered at first surgery, which may affect the conduct of reoperation.

References

1. Nishimura RA, Otto CM, Bonow RO, et al. 2014 AHA/ACC guideline for the management of patients with valvular heart disease: executive summary. A report of the American College of Cardiology/American Heart Association Task Force on Practice Guidelines. *J Am Coll Cardiol.* 2014;63:2438-2488.
2. Habib G, Lancellotti P, Antunes MJ, et al. 2015 ESC Guidelines for the management of infective endocarditis: the Task Force for the Management of Infective Endocarditis of the European Society of Cardiology (ESC). Endorsed by the European Association for Cardio-Thoracic Surgery (EACTS) and the European Association of Nuclear Medicine (EANM). *Eur Heart J.* 2015;36:3075-3128.
3. Pibarot P, Dumesnil JG. Prosthetic heart valves: selection of the optimal prosthesis and long-term management. *Circulation.* 2009;119:1034-1048.
4. Pepper J, Cheng D, Stanbridge R, et al. Stentless versus stented bioprosthetic aortic valves: A consensus statement of the International Society of Minimally Invasive Cardiothoracic Surgery (ISMICS) 2008. *Innovations (Phila).* 2009;4:49-60.
5. Johnston JA, Cluxton RJ Jr., Heaton PC, Guo JJ, Moomaw CJ, Eckman MH. Predictors of warfarin use among Ohio Medicaid patients with new-onset nonvalvular atrial fibrillation. *Arch Intern Med.* 2003;163:1705-1710.
6. Grunkemeier GL, Li HH, Naftel DC, Starr A, Rahimtoola SH. Long-term performance of heart valve prostheses. *Curr Probl Cardiol.* 2000;25:73-154.
7. Chiang YP, Chikwe J, Moskowitz AJ, Itagaki S, Adams DH, Egorova NN. Survival and long-term outcomes following bioprosthetic vs mechanical aortic valve replacement in patients aged 50 to 69 years. *JAMA.* 2014;312:1323-1329.
8. Chikwe J, Chiang YP, Egorova NN, Itagaki S, Adams DH. Survival and outcomes following bioprosthetic vs mechanical mitral valve replacement in patients aged 50 to 69 years. *JAMA.* 2015;313:1435-1442.

9. Hammermeister K, Sethi GK, Henderson WG, Grover FL, Oprian C, Rahimtoola SH. Outcomes 15 years after valve replacement with a mechanical versus a bioprosthetic valve: final report of the Veterans Affairs randomized trial. *J Am Coll Cardiol*. 2000;36:1152-1158.

10. McClure RS, McGurk S, Cevasco M, et al. Late outcomes comparison of nonelderly patients with stented bioprosthetic and mechanical valves in the aortic position: a propensity-matched analysis. *J Thorac Cardiovasc Surg*. 2014;148:1931-1939.

11. Oxenham H, Bloomfield P, Wheatley DJ, et al. Twenty year comparison of a Bjork- Shiley mechanical heart valve with porcine bioprostheses. *Heart*. 2003;89:715-721.

12. Stassano P, Di Tommaso L, Monaco M, et al. Aortic valve replacement: a prospective randomized evaluation of mechanical versus biological valves in patients ages 55 to 70 years. *J Am Coll Cardiol*. 2009;54:1862-1868.

13. LaPar DJ, Yang Z, Stukenborg GJ, et al. Outcomes of reoperative aortic valve replacement after previous sternotomy. *J Thorac Cardiovasc Surg*. 2010;139:263-272.

14. Breglio A, Anyanwu A, Itagaki S, Polanco A, Adams DH, Chikwe J. Does prior coronary bypass surgery present a unique risk for reoperative valve surgery? *Ann Thorac Surg*. 2013;95:1603-1608.

CHAPTER 53

Antithrombotic Therapy for Valvular Heart Disease

Jonathan Afilalo

QUESTIONS

DIRECTIONS: Choose the one best response to each question.

53-1. A 62-year-old man with a prior history of idiopathic dilated cardiomyopathy was admitted to the cardiology unit with advanced heart failure and severe functional mitral regurgitation. During his admission, the patient suffered from recurrent pulmonary edema complicated by intractable hemodynamic instability. After discussing the case with the heart team, the patient underwent percutaneous edge-to-edge repair for mitral regurgitation using the MitraClip device. Which of the following antithrombotic regimens would you recommend to reduce this patient's risk of thromboembolic events post-procedure?

A. Warfarin indefinitely
B. Apixaban indefinitely
C. Aspirin for 6 months along with clopidogrel for 30 days
D. Warfarin indefinitely along with aspirin for 6 months
E. No specific antithrombotic therapy is recommended

53-2. A 75-year-old woman with a prior history of rheumatic heart disease and stage 5 chronic kidney disease presented to the emergency department following a fall complicated by a femoral neck fracture. She denied any history of falls prior to this event, and she had been generally very active and well. Her physical examination revealed an irregularly irregular pulse and a metallic click best heard at the apex. After reviewing her old medical notes, you noticed that the patient underwent a successful mechanical mitral valve replacement (MVR) surgery 15 years ago for which she was taking warfarin. The patient was subsequently evaluated by the orthopedic team, and the plan was to proceed with hip arthroplasty surgery. Which of the following antithrombotic regimens would you recommend during the perioperative period?

A. Stop warfarin 2 to 4 days before surgery, start intravenous unfractionated heparin when the INR falls to < 2.0, and restart warfarin 12 to 24 hours after surgery if bleeding risk allows
B. Stop warfarin 2 to 4 days before surgery, start low molecular weight heparin when the INR falls to < 2.0, and restart warfarin 12 to 24 hours after surgery if bleeding risk allows
C. Stop warfarin 2 to 4 days before surgery and restart warfarin 12 to 24 hours after surgery if bleeding risk allows
D. Do *not* stop warfarin (maintain therapeutic INR), and proceed with hip surgery because the patient's risk for thromboembolic events is very high
E. Cancel the hip surgery and manage the patient conservatively

53-3. A 55-year-old man with a prior history of mechanical MVR, hypertension, and dyslipidemia was admitted to the cardiac unit for a NSTEMI in the anterior territory. The patient underwent coronary angiography, and a drug-eluting stent was deployed in the proximal left anterior descending artery. The patient was discharged on triple therapy with warfarin, aspirin, and clopidogrel. Twelve months later, the patient returned to your clinic as part of follow-up and stated that he had been feeling very well since discharge and denied any cardiovascular symptoms or bleeding events. Which of the following antithrombotic regimens would you recommend at this time?

A. Warfarin only
B. Apixaban only
C. Aspirin and clopidogrel
D. Warfarin and clopidogrel
E. Apixaban and aspirin

53-4. You receive a phone call for an urgent consultation regarding a 31-year-old pregnant woman who was recently found to be pregnant. The patient had a mechanical mitral valve prosthesis implanted 5 years ago and was taking warfarin with a therapeutic INR up to this time. Which of the following anticoagulation regimens would *not* be an acceptable option for this patient?

A. Warfarin for the first 36 weeks with a switch to heparin

B. Low molecular weight heparin restricted to the first 6 to 12 weeks, followed by warfarin up to 36 weeks, with a switch to heparin

C. Intravenous unfractionated heparin restricted to the first 6 to 12 weeks, followed by warfarin up to 36 weeks, with a switch to heparin

D. Warfarin restricted to the first 6 to 12 weeks, followed by low molecular weight heparin up to 36 weeks, with a switch to heparin

E. Unfractionated or low molecular weight heparin throughout the pregnancy

53-5. After extensive discussion with the patient described in Question 53-4, since she had an older-generation mechanical mitral valve prosthesis and was taking only 4 mg/d of warfarin, the decision was to continue warfarin throughout the pregnancy (up to 36 weeks). The patient, who is now in her second trimester, had been taking warfarin with an INR of 2.8 and a time in the therapeutic range of 80%. You receive a phone call from her perinatologist seeking advice on the best anticoagulation management at this stage. Which of the following recommendations would be appropriate for the management of this patient?

A. Weekly INR with 2.0 to 3.0 target

B. Weekly INR with 2.5 to 3.5 target

C. Add aspirin and weekly INR with 2.0 to 3.0 target

D. Add aspirin and weekly INR with 2.5 to 3.5 target

E. Add aspirin and weekly INR with 3.0 to 4.0 target

53-6. A 64-year-old man with a prior history of a mechanical aortic valve replacement surgery presented to the emergency department complaining of acute dyspnea. The physical examination revealed a BP of 90/55 mm Hg, bilateral pulmonary crackles, and a harsh 5/6 systolic murmur over the aortic area; the aortic click was not audible. Upon reviewing the patient's old chart, he had been noted to have a softer 2/6 systolic murmur and audible aortic click since his valve replacement surgery. A chest x-ray confirmed the presence of florid alveolar edema and showed a well-positioned mechanical aortic valve prosthesis. The patient was intubated and underwent an urgent transesophageal echocardiogram, which revealed a large thrombus on the aortic valve prosthesis, associated with significant outflow obstruction. Which of the following is the most appropriate next step?

A. Emergency surgery

B. Admission to the cardiovascular ICU for stabilization and surgery in 2 to 3 days

C. Intravenous unfractionated heparin with half-dose fibrinolysis

D. Intravenous unfractionated heparin with fibrinolysis in 1 hour if the patient deteriorates

E. Low molecular weight heparin without fibrinolysis

53-7. You receive a phone call from a family physician seeking advice on the best anticoagulation regimen for 64-year-old woman with a prior history of a mechanical MVR 15 years ago. A couple of years ago, aspirin (81 mg) was added to warfarin by the family physician for a suspected diagnosis of stable angin Which of the following antithrombotic regimens would you recommend at this time?

A. Stop aspirin and continue with warfarin alone

B. Continue with the current regimen (warfarin and aspirin)

C. Switch warfarin to apixaban and stop aspirin

D. Switch warfarin to apixaban and continue aspirin

E. Increase the dose of aspirin to 320 mg daily

53-8. A 27-year-old woman at 36 weeks' gestation, with no significant prior medical history, was admitted to the acute antenatal care unit with symptoms suggestive of acute decompensated heart failure. Upon further questioning, the patient stated that she had had a febrile illness a couple of weeks ago and since then had been feeling generally unwell. An echocardiography was obtained and revealed a myxomatous mitral valve with a mobile vegetation complicated by severe mitral regurgitation. The patient was stabilized on medical therapy and underwent an induced delivery. A few weeks after delivery, the patient experienced recurrent heart failure symptoms and underwent MVR with a bioprosthetic valve, in view of her wishes for future pregnancies. Which of the following antithrombotic regimens would you recommend during the first 3 months after MVR?

A. Warfarin with a target INR between 2.0 and 3.0

B. Warfarin with a target INR between 2.5 and 3.5

C. Warfarin with a target INR between 3.0 and 4.0

D. Apixaban alone

E. Clopidogrel and aspirin

53-9. The patient described in Question 53-8 returned to your clinic 3 months after her bioprosthetic MVR as part of the routine follow-up. Which of the following antithrombotic regimens would you recommend at this time?

A. Stop warfarin

B. Continue warfarin

C. Continue warfarin and prescribe low-dose aspirin

D. Stop warfarin and prescribe low-dose aspirin

E. Switch warfarin to apixaban

53-10. An 85-year-old man with a past medical history of coronary artery disease, arterial hypertension, dyslipidemia, type 2 diabetes mellitus, and severe COPD was diagnosed with severe symptomatic aortic valve stenosis following admission to the cardiology ward with heart failure. Based on his predicted risk of operative mortality, the patient was deemed high risk for surgical aortic valve replacement and underwent transcatheter aortic valve replacement (TAVR). Which of the following antithrombotic regimens would you recommend after TAVR?

A. Warfarin for the first 3 months followed by aspirin indefinitely
B. Aspirin only
C. Clopidogrel for the first 6 months along with lifelong low-dose aspirin
D. Clopidogrel for the first 6 months along with lifelong high-dose aspirin
E. Clopidogrel for the first 12 months along with lifelong low-dose aspirin

53-1. **The answer is C.** *(Hurst's The Heart, 14th Edition, Chap. 53)* Following percutaneous edge-to-edge repair for mitral regurgitation using the MitraClip device, aspirin (325 mg/d) is recommended for 6 months along with clopidogrel (75 mg/d) for 30 days after the procedure.[1]

53-2. **The answer is A.** *(Hurst's The Heart, 14th Edition, Chap. 53)* For patients with a mechanical mitral valve, bridging anticoagulation with intravenous unfractionated heparin or subcutaneous low molecular weight heparin is recommended to reduce the risk of adverse effects.[2] Warfarin is stopped 2 to 4 days before surgery. When the INR falls to < 2.0, intravenous heparin infusion or weight-adjusted low molecular weight heparin (twice daily) is initiated. This is stopped 4 to 6 hours (for unfractionated heparin) or 12 hours (for low molecular weight heparin) before surgery. Once bleeding risk allows (usually 12 to 24 hours after surgery), warfarin is restarted. The use of low molecular weight heparin is contraindicated in those with severe renal failure, as in this case (option B).

53-3. **The answer is D.** *(Hurst's The Heart, 14th Edition, Chap. 53)* After 12 months, stable coronary patients may be managed with oral anticoagulants alone. But in the case of mechanical valves, the addition of low-dose aspirin to anticoagulant therapy has been shown to be beneficial in the long term and is recommended. In select cases such as left main stenting, proximal bifurcation stenting, or proximal LAD stenting, clopidogrel 75 mg/d may be preferred over low-dose aspirin for the long-term treatment.

53-4. **The answer is D.** *(Hurst's The Heart, 14th Edition, Chap. 53)* Pregnancy with a mechanical heart valve constitutes the WHO risk class III (significantly increased risk of maternal mortality or severe morbidity).[3] There is no ideal anticoagulation regimen. Anticoagulation options are (1) VKA (warfarin) throughout pregnancy with a switch to heparin at 36 weeks; (2) unfractionated or low molecular weight heparin restricted to the first 6 to 12 weeks, followed by warfarin up to 36 weeks, with a switch to heparin; and (3) unfractionated or low molecular weight heparin throughout the pregnancy.[2-5] Warfarin is more efficacious than heparin for thromboprophylaxis, but it is associated with an increased risk of embryopathy, particularly between weeks 6 and 12 of gestation.[6] Warfarin therapy throughout pregnancy is recommended for patients with a daily dose requirement of < 5 mg/d and for those who at are at very high risk of thromboembolism (older generation mitral valve prosthesis or those with previous history of thromboembolism).[2]

53-5. **The answer is D.** *(Hurst's The Heart, 14th Edition, Chap. 53)* Current guidelines recommend frequent monitoring of anticoagulation therapy during pregnancy irrespective of the antithrombotic regimen chosen.[2,3,5] INR should be measured weekly. For mechanical MVR, older-generation AVR, and those with risk factors for thromboembolism, the target INR should be 3 (range 2.5 to 3.5). For patients with a bileaflet aortic valve and no risk factors for thromboembolism, the recommended target INR is 2.5 (range 2 to 3). Low-dose aspirin (75 to 100 mg/d) is recommended for pregnant patients with either mechanical or bioprosthetic valves in the second and third trimesters.

53-6. **The answer is A.** *(Hurst's The Heart, 14th Edition, Chap. 53)* The ACC/AHA valvular heart disease guidelines recommend emergency surgery (class 1 recommendation) for left-sided prosthetic heart vale thrombosis with moderate to severe (NYHA 3-4) symptoms. Emergency surgery is also preferred in patients with a mobile or large thrombus (> 0.8 cm^2). For patients with mild symptoms (NYHA 1 to 2) of recent onset (< 14 d) and small thrombus burden (< 0.8 cm^2), an initial trial with intravenous infusion of unfractionated heparin may be given. If this is unsuccessful, fibrinolytic therapy is recommended.

53-7. The answer is B. *(Hurst's The Heart, 14th Edition, Chap. 53)* A systematic review found that adjunctive therapy with aspirin in addition to oral anticoagulation was associated with a reduction in overall mortality and thromboembolic events among patients with mechanical heart valves at the cost of increased bleeding.[7] This increased risk of bleeding was not seen among low-dose aspirin trials (aspirin 100 mg/d) (OR: 0.96, 95% CI: 0.60 to 1.55, $P = 0.87$). On the other hand, the effectiveness of low-dose aspirin (100 mg/d) was similar to that of higher-dose aspirin. Accordingly, the addition of low-dose aspirin (< 100 mg) is recommended by the American College of Cardiology and the American Heart Association for all patients with mechanical valves.[2] The newer oral anticoagulants (dabigatran, apixaban, rivaroxaban) are not indicated for atrial fibrillation associated with rheumatic MS, mechanical or bioprosthetic heart valve, or after mitral valve repair.[2,8]

53-8. The answer is A. *(Hurst's The Heart, 14th Edition, Chap. 53)* Thromboembolic risk associated with bioprosthetic valves appears to be greatest in the first 3 months after implantation.[9] The risk is greater after mitral valve surgery. Based on this risk, antithrombotic therapy with a vitamin K antagonist is recommended for the first 3 months after bioprosthetic MVR to achieve an INR of 2.5 (range 2.0 to 3.0).[2,10]

53-9. The answer is D. *(Hurst's The Heart, 14th Edition, Chap. 53)* After 3 months, the tissue valve and the repaired valve can be treated as native valve and anticoagulation discontinued. After the first 3 months, low-dose aspirin (75 to 100 mg/d), should be continued indefinitely for bioprosthetic AVR or MVR and mitral valve repair patients[2] because this is associated with a reduction in thromboembolic events compared with no antithrombotic treatment.[11]

53-10. The answer is C. *(Hurst's The Heart, 14th Edition, Chap. 53)* For patients undergoing TAVR, clopidogrel 75 mg daily is recommended for the first 6 months after the procedure, along with lifelong low-dose aspirin (75 to 100 mg daily).[2]

References

1. Feldman T, Foster E, Glower DG, et al. Percutaneous repair or surgery for mitral regurgitation. *N Engl J Med.* 2011;364:1395-1406.
2. Nishimura RA, Otto CM, Bonow RO, et al. 2014 AHA/ACC guideline for the management of patients with valvular heart disease: a report of the American College of Cardiology/American Heart Association Task Force on Practice Guidelines. *J Am Coll Cardiol.* 2014;63:2438-2488.
3. Regitz-Zagrosek V, Blomstrom Lundqvist C, Borghi C, et al. ESC guidelines on the management of cardiovascular diseases during pregnancy: the Task Force on the Management of Cardiovascular Diseases during Pregnancy of the European Society of Cardiology (ESC). *Eur Heart J.* 2011;32:3147-3197.
4. Ayad SW, Hassanein MM, Mohamed EA, et al. Maternal and fetal outcomes in pregnant women with a prosthetic mechanical heart valve. *Clin Med Insights Cardiol.* 2016;10:11-17.
5. Bates SM, Greer IA, Middeldorp S, et al. VTE, thrombophilia, antithrombotic therapy, and pregnancy: Antithrombotic Therapy and Prevention of Thrombosis, 9th ed. American College of Chest Physicians Evidence-Based Clinical Practice Guidelines. *Chest.* 2012;141:e691S-e736S.
6. Chan WS, Anand S, Ginsberg JS. Anticoagulation of pregnant women with mechanical heart valves: a systematic review of the literature. *Arch Intern Med.* 2000;160:191-196.
7. Massel DR, Little SH. Antiplatelet and anticoagulation for patients with prosthetic heart valves. *Cochrane Database Syst Rev.* 2013:CD003464.
8. January CT, Wann LS, Alpert JS, et al. 2014 AHA/ACC/HRS guideline for the management of patients with atrial fibrillation: a report of the American College of Cardiology/American Heart Association Task Force on Practice Guidelines and the Heart Rhythm Society. *Circulation.* 2014;130:e199-e267.
9. Heras M, Chesebro JH, Fuster V, et al. High risk of thromboemboli early after bioprosthetic cardiac valve replacement. *J Am Coll Cardiol.* 1995;25:1111-1119.
10. Vahanian A, Alfieri O, Andreotti F, et al. Joint Task Force on the Management of Valvular Heart Disease of the European Society of Cardiology (ESC); European Association for Cardiothoracic Surgery (EACTS) Guidelines on the management of valvular heart disease (version 2012). *Eur Heart J.* 2012;33: 2451-2496.
11. David TE, Ho WI, Christakis GT. Thromboembolism in patients with aortic porcine bioprostheses. *Ann Thorac Surg.* 1985;40:229-233.

CHAPTER 54

Management of Mixed Valvular Heart Disease

Jonathan Afilalo

QUESTIONS

DIRECTIONS: Choose the one best response to each question.

54-1. The general rule for treating secondary tricuspid regurgitation (TR) is to optimize therapy for the underlying cause. Which of the following TR outcomes may be observed after correction of underlying mitral or aortic valve disease?

A. Improvement of TR
B. Worsening of TR
C. No change in TR
D. De novo TR
E. All of the above

54-2. Most TR is secondary to overload caused by left-sided heart disease or by lung disease. Which of the following statements about tricuspid intervention during left-sided surgery is *true*?

A. TR surgery reduces postoperative TR but not RV dilatation
B. TR surgery reduces mortality in this setting
C. TR surgery reduces the risk of postoperative conduction abnormalities
D. 10-year survival is similar for mechanical prostheses versus bioprostheses
E. All of the above

54-3. A 62-year-old man with a history of mitral valve replacement (MVR) 2 years ago presents with increasing leg edema and abdominal girth. A holosystolic murmur is heard at the lower sternal border, with large visible "v" waves noted in the jugular venous pulsation. Echocardiography reveals a normally functioning mitral bioprosthesis, but there is severe functional TR, which was preoperatively

graded as mild-to-moderate TR. Which of the following factors may contribute to the variable response of the TR after correction of the mitral valve disease?

A. Right ventricular size and function
B. Pulmonary arterial hemodynamics
C. The underlying etiology of the left-sided valve disease
D. Atrial fibrillation
E. All of the above

54-4. A meta-analysis reviewed the fate of moderate-to-severe MR in a large pool of patients having undergone transcatheter aortic valve replacement (TAVR).[16] In what proportion of patients did the MR severity improve post-TAVR?

A. 10%
B. 30%
C. 50%
D. 70%
E. 90%

54-5. A 90-year-old woman with a history of TAVR 12 months ago presents for routine echocardiographic follow-up. She is feeling well, and her functional class has improved from NYHA III pre-TAVR to NYHA I at the present time. The echocardiogram reveals only trace MR, whereas it was graded as "at least moderate" before TAVR. Which of the following factors may contribute to the MR improvement after TAVR?

A. Secondary MR etiology
B. Aortic mean gradient > 40 mm Hg
C. Sinus rhythm
D. None of the above
E. All of the above

54-6. Irrespective of etiology, it is unusual for mixed aortic valve disease to have equal components of aortic stenosis (AS) and regurgitation (AR). Which of the following statements is *true*?

A. In cases of moderate combined AS/AR, the AS pressure gradients should be lower than expected for isolated moderate AS

B. In cases of moderate combined AS/AR, the LV behaves much more as it would in pure AR

C. In cases of moderate combined AS/AR, outcomes resemble those of AR

D. None of the above

E. All of the above

54-7. Which of the following statements about mixed aortic valve disease, particularly moderate combined AS/AR, is *true*?

A. The outcome compares best with that of severe AS

B. The outcome is substantially worse than moderate AS

C. The outcome is substantially worse than moderate AR

D. Aortic valve replacement should be performed at symptom onset

E. All of the above

54-8. A 51-year-old woman with a prior history of diet-controlled type 2 diabetes and COPD was referred by her GP to the cardiology clinic because of a heart murmur. She was very active and reported no cardiovascular symptoms. A physical examination revealed "a mixed murmur" as described by the examiner. A transthoracic echocardiogram revealed rheumatic valve changes with commissural fusion and diastolic doming of the mitral valve leaflets, and an MVA of 1.1 cm². In addition, there was moderate aortic regurgitation, a left ventricular ejection fraction (LVEF) of 65%, and a left ventricular end systolic dimension of 37 mm. Which of the following statements about the combination of MS and AR is *true*?

A. It is seen almost always in the setting of senile degenerative calcific valvular disease

B. It may lead to underestimation of AR severity during physical examination but not during imaging

C. It may lead to underestimation of AR severity during imaging but not during physical examination

D. It may lead to underestimation of AR severity both during physical examination and during imaging.

E. None of the above

54-9. A 53-year-old woman with no prior medical history was referred for cardiology consultation for a 6-month history of dyspnea on exertion. A physical examination revealed a soft systolic murmur best heard at the apex. A transthoracic echocardiogram revealed rheumatic valve changes with commissural fusion and diastolic doming of the mitral valve leaflets, an MVA of 1.8 cm², and a diastolic pressure half time of 130 ms. In addition, there was significant MR, LVEF of 66%, and LVESD of 35 mm. Which of the following is the best next step in the management of this patient?

A. Immediate admission for IV vasodilators

B. Invasive hemodynamics

C. Elective mitral valve repair

D. Elective mitral valve replacement

E. Elective balloon mitral valvotomy (BMV)

54-10. A 50-year-old woman with a prior history of acute rheumatic fever at the age of 11 was referred for cardiology consultation for a 3-month history of dyspnea on minimal exercise. Physical examination revealed a loud first heart sound and a middiastolic rumble. A transthoracic echocardiogram was performed and revealed rheumatic valve changes with commissural fusion and diastolic doming of the mitral valve leaflets, an MVA of 0.9 cm², and a diastolic pressure half time of 230 ms. In addition, there was moderate MR, LVEF of 62%, and LVESD of 39 mm. Which of the following is the best next step in the management of this patient?

A. IV vasodilators

B. IV beta-blockers

C. Invasive hemodynamics

D. MVR

E. BMV

ANSWERS

54-1. The answer is E. *(Hurst's The Heart, 14th Edition, Chap. 54)* Although it has long been hoped that correction of the hemodynamic load associated with underlying mitral or aortic valve disease would improve secondary TR, observed results remain unpredictable, with TR sometimes improving (option A), sometimes worsening (option B), sometimes remaining unchanged (option C), and sometimes even arising de novo following left-sided valve surgery (option D).[1-6] All of the options are thus possible TR outcomes after correction of underlying mitral or aortic valve disease. Therefore the best answer is option E.

54-2. The answer is D. *(Hurst's The Heart, 14th Edition, Chap. 54)* It seems clear that tricuspid intervention during left-sided surgery reduces postoperative TR and RV dilatation (option A is thus not correct). However, it has been difficult to show that TR surgery reduces mortality (option B is thus not correct).[5,7-14] Although tricuspid repair reduces postoperative heart failure and TR, it has increased the risk of postoperative conduction abnormalities (option C is thus not correct), requiring permanent pacemaker implantation in some but not all reports. In a large meta-analysis, 10-year survival (about 60%) was nearly identical for bioprostheses versus mechanical prostheses, and this is the correct answer (option D).[15]

54-3. The answer is E. *(Hurst's The Heart, 14th Edition, Chap. 54)* The variable response of TR to correction of left-sided valve disease is in part related to the causes and effects of the left-sided valve disease and its correction. Predictors of TR progression after left-sided valve surgery include: advanced age, right ventricular dilation and dysfunction (option A), tricuspid annular dilation, persistent pulmonary hypertension after surgery (option B), rheumatic or ischemic mitral valve disease etiology (option C), and atrial fibrillation (option D). All of the options are correct, and therefore the best answer is option E.

54-4. The answer is C. *(Hurst's The Heart, 14th Edition, Chap. 54)* In high-risk AS patients, the presence of MR must be considered in the decision of SAVR versus TAVR because the MR is not addressed directly at the time of TAVR but can be repaired at the time of SAVR. Thus it would be important to be able to predict the fate of MR following TAVR in making AVR decisions. In a meta-analysis of observational and randomized studies,[16] MR severity improved in 50% of patients over a median follow-up of 180 days after TAVR. Other studies have shown variable results.[17-29] Options A, B, D, and E are therefore not correct.

54-5. The answer is E. *(Hurst's The Heart, 14th Edition, Chap. 54)* Although the outcome of MR following TAVR still remains difficult to predict, Toggweiler and coworkers[24] found that MR was more likely to improve when it was secondary (option A), when there was an aortic mean gradient > 40 mm Hg (option B), and when atrial fibrillation was absent (eg, sinus rhythm, option C). All of the options are correct, and therefore the best answer is option E.

54-6. The answer is D. *(Hurst's The Heart, 14th Edition, Chap. 54)* In cases of moderate combined AS/AR, the LV behaves much more as it would in pure AS rather than in AR (option B is thus not correct), and outcomes resemble those of AS (option C is thus not correct).[30] Aortic regurgitation causes increased systolic flow through the moderately stenotic valve, thereby increasing jet velocity, pressure gradient, and in tandem, pressure overload on the LV (option A is thus not correct). In turn, the patient and his or her LV respond primarily to the pressure overloads. All of the options are incorrect, and therefore the best answer is option D.

54-7. The answer is E. *(Hurst's The Heart, 14th Edition, Chap. 54)* The outcome for moderate combined AS/AR compares best with that of severe AS (option A), and substantially worse than moderate AS or moderate AR (options B and C).[31] Thus the management of mixed

AS/AR should follow the guideline strategy for managing patients with pure AS. Aortic valve replacement should be performed at symptom onset (option D) and might be considered for patients with jet velocity exceeding 5 m/s or patients with abnormal exercise tolerance tests. All of the options are correct, and therefore the best answer is option E.

54-8. The answer is D. *(Hurst's The Heart, 14th Edition, Chap. 54)* The combination of MS and AR is seen almost always in the setting of rheumatic heart disease (and not in the setting of senile degenerative calcific valvular disease—option A). It may be confusing, especially by understating the severity of AR.[32] Because MS limits LV inflow, total LV volumes and the manifestations of volume overload for any degree of AR are lessened, potentially causing underestimation of AR severity both during physical examination and during imaging. Options B, C, and E are therefore not correct.

54-9. The answer is B. *(Hurst's The Heart, 14th Edition, Chap. 54)* Mixed mitral stenosis (MS) and mitral regurgitation (MR) usually occurs in the context of rheumatic heart disease. The management dilemma often presented to clinicians is whether the presence of symptoms in a patient with moderate MS and moderate MR is the result of the valve disease, because neither lesion by itself would probably cause symptoms. Further, if the valve is causing symptoms, current guidelines are unclear with respect to management. Thus although symptom onset in VHD is almost always a cause for mechanical intervention, moderate disease is not (options C, D, and E are therefore not correct). In such cases, invasive hemodynamics performed at rest or during exercise often clarifies the issue. If exercise generates filling pressures that are high enough to cause the patient's symptoms, it is highly likely that MS/MR is the cause of both the clinical and the hemodynamic consequences. This patient, with a history of exertional dyspnea and a moderate VHD, is relatively stable and therefore does not required immediate admission for IV vasodilators (option A).

54-10. The answer is D. *(Hurst's The Heart, 14th Edition, Chap. 54)* This patient is symptomatic, and symptom onset in VHD is almost always a cause for mechanical intervention. Therefore, there is no role for IV vasodilators (option A) and beta-blockers (option B) in this case. Although invasive hemodynamics may be considered in cases of discordance between the clinical presentation and the echo data, this would not be the best next step in the management of this symptomatic patient with severe MS (option C). Balloon mitral valvotomy (BMV) is usually contraindicated because it may worsen MR (option E), and therefore MVR is indicated for relief of symptoms.

References

1. Kwak JJ, Kim YJ, Kim MK, et al. Development of tricuspid regurgitation late after left-sided valve surgery: a single-center experience with long-term echocardiographic examinations. *Am Heart J.* 2008;155:732-737.
2. Matsunaga A, Duran CM. Progression of tricuspid regurgitation after repaired functional ischemic mitral regurgitation. *Circulation.* 2005;112:1453-1457.
3. Matsuyama K, Matsumoto M, Sugita T, Nishizawa J, Tokuda Y, Matsuo T. Predictors of residual tricuspid regurgitation after mitral valve surgery. *Ann Thorac Surg.* 2003;75:1826-1828.
4. Izumi C, Iga K, Konishi T. Progression of isolated tricuspid regurgitation late after mitral valve surgery for rheumatic mitral valve disease. *J Heart Valve Dis.* 2002;11:353-356.
5. Dreyfus GD, Corbi PJ, Chan KM, Bahrami T. Secondary tricuspid regurgitation or dilatation: which should be the criteria for surgical repair? *Ann Thorac Surg.* 2005;79:127-132.
6. Mahesh B, Wells F, Nashef S, Nair S. Role of concomitant tricuspid surgery in moderate functional tricuspid regurgitation in patients undergoing left heart valve surgery. *Eur J Cardiothorac Surg.* 2013;43(1): 2-8.
7. Chan V, Burwash IG, Lam BK, et al. Clinical and echocardiographic impact of functional tricuspid regurgitation repair at the time of mitral valve replacement. *Ann Thorac Surg.* 2009;88(4):1209-1215.
8. Calafiore AM, Gallina S, Iacò AL, et al. Mitral valve surgery for functional mitral regurgitation: should moderate-or-more tricuspid regurgitation be treated? A propensity score analysis. *Ann Thorac Surg.* 2009;87(3):698-703.
9. Navia JL, Brozzi NA, Klein AL, et al. Moderate tricuspid regurgitation with left-sided degenerative heart valve disease: to repair or not to repair? *Ann Thorac Surg.* 2012; 93:59-69.

10. Kim JB, Yoo DG, Kim GS, et al. Mild-to-moderate functional tricuspid regurgitation in patients undergoing valve replacement for rheumatic mitral disease: the influence of tricuspid valve repair on clinical echocardiographic outcomes. *Heart*. 2012;98(1):24-30.

11. Chikwe J, Itagaki S, Anyanwu A, Adams D. Impact of concomitant tricuspid annuloplasty on tricuspid regurgitation, right ventricular function, and pulmonary artery hypertension after repair of mitral valve prolapse. *J Am Coll Cardiol*. 2015;65(18):1931-1938.

12. Benedetto U, Melina G, Angeloni E, et al. Prophylactic tricuspid annuloplasty in patients with dilated tricuspid annulus undergoing mitral valve surgery. *J Thorac Cardiovasc Surg*. 2012;143(3):632-638.

13. Yilmaz O, Suri RM, Dearani JA, et al. Functional tricuspid regurgitation at the time of mitral valve repair for degenerative leaflet prolapse: the case for a selective approach. *J Thorac Cardiovasc Surg*. 2011;142(3):608-613.

14. Kusajima K, Fujita T, Hata H, Shimahara Y, Miura S, Kobayashi J. Long-term echocardiographic follow-up of untreated 2+ functional tricuspid regurgitation in patients undergoing mitral valve surgery. *Interact Cardiovasc Thorac Surg*. 2016 Jul;23(1):96-103. https://www.ncbi.nlm.nih.gov/pubmed/26993477.

15. Kunadian B, Vijayalakshmi K, Balasubramanian S, Dunning J. Should the tricuspid valve be replaced with a mechanical or biological valve? *Interact Cardiovasc Thorac Surg*. 2007;6(4):551-557.

16. Nombela-Franco L, Ribeiro HB, Urena M, et al. Significant mitral regurgitation left untreated at the time of aortic valve replacement. *J Am Coll Cardiol*. 2014;63(24):2643-2658.

17. Tzikas A, Piazza N, van Dalen BM, et al. Changes in mitral regurgitation after transcatheter aortic valve implantation. *Catheter Cardiovasc Interv*. 2010;75:43-49.

18. Gotzmann M, Lindstaedt M, Bojara W, Mügge A, Germing A. Hemodynamic results and changes in myocardial function after transcatheter aortic valve implantation. *Am Heart J*. 2010;159:926-932.

19. Masson JB, Lee M, Boone RH, et al. Impact of coronary artery disease on outcomes after transcatheter aortic valve implantation. *Catheter Cardiovasc Interv*. 2010;76:165-173.

20. Durst R, Avelar E, McCarty D, et al. Outcome and improvement predictors of mitral regurgitation after transcatheter aortic valve implantation. *J Heart Valve Dis*. 2011;20:272-281.

21. De Chiara B, Moreo A, De Marco F, et al. Influence of CoreValve revalving system implantation on mitral valve function: an echocardiographic study in selected patients. *Catheter Cardiovasc Interv*. 2011;78:638-644.

22. Samim M, Stella PR, Agostoni P, et al. Transcatheter aortic implantation of the Edwards-SAPIEN bioprosthesis: insights on early benefit of TAVR on mitral regurgitation. *Int J Cardiol*. 2011;152:124-126.

23. Hekimian G, Detaint D, Messika-Zeitoun D, et al. Mitral regurgitation in patients referred for transcatheter aortic valve implantation using the Edwards Sapien prosthesis: mechanisms and early post procedural changes. *J Am Soc Echocardiogr*. 2012;25:160-165.

24. Toggweiler S, Boone RH, Rodés-Cabau J, et al. Transcatheter aortic valve replacement: outcomes of patients with moderate or severe mitral regurgitation. *J Am Coll Cardiol*. 2012;59:2068-2074.

25. D'Onofrio A, Gasparetto V, Napodano M, et al. Impact of preoperative mitral valve regurgitation on outcomes after transcatheter aortic valve implantation. *Eur J Cardiothorac Surg*. 2012;41:1271-1276.

26. Hutter A, Bleiziffer S, Richter V, et al. Transcatheter aortic valve implantation in patients with concomitant mitral and tricuspid regurgitation. *Ann Thorac Surg*. 2013;95:77-84.

27. Giordana F, Capriolo M, Frea S, et al. Impact of TAVR on mitral regurgitation: a prospective echocardiographic study. *Echocardiography*. 2013;30:250-257.

28. Barbanti M, Webb J, Hahn RT, et al. Impact of preoperative moderate/severe mitral regurgitation on 2-year outcome after transcatheter and surgical aortic valve replacement: insight from the PARTNER (Placement of AoRTic TraNscathetER Valve) Trial Cohort A. *Circulation*. 2013;128:2776-2784.

29. Bedogni F, Latib A, Brambilla N, et al. Interplay between mitral regurgitation and transcatheter aortic valve replacement with the CoreValve revalving system: a multicenter registry. *Circulation*. 2013;128:2145-2153.

30. Zilberszac R, Gabriel H, Schemper M, et al. Outcome of combined stenotic and regurgitant aortic valve disease. *J Am Coll Cardiol*. 2013;61(14):1489.

31. Egbe AC, Luis SA, Padang R, et al. Outcomes in moderate mixed aortic valve disease: is it time for a paradigm shift? *J Am Coll Cardiol*. 2016;67(20):232.

32. Gash AK, Carabello BA, Kent RL, Frazier JA, Spann JF. Left ventricular performance in patients with coexistent mitral stenosis and aortic insufficiency. *J Am Coll Cardiol*. 1984;3(3):703-711.

SECTION 9

Congenital Heart Disease

CHAPTER 55

Mendelian Basis of Congenital and Other Cardiovascular Diseases

Ravi Karra

DIRECTIONS: Choose the one best response to each question.

55-1. A 54-year-old man presents to your office to establish care. His family history is notable for hypertrophic cardiomyopathy in his grandfather, paternal uncle, and sister. His father and his two other brothers are unaffected. He has previously undergone genetic testing and is a carrier for a mutation in the *MYH6* gene that is associated with hypertrophic cardiomyopathy. He is otherwise healthy and denies any functional limitation. His electrocardiogram and echocardiogram are essentially normal. Which of the following concepts explains your patient's lack of a phenotype?

A. Low expressivity
B. Variable penetrance
C. Genetic heterogeneity
D. Spontaneous mutation to a wild type allele
E. The allele is recessive

55-2. A 62-year-old woman presents to your office to establish care. Her past medical history is notable for aortic valve replacement with arch repair for a thoracic aortic aneurysm. Her exam is notable for short stature and low-set ears. She was unable to have children despite trying to become pregnant. Karyotype analysis would likely reveal which of the following?

A. Trisomy 21
B. Trisomy 18
C. Trisomy 13
D. Monosomy of the X chromosome
E. A deletion in the long arm of chromosome 22

55-3. A 45-year-old man presents to your office with exertional dyspnea and palpitations. His exam is notable for brown spots around his lips and eyes. His past medical history is notable for resection of a pituitary adenoma. His cardiac MRI is shown in Figure 55-1. This patient likely has a mutation in which of the following genes?

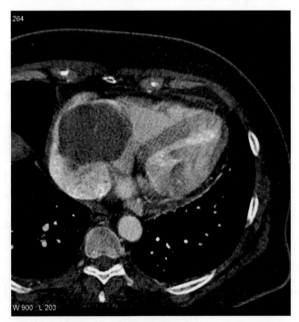

FIGURE 55-1 Cardiac MRI for the patient in Question 55-3. (Case courtesy of A. Prof Frank Gaillard, Radiopaedia.org, rID: 8544)

A. *JAG1*
B. *TBX5*
C. *NKX2.5*
D. *PTPN11*
E. *PRKRA1A*

55-4. You are asked to consult on a 45-year-old man admitted to the neurology service with a stroke. His past medical history includes hypertrophic cardiomyopathy and chronic kidney disease with proteinuria. His family history is notable for multiple family members on his maternal side with enlarged hearts, including his uncle and grandfather. His physical exam suggests normal filling pressures, no inducible obstruction, and right arm weakness. An ECG shows normal sinus rhythm with left ventricular hypertrophy, and an echocardiogram shows hyperdynamic ventricular function with concentric hypertrophy. Which of the following tests would be useful for diagnosing his underlying disorder?

A. Genetic testing for sarcomeric mutations
B. Measurement of α-Gal A levels
C. Genetic testing for *PRKAG2* mutations
D. Genetic testing for *FRDA* mutations
E. A cardiac MRI to evaluate for iron overload

55-5. A 43-year-old woman presents to your clinic for a second opinion regarding her dilated cardiomyopathy. Outside records reveal an ejection fraction of 35% with left ventricular dilation. Clinically, she is well-compensated and on maximally tolerated guideline-directed therapy for her heart failure. Her course has been uncomplicated, and she has no history of arrhythmia. Her past medical history is otherwise unremarkable, but her family history is notable for multiple family members with a similar cardiomyopathy on her maternal side. In which of the following genes is she most likely to have a mutation?

A. *TTN*
B. *LMNA*
C. *CRYAB*
D. *DMD*
E. *SCN5A*

55-6. A 17-year-old basketball player presents to your office for syncopal events. The events have been occurring more often over the past several months. Her exam is unremarkable. Her ECG is notable for an epsilon wave. Cardiac MRI shows a thin right ventricle with prominent fatty infiltration. Which of the following hereditary conditions is she most likely to have?

A. Hypertrophic cardiomyopathy
B. Catecholaminergic polymorphic ventricular tachycardia (CPVT)
C. Arrhythmogenic right ventricular cardiomyopathy (ARVC)
D. Emery–Dreifuss syndrome
E. Brugada syndrome

55-7. A 25-year-old man from Thailand presents to your office for evaluation of recurrent syncopal episodes. The episodes have no prodrome. He has a family history of these episodes, with numerous family members on his paternal side having suffered sudden death, either as infants or as young adults. His ECG is shown in Figure 55-2. A physical examination is unremarkable. In which of the following genes does he most likely have a mutation?

A. *KCNQ1*
B. *KCNH2*
C. *KCNJ2*
D. *DSP*
E. *SCN5A*

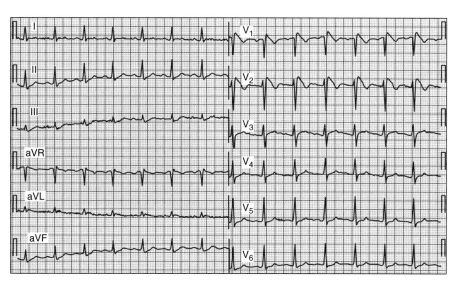

FIGURE 55-2 ECG for patient in Question 55-7.

55-8. A 23-year-old woman is referred for evaluation after an abnormal lipid check at an employee health screening fair. Family history is notable for premature coronary artery disease on both sides of her family. She says that her family is known to have a mutation in a gene that affects cholesterol, but she cannot remember the name of the gene. Which of the following mutations is she *unlikely* to have?

A. Loss of function mutations in *LDLR*
B. A mutation of *APOB* that leads to a decreased affinity of APOB for the LDL receptor
C. A mutation of *PSCK9* that causes increased clearance of the LDL receptor
D. A mutation in the *LDLRAP1* that decreases LDL clearance
E. A mutation in *ABCA1* that promotes free cholesterol transport to the extracellular space

55-9. Mutations to which of the following genes are *not* associated with primary pulmonary hypertension (PPH)?

A. *BMPR2*
B. *ACVRL1*
C. *KCNA5*
D. *FBN1*
E. *KCNK3*

55-10. A 35-year-old man is referred to you for management of a thoracic aortic aneurysm. He has a family history of aortic aneurysms and is positive for a genetic mutation in the *FBN1* gene. Which of the following is *not* likely to be observed in this patient?

A. Dislocated lens
B. Aortic regurgitation
C. Arachnodactyly
D. Bifid uvula
E. Mitral regurgitation

55-1. The answer is B. *(Hurst's The Heart, 14th Edition, Chap. 55)* This patient carries a disease allele but does not have signs or symptoms of the disease, suggesting that the allele is not fully penetrant (option B). Expressivity refers to variable degrees of disease severity in carriers of the disease allele, but all carriers exhibit some signs of the disease (option A). Genetic heterogeneity refers to different disease alleles at different loci that can result in the same phenotypic disease (option C). For instance, multiple mutations in different genes can result in hypertrophic cardiomyopathy. The pattern of inheritance here is consistent with an autosomal dominant allele (option E). Like your patient, his father is likely to also carry the disease allele but not have phenotypic disease. This patient tested positive for the disease allele, so spontaneous mutation to a wild type allele is unlikely (option D).

55-2. The answer is D. *(Hurst's The Heart, 14th Edition, Chap. 55)* This patient has Turner syndrome, which is associated with monosomy of the X chromosome (option D). Patients with Turner syndrome can have a bicuspid aortic valve, often associated with aortic aneurysms.[1] Trisomy 21 is associated with Down syndrome (option A). Trisomy 18 is associated with Edwards syndrome (option B). Trisomy 13 is associated with Patau syndrome (option C). A deletion in the long arm of chromosome 22 is associated with DiGeorge syndrome (option E).

55-3. The answer is E. *(Hurst's The Heart, 14th Edition, Chap. 55)* This patient has Carney complex, manifested by the atrial myxoma shown in the cardiac MRI, lentigines, and endocrine tumors. The Carney complex is associated with mutations in *PRKRA1A* (option E). Mutations in *JAG1* are associated with Alagille syndrome (option A). Mutations in *PTPN11* are associated with Noonan syndrome (option D). Mutations of the cardiac transcription factors *NKX2.5* and *TBX5* are associated with VSDs and Holt–Oram syndrome, respectively (options B and C).

55-4. The answer is B. *(Hurst's The Heart, 14th Edition, Chap. 55)* This patient likely has Fabry's disease. Fabry's disease is an X-linked disorder (note that only males on his maternal side are affected) that involves the heart and kidneys. The diagnosis is established by measuring α-Gal A levels and activity in leukocytes (option B). Fabry's disease is associated with transient ischemic attacks and stroke. Fabry's disease is an example of one of the many disorders that can cause hypertrophic cardiomyopathy, such as glycogen storage diseases with *PRKAG2* mutations and Friedrich's ataxia with mutations in the *FRDA* locus (options C and D). Iron overload is seen in hemochromatosis, but this usually manifests as a dilated cardiomyopathy (option E). Sarcomeric gene mutations are associated with hypertrophic cardiomyopathy (option A).

55-5. The answer is A. *(Hurst's The Heart, 14th Edition, Chap. 55)* This patient has an isolated hereditary dilated cardiomyopathy. Up to 25% of these cardiomyopathies are associated with a mutation in the sarcomeric gene *TTN* (option A).[2] Cardiomyopathies involving sarcomeric genes tend to be isolated cardiomyopathies without other organ systems being involved. Mutations in *DMD* (option D) and *CRYAB* (option C), by contrast, are also associated with skeletal myopathies. Hereditary cardiomyopathies due to mutation in *LMNA* (option B) and *SCN5A* (option E) tend to be associated with arrhythmias.

55-6. The answer is C. *(Hurst's The Heart, 14th Edition, Chap. 55)* This patient most likely has ARVC with involvement of the right ventricle and fatty dysplasia of the right ventricle (option C). Hypertrophic cardiomyopathy would be noted by a thickened ventricle by cardiac MRI (option A). CPVT is marked by arrhythmias without structural changes to the right ventricle (option B). Emery-Dreifuss is due to a mutation in the *LMNA* gene that results in cardiac arrhythmia and depressed left ventricular function (option D). Brugada syndrome results in sudden death and cardiomyopathy (option E).

55-7. The answer is E. *(Hurst's The Heart, 14th Edition, Chap. 55)* This patient likely has Brugada syndrome. His ECG has a typical pattern with ST elevations in the right precordial leads. *KCNQ1, KCNH2, KCNJ2* are all related to long-QT syndromes (options A to C). Mutations in desmoplakin (*DSP*) are related to ARVC (option D). Mutations in *SCN5A* can cause Brugada syndrome, LQT3, and other conduction defects (option E).

55-8. The answer is E. *(Hurst's The Heart, 14th Edition, Chap. 55)* Monogenic syndromes that can lead to premature coronary atherosclerosis include familial hypercholesterolemia, fish eye disease, and Tangier disease. Mutations of the *LDLR, APOB, PSCK9,* and *LDLRAP1* all can result in familial hypercholesterolemia (options A through D). Mutations of *ABCA1* can cause Tangier disease, by reducing the efflux of free cholesterol to the extracellular space (option E).

55-9. The answer is D. *(Hurst's The Heart, 14th Edition, Chap. 55)* Primary pulmonary hypertension is a familial disease with an autosomal dominant mode of inheritance in 5% to 10% of the cases. PPH is a genetically heterogenous disease. Mutations in bone morphogenic protein receptor type II (*BMPR2*), mapped to chromosome 2q31–33, are responsible for approximately 50% of the familial PPH and 10% to 15% of the sporadic cases (option A).[3,4] Mutations in *ACVRL1*, which codes for a type I receptor of the TGF-β family, cause an autosomal-dominant vascular disorder characterized by pulmonary hypertension, hereditary hemorrhagic telangiectasia (HHT), and visceral arteriovenous malformations (option B).[5] Likewise, mutations in *SMAD9, ENG* encoding endoglin, *CAV1* encoding caveolin 1, *KCNA5* and *KCNK3*, both encoding potassium channels, and *EIF2AK4*, coding for eukaryotic translation initiation factor 2 alpha kinase 4, are causes of PPH (options C and E).[6-8] Mutations in *FBN1* are associated with Marfan syndrome (option D).

55-10. The answer is D. *(Hurst's The Heart, 14th Edition, Chap. 55)* Marfan syndrome is associated with cardiovascular abnormalities, including aortic aneurysm and dissection, aortic regurgitation, and mitral regurgitation (options B and E). In addition to cardiovascular abnormalities, Marfanoid habitus (increased height, disproportionately long limbs and digits), lens dislocation or subluxation, arachnodactyly, thoracic abnormalities, and increased joint laxity are common clinical features (options A and C). Bifid uvula is a classic feature of Loeys–Dietz syndrome (option D).[9]

References

1. Gravholt CH. Clinical practice in Turner syndrome. *Nat Clin Pract Endocrinol Metab.* 2005;1(1):41-52.
2. Herman DS, Lam L, Taylor MR, et al. Truncations of titin causing dilated cardiomyopathy. *N Engl J Med.* 2012;366(7):619-628.
3. Deng Z, Morse JH, Slager SL, et al. Familial primary pulmonary hypertension (gene PPH1) is caused by mutations in the bone morphogenetic protein receptor-II gene. *Am J Hum Genet.* 2000;67(3):737-744.
4. International PPHC, Lane KB, Machado RD, et al. Heterozygous germline mutations in BMPR2, encoding a TGF-beta receptor, cause familial primary pulmonary hypertension. *Nat Genet.* 2000;26(1):81-84.
5. Harrison RE, Flanagan JA, Sankelo M, et al. Molecular and functional analysis identifies ALK-1 as the predominant cause of pulmonary hypertension related to hereditary haemorrhagic telangiectasia. *J Med Genet.* 2003;40(12):865-871.
6. Tuder RM, Archer SL, Dorfmuller P, et al. Relevant issues in the pathology and pathobiology of pulmonary hypertension. *J Am Coll Cardiol.* 2013;62(25 Suppl):D4-D12.
7. Machado RD, Southgate L, Eichstaedt CA, et al. Pulmonary arterial hypertension: a current perspective on established and emerging molecular genetic defects. *Hum Mutat.* 2015;36(12):1113-1127.
8. Vonk-Noordegraaf A, Haddad F, Chin KM, et al. Right heart adaptation to pulmonary arterial hypertension: physiology and pathobiology. *J Am Coll Cardiol.* 2013;62(25 Suppl):D22-D33.
9. Loeys BL, Schwarze U, Holm T, et al. Aneurysm syndromes caused by mutations in the TGF-beta receptor. *N Engl J Med.* 2006;355(8):788-798.

CHAPTER 56

Congenital Heart Disease in Adolescents and Adults

Ravi Karra

DIRECTIONS: Choose the one best response to each question.

56-1. A 56-year-old man with a nonrestrictive VSD develops worsening exercise intolerance, pulmonary hypertension, and cyanosis. Which of the following is *not true* of the Eisenmenger syndrome?

A. Survival in patients with Eisenmenger physiology is reduced compared to healthy control subjects
B. Patients with Eisenmenger physiology are susceptible to *in situ* pulmonary arterial thrombosis
C. The risk for hyperviscosity is low, with a hemoglobin < 20 g/dL
D. A pulmonary vasodilator may be indicated
E. Closure of the VSD is indicated

56-2. Which of the following patients *does not* require prophylactic antibiotics prior to bacteremic procedures, such as dental surgery?

A. A 54-year-old man with a mechanical mitral valve prosthesis
B. A 43-year-old woman with repaired patent ductus arteriosus
C. A 43-year-old woman with Eisenmenger complex
D. A 32-year-old man with tricuspid atresia treated with a Fontan conduit
E. A 31-year-old man with a history of infective endocarditis.

56-3. A 31-year-old woman with a history of mechanical mitral valve replacement presents to your office for pregnancy counseling. She has excellent functional capacity. Echocardiography reveals normal ventricular function and a well-functioning mechanical mitral valve. Her medications are notable only for warfarin 3 mg daily. Her INR has been stable on this dose for the past several years. Which of the following would be appropriate advice?

A. If she were to become pregnant, termination of the pregnancy would be recommended
B. She could continue with warfarin during the second and third trimesters of pregnancy
C. She should undergo caesarean section
D. She would have an increased risk for miscarriage
E. None of the above

56-4. A 24-year-old woman presents to your office to establish care. She has a past medical history notable for atrial septal defect (ASD) but does *not* bring prior records. She denies any history of valvular disease. Her ECG shows RSR' and a rightward axis. She is physically fit and exercises regularly without limitation. She wants to know about her prognosis. Which of the following would you tell her?

A. Pregnancy is contraindicated at this stage.
B. She most likely has a primum defect
C. Antimicrobial prophylaxis against endocarditis is recommended with dental procedures
D. She is potentially at risk for right ventricular (RV) failure, pulmonary hypertension, and tricuspid regurgitation over time
E. Systemic anticoagulation is indicated to prevent paradoxical emboli

56-5. A 56-year-old man presents to your office for hypertension. On exam, you note a very loud holosystolic murmur at the lower sternal border. He exercises regularly without limitation. Echocardiography reveals a small restrictive perimembranous VSD and suggests normal pulmonary pressures. Which of the following is the next best step in management?

A. Prophylactic closure
B. Recommendation for antimicrobial prophylaxis against endocarditis with invasive procedures
C. Continued observation
D. A and B
E. None of the above

56-6. A 48-year-old man presents to your office to establish care. He has a history of tetralogy of Fallot repaired with anterior ventriculotomy followed by VSD repair and a pericardial transannular patch. Over his lifetime, which of the following is this patient *not* at risk for?

A. Ventricular arrhythmias
B. Progressive pulmonary regurgitation
C. Eisenmenger physiology
D. A and B
E. B and C

56-7. A 25-year-old with pulmonic stenosis presents to your clinic. She has excellent exercise capacity and is otherwise healthy. Routine echocardiography confirms pulmonic stenosis with dysplastic leaflets and no evidence for infundibular stenosis. The peak gradient across the valve is 45 mm Hg, and the mean gradient is 35 mm Hg. Which of the following would be the next best steps in her management?

A. Continued surveillance
B. Recommendations for endocarditis prophylaxis with bacteremic procedures
C. Percutaneous balloon valvuloplasty
D. Exercise stress testing
E. C and D

56-8. A 42-year-old man presents for evaluation of shortness of breath and chest pain. Physical examination is notable for a harsh late peaking crescendo-decrescendo murmur at the upper sternal border that obscures S2. There is also an early diastolic decrescendo murmur at the mid-right sternal border. An echocardiogram reveals severe aortic stenosis, moderate aortic regurgitation, and a bicuspid aortic valve. Which of the following is also associated with the presence of a bicuspid aortic valve?

A. Perimembranous VSD
B. Parachute mitral valve
C. Dilated ascending aorta
D. Mitral stenosis
E. None of the above

56-9. A 25-year-old man presents for evaluation of hypertension. A physical examination reveals a systolic blood pressure of the right arm of 180 mm Hg and a left lower leg systolic pressure of 150 mm Hg. Which of the following is *not true* of this patient's likely condition?

A. He is at increased risk for intracranial aneurysms
B. Correction of his lesion will cure his hypertension
C. Even with treatment, he would be at risk for atherosclerotic heart disease, heart failure, and stroke
D. He is at increased risk to have a bicuspid aortic valve
E. None of the above

56-10. A 43-year-old woman presents to establish care. She has a history of isolated congenitally corrected transposition of the great arteries (TGA). Which of the following complications is she at increased risk for?

A. Atrioventricular (AV) conduction disturbances
B. Dysfunction of the systemic ventricle
C. Aortic stenosis
D. Aortic dissection
E. A and B

56-1. **The answer is E.** *(Hurst's The Heart, 14th Edition, Chap. 56)* This patient has the Eisenmenger complex (a reversed shunt in the presence of a nonrestrictive VSD). Survival in patients with Eisenmenger syndrome is reduced by approximately 20 years compared with healthy control subjects (option A).[1,2] Shunt correction is contraindicated once shunt reversal occurs (option E). Cyanosis is associated with multiple complications, including *in situ* pulmonary arterial thrombosis, hyperviscosity (rarely with a hemoglobin < 20 g/dL), pulmonary arterial atherosclerosis, increased susceptibility to gout, and a heightened risk for infective endocarditis (options B and C).[3-5] Promising advances have occurred over the past decade in the treatment of patients with pulmonary hypertension with pulmonary vasodilators. In the Bosentan Randomized Trial of Endothelin Antagonist Therapy-5 (BREATHE-5) trial, patients with Eisenmenger syndrome who were treated with Bosentan had a significant decrease in pulmonary vascular resistance and systemic vascular resistance, and a significant increase in 6-minute walk distance (option D).[6,7]

56-2. **The answer is B.** *(Hurst's The Heart, 14th Edition, Chap. 56)* Certain subgroups are considered at higher risk for infective endocarditis. Guidelines from the European Society of Cardiology and the AHA/ACC on the prevention of infective endocarditis place patients with prosthetic valves, cyanosis, and systemic or pulmonary artery conduits, as well as patients with previous endocarditis, into a high-risk subgroup (options A, C, D, and E).[8,9] Most other congenital cardiac conditions are in a moderate-risk category, except for patients who have undergone surgical or transcatheter repair of ASD, VSD, or PDA (without residua beyond 6 months), who are considered low risk provided there are no sequelae (eg, aortic valve prolapse, aortic regurgitation) (option B).

56-3. **The answer is B.** *(Hurst's The Heart, 14th Edition, Chap. 56)* Pregnancy results in considerable hemodynamic stress on the heart, and delivery is associated with large fluid shifts. Patients with left ventricular dysfunction, stenotic lesions, cyanotic heart disease, and aortic disease tend to have the highest risk for complications during pregnancy (options A and D). For most patients with cardiovascular disease, vaginal delivery is preferred because it results in less blood loss than caesarean section (option C). Pregnant women are inherently hypercoagulable, and their risk of valve thrombosis is increased, thus necessitating appropriate anticoagulation. Oral warfarin accomplishes this task well and is associated with a lower maternal risk, but it is teratogenic to fetuses, especially in the first trimester; the risk of teratogenicity is low after the eighth week of gestation.[10] Therefore, warfarin is recommended by the ACC/AHA guidelines in the second and third trimesters of pregnancy (option B).[11]

56-4. **The answer is D.** *(Hurst's The Heart, 14th Edition, Chap. 56)* Based on the presentation, this patient likely has a secundum ASD. The ECG usually demonstrates a characteristic RSR' complex in the anterior precordial leads with a rightward QRS axis in patients with secundum-type defects and left-axis deviation in those with primum-type ASD (option B). ASDs tend to be well tolerated initially, as in this patient. Thus, pregnancy is not contraindicated (option A). Progressive symptoms of dyspnea on exertion and palpitations often occur in adulthood and are caused by increasing right-sided chamber enlargement, pulmonary hypertension, RV failure, tricuspid regurgitation, and atrial arrhythmias (option D). Patients with large ASDs causing left-to-right shunts develop RV volume overload, which is relatively well tolerated for the first two decades. The risk of infective endocarditis is low unless the patient has coexistent valvular disease (eg, cleft mitral valve) (option C). Paradoxical emboli can occur but are rare, and preventive anticoagulation is not indicated (option E).

56-5. The answer is C. *(Hurst's The Heart, 14th Edition, Chap. 56)* This patient has a small restrictive VSD. For small restrictive defects or defects that have closed partially with time, the pulmonary vascular resistance is not significantly elevated, and the left-to-right shunt magnitude is mild (Qp:Qs ratio ≤ 1.5:1). The intensity of the precordial holosystolic murmur is inversely related to the size of the defect; therefore, a disturbingly loud and harsh precordial holosystolic murmur in a patient with VSD should be viewed as a reassuring sign, not a cause for alarm. Although antibiotics for endocarditis prophylaxis are no longer recommended by the ACC/AHA guidelines, patients are at increased risk for endocarditis.[11] Small restrictive defects of the muscular or membranous septum may be watched conservatively without the need for operative intervention (option C).

56-6. The answer is C. *(Hurst's The Heart, 14th Edition, Chap. 56)* The four characteristic findings in TOF are (1) a malaligned VSD, (2) RV outflow or pulmonary valve or artery stenosis or atresia, (3) a dextraposed over-riding aorta, and (4) RV hypertrophy. Surgical treatment of tetralogy of Fallot is one of the major advances in cardiac surgery. The first generation of intracardiac repairs was performed via a large anterior ventriculotomy and often included incision of the pulmonary valve annulus and placement of a transannular patch made of pericardium or synthetic material. This technique successfully relieved the outflow tract obstruction but resulted in pulmonary valvular incompetence and severe pulmonary regurgitation. Over time, this can lead to RV failure (option B). Ventricular arrhythmias are more likely to occur following such repairs, and they often arise from the region of the transannular patch or ventriculotomy suture lines (option A). This patient has been repaired and no longer has shunting, so he is not at risk for Eisenmenger physiology (option C).

56-7. The answer is A. *(Hurst's The Heart, 14th Edition, Chap. 56)* Mild and moderate degrees of pulmonary stenosis (peak gradient ≤ 50 mm Hg) are well tolerated and generally do not require surgical or percutaneous intervention (option A).[12] Asymptomatic patients with severe pulmonary stenosis and a peak gradient ≥ 60 mm Hg or a mean gradient ≥ 40 should undergo intervention to reduce the severity of the stenosis. Symptomatic patients with a peak gradient ≥ 50 mm Hg or a mean gradient ≥ 30 mm Hg should undergo intervention (option C).[13] Infective endocarditis of the pulmonary valve is rare; endocarditis prophylaxis during bacteremic procedures is not recommended (option B).[13]

56-8. The answer is C. *(Hurst's The Heart, 14th Edition, Chap. 56)* Options A, B, and D are associated with subvalvular aortic stenosis and the Shone complex. Patients with bicuspid aortic valves often have abnormalities of the aorta similar to patients with Marfan syndrome. The ascending aorta in patients with BAV gradually dilates at a mean of 0.9 mm/year (option C).[14] The risk of dissection in patients with BAV is estimated to be five to nine times that of the general population and is highest in patients with concomitant coarctation.[15,16] Patients with a BAV and ≥ 55-mm aortic root diameter should be referred for surgical aortic root wrapping or replacement.[11]

56-9. The answer is B. *(Hurst's The Heart, 14th Edition, Chap. 56)* This patient is likely to have coarctation of the aorta. A normal patient should have a 5- to 10-mm Hg increase in systolic blood pressure in the lower extremities compared with the upper extremities. Absence of this increase or the presence of a decrease in the lower extremities should arouse suspicion of coarctation. A BAV is present in about half of cases (option D). Intracranial aneurysms, often in the circle of Willis, have been detected in up to 10% of patients (option A).[17] Patients with successfully treated coarctation often continue to have systemic arterial hypertension despite the absence of significant residual coarctation.[18,19] Patients who undergo repair in childhood demonstrate very good long-term survival up to 60 years.[20] Late repair (> 14 years of age) is associated with higher rates of hypertension and decreased survival (option B).[21] Patients with hypertension after late repair are at an increased risk of developing heart failure, atherosclerosis, stroke, and progressive aortic disease (option C).

56-10. The answer is E. *(Hurst's The Heart, 14th Edition, Chap. 56)* Congenitally corrected TGA is characterized by AV and ventriculoarterial discordance. From a circulatory oxygenation standpoint, these patients are "congenitally corrected," essentially "two wrongs make a right," and the pulmonary and systemic circulations run in series, not in parallel, as with dextro-TGA. There is ventricular inversion, and the respective AV valves follow the ventricles. Therefore, the systemic right ventricle (RV) is transposed to the left, and the tricuspid valve goes with it. The left atrium empties into the RV, which then pumps to the leftward and usually anterior aorta. Because the RV is the systemic ventricle, the RV is susceptible to failure over time (option B). The left ventricle (LV) and mitral valve are dextraposed, and the pulmonary artery emerges posteriorly from the LV. Fewer than 10% of patients are free of associated abnormalities, which include VSD (membranous or muscular) in up to 80%, pulmonic stenosis (valvular or subvalvular) in up to 70%, and tricuspid valve abnormalities (usually Ebstein anomaly) in 33% (options C and D).[22] Furthermore, these patients have an increased incidence of AV conduction problems and complete heart block with age (option A).[23]

References

1. Diller GP, Dimopoulos K, Broberg CS, et al. Presentation, survival prospects, and predictors of death in Eisenmenger syndrome: a combined retrospective and case-control study. *Eur Heart J.* 2006;27(14):1737-1742.

2. Dimopoulos K, Diller GP, Koltsida E, et al. Prevalence, predictors, and prognostic value of renal dysfunction in adults with congenital heart disease. *Circulation.* 2008;117(18):2320-2328.

3. Silversides CK, Granton JT, Konen E, et al. Pulmonary thrombosis in adults with Eisenmenger syndrome. *J Am Coll Cardiol.* 2003;42(11):1982-1987.

4. Perloff JK, Rosove MH, Child JS, Wright GB. Adults with cyanotic congenital heart disease: hematologic management. *Ann Intern Med.* 1988;109(5):406-413.

5. Perloff JK, Latta H, and Barsotti P. Pathogenesis of the glomerular abnormality in cyanotic congenital heart disease. *Am J Cardiol.* 2000;86(11):1198-1204.

6. Galie N, Beghetti M, Gatzoulis MA, et al. Bosentan therapy in patients with Eisenmenger syndrome: a multicenter, double-blind, randomized, placebo-controlled study. *Circulation.* 2006;114(1):48-54.

7. Apostolopoulou SC, Manginas A, Cokkinos DV, and Rammos S. Long-term oral bosentan treatment in patients with pulmonary arterial hypertension related to congenital heart disease: a 2-year study. *Heart.* 2007;93(3):350-354.

8. Nishimura RA, Carabello BA, Faxon DP, et al. ACC/AHA 2008 Guideline update on valvular heart disease: focused update on infective endocarditis: a report of the American College of Cardiology/American Heart Association Task Force on Practice Guidelines endorsed by the Society of Cardiovascular Anesthesiologists, Society for Cardiovascular Angiography and Interventions, and Society of Thoracic Surgeons. *J Am Coll Cardiol.* 2008;52(8):676-685.

9. Horstkotte D, Follath F, Gutschik E, et al. Guidelines on prevention, diagnosis and treatment of infective endocarditis executive summary; the Task Force on Infective Endocarditis of the European Society of Cardiology. *Eur Heart J.* 2004;25(3):267-276.

10. Schaefer C, Hannemann D, Meister R, et al. Vitamin K antagonists and pregnancy outcome. A multicentre prospective study. *Thromb Haemost.* 2006;95(6):949-957.

11. Nishimura RA, Otto CM, Bonow RO, et al. 2017 AHA/ACC focused update of the 2014 AHA/ACC Guideline for the Management of Patients with Valvular Heart Disease: a report of the American College of Cardiology/American Heart Association Task Force on Clinical Practice Guidelines. *J Am Coll Cardiol.* 2017;70(2):252-289.

12. Khairy P, Harris L, Landzberg MJ, et al. Implantable cardioverter-defibrillators in tetralogy of Fallot. *Circulation.* 2008;117(3):363-370.

13. Warnes CA, Williams RG, Bashore TM, et al. ACC/AHA 2008 guidelines for the management of adults with congenital heart disease: a report of the American College of Cardiology/American Heart Association Task Force on Practice Guidelines (Writing Committee to Develop Guidelines on the Management of Adults with Congenital Heart Disease). Developed in collaboration with the American Society of Echocardiography, Heart Rhythm Society, International Society for Adult Congenital Heart Disease, Society for Cardiovascular Angiography and Interventions, and Society of Thoracic Surgeons. *J Am Coll Cardiol.* 2008;52(23):e143-e263.

14. Ferencik M, Pape LA. Changes in size of ascending aorta and aortic valve function with time in patients with congenitally bicuspid aortic valves. *Am J Cardiol.* 2003;92(1):43-46.

15. Nistri S, Sorbo MD, Marin M, et al. Aortic root dilatation in young men with normally functioning bicuspid aortic valves. *Heart.* 1999;82(1):19-22.

16. Roberts CS, Roberts WC. Dissection of the aorta associated with congenital malformation of the aortic valve. *J Am Coll Cardiol.* 1991;17(3):712-716.

17. Connolly HM, Huston J 3rd, Brown RD Jr., et al. Intracranial aneurysms in patients with coarctation of the aorta: a prospective magnetic resonance angiographic study of 100 patients. *Mayo Clin Proc.* 2003;78(12):1491-1499.

18. Stewart AB, Ahmed R, Travill CM, Newman CG. Coarctation of the aorta life and health 20-44 years after surgical repair. *Br Heart J.* 1993;69(1):65-70.

19. O'Sullivan JJ, Derrick G, Darnell R. Prevalence of hypertension in children after early repair of coarctation of the aorta: a cohort study using casual and 24 hour blood pressure measurement. *Heart.* 2002;88(2):163-166.

20. Choudhary P, Canniffe C, Jackson DJ, et al. Late outcomes in adults with coarctation of the aorta. *Heart.* 2015;101(15):1190-1195.

21. Beauchesne LM, Connolly HM, Ammash NM, Warnes CA. Coarctation of the aorta: outcome of pregnancy. *J Am Coll Cardiol.* 2001;38(6):1728-1733.

22. Lundstrom U, Bull C, Wyse RK, Somerville J. The natural and "unnatural" history of congenitally corrected transposition. *Am J Cardiol.* 1990;65(18):1222-1229.

23. Graham TP, Jr., Bernard YD, Mellen BG, et al. Long-term outcome in congenitally corrected transposition of the great arteries: a multi-institutional study. *J Am Coll Cardiol.* 2000;36(1):255-261.

SECTION 10

Myocardial, Pericardial, and Endocardial Diseases

CHAPTER 57

Classification of Cardiomyopathies

Ravi Karra

DIRECTIONS: Choose the one best response to each question.

57-1. Which of the following is *true* about the American Heart Association (AHA) classification of cardiomyopathies?

A. Primary cardiomyopathies are limited to cardiomyopathies with systolic dysfunction
B. Secondary cardiomyopathies are cardiomyopathies that are associated with a systemic, multiorgan disorder
C. A patient with hypertrophic cardiomyopathy (HCM) that results in a dilated phenotype would be considered to have a mixed cardiomyopathy
D. Ion channel disorders are *not* considered to be primary cardiomyopathies
E. None of the above

57-2. Which of the following is *not true* of the 2008 European Society of Cardiology (ESC) classification of cardiomyopathy?

A. Ion channelopathies are *not* included in the classification of cardiomyopathies
B. Familial cardiomyopathies are defined by the occurrence of a phenotype in more than one family member that could be caused by the same genetic mutation
C. Arrhythmogenic right ventricular cardiomyopathy (ARVC) is considered a distinct cardiomyopathy, different from dilated cardiomyopathy, HCM, and restrictive cardiomyopathy
D. The genetic basis of cardiomyopathy is emphasized over morphofunctional features in the classification
E. None of the above are true

57-3. Which of the following is *true* regarding the 2013 World Heart Foundation classification?

A. The five attributes to determine classification include morphofunctional phenotype, organ system involvement, genetic pattern of inheritance, etiology, and stage
B. The classification system allows for specific genotypes to be annotated
C. Familial cardiomyopathy should be diagnosed when two or more family members are affected
D. Assessment of functional status incorporates the AHA staging system as well as the New York Heart Association (NYHA) classification system
E. All of the above are true

57-4. A 47-year-old has HCM that progressed from the hypertrophic phenotype to the dilated phenotype. Under the MOGES classification, his M phenotype would be:

A. M_H
B. M_D
C. M_{H+D}
D. M_R
E. None of the above

57-5. The patient in Question 57-4 has an 8-year-old daughter. Genetic testing confirms she is also a carrier for the same sarcomeric mutation. A screening echocardiogram shows no structural abnormalities, and she is otherwise healthy. Which of the following is the best way to describe her morphofunctional description under the MOGES system?

A. MOGES is *not* applicable since she does not have structural abnormalities
B. M_H
C. $M_{E[H]}$
D. $M_{0[H]}$
E. None of the above

57-6. A 34-year-old man presents with 2 weeks of new-onset shortness of breath, paroxysmal nocturnal dyspnea, orthopnea, and pedal edem. He is short of breath with moderate exertion. Prior to experiencing these symptoms, he had an upper respiratory tract illness. He has no family history for cardiomyopathy. Cardiac MRI shows a dilated left ventricle with an ejection fraction of 25%, and a scar pattern consistent with a viral myocarditis. Which of the following is the correct MOGES classification for this patient?

A. $M_D\ O_{H+L}\ G_N\ E_V\ S_{C-II}$
B. $M_D\ O_H\ G_N\ E_V\ S_{C-II}$
C. $M_E\ O_{H+L}\ G_N\ E_V\ S_{C-II}$
D. $M_E\ O_{H+L}\ G_N\ E_V\ S_{B-II}$
E. $M_E\ O_H\ G_o\ E_V\ S_{B-II}$

57-7. A 32-year-old woman transfers her care to you. She feels well and denies any cardiopulmonary limitation. She had been previously seen by a cardiologist and was assigned a MOGES classification of $M_0\ O_0\ G_{AD}\ E_{G-LMNA}\ S_{A-I}$. Which of the following is this patient at risk for?

A. Arrhythmias
B. Stroke
C. Pulmonary hypertension
D. Respiratory failure
E. None of the above

57-8. A 64-year-old man has a MOGES classification of $M_D\ O_0\ G_{AD}\ E_{G-N-}\ S_{D-IV}$. Which of the following is *true* about this patient?

A. He has HCM
B. He has asymptomatic left ventricular dysfunction
C. He has a suspected genetic etiology, but the genetic defect is not known
D. He has a familial etiology that follows an autosomal recessive pattern of inheritance
E. None of the above

57-9. What is the significance of the color code of MOGES classification?

A. Asymptomatic carriers of a mutation
B. Known significance of a mutation
C. Morphofunctional phenotype
D. Functional status
E. None of the above

57-10. A 37-year-old man has a MOGES classification of $M_D\ O_{Lu}\ G_N\ E_{AI-Sarcoid}\ S_{B-I}$. Which of the following is *true* about this patient?

A. He has asymptomatic left ventricular dysfunction
B. He has a cardiomyopathy secondary to sarcoidosis
C. He has only cardiac involvement
D. A and B
E. None of the above

57-1. **The answer is B.** (*Hurst's The Heart, 14th Edition, Chap. 57*) The AHA classification emphasizes the mechanism for cardiomyopathy, not the morphology.[1] Under the AHA classification, cardiomyopathies are not limited to disorders of systolic dysfunction (option A). Cardiomyopathies were divided into two major groups based on predominant organ involvement. The *primary* cardiomyopathies were those solely or predominantly confined to heart muscle. The primary cardiomyopathies were further categorized into genetic, acquired, and mixed varieties and represented the novelty of the AHA classification (Figure 57-1). Ion channel disorders are included as genetic cardiomyopathies (Figure 57-1) (option D). Thus, a patient with HCM would have a primary genetic cardiomyopathy (option C). The *secondary* cardiomyopathies showed pathologic myocardial involvement as part of systemic (multiorgan) disorders (option B).

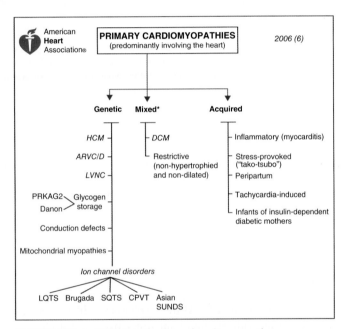

FIGURE 57-1 AHA classification of cardiomyopathy. (Reproduced with permission from Maron BJ, Towbin JA, Thiene G, et al. Contemporary definitions and classification of the cardiomyopathies: an American Heart Association Scientific Statement from the Council on Clinical Cardiology, Heart Failure and Transplantation Committee; Quality of Care and Outcomes Research and Functional Genomics and Translational Biology Interdisciplinary Working Groups; and Council on Epidemiology and Prevention, *Circulation.* 2006 Apr 11;113(14):1807-1816.)

57-2. **The answer is D.** (*Hurst's The Heart, 14th Edition, Chap. 57*). The 2008 ESC classification of cardiomyopathy emphasizes morphofunctional features over the genetic features and thus differs from the AHA classification (Figure 57-2) (option D).[2] Morphofunctional categories include dilated cardiomyopathy, HCM, restrictive cardiomyopathy, ARVC, and idiopathic cardiomyopathy (option C). After morphofunctional classification, cardiomyopathies are classified as familial/genetic or nonfamilial/nongenetic. Familial cardiomyopathies are defined by the occurrence of a phenotype in more than one family member that could be caused by the same genetic mutation (option B). Ion channelopathies, a genetic subtype included in the AHA classification of primary cardiomyopathy, were not accepted as cardiomyopathy in the ESC classification because genes encoding for ion channels might not be associated with overt myocardial dysfunction (option A).

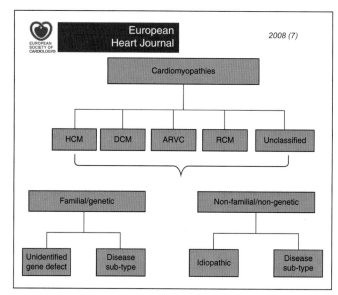

FIGURE 57-2 ESC classification of cardiomyopathy. (Reproduced with permission from Elliott P, Andersson B, Arbustini E, et al. Classification of the cardiomyopathies: a position statement from the European Society of Cardiology Working Group on Myocardial and Pericardial Diseases, *Eur Heart J.* 2008 Jan;29(2):270-276.)

57-3. **The answer is E.** *(Hurst's The Heart, 14th Edition, Chap. 57).* The WHF classification system builds on the AHA and ESC systems and is influenced by the TNM convention used in oncology.[3] The five attributes used for classification include morphofunctional phenotype, organ system involvement, genetic pattern of inheritance, etiology, and stage (option A). The system is versatile and even allows for the annotation of specific mutations along with clinical relevant phenotypes such as ventricular morphology and functional status, using the AHA and NYHA staging conventions (options B and D).

57-4. **The answer is C.** *(Hurst's The Heart, 14th Edition, Chapter 57)* Unlike previous classifications, the mixed or overlapping phenotypes can be easily presented in the MOGES classification system, such as HCM that evolves into dilated congestive phenotype (M_{H+D}) or HCM presenting with predominant restrictive pattern (M_{H+R}) (option C). Option A refers to a purely hypertrophic phenotype; option B refers to a purely dilated phenotype; and option D refers to a purely restrictive phenotype.

57-5. **The answer is D.** *(Hurst's The Heart, 14th Edition, Chap. 57).* Under the MOGES system, M allows the description of *early* phenotypes (M_E), such as when the diagnostic criteria for the suspected clinical phenotype (such as DCM or HCM) are not fulfilled and imaging data indicate an increased LV diameter and borderline LV function ($M_{E[D]}$) or possible LV hypertrophy ($M_{E[H]}$) (option C). Clinically healthy mutation carriers are described as $M_{0[H]}$ or $M_{0[D]}$ (0 is for zero) (options A and D). In this case, D and H refer to the phenotype of affected probands (option B).

57-6. **The answer is B.** *(Hurst's The Heart, 14th Edition, Chap. 57).* The MOGES classification system is provided in Figure 57-3. He has a dilated cardiomyopathy, so he is M_D (options A, B). His organ involvement is the heart only, so he is O_H (options B and E). He has no family history and a history was taken, so he is G_N (options A through D). The etiology is likely viral, so he is E_V. Finally, he is stage C and has class II symptoms, indicated by S_{C-II} (options A through C).

SUBSCRIPT NOTATION	M MORPHO-FUNCTIONAL PHENOTYPE	O ORGAN/SYSTEM INVOLVEMENT	G GENETIC INHERITANCE PATTERN	E ETIOLOGY	S STAGE
	D Dilated	H Heart	N Family history negative	G Genetic cause	ACC-AHA stage represented as letter A, B, C, D
	H Hypertrophic	*LV=left ventricle*	U Family history unknown	OC Obligate carrier	
	R Restrictive	*RV=right ventricle*	AD Autosomal dominant	ONC Obligate non-carrier	NA not applicable
	R EMF	*RLV=biventricular*	AR Autosomal recessive	DN De novo	
	Endomyocardial fibrosis	M Muscle (skeletal)	XLD X-linked dominant	Neg Genetic test negative for the known familial mutation	NU not used
	LV=left ventricle	N Nervous	XLR X-linked recessive	N Genetic defect not identified	
	RV=right ventricle	C Cutaneous	XL X-linked	O No genetic test, any reason*	*followed by*
	RLV=biventricular	E Eye, Ocular	M Matrilineal	G-A-TTR Genetic amyloidosis	NYHA class represented as Roman numeral I, II, III, IV
	A ARVC	A Auditory	O Family history not investigated*	G-HFE Hemochromatosis	
	M=major	K Kidney	Undet Inheritance still undetermined	*Non-genetic etiologies:*	
	m=minor	G Gastrointestinal	S Phenotypically Sporadic (apparent or real)	M Myocarditis	
	c=category	Li Liver		V Viral infection (add the virus identified in affected heart)	
	LV= left ventricle	Lu Lung			
	RV=right ventricle	S Skeletal		AI Autoimmune/immune-mediate; suspected (AI-S), proven (AI-P)	
	RLV=biventricular	O Absence of organ/system involvement*, e.g. in family members who are healthy mutation carriers; the mutation is specified in E and inheritance in G		A Amyloidosis (add type: A-K, A-L, A-SAA)	
	NC LVNC			I Infectious, non viral (add the infectious agent)	
	E Early, with type in parentheses			T Toxicity (add cause/drug)	
	NS Nonspecific phenotype			Eo Hypereosinophilic heart disease	
	NA Information non available			O Other	
	O Unaffected*				

FIGURE 57-3 MOGES system for classification of cardiomyopathies. (Reproduced with permission from Arbustini E, Narula N, Tavazzi L, et al. The MOGE(S) classification of cardiomyopathy for clinicians, *J Am Coll Cardiol.* 2014 Jul 22;64(3):304-318.)

57-7. **The answer is A.** (*Hurst's The Heart, 14th Edition, Chap. 57*). This patient is a carrier for a mutation in LMNA. Although she has not developed a morphofunctional phenotype, patients with cardiac laminopathies are at risk for arrhythmias, both ventricular and supraventricular (option A). The other options reflect risks associated with cardiomyopathy in general.

57-8. **The answer is C.** (*Hurst's The Heart, 14th Edition, Chap. 57*) This patient has a dilated cardiomyopathy (M_D) with NYHA class IV symptoms (S_{D-IV}) (options A and B). The patient is believed to have a genetic etiology with an autosomal dominant pattern of inheritance (G_{AD}). However, the genetic defect is not known (E_{G-N-}) (options C and D).

57-9. **The answer is B.** (*Hurst's The Heart, 14th Edition, Chap. 57*) The color code describes possible and probable pathologic genetic mutations in red; genetic variants of unknown significance in yellow; and single-nucleotide polymorphisms with possible functional significance in green (option B). The others options are a part of the MOGES system but do not use color.

57-10. **The answer is D.** (*Hurst's The Heart, 14th Edition, Chap. 57*) This patient has a dilated cardiomyopathy (M_D) secondary to sarcoidosis ($E_{AI-Sarcoid}$) (options A and B). His sarcoid also involves his lungs (O_{Lu}) (option C). He has stage B heart failure and NYHA class I symptoms and therefore has asymptomatic left ventricular dysfunction (option A).

References

1. Maron BJ, Towbin JA, Thiene G, et al. Contemporary definitions and classification of the cardiomyopathies: an American Heart Association scientific statement from the Council on Clinical Cardiology, Heart Failure and Transplantation Committee; Quality of Care and Outcomes Research and Functional Genomics and Translational Biology Interdisciplinary Working Groups; and Council on Epidemiology and Prevention. *Circulation.* 2006;113(14):1807-1816.

2. Elliott P, Andersson B, Arbustini E, et al. Classification of the cardiomyopathies: a position statement from the European Society of Cardiology Working Group on Myocardial and Pericardial Diseases. *Eur Heart J.* 2008;29(2):270-276.

3. Arbustini E, Narula N, Dec GW, et al. The MOGE(S) classification for a phenotype-genotype nomenclature of cardiomyopathy: endorsed by the World Heart Federation. *J Am Coll Cardiol.* 2013;62(22):2046-2072.

CHAPTER 58

Dilated Cardiomyopathy

Ravi Karra

QUESTIONS

DIRECTIONS: Choose the one best response to each question.

58-1. A 42-year-old man presents to your clinic to establish care for a newly diagnosed dilated cardiomyopathy (DCM). His previous evaluation is notable for the absence of coronary artery disease. Review of his family history reveals that his father also had DCM and his sister has DCM. Which of the following is *not true* about familial DCM?

A. DCM is familial in more than 60% of cases
B. This patient has an X-linked cardiomyopathy allele
C. The most common cause of familial DCM is mutations to sarcomeric genes
D. Of the nuclear envelope genes, mutations to LMNA most often result in DCM
E. Most DCM genes also cause other types of cardiomyopathy

58-2. A 43-year-old woman is found to have a mutation of *LMNA2* associated with DCM. An echocardiogram reveals an ejection fraction of 40%. Which of the following is *true* of cardiac laminopathies that occur due to mutations of *LMNA2*?

A. Conduction system disease often presents prior to DCM
B. Progression of the PR interval is associated with cardiac laminopathies due to mutations of *LMNA2*
C. Patients with cardiac laminopathies due to mutations of *LMNA2* are at high risk for ventricular tachycardia and sudden death
D. Prophylactic ICD implantation would be indicated for this patient if she demonstrated nonsustained ventricular tachycardia on ambulatory ECG monitoring
E. All of the above

58-3. A 24-year-old woman with systemic scleroderma develops exertional dyspnea associated with pedal edema, paroxysmal nocturnal dyspnea, and orthopnea. Which of the following is *not* an associated cardiac manifestation of scleroderma?

A. Hypertrophic cardiomyopathy
B. Pericardial effusion
C. Left ventricular (LV) systolic and diastolic dysfunction
D. Pulmonary hypertension
E. Interstitial fibrosis

58-4. A 37-year-old woman presents with new-onset shortness of breath and orthopnea. She is noted to have an ejection fraction of 30%. Her history is remarkable for having recently delivered a baby boy 4 months ago. Which of the following is needed for a diagnosis of peripartum cardiomyopathy?

A. The cardiomyopathy must be an idiopathic condition
B. The onset of the cardiomyopathy must be related to the timing of pregnancy
C. There should be no preexisting heart disease
D. There must be LV dysfunction
E. All of the above

58-5. A 54-year-old man is admitted for a newly diagnosed cardiomyopathy. His past medical history is notable for heavy alcohol use. Which of the following is *true* of an alcohol-induced cardiomyopathy?

A. Administration of thiamine can reverse the cardiomyopathy
B. A daily alcohol intake of > 80 grams per day (3 drinks) for five years prior to diagnosis is associated with cardiomyopathy
C. A hypertrabeculated phenotype
D. Occurrence of atrial fibrillation is associated with poorer outcomes
E. None of the above

58-6. You are asked to provide a preoperative risk assessment for a 38-year-old man with cirrhosis who is scheduled for transjugular intrahepatic portosystemic shunt (TIPS). Which of the following is *true* of cirrhotic cardiomyopathy?

A. During the early phase of cardiomyopathy, diastolic dysfunction is apparent

B. QT prolongation is present in more than 50% of cases

C. Diastolic dysfunction predicts death after TIPS implantation

D. Latent heart failure is often unmasked by stressors

E. All of the above

58-7. You are asked to consult on the oncology ward for a possible chemotherapy-related cardiomyopathy. Which of the following is *not true* about chemotherapy-related cardiomyopathies?

A. Anthracyclines are associated with type 1 myocardial damage

B. Trastuzumab is associated with type 2 myocardial damage

C. Cyclophosphamide is associated with a hemorrhagic myocarditis

D. Sumatinib is associated with hypertension

E. The incidence of cardiomyopathy increases when trastuzumab is used without an anthracycline

58-8. Which of the following is associated with a reversible cardiomyopathy?

A. Alcohol-induced cardiomyopathy

B. Tachycardia-induced cardiomyopathy

C. Takotsubo cardiomyopathy

D. Viral myocarditis

E. All of the above

58-9. A 37-year-old man is admitted for a new-onset cardiomyopathy. His EKG shows frequent premature ventricular contractions (PVCs). Which of the following is *not* associated with a PVC-induced cardiomyopathy?

A. More than 10,000 PVCs per day are associated with LV dilation

B. More than 20,000 PVCs per day are associated with reduced ejection fraction

C. For patients with a PVC-induced cardiomyopathy, successful termination of the PVCs can reverse the cardiomyopathy

D. Therapy for frequent PVCs in patients with idiopathic LV dysfunction modifies clinical outcomes

E. PVC-induced cardiomyopathy can occur in children

58-10. Which of the following is *not* associated with a mitochondrial cardiomyopathy?

A. Hypertrophic phenotype

B. Dilated phenotype

C. Maternal inheritance

D. Autosomal inheritance

E. Clinical manifestations tend to be restricted to the heart

58-1. **The answer is B.** *(Hurst's The Heart, 14th Edition, Chap. 58)* In more than 60% of cases of DCM, the disease is familial, as proven by clinical family screening demonstrating that more than one member is affected or shows traits that predict the development of the disease (option A).[1,2] This patient likely has an autosomal dominant allele. This patient's father is affected, and because he did not inherit an X chromosome from his father, the disease allele cannot be X-linked (option B). Sarcomere genes (*TTN, MYH7, MYBPC3, TNNT2, TNNI3, MYL2, MYL3*) are mutated in 25% to 30% of DCM patients (option C).[3] Nuclear envelope genes (*LMNA, EMD, SYNE1, TMPO*) are mutated in about 7% to 10% of cases, with *LMNA* mutations accounting for the majority of DCM in this subgroup (option D).[4] Most DCM genes also cause other types of cardiomyopathy (HCM, restrictive cardiomyopathy, and arrhythmogenic right ventricular cardiomyopathy (option E).

58-2. **The answer is E.** *(Hurst's The Heart, 14th Edition, Chap. 58)* The development of conduction system disease usually precedes the appearance of the DCM (option A). The natural history is characterized by a long asymptomatic phase in which regular and slowly progressive LV dilation or dysfunction is demonstrated (option B).[5] The high risk of life-threatening ventricular arrhythmias is one of the characteristics of cardiolaminopathies, and such arrhythmias may manifest even in mildly dilated and dysfunctioning hearts.[6,7] Recent guidelines on the primary prevention of sudden cardiac death (SCD) recommend ICD implantation in patients with DCM and a confirmed disease-causing *LMNA* mutation and such clinical risk factors (Class IIa level B) as nonsustained ventricular tachycardia during ambulatory ECG monitoring, LV ejection fraction (LVEF) < 45% on initial evaluation, male gender, and nonmissense mutations (insertion, deletion, truncation, or mutations affecting splicing) (options C and D).

58-3. **The answer is A.** *(Hurst's The Heart, 14th Edition, Chap. 58)* The heterogeneous cardiac manifestations of scleroderma include myocarditis, pericarditis, and pericardial effusion (option B); conduction disturbances; LV systolic and diastolic dysfunction (option C); valve dysfunction; myocardial ischemia and coronary artery disease; and pulmonary hypertension (option D).[8] Histologically, scleroderma is associated with fibrosis (option E). Hypertrophic cardiomyopathy is not typically associated with scleroderma (option A).

58-4. **The answer is E.** *(Hurst's The Heart, 14th Edition, Chap. 58)* Criteria for diagnosing peripartum cardiomyopathy include: (1) idiopathic condition (no detectable cause of HF) (option A); (2) temporal appearance (the last month of pregnancy or during the first 5 months postpartum according to NHLBI and toward the end of pregnancy or in the months following delivery according to ESC (option B); (3) the absence of preexisting known heart disease (option C); and (4) the presence of LV dysfunction (option D).

58-5. **The answer is B.** *(Hurst's The Heart, 14th Edition, Chap. 58)* The three criteria for diagnosing alcoholic cardiomyopathy include DCM phenotype, absence of other known and detectable causes of DCM (option C), and a long history of heavy alcohol intake. The toxic effect is expected for daily alcohol consumption over 80 g (three or more standard-sized drinks per day) lasting 5 years or more before the onset or diagnosis (option B).[9] Atrial fibrillation, QRS width > 120 ms, and the absence of β-blocker therapy identify patients with a poor outcome (option D). Thiamine deficiency (beriberi) is no longer confused with alcoholic cardiomyopathy; the former fully responds to thiamine administration, whereas the latter does not (option A).

58-6. **The answer is E.** *(Hurst's The Heart, 14th Edition, Chap. 58)* According to the 2005 World Congress of Gastroenterology, cirrhotic cardiomyopathy is defined by "chronic cardiac dysfunction in patients with cirrhosis characterized by impaired contractile responsiveness to stress and/or altered diastolic relaxation with electrophysiological abnormalities in the absence of other known cardiac disease."[10] The impaired diastolic relaxation is more common in early phases, whereas systolic dysfunction and LV dilation are manifest in advanced phases (option A); electrophysiological abnormalities include prolongation of QT interval in more than 50% of cases (option B), electromechanical dyssynchrony, and chronotropic and/or inotropic incompetence.[11] In the complex pathophysiology of cirrhosis-related cardiac and hemodynamic changes, diastolic dysfunction seems to predict death after TIPS implantation (option C).[12] Patients with cirrhosis often demonstrate hyperdynamic circulation and increased cardiac output, decreased systemic vascular resistance, and increased compliance of the arterial vessels. This combination of hemodynamic conditions corresponds to latent left HF where any stressor may clinically unmask the LV dysfunction (option D).

58-7. **The answer is E.** *(Hurst's The Heart, 14th Edition, Chap. 58)* Heart muscle toxicity is generally characterized as *nonreversible injury* (type 1) as a result of the presence of structural damage (prototyped by the anthracycline or high-dose cyclophosphamide DCM in acute and chronic forms) and potentially reversible (on cessation of therapy) dysfunction (type 2) in the absence of structural abnormalities, as with targeted therapies (ie, trastuzumab, sunitinib, lapatinib) (options A and B). The 3-year cumulative incidence of cardiomyopathy is 6.6% when trastuzumab is used with anthracyclines and 5.1% when used without anthracyclines (option E).[13] Myocarditis is a rare complication described in patients treated for cancer (ie, cyclophosphamide and hemorrhagic myocarditis) (option C). Hypertension is the most common cardiovascular complication associated with vascular endothelial growth factor inhibitors (option D).

58-8. **The answer is E.** *(Hurst's The Heart, 14th Edition, Chap. 58).* All of the above are associated with a reversible cardiomyopathy (options A through D), although reversal of the cardiomyopathy is not guaranteed with cessation of the cause.

58-9. **The answer is D.** *(Hurst's The Heart, 14th Edition, Chap. 58)* A dose-response relationship has been demonstrated in serial evaluations of LV function among 239 consecutive patients with frequent PVCs and no obvious cardiac disease; > 20,000 PVCs per 24 hours were associated with subclinical deterioration in LVEF whereas >10,000 PVCs per 24 hours showed LV dilation without a change in LVEF (options A and B).[14] For patients with a PVC-induced cardiomyopathy, successful termination of the PVCs can reverse the cardiomyopathy (option C). Randomized trials are ongoing, aimed at assessing whether therapy for frequent PVCs in patients with idiopathic LV dysfunction modifies clinical outcomes (option D). In children, the proportion of PVC-induced cardiomyopathy seems higher than previously expected, especially because ectopy tends to persist throughout follow-up (option E).

58-10. **The answer is E.** *(Hurst's The Heart, 14th Edition, Chap. 58)* Mitochondrial cardiomyopathies can be caused by mutations both in mitochondrial DNA genes (maternal inheritance) and in nuclear genes (Mendelian inheritance: no male passes down the disease to children) coding mitochondrial proteins (options C and D). They are characterized by either a hypertrophic phenotype evolving through dilated and dysfunctional hearts or DCM (options A and B). They are commonly observed in families in which mutation carriers also express noncardiac traits, such as hearing loss, palpebral ptosis, myopathy, renal failure, cryptogenic stroke, diabetes, optic neuritis, and/or retinitis pigmentosa (option E).

References

1. Pinto YM, Elliott PM, Arbustini E, et al. Proposal for a revised definition of dilated cardiomyopathy, hypokinetic non-dilated cardiomyopathy, and its implications for clinical practice: a position statement of the ESC Working Group on Myocardial and Pericardial Diseases. *Eur Heart J.* 2016;37(23):1850-1858.
2. Charron P, Arad M, Arbustini E, et al. Genetic counselling and testing in cardiomyopathies: a position statement of the European Society of Cardiology Working Group on Myocardial and Pericardial Diseases. *Eur Heart J.* 2010;31(22):2715-2726.

3. Lakdawala NK, Funke BH, Baxter S, et al. Genetic testing for dilated cardiomyopathy in clinical practice. *J Card Fail.* 2012;18(4):296-303.

4. Hirtle-Lewis M, Desbiens K, Ruel I, et al. The genetics of dilated cardiomyopathy: a prioritized candidate gene study of LMNA, TNNT2, TCAP, and PLN. *Clin Cardiol.* 2013;36(10):628-633.

5. Brodt C, Siegfried JD, Hofmeyer M, et al. Temporal relationship of conduction system disease and ventricular dysfunction in LMNA cardiomyopathy. *J Card Fail.* 2013;19(4):233-239.

6. van Rijsingen IA, Arbustini E, Elliott PM, et al. Risk factors for malignant ventricular arrhythmias in lamin A/C mutation carriers: a European cohort study. *J Am Coll Cardiol.* 2012;59(5):493-500.

7. Anselme F, Moubarak G, Savoure A, et al. Implantable cardioverter-defibrillators in lamin A/C mutation carriers with cardiac conduction disorders. *Heart Rhythm.* 2013;10(10):1492-1498.

8. Boueiz A, Mathai SC, Hummers LK, Hassoun PM. Cardiac complications of systemic sclerosis: recent progress in diagnosis. *Curr Opin Rheumatol.* 2010;22(6):696-703.

9. Fauchier L, Babuty D, Poret P, et al. Comparison of long-term outcome of alcoholic and idiopathic dilated cardiomyopathy. *Eur Heart J.* 2000;21(4):306-314.

10. Ruiz-del-Arbol L, Serradilla R. Cirrhotic cardiomyopathy. *World J Gastroenterol.* 2015;21(41):11502-11521.

11. Milic S, Lulic D, Stimac D, Ruzic A, Zaputovic L. Cardiac manifestations in alcoholic liver disease. *Postgrad Med J.* 2016;92(1086):235-239.

12. Ruiz-del-Arbol L, Achecar L, Serradilla R, et al. Diastolic dysfunction is a predictor of poor outcomes in patients with cirrhosis, portal hypertension, and a normal creatinine. *Hepatology.* 2013;58(5):1732-1741.

13. Abdel-Qadir H, Amir E, Thavendiranathan P. Prevention, detection, and management of chemotherapy-related cardiac dysfunction. *Can J Cardiol.* 2016;32(7):891-899.

14. Niwano S, Wakisaka Y, Niwano H, et al. Prognostic significance of frequent premature ventricular contractions originating from the ventricular outflow tract in patients with normal left ventricular function. *Heart.* 2009;95(15):1230-1237.

CHAPTER 59

Hypertrophic Cardiomyopathies

Ravi Karra

QUESTIONS

DIRECTIONS: Choose the one best response to each question.

59-1. A 25-year-old woman seeks to establish care for hypertrophic cardiomyopathy (HCM). Her family history is notable for multiple affected family members. Which of the following is *not true* regarding the genetics of HCM?

A. She is most likely to have a mutation of a sarcomeric protein
B. 5% to 10% of cases are caused by metabolic or storage disorders
C. Missense single nucleotide variants of *MYH7* are associated with a dominant negative effect
D. Nonsense mutations of MYBC3 are associated with haploinsufficiency
E. Unaffected family members cannot have the causal mutation

59-2. You are asked to be an expert witness at a trial for an 18-year-old man who experienced sudden death while playing basketball. Which of the following autopsy findings are *not* consistent with a diagnosis of HCM?

A. Asymmetric septal hypertrophy with a small left ventricular cavity
B. If left ventricular outflow tract obstruction was present, plaque may be located on the upper septal area
C. Mitral valve abnormalities are rarely present
D. Epicardial arteries can follow an intramural course
E. Histopathologic examination shows cardiomyocyte hypertrophy and disarray

59-3. A 24-year-old woman with HCM is on a maximally tolerated dose of beta-blocker and continues to have class III exertional dyspnea. Which of the following are causes of diastolic dysfunction in patients with HCM?

A. Impairment of ventricular relaxation
B. Increased chamber stiffness
C. Insufficient coronary blood flow
D. Compromised myocardial energy metabolism
E. All of the above

59-4. Which of the following physical examination findings are *not* associated with HCM with obstruction?

A. Pulsus alternans
B. Bifid apical impulse
C. Decrease in murmur quality going from sitting to standing
D. Decrease in the murmur when raising the legs
E. Amyl nitrite will increase the murmur

59-5. A 27-year-old man presents to your office for exertional syncope and shortness of breath. Which of the following would be consistent with a diagnosis of sarcomeric HCM?

A. Left ventricular wall thickness > 10 mm
B. Diffuse subendocardial late gadolinium enhancement on cardiac MRI
C. Systolic anterior motion (SAM) of the mitral valve apparatus to cause obstruction
D. Short PR interval, pre-excitation, and extreme left ventricular hypertrophy (LVH) on ECG
E. Increased serum creatine phosphokinase (CPK) and lactate

59-6. Your patient with HCM is in the cardiac catheterization laboratory for hemodynamic assessment and has the tracing shown in Figure 59-1. Which of the following maneuvers can elicit this phenomenon?

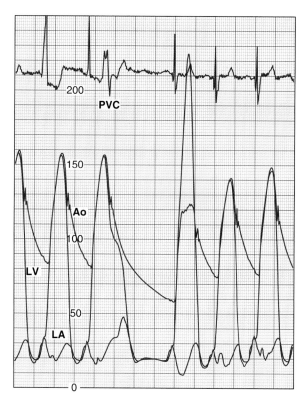

FIGURE 59-1 Invasive hemodynamic tracings for question 59-6.

A. Valsalva
B. Norepinephrine infusion
C. Isooproterenol infusion
D. A and C
E. A and B

59-7. Your patient with HCM has several questions about his risk for sudden death (SCD). Which of the following features are *not* associated with an increased risk of SCD with HCM?

A. History of prior cardiac arrest or spontaneous sustained ventricular tachycardia
B. A family history of premature SCD in a first-degree relative with HCM
C. Nonsustained ventricular tachycardia on ambulatory testing
D. Hypertensive blood pressure response to exercise
E. Extreme LVH > 30 mm

59-8. A 32-year-old man presents for exertional dyspnea. His echocardiogram is diagnostic of hypertrophic obstructive cardiomyopathy (HOCM). He is currently *not* taking any medications. Which of the following could be recommended?

A. Fluid restriction
B. Initiation of a beta-blocker
C. Verapamil
D. Alcohol septal ablation
E. Surgical myectomy

59-9. A 44-year-old woman with HOCM continues to have class 3 shortness of breath despite maximal medical therapy. Which of the following are indications for myectomy?

A. An LV outflow tract obstructive gradient ≥ 50 mm Hg
B. New York Heart Association functional class III-IV symptoms despite maximal medical therapy
C. Recurrent exertional syncope despite maximally tolerated drug therapy
D. A and B
E. All of the above

59-10. A 44-year-old woman with HOCM continues to have class III shortness of breath despite maximal medical therapy and is interested in myectomy. Which of the following is *not true* regarding complications of myectomy?

A. In large-volume centers, the operative mortality for septal myectomy is < 1%
B. Complications of surgical myectomy (AV nodal block, ventricular septal defect, and aortic regurgitation) of surgery are uncommon
C. The major complication of alcohol septal ablation is complete heart block
D. The risk for complete heart block following alcohol septal ablation is increased if right bundle branch block is present prior to the ablation procedure
E. A maximum LV wall thickness < 16 mm at the point of leaflet-septal contact is a risk factor for ventriculoseptal defects in both alcohol septal ablation and myectomy

59-1. **The answer is E.** (*Hurst's The Heart, 14th Edition, Chap. 59*) The majority of mutations that cause HCM involve sarcomeric proteins. Between 75% and 80% involve cardiac myosin heavy chain (*MYH7*) and cardiac myosin binding protein C (*MYBPC3*). Mutations in cardiac troponin T (*TNNT2*), troponin I (*TNNI3*), α-tropomyosin (*TPM1*), myosin light chains (*MYL2, MYL3*), and cardiac actin (*ACTC1*) account for 15% to 20% of mutation-positive individuals (option A).[1] A further 5% to 10% of cases are caused by metabolic or storage disorders (eg, Anderson-Fabry disease, mitochondrial disorders, glycogen storage diseases), neuromuscular disorders, chromosome abnormalities, and genetic syndromes such as cardio-facial-cutaneous syndromes, including Noonan and LEOPARD syndromes (option B).[2] Two pathogenic mechanisms are thought to account for disease associated with mutations in cardiac sarcomere proteins. Missense single nucleotide variants (a nucleotide change that results in an amino acid being substituted by another amino acid in the protein) predominantly lead to a *dominant negative effect* (described as a "poison peptide" mechanism) in which the mutated protein is not destroyed but rather integrates into the sarcomere, leading to the disease phenotype; this is thought to be characteristic of *MYH7* variants (option C). Alternatively, nonsense single nucleotide variants or small frameshift insertion-deletions can introduce a premature stop codon and cause haploinsufficiency as a result of nonsense mRNA-mediated decay or proteolysis of a truncated (just partially translated) protein. This mechanism is believed to be typical of the majority of *MYBPC3* disease-causing mutations (option D).[3] HCM is characterized by variable intra- and interfamilial expression and incomplete and age-dependent clinical penetrance. Thus, unaffected family members can be carriers of the causal mutation (option E).[4]

59-2. **The answer is C.** (*Hurst's The Heart, 14th Edition, Chap. 59*) Gross examination of the heart in patients with HCM demonstrates asymmetric septal hypertrophy with a small left ventricular cavity (option A).[5] The mural endocardium may be thickened by fibrous tissue, and if left ventricular outflow tract obstruction is present, there is often a plaque located on the upper septal area where the mitral valve repeatedly has come in contact with the septum (option B). The mitral valve itself may be abnormal, with elongation of the mitral chordae and anterior displacement of hypertrophied papillary muscles. Abnormal attachments of the mitral valve chordae into the septum, insertion of the papillary muscle head directly into the mitral leaflets, myocardial clefts, and increased ventricular trabeculation are also common (option C).[6] Although the epicardial coronary arteries are usually normal, they can follow an intramural course and be compressed during ventricular systole (option D).[7] The classic histopathologic appearance of HCM consists of cardiomyocyte hypertrophy and disarray, interstitial and replacement fibrosis, and dysplastic arterioles (option E).[8]

59-3. **The answer is E.** (*Hurst's The Heart, 14th Edition, Chap. 59*) Diastolic dysfunction arises from multiple factors that affect both ventricular relaxation and chamber stiffness (options A and B).[9] Patients with HCM have increased oxygen demand as a result of ventricular hypertrophy and abnormal loading conditions but also have compromised coronary blood flow to the LV myocardium because of abnormally small and partially obliterated intramural coronary arteries (option C). In addition, myocardial energy metabolism is compromised as a result of inefficient cardiomyocyte contraction and is an early feature of the disease in carriers of sarcomeric protein mutation (option D).[10]

59-4. **The answer is A.** (*Hurst's The Heart, 14th Edition, Chap. 59*) The classic carotid pulsation is brisk with a spike-and-dome pattern, characterized by a rapid rise (percussion wave) followed by a midsystolic drop that is, in turn, followed by a secondary wave (tidal wave). Pulsus alternans is alternating strong and weak beats, often associated with severe LV dysfunction (option A). The apical impulse is almost always abnormal in patients with HCM. Typically, it is a sustained systolic thrust that continues throughout most of systole and can be bifid as a result of a forceful atrial systole (option B). From the standing position to a prompt squat, the murmur will markedly decrease in intensity as a result of increases in afterload and preload (option C). Other maneuvers that are used to change the intensity of the murmur include leg-raising to increase preload (and thereby decrease the intensity of the murmur) and inhaling amyl nitrite to decrease afterload (options D and E).

59-5. **The answer is C.** (*Hurst's The Heart, 14th Edition, Chap. 59*) Increased LV wall thickness measured by any imaging technique is the basis for the diagnosis of HCM. In adults, a wall thickness ≥ 15 mm at end-diastole in one or more myocardial segments and, in children, a wall thickness more than two standard deviations greater than the predicted mean are sufficient to make the diagnosis (option A). Diffuse subendocardial late gadolinium enhancement on cardiac MRI is suggestive of amyloid. HCM typically has midwall late gadolinium enhancement or late gadolinium enhancement at the insertion zones of the right ventricle (RV) in the septum (option B). Dynamic LV outflow tract obstruction (LVOTO) is characterized by SAM of the mitral valve apparatus and an open ventricular chamber. Most patients have SAM of the anterior leaflet, but it also occurs with the posterior leaflet.[11] Short PR interval, pre-excitation, and extreme LVH on ECG are more consistent with Danon's disease or glycogen storage disease (option D). Increased serum CPK and lactate tend to go along with mitochondrial myopathies (option E).

59-6. **The answer is D.** (*Hurst's The Heart, 14th Edition, Chap. 59*) Figure 59-1 shows the Brockenbrough phenomenon—the hallmark of latent obstruction. After a premature contraction, an increase in the contractility of the ventricle results in a marked increase in the degree of dynamic obstruction. This is seen as an increase in the outflow gradient and a decrease in the aortic pulse pressure after the pause. When there is little resting obstruction, provocation using the Valsalva maneuver or infusion of isoproterenol can be performed in the catheterization laboratory (options A and C). Norepinephrine infusion would increase afterload and is unlikely to increase obstruction (option B).

59-7. **The answer is D.** (*Hurst's The Heart, 14th Edition, Chap. 59*) Several clinical features are associated with a high risk for SCD in patients with HCM.[12] Patients who have had a prior cardiac arrest or spontaneous sustained ventricular tachycardia are at highest risk (option A). A family history of premature SCD in a first-degree relative with HCM portends a high risk, particularly if there are multiple occurrences (option B). Other risk markers include recent unexplained syncope, nonsustained ventricular tachycardia (option C), hypotensive blood pressure response to exercise (option D), and extreme LV hypertrophy (> 30 mm) (option E).

59-8. **The answer is B.** (*Hurst's The Heart, 14th Edition, Chap. 59*). Patients with LVOTO should maintain hydration at all times, avoid excessive alcohol consumption, and maintain a healthy weight (option A).[12] Medical therapy should be considered the first-line therapy for the relief of symptoms in patients with obstructive HCM. Beta-adrenergic blocking agents are usually the drugs of choice. Theoretic actions of beta-blockers include decreased heart rate response to exercise, relief of angina by a decrease in myocardial oxygen demand, and improvement in diastolic filling time (option B). Nondihydropyrine calcium channel blockers—specifically, verapamil and diltiazem—are also of value in the treatment of HCM, particularly if beta-blockers are contraindicated or ineffective (option C). A trial of medical therapy should be offered before considering alcohol septal ablation or surgical myectomy (options D and E).

59-9. **The answer is E.** (*Hurst's The Heart, 14th Edition, Chap. 59*) For patients who have an LV outflow tract obstructive gradient ≥ 50 mm Hg (option A), moderate-to-severe symptoms (New York Heart Association functional class III-IV) (option B), or recurrent exertional syncope despite maximally tolerated drug therapy (option C), other treatment options such as septal myectomy, septal ablation, or dual-chamber pacing should be considered.[12]

59-10. **The answer is D.** (*Hurst's The Heart, 14th Edition, Chap. 59*) In large-volume centers, the operative mortality for septal myectomy is < 1% (option A).[13] Complications of myectomy

(AV nodal block, ventricular septal defect, and aortic regurgitation) of surgery are uncommon (option B).[12] The major complication of alcohol septal ablation is complete heart block, which, with small doses of alcohol and guidance with myocardial contrast echocardiography, occurs in 7% to 20% of patients (option C). The risk for heart block is increased in patients with a preexisting LBBB (option D). A maximum LV wall thickness < 16 mm at the point of leaflet-septal contact is a risk factor for ventriculoseptal defects in both alcohol septal ablation and myectomy.[12]

References

1. Van Driest SL, Ommen SR, Tajik AJ, Gersh BJ, Ackerman MJ. Sarcomeric genotyping in hypertrophic cardiomyopathy. *Mayo Clin Proc.* 2005;80(4):463-469.

2. Elliott P, Charron P, Blanes JR, et al. European Cardiomyopathy Pilot Registry: EURObservational Research Programme of the European Society of Cardiology. *Eur Heart J.* 2016;37(2):164-173.

3. Lopes LR, Elliott PM. A straightforward guide to the sarcomeric basis of cardiomyopathies. *Heart.* 2014;100(24):1916-1923.

4. Maron BJ, Maron MS, Semsarian C. Genetics of hypertrophic cardiomyopathy after 20 years: clinical perspectives. *J Am Coll Cardiol.* 2012;60(8):705-715.

5. Davies MJ, Pomerance A, Teare RD. Pathological features of hypertrophic obstructive cardiomyopathy. *J Clin Pathol.* 1974;27(7):529-535.

6. Klues HG, Proschan MA, Dollar AL, et al. Echocardiographic assessment of mitral valve size in obstructive hypertrophic cardiomyopathy. Anatomic validation from mitral valve specimen. *Circulation.* 1993;88(2):548-555.

7. Tavora F, Cresswell N, Li L, et al. Morphologic features of exertional versus nonexertional sudden death in patients with hypertrophic cardiomyopathy. *Am J Cardiol.* 2010;105(4):532-537.

8. Varnava AM, Elliott PM, Baboonian C, et al. Hypertrophic cardiomyopathy: histopathological features of sudden death in cardiac troponin T disease. *Circulation.* 2001;104(12):1380-1384.

9. Nihoyannopoulos P, Karatasakis G, Frenneaux M, McKenna WJ, Oakley CM. Diastolic function in hypertrophic cardiomyopathy: relation to exercise capacity. *J Am Coll Cardiol.* 1992;19(3):536-540.

10. Crilley JG, Boehm EA, Blair E, et al. Hypertrophic cardiomyopathy due to sarcomeric gene mutations is characterized by impaired energy metabolism irrespective of the degree of hypertrophy. *J Am Coll Cardiol.* 2003;41(10):1776-1782.

11. Cardim N, Galderisi M, Edvardsen T, et al. Role of multimodality cardiac imaging in the management of patients with hypertrophic cardiomyopathy: an expert consensus of the European Association of Cardiovascular Imaging Endorsed by the Saudi Heart Association. *Eur Heart J Cardiovasc Imaging.* 2015;16(3):280.

12. Authors/Task Force members, Elliott PM, Anastasakis A, et al. 2014 ESC guidelines on diagnosis and management of hypertrophic cardiomyopathy: the Task Force for the Diagnosis and Management of Hypertrophic Cardiomyopathy of the European Society of Cardiology (ESC). *Eur Heart J.* 2014;35(39):2733-2779.

13. Woo A, Williams WG, Choi R, et al. Clinical and echocardiographic determinants of long-term survival after surgical myectomy in obstructive hypertrophic cardiomyopathy. *Circulation.* 2005;111(16):2033-2041.

CHAPTER 60

Left Ventricular Noncompaction

Ravi Karra

DIRECTIONS: Choose the one best response to each question.

60-1. Which of the following imaging findings is consistent with a diagnosis of left ventricular noncompaction (LVNC)?

A. A ratio of noncompacted myocardium to compact myocardium > 2 in the parasternal short axis by echocardiography

B. A ratio of noncompacted myocardium to compact myocardium > 2.3 in the horizontal long axis by cardiac MRI

C. A ratio of noncompacted myocardium to compact myocardium > 1 in at least two segments of short axis images by multidetector CT

D. All of the above

E. A and B

60-2. A 57-year-old man presents to your clinic to follow up a negative cardiac MRI (CMR) stress test for nonspecific chest pain. He was noted to have an increased ratio of noncompact to compact myocardium with normal left ventricular (LV) function. He is otherwise healthy. Which of the following is *not true* about compact and trabecular myocardium in the normal population?

A. The compacted layer but not the trabeculated layer is thicker in men than in women

B. The compacted layer thickens, whereas the trabeculated layer thins with systole

C. Trabeculated LV segments show increased systolic thinning of trabeculated layers and greater thickening of the compact segments with age

D. There are sex-specific differences in the trabeculated/compacted ratio at end systole or end diastole

E. In end systole, the trabeculated/compacted ratio is lower in older (50–79 years) subjects than in younger (20–49 years) subjects

60-3. Which of the following is *not true* regarding the proposed pathogenesis of LVNC?

A. LVNC may be the result of abnormal cardiac development

B. Polymorphisms of genes affecting the Notch pathway are associated with LVNC

C. The causes of interruption of myocardial compaction during cardiac development are unknown

D. LVNC is always inherited and never acquired

E. LVNC can be regarded as an isolated entity or as one of the traits that may recur in other cardiac and noncardiac diseases

60-4. A 32-year-old woman with a history of Barth syndrome in her family is pregnant with a boy. She wants to know about the risks of Barth syndrome if her son is affected. Which of the following is *true* of Barth syndrome?

A. Barth syndrome is not transmitted from mother to son

B. Barth syndrome is due to a mutation of the *MIB1* gene

C. Hypertrophic cardiomyopathy does not occur with Barth syndrome

D. Among children with a dilated cardiomyopathy (DCM), reverse remodeling can occur with normalization of heart function

E. Arrhythmias are uncommon

60-5. Which of the following is *not true* about the genetic basis for LVNC?

A. LVNC can result from mutations to genes that encode sarcomeric proteins

B. The same mutations that cause LVNC can result in hypertrophic cardiomyopathy (HCM), dilated cardiomyopathy (DCM), and restrictive cardiomyopathy (RCM)

C. LVNC can be seen in patients with neuromuscular disorders

D. LVNC has been associated with mutations of ion channels

E. All of the above are true

60-6. A 34-year-old athlete is referred to you for palpitations. CMR showed a LVNC phenotype with normal left ventricular function. Which of the following is *true* of acquired LVNC?

A. LVNC is a rare finding among athletes

B. The majority of women who develop LVNC during pregnancy will have a regression of trabeculation after delivery

C. Patients with siderosis and LVNC have preferential accumulation of iron in the compact layer

D. LVNC is rare among patients with bicuspid aortic valve disease

E. Patients with acquired LVNC are likely to have an underlying familial syndrome

60-7. Which of the following is a typical finding in the evaluation of LVNC?

A. An abnormal ECG

B. A ratio of > 2:1 of noncompacted to compacted layer at end diastole by echo

C. Myocardial fibrosis is identified by late gadolinium enhancement during CMR

D. Elevation of troponin in the serum

E. All of the above are typical findings

60-8. A 45-year-old man presents for evaluation of LVNC. He is asymptomatic but was found to incidentally have an ejection fraction of 35% and LVNC. Which of the following is *true* about the prognosis for patients with LVNC?

A. Asymptomatic patients or individuals with LVNC and normal LV function have a poor prognosis

B. Patients presenting with heart failure (New York Heart Association class III or IV), sustained ventricular arrhythmias, or left atrial dilation have a favorable prognosis

C. A right bundle branch block is associated with a good prognosis

D. Prognosis depends on the severity of the underlying cardiac disease rather than the trabecular anatomy of the LV

E. None of the above are true

60-9. Which of the following is *not* indicated in patients with Barth syndrome?

A. Consideration of aspirin with severe LV dysfunction

B. Inclusion of uncooked cornstarch in the diet to prevent muscle protein loss

C. Avoidance of succinylcholine

D. Use of prophylactic antibiotics in high-risk clinical situations

E. Empiric administration of warfarin with a goal INR of 2-3

60-10. Which of the following is *true* regarding the epidemiology of LVNC?

A. The incidence of LVNC in children is less than 0.1 per 100,000.

B. Approximately 10% of pediatric cardiomyopathies are associated with LVNC

C. LVNC is more common in women than in men

D. A and B

E. A and C

60-1. **The answer is E.** *(Hurst's The Heart, 14th Edition, Chap. 60)* A ratio of noncompacted myocardium to compact myocardium > 2 by echocardiography is consistent with a diagnosis of LVNC (option A).[1] A ratio of noncompacted myocardium to compact myocardium > 2.3 in the horizontal long axis by cardiac MRI is consistent with a diagnosis of LVNC (option B).[2] A ratio of noncompacted myocardium to compact myocardium >2.2 in at least 2 segments of short axis images by cardiac CT is consistent with a diagnosis of LVNC (option C).[2]

60-2. **The answer is D.** *(Hurst's The Heart, 14th Edition, Chap. 60)* CMR studies in normal adult volunteers demonstrated the following sex- and age-related differences: (1) the compacted but not the trabeculated layer is thicker in men than in women (option A); (2) the compacted layer thickens, whereas the trabeculated layer thins with systole (option B); (3) trabeculated LV segments show increased systolic thinning of trabeculated layers and greater thickening of the compact segments ($P < .05$) with age (option C); (4) total wall thickening is neither sex nor age dependent; (5) there were no sex-specific differences in the trabeculated/compacted ratio at end systole or end diastole (option D); and (6) in end systole, the trabeculated/compacted ratio was lower in older (50–79 years) subjects than in younger (20–49 years) subjects ($P < .05$) (option E).[3] Overall, the application of current diagnostic criteria demonstrates that LVNC may occur in a relevant proportion of healthy individuals.

60-3. **The answer is D.** *(Hurst's The Heart, 14th Edition, Chap. 60)* The most cited pathogenetic hypothesis for LVNC is embryogenic arrest of the normal process of trabecular maturation during early intrauterine life when the heart undergoes cardiac chamber maturation (option A).[4] However, LVNC can be heritable or acquired. For example, patients with cardiomyopathies may develop LVNC during the course of their disease (option D).[5,6] While many signaling pathways have been linked to compaction during heart development, only mutations of the *MIB1* gene have been linked to LVNC. The *MIB1* gene encodes a ubiquitin ligase that regulates endocytosis of Notch ligands.[7] To date, mutations in this gene have been reported in individuals with LVNC in two Spanish families (option B).[8] The causes of interruption of myocardial compaction are unknown (option D). LVNC can be regarded as an isolated entity or as one of the traits that may recur in other cardiac and noncardiac diseases. For example, LVNC is associated with tafazzinopathies [caused by mutations in the *TAZ* (*Tafazzin*, or *G4.5*) gene] (option E).[9]

60-4. **The answer is D.** *(Hurst's The Heart, 14th Edition, Chap. 60)* Barth syndrome should be suspected in all male infants with heart failure, DCM, and LVNC, especially when associated with other markers of disease. Barth syndrome is a rare X-linked recessive disorder characterized by cardiomyopathy, neutropenia, skeletal myopathy, prepubertal growth delay, and distinctive facial characteristics. As an X-linked disorder, the mutation is passed from mother to son (option A). While mutations of *MIB1* have been associated with LVNC, Barth syndrome is caused by mutations in the *G4.5* gene (*TAZ*) (option B).[9-11] LVNC is commonly associated with LV dilation and dysfunction at onset.[9] Less commonly, Barth cardiomyopathy may present with a hypertrophic or hypertrophic-dilated phenotype (option C). Heart involvement occurs in almost all children before the age of 5 years. Thereafter, the cardiomyopathy may demonstrate an intermittent course during which the heart can undergo remodeling. Improvement can be observed after infancy, with possible stabilization after the toddler years (option D).[12] Overall, however, cardiac function varies and tends to decline over time. Arrhythmias, both supraventricular and ventricular, are more commonly reported in adolescents and young adults than in infants.[9]

60-5. **The answer is E.** *(Hurst's The Heart, 14th Edition, Chap. 60)* LVNC can result from a diverse set of mutations, including to sarcomeric proteins (option A), ion channels (option D), and neuromuscular disease loci (option C). Mutations to the sarcomeric proteins ACTC1 (cardiac actin alpha) and MHY7 can cause DCM, RCM, and HCM (option B).[13,14]

60-6. The answer is B. *(Hurst's The Heart, 14th Edition, Chap. 60)* The proportion of athletes who develop LVNC under intensive exercise is relevant (about 10%) (option A).[15] Among pregnant women with LVNC, 69.2% showed complete resolution of LV trabeculations over a mean duration of 8.1 ± 4.2 months (option B).[16] Although LVNC can be associated with disorders of red blood cells, in patients with myocardial iron overload and siderosis, a preferential distribution of intramyocyte iron in the compacted or noncompacted layers has not been observed (option C).[17] A high prevalence of LVNC is reported in patients fulfilling the echocardiographic criteria for bicuspid aortic valve (BAV). Specifically, in one study, 12 (11.0%) of 109 patients with BAV fulfilled the criteria for LVNC, with nine of the 12 patients being men. Although the pathophysiologic basis of LVNC in patients with BAV is unclear, special attention should be given to the evaluation of LV trabecular anatomy.[18] All these acquired conditions of LVNC demonstrate that a unique pathogenetic hypothesis of embryogenic defect is unlikely to explain acquired, late-onset, transient LVNC (option E).

60-7. The answer is A. *(Hurst's The Heart, 14th Edition, Chap. 60)* Although a normal ECG finding is rare in LVNC and is observed in a minority of patients (from 6% to 13%), there are no changes specific to LVNC (option A).[19] A ratio of > 2:1 of noncompacted to compacted layer at end systole by echo is characteristic of LVNC (option B). Myocardial fibrosis is not a criterion for the diagnosis of LVNC (option C). There are no specific biomarkers for LVNC (option D).

60-8. The answer is D. *(Hurst's The Heart, 14th Edition, Chap. 60)* Prognosis in LVNC depends on the clinical presentation. Asymptomatic patients or individuals with LVNC and normal LV function have a good prognosis (option A).[20] Alternatively, patients presenting with heart failure (New York Heart Association class III or IV), sustained ventricular arrhythmias, or left atrial dilation have an unfavorable prognosis (option B).[20,21] Adverse outcomes of isolated LVNC occur in patients with advanced heart failure, dilated left heart with systolic dysfunction, reduced systolic blood pressure, pulmonary hypertension, and right bundle branch block (option C).[20] In summary, prognosis depends on the severity of the underlying cardiac disease rather than the trabecular anatomy of the LV (option D).

60-9. The answer is E. *(Hurst's The Heart, 14th Edition, Chap. 60)* Patients diagnosed with Barth syndrome with heart failure should receive standard medications as per guidelines. Aspirin can eventually be added to decrease the risk of stroke in patients with severe LV dysfunction (option A). Empiric warfarin in the absence of thromboembolic events is not recommended (option E). The monitoring of arrhythmias and related prevention strategies should be maintained over the course of the patient's life. Disease-specific treatments can include the administration of granulocyte colony-stimulating factor either routinely or in high-risk clinical situations (eg, infections, surgery) along with prophylactic antibiotics (option D). Diets should include the administration of uncooked cornstarch to prevent muscle protein loss overnight (option B). Succinylcholine, a nondepolarizing neuromuscular blocker that could have a prolonged effect, should be avoided (option C).[12]

60-10. The answer is D. *(Hurst's The Heart, 14th Edition, Chap. 60)* The precise proportion of LVNC remains elusive. Data on the annual incidence of LVNC in children report values < 0.1 per 100,000 (option A).[22] Isolated LVNC accounted for 9.2% of all cases in a population-based retrospective cohort study of primary cardiomyopathies in Australian children.[23] This prevalence was close to that recorded in the Texas Children's Hospital echocardiography database (9.5%) (option B).[24] As for sex, LVNC is reported to be more common in men (56% to 82%) than in women (option C).[25-28]

References

1. Jenni R, Oechslin E, Schneider J, Attenhofer Jost C, Kaufmann PA. Echocardiographic and pathoanatomical characteristics of isolated left ventricular non-compaction: a step towards classification as a distinct cardiomyopathy. *Heart.* 2001;86(6):666-671.

2. Belanger AR, Miller MA, Donthireddi UR, Najovits AJ, Goldman ME. New classification scheme of left ventricular noncompaction and correlation with ventricular performance. *Am J Cardiol.* 2008;102(1):92-96.

3. Dawson DK, Maceira AM, Raj VJ, et al. Regional thicknesses and thickening of compacted and trabeculated myocardial layers of the normal left ventricle studied by cardiovascular magnetic resonance. *Circ Cardiovasc Imaging.* 2011;4(2):139-146.

4. Arbustini E, Narula N, Dec GW, et al. The MOGE(S) classification for a phenotype-genotype nomenclature of cardiomyopathy: endorsed by the World Heart Federation. *J Am Coll Cardiol.* 2013;62(22):2046-2072.

5. Bleyl SB, Mumford BR, Brown-Harrison MC, et al. Xq28-linked noncompaction of the left ventricular myocardium: prenatal diagnosis and pathologic analysis of affected individuals. *Am J Med Genet.* 1997;72(3):257-265.

6. Statile CJ, Taylor MD, Mazur W, et al. Left ventricular noncompaction in Duchenne muscular dystrophy. *J Cardiovasc Magn Reson.* 2013;15:67.

7. Hansson EM, Lanner F, Das D, et al. Control of Notch-ligand endocytosis by ligand-receptor interaction. *J Cell Sci.* 2010;123(Pt 17):2931-2942.

8. Luxan G, Casanova JC, Martinez-Poveda B, et al. Mutations in the NOTCH pathway regulator MIB1 cause left ventricular noncompaction cardiomyopathy. *Nat Med.* 2013;19(2):193-201.

9. Bleyl SB, Mumford BR, Thompson V, et al. Neonatal, lethal noncompaction of the left ventricular myocardium is allelic with Barth syndrome. *Am J Hum Genet.* 1997;61(4):868-872.

10. Chen R, Tsuji T, Ichida F, et al. Mutation analysis of the G4.5 gene in patients with isolated left ventricular noncompaction. *Mol Genet Metab.* 2002;77(4):319-325.

11. Karkucinska-Wieckowska A, Trubicka J, Werner B, et al. Left ventricular noncompaction (LVNC) and low mitochondrial membrane potential are specific for Barth syndrome. *J Inherit Metab Dis.* 2013;36(6):929-937.

12. Ferreira C, Thompson R, Vernon H. Barth syndrome. *GeneReviews®* [Internet]. 2014.

13. Greenway SC, McLeod R, Hume S, et al. Exome sequencing identifies a novel variant in ACTC1 associated with familial atrial septal defect. *Can J Cardiol.* 2014;30(2):181-187.

14. Hoedemaekers YM, Caliskan K, Majoor-Krakauer D, et al. Cardiac beta-myosin heavy chain defects in two families with non-compaction cardiomyopathy: linking non-compaction to hypertrophic, restrictive, and dilated cardiomyopathies. *Eur Heart J.* 2007;28(22):2732-2737.

15. Jacquier A, Thuny F, Jop B, et al. Measurement of trabeculated left ventricular mass using cardiac magnetic resonance imaging in the diagnosis of left ventricular non-compaction. *Eur Heart J.* 2010;31(9):1098-1104.

16. Gati S, Papadakis M, Papamichael ND, et al. Reversible de novo left ventricular trabeculations in pregnant women: implications for the diagnosis of left ventricular noncompaction in low-risk populations. *Circulation.* 2014;130(6):475-483.

17. Wood JC. Cardiac iron across different transfusion-dependent diseases. *Blood Rev.* 2008;22 Suppl 2: S14-S21.

18. Agarwal A, Khandheria BK, Paterick TE, et al. Left ventricular noncompaction in patients with bicuspid aortic valve. *J Am Soc Echocardiogr.* 2013;26(11):1306-1313.

19. Steffel J, Kobza R, Oechslin E, Jenni R, Duru F. Electrocardiographic characteristics at initial diagnosis in patients with isolated left ventricular noncompaction. *Am J Cardiol.* 2009;104(7):984-989.

20. Tian T, Liu Y, Gao L, et al. Isolated left ventricular noncompaction: clinical profile and prognosis in 106 adult patients. *Heart Vessels.* 2014;29(5):645-652.

21. Caliskan K, Michels M, Geleijnse ML, et al. Frequency of asymptomatic disease among family members with noncompaction cardiomyopathy. *Am J Cardiol.* 2012;110(10):1512-1517.

22. Ichida F. Left ventricular noncompaction. *Circ J.* 2009;73(1):19-26.

23. Nugent AW, Daubeney PE, Chondros P, et al. The epidemiology of childhood cardiomyopathy in Australia. *N Engl J Med.* 2003;348(17):1639-1646.

24. Pignatelli RH, McMahon CJ, Dreyer WJ, et al. Clinical characterization of left ventricular noncompaction in children: a relatively common form of cardiomyopathy. *Circulation.* 2003;108(21):2672-2678.

25. Ritter M, Oechslin E, Sutsch G, et al. Isolated noncompaction of the myocardium in adults. *Mayo Clin Proc.* 1997;72(1):26-31.

26. Oechslin E, Jenni R. Left ventricular non-compaction revisited: a distinct phenotype with genetic heterogeneity? *Eur Heart J.* 2011;32(12):1446-1456.

27. Zarrouk-Mahjoub S, Finsterer J. Noncompaction with valve abnormalities is rarely associated with neurologic or genetic disease. *Int J Cardiol.* 2016;202:627-628.

28. Ichida F, Hamamichi Y, Miyawaki T, et al. Clinical features of isolated noncompaction of the ventricular myocardium: long-term clinical course, hemodynamic properties, and genetic background. *J Am Coll Cardiol.* 1999;34(1):233-240.

CHAPTER 61

Restrictive Heart Diseases

Ravi Karra

DIRECTIONS: Choose the one best response to each question.

61-1. Which of the following echocardiographic findings are associated with restrictive physiology?

A. An increased ratio of early diastolic filling to atrial filling (≥ 2)
B. Decreased E-deceleration time (< 160 ms)
C. Increased isovolumetric relaxation time
D. A and B
E. B and C

61-2. Which of the following features are consistent with the European Society of Cardiology and American Heart Association definitions of restrictive cardiomyopathy?

A. Normal or reduced diastolic volumes of one or both ventricles
B. Increased ventricular wall thickness
C. Normal or reduced systolic volumes of one or both ventricles
D. A and B
E. A and C

61-3. A 43-year-old woman is admitted to your care for acute decompensated heart failure with preserved ejection fraction. The family history is notable for restrictive cardiomyopathy. She has experienced a nearly 25-pound weight gain, is orthopneic, and is short of breath at rest. Which of the following would you *not* expect to observe during her physical examination?

A. Prominent jugular venous pulse and X and Y descents
B. Ascites
C. Crescendo-decrescendo murmur that worsens with Valsalva
D. A filling sound
E. Diminished pulse pressure

61-4. Which of the following findings favor a diagnosis of constrictive pericarditis over restrictive cardiomyopathy?

A. Elevated NT-proBNP
B. Kussmaul's sign
C. Shift of the septum with respiration by echocardiogram
D. Higher lateral e´ velocity compared to the medial e´
E. Prominent y descent on the jugular venous waveform

61-5. Which of the following is *true* regarding the genetic basic of RCM?

A. Most cases are autosomal recessive
B. Mutations of *TNNI3* are associated with RCM
C. EMB demonstrating immunoreactive granulofilamentous material accumulated within myocytes is indicative of a typical RCM desminopathy
D. B and C
E. None of the above are true

61-6. A 32-year-old woman presents to your clinic for volume overload. Her examination is notable for an elevated jugular venous pressure with prominent y descent. Her neck is also notable for the finding in Figure 61-1. She also has ascites marked peripheral edema. Echocardiography shows a RCM. Family history is notable for family members with the same condition. Which of the following genes are associated with this condition?

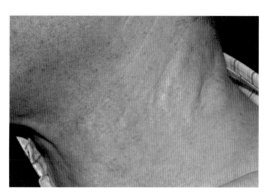

FIGURE 61-1 Neck of the patient in question 61-6.

A. *MYH6*
B. *MYBC3*
C. *ABCC6*
D. *TNNI3*
E. *TNNT2*

61-7. Which of the following is *not* characteristic of cardiac involvement of hereditary hemochromatosis (HH)?

A. Serum ferritin > 300 ng/mL
B. Low voltage on ECG
C. Longer T2* times with cardiac MRI are associated with a better prognosis
D. Diastolic dysfunction occurs early and is followed by reduced systolic function later in the disease
E. Lower early (E′) diastolic velocity by echocardiography

61-8. A 65-year-old man presents to your office for evaluation of cardiac amyloidosis. He had been having shortness of breath, and a cardiac MRI was suggestive of amyloid deposition. Which of the following would *not* be indicated to resolve the cause of his amyloid?

A. Endomyocardial biopsy (EMB) with mass spectrometry of the sample
B. Serum protein electrophoresis
C. Serum free light chains
D. No further testing, and referral for palliation
E. Pro-BNP levels

61-9. A 54-year-old woman presents with cutaneous flushing, diarrhea, bronchospasm with wheezing and shortness of breath, and volume overload. You suspect carcinoid heart disease. Which of the following is indicated to make a diagnosis?

A. Coronary angiography
B. Serum serotonin, platelet serotonin, and urinary 5-hydroxyindoleacetic acid levels
C. Serum ACE level
D. Cardiopulmonary exercise testing
E. Fecal evaluation for ova and parasites

61-10. A 73-year-old woman is diagnosed with AL amyloid complicated by cardiac involvement. She is referred to you for cardiac clearance prior to treatment consideration. Which of the following has prognostic value for this patient?

A. Serum NT-proBNP
B. Cardiac troponin T
C. Evaluation of NYHA functional class
D. A and B
E. All of the above

61-1. The answer is D. *(Hurst's The Heart, 14th Edition, Chap. 61)* Restrictive physiology describes a pattern of ventricular filling in which increased myocardial stiffness causes a precipitous elevation of ventricular pressure matched by a limited increase in volume; the resultant diastolic dysfunction is characterized by a pattern of mitral inflow Doppler velocities with an increased ratio of early diastolic filling to atrial filling (≥ 2) (option A), decreased E-deceleration time (< 160 ms) (option B), and decreased isovolumetric relaxation time (option C).

61-2. The answer is E. *(Hurst's The Heart, 14th Edition, Chap. 61)* According to the definition of the European Society of Cardiology (ESC), "Restrictive cardiomyopathies are defined as restrictive ventricular physiology in the presence of normal or reduced diastolic volumes of one or both ventricles, normal or reduced systolic volumes, and normal ventricular wall thickness."[1] According to the definition of the American Heart Association (AHA), "Primary restrictive non-hypertrophied cardiomyopathy is a rare form of heart muscle disease and a cause of heart failure that is characterized by normal or decreased volume of both ventricles associated with biatrial enlargement, normal left ventricular (LV) wall thickness and atrioventricular (AV) valves, impaired ventricular filling with restrictive physiology, and normal (or near normal) systolic function."[2] Both definitions emphasize restrictive ventricular physiology, normal or reduced volume of one or both ventricles, and normal wall thickness.

61-3. The answer is C. *(Hurst's The Heart, 14th Edition, Chap. 61)* A physical examination of patients with RCM reflects the elevated systemic and pulmonary venous pressures, with prominent jugular venous pulse and X and Y descents. In the advanced course of the disease, the pulse volume is low, the stroke volume declines, and the heart rate increases. A systolic murmur and filling sound reflect AV valve regurgitation and fast early diastolic filling; a fourth heart sound (S4) can be present. Hepatomegaly, ascites, and peripheral edema are common in decompensated patients. A crescendo-decrescendo murmur that worsens with Valsalva is more consistent with a diagnosis of hypertrophic obstructive cardiomyopathy.

61-4. The answer is C. *(Hurst's The Heart, 14th Edition, Chap. 61)* It is crucial to distinguish between RCM and constrictive pericarditis (CP) because RCM typically responds only to medical management and carries a poor prognosis, whereas CP may be curable by pericardiectomy and represents a potentially reversible cause of heart failure.[3] Two-dimensional echocardiography, M-mode, and Doppler blood-flow evaluation including respiratory-related ventricular septal shift (option C), preserved or increased medial mitral annular e′ velocity (option D), and prominent hepatic vein expiratory diastolic flow reversal are independently associated with the diagnosis of CP.[4-6] NT-proBNP levels are significantly higher in RCM than in CP (option A).[7] Kussmaul's sign can be observed in CP or RCM (option B). CP is associated with a prominent x descent and y descent, while RCM is associated a prominent y descent but a blunted x descent (option E).

61-5. The answer is C. *(Hurst's The Heart, 14th Edition, Chap. 61)* Familial RCM demonstrates autosomal dominant inheritance in the majority of cases (option A). The *TNNI3* gene that encodes the thin filament troponin I is the most common disease gene responsible for RCM (option B).[8] The typical RCM desminopathy is easily diagnosed by EMB demonstrating desmin immunoreactive granulofilamentous material accumulated within myocytes (option C).[9]

61-6. The answer is C. *(Hurst's The Heart, 14th Edition, Chap. 61)* This patient has pseudoxanthoma elasticum (PXE). PXE is a rare autosomal recessive systemic disease of the connective tissue that affects the extracellular matrix of multiple organs. PXE involves the cutaneous, ocular, and cardiovascular systems.[10,11] The cutaneous lesions typically occur in flexural areas (Figure 61-1), and the fundi may show angioid streaks radiating out from the optic discs, subretinal neovascularization, and/or hemorrhage. The cardiovascular manifestations are characterized by the development of arterial calcifications, premature coronary artery disease, peripheral vascular disease, and RCM.[12-17] PXE is caused by homozygous or compound heterozygous mutations in the *ABCC6* (ATP-binding cassette subfamily C member 6) gene that encodes a transmembrane adenosine triphosphate (ATP)-driven organic anion transporter (option C). Options A, B, D, and E are sarcomeric genes for which mutations are associated with hypertrophic cardiomyopathy and dilated cardiomyopathy.

61-7. **The answer is B.** *(Hurst's The Heart, 14th Edition, Chap. 61)* The cardiac phenotype of HH is characterized by early LV diastolic dysfunction with evolution through LV systolic dysfunction and dilation (option D). The diagnosis of HH is established by genetic testing in patients with elevated serum ferritin (> 300 ng/mL) and transferrin saturation values (> 55%) (option A). The ECG is nonspecific and does not significantly contribute to the diagnosis of HH cardiomyopathy; low QRS complex voltage and nonspecific repolarization abnormalities are uncommon in early phases; conduction disease may be present (option B). With cardiac MRI, the T2* method is highly sensitive and specific and is especially useful for detecting, grading, and monitoring iron deposition.[18-20] Patients demonstrating a T2* higher than 20 ms are at low risk for developing heart failure (HF); T2* between 10 and 20 ms indicates the presence of cardiac iron deposition and an intermediate risk of HF; and a T2* less than 10 ms indicates high risk of HF and a need for immediate chelation therapy.[21] Other modalities can suggest HH as well. In a multivariable analysis, echocardiographic spectral tissue Doppler lower early (E′) diastolic velocity was independently associated with hemochromatosis.[22]

61-8. **The answer is D.** *(Hurst's The Heart, 14th Edition, Chap. 61)* The gigantic scientific achievements in advancing our understanding of the biomolecular bases of amyloidogenic processes, and the development of novel drugs that target the different types of amyloidosis, are rapidly helping to change the fate of those with an ominous disease that until recently was hopeless and that is now a prototype of a successful model of precision and personalized medicine (option D). In the patient with unexplained LV hypertrophy and clinical suspicion for amyloidosis, biochemical testing should include evaluation for monoclonal protein production, serum immunofixation and electrophoresis, and serum free light chain assay (options B and C).[23-26] EMB has the dual advantage of being able to demonstrate amyloid deposition and to allow for the immune characterization of amyloidogenic protein. Recently, mass spectrometry–based proteomics have been introduced as a valuable tool for amyloid typing, with the advantage of not being antibody dependent. This can be performed on whole tissues or after laser capture microdissection of Congo red–positive areas (option A).[27] A high concentration of NT-proBNP allows the detection of AL amyloidosis at presymptomatic stages with a diagnostic sensitivity of 100%. Thus, screening with NT-proBNP has been advocated in patients at risk of developing AL amyloidosis (ie, patients followed by hematologists for monoclonal gammopathy of undetermined significance and altered circulating free light chain ratio).[28] Further, serum NT-proBNP levels are prognostic (option E).

61-9. **The answer is B.** *(Hurst's The Heart, 14th Edition, Chap. 61)* Carcinoid heart disease (Hedinger syndrome) is a rare condition that affects the right side of the heart in up to 60% of patients with neuroendocrine tumors (NETs) and systemic carcinoid syndrome (CS).[29] CS is caused by vasoactive substances secreted by NET cells; 5-hydroxytryptamine (serotonin) is the predominant peptide, followed by prostaglandins, histamine, bradykinin, tachykinins, and transforming growth factor-β (TGF-β). Both the tachykinins and TGF-β display profibrogenic properties inducing fibromyxoid plaques that affect the right ventricular endocardium, the ventricular side of the tricuspid valve apparatus (leaflets, chordae, and papillary muscles), the ventricular site of the pulmonary valve, and less commonly, the pulmonary artery. Serum serotonin, platelet serotonin, and urinary 5-hydroxyindoleacetic acid levels are elevated (option B).[30] The other options provided are helpful to exclude other causes of heart failure such as coronary artery disease (option A), shortness of breath (option D), sarcoid (option C), and diarrhea (option E). However, none of these are specific to the diagnosis of carcinoid.

61-10. **The answer is E.** (*Hurst's The Heart, 14th Edition, Chap. 61*) With AL amyloid, the criteria for evaluating both hematologic response (decreased amyloidogenic light chains) and organ response (improvement of organ function) are well established and graded. Treatment options depend on eligibility for autologous stem cell transplantation as well as on individual criteria to evaluate the tolerability of chemotherapeutic agents, including novel agent-based treatments with proteasome inhibitors, such as bortezomib, or immunomodulatory drugs such as thalidomide, lenalidomide, and pomalidomide.[31] Elevated cardiac biomarkers (NT-proBNP > 5000 ng/L, cardiac troponin T > 0.06 ng/mL) are considered exclusion criteria for stem cell transplantation (options A and B).[32] Standard chemotherapy requires dose reductions in stage IIIb patients (option C). Non-chemotherapy approaches to the treatment of AL amyloidosis are now rapidly expanding.

References

1. Elliott P, Andersson B, Arbustini E, et al. Classification of the cardiomyopathies: a position statement from the European Society of Cardiology Working Group on Myocardial and Pericardial Diseases. *Eur Heart J.* 2008;29(2):270-276.
2. Maron BJ, Towbin JA, Thiene G, et al. Contemporary definitions and classification of the cardiomyopathies: an American Heart Association scientific statement from the Council on Clinical Cardiology, Heart Failure and Transplantation Committee; Quality of Care and Outcomes Research and Functional Genomics and Translational Biology Interdisciplinary Working Groups; and Council on Epidemiology and Prevention. *Circulation.* 2006;113(14):1807-1816.
3. Syed FF, Schaff HV, Oh JK. Constrictive pericarditis—a curable diastolic heart failure. *Nat Rev Cardiol.* 2015;12(12):682.
4. Klein AL, Abbara S, Agler DA, et al. American Society of Echocardiography clinical recommendations for multimodality cardiovascular imaging of patients with pericardial disease: endorsed by the Society for Cardiovascular Magnetic Resonance and Society of Cardiovascular Computed Tomography. *J Am Soc Echocardiogr.* 2013;26(9):965-1012 e15.
5. Oh JK, Hatle LK, Seward JB, et al. Diagnostic role of Doppler echocardiography in constrictive pericarditis. *J Am Coll Cardiol.* 1994;23(1):154-162.
6. Veress G, Feng D, Oh JK. Echocardiography in pericardial diseases: new developments. *Heart Fail Rev.* 2013;18(3):267-275.
7. Parakh N, Mehrotra S, Seth S, et al. NT pro B type natriuretic peptide levels in constrictive pericarditis and restrictive cardiomyopathy. *Indian Heart J.* 2015;67(1):40-44.
8. Mogensen J, Hey T, Lambrecht S. A systematic review of phenotypic features associated with cardiac troponin I mutations in hereditary cardiomyopathies. *Can J Cardiol.* 2015;31(11):1377-1385.
9. Arbustini E, Pasotti M, Pilotto A, et al. Desmin accumulation restrictive cardiomyopathy and atrioventricular block associated with desmin gene defects. *Eur J Heart Fail.* 2006;8(5):477-483.
10. Uitto J, Pulkkinen L, Ringpfeil F. Molecular genetics of pseudoxanthoma elasticum: a metabolic disorder at the environment-genome interface? *Trends Mol Med.* 2001;7(1):13-17.
11. Uitto J, Jiang Q. Pseudoxanthoma elasticum-like phenotypes: more diseases than one. *J Invest Dermatol.* 2007;127(3):507-510.
12. Nitschke Y, Baujat G, Botschen U, et al. Generalized arterial calcification of infancy and pseudoxanthoma elasticum can be caused by mutations in either ENPP1 or ABCC6. *Am J Hum Genet.* 2012;90(1):25-39.
13. Musumeci MB, Semprini L, Casenghi M, et al. Restrictive cardiomyopathy and pseudoxanthoma elasticum skin lesions. *J Cardiovasc Med (Hagerstown).* 2016;17 Suppl 2:e193-e195.
14. Navarro-Lopez F, Llorian A, Ferrer-Roca O, Betriu A, Sanz G. Restrictive cardiomyopathy in pseudoxanthoma elasticum. *Chest.* 1980;78(1):113-115.
15. Stollberger C, Finsterer J. Extracardiac medical and neuromuscular implications in restrictive cardiomyopathy. *Clin Cardiol.* 2007;30(8):375-380.
16. Combrinck M, Gilbert JD, Byard RW. Pseudoxanthoma elasticum and sudden death. *J Forensic Sci.* 2011;56(2):418-422.
17. Lebwohl M, Halperin J, Phelps RG. Brief report: occult pseudoxanthoma elasticum in patients with premature cardiovascular disease. *N Engl J Med.* 1993;329(17):1237-1239.
18. Wood JC. Use of magnetic resonance imaging to monitor iron overload. *Hematol Oncol Clin North Am.* 2014;28(4):747-764, vii.
19. Anderson LJ, Holden S, Davis B, et al. Cardiovascular T2-star (T2*) magnetic resonance for the early diagnosis of myocardial iron overload. *Eur Heart J.* 2001;22(23):2171-2179.

20. Barrera Portillo MC, Uranga Uranga M, Sanchez Gonzalez J, et al. [Liver and heart T2* measurement in secondary haemochromatosis]. *Radiologia.* 2013;55(4):331-339.

21. Pepe A, Positano V, Santarelli MF, et al. Multislice multiecho T2* cardiovascular magnetic resonance for detection of the heterogeneous distribution of myocardial iron overload. *J Magn Reson Imaging.* 2006;23(5):662-668.

22. Davidsen ES, Hervig T, Omvik P, Gerdts E. Left ventricular long-axis function in treated haemochromatosis. *Int J Cardiovasc Imaging.* 2009;25(3):237-247.

23. Wechalekar AD, Gillmore JD, Hawkins PN. Systemic amyloidosis. *Lancet.* 2016;387(10038):2641-2654.

24. Gertz MA, Dispenzieri A, Sher T. Pathophysiology and treatment of cardiac amyloidosis. *Nat Rev Cardiol.* 2015;12(2):91-102.

25. Rapezzi C, Lorenzini M, Longhi S, et al. Cardiac amyloidosis: the great pretender. *Heart Fail Rev.* 2015;20(2):117-124.

26. Muchtar E, Buadi FK, Dispenzieri A, Gertz MA. Immunoglobulin light-chain amyloidosis: from basics to new developments in diagnosis, prognosis and therapy. *Acta Haematol.* 2016;135(3):172-190.

27. Brambilla F, Lavatelli F, Di Silvestre D, et al. Reliable typing of systemic amyloidoses through proteomic analysis of subcutaneous adipose tissue. *Blood.* 2012;119(8):1844-1847.

28. Bellavia D, Pellikka PA, Al-Zahrani GB, et al. Independent predictors of survival in primary systemic (Al) amyloidosis, including cardiac biomarkers and left ventricular strain imaging: an observational cohort study. *J Am Soc Echocardiogr.* 2010;23(6):643-652.

29. Fox DJ, Khattar RS. Carcinoid heart disease: presentation, diagnosis, and management. *Heart.* 2004;90(10):1224-1228.

30. Pape UF, Perren A, Niederle B, et al. ENETS Consensus Guidelines for the management of patients with neuroendocrine neoplasms from the jejuno-ileum and the appendix including goblet cell carcinomas. *Neuroendocrinology.* 2012;95(2):135-156.

31. Jelinek T, Kufova Z, Hajek R. Immunomodulatory drugs in AL amyloidosis. *Crit Rev Oncol Hematol.* 2016;99:249-260.

32. Palladini G, Merlini G. What is new in diagnosis and management of light chain amyloidosis? *Blood.* 2016;128(2):159-168.

CHAPTER 62

Arrhythmogenic Cardiomyopathy

Jacqueline Joza

QUESTIONS

DIRECTIONS: Choose the one best response to each question.

62-1. A 35-year-old man experiences a sudden-onset syncope while playing soccer, and you are consulted by the emergency department. All of the following represent *major* criteria from the updated Task Force criteria for arrhythmogenic right ventricular cardiomyopathy (ARVC) *except*:

A. Regional right ventricular akinesia on transthoracic echo
B. Inverted T waves in leads V1 and V2 in the absence of complete right bundle branch block
C. Nonsustained ventricular tachycardia with LBBB morphology and superior axis
D. Identification of a pathogenic mutation
E. Epsilon wave

62-2. Which of the following regarding the prevalence of ARVC in the general population and the prevalence of clinical manifestations in men versus women respectively is *correct*?

A. 1/1000 – 1/5000; males > females 5:1
B. 1/5000 – 1/10,000; males > females 5:1
C. 1/1000 – 1/5000; males > females 3:1
D. 1/1000 – 1/5000; females > males 3:1
E. 1/5000 – 1/10,000; females > males 5:1

62-3. Classic right-sided ARVC is a genetic disease of the intercalated disks. Which of the following regarding intercalated disks is *incorrect*?

A. Intercalated disks are the units of electromechanical continuity between cardiac myocytes
B. The sarcomere constitutes a component of the intercalated disk

C. Gap junctions constitute a component of the intercalated disk
D. Adherens junctions constitute a component of the intercalated disk
E. Desmosomes constitute a component of the intercalated disk

62-4. A 30-year-old man presents to your clinic with bilateral lower extremity edema that has been progressive over the last few months. His physical exam reveals an elevated jugular venous pressure. In what percentage of ARVC cases do patients present with this physical finding?

A. 5% to 10%
B. 20% to 30%
C. 30% to 40%
D. 50% to 60%
E. 70% to 80%

62-5. A 25-year-old man presents to the hospital with rapid-onset palpitations. These lasted for approximately 10 minutes and were associated with dizziness. No documentation of a sustained arrhythmia was noted on monitoring, but he is noted to have frequent premature ventricular contractions of RBBB morphology, superior axis, and negativity in lead I. On physical exam, you note thickening of the skin on the palms of his hands. A transthoracic echocardiogram is performed and reveals left ventricular (LV) dilatation and dyskinesia. This constellation of findings is *most* consistent with:

A. Anderson–Tawil syndrome
B. Naxos disease
C. Brugada syndrome
D. Catecholaminergic polymorphic ventricular tachycardia
E. Caravajal syndrome

62-6. After you suspect ARVC in a 40-year-old woman, a cardiac MRI is performed. The conclusion in the final report notes, "an affected triangle of dysplasia, a pattern most consistent with ARVC. Correlate clinically." The *triangle of dysplasia* refers to the combination of which of the following structures?

A. Epicardial subtricuspid region, cavotricuspid isthmus, and right ventricular (RV) outflow tract
B. Left, right, and noncoronary cusps of the aortic valve
C. RV apex, interventricular septum, and LV apex
D. Epicardial subtricuspid region, RV basal anterior wall, and posterolateral left ventricle
E. Basal mitral valve region, RV basal anterior wall, and LV apex

62-7. A 45-year-old woman has a diagnosis of nonischemic cardiomyopathy, with signs and symptoms of predominantly right-sided heart failure. You suspect ARVC based on a few minor criteria. She cannot undergo a cardiac MRI due to significant renal dysfunction. Genetic testing does *not* reveal any relevant mutations. You consider endomyocardial biopsy. Which of the following statements is *incorrect* about the use of endomyocardial biopsy in patients with suspected ARVC?

A. The loss of normal RV myocardium with evidence of fibrofatty infiltration supports the diagnosis
B. The risk of cardiac perforation is equivalent for RV septal wall and RV free wall biopsies
C. RV septal wall or LV biopsies are not usually helpful
D. There is a high rate of false negatives and low sensitivity
E. The diagnostic yield may be improved by using electro-anatomic voltage mapping to guide biopsy

62-8. You refer your patient with probable ARVC to a specialized center for genetic testing. Which of the following statements is *incorrect*?

A. The predominant inheritance pattern is autosomal recessive with variable penetrance and expressivity, although an autosomal dominant pattern has been described
B. Class I recommendation for mutation-specific screening of family members following the identification of a pathogenic mutation in the proband
C. Class IIa recommendation for genetic testing of confirmed cases of ARVC
D. Class IIb recommendation for genetic testing of borderline cases of ARVC
E. Class III recommendation for genetic testing of patients who fulfill only a single minor Task Force criterion

62-9. All of the following put a clinically confirmed ARVC patient at a higher risk for sudden cardiac death *except*:

A. Unexplained syncope
B. Older age
C. Left ventricular dysfunction
D. Presence of heart failure
E. Sustained ventricular arrhythmias

62-10. A 25-year-old man presents with frequent premature ventricular contractions (PVCs). Twenty-four-hour Holter monitoring reveals a PVC burden of 18%. The morphology of the PVCs is consistent with a left bundle branch pattern with a transition at V5, with an inferior access suggesting an origin at the right ventricular outflow tract (RVOT). Which of the following is more suggestive of ARVC as opposed to RVOT-ventricular tachyardia (VT)?

A. Good response to verapamil
B. Endocardial ablation suppresses the arrhythmia
C. RVOT-VT is difficult to induce by programmed ventricular stimulation
D. QRS duration during VT is shorter (< 120 ms in lead I)
E. A single VT morphology with LBBB pattern and an inferior axis is commonly recorded

62-1. The answer is B. *(Hurst's The Heart, 14th Edition, Chap. 62)* Inverted T waves in the right precordial leads must be present past V2 to constitute a major criterion: including V1, V2, and V3 or beyond in patients > 14 years of age in the absence of complete right bundle branch block. Otherwise, inverted T waves in leads V1 and V2 only is a *minor* finding. Originally dating back to 1994, the Task Force criteria for ARVC were modified in 2010 to improve the diagnosis and management of ARVC. The criteria were aimed at facilitating the recognition and interpretation of the clinical and pathologic features of ARVC, and the modified criteria incorporated new knowledge on the genetic basis of the disease, improving diagnostic sensitivity and maintaining diagnostic specificity. The structural, histologic, ECG, arrhythmic, and genetic features are structured in major and minor criteria. The Task Force document formally introduced the biventricular variant and the left dominant variant.[1] Options A and C through E represent major criteria from the updated Task Force criteria. A definite diagnosis requires two major, or one major and two minor, or four minor criteria from different categories to be fulfilled.

62-2. The answer is C. *(Hurst's The Heart, 14th Edition, Chap. 62)* The prevalence of ARVC is estimated to range from 1 in 1000 to 1 in 5000 in the general population.[2-5] A small proportion of patients progress to LV dysfunction; in these patients, the clinical hallmark remains ventricular arrhythmias.[6] The prevalence of clinical manifestations of the disease is higher in males than in females (3:1).[7-8] The disease usually manifests in young adults; of 439 index patients described by Groeneweg et al,[7] only 4 presented before the age of 13 years, while none presented before the age of 10 years. The reason could be related to the completion of intercalated disk maturation or the need for prolonged exposure to exercise before the disease becomes manifest.[7]

62-3. The answer is B. *(Hurst's The Heart, 14th Edition, Chap. 62)* Intercalated disks are highly specialized cell-cell junctions; they are the units of electromechanical continuity between cardiac myocytes (option A)[9] and are constituted of gap junctions (option C), adherens junctions (option D), and desmosomes (option E). In *dilated* cardiomyopathy, genetic abnormalities in the sarcomere may be causal for disease (option B). *Gap junctions* (nexus, communicating junctions) are located in the lateral parts of the intercalated disks and mediate ionic traffic between the adjacent cells and provide the basis for functional cell coupling. Key structural proteins are connexins; the connexins predominantly expressed by cardiac myocytes are Cx43, Cx40, and Cx45. *Adherens junctions* (fasciae adhaerentes) are located in the transverse parts of the intercalated disks where the actin filaments of the sarcomeres are anchored and connected with the plasma membrane. This anchorage provides the intercellular "mechanical continuity" between the myocytes supporting the transmission of force between cells and synchronous contraction and relaxation. *Desmosomes* (maculae adhaerentes) are located in both the transverse and lateral parts of the intercalated disks: they reinforce the adherens junctions and fix adjacent cells. Desmosomes bind desmin on the intracellular side, span the cell membrane, and bind adjacent desmosomes on the extracellular side. Desmosome-forming proteins include plakophilin-2 (PKP2), desmoglein 2 (DSG2), desmocollin 2 (DSC2), plakoglobin (JUP), and desmoplakin (DSP).

62-4. The answer is A. *(Hurst's The Heart, 14th Edition, Chap. 62)* It is relatively uncommon for patients with ARVC to present with symptoms of right heart failure. Those with ARVC typically present between the second and fifth decades of life.[10] Symptoms are heterogeneous but most commonly reflect the presence of ventricular arrhythmias, which can range from isolated premature ventricular contractions to sustained ventricular tachycardia. Supraventricular arrhythmias also occur in 14% of ARVC patients, with atrial fibrillation being the most frequently reported.[11] In a study of 129 probands, symptoms on presentation included palpitations in 56%, dizziness in 29%, syncope in 26%, chest pain in 19%, and cardiac arrest in 22%.[12] Symptoms related to right heart failure are present in 6% (option A).[13] These findings are consistent with other studies.[4,10,14-15]

62-5. **The answer is E.** *(Hurst's The Heart, 14th Edition, Chap. 62)* Naxos disease (option B) and Carvajal syndrome (option E) are distinctive forms of ARVC that are inherited in an autosomal recessive manner in association with extracardiac manifestations, including wooly hair and plantopalmar keratoderma (thickening of the skin on the palms and soles).[16] Carvajal syndrome is a variant of Naxos disease with predominant LV involvement (option E) as noted in the question stem. Premature ventricular contractions with a right bundle branch morphology typically originate from the left ventricle, and with a superior axis and negativity in lead I they suggest an anterolateral LV origin. Anderson–Tawil syndrome, or long QT type 7 (option A), is characterized by periodic paralysis, ventricular arrhythmias, and prolonged QT interval (specifically polymorphic ventricular tachycardia and premature ventricular contractions), and anomalies including low-set ears, widely spaced eyes, small mandible, fifth-digit clinodactyly, syndactyly, short stature, and scoliosis. Brugada syndrome (option C) can mimic ARVC because both conditions may demonstrate RV conduction delay, and mutations typically recurrent in Brugada syndrome have been found in ARVC patients and vice versa. The demonstration of the presence of structural abnormalities supports the diagnosis of ARVC. Catecholaminergic polymorphic ventricular tachycardia (option D) is another inherited arrhythmia characterized by episodic syncope that occurs during exercise or acute emotion in individuals without structural cardiac abnormalities; the underlying cause is the onset of fast ventricular tachycardia (bidirectional or polymorphic).

62-6. **The answer is D.** *(Hurst's The Heart, 14th Edition, Chap. 62)* The triangle of dysplasia involves the epicardial subtricuspid region, RV basal anterior wall, and posterolateral LV, with the RV apex being mostly spared.[17] Historically, the *triangle of dysplasia* referred to the RV apex, the RV inflow tract, and the outflow tract and was thought only to be present in advanced stages of the disease.[17-18] Although cardiac MRI has emerged as the preferred imaging modality for ARVC, it is also one of the most common reasons for misdiagnosis. Common pitfalls include misinterpretation of variants of normal RV wall motion and inaccurate interpretation of intramyocardial fat infiltration.[19] It is important to note that in pediatric ARVC patients, intramyocardial fat infiltration and myocardial fibrosis are uncommon findings by CMRI.[20]

62-7. **The answer is B.** *(Hurst's The Heart, 14th Edition, Chap. 62)* An increased risk of cardiac perforation and tamponade is present with a biopsy at the RV free wall. Endomyocardial biopsy is rarely performed but may be helpful in establishing a diagnosis of ARVC when the etiology of cardiomyopathy or structural changes are unclear. The American College of Cardiology/American Heart Association consensus guidelines give a Class IIa (level of evidence C) indication for endomyocardial biopsy in patients with heart failure when a specific diagnosis is suspected that would influence therapy.[21] The demonstration of fibrofatty infiltration with loss of normal RV myocardium supports the diagnosis (option A).[22-23] There is a high rate of false negatives and low sensitivity as a result of the patchy nature of disease and the predilection for specific areas of the RV (option D).[23] Thus, conventional RV septal wall or LV biopsies are not helpful because these areas are commonly spared. Diagnostic yield may be improved by using electroanatomic voltage mapping to guide biopsy (option E).[24]

62-8. **The answer is A.** *(Hurst's The Heart, 14th Edition, Chap. 62)* The predominant inheritance pattern is autosomal dominant with variable penetrance and expressivity, although an autosomal recessive inheritance pattern has been described with the cardiocutaneous syndromes of Naxos disease and Carvajal syndrome (option A).[16] Approximately 60% of probands will have an identifiable pathogenic mutation.[7] Identification of a pathogenic mutation on genetic testing is a major criterion for the diagnosis of ARVC.[22] Currently, one of the major roles of genetic testing in ACM is for mutation-specific screening of family members following the identification of a pathogenic mutation in the proband (option B). The Heart Rhythm Society and European Heart Rhythm Association expert consensus guidelines give this indication a Class I recommendation.[25] Although genetic testing may be useful for confirmed cases (Class IIa)(option C) or considered for borderline cases (Class IIb)(option D), it is not recommended (Class III)(option E) for those fulfilling only a single minor Task Force criterion.[25] The clinical genetic and molecular workup in the proband and his or her family should be performed as in other familial cardiomyopathies and include clinical and genetic screening of first-degree relatives. A positive family history of ARVC is a risk factor for disease, with over a third of family members of affected individuals developing disease.[7,26-27] The cumulative 5-year and 10-year probabilities of developing ARVC in first-degree family members are 7% and 21%, respectively, with siblings of probands having a threefold higher risk compared to parents or children.[26] Pathogenic mutations are identified in 36% to 72% of selected family members, and up to 40% of these individuals will fulfill Task Force criteria for ARVC.[7,28] Disease will still occur in 18% of those who are mutation negative.[7] Also, the presence of symptoms or the occurrence of more than one genetic variant in family members increases the likelihood of Task Force criteria–confirmed disease.[7,26,28] The constellation of findings highlights the complexity of the genetics of ARVC and firmly supports the screening of family members of affected individuals.

62-9. **The answer is B.** (*Hurst's The Heart, 14th Edition, Chap. 62*) There are no prospective, randomized clinical trials to identify who has the highest risk for sudden cardiac death (SCD) and would benefit most from an implantable cardioverter-defibrillator (ICD). However, based on observational studies in ARVC patients, a history of prior cardiac arrest, sustained ventricular arrhythmias (option E), unexplained syncope (option A), *younger* age (option B), extensive RV dysfunction, LV dysfunction (option C), and the presence of heart failure (option D) are independently associated with subsequent ventricular arrhythmias.[29-37] In a study of patients receiving ICDs for definite or probable ARVC, 48% received an appropriate ICD therapy during a mean follow-up of 5 years.[38] The only independent predictors of ICD therapy were the presence of nonsustained VT and inducibility at electrophysiology study. The role of electrophysiology study for risk stratification is unclear because studies provide conflicting evidence.[31,33,38,39]

62-10. **The answer is D.** (*Hurst's The Heart, 14th Edition, Chap. 62*) Differential diagnoses of ARVC include idiopathic RV outflow tract VT (RVOT-VT), sarcoidosis, myocarditis, dilated cardiomyopathy, Brugada syndrome, athlete's heart, RV infarction, Chagas disease in endemic areas, pulmonary hypertension, and congenital heart disease. Idiopathic RVOT-VT should be differentiated from early ARVC, when gross structural abnormalities are absent. Differential diagnosis is based on clinical data (Task Force criteria), pathology data (endomyocardial biopsy), and imaging data such as echocardiography and cardiac MRI or positron emission tomography demonstrating or excluding scars and inflammation.[40,41] In general, in RVOT-VT: (1) Twelve-lead surface ECG and SAECG are normal during sinus rhythm, (2) A single VT morphology with LBBB pattern and an inferior axis is commonly recorded (option E),[42] (3) QRS duration during VT is *longer* ($\geq$ 120 ms in lead I) (option D),[43] (4) a notched QRS and precordial transition in lead V6 recur in ARVC but not in RVOT-VT,[44] (5) RVOT-VT is difficult to induce by programmed ventricular stimulation (option C),[41] (6) patients with idiopathic RVOT-VT are good responders to verapamil (option A),[41] and (7) endocardial ablation suppresses the arrhythmia in RVOT-VT (option B).[41]

References

1. Marcus FI, McKenna WJ, Sherrill D, et al. Diagnosis of arrhythmogenic right ventricular cardiomyopathy/dysplasia: proposed modification of the Task Force Criteria. *Eur Heart J.* 2010;31:806-814.

2. Haugaa KH, Haland TF, Leren IS, Saberniak J, Edvardsen T. Arrhythmogenic right ventricular cardiomyopathy, clinical manifestations, and diagnosis. *Europace.* 2016;18:965-972.

3. Basso C, Corrado D, Marcus FI, Nava A, Thiene G. Arrhythmogenic right ventricular cardiomyopathy. *Lancet.* 2009;373:1289-1300.

4. Marcus FI, Zareba W, Calkins H, et al. Arrhythmogenic right ventricular cardiomyopathy/dysplasia clinical presentation and diagnostic evaluation: results from the North American Multidisciplinary Study. *Heart Rhythm.* 2009;6:984-992.

5. Peters S, Trummel M, Meyners W. Prevalence of right ventricular dysplasia-cardiomyopathy in a non-referral hospital. *Int J Cardiol.* 2004;97:499-501.

6. Sen-Chowdhry S, Morgan RD, Chambers JC, McKenna W. Arrhythmogenic cardiomyopathy: etiology, diagnosis, and treatment. *Annu Rev Med.* 2010;61:233-253.

7. Groeneweg JA, Bhonsale A, James CA, et al. Clinical presentation, long-term follow-up, and outcomes of 1001 arrhythmogenic right ventricular dysplasia/cardiomyopathy patients and family members. *Circ Cardiovasc Genet.* 2015;8:437-446.

8. Calkins H. Arrhythmogenic right ventricular dysplasia/cardiomyopathy—three decades of progress. *Circ J.* 2015;79:901-913.

9. Calore M, Lorenzon A, De Bortoli M, Poloni G, Rampazzo A. Arrhythmogenic cardiomyopathy: a disease of intercalated discs. *Cell Tissue Res.* 2015;360:491-500.

10. Dalal D, Nasir K, Bomma C, et al. Arrhythmogenic right ventricular dysplasia: a United States experience. *Circulation.* 2005;112:3823-3832.

11. Camm CF, James CA, Tichnell C, et al. Prevalence of atrial arrhythmias in arrhythmogenic right ventricular dysplasia/cardiomyopathy. *Heart Rhythm.* 2013;10:1661-1668.

12. Krahn AD, Healey JS, Gerull B, et al. The Canadian Arrhythmogenic Right Ventricular Cardiomyopathy Registry: rationale, design, and preliminary recruitment. *Can J Cardiol.* 2016;32(12):1396-1401.

13. Hulot JS, Jouven X, Empana JP, Frank R, Fontaine G. Natural history and risk stratification of arrhythmogenic right ventricular dysplasia/cardiomyopathy. *Circulation.* 2004;110:1879-1884.

14. te Riele AS, James CA, Rastegar N, et al. Yield of serial evaluation in at-risk family members of patients with ARVD/C. *J Am Coll Cardiol.* 2014;64:293-301.

15. Sen-Chowdhry S, Syrris P, Ward D, Asimaki A, Sevdalis E, McKenna WJ. Clinical and genetic characterization of families with arrhythmogenic right ventricular dysplasia/cardiomyopathy provides novel insights into patterns of disease expression. *Circulation.* 2007;115:1710-1720.

16. Protonotarios N, Tsatsopoulou A. Naxos disease and Carvajal syndrome: cardiocutaneous disorders that highlight the pathogenesis and broaden the spectrum of arrhythmogenic right ventricular cardiomyopathy. *Cardiovasc Pathol.* 2004;13:185-194.

17. Te Riele AS, James CA, Philips B, et al. Mutation-positive arrhythmogenic right ventricular dysplasia/cardiomyopathy: the triangle of dysplasia displaced. *J Cardiovasc Electrophysiol.* 2013;24:1311-1320.

18. Marcus FI, Fontaine GH, Guiraudon G, et al. Right ventricular dysplasia: a report of 24 adult cases. *Circulation.* 1982;65:384-398.

19. Rastegar N, Burt JR, Corona-Villalobos CP, et al. Cardiac MR findings and potential diagnostic pitfalls in patients evaluated for arrhythmogenic right ventricular cardiomyopathy. *Radiographics.* 2014;34: 1553-1570.

20. Etoom Y, Govindapillai S, Hamilton R, et al. Importance of CMR within the Task Force Criteria for the diagnosis of ARVC in children and adolescents. *J Am Coll Cardiol.* 2015;65:987-995.

21. Yancy CW, Jessup M, Bozkurt B, et al. 2013 ACCF/AHA guideline for the management of heart failure: a report of the American College of Cardiology Foundation/American Heart Association Task Force on Practice Guidelines. *J Am Coll Cardiol.* 2013;62:e147-e239.

22. Marcus FI, McKenna WJ, Sherrill D, et al. Diagnosis of arrhythmogenic right ventricular cardiomyopathy/dysplasia: proposed modification of the Task Force Criteria. *Eur Heart J.* 2010;31:806-814.

23. Basso C, Ronco F, Marcus F, et al. Quantitative assessment of endomyocardial biopsy in arrhythmogenic right ventricular cardiomyopathy/dysplasia: an in vitro validation of diagnostic criteria. *Eur Heart J.* 2008;29:2760-2771.

24. Avella A, d'Amati G, Pappalardo A, et al. Diagnostic value of endomyocardial biopsy guided by electroanatomic voltage mapping in arrhythmogenic right ventricular cardiomyopathy/dysplasia. *J Cardiovasc Electrophysiol.* 2008;19:1127-1134.

25. Ackerman MJ, Priori SG, Willems S, et al. HRS/EHRA expert consensus statement on the state of genetic testing for the channelopathies and cardiomyopathies: this document was developed as a partnership between the Heart Rhythm Society (HRS) and the European Heart Rhythm Association (EHRA). *Europace.* 2011;13:1077-1109.

26. Te Riele AS, James CA, Groeneweg JA, et al. Approach to family screening in arrhythmogenic right ventricular dysplasia/cardiomyopathy. *Eur Heart J.* 2016;37:755-763.

27. Hamid MS, Norman M, Quraishi A, et al. Prospective evaluation of relatives for familial arrhythmogenic right ventricular cardiomyopathy/dysplasia reveals a need to broaden diagnostic criteria. *J Am Coll Cardiol.* 2002;40:1445-1450.

28. Quarta G, Muir A, Pantazis A, et al. Familial evaluation in arrhythmogenic right ventricular cardiomyopathy: impact of genetics and revised task force criteria. *Circulation.* 2011;123:2701-2709.

29. Hulot JS, Jouven X, Empana JP, Frank R, Fontaine G. Natural history and risk stratification of arrhythmogenic right ventricular dysplasia/cardiomyopathy. *Circulation.* 2004;110:1879-1884.

30. Link MS, Laidlaw D, Polonsky B, et al. Ventricular arrhythmias in the North American multidisciplinary study of ARVC: predictors, characteristics, and treatment. *J Am Coll Cardiol.* 2014;64:119-125.

31. Link MS, Wang PJ, Haugh CJ, et al. Arrhythmogenic right ventricular dysplasia: clinical results with implantable cardioverter defibrillators. *J Interv Card Electrophysiol.* 1997;1:41-48.

32. Roguin A, Bomma CS, Nasir K, et al. Implantable cardioverter-defibrillators in patients with arrhythmogenic right ventricular dysplasia/cardiomyopathy. *J Am Coll Cardiol.* 2004;43:1843-1852.

33. Corrado D, Calkins H, Link MS, et al. Prophylactic implantable defibrillator in patients with arrhythmogenic right ventricular cardiomyopathy/dysplasia and no prior ventricular fibrillation or sustained ventricular tachycardia. *Circulation.* 2010;122:1144-1152.

34. Pinamonti B, Dragos AM, Pyxaras SA, et al. Prognostic predictors in arrhythmogenic right ventricular cardiomyopathy: results from a 10-year registry. *Eur Heart J.* 2011;32:1105-1113.

35. Saguner AM, Vecchiati A, Baldinger SH, et al. Different prognostic value of functional right ventricular parameters in arrhythmogenic right ventricular cardiomyopathy/dysplasia. *Circ Cardiovasc Imaging.* 2014;7:230-239.

36. Peters S. Long-term follow-up and risk assessment of arrhythmogenic right ventricular dysplasia/cardiomyopathy: personal experience from different primary and tertiary centres. *J Cardiovasc Med (Hagerstown).* 2007;8:521-526.

37. Lemola K, Brunckhorst C, Helfenstein U, Oechslin E, Jenni R, Duru F. Predictors of adverse outcome in patients with arrhythmogenic right ventricular dysplasia/cardiomyopathy: long term experience of a tertiary care centre. *Heart.* 2005;91:1167-1172.

38. Bhonsale A, James CA, Tichnell C, et al. Incidence and predictors of implantable cardioverter-defibrillator therapy in patients with arrhythmogenic right ventricular dysplasia/cardiomyopathy undergoing implantable cardioverter-defibrillator implantation for primary prevention. *J Am Coll Cardiol.* 2011;58:1485-1496.

39. Corrado D, Leoni L, Link MS, et al. Implantable cardioverter-defibrillator therapy for prevention of sudden death in patients with arrhythmogenic right ventricular cardiomyopathy/dysplasia. *Circulation.* 2003;108:3084-3091.

40. Corrado D, Basso C, Leoni L, et al. Three-dimensional electroanatomical voltage mapping and histologic evaluation of myocardial substrate in right ventricular outflow tract tachycardia. *J Am Coll Cardiol.* 2008;51:731-731.

41. John RM, Stevenson WG. Outflow tract premature ventricular contractions and ventricular tachycardia: the typical and the challenging. *Card Electrophysiol Clin.* 2016;8:545-554.

42. Liao Z, Zhan X, Wu S, et al. Idiopathic ventricular arrhythmias originating from the pulmonary sinus cusp: prevalence, electrocardiographic/electrophysiological characteristics, and catheter ablation. *J Am Coll Cardiol.* 2015;66:2633-2644.

43. Ainsworth CD, Skanes AC, Klein GJ, Gula LJ, Yee R, Krahn AD. Differentiating arrhythmogenic right ventricular cardiomyopathy from right ventricular outflow tract ventricular tachycardia using multilead QRS duration and axis. *Heart Rhythm.* 2006;3:416-423.

44. Hoffmayer KS, Machado ON, Marcus GM, et al. Electrocardiographic comparison of ventricular arrhythmias in patients with arrhythmogenic right ventricular cardiomyopathy and right ventricular outflow tract tachycardia. *J Am Coll Cardiol.* 2011;58:831-838.

CHAPTER 63

Myocarditis

Ravi Karra

QUESTIONS

DIRECTIONS: Choose the one best response to each question.

63-1. A 42-year-old man presents with two weeks of dyspnea on exertion, pedal edema, and orthopnea. One month ago, he had a mild febrile illness. Echocardiography confirms reduced left ventricular (LV) systolic dysfunction. Serologies are suggestive of a viral myocarditis secondary to coxsackievirus B3. Which of the following is *not true* regarding coxsackie-mediated viral myocarditis?

A. Myocardial infection is initiated by the transmembrane coxsackievirus-adenovirus receptor (CAR)
B. Cell damage is induced by direct cytotoxicity and is mediated by viral proteinases
C. Patients with defects of dystrophin and dysferlin demonstrate increased susceptibility to myocardial CV-B3 infection
D. The early innate immune response results in direct myocyte injury
E. All of the above are true

63-2. Which of the following is *not* associated with a poor outcome after a diagnosis of viral myocarditis?

A. New York Heart Association (NYHA) classes III to IV symptoms at 6 months
B. Biventricular dysfunction at the time of diagnosis
C. The presence of late gadolinium enhancement (LGE)
D. High rate of cardiomyocyte apoptosis on biopsy
E. Presentation with heart failure symptoms

63-3. A 67-year-old woman received an orthotopic heart transplant 6 months ago. She presents with generalized malaise and new-onset heart failure. Echocardiography confirms allograft dysfunction, and serum PCR demonstrates human cytomegalovirus (HCMV) viremia. Which of the following is *true* regarding HCMV myocarditis?

A. Myocardial infection with HCMV is usually observed in immunocompetent hosts
B. Myocardial pathology is notable for an infiltrate by eosinophils
C. Viral infection is restricted to myocytes
D. In immunosuppressed patients, infection often occurs by reactivation of a latent infection
E. First-line treatment is with acyclovir

63-4. A 43-year-old woman presents with new-onset heart failure, generalized myalgias, and periorbital swelling. A careful history indicates that she has a predilection for eating raw pork. Which of the following is *not true* regarding *Trichinella* myocarditis?

A. Infection of striated muscles occurs in the first phase of infection
B. A complete blood count can show hypereosinophilia
C. A muscle biopsy would show larvae
D. Treatment is albendazole
E. All of the above

63-5. Which of the following is *true* of cardiac MRI (CMR) findings of acute myocarditis?

A. CMR findings are diagnostic but not prognostic
B. LGE is present in a noncoronary distribution
C. CMR would show decreased myocardial edema
D. Early gadolinium enhancement is normal
E. The presence of a pericardial effusion increases the diagnostic accuracy of CMR for myocarditis

63-6. A 20-year-old college student presents with acute decompensated heart failure. His history is notable for a recent study abroad in South America. Which of the following is *true* for Chagas myocarditis?

A. The causal agent is *T. gondii*
B. Myocarditis is part of the acute phase
C. The chronic phase can lead to chronic cardiomyopathy
D. Treatment is with trimethoprim-sulfamethoxazole
E. Both B and C are correct

63-7. A 48-year-old woman from Wisconsin presents with syncopal episodes. Approximately three weeks earlier she had been camping and noted a bulls-eye rash. Which of the following is *true* of Lyme carditis?

A. Lyme carditis typically manifests at the same time as erythema migrans
B. Atrioventricular block can occur within a week of infection
C. Patients often recall erythema migrans at the time of presentation
D. Myopericarditis results in focal wall motion abnormalities
E. Both A and D are correct

63-8. A 38-year-old man presents with acute cardiogenic shock and incessant ventricular arrhythmias. After he is stabilized with mechanic circulatory support, an endomyocardial biopsy is performed. The results are shown in Figure 63-1. Which of the following is *true* of this condition?

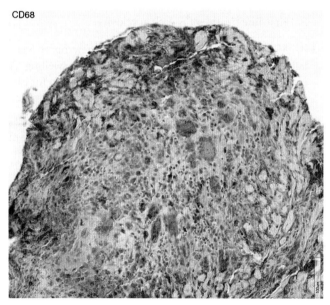

CD68

FIGURE 63-1 Biopsy from patient in question 63-8 after staining with anti-CD68.

A. The prognosis is excellent
B. Treatment with muromonab-CD3 may be of benefit
C. Following transplantation, recurrence in the donor heart can occur
D. Mechanical support often requires biventricular support
E. Both C and D are correct

63-9. A 47-year-old woman presents with wheezing and syncope. A chest x-ray shows hilar lymphadenopathy, and an echocardiogram reveals left ventricular dysfunction. Which of the following is *not true* about sarcoidosis?

A. The pathologic hallmark is noncaseating epithelioid granulomas in the affected tissues
B. Endomyocardial biopsy is both sensitive and specific for diagnosing cardiac sarcoidosis
C. Patients with cardiac sarcoid and normal LV ejection fraction (LVEF) continue to be at risk for arrhythmia
D. LGE by cardiac MRI corresponds with biopsy findings of granuloma
E. Cardiac PET can be used to assess arrhythmogenic risk

63-10. Which of the following is *true* of cardiac involvement with hypereosinophilic syndrome (HES)?

A. Affected patients often present with acute decompensated heart failure during the acute necrotic stage
B. During the thrombotic phase, oral anticoagulation is appropriate to prevent major embolic events
C. Late cardiac involvement results in a restrictive cardiomyopathy
D. Both B and C are true
E. All of the above

63-1. The answer is D. *(Hurst's The Heart, 14th Edition, Chap. 63)* The cardiotropic coxsackievirus B3 (CV-B3) is one of the most common causes of myocarditis.[1] The myocardial infection is initiated by the transmembrane CAR; the ablation of CAR blocks viral affliction of myocardial cells and inflammation in the myocardium in experimental models (option A).[2] In CV-B3–infected myocytes, the cell damage is induced by direct cytotoxicity and mediated by viral proteinases (option B).[3] Patients with defects of dystrophin and dysferlin demonstrate increased susceptibility to myocardial CV-B3 infection by enhancing viral propagation to adjacent cardiomyocytes and disrupting membrane repair function (option C).[4-6] In viral infections, the early innate immune response provides the first defense mechanism and is mediated by cytokines. However, the late adaptive immune response contributes to the myocardial lymphocyte infiltration that must clear virus-infected cardiac myocytes in CV-B3 myocarditis and endothelial cells in parvovirus B19 myocarditis. Although this mechanism clears the virus, it also results in myocyte injury (option D).

63-2. The answer is D. *(Hurst's The Heart, 14th Edition, Chap. 63)* Predictors of outcome vary in different myocardial biopsy studies. Persistence of New York Heart Association (NYHA) classes III to IV, left atrium enlargement, and improvement in LVEF at 6 months emerged as independent predictors of long-term outcome in one study (option A).[7] Biventricular dysfunction at diagnosis was the main predictor of death/transplantation in another study (option B).[8] High rates of cardiomyocyte apoptosis were associated with functional recovery at 1 year (option D).[9] The presence of LGE emerged as the best independent predictor of all-cause and cardiac mortality, whereas the initial presentation with heart failure was a predictor of incomplete long-term recovery (options C and E).[10]

63-3. The answer is D. *(Hurst's The Heart, 14th Edition, Chap. 63)* Myocardial infection with HCMV is more commonly observed in immunocompromised hosts (option A). The myocardial pathology is characterized by T-cell inflammatory infiltrate and by the presence of typical intranuclear amphophilic inclusion bodies that specifically immune-stain with anti-HCMV antibodies (option B). The virus infects both myocytes and endothelial cells (option C). Children become infected early in life in developing countries, whereas up to 80% of the adult population is infected in developed nations. The course of primary infection is usually mild or asymptomatic in immunocompetent hosts as HCMV establishes a latent but persistent infection reflecting the inability of the immune system to clear the infection; immune evasion mechanisms allow infected cells to escape both innate and adaptive effector immunity.[11] In immunosuppressed patients (eg, solid organ or bone marrow transplantation recipients), the infection can be reactivated to result in systemic and organ infection; the heart is a possible target for tissue infection, especially in heart transplant recipients (option D). For herpes simplex virus types 1 and 2 and for varicella-zoster virus, acyclovir (or its prodrug valacyclovir) and famciclovir have greatly reduced the burden of disease and have demonstrated a remarkable safety record. Ganciclovir and valganciclovir remain the drugs of choice for HCMV infection in immunocompromised hosts (option E).[12,13]

63-4. The answer is A. *(Hurst's The Heart, 14th Edition, Chap. 63)* Eosinophilic myocarditis is a possible complication in patients with trichinosis, a zoonosis caused by nematodes of the genus *Trichinella*. *Trichinella* is endemic in the areas with unregulated slaughter of pigs and particularly in areas where these are in contact with wild animals.[14,15] Symptoms of trichinosis occur in two stages. Intestinal infection is the first stage and develops 1 to 2 days after consuming contaminated meat. The most common symptoms are nausea, diarrhea, abdominal cramps, and fever. The second stage corresponds to larval invasion of muscles and starts after about 7 to 15 days (option A). The diagnosis of trichinellosis should be based on clinical findings; pathology findings of muscle and/or EMB detecting larvae; laboratory findings of specific antibody response by indirect immunofluorescence, ELISA, or Western blot; hypereosinophilia (1000 eosinophils/mL) and/or increased total IgE levels; increased levels of muscle enzymes; and investigation of the possible source and origin of infection (options B and C).[14-16] When the diagnosis is proven, the treatment is based on antihelminthic drugs, such as albendazole or mebendazole, and supportive therapy in patients with heart failure (option D).[15]

63-5. **The answer is B.** *(Hurst's The Heart, 14th Edition, Chap. 63)* CMR provides a detailed morphofunctional description of ventricular involvement and offers important prognostic information.[17] There is a substantially lower risk of events in patients with suspected myocarditis but normal CMR findings (option A).[18] According to the Lake Louise CMR criteria, acute myocarditis is associated with (1) increased regional or global myocardial signal intensity in T2-weighted images (indicating myocardial edema); (2) increased global myocardial early gadolinium enhancement (EGE) ratio between myocardium and skeletal muscle in T1-weighted images (supporting hyperemia/capillary leakage); and (3) at least one focal lesion with nonischemic distribution in LGE T1-weighted images (suggestive of cell injury/necrosis) (options B through D).[17] The diagnostic accuracy does not increase with the addition of pericardial effusion (option E).[19]

63-6. **The answer is E.** *(Hurst's The Heart, 14th Edition, Chap. 63)* Chagas disease (CD) is caused by the protozoan parasite *T. cruzi* (option A).[20] In the acute phase, the disease can manifest with myocarditis, conduction system abnormalities, and pericarditis (option B). In untreated patients, the disease progresses to the chronic phase.[21,22] In the chronic phase, illness can be severe, with LV dilation and dysfunction, aneurysm, congestive heart failure, thromboembolism, ventricular arrhythmias, and sudden cardiac death, which is the leading cause of death in patients with Chagas heart disease (option C).[23] Two antiparasitic drugs are available for the treatment of CD: benznidazole and nifurtimox (option D).[23,24]

63-7. **The answer is C.** *(Hurst's The Heart, 14th Edition, Chap. 63)* Lyme carditis is rare and typically manifests 2 to 5 weeks after the erythema migrans (option A). Patients who develop Lyme disease may first manifest atrioventricular block at 14 days (range, 2–24 days) after the onset; only one-third of patients recall the erythema migrans (options B and C).[25,26] Myopericarditis can present with chest pain, dyspnea, or syncope, and the signs and symptoms of Lyme myopericarditis can mimic acute coronary syndrome, with ECG ST-segment alterations and elevated peripheral blood cardiac biomarkers.[26] In such cases, echocardiography demonstrates diffuse ventricular hypokinesis rather than the focal wall motion abnormalities expected with an acute coronary syndrome (option D).[25]

63-8. **The answer is E.** *(Hurst's The Heart, 14th Edition, Chap. 63).* The biopsy in Figure 63-1 shows giant cells consistent with a diagnosis of giant cell myocarditis. GCM carries a poor prognosis, with a median survival of 5.5 months from the onset of symptoms; in one report, 89% of patients either died or required cardiac transplantation, and another report showed 1-year survival of 30% to 69% (option A).[27,28] Mechanical circulatory support for bridge to recovery is rare, whereas it is more commonly used as bridge to transplant; biventricular support is often required (option D).[29,30] Heart failure treatment includes standard regimen with beta-blockers, angiotensin-converting enzyme inhibitors, angiotensin receptor blockers, and aldosterone antagonists as per guidelines.[31,32] The management of GCM has also included the use of muromonab-CD3, pulse steroids, and varying combinations of azathioprine, cyclosporine, and prednisone monitored with surveillance EMB (option B). Post-transplant survival is similar to that of patients who underwent heart transplantation for other diseases; however, GCM may recur in 10% to 50% of transplanted hearts (option C).[27,28,33]

63-9. **The answer is B.** *(Hurst's The Heart, 14th Edition, Chap. 63)* Sarcoidosis is a chronic multisystem inflammatory disease of unknown etiology that carries the pathologic hallmark of noncaseating epithelioid granulomas in the affected tissues (option A).[34] CMR offers a high sensitivity and specificity for the assessment of cardiac involvement.

Whereas T2 hyper-enhancement identifies early edema, the LGE in a nonvascular distribution supports myocardial scarring. LGE correlates with cardiac biopsy findings of granulomatous inflammation (option D).[35,36] In patients with preserved LVEF and extracardiac sarcoidosis, major adverse cardiac events, including death and ventricular tachycardia, are associated with a greater LGE and right ventricular involvement; preserved LVEF does not exclude the risk for adverse events (option C).[37] Additionally, PET studies have proved to be clinically useful for diagnostic and prognostic information, especially for the risk of ventricular arrhythmias in patients with cardiac sarcoidosis. The presence of focal perfusion defects (rubidium-82 imaging in this report) and FDG uptake identified a higher risk of death or ventricular tachycardia (option E).[38] Although EMB has low sensitivity (19%–32%) as a result of the inherent sampling limitation for focal epithelioid granulomas, it offers high specificity for the diagnosis (option B).[39]

63-10. **The answer is D.** *(Hurst's The Heart, 14th Edition, Chap. 63)* Cardiac involvement is a major cause of morbidity and mortality in HES.[40] The cardiac pathology is divided into three stages: (1) an acute necrotic stage, (2) a thrombotic stage, and (3) a fibrotic stage. The early, acute necrotic stage is characterized by eosinophilic and lymphocyte infiltration; in the myocardial interstitium, eosinophils undergo degranulation with release of biologically active factors that cause myocyte injury. Clinical presentation may comprise nonspecific manifestations. Patients may *infrequently* present with acute heart failure or cardiogenic shock at onset (option A).[41] In the thrombotic stage, mural thrombi develop on the endocardium. Thromboembolic complications occur in up to 30% of patients; oral anticoagulation is appropriate to prevent major embolic events (option B). In the scarring, fibrotic stage, both ventricles and subvalvular structures of the AV valves are involved. The functional phenotype is typically restrictive as in endomyocardial fibrosis (option C).

References

1. Garmaroudi FS, Marchant D, Hendry R, et al. Coxsackievirus B3 replication and pathogenesis. *Future Microbiol.* 2015;10(4):629-653.

2. Shi Y, Chen C, Lisewski U, et al. Cardiac deletion of the Coxsackievirus-adenovirus receptor abolishes Coxsackievirus B3 infection and prevents myocarditis in vivo. *J Am Coll Cardiol.* 2009;53(14):1219-1226.

3. Jagdeo JM, Dufour A, Fung G, et al. Heterogeneous nuclear ribonucleoprotein M facilitates enterovirus infection. *J Virol.* 2015;89(14):7064-7078.

4. Wang C, Wong J, Fung G, et al. Dysferlin deficiency confers increased susceptibility to coxsackievirus-induced cardiomyopathy. *Cell Microbiol.* 2015;17(10):1423-1430.

5. Badorff C, Lee GH, Lamphear BJ, et al. Enteroviral protease 2A cleaves dystrophin: evidence of cytoskeletal disruption in an acquired cardiomyopathy. *Nat Med.* 1999;5(3):320-326.

6. Xiong D, Lee GH, Badorff C, et al. Dystrophin deficiency markedly increases enterovirus-induced cardiomyopathy: a genetic predisposition to viral heart disease. *Nat Med.* 2002;8(8):872-877.

7. Anzini M, Merlo M, Sabbadini G, et al. Long-term evolution and prognostic stratification of biopsy-proven active myocarditis. *Circulation.* 2013;128(22):2384-2394.

8. Caforio AL, Calabrese F, Angelini A, et al. A prospective study of biopsy-proven myocarditis: prognostic relevance of clinical and aetiopathogenetic features at diagnosis. *Eur Heart J.* 2007;28(11):1326-1333.

9. Abbate A, Sinagra G, Bussani R, et al. Apoptosis in patients with acute myocarditis. *Am J Cardiol.* 2009;104(7):995-1000.

10. Grun S, Schumm J, Greulich S, et al. Long-term follow-up of biopsy-proven viral myocarditis: predictors of mortality and incomplete recovery. *J Am Coll Cardiol.* 2012;59(18):1604-1615.

11. Poole E, Sinclair J. Sleepless latency of human cytomegalovirus. *Med Microbiol Immunol.* 2015;204(3):421-429.

12. Field HJ, Vere Hodge RA. Recent developments in anti-herpesvirus drugs. *Br Med Bull.* 2013;106:213-249.

13. Owers DS, Webster AC, Strippoli GF, Kable K, Hodson EM. Pre-emptive treatment for cytomegalovirus viraemia to prevent cytomegalovirus disease in solid organ transplant recipients. *Cochrane Database Syst Rev.* 2013(2):CD005133.

14. Murrell KD, Pozio E. Worldwide occurrence and impact of human trichinellosis, 1986-2009. *Emerg Infect Dis.* 2011;17(12):2194-2202.

15. Gottstein B, Pozio E, Nockler K. Epidemiology, diagnosis, treatment, and control of trichinellosis. *Clin Microbiol Rev.* 2009;22(1):127-145, Table of Contents.

16. Okello AL, Burniston S, Conlan JV, et al. Prevalence of endemic pig-associated zoonoses in Southeast Asia: a review of findings from the Lao People's Democratic Republic. *Am J Trop Med Hyg.* 2015;92(5):1059-1066.

17. Friedrich MG, Sechtem U, Schulz-Menger J, et al. Cardiovascular magnetic resonance in myocarditis: a JACC white paper. *J Am Coll Cardiol.* 2009;53(17):1475-1487.

18. Schumm J, Greulich S, Wagner A, et al. Cardiovascular magnetic resonance risk stratification in patients with clinically suspected myocarditis. *J Cardiovasc Magn Reson.* 2014;16:14.

19. Lurz P, Eitel I, Klieme B, et al. The potential additional diagnostic value of assessing for pericardial effusion on cardiac magnetic resonance imaging in patients with suspected myocarditis. *Eur Heart J Cardiovasc Imaging.* 2014;15(6):643-650.

20. Malik LH, Singh GD, Amsterdam EA. The epidemiology, clinical manifestations, and management of Chagas heart disease. *Clin Cardiol.* 2015;38(9):565-569.

21. Garcia MN, Woc-Colburn L, Aguilar D, Hotez PJ, Murray KO. Historical perspectives on the epidemiology of human Chagas disease in Texas and recommendations for enhanced understanding of clinical Chagas disease in the southern United States. *PLoS Negl Trop Dis.* 2015;9(11):e0003981.

22. Nouvellet P, Dumonteil E, Gourbiere S. The improbable transmission of Trypanosoma cruzi to human: the missing link in the dynamics and control of Chagas disease. *PLoS Negl Trop Dis.* 2013;7(11):e2505.

23. Rassi A, Jr., Rassi SG, Rassi A. Sudden death in Chagas' disease. *Arq Bras Cardiol.* 2001;76(1):75-96.

24. Bestetti RB, Cardinalli-Neto A. Antitrypanosomal therapy for chronic Chagas' disease. *N Engl J Med.* 2011;365(13):1258-1259; author reply 9.

25. Robinson ML, Kobayashi T, Higgins Y, Calkins H, Melia MT. Lyme carditis. *Infect Dis Clin North Am.* 2015;29(2):255-268.

26. Forrester JD, Mead P. Third-degree heart block associated with Lyme carditis: review of published cases. *Clin Infect Dis.* 2014;59(7):996-1000.

27. Cooper LT, Jr., Berry GJ, Shabetai R. Idiopathic giant-cell myocarditis—natural history and treatment. Multicenter Giant Cell Myocarditis Study Group Investigators. *N Engl J Med.* 1997;336(26):1860-1866.

28. Kandolin R, Lehtonen J, Salmenkivi K, et al. Diagnosis, treatment, and outcome of giant-cell myocarditis in the era of combined immunosuppression. *Circ Heart Fail.* 2013;6(1):15-22.

29. Murray LK, Gonzalez-Costello J, Jonas SN, et al. Ventricular assist device support as a bridge to heart transplantation in patients with giant cell myocarditis. *Eur J Heart Fail.* 2012;14(3):312-318.

30. Seeburger J, Doll N, Doll S, Borger MA, Mohr FW. Mechanical assist and transplantation for treatment of giant cell myocarditis. *Can J Cardiol.* 2010;26(2):96-97.

31. Yancy CW, Jessup M, Bozkurt B, et al. 2013 ACCF/AHA guideline for the management of heart failure: a report of the American College of Cardiology Foundation/American Heart Association Task Force on Practice Guidelines. *J Am Coll Cardiol.* 2013;62(16):e147-239.

32. Cooper LT, Jr., Hare JM, Tazelaar HD, et al. Usefulness of immunosuppression for giant cell myocarditis. *Am J Cardiol.* 2008;102(11):1535-1539.

33. Maleszewski JJ, Orellana VM, Hodge DO, et al. Long-term risk of recurrence, morbidity and mortality in giant cell myocarditis. *Am J Cardiol.* 2015;115(12):1733-1738.

34. Sekhri V, Sanal S, Delorenzo LJ, Aronow WS, Maguire GP. Cardiac sarcoidosis: a comprehensive review. *Arch Med Sci.* 2011;7(4):546-554.

35. Yoshida A, Ishibashi-Ueda H, Yamada N, et al. Direct comparison of the diagnostic capability of cardiac magnetic resonance and endomyocardial biopsy in patients with heart failure. *Eur J Heart Fail.* 2013;15(2):166-175.

36. Ise T, Hasegawa T, Morita Y, et al. Extensive late gadolinium enhancement on cardiovascular magnetic resonance predicts adverse outcomes and lack of improvement in LV function after steroid therapy in cardiac sarcoidosis. *Heart.* 2014;100(15):1165-1172.

37. Murtagh G, Laffin LJ, Beshai JF, et al. Prognosis of myocardial damage in sarcoidosis patients with preserved left ventricular ejection fraction: risk stratification using cardiovascular magnetic resonance. *Circ Cardiovasc Imaging.* 2016;9(1):e003738.

38. Mc Ardle BA, Birnie DH, Klein R, et al. Is there an association between clinical presentation and the location and extent of myocardial involvement of cardiac sarcoidosis as assessed by (1)(8)F-fluorodoexyglucose positron emission tomography? *Circ Cardiovasc Imaging.* 2013;6(5):617-626.

39. Lagana SM, Parwani AV, Nichols LC. Cardiac sarcoidosis: a pathology-focused review. *Arch Pathol Lab Med.* 2010;134(7):1039-1046.

40. Kleinfeldt T, Nienaber CA, Kische S, et al. Cardiac manifestation of the hypereosinophilic syndrome: new insights. *Clin Res Cardiol.* 2010;99(7):419-427.

41. Ginsberg F, Parrillo JE. Eosinophilic myocarditis. *Heart Fail Clin.* 2005;1(3):419-429.

CHAPTER 64

The Athlete and the Cardiovascular System

Mark J. Eisenberg

QUESTIONS

DIRECTIONS: Choose the one best response to each question.

64-1. A 56-year-old woman presents for an exercise stress test. She completes 10.2 METS. The acute response to aerobic exercise includes increases in all of the following *except*:

A. Maximum oxygen consumption
B. Cardiac output
C. Stroke volume
D. Systolic blood pressure
E. Peripheral vascular resistance

64-2. A 29-year-old professional athlete is referred to you with left ventricle (LV) hypertrophy on his echocardiogram. Which criteria favor hypertrophic cardiomyopathy (HCM) or dilated cardiomyopathy over the athletic heart syndrome?

A. LV wall thickness ≥ 16 mm
B. LV hypertrophy with an unusual distribution (heterogeneous, asymmetric, or sparing the anterior septum)
C. Persistence of hypertrophy after physical deconditioning
D. LV end-diastolic diameter > 70 mm
E. All of the above

64-3. A 29-year-old Olympic canoeist is referred to you by her family physician with an abnormal ECG pattern. Which ECG abnormality is *not* commonly seen on the ECGs of elite endurance athletes?

A. Incomplete left bundle branch block
B. Early repolarization
C. Increased QRS voltages with diffuse T-wave inversion and deep Q waves

D. Mildly increased P-wave amplitude
E. Increased voltages consistent with right ventricular and LV hypertrophy

64-4. An endurance runner is referred to you by his family physician after a routine ECG shows an arrhythmia. Which of the following arrhythmias are *not* commonly noted among elite athletes?

A. Sinus arrhythmia and sinus bradycardia
B. First-degree and Mobitz type II second-degree AV block
C. Frequent premature beats and couplets
D. Nonsustained ventricular tachycardia
E. Junctional rhythm

64-5. A 22-year-old college football player has a cardiac arrest and sudden death during a championship game. Which of the following statements is *not true* about sudden death in athletes?

A. Sudden death occurs with an incidence of 1 to 2 per 100,000 athletes (12 to 35 years of age) per year
B. The frequency of sudden death is fourfold lower in female athletes
C. In athletes younger than 35 years, inherited diseases such as HCM, arrhythmogenic right ventricular cardiomyopathy, and congenital coronary artery abnormalities of wrong sinus origin are the most common causes of sudden death
D. In athletes older than 35 years, atherosclerotic coronary artery disease is the most common cause of death
E. All of the above are true

64-6. A 17-year-old athlete is referred to you for assessment after a cardiac arrest requiring resuscitation during a high school basketball game. Which of the following statements is *true* about HCM?

A. HCM is the single most common cause of sudden cardiac arrest in athletes in the United States

B. HCM accounts for about one-third of sport-related sudden fatalities

C. HCM is a genetically transmitted disease characterized by genotypic and phenotypic heterogeneity

D. LV hypertrophy is characteristically asymmetric with a variety of patterns of wall thickening

E. All of the above are true

64-7. Which of the following statements is *not true* regarding arrhythmogenic right ventricular cardiomyopathy?

A. Arrhythmogenic right ventricular cardiomyopathy is an inherited heart muscle disorder characterized pathologically by fibrofatty replacement of right ventricular myocardium

B. It is an uncommon cause of sudden death on the athletic field in the United States

C. Clinical manifestations include ECG depolarization and repolarization abnormalities commonly localized to right precordial leads

D. Myocardial aneurysms are localized to the posterobasal, apical, and outflow tract regions

E. Sudden death during physical exercise is likely related to hemodynamic factors, increased right ventricular volume and wall stress, and enhanced sympathetic tone that culminate in ventricular fibrillation

64-8. A 15-year-old lacrosse player who recently had a normal history and physical with his family physician collapses during a game. Which of the following statements is *true* regarding sudden death in athletes with no evidence of structural heart disease?

A. Approximately 10% of young athletes who die suddenly with exercise have no evidence of structural heart diseases

B. Sudden death may be due to ventricular pre-excitation

C. Sudden death may be due to inherited cardiac ion channelopathies, including long QT syndrome, short QT syndrome, and Brugada syndrome

D. Sudden death may be due to catecholaminergic polymorphic ventricular tachycardia

E. All of the above are true

64-9. An amateur boxer collapses shortly after being punched in the chest. Which of the following statements is *not true* about commotio cordis?

A. The most common sports associated with commotio cordis deaths in the United States are those in which projectiles are integral to the game

B. Collapse is almost never instantaneous and is usually delayed to 10 to 20 seconds after the chest blow

C. The most common cardiac arrhythmia documented soon after collapse is generally ventricular fibrillation

D. Survival from commotion cordis has increased to > 50% as a result of more rapid response times and access to external defibrillation as well as greater public awareness

E. The cellular determinants of VF induced by chest wall blows likely include ion channel activation caused by increased LV pressure

64-10. Which of the following is *not true* with respect to the routine use of ECGs during athlete screening in the United States?

A. Routine use of ECG screening has not been supported because of the large number of athletes to be screened

B. Routine use of ECG screening has not been supported because of the low incidence of events

C. Routine use of ECG screening has not been supported because of the substantial number of expected false-negative and false-positive results

D. Routine use of ECG screening has not been supported because of the need for repetitive ECG screening during adolescence

E. Routine use of ECGs is mandated as part of athlete screening in the United States

64-1. The answer is E. (*Hurst's The Heart, 14th Edition, Chap. 64*) The acute response to training for such athletic activities as cross-country skiing, long-distance running, swimming, or bicycling includes substantial increases in maximum oxygen consumption (option A), cardiac output (option B), stroke volume (option C), and systolic blood pressure (option D), associated with decreased (*not increased*) peripheral vascular resistance (option E).[1] With several weeks of endurance training, the chronic adaptations to training include increased maximal oxygen uptake from augmented stroke volume and cardiac output and increased arteriovenous oxygen difference. The response to endurance exercise predominantly produces a volume load on the left ventricle.

64-2. The answer is E. (*Hurst's The Heart, 14th Edition, Chap. 64*) Differentiating the physiologic changes resulting from habitual exercise in the athletic heart syndrome with HCM or dilated cardiomyopathy represents a challenge to the clinician. Physiologic cardiac adaptation from regular exercise leads to an increase in left ventricle (LV) wall thickness. This can be difficult to distinguish from the pathologic changes of HCM. Criteria favoring HCM include a high degree of LV hypertrophy (wall thickness ≥ 16 mm) (option A) with an unusual distribution (heterogeneous, asymmetric, or sparing the anterior septum) (option B), a small LV cavity (< 45 mm), the presence of striking electrocardiogram (ECG) abnormalities, and the persistence of hypertrophy after physical deconditioning (option C). Although many athletes have increased intracavitary dimensions, LV end-diastolic diameter > 70 mm is distinctly unusual as a manifestation of the athlete's heart (option D). LV wall thickness > 12 mm is unusual even in highly trained athletes but is not uncommon in elite rowers and cyclists. LV wall thickness ≥ 16 mm raises the possibility of HCM. Hypertrophy (> 12 mm) above the normal range is distinctly uncommon in female athletes. Athletes with LV wall hypertrophy may have increased cavity dimensions, which are rarely present in diseases with pathologic wall thickening.[1]

64-3. The answer is A. (*Hurst's The Heart, 14th Edition, Chap. 64*) A spectrum of abnormal 12-lead ECG patterns is present in up to one-half of trained athletes, more commonly in men and in endurance athletes.[2-7] The most commonly observed alterations include early repolarization patterns (option B), increased QRS voltages, diffuse T-wave inversion, and deep Q waves (option C). ECGs in endurance athletes can show mildly increased P-wave amplitude (option D), suggesting atrial enlargement, incomplete right (*not left*) bundle branch block (option E), and increased voltages consistent with right ventricular and LV hypertrophy.[2-7] Among endurance athletes, voltage criteria for right ventricular hypertrophy are present in a substantial proportion. Abnormal and bizarre ECG patterns suggestive of cardiac disease are noted in a minority of elite athletes.[2-7] Most such ECGs represent only extreme manifestations of physiologic athlete's heart. A significant minority of asymptomatic elite athletes show distinctly abnormal ECG patterns usually associated with precordial T-wave inversions but without evidence of cardiac disease.[8] Many uncommon ECG findings in athletes are not considered normal variants and require further evaluation.

64-4. The answer is B. (*Hurst's The Heart, 14th Edition, Chap. 64*) Arrhythmias commonly noted in athletes include sinus arrhythmia, sinus bradycardia (option A), and junctional rhythm (option E). They are often accompanied by other manifestations of enhanced parasympathetic tone. Atrioventricular (AV) conduction delays with first-degree and Wenckebach or Mobitz type I (*not Mobitz type II*) second-degree AV block (option B) are common in endurance athletes and attributable to enhanced vagal tone and withdrawal of sympathetic tone at rest.[8] Ambulatory monitoring of athletes has demonstrated ventricular arrhythmias, including frequent premature beats, couplets (option C), and nonsustained ventricular tachycardia (option D). These arrhythmias can be within the spectrum of physiologic athlete's heart.[8] Such arrhythmias are generally not associated with symptoms or an increased risk of sudden cardiac death, and they are generally reduced with exercise or deconditioning.[9]

64-5. **The answer is B.** *(Hurst's The Heart, 14th Edition, Chap. 64)* The underlying cardiovascular conditions that predispose to the rare and tragic sudden deaths in young athletes are known.[10-16] Available population-based data show that these events occur with an incidence of 1 to 2 per 100,000 athletes (12–35 years of age) per year (option A) with the frequency eightfold lower *(not fourfold lower)* in female athletes (option B).[10-16] In athletes younger than 35 years, inherited diseases such as HCM, arrhythmogenic right ventricular cardiomyopathy, and congenital coronary artery abnormalities of wrong sinus origin are the most common causes of sudden death (option C). In athletes older than 35 years, atherosclerotic coronary artery disease is the most common cause of death (option D).[10-16]

64-6. **The answer is E.** *(Hurst's The Heart, 14th Edition, Chap. 64)* Hypertrophic cardiomyopathy is the single most common cause of sudden cardiac arrest in athletes in the United States in which a definitive cardiac diagnosis can be made postmortem (option A). HCM accounts for about one-third of sport-related sudden fatalities (option B).[10-16] HCM is a genetically transmitted disease characterized by genotypic and phenotypic heterogeneity (option C). Usually, the characteristic hypertrophied, nondilated LV with increased wall thickness manifests during adolescence.[10] LV hypertrophy is characteristically asymmetric with a variety of patterns of wall thickening (option D).[17]

64-7. **The answer is E.** *(Hurst's The Heart, 14th Edition, Chap. 64)* Arrhythmogenic right ventricular cardiomyopathy is an inherited heart muscle disorder characterized pathologically by fibrofatty replacement of right ventricular myocardium (option A).[18-22] It represents the leading cause of sudden death on the athletic field in the Veneto region of Italy, accounting for approximately 25% of cardiovascular sudden death in young competitive athletes, but it is distinctly uncommon in the United States (5% of athlete deaths) (option B).[18-22] Clinical manifestations include ECG depolarization and repolarization abnormalities commonly localized to right precordial leads (option C). These include inverted T waves in V1-V3 in most patients with arrhythmogenic right ventricular cardiomyopathy. Less commonly, distinctive depolarization waves known as epsilon waves are seen after the QRS complex in the ST segment on the ECG. Cardiac imaging techniques demonstrate right ventricular global or regional morphologic and functional abnormalities.[18-22] Commonly, premature ventricular contractions or sustained monomorphic ventricular tachycardia with left bundle morphology originate from the right ventricle and are associated with exercise.[17-22] Myocardial aneurysms are localized to the posterobasal, apical, and outflow tract regions (option D), resulting in the clinical characterization of these regions as the triangle of dysplasia. Sudden death during physical exercise is likely related to hemodynamic factors, increased right ventricular volume and wall stress, and enhanced sympathetic tone that culminate in ventricular tachycardia *(not ventricular fibrillation)* (option E).[18-23] Physical exercise can acutely increase right ventricular afterload and cavity enlargement, which in turn can trigger ventricular arrhythmias by stretching the diseased right ventricular musculature.[18-23]

64-8. **The answer is E.** *(Hurst's The Heart, 14th Edition, Chap. 64)* Approximately 10% of young athletes who die suddenly with exercise have no evidence of structural heart diseases (option A). In many such patients, the cause of sudden death is likely a primary electrical heart disease. These include primary electrical abnormalities such as ventricular pre-excitation (Wolff-Parkinson-White syndrome) (option B) and inherited cardiac ion channelopathies, including long QT syndrome, short QT syndrome, Brugada syndrome (option C), and catecholaminergic polymorphic ventricular tachycardia (option D).[24] These primary electrical abnormalities and other conditions predisposing to athletic sudden death have ECG changes.[10-16]

64-9. **The answer is B.** *(Hurst's The Heart, 14th Edition, Chap. 64)* In the absence of underlying cardiovascular disease, blunt nonpenetrating chest blows[25-32] during athletic or recreational activities that cause sudden cardiac death are known as commotio cordis. Although first noted a century ago, it is only in the last 15 to 20 years that commotio cordis has been recognized as a not-uncommon occurrence in youth sports, and it is now regarded as the second leading cause of sudden cardiac death in young athletes, with global recognition.[25-32] The most common sports associated with commotio cordis deaths in the United States are those in which projectiles are integral to the game (eg, baseball, softball, ice hockey, football, lacrosse) (option A). Ages of victims range from 1 to 50 years, although the mean age of individuals experiencing commotio cordis is 14 years, with 30% of individuals older than 18 years. Collapse *is usually instantaneous*, although occasionally delayed 10 to 20 seconds after the chest blow (option B). Cardiac arrhythmias documented soon after collapse are generally ventricular fibrillations (VF) (option C); however, as the time to first documented arrhythmia increases, asystole is more frequently evident. Early reports of resuscitated commotio cordis showed poor survival, although more recently, survival from these events has increased markedly to more than 50% as a result of more rapid response times and access to external defibrillation as well as greater public awareness of this condition (option D).[25-32] The mechanism by which commotio cordis occurs is complex and largely unresolved, and a porcine model was developed for study of this syndrome, which demonstrated that the immediate cause of collapse was VF.[25-32] The use of this model has allowed the definition of several important determinants of VF following a chest blow, including, most importantly, an impact delivered directly over the heart and the timing within the vulnerable phase of repolarization (a narrow 10- to 30-millisecond window just prior to the T-wave peak, equivalent to only 1% to 2% of the cardiac cycle) associated with peak LV pressure caused by the blow, although a wide range of individual vulnerability to VF is evident in the model.[25-32] Furthermore, impact velocity appears to have a Gaussian distribution, with a velocity of 40 mph most likely to trigger VF. In addition, hardness and reduced diameter of the impact object have been correlated directly with the risk of VF.[25-32] Sudden cardiac death in commotio cordis appears to be a primary electrical event. The cellular determinants of VF induced by chest wall blows likely include ion channel activation caused by increased LV pressure (option E).[25-29] The potassium–adenosine triphosphate ion channel mediates the initiation of VF in the swine model and has also been shown to be activated by atrial stretch.[25-29] It is possible that more stretch-activated ion channels are also involved.

64-10. **The answer is E.** (*Hurst's The Heart, 14th Edition, Chap. 64*) The routine use of ECGs is *not* mandated as part of athlete screening in the United States (option E). On many occasions, AHA consensus expert panels have evaluated and decided not to support mandatory national athlete screening in the United States with routine use of ECGs.[33-36] Indeed, sudden cardiovascular deaths in athletes are rare (albeit tragic) events insufficient in number to be judged as a major public health problem or justify a change in national health care policy. The most frequently cited obstacles to mandatory national screening of trained athletes are: (1) the large number of athletes to be screened nationally on an annual basis (ie, about 10 to 12 million) (option A); (2) the low incidence of events (option B); (3) the substantial number of expected false-negative and false-positive results in the range of 5% to 20%, depending on the specific ECG criteria used (option C); (4) cost-effectiveness considerations (ie, extensive resources and expenses required vs few events in absolute numbers); (5) liability issues for physicians (ie, charged with both enforcement and the sole responsibility for disqualifying athletes from competition); (6) the lack of resources or physicians dedicated to performing examinations and interpreting ECGs, in contrast to the long-standing sports medicine program in Italy; (7) the influence of observer variability, technical considerations, and the impact of ethnicity/race on the interpretation of ECGs, particularly important for multicultural athlete populations such as those in the United States; (8) the need for repetitive (ie, annual) ECG screening during adolescence (option D), given the possibility of developing phenotypic evidence of cardiomyopathies during this time period or later; (9) the logistical challenges and cost related to second-tier confirmatory screening with imaging and other testing, should primary evaluations raise the suspicion of cardiac disease; and (10) the recognition that even with testing, screening cannot be expected to identify all athletes with important cardiovascular abnormalities, and a significant false-negative rate can be expected.[32-44]

References

1. Baggish AL, Wood MJ. Athlete's heart and cardiovascular care of the athlete: scientific and clinical update. *Circulation*. 2011;123(23):2723-2735.

2. Chandra N, Bastiaenen R, Papadakis M, et al. Prevalence of electrocardiographic anomalies in young individuals: relevance to a nationwide cardiac screening program. *J Am Coll Cardiol*. 2014;63(19):2028-2034.

3. Sheikh N, Papadakis M, Ghani S, et al. Comparison of electrocardiographic criteria for the detection of cardiac abnormalities in elite black and white athletes. *Circulation*. 2014;129(16):1637-1649.

4. Calore C, Zorzi A, Sheikh N, et al. Electrocardiographic anterior T-wave inversion in athletes of different ethnicities: differential diagnosis between athlete's heart and cardiomyopathy. *Eur Heart J*. November 17, 2015. Epub ahead of print.

5. Corrado D, Pelliccia A, Heidbuchel H, et al. Recommendations for interpretation of 12-lead electrocardiogram in the athlete. *Eur Heart J*. 2010;31(2):243-259.

6. Uberoi A, Stein R, Perez MV, et al. Interpretation of the electrocardiogram of young athletes. *Circulation*. 2011;124(6):746-757.

7. Drezner JA, Ackerman MJ, Anderson J, et al. Electrocardiographic interpretation in athletes: the "Seattle criteria." *Br J Sports Med*. 2013;47(3):122-124.

8. Pelliccia A, Maron BJ, Culasso F, et al. Clinical significance of abnormal electrocardiographic patterns in trained athletes. *Circulation*. 2000;102:278-284.

9. Zipes DP, Link MS, Ackerman MJ, Kovacs RJ, Myerburg RJ, Estes NA 3rd. Eligibility and disqualification recommendations for competitive athletes with cardiovascular abnormalities: Task Force 9: arrhythmias and conduction defects: a scientific statement from the American Heart Association and American College of Cardiology. *J Am Coll Cardiol*. 2015;66(21):2412-2423.

10. Maron BJ. Sudden death in young athletes. *N Engl J Med*. 2003;349:1064-1075.

11. Maron BJ, Doerer JJ, Haas TS, et al. Sudden deaths in young competitive athletes: analysis of 1866 deaths in the United States, 1980-2006. *Circulation*. 2009;119(8): 1085-1092.

12. Maron BJ, Zipes DP, Kovacs RJ. Eligibility and disqualification recommendations for competitive athletes with cardiovascular abnormalities: preamble, principles, and general considerations: a scientific statement from the American Heart Association and American College of Cardiology. *J Am Coll Cardiol*. 2015;21:2343-2349.

13. Corrado D, Basso C, Schiavon M, et al. Screening for hypertrophic cardiomyopathy in young athletes. *N Engl J Med*. 1998;339:364-369.

14. Corrado D, Basso C, Rizzoli G, et al. Does sports activity enhance the risk of sudden death in adolescents and young adults? *J Am Coll Cardiol*. 2003;42:1959-1963.

15. Priori SG, Aliot E, Blomstrom-Lundqvist C, et al. Task force report on sudden cardiac death of the European Society of Cardiology. *Eur Heart J*. 2001;22:1374-1450.

16. Basso C, Calabrese F, Corrado D, et al. Postmortem diagnosis in sudden cardiac death victims: macroscopic, microscopic and molecular findings. *Cardiovasc Res*. 2001;50:290-300.

17. Maron BJ. Hypertrophic cardiomyopathy; a systemic review. *JAMA*. 2002;287:1308-1320.

18. Jain R, Dalal D, Daly A, et al. Prevalence and pathophysiologic attributes of ventricular dyssynchrony in arrhythmogenic right ventricular dysplasia/cardiomyopathy. *J Am Coll Cardiol*. 2009;54(5):445-451.

19. Tandri H, Macedo R, Calkins H, et al. Multidisciplinary study of right ventricular dysplasia investigators. Role of magnetic resonance imaging in arrhythmogenic right ventricular dysplasia: insights from the North American arrhythmogenic right ventricular dysplasia (ARVD/C) study. *Am Heart J*. 2008;155(1):147-153.

20. Corrado D, Basso C, Thiene G, et al. Spectrum of clinicopathologic manifestations of arrhythmogenic right ventricular cardiomyopathy/dysplasia: a multicenter study. *J Am Coll Cardiol*. 1997;30:1512-1520.

21. Corrado D, Leoni L, Link MS, et al. Implantable cardioverter-defibrillator therapy for prevention of sudden death in patients with arrhythmogenic right ventricular cardiomyopathy/dysplasia. *Circulation*. 2003;108:3084-3091.

22. Nava A, Bauce B, Basso C, et al. Clinical profile and long-term follow-up of 37 families with arrhythmogenic right ventricular cardiomyopathy. *J Am Coll Cardiol*. 2000; 36:2226-2233.

23. Corrado D, Wichter T, Link MS, et al. Treatment of arrhythmogenic right ventricular cardiomyopathy/dysplasia: an international task force consensus statement. *Eur Heart J*. 2015;36(46):3227-3237.

24. Krahn AD, Healey JS, Chauhan V, et al. Systematic assessment of patients with unexplained cardiac arrest: cardiac arrest survivors with preserved ejection fraction registry (CASPER). *Circulation*. 2009;120(4):278-285.

25. Link MS. Commotio cordis. *Circ Arrhythm Electrophysiol*. 2012;5:425-432.

26. Maron BJ, Estes NA Commotio cordis. *N Engl J Med*. 2010;362:917-927.

27. Maron BJ, Haas TS, Ahluwalia A, Garberich RF, Estes NAM III, Link MS. Increasing survival rate from commotio cordis. *Heart Rhythm*. 2013;10:219-223.

28. Alsheikh-Ali AA, Madias C, Supran S, Link MS. Marked variability in susceptibility to ventricular fibrillation in an experimental commotio cordis model. *Circulation*. 2010;122:2499-2504.

29. Kalin J, Madias C, Alsheikh-Ali AA, Link MS. Reduced diameter spheres increases the risk of chest blow-induced ventricular fibrillation (commotio cordis). *Heart Rhythm*. 2011;8:1578-1581.

30. Maron BJ, Ahluwalia A, Haas TS, Semsarian C, Link MS, Estes NAM III. Global epidemiology and demographics. *Heart Rhythm*. 2011;8(12):1969-1971.

31. Weinstock J, Maron BJ, Song C, et al. Failure of commercially available chest wall protectors to prevent sudden cardiac death induced by chest wall blows in an experimental model of commotio cordis. *Pediatrics*. 2006;117(4):e656-e662.

32. Link MS, Estes NA 3rd, Maron BJ. Eligibility and disqualification recommendations for competitive athletes with cardiovascular abnormalities: Task Force 13: commotio cordis: a scientific statement from the American Heart Association and American College of Cardiology. *J Am Coll Cardiol*. 2015;66(21):2439-2443.

33. Corrado D, Basso C, Pavei A, et al. Trends in sudden cardiovascular death in young competitive athletes after implementation of preparticipation screening program. *JAMA*. 2006;296:1593-1601.

34. Maron BJ, Friedman RA, Kligfield P, et al. Assessment of the 12-lead electrocardiogram as a screening test for detection of cardiovascular disease in general healthy populations of young people (12-22 years of age). *Circulation*. 2014;130:1303-1334.

35. Maron BJ, Thompson PD, Ackerman MJ, et al. Recommendations and considerations related to preparticipation screening for cardiovascular abnormalities in competitive athletes: update 2007. A scientific statement from the American Heart Association, Nutrition, Physical Activity, and Metabolism Council. *Circulation*. 2007;115:1643-1655.

36. Maron BJ, Thompson PD, Puffer JC, et al. Cardiovascular preparticipation screening of competitive athletes: a statement for health professionals from the Sudden Death Committee (Clinical Cardiology) and Congenital Cardiac Defects Committee (Cardiovascular Diseases in the Young) American Heart Association. *Circulation*. 1996;94:850-856.

37. Pelliccia A, Zipes DP, Maron BJ. Bethesda Conference #36 and the European Society of Cardiology consensus recommendations revisited: a comparison of U.S. and European criteria for eligibility and disqualification of competitive athletes with cardiovascular abnormalities. *J Am Coll Cardiol*. 2008;52: 1990-1996.

38. Corrado D, Pelliccia A, Bjørnstad HH, et al. Cardiovascular pre-participation screening of young competitive athletes for prevention of sudden death: proposal for a common European protocol. Consensus statement of the Study Group of Sport Cardiology of the Working Group of Cardiac Rehabilitation and Exercise Physiology and the Working Group of Myocardial and Pericardial Diseases of the European Society of Cardiology. *Eur Heart J*. 2005;26:516-524.

39. Corrado D, Basso C, Pavei A, Michieli P, Schiavon M, Thiene G. Trends in sudden cardiovascular death in young competitive athletes after implementation of a preparticipation screening program. *JAMA*. 2006;296:1593-1601.

40. Baggish AL, Hutter AM, Wang F, et al. Cardiovascular screening in college athletes with and without electrocardiography. *Ann Intern Med*. 2010;152:269-275.

41. Malhotra R, West JJ, Dent J, et al. Cost and yield of adding electrocardiography to history and physical in screening division I intercollegiate athletes: a 5-year experience. *Heart Rhythm*. 2011;8:721-727.

42. Magalski A, McCoy M, Zabel M, et al. Cardiovascular screening with electrocardiography and echocardiography in collegiate athletes. *Am J Med*. 2011;124:511-518.

43. Weiner RB, Hutter AM, Wang F, et al. Performance of the 2010 European Society of Cardiology criteria for ECG interpretation in athletes. *Heart*. 2011;97:1573-1577.

44. Rowin EJ, Maron BJ, Appelbaum E, et al. Significance of false negative electrocardiograms in preparticipation screening of athletes for hypertrophic cardiomyopathy. *Am J Cardiol*. 2012;110:1027-1032.

CHAPTER 65

Cardiovascular Disease in the Elderly: Pathophysiology and Clinical Implications

Mark J. Eisenberg

QUESTIONS

DIRECTIONS: Choose the one best response to each question.

65-1. Which of the following is *not* an effect of aging on the gross anatomy of the heart?

A. Endocardial thickening and sclerosis
B. Increased left atrial size
C. Valvular fibrosis and sclerosis
D. Decreased epicardial fat
E. All of the above

65-2. Which of the following is a cardiovascular effect associated with aging?

A. Thrombosis
B. Bleeding complications with antiplatelet, anticoagulant, and fibrinolytic agents
C. Sarcopenia
D. Altered pharmacodynamics
E. All of the above

65-3. Which of the following statements about multimorbidity is *true*?

A. The most common pattern of multimorbidity is the coexistence of a cardiometabolic condition and osteoarthritis
B. The dyad of hypertension and hyperlipidemia is rare among Medicare beneficiaries

C. Over 50% of Medicare beneficiaries with HF, stroke, or AF have more than seven chronic conditions
D. Noncardiovascular conditions account for almost a quarter of readmissions after HF or MI in older adults
E. All of the above

65-4. Which of the following statements about polypharmacy is *false*?

A. Polypharmacy is defined as concomitant use of three or more medications
B. About 40% of community-dwelling older adults take at least five medications
C. About 20% of community-dwelling older adults take medications that may exacerbate coexisting conditions
D. Medications used to treat arthritis can antagonize the effects of many cardiovascular medications
E. All of the above

65-5. Which of the following statements about frailty is *false*?

A. Frailty is characterized by reduced physiologic reserve in multiple organ systems to maintain homeostasis after a stressful event
B. After functional decline, frailty is considered the second most problematic manifestation of aging
C. When using a comprehensive definition of frailty, more than 50% of the general population is affected
D. Persons with three or more criteria from the *frailty phenotype* are considered frail
E. None of the above statements are false

65-6. Which of the following statements about cognitive impairment is *true*?

A. Dementia affects 25% of adults age 70 years or older in the United States

B. The prevalence of dementia increases from 5% in patients age 71 to 79 years to 37% in those over 90 years of age

C. Mild cognitive impairment is present in 52% of people ≥ 70 years old

D. The prevalence of cognitive impairment is higher in older adults undergoing CABG than in those who are hospitalized with HF

E. Large cerebral infarcts, grey matter lesions, lacunes, and microinfarcts are some of the cerebrovascular pathologies associated with dementia

65-7. Which of the following statements is *true* about the effects of aging on the risk of heart failure (HF)?

A. The high prevalence of HF in elderly patients is *not* solely related to improved survival from acute MI and other CVDs

B. The exponential rise in HF among older people is due to a gradual erosion in cardiovascular reserve

C. The effects of normal aging alter the four major determinants of cardiac output

D. A healthy 90-year-old person has the exercise capacity and cardiovascular reserve equivalent to a younger person with New York Heart Association functional class III HF.

E. All of the above

65-8. Which of the following statements about the use of intravenous antiplatelet therapy in older adults is *false*?

A. Patients at a higher risk of reinfarction tend to benefit the most from intravenous antiplatelet therapy

B. It is difficult to say whether intravenous antiplatelet therapy is beneficial to older adults because few studies have enrolled patients older than 75

C. Current guidelines recommend avoiding intravenous antiplatelet therapy in STEMI patients ≥ 85 years of age

D. The use of glycoprotein IIb/IIIa should be limited to older persons with high thrombosis risk and low bleeding risk

E. All of the above

65-9. Which of the following statements about aortic stenosis (AS) is *true*?

A. The prevalence of AS in patients older than 80 years of age is higher than 20%

B. More than 90% of all aortic valve procedures are performed in the geriatric population

C. AS is an uncommon valvular abnormality in both young and older patients

D. Symptoms of AS are known to be especially prominent in elderly patients with a sedentary lifestyle

E. Older individuals with severe AS are less likely to exhibit delayed upstroke of the carotid pulse wave

65-10. Sinus node pacemaker cells degenerate progressively with age. By age 75, approximately what percentage of sinus node pacemaker cells continue to function normally?

A. 5%

B. 10%

C. 20%

D. 30%

E. 50%

65-1. **The answer is D.** (*Hurst's The Heart, 14th Edition, Chap. 65*) The effects of aging on the gross anatomy of the heart are: increased left ventricular wall thickness and decreased cavity size, endocardial thickening and sclerosis (option A), increased left atrial size (option B), valvular fibrosis and sclerosis (option C), and increased (*not decreased*) epicardial fat (option D).

65-2. **The answer is E.** (*Hurst's The Heart, 14th Edition, Chap. 65*) With increasing age, changes in the hemostatic system shift the intrinsic balance between thrombosis and fibrinolysis in the direction of thrombosis (option A). As a result, older adults are at increased risk for both venous thromboembolic disease (ie, deep venous thrombosis and pulmonary embolism) and thrombosis in the arterial system, including myocardial infarction (MI), left atrial appendage thrombus in AF, and stroke. Despite these changes, and perhaps paradoxically, older adults are also at increased risk for bleeding complications with all antiplatelet, anticoagulant, and fibrinolytic agents (option B), as exemplified by the increased incidence of intracranial hemorrhage in older adults receiving prasugrel or fibrinolytic agents. In addition, age-associated declines in muscular mass (sarcopenia) and bone mass (osteopenia) contribute to reductions in exercise tolerance, adversely affect balance, and predispose to injurious falls (option C). Further, aging is associated with altered pharmacokinetics and pharmacodynamics of almost all medications (option D), so that drug dosages tested in clinical trials involving predominantly younger and healthier patients may not be appropriate for the majority of older adults.

65-3. **The answer is A.** (*Hurst's The Heart, 14th Edition, Chap. 65*) Multimorbidity often involves CVD—the coexistence of a cardiometabolic condition and osteoarthritis was the most common multimorbidity pattern in several population-based studies (option A).[1] Among Medicare beneficiaries, the dyad of hypertension and hyperlipidemia was most prevalent (53%) (option B), and other common conditions were ischemic heart disease, diabetes, and arthritis.[2,3] In addition, over 50% of Medicare beneficiaries with HF, stroke, or AF have more than five chronic conditions (option C).[4] Prevalent noncardiovascular conditions include arthritis, anemia, chronic kidney disease, cataracts, chronic obstructive pulmonary disease, dementia, and depression.[3] Furthermore, noncardiovascular conditions account for almost half of readmissions after HF or MI in older adults (option D).[5] Therefore, identifying common patterns of multimorbidity may guide clinical decisions by helping clinicians to prioritize interventions that are most likely to have a positive impact on overall outcomes.

65-4. **The answer is A.** (*Hurst's The Heart, 14th Edition, Chap. 65*) *Polypharmacy* is typically defined as concomitant use of five or more medications (option A).[6] The use of prescription medications and the prevalence of polypharmacy have increased markedly over the past decade.[7] The number of chronic conditions and prescribing practices aligned with disease-based guidelines are directly correlated with polypharmacy.[6,8] Approximately 40% of community-dwelling older adults take at least five medications (option B),[6] and 20% take medications that may exacerbate coexisting conditions (option C).[9] For example, arthritis is often treated with nonsteroidal anti-inflammatory drugs, which antagonize the effects of many cardiovascular medications (ACEIs, ARBs, diuretics) and also increase the risk for MI, HF, and worsening renal function (option D). The number of medications and treatment complexity are associated with nonadherence, drug-related adverse events, financial burden, and caregiver stress.[6,10-16]

65-5. **The answer is B.** (*Hurst's The Heart, 14th Edition, Chap. 65*) *Frailty* is a geriatric syndrome that is characterized by a reduced physiologic reserve in multiple organ systems (eg, the brain or the endocrine, immune, musculoskeletal, or cardiovascular systems) to maintain homeostasis after a stressful event and an increased vulnerability to adverse health outcomes (option A).[17] It is the most problematic manifestation of aging and contributes substantially to the heterogeneity in the health status of the aging population (option B). Several criteria for diagnosing frailty have been developed, yielding varying prevalence estimates in the general population, from < 5% using a specific physical performance-based definition to > 50% using a more comprehensive definition (option C).[18] The *frailty phenotype*, derived from the Cardiovascular Health Study, is a widely accepted method for classifying older adults into robust, prefrail, or frail categories based on unintentional weight loss, weak handgrip strength, exhaustion, slow gait speed, and low physical activity.[19] Persons with three or more of these criteria are considered frail (option D); those with one or two criteria are considered prefrail.

65-6. **The answer is B.** *(Hurst's The Heart, 14th Edition, Chap. 65)* Dementia affects 14% of adults age 70 years or older in the United States (option A), and the prevalence increases with age, from 5% in patients age 71 to 79 years to 37% in those over 90 years of age (option B).[20] Mild cognitive impairment, a less severe form of cognitive limitation with relative preservation of functional status, is present in 22% of people ≥ 70 years old (option C).[21] The annual rate of progression from mild cognitive impairment to dementia is estimated to be about 12%.[21] The prevalence of cognitive impairment in older adults with CVD is higher than that in the general population: 35% in patients undergoing coronary artery bypass graft (CABG) surgery[22] and 47% in hospitalized patients with HF (option D).[23] The underlying mechanisms include hypoperfusion, oxidative stress, and inflammation, which lead to diverse cerebrovascular pathologies, including large cerebral infarcts, white matter lesions, lacunes, microinfarcts, and microbleeds (option E).[24]

65-7. **The answer is E.** *(Hurst's The Heart, 14th Edition, Chap. 65)* Although the high prevalence of HF in elderly patients is partly related to improved survival from acute MI and other CVDs, other age-related factors contribute to the development of HF, including long-standing hypertension (option A) (present in 75% of patients with HF), vascular stiffness, left ventricular diastolic dysfunction, sinus node dysfunction, progressive valvular heart disease, coronary ischemia, and reduced responsiveness to β-adrenergic stimulation.[25] As a result, a gradual erosion in cardiovascular reserve with age results in an exponential rise in HF among older persons (option B). Studies in healthy older adults have confirmed that the effects of normal aging lead to altered preload, afterload, heart rate, and contractility—the four major determinants of cardiac output (option C)—thus resulting in a progressive decline in peak cardiopulmonary performance, even in the absence of clinically evident CVD.[26] Stated another way, an otherwise healthy 90-year-old person is likely to have exercise capacity and cardiovascular reserve equivalent to a younger person with New York Heart Association functional class III HF (option D).

65-8. **The answer is C.** *(Hurst's The Heart, 14th Edition, Chap. 65)* The role of intravenous antiplatelet therapy in ACS is difficult to define, both for younger and older patients. Glycoprotein IIb/IIIa inhibitors appear to reduce reinfarction and overall infarct size at the time of NSTE-ACS, with patients at higher risk deriving the most benefit (option A), but few studies have enrolled patients over age 75 (option B), and the risk of bleeding complications increases with age.[25,27] One study of ACS patients demonstrated higher event rates in octogenarians randomized to glycoprotein IIb/IIIa inhibitor therapy,[28] and current guidelines recommend avoiding these medications entirely in the setting of fibrinolytic therapy for STEMI in patients ≥75 years of age (option C).[29] Because these drugs are associated with greater bleeding risks in the elderly, the use of glycoprotein IIb/IIIa inhibitors should probably be limited to select older individuals with high thrombosis risk and low bleeding risk (option D). The intravenous platelet inhibitor cangrelor has a different mechanism of action than the glycoprotein IIb/IIIa inhibitors, and clinical trials evaluating cangrelor demonstrated similar benefits among patients older and younger than age 75 years.[30] However, the magnitude of the bleeding risk associated with cangrelor remains unclear;[31] thus, the safety of this drug in elderly patients requires further study.

65-9. **The answer is E.** *(Hurst's The Heart, 14th Edition, Chap. 65)* The prevalence of symptomatic aortic stenosis (AS) increases from 0.2% in patients under age 60 to nearly 10% in those

≥80 years of age (option A).[25,32] As a result, over 70% of all aortic valve procedures are performed in the geriatric population (option B), and AS is the most common valvular abnormality requiring surgical or percutaneous intervention (option C). Symptoms may not be as prominent in elderly patients with sedentary lifestyles (option D), resulting in delayed presentation or incidental diagnosis of severe AS at the time of presentation for other medical problems.[25] In addition, although physical findings are generally similar in younger and older patients, older patients with severe AS are less likely to exhibit delayed upstroke of the carotid pulse wave (pulsus tardus et parvus) as a result of increased arterial stiffness (option E).

65-10. The answer is B. *(Hurst's The Heart, 14th Edition, Chap. 65)* The progressive degeneration of sinus node pacemaker cells results in only 10% continuing to function normally by age 75 (option B).[25] Similar processes occur in the tissues surrounding the sinus node and within the conduction pathways, contributing to the development of sinoatrial exit block or atrioventricular nodal block.

References

1. Violan C, Foguet-Boreu Q, Flores-Mateo G, et al. Prevalence, determinants and patterns of multimorbidity in primary care: a systematic review of observational studies. *PLoS One.* 2014;9(7):e102149.

2. Goodman RA, Ling SM, Briss PA, Parrish RG, Salive ME, Finke BS. Multimorbidity patterns in the United States: implications for research and clinical practice. *J Gerontol A Biol Sci Med Sci.* 2016;71(2): 215-220.

3. Arnett DK, Goodman RA, Halperin JL, Anderson JL, Parekh AK, Zoghbi WA. AHA/ACC/HHS strategies to enhance application of clinical practice guidelines in patients with cardiovascular disease and comorbid conditions: from the American Heart Association, American College of Cardiology, and U.S. Department of Health and Human Services. *J Am Coll Cardiol.* 2014;64(17):1851-1856.

4. Centers for Medicare and Medicaid Services. *Chronic Conditions among Medicare Beneficiaries, Chartbook.* 2012 Edition. Baltimore, MD: Centers for Medicare and Medicaid Services; 2012.

5. Dharmarajan K, Hsieh AF, Lin Z, et al. Diagnoses and timing of 30-day readmissions after hospitalization for heart failure, acute myocardial infarction, or pneumonia. *JAMA.* 2013;309(4):355-363.

6. Centers for Disease Control and Prevention. Health, United States, 2013. With special feature on prescription drugs. http://www.cdc.gov/nchs/data/hus/hus13.pdf. Accessed January 13, 2016.

7. Bajcar JM, Wang L, Moineddin R, Nie JX, Tracy CS, Upshur RE. From pharmacotherapy to pharmacoprevention: trends in prescribing to older adults in Ontario, Canada, 1997-2006. *BMC Fam Pract.* 2010;11:75.

8. Tinetti ME, McAvay G, Trentalange M, Cohen AB, Allore HG. Association between guideline recommended drugs and death in older adults with multiple chronic conditions: population based cohort study. *BMJ.* 2015;351:h4984.

9. Lorgunpai SJ, Grammas M, Lee DS, McAvay G, Charpentier P, Tinetti ME. Potential therapeutic competition in community-living older adults in the U.S.: use of medications that may adversely affect a coexisting condition. *PLoS One.* 2014;9(2):e89447.

10. Boyd CM, Darer J, Boult C, Fried LP, Boult L, Wu AW. Clinical practice guidelines and quality of care for older patients with multiple comorbid diseases: implications for pay for performance. *JAMA.* 2005;294(6):716-724.

11. Lorgunpai SJ, Grammas M, Lee DS, McAvay G, Charpentier P, Tinetti ME. Potential therapeutic competition in community-living older adults in the U.S.: use of medications that may adversely affect a coexisting condition. *PLoS One.* 2014;9(2):e89447.

12. Hakkarainen KM, Hedna K, Petzold M, Hagg S. Percentage of patients with preventable adverse drug reactions and preventability of adverse drug reactions: a meta-analysis. *PLoS One.* 2012;7(3):e33236.

13. Tache SV, Sonnichsen A, Ashcroft DM. Prevalence of adverse drug events in ambulatory care: a systematic review. *Ann Pharmacother.* 2011;45(7-8):977-989.

14. Willson MN, Greer CL, Weeks DL. Medication regimen complexity and hospital readmission for an adverse drug event. *Ann Pharmacother.* 2014;48(1):26-32.

15. Choudhry NK, Fischer MA, Avorn J, et al. The implications of therapeutic complexity on adherence to cardiovascular medications. *Arch Intern Med.* 2011;171(9):814-822.

16. Giovannetti ER, Wolff JL, Xue QL, et al. Difficulty assisting with health care tasks among caregivers of multimorbid older adults. *J Gen Intern Med.* 2012;27(1):37-44.

17. Clegg A, Young J, Iliffe S, Rikkert MO, Rockwood K. Frailty in elderly people. *Lancet.* 2013;381(9868):752-762.

18. Collard RM, Boter H, Schoevers RA, Oude Voshaar RC. Prevalence of frailty in community-dwelling older persons: a systematic review. *J Am Geriatr Soc.* 2012;60(8):1487-1492.

19. Fried LP, Tangen CM, Walston J, et al. Frailty in older adults: evidence for a phenotype. *J Gerontol A Biol Sci Med Sci.* 2001;56(3):M146-156.

20. Plassman BL, Langa KM, Fisher GG, et al. Prevalence of dementia in the United States: the Aging, Demographics, and Memory Study. *Neuroepidemiology.* 2007;29(1-2):125-132.

21. Plassman BL, Langa KM, Fisher GG, et al. Prevalence of cognitive impairment without dementia in the United States. *Ann Intern Med.* 2008;148(6):427-434.

22. Silbert BS, Scott DA, Evered LA, Lewis MS, Maruff PT. Preexisting cognitive impairment in patients scheduled for elective coronary artery bypass graft surgery. *Anesth Analg.* 2007;104(5):1023-1028.

23. Dodson JA, Truong TT, Towle VR, Kerins G, Chaudhry SI. Cognitive impairment in older adults with heart failure: prevalence, documentation, and impact on outcomes. *Am J Med.* 2013;126(2):120-126.

24. Iadecola C. The pathobiology of vascular dementia. *Neuron.* 2013;80(4):844-866.

25. Rich MW, Stolker JM. Diagnosis and management of heart disease in the elderly. In: Arenson C, Busby-Whitehead J, Brummel-Smith K, O'Brien JG, Palmer MH, Reichel W, eds. *Reichel's Care of the Elderly: Clinical Aspects of Aging.* 7th ed. New York, NY: Cambridge University Press; 2016.

26. Fleg JL, Morrell CH, Bos AG, et al. Accelerated longitudinal decline of aerobic capacity in healthy older adults. *Circulation.* 2005;112(5):674-682.

27. Iakovou I, Dangas G, Mehran R, et al. Comparison of effect of glycoprotein IIb/IIIa inhibitors during percutaneous coronary interventions on risk of hemorrhagic stroke in patients > or = 75 years of age versus those < 75 years of age. *Am J Cardiol.* 2003;92(9):1083-1086.

28. PURSUIT Trial Investigators. Inhibition of platelet glycoprotein IIb/IIIa with eptifibatide in patients with acute coronary syndromes. *N Engl J Med.* 1998;339(7):436-443.

29. O'Gara PT, Kushner FG, Ascheim DD, et al. 2013 ACCF/AHA guideline for the management of ST-elevation myocardial infarction. *Circulation.* 2013;127(4):e362-425.

30. Bhatt DL, Stone GW, Mahaffey KW, et al. Effect of platelet inhibition with cangrelor during PCI on ischemic events. *N Engl J Med.* 2013;368(14):1303-1313.

31. Serebruany VL, Aradi D, Kim MH, Sibbing D. Cangrelor infusion is associated with an increased risk for bleeding: meta-analysis of randomized trials. *Int J Cardiol.* 2013;169(3):225-228.

32. Otto CM, Prendergast B. Aortic-valve stenosis: from patients at risk to severe valve obstruction. *N Engl J Med.* 2014;371(8):744-756.

CHAPTER 66

Pericardial Diseases

Patrick R. Lawler

QUESTIONS

DIRECTIONS: Choose the one best response to each question.

66-1. Which of the following is *correct* regarding the normal anatomy and physiology of the pericardium?

A. It allows great distention of the cardiac chambers and increased cardiac filling
B. Congenital absence or surgical removal of the pericardium is fatal
C. The human pericardium consists of two distinct layers, the inner serosa and the outer fibrosa
D. Most of the innervation of the pericardium occurs via the vagus nerves
E. All of the above

66-2. A 49-year-old man presents to clinic with pleuritic chest pain, myalgia, and fever. Which of the following findings is *not* a diagnostic criterion for acute pericarditis?

A. New widespread ST elevation or PR depression on ECG
B. Sharp chest pain that is worse on inspiration
C. Fever > 38°C
D. Pericardial friction rub
E. New or worsening pericardial effusion

66-3. A 63-year-old woman presents with recurrent pericardial disease. Which of the following is a Class I level A recommendation on the proper diagnosis and management of pericardial diseases?

A. Corticosteroids should be prescribed as first choice in patients with acute pericarditis
B. Vasodilators and diuretics are recommended in the presence of cardiac tamponade
C. An absolute contraindication to draining a pericardial effusion includes a suspicion of bacterial etiology

D. Colchicine is a first-choice drug to be used as an adjunct to aspirin/NSAIDs to treat and prevent recurrent episodes of pericarditis
E. None of the above

66-4. Which of the following is *not* a recommended therapeutic option for recurrent pericarditis?

A. High-dose prednisone (1.0 to 1.5 mg/kg/d)
B. Triple therapy of aspirin, colchicine, and corticosteroids
C. Pericardiectomy
D. Low-dose prednisone for patients on oral anticoagulants
E. Aspirin/NSAID and colchicine

66-5. A 40-year-old woman presents to the emergency room with chest pain, fever, and night sweats. She has recently returned from travelling in India and has lost 10 pounds. Which of the following findings is *not* consistent with a diagnosis of tuberculous pericarditis with pericardial effusion?

A. Lack of signs and symptoms of pulmonary tuberculosis
B. Presence of pulsus paradoxus
C. Electrical alternans on ECG
D. Negative acid-fast bacilli staining and mycobacterium cultures on pericardial fluid
E. Elevated C-reactive protein

66-6. Which of the following clinical presentations is consistent with cardiac tamponade?

A. Pulmonary edema
B. Impaired ventricular diastolic filling
C. Third heart sound
D. Decreased central venous pressure
E. All of the above

66-7. A 63-year-old man is brought to the emergency room with altered level of consciousness and is found to be tachycardic and hypotensive. Echocardiography reveals a large pericardial effusion with echocardiographic evidence of tamponade. Which of the following is *not* appropriate in the subsequent management of this patient with cardiac tamponade?

A. If a pericardial catheter is placed, removal of the intrapericardial catheter when the output is < 90 mL over a 24-hour period

B. Prompt needle pericardiocentesis to aspirate all the pericardial fluid

C. Pericardiocentesis should be guided by echocardiography to prevent tissue injury

D. If a pericardial catheter is placed, reassessment of effusion size and areas of loculation before catheter removal

E. All of the above are correct

66-8. Which of the following statements about constrictive pericarditis is *correct*?

A. It is twice as prevalent in women as in men (2:1 ratio)

B. The thickened pericardium has decreased compliance, resulting in ventricular interdependence

C. Orthopnea and paroxysmal nocturnal dyspnea are typically observed

D. Patients often present with features of left-heart failure

E. None of the above

66-9. Which of the following is most likely to provide definitive treatment for symptomatic patients with constrictive pericarditis?

A. Anti-inflammatory therapy

B. Pericardiocentesis

C. Pericardiectomy

D. Close follow-up

E. None of the above

66-10. A 55-year-old woman presents to your clinic with vague chest pain and dyspnea. A chest radiograph reveals a mass in the right costophrenic angle. CT of the chest suggests a pericardial cyst. Which of the following is *correct*?

A. Pericardial cysts are smooth, thin-walled structures usually filled with pus

B. The recommended therapeutic course is observation of the patient

C. Pericardial cysts are usually symptomatic and tend to increase in size over time

D. The patient's symptoms are likely unrelated to the cyst

E. Percutaneous drainage of the cyst is recommended for asymptomatic patients

66-1. The answer is C. *(Hurst's The Heart, 14th Edition, Chap. 66)* The human pericardium has two distinct layers; the serosa is composed of a single column of mesothelial cells that surrounds all four cardiac chambers and the proximal great vessels and reflects on itself to form the inner surface of the fibrosa, a fibrocollagenous structure (option C). This monolayer of serosal cells covering the surface of the heart and epicardial fat is also called the visceral pericardium, whereas the fibrosa and the reflection of the serosa make the parietal pericardium.

Most of the innervation of the pericardium occurs via the phrenic nerves (C4–C6), which course anteriorly (option D); this is particularly relevant during pericardiectomy. No adverse consequences follow congenital absence or surgical removal of the pericardium (option B). However, the pericardium serves many important (although subtle) functions. It limits distension of the cardiac chambers and facilitates the interaction and coupling of the ventricles and atria (option A). Limitation of cardiac filling volumes by the pericardium may also limit cardiac output and oxygen delivery during exercise.

66-2. The answer is C. *(Hurst's The Heart, 14th Edition, Chap. 66)* The clinical diagnosis of acute pericarditis is established when two of four clinical criteria are satisfied (Table 66-1). Acute pericarditis is usually characterized by sharp retrosternal pain (option B) that is aggravated by lying down and relieved by sitting up; its onset is often heralded by a prodrome of fever, malaise, and myalgia. The most specific physical sign can be the presence of a pericardial friction rub (option D), which is identifiable in no more than a third of cases. Within a few hours of the onset of chest pain, typical ECG changes include ST-segment elevations and depression of the PR segment (except in lead aVR), which can persist for hours or days (option A). This is the first ECG stage of pericarditis, followed by normalization of the ST segments (stage 2), T-wave inversions (stage 3), and finally, normalization again (stage 4). This is different from myocardial infarction, wherein T-wave inversions often begin while the ST segments are still elevated. In addition, echocardiographic identification of pericardial effusion confirms the clinical diagnosis of acute pericarditis (option E). Elevated fever (option C) is a major indicator of poor prognosis but is not a diagnostic criterion.

TABLE 66-1 **Definition and Diagnostic Criteria for Acute Pericarditis**

Inflammatory pericardial syndrome to be diagnosed with at least 2 of the 4 following criteria:
(1) pericarditic chest pain
(2) pericardial rubs
(3) new widespread ST elevation or PR depression on ECG
(4) pericardial effusion (new or worsening)
Additional supporting findings:
Elevation of markers of inflammation (ie, C-reactive protein, erythrocyte sedimentation rate, and white blood cell count);
Evidence of pericardial inflammation by an imaging technique (computed tomography, cardiac magnetic resonance).

66-3. The answer is D. *(Hurst's The Heart, 14th Edition, Chap. 66)* Treatment of pericardial disease is challenging because there is a paucity of randomized, placebo-controlled trials that identify appropriate therapy and help with clinical decision making. Table 66-2 summarizes the main recommendations of the 2015 ESC guidelines.[1] Colchicine is a first-line therapy to be used as adjunct to aspirin/NSAIDs or corticosteroids to treat and prevent pericarditis, either in acute or recurrent cases (Class I recommendation, level of evidence: A) (option D). Corticosteroids should not be prescribed as first choice in patients with acute pericarditis, given the risk of recurrence (Class III recommendation, level of evidence: C) (option A). The essential indications to drain a pericardial effusion include: cardiac tamponade (therapeutic pericardiocentesis), a suspicion of bacterial or neoplastic etiology,

TABLE 66-2 Summary of the 2015 European Society of Cardiology Guidelines on the Diagnosis and Management of Pericardial Diseases

	Indication	Evidence
Acute and recurrent pericarditis		
A triage is recommended to identify high-risk patients who should be admitted to hospital. Low-risk patients can be managed as outpatients.	Class I	Level B
Colchicine is now a first-choice drug to be used as adjunct to aspirin/NSAID or corticosteroids to treat and prevent pericarditis either in acute or recurrent pericarditis (weight-adjusted doses are recommended without a loading dose; eg, 0.5 mg twice a day for 3 months in acute pericarditis and 6 months in recurrent pericarditis; colchicine should be given only as 0.5 mg once for patients > 70 kg).	Class I	Level A
Levels of C-reactive protein are useful to guide the treatment duration and assess the response to treatment in acute and recurrent pericarditis; anti-inflammatory therapy should be maintained until symptom resolution and C-reactive protein normalization.	Class IIa	Level C
Corticosteroids should not be prescribed as first choice in patients with acute pericarditis since it may favor chronicization.	Class III	Level C
Pericardial effusion		
The essential indications to drain a pericardial effusion include: (1) cardiac tamponade (therapeutic pericardiocentesis), (2) a suspicion of bacterial or neoplastic aetiology, and (3) persistent moderate to large pericardial effusion without response to medical therapy.	Class I	Level C
A triage system is proposed also for the management of pericardial effusion and is essentially based on the following: (1) recognize cardiac tamponade and possible bacterial of neoplastic etiologies, (2) exclude concomitant pericarditis or treat as pericarditis, (3) identify associated underlying diseases, and (4) if chronic and large (> 20 mm), consider pericardial drainage to prevent cardiac tamponade during follow-up.	Class I	Level C
Treatment of pericardial effusions should be tailored as much as possible to the underlying etiology.	Class I	Level C
Cardiac tamponade		
In a patient with clinical suspicion of cardiac tamponade, echocardiography is recommended as the first imaging technique to evaluate the size, location, and degree of hemodynamic impact of the pericardial effusion.	Class I	Level C
Urgent pericardiocentesis or cardiac surgery is recommended to treat cardiac tamponade.	Class I	Level C
A judicious clinical evaluation including echocardiographic findings is recommended to guide the timing of pericardiocentesis.	Class I	Level C
Vasodilators and diuretics are not recommended in the presence of cardiac tamponade.	Class III	Level C
Constrictive pericarditis		
CT and CMR are indicated for the evaluation of a suspected constrictive pericarditis as second-level imaging techniques after echocardiography.	Class I	Level C
Cardiac catheterization is indicated only in complex cases when noninvasive imaging does not provide a clear-cut diagnosis or provides conflicting results.	Class I	Level C
The mainstay of therapy for chronic constriction is radical pericardiectomy, but it is acknowledged that there is a need to assess the possible presence of pericardial inflammation (eg, elevation of C-reactive protein, pericardial inflammation on CT/CMR) as precipitating cause in new-onset cases in order to treat with empiric anti-inflammatory therapy.	Class I	Level C
Diagnostic workup of pericardial diseases		
First diagnostic evaluation in a patient with a clinical suspicion of pericardial disease should include: focused history and physical examination, ECG, chest x-ray, and routine blood tests, including markers of myocardial inflammation and lesion and renal function.	Class I	Level C
Echocardiography is the first essential diagnostic imaging tool, whereas CT and CMR are second-level imaging techniques for specific indications.	Class I	Level C
Additional diagnostic testing should be targeted and clinically guided.	Class I	Level C
Main specific forms		
Tuberculosis		
Empiric antituberculous therapy is only recommended in countries where tuberculosis is endemic and the disease is highly probable in the setting of a patient with pericarditis and pericardial effusion.	Class I	Level C
In cases with an established diagnosis of tuberculous pericarditis, standard antituberculous therapy is recommended for 6 months and prevents the evolution to constrictive pericarditis.	Class I	Level C
In patients with tuberculous pericarditis with features of constriction and not responding to antituberculous therapy, pericardiectomy is recommended after 4–8 weeks of medical therapy.	Class I	Level C

(Continued)

TABLE 66-2 Summary of the 2015 European Society of Cardiology Guidelines on the Diagnosis and Management of Pericardial Diseases (*Continued*)

	Indication	Evidence
Neoplastic pericardial diseases		
The definite diagnosis of neoplastic pericardial disease relies on the evidence of neoplastic cells on cytology of pericardial fluid.	Class I	Level B
Pericardial biopsy should be considered for the final etiologic diagnosis in selected cases.	Class IIa	Level B
Tumor markers in pericardial fluid may be helpful to differentiate a benign vs a malignant pericardial effusion.	Class IIa	Level B
In cases with a confirmed diagnosis of neoplastic pericardial disease, systemic antineoplastic treatment is indicated.	Class I	Level B
Extended pericardial drainage is recommended to prevent recurrent cardiac tamponade and pericardial effusion and to provide a way for intrapericardial therapy.	Class I	Level B
Intrapericardial therapy with cytostatic agents should be considered to treat neoplastic pericardial disease.	Class IIa	Level B

Abbreviations: CMR, cardiac magnetic resonance; CT, computed tomography; ECG, electrocardiography; NSAID, nonsteroidal anti-inflammatory drugs.

and persistent moderate to large pericardial effusion without response to medical therapy (Class I recommendation, level of evidence: C) (option C). Vasodilators and diuretics are not recommended in the presence of cardiac tamponade (Class III recommendation, level of evidence: C) (option B).

66-4. **The answer is A.** (*Hurst's The Heart, 14th Edition, Chap. 66*) Recurrent pericarditis is one of the most troublesome complications of pericarditis, occurring in one-third of cases. The mainstay of therapy for recurrences is similar to that for acute pericarditis: aspirin or an NSAID plus colchicine at the same doses that are recommended for acute pericarditis (option E). Corticosteroids should be considered as a second-line therapy for patients with contraindications for or failure of aspirin/NSAIDs or patients with specific indications (eg, pregnant patients, patients with a systemic inflammatory disease already on corticosteroids, patients with renal failure, patients on oral anticoagulant therapies to avoid interference with aspirin/NSAIDs) (option D). If used, low to moderate doses (eg, prednisone 0.2 to 0.5 mg/kg/d or equivalent) are indicated because high doses (eg, prednisone 1.0 to 1.5 mg/kg/d) are associated with a high rate of severe side effects (up to 25%) with more drug withdrawals, drug-related hospitalization, and recurrences (option A). In more difficult cases, aspirin or NSAID, colchicine, and corticosteroids may be used together as a triple therapy to achieve better control of symptoms (option B).[2] After failure of medical therapy, pericardiectomy can be considered (option C), although it should be performed in centers with specific expertise in such surgery to achieve the best outcomes.[3]

66-5. **The answer is D.** (*Hurst's The Heart, 14th Edition, Chap. 66*) Tuberculosis is a major cause of pericarditis in nonindustrialized countries but an uncommon cause in developed countries with a low prevalence of tuberculosis. Tuberculous pericarditis results from hematogenous spread of primary tuberculosis or from the breakdown of infected mediastinal lymph nodes, with the result that affected individuals generally lack the typical symptoms and signs of pulmonary tuberculosis (option A). Early signs include fever, weight loss, and night sweats. Essentially, all causes of pericarditis can manifest as pericardial effusion. In developing countries, tuberculosis continues to be the predominant etiology, accounting for 50% to 60% of cases.[4] Findings suggestive of pericardial effusion with tamponade physiology (that are nonspecific to tuberculous pericardial disease, however) include an elevated pulsus paradoxus (option B) and ECG findings of low QRS voltage and electrical alternans (option C). Bacterial and mycobacterial cultures should be performed if bacterial infection or tuberculosis is suspected, respectively. However, TB is a slow-growing organism, and cultures can take weeks to become positive. Acid-fast bacilli staining (option D), adenosine deaminase, pericardial lysozyme, and interferon-γ levels, as well polymerase chain reaction testing, should be added in the evaluation of tuberculous pericarditis. Nonspecific blood markers of inflammation, such as the erythrocyte sedimentation rate, C-reactive protein (option E), and white blood cell count, usually increase in cases of pericarditis and can support the diagnosis.

66-6. **The answer is B.** *(Hurst's The Heart, 14th Edition, Chap. 66)* Cardiac tamponade corresponds to a corollary of hemodynamic derangements that are secondary to increased intrapericardial pressure. As intrapericardial pressure rises in patients with cardiac tamponade, elevated pericardial pressure is transmitted to all four chambers, affecting diastolic filling. Inspection of the jugular veins will show elevation in central venous pressure (option D); venous distention may or may not be present. Analysis of the venous wave contour will reveal absence or blunting of the *y* descent, representing impaired ventricular diastolic filling (option B).

Cardiac auscultation might reveal distant heart sounds. Because early diastolic filling is profoundly impaired, a third heart sound should not be present (option C); its occurrence suggests an alternative diagnosis. For unclear reasons, tamponade does not usually lead to pulmonary edema (option A); the lungs are often clear on auscultation in patients with isolated cardiac tamponade. Rather, hemodynamic compromise is the more striking finding.

66-7. **The answer is A.** *(Hurst's The Heart, 14th Edition, Chap. 66)* Cardiac tamponade is a cardiac emergency and should be treated with prompt needle pericardiocentesis (option B) unless it is caused by aortic dissection. The goal should be aspiration of all pericardial fluid. The procedure should be done with transthoracic echocardiographic guidance by an experienced operator (option C). During echo-guided pericardiocentesis, the largest collection of fluid in closest proximity to the chest wall should be identified, defining the optimal site for needle entry. Echocardiography also confirms the absence of interposed lung or liver tissue. Complications include cardiac or coronary perforation, hemothorax or liver injury, pneumothorax, and pneumopericardium. The daily output of pericardial fluid is recorded. The pigtail catheter should not be removed until the output is < 30 mL over a 24-hour period (option A). Before the intrapericardial catheter is removed, a limited echocardiogram is often repeated to reassess the effusion size and areas of loculation (option D).

66-8. **The answer is B.** *(Hurst's The Heart, 14th Edition, Chap. 66)* Constrictive pericarditis results from inflammation and/or scarring of the pericardium, leading to impairment of cardiac filling. The disease also appears to favor men over women (2:1 ratio) (option A). Given the abnormal pericardial compliance, diastolic filling is significantly impaired in patients with constrictive pericarditis (steeper increase in pressure per change in volume in the pressure–volume curve). As a consequence, cardiac filling pressures increase, and cardiac output falls as stroke volume decreases. The thickened pericardium has limited expansion, and cardiac chambers "compete" for pericardial space during diastolic filling. With respiration, an increase in preload in one ventricle occurs at the expense of filling in the other (ventricular interdependence) (option B). Patients with constrictive pericarditis typically present with features of right-sided heart failure (option D), manifested by elevated venous pressure, ascites, and leg edema. Orthopnea and paroxysmal nocturnal dyspnea are not usually observed and suggest another etiology (option C).

66-9. **The answer is C.** *(Hurst's The Heart, 14th Edition, Chap. 66)* Although patients presenting with constrictive pericarditis and evidence of active pericardial inflammation (either by CMR or elevated inflammatory markers) might respond to anti-inflammatory therapy (Class IIb recommendation; level of evidence: C) (option A), therapeutic pericardiectomy is the recommended treatment for symptomatic patients with constrictive pericarditis (Class I recommendation; level of evidence: C) (option C). Pericardiectomy is the surgical removal of the pericardium, and the procedure is applicable to all variants of pericardial disease. Some patients presenting with cardiac tamponade demonstrate features of constrictive pericarditis immediately after pericardiocentesis is performed and tamponade relieved, such as in the case of those with effusive constrictive pericarditis. In such cases, therapy should be focused on treating active inflammation; a subset of patients might develop chronic constrictive pericarditis and require pericardiectomy following the pericardiocentesis (option B). Therefore, close follow-up of patients with effusive-constrictive pericarditis is recommended (option D).

66-10. **The answer is B.** *(Hurst's The Heart, 14th Edition, Chap. 66)* Pericardial cysts are smooth, thin-walled structures filled with clear fluid (hence the term spring water cysts) (option A). Patients with pericardial cysts are usually asymptomatic, and the cysts tend not to increase in size (option C). Some patients with pericardial cysts complain of atypical chest pain or dyspnea, most likely as a result of compression of contiguous structures (option D). For patients with symptoms related to the pericardial cyst, percutaneous drainage or surgical removal can be performed (option E).[5] However, given the risks associated with both procedures and the benign, well-tolerated course of the disease, observation is likely most appropriate for the majority of patients with pericardial cysts (option B).

References

1. Adler Y, Charron P, Imazio M, et al. 2015 ESC guidelines for the diagnosis and management of pericardial diseases: the Task Force for the Diagnosis and Management of Pericardial Diseases of the European Society of Cardiology (ESC) endorsed by the European Association for Cardio-Thoracic Surgery (EACTS). *Eur Heart J.* 2015;36(42):2921-2964.
2. Imazio M, Lazaros G, Brucato A, Gaita F. Recurrent pericarditis: new and emerging therapeutic options. *Nat Rev Cardiol.* 2016;13(2):99-105.
3. Khandaker MH, Schaff HV, Greason KL, et al. Pericardiectomy vs medical management in patients with relapsing pericarditis. *Mayo Clin Proc.* 2012;87(11):1062-1070.
4. Syed FF, Ntsekhe M, Mayosi BM. Tailoring diagnosis and management of pericardial disease to the epidemiological setting. *Mayo Clin Proc.* 2010;85(9):866.
5. Najib MQ, Chaliki HP, Raizada A, Ganji JL, Panse PM, Click RL. Symptomatic pericardial cyst: a case series. *Eur J Echocardiogr.* 2011;12(11):E43.

CHAPTER 67

Infective Endocarditis

Patrick R. Lawler

QUESTIONS

DIRECTIONS: Choose the one best response to each question.

67-1. Which of the following statements about infective endocarditis (IE) is *correct*?

A. In developed countries, rheumatic heart disease is the most frequent predisposing cardiac condition for IE

B. The median age of patients with IE has gradually decreased since the preantibiotic era

C. Antibiotics are sufficient treatment for catheter-related bloodstream infections

D. The majority of IE cases in injection drug users involve the right heart

E. Antibiotic prophylaxis before cardiovascular device implantation does not prevent infectious complications

67-2. The pathogenesis of IE includes all of the following *except*:

A. Osler nodes and Janeway lesions are systemic manifestations of immunologically induced vasculitis

B. Bacteria adhere to damaged endothelium by binding extracellular matrix components

C. Host endothelial damage is the key predisposing insult

D. Bacterial proliferation creates dense vegetations on sites of injury

E. Infected emboli can result in satellite areas of infection

67-3. A 65-year-old man receiving hemodialysis for the past 6 months is seen in clinic. He has a fever of 38.5°C and has lost weight. A new heart murmur is auscultated. Which of the following is *not correct* regarding native valve endocarditis (NVE)?

A. *Staphylococcus aureus* is an independent predictor of favorable prognosis in IE

B. Patients on dialysis are at an increased risk for NVE

C. Streptococcal NVE can usually be treated with penicillin monotherapy

D. Enterococcal IE can result from indwelling central venous catheters

E. None of the above are incorrect

67-4. A 56-year-old man presents to clinic with persistent fever, night sweats, and back pain. His past medical history is unremarkable, but a heart murmur is auscultated. Which of the following signs and symptoms is a *major* criterion for the diagnosis of IE according to the modified Duke criteria?

A. Roth spots
B. Osler nodes
C. Positive blood culture
D. Splinter hemorrhages
E. Glomerulonephritis

67-5. Which of the following statements about the modified Duke criteria is *correct*?

A. *Definite* IE is established by evidence of one major criterion

B. The modified Duke criteria account for culture-negative IE

C. Patients with *possible* IE should not be treated until diagnosis is confirmed

D. *Possible* IE is established by evidence of two minor criteria

E. *Definite* IE is established by evidence of one major and one minor criterion

67-6. A 67-year-old woman is brought to the emergency room tachycardic and hypotensive. She reports feeling unwell for the past several weeks with persistent fever. She has a history of intravenous drug use, and the physical examination reveals a heart murmur and some cognitive impairment. A transthoracic echocardiogram confirms the presence of valvular vegetations. Which of the following is *true* regarding the patient's risk for acute complications of IE?

A. Lack of a widened pulse pressure decreases the likelihood that the patient developed heart failure
B. The brain and the spleen are the most common sites of embolization in IE related to intravenous drug use
C. Patients with definite IE should be screened for intracranial mycotic aneurysms because there are no associated signs or symptoms
D. Periannular extension of infection should be considered when there is persistent fever and bacteremia despite antibiotic therapy
E. All of the above are correct

67-7. A 68-year-old male patient is suspected of having native valve endocarditis. Which of the following is *true* regarding blood culture collection and antibiotic initiation?

A. Initial IV antibiotic therapy with nafcillin and gentamicin should continue until the causative organism is identified
B. Antiplatelet therapy to prevent embolic complications is needed until antibiotic therapy can be initiated
C. Outpatient oral antibiotic therapy with ampicillin is recommended until the pathogen is identified
D. No treatment should be initiated until blood cultures confirm the causative organism
E. None of the above are appropriate treatments

67-8. After several weeks of treatment with parenteral antibiotics, a 60-year-old female patient with native valve endocarditis is *not* improving, and other therapeutic options are considered. Which of the following constitutes a Class I indication for surgery?

A. The patient suffered a major intracranial hemorrhage
B. The patient has a mobile vegetation > 10 mm in size
C. The patient has persistent bacteremia and fever even after seven days of appropriate antibiotics
D. The patient is an IV drug user
E. All of the above

67-9. All of the following are associated with unfavorable prognosis in patients with infective endocarditis *except*:

A. Female gender
B. Diabetes mellitus
C. Serum creatinine > 2.0 mg/dL
D. *Staphylococcus aureus* infection
E. Low Acute Physiology and Chronic Health Evaluation (APACHE) II score

67-10. For which of the following procedures would it be *inappropriate* to use antibiotic prophylaxis for the prevention of IE?

A. Heart valve replacement
B. GI/genitourinary tract procedures
C. Tonsillectomy
D. Dental procedures involving gingival tissue
E. Surgical procedures that involve infected skin

67-1. **The answer is D.** *(Hurst's The Heart, 14th Edition, Chap. 67)* Infective endocarditis (IE) is a disease caused by a microbial infection involving the endothelial lining of intracardiac structures such as the heart valves. In developing countries, rheumatic heart disease remains the most frequent predisposing cardiac condition (option A). However, the epidemiologic features of IE in developed countries have changed considerably in recent decades. The aging of the population has been paralleled by increases in the prevalence of degenerative heart valve disease and in the use of prosthetic heart valves and other intracardiac devices. The median age of patients with IE has gradually increased from 30 to 40 years in the preantibiotic era to 47 to 69 years in the late 20th century (option B). IE is also a dreaded complication of injection (intravenous) drug use. The distinctive feature of IE in intravenous drug users is that it often involves the right heart (option D), with 60% to 70% of cases involving the tricuspid valve. The tricuspid valve may be particularly susceptible to bacterial infection as a result of chronic degenerative changes caused by the repetitive injection of irritants (eg, talcum) into peripheral veins. In the case of catheter-related bloodstream infections, treatment with antibiotics alone yields poor results (option C), and removal of infected catheters or grafts is necessary in most circumstances. A retrospective analysis of patients undergoing pacemaker implantation suggests that antibiotic prophylaxis before device implantation can prevent infectious complications (option E).

67-2. **The answer is A.** *(Hurst's The Heart, 14th Edition, Chap. 67)* Normal vascular endothelium resists colonization by bacteria. Damaged vascular endothelium can be colonized by circulating bacteria. The hallmark of IE is persistent endocardial or endovascular infection causing continuous bacteremia. There are substantial experimental data to suggest that host endothelial damage is the key predisposing insult (option C), with subsequent platelet and fibrin deposition and creation of a receptive milieu for bacterial colonization during episodes of transient bacteremia. Bacteria that have entered the bloodstream must be able to adhere to the damaged endothelium, exposed extracellular matrix, or areas of fibrin deposition.[1] This adherence is mediated by microbial surface components recognizing adhesive matrix molecules (option B), which, in turn, recognize a variety of host proteins such as fibronectin, collagen, and integrins. Once adherent, repetitive cycles of bacterial proliferation, fibrin-platelet deposition, and host tissue destruction create an infected vegetation (option D), within which bacteria can reach extremely high concentrations. The various systemic manifestations of IE are the result of showers of bacteria-laden emboli that often result in satellite areas of infection with subsequent abscess formation (option E). Janeway lesions are the result of infected emboli, whereas Osler nodes are the result of immunologically induced vasculitis (option A).

67-3. **The answer is A.** *(Hurst's The Heart, 14th Edition, Chap. 67)* A wide range of microorganisms can cause IE, but only a few species account for the vast majority of cases. Streptococci and staphylococci are the cause of > 80% of IE cases in which a responsible organism is identified. Meanwhile, the *Enterococcus* species are responsible for 5% to 18% of cases of native valve IE. The incidence of enterococcal endocarditis appears to be rising, likely as a result of the increased genitourinary and GI instrumentation in older adults and the increased use of indwelling central venous catheters and prosthetic implants (option D). Although only a fraction of patients with *Staphylococcus aureus* bacteremia will develop NVE, populations at increased risk include patients on dialysis (option B), patients with type 1 diabetes, burn victims, persons with HIV, and IDU. *Staphylococcus aureus* as a causative organism is an independent predictor of poor prognosis in IE (option A) and is associated with a 25% to 30% mortality. In contrast, viridans streptococci are usually highly sensitive to penicillin, as defined by a minimum inhibitory concentration of < 0.1 µg/mL, and thus they can often be eradicated with penicillin monotherapy (option C).

67-4. The answer is C. (*Hurst's The Heart, 14th Edition, Chap. 67*) Although the history and physical examination are useful, the diagnosis of IE rests on the ability to demonstrate endocardial involvement and persistent bacteremia. Along with the clinical and echocardiographic features, the microbiology is the foundation for the modified Duke criteria and constitutes a major criterion for the diagnosis of IE (option C). Minor criteria include classic IE-related findings such as mucosal or conjunctival petechiae, splinter hemorrhages of the nail beds (option D), Janeway lesions, Osler nodes (option B), Roth spots (option A), and urinary red cell casts suggestive of glomerulonephritis (option E). Definitions of specific criteria and terms used in the modified Duke criteria are detailed in Table 67-1.

TABLE 67-1 **Definition of Terms Used in the Proposed Modified Duke Criteria for the Diagnosis of Infective Endocarditis**

Major criteria
Blood culture positive for IE
Typical microorganisms consistent with IE from 2 separate blood cultures:
Viridans streptococci, *Streptococcus bovis*, HACEK group, *Staphylococcus aureus*; or
Community-acquired enterococci in the absence of a primary focus; or
Microorganisms consistent with IE from persistently positive blood cultures, defined as follows:
At least 2 positive cultures of blood samples drawn more than 12 h apart; or
All of 3 or a majority of greater than 4 separate cultures of blood (with first and last sample drawn at least 1 h apart)
Single positive blood culture for *Coxiella brunetti* or anti–phase 1 IgG antibody titer > 1:800
Evidence of endocardial involvement
Echocardiogram positive for IE (TEE recommended in patients with prosthetic valves, rated at least "possible IE" by clinical criteria, or complicated IE [paravalvular abscess]; TTE as first test in other patients), defined as follows:
Oscillating intracardiac mass on valve or supporting structures, in the path of regurgitant jets, or on implanted material in the absence of an alternative anatomic explanation; or
Abscess; or
New partial dehiscence of prosthetic valve
New valvular regurgitation (worsening or changing of pre-existing murmur not sufficient)
Minor criteria
Predisposition, predisposing heart condition, or injection drug use
Fever, temperature > 100.4°F (38°C)
Vascular phenomena, major arterial emboli, septic pulmonary infarcts, mycotic aneurysm, intracranial hemorrhage, conjunctival hemorrhages, and Janeway lesions
Immunologic phenomena; glomerulonephritis, Osler nodes, Roth spots, and rheumatoid factor
Microbiologic evidence: positive blood culture but does not meet a major criterion,[a] or serologic evidence of active infection with organism consistent with IE
Echocardiographic minor criteria eliminated

Abbreviations: HACEK, *Haemophilus* species, *Actinobacillus, Cardiobacterium hominis, Eikenella corrodens,* and *Kingella* species; IE, infective endocarditis; Ig, immunoglobulin; TEE, transesophageal echocardiography; TTE, transthoracic echocardiography.

[a]Excludes single positive cultures for coagulase-negative staphylococci and organisms that do not cause endocarditis.

Reproduced with permission from Li JS, Sexton DJ, Mick N, et al. Proposed modifications to the Duke criteria for the diagnosis of infective endocarditis, *Clin Infect Dis.* 2000 Apr;30(4):633-638.

67-5. The answer is B. (*Hurst's The Heart, 14th Edition, Chap. 67*) In 1994, Durack and colleagues published the Duke criteria[2] for the diagnosis of IE that incorporated clinical factors as well as echocardiographic data. These criteria were revised in 2000 to increase the sensitivity for detection of cases related to *Staphylococcus aureus* bacteremia, and to account for culture-negative IE (option B).[3] A diagnosis of definite IE is established clinically by evidence of two major criteria, one major plus three minor criteria, or five minor criteria (options A and E). Patients identified with possible IE (one major criterion plus one minor criterion or three minor criteria) (option D) should be treated for IE until the diagnosis is satisfactorily excluded (option C). Application of these criteria in clinical practice will capture the vast majority of cases of IE and render quite remote the possibility of missing a potential case.

67-6. **The answer is D.** (*Hurst's The Heart, 14th Edition, Chap. 67*) Complication rates with IE have remained relatively unchanged despite advances in diagnosis and antimicrobial therapy. Heart failure is the most frequent major complication of IE, but examination findings may be masked by its severity. Although a widened pulse pressure can suggest aortic insufficiency complicating IE, this finding is nonspecific (option A). Embolization is a frequent complication of IE. The brain and the spleen are the most common sites of embolization in left-sided IE, whereas septic pulmonary emboli are common in right-sided IE related to intravenous drug use (option B). Mycotic aneurysms (MAs) represent a small but extremely dangerous subset of embolic complications. The presenting symptoms of intracranial MAs are highly variable and can range from a localized headache to dense neurologic deficits resulting from sudden intracranial hemorrhage. Routine screening of patients with definite IE for the presence of intracranial MAs is not currently recommended (option C), and neurologic imaging is reserved for symptomatic patients. Extension or spread of infection beyond the valve annulus is a potentially very dangerous development that usually presages the need for surgical therapy. Findings such as persistent fever and bacteremia despite antibiotic therapy, heart failure, or new conduction block should raise an immediate suspicion for this complication (option D).

67-7. **The answer is A.** (*Hurst's The Heart, 14th Edition, Chap. 67*) Rapid institution of appropriate parenteral antibiotic therapy is the single most important initial intervention in the treatment of suspected or proven IE (option D). The lesions of IE are extremely difficult to eradicate because the infection exists in a sequestered area of impaired host defense. Thus IE requires weeks of parenteral antibiotic therapy, preferably with a drug that has bactericidal activity against the offending organism. Initial empiric antibiotic therapy (ie, before blood culture results are available) should cover *Staphylococcus aureus* and the many species of streptococci that can cause IE, with consideration of *E faecalis* in certain circumstances. Thus, a combination of a β-lactamase–resistant penicillin (nafcillin)—or vancomycin for penicillin-allergic patients—and gentamicin is often used (option A). Patients should remain in an inpatient setting during the initial phase of treatment when complications are most likely to occur, after which appropriate patients can be considered for outpatient parenteral antibiotic therapy (option C). There are no clinical studies that support the use of either antiplatelet or antithrombin agents to prevent embolic complications or hasten antibiotic cure (option B). Moreover, small uncontrolled studies suggest that antithrombin therapy actually increases the risk of intracranial hemorrhage after CNS embolization.

67-8. **The answer is C.** (*Hurst's The Heart, 14th Edition, Chap. 67*) The decision for surgical intervention in the treatment of IE can be extremely challenging. The most recent American College of Cardiology/American Heart Association guidelines for surgery in IE are summarized in Table 67-2. Surgery is reasonable for patients with recurrent emboli and persistent vegetations and for patients with persistent bacteremia despite several days (5–7 days) of appropriate antibiotic therapy in the absence of a metastatic focus of infection (option C). Surgery to prevent embolization can be considered for treatment of large (> 1.0 cm), mobile vegetations, particularly in high-volume cardiac surgical centers with expertise in primary valve repair (Class II indication) (option B). It is reasonable to avoid surgery when possible in patients who are IV drug users (Class IIa indication). In cases with intracerebral hemorrhage, the neurologic prognosis is worse, and surgery is usually postponed for at least 1 month (option A).

TABLE 67-2 Indications for Surgery for Native Valve Endocarditis

Class I

1. Early surgery (during initial hospitalization and before completion of a full course of antibiotics) is indicated in patients with IE who present with valve dysfunction resulting in symptoms of heart failure. CLASS I

2. Early surgery should be considered particularly in patients with IE caused by fungal or highly resistant organisms (eg, vancomycin-resistant *Enterococcus*, multidrug-resistant gram-negative bacilli). CLASS I

3. Early surgery is indicated in patients with IE complicated by heart block, annular or cardiac or aortic abscess, or destructive penetrating lesions. CLASS I

4. Early surgery is indicated for evidence of persistent infection (manifested by persistent bacteremia or fever lasting > 5-7 days and provided that other sites of infection and fever have been excluded) after the start of appropriate antibiotics. CLASS I

Class II

5. Early surgery is reasonable in patients who present with recurrent emboli and persistent or enlarging vegetations despite appropriate antibiotic therapy. CLASS IIa

6. Early surgery is reasonable in patients with severe valve regurgitation and mobile vegetations > 10 mm. CLASS IIa

7. Early surgery may be considered in patients with mobile vegetations > 10 mm, particularly when involving the anterior leaflet of the mitral valve and associated with other relative indications for surgery. CLASS IIb

Valve Surgery in Patients with Right-Sided IE

1. Surgical intervention is reasonable for patients with certain complications (eg, heart failure, recurrent emboli, resistant organisms). CLASS IIa

2. Valve repair rather than replacement should be performed when feasible. CLASS I

3. If valve replacement is performed, then an individualized choice of prosthesis by the surgeon is reasonable. CLASS IIa

4. If is reasonable to avoid surgery when possible in patients who are IV drug users. CLASS IIa

Valve Surgery in Patients with Prior Emboli/Hemorrhage/Stroke

1. Valve surgery may be considered in IE patients with stroke or subclinical cerebral emboli and residual vegetation without delay if intracranial hemorrhage has been excluded by imaging studies and neurologic damage is not severe. CLASS IIb

2. In patients with major ischemic stroke or intracranial hemorrhage, it is reasonable to delay valve surgery for at least 4 weeks. CLASS IIa

Abbreviations: IE, infective endocarditis; IV, intravenous.
Data from Baddour LM, Wilson WR, Bayer AS, et al. Infective endocarditis in adults: diagnosis, antimicrobial therapy, and management of complications: a scientific statement for healthcare professionals from the American Heart Association, *Circulation*. 2015 Oct 13;132(15):1435-1486.

67-9. **The answer is E.** (*Hurst's The Heart, 14th Edition, Chap. 67*) Patients with IE are an extremely heterogeneous group, with varying comorbidities, causative organisms, and complications. Accurate prognostic classification may help inform individual treatment decisions. Chu and colleagues analyzed 267 consecutive cases of definite IE and found the following factors to be independently predictive of death: diabetes mellitus (option B), *Staphylococcus aureus* as the causative organism (option D), an embolic event, and increased Acute Physiology and Chronic Health Evaluation (APACHE) II score.[4] In a separate analysis, a group found that in addition to age, female sex (option A), serum creatinine > 2.0 mg/dL (option C), moderate or severe heart failure, and vegetation length > 1.5 cm were independent predictors of 1-year mortality.

67-10. **The answer is B.** (*Hurst's The Heart, 14th Edition, Chap. 67*) The specific procedures for which antibiotic prophylaxis is recommended in the absence of an intercurrent infection are listed in Table 67-3. Briefly, antibiotic prophylaxis is recommended for all dental procedures that involve manipulation of gingival tissue or the periapical region of teeth or perforation of the oral mucosa (option D). It is likewise recommended for invasive procedures of the respiratory tract that involve incision or biopsy of the respiratory mucosa, such as tonsillectomy (option C), and surgical procedures that involve infected skin (option E), skin structure, or musculoskeletal tissue. All patients who undergo heart valve replacement (option A) or who receive an intravascular graft or intracardiac device should receive

TABLE 67-3 Procedures for Which Antibiotic Prophylaxis Is Recommended for High-Risk Patients

A. Dental: All dental procedures that involve manipulation of gingival tissue or the periapical region of teeth or perforation of the oral mucosa. The following procedures and events do not need antibiotic prophylaxis: routine anesthetic injections through noninfected tissue, taking dental radiographs, placement of removable prosthodontic or orthodontic appliances, adjustment of orthodontic appliances, placement of orthodontic brackets, shedding of deciduous teeth, and bleeding from trauma to the lips or oral mucosa.

B. Respiratory tract: Invasive procedures of the respiratory tract that involve incision or biopsy of the respiratory mucosa, such as tonsillectomy or adenoidectomy. Routine prophylaxis for bronchoscopy is not recommended unless the procedure involves incision of the respiratory tract mucosa.

C. Infected skin or musculoskeletal: Surgical procedures that involve infected skin, skin structure, or musculoskeletal tissue.

Data from Baddour LM, Wilson WR, Bayer AS, et al. Infective endocarditis in adults: diagnosis, antimicrobial therapy, and management of complications: a scientific statement for healthcare professionals from the American Heart Association, *Circulation.* 2015 Oct 13;132(15):1435-1486.

periprocedural prophylaxis with an antistaphylococcal agent. The revised guidelines stipulate that antibiotic prophylaxis solely to prevent IE is no longer recommended for GI/genitourinary tract procedures (option B), for no published data demonstrate a conclusive link between these procedures and the development of IE.

References

1. Moreillon P, Que YA, Bayer AS. Pathogenesis of streptococcal and staphylococcal endocarditis. *Infect Dis Clin North Am.* 2002;16:297-318.
2. Durack DT, Lukes AS, Bright DK. New criteria for diagnosis of infective endocarditis: utilization of specific echocardiographic findings. Duke Endocarditis Service. *Am J Med.* 1994;96:200-209.
3. Li JS, Sexton DJ, Mick N, et al. Proposed modifications to the Duke criteria for the diagnosis of infective endocarditis. *Clin Infect Dis.* 2000;30:633-638.
4. Chu VH, Cabell CH, Benjamin DK Jr, et al. Early predictors of in-hospital death in infective endocarditis. *Circulation.* 2004;109:1745-1749.

SECTION 11

Heart Failure

CHAPTER 68

Pathophysiology of Heart Failure

Ravi Karra

QUESTIONS

DIRECTIONS: Choose the one best response to each question.

68-1. Which of the following is *true* of heart failure with preserved ejection fraction (HFpEF)?

A. HFpEF only affects a minority of patients with heart failure
B. HFpEF is defined as having a left ventricular ejection fraction (LVEF) > 55%
C. Therapies that are effective for heart failure with reduced ejection fraction (HFrEF) are not as effective for HFpEF
D. Diagnostic criteria for HFpEF are well defined
E. None of the above are true

68-2. Which of the following molecular changes are associated with a failing heart?

A. α-MHC is upregulated and β-MHC is downregulated
B. Action potential duration is shortened in patients with HF
C. Ca^{2+} uptake and release are dysregulated
D. Oxidative phosphorylation is increased
E. All of the above

68-3. Which of the following is *true* of neurohormonal activation with heart failure?

A. The sympathetic nervous system is activated early in the disease process
B. The renin-angiotensin-aldosterone system (RAAS) is activated
C. Neurohormonal activation results in sodium and water retention
D. Persistent neurohormonal activation can lead to myocyte death
E. All of the above are true

68-4. Which of the following is *true* of changes to signaling pathways with HFrEF?

A. β-adrenergic receptors are desensitized and uncoupled
B. Angiotensin II levels are elevated
C. Elevated arginine vasopressin (AVP) levels are associated with poor outcomes
D. The inflammasome is activated
E. All of the above

68-5. Which of the following is *true* of natriuretic peptide signaling in HFrEF?

A. Atrial natriuretic peptide (ANP) is only produced by the atria
B. NT-proBNP is the uncleaved precursor to BNP
C. Neprilysin inhibitors inhibit the degradation of natriuretic peptides
D. BNP guided therapy improves heart failure outcomes
E. C and D

68-6. Which of the following is *not true* of myocardial remodeling in HFrEF?

A. The force-frequency relationship is preserved
B. The Frank–Starling curve flattens
C. Left ventricular (LV) elasticity is reduced
D. The LV eventually becomes more sensitive to afterload than to preload
E. Cardiomyocytes adopt a more fetal-like state

68-7. Which of the following is *true* of diastolic function in patients with HFpEF?

A. The LV relaxation constant tau (τ) is decreased
B. E/A reversal is observed on echocardiographic assessment of the transmitral flow velocity pattern
C. Impaired LV relaxation can lead to exercise intolerance
D. LV elastance is decreased
E. C and D

68-8. Which of the following is *true* regarding the molecular basis for HFpEF?

A. Ca^{2+} uptake into the sarcoplasmic reticulum (SR) is increased

B. β-adrenergic signaling is increased

C. Protein kinase A activity is increased

D. Increased deposition of extracellular matrix (ECM) contributes to diastolic stiffness

E. There is increased phosphorylation of titin

68-9. A 68-year-old man with advanced class IV HFrEF is more and more volume overloaded, although his weight has remained the same. Which of the following is *true* of cardiac cachexia?

A. Cachexia may be related to altered nutritional absorption

B. Decreased levels of TNF-α are associated with sarcopenia and fat

C. Adiponectin levels are decreased

D. High cholesterol is associated with an adverse prognosis

E. LV mass increases

68-10. A 68-year-old man is admitted to the inpatient cardiology ward with acute decompensated heart failure. His serum creatinine is nearly double that of his baseline value. Which of the following is *not true* regarding cardiorenal interaction?

A. Neurohormonal activation leads to excessive salt and water retention by the kidney

B. Cardiac output correlates well with the estimated glomerular filtration rate at baseline

C. Increased renal venous pressures result in a decreased perfusion gradient across the glomerular capillary network

D. Right ventricular dysfunction may contribute to cardiorenal syndrome by impeding LV filling

E. All of the above are true

ANSWERS

68-1. The answer is C. (*Hurst's The Heart, 14th Edition, Chap. 68*) Approximately half of heart failure (HF) patients have HFrEF and half have HFpEF (option A). A diagnosis of HFpEF is typically based on the ejection fraction of the left ventricle (LV) on cardiac imaging. The cutoff LVEF by which to distinguish HFrEF from HFpEF is not well established, but clinical trials (the same trials that have either supported or refuted a specific HF therapy for use) have used LVEF ≤ 35% to 40% to define HFrEF and LVEF ≥ 40% to 50% to define HFpEF (options B and D).[1-8] It is important to distinguish between HFpEF and HFrEF because therapies that have a proven mortality and morbidity benefit in patients with HFrEF do not appear to be effective in patients with HFpEF, and to some extent these conditions may have fundamentally different pathophysiologic mechanisms and phenotypes (option C).[4,5,7,9,10]

68-2. The answer is C. (*Hurst's The Heart, 14th Edition, Chap. 68*) Two myosin heavy-chain (MHC) isoforms are present in the mammalian heart, α- and β-MHC. The α-MHC is cardiac specific and is more enzymatically active. The less active β-MHC is present in the heart and in slow-twitch skeletal muscle. The distribution of α- and β-MHC is developmentally and hormonally regulated. Mechanical stress, such as pressure overload, induces an α- to β-MHC transition in the ventricles of experimental animals, thus imparting a slower but more economical type of work for the overloaded heart (option A). A common feature of both animal and human models of HF is prolongation of the action potential (option B). Both decreased sodium influx and potassium efflux are contributory and are mediated by reduced activity of the myocardial membrane (also known as sarcolemma) sodium and potassium channels, respectively. Key defects in SR Ca^{2+} uptake and release are present in HF, including dysregulation of RyR, RyR2/Ca^{2+} release channel macromolecular complexes, and the SR calcium transport proteins, especially the sarcoplasmic-endoplasmic reticulum calcium ATPase (SERCA) and phospholamban, a reversible inhibitor of cardiac SR Ca^{2+}-ATPase activity.[11] Many abnormalities and inefficiencies in myocardial energy metabolism have been shown to occur in HF; these include altered energy substrate with an increased dependence on glucose, decreased oxidative phosphorylation, and high-energy phosphate and mitochondrial dysfunction (option D).[12]

68-3. The answer is E. (*Hurst's The Heart, 14th Edition, Chap. 68*) The neurohormonal system is one of the first activated responses to myocardial injury or to changes in cardiac loading. Decreased cardiac output (any combination of decreased blood pressure, pulse pressure, and perfusion) is sensed by various mechanoreceptors throughout the body, including the LV, carotid sinus, aortic arch, and afferent renal arterioles. When there is diminished activation of these receptors, as in HF, the neurohormonal system is activated in an attempt to maintain cardiac output and vital organ perfusion. The sympathetic nervous system is activated early, followed by the RAAS (options A and B). Nonosmotic release of AVP (also known as vasopressin or antidiuretic hormone) and underfilling of renal arterial bed result in sodium and water retention (option C).[13] Heightened peripheral vasoconstriction, increased myocardial contractility and heart rate, and increased blood volume restore cardiac output and arterial pressure in the short term. However, sustained and unopposed neurohormonal activation has many important adverse consequences at the cellular level, including facilitation of myocyte hypertrophy, collagen synthesis, and fibrosis, as well as promoting apoptosis and return to fetal isoforms of contractile proteins.[14-18] Cardiac myocyte necrosis also occurs in response to pathophysiologic levels of endogenous and low-dose exogenous angiotensin II infusion (option D).[19]

68-4. The answer is E. (*Hurst's The Heart, 14th Edition, Chap. 68*) The β-adrenergic receptor abnormalities in HF appear to be caused by desensitization and uncoupling of the β1-receptor produced by local rather than systemic alterations in catecholamines (option A). The RAAS plays a pivotal role in the pathogenesis of HF, and consistent benefit has been derived from ACE inhibitor, angiotensin II receptor blocker (ARB), and aldosterone antagonist therapy in HF patients.[20] Mechanisms responsible for the release of renin from the renal cortex have been exhaustively studied; they include increased sympathetic drive in the kidneys, β-adrenergic receptor activation, and actual or perceived hypovolemia with hyponatremia or hypochloremia at the level of renal macula densa or arteriole.[21-23] Renin proteolytic enzyme has little biologic activity, but it interacts with angiotensinogen to split off two amino acids to form angiotensin I. This is then cleaved by ACE (distributed widely in the vascular system, especially the lungs) to produce angiotensin II, a peptide with a vast range of biologic activities (option B). HF is often characterized by water retention in excess of sodium retention, leading to hyponatremia. The hyponatremia is caused in part by the nonosmotic release of AVP (also known as vasopressin or antidiuretic hormone) from the neurosecretory cells located in the hypothalamus; AVP acts on the kidneys to reduce free water clearance and to promote vasoconstriction. Hyponatremia is a powerful predictor of poor outcomes in HF, and elevated AVP levels in HF patients are associated with severe HF (option C). The inflammasome is a macromolecular structure that plays a central role in the inflammatory response to injury by first sensing the injury and then amplifying the inflammatory response by activating powerful cytokines. This activation of the inflammasome in the heart in the setting of injury may promote adverse ventricular remodeling and HF (option D).[24]

68-5. The answer is C. *(Hurst's The Heart, 14th Edition, Chap. 68)* ANP and BNP are often increased in patients with HF, and this has been leveraged to assist in the diagnosis of acute HF.[25] ANP is a 28-amino-acid peptide that is normally synthesized and stored in the atria and to some extent in the ventricles (option A). It is released into the circulation during atrial distension. BNP is synthesized mainly by the ventricles and is released with LV dysfunction or early HF after cleavage (presumably by a protease, corin or furin) from the propeptide to BNP and NT-proBNP (option B).[26] Recently, drugs designed to inhibit the degradation of natriuretic peptides (neutral endopeptidase or neprilysin inhibitor), among other effects, have been combined with ARBs (sacubitril/valsartan) and have shown mortality and morbidity benefit in HF (option C).[27] The powerful prognostic role of BNP in patients with HF has raised hope that BNP-guided HF therapy can improve outcomes. However, the recently completed GUIDE-IT study failed to show any benefit in using BNP values to guide HF treatment.[28]

68-6. The answer is A. *(Hurst's The Heart, 14th Edition, Chap. 68)* The failing heart undergoes several physiologic and structural changes termed *remodeling*. Normally, an increase in the frequency of stimulation and heart rate is accompanied by an increased rate of force development, a decreased duration of contraction, and an enhanced rate of relaxation (Bowditch effect). This tends to preserve or increase contractile force while preserving diastolic filling time. In the setting of HF, an increase in stimulation and heart rate is accompanied by a decrease in the rate of myocardial performance (option A). In systolic LV dysfunction, the extent of shortening for a given diastolic fiber length and afterload is reduced. Thus, in end-stage HF in the intact circulation, the Frank–Starling curve flattens (option B). Furthermore, the dilated LV can lose elasticity, like an overstretched elastic band (option C). As a result, the failing heart gradually becomes less sensitive to preload (EDV and fiber length) and more sensitive to afterload stress (option D). Finally, reprogramming of the cardiac myocytes occurs, resulting in a more fetal-like state (option E).

68-7. The answer is C. *(Hurst's The Heart, 14th Edition, Chap. 68)* Tau (t) is the time constant of relaxation that describes the rate of LV pressure changes during isovolemic relaxation. Normally, tau is < 40 milliseconds, and the larger the tau, the more impaired is the relaxation (option A). Echocardiography can be used to assess diastolic indices. Commonly, the ratio of early (E) filling to the atrial filling (A) across the mitral valve in diastole is used. Depending on the degree of diastolic dysfunction the E/A ratio can be reversed or pseudo-normalized (Figure 68-1). Thus, the E/A ratio by itself cannot determine diastolic dysfunction (option B). In the setting of impaired LV relaxation, there is evidence of chronotropic incompetence and impaired myocardial reserve during exercise as well as an increase in

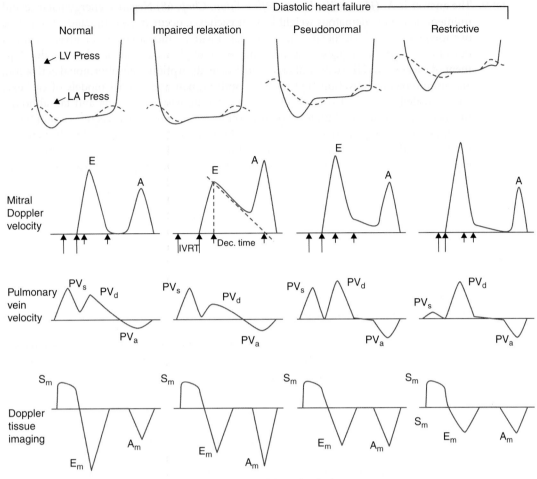

FIGURE 68-1 Doppler echocardiographic evidence of diastolic dysfunction.

Abbreviations: Am = atrial mitral annulus velocity; Em = early mitral annulus velocity; IVRT = isovolemic relaxation time; LA = left atrium; LV = left ventricle; PVa = atrial pulmonary vein flow velocity; PVd = diastolic pulmonary vein flow velocity; PVs = systolic pulmonary vein flow velocity; Sm = systolic mitral annulus velocity. (Reproduced with permission from Faggiano P, Vizzardi E, Pulcini E, et al. The study of left ventricular diastolic function by Doppler echocardiography: the essential for the clinician, *Heart international.* 2007;3(1-2):42-50.)

LV diastolic pressures when heart rate and blood pressure increase in response to exercise (option C).[29,30] With increased stiffness of the LV or impaired elastance, there is an increase in LA pressures, pulmonary venous pressure, and congestion. Elastance is the ability of the LV to stretch and recoil with the distending intraventricular force on the myocardium. Elastance is the inverse of compliance, and elastance is defined as dP/dV. With diastolic dysfunction, there is a larger LV pressure for a given change in volume (option D).

68-8. **The answer is D.** *(Hurst's The Heart, 14th Edition, Chap. 68)* For the myofiber to lengthen during diastole, the actin-myosin cross-bridges have to detach in an active, ATP-dependent process. This process involves close and rapid regulation of cytosolic Ca^{2+}. In animal models of HFpEF, there appears to be reduced Ca^{2+} reuptake into the SR via decreased SERCA activity, impaired β-adrenergic signaling leading to reduced protein kinase A activity, increased protein kinase C via protein phosphatases, and elevated catecholamine activation (options A, B, and C).[31,32] Extracellular matrix surrounding myofibers contains fibrillar proteins such as collagen type I and III, elastin, proteoglycans, and the basement membrane proteins laminin and fibronectin and contributes significantly to LV diastolic stiffness (option D).[33] Another factor affecting LV diastolic stiffness is titin, a large protein that acts as a spring in the heart's scaffolding. Change in titin isoforms or decreased phosphorylation of titin can raise the resting tension of biopsied human myocytes (option E).[34,35]

68-9. The answer is A. *(Hurst's The Heart, 14th Edition, Chap. 68)* Negative energy balance and unintentional, nonedematous weight loss, or cachexia, occur in an estimated 13% to 35% of patients with HF.[36] Cachexia is also associated with an increased risk of adverse clinical outcomes.[37,38] Studies suggest that there may be multiple factors involved in the development of cachexia in HF, such as altered nutritional absorption, neurohormonal activation, and immunologic activation (option A).[39] Both human and animal models of cachexia have revealed that elevated levels of TNF-α correlate with sarcopenia and fat, although the mechanism is not well understood (option B).[39,40] Adipose tissue secretes a number of cytokines, including adiponectin. Elevated adiponectin level is associated with increased mortality and is probably a marker of wasting (option C).[41] Moreover, low rather than high cholesterol levels are associated with a poor outcome in patients with chronic HF (option D). In HF, whole-body protein synthesis seems to be suppressed, and breakdown of myofibrillar protein, principally leg skeletal muscle, is increased. A significant decrease in LV mass also occurs in patients with cardiac cachexia (option E).[42]

68-10. The answer is B. *(Hurst's The Heart, 14th Edition, Chap. 68)* The interaction between the heart and the kidney is bidirectional, with the heart affecting the renal function and the kidneys affecting the cardiac function.[43] A number of mechanisms may be involved, including neurohormonal activation, reduced renal perfusion, and increased renal venous pressures. Activation of the neurohormonal system, including the activation of the sympathetic nervous system and RAAS system, release of vasopressin, and ET-1 lead to excessive salt and water retention and vasoconstriction and overwhelm the counter-regulatory systems (option A). However, such vasoconstriction also results in increased afterload and reduces cardiac output. Decreased cardiac output can further contribute to reduced renal perfusion in a vicious cycle. However, the relationship between decreased cardiac output and decreased renal perfusion may not be a simple one; evidence suggests that an invasive measure of cardiac output does not correlate well with estimated glomerular filtration rate at baseline, and a change in cardiac output did not correlate with a change in renal function at moderate cardiac dysfunction, but may correlate in severely reduced cardiac output states (option B).[44] More importantly, both animal and human models have shown that increased renal venous pressures resulting in a decreased perfusion gradient across the glomerular capillary network in accordance with the Poiseuille law may cause a reduction in renal function (option C).[45-49] Right ventricular dilation and systolic dysfunction have also been suggested as other mechanisms of cardiorenal syndrome through elevated central venous pressure as well as interventricular interaction impeding LV filling caused by increased right-sided pressures (option D).[50]

References

1. SOLVD Investigators, Yusuf S, Pitt B, et al. Effect of enalapril on survival in patients with reduced left ventricular ejection fractions and congestive heart failure. *N Engl J Med*. 1991;325(5):293-302.
2. Effect of metoprolol CR/XL in chronic heart failure: Metoprolol CR/XL Randomised Intervention Trial in Congestive Heart Failure (MERIT-HF). *Lancet*. 1999;353(9169):2001-2007.
3. Pitt B, Pfeffer MA, Assmann SF, et al. Spironolactone for heart failure with preserved ejection fraction. *N Engl J Med*. 2014;370(15):1383-1392.
4. Massie BM, Carson PE, McMurray JJ, et al. Irbesartan in patients with heart failure and preserved ejection fraction. *N Engl J Med*. 2008;359(23):2456-2467.
5. Yusuf S, Pfeffer MA, Swedberg K, et al. Effects of candesartan in patients with chronic heart failure and preserved left-ventricular ejection fraction: the CHARM-Preserved Trial. *Lancet*. 2003;362(9386):777-781.
6. Redfield MM, Chen HH, Borlaug BA, et al. Effect of phosphodiesterase-5 inhibition on exercise capacity and clinical status in heart failure with preserved ejection fraction: a randomized clinical trial. *JAMA*. 2013;309(12):1268-1277.
7. Redfield MM, Anstrom KJ, Levine JA, et al. Isosorbide mononitrate in heart failure with preserved ejection fraction. *N Engl J Med*. 2015;373(24):2314-2324.
8. Kelly JP, Mentz RJ, Mebazaa A, et al. Patient selection in heart failure with preserved ejection fraction clinical trials. *J Am Coll Cardiol*. 2015;65(16):1668-1682.
9. Hernandez AF, Hammill BG, O'Connor CM, et al. Clinical effectiveness of beta-blockers in heart failure: findings from the OPTIMIZE-HF (Organized Program to Initiate Lifesaving Treatment in Hospitalized Patients with Heart Failure) registry. *J Am Coll Cardiol*. 2009;53(2):184-192.

10. Cleland JG, Tendera M, Adamus J, et al. The perindopril in elderly people with chronic heart failure (PEP-CHF) study. *Eur Heart J.* 2006;27(19):2338-2345.

11. Marks AR. Calcium cycling proteins and heart failure: mechanisms and therapeutics. *J Clin Invest.* 2013;123(1):46-52.

12. Ardehali H, Sabbah HN, Burke MA, et al. Targeting myocardial substrate metabolism in heart failure: potential for new therapies. *Eur J Heart Fail.* 2012;14(2):120-129.

13. Chen HH, Schrier RW. Pathophysiology of volume overload in acute heart failure syndromes. *Am J Med.* 2006;119(12 Suppl 1):S11-S16.

14. Dube P, Weber KT. Congestive heart failure: pathophysiologic consequences of neurohormonal activation and the potential for recovery: part I. *Am J Med Sci.* 2011;342(5):348-351.

15. Dube P, Weber KT. Congestive heart failure: pathophysiologic consequences of neurohormonal activation and the potential for recovery: part II. *Am J Med Sci.* 2011;342(6):503-506.

16. Hunter JJ, Chien KR. Signaling pathways for cardiac hypertrophy and failure. *N Engl J Med.* 1999;341(17):1276-1283.

17. Weber KT, Brilla CG. Pathological hypertrophy and cardiac interstitium. Fibrosis and renin-angiotensin-aldosterone system. *Circulation.* 1991;83(6):1849-1865.

18. Creemers EE, Pinto YM. Molecular mechanisms that control interstitial fibrosis in the pressure-overloaded heart. *Cardiovasc Res.* 2011;89(2):265-272.

19. Tan LB, Jalil JE, Pick R, Janicki JS, Weber KT. Cardiac myocyte necrosis induced by angiotensin II. *Circ Res.* 1991;69(5):1185-1195.

20. Yancy CW, Jessup M, Bozkurt B, et al. 2013 ACCF/AHA guideline for the management of heart failure: a report of the American College of Cardiology Foundation/American Heart Association Task Force on Practice Guidelines. *J Am Coll Cardiol.* 2013;62(16):e147-239.

21. Bock HA, Hermle M, Brunner FP, Thiel G. Pressure dependent modulation of renin release in isolated perfused glomeruli. *Kidney Int.* 1992;41(2):275-280.

22. Kopp U, DiBona GF. Interaction of renal beta 1-adrenoceptors and prostaglandins in reflex renin release. *Am J Physiol.* 1983;244(4):F418-424.

23. Lorenz JN, Weihprecht H, Schnermann J, Skott O, Briggs JP. Renin release from isolated juxtaglomerular apparatus depends on macula densa chloride transport. *Am J Physiol.* 1991;260(4 Pt 2):F486-493.

24. Toldo S, Mezzaroma E, Mauro AG, et al. The inflammasome in myocardial injury and cardiac remodeling. *Antioxid Redox Signal.* 2015;22(13):1146-1161.

25. Maisel AS, Krishnaswamy P, Nowak RM, et al. Rapid measurement of B-type natriuretic peptide in the emergency diagnosis of heart failure. *N Engl J Med.* 2002;347(3):161-167.

26. Kim HN, Januzzi JL, Jr. Natriuretic peptide testing in heart failure. *Circulation.* 2011;123(18):2015-2019.

27. McMurray JJ, Packer M, Desai AS, et al. Angiotensin-neprilysin inhibition versus enalapril in heart failure. *N Engl J Med.* 2014;371(11):993-1004.

28. Felker GM, Anstrom KJ, Adams KF, et al. Effect of natriuretic peptide-guided therapy on hospitalization or cardiovascular mortality in high-risk patients with heart failure and reduced ejection fraction: a randomized clinical trial. *JAMA.* 2017;318(8):713-720.

29. Borlaug BA, Melenovsky V, Russell SD, et al. Impaired chronotropic and vasodilator reserves limit exercise capacity in patients with heart failure and a preserved ejection fraction. *Circulation.* 2006;114(20):2138-2147.

30. Kawaguchi M, Hay I, Fetics B, Kass DA. Combined ventricular systolic and arterial stiffening in patients with heart failure and preserved ejection fraction: implications for systolic and diastolic reserve limitations. *Circulation.* 2003;107(5):714-720.

31. Perrino C, Naga Prasad SV, Mao L, et al. Intermittent pressure overload triggers hypertrophy-independent cardiac dysfunction and vascular rarefaction. *J Clin Invest.* 2006;116(6):1547-1560.

32. Braz JC, Gregory K, Pathak A, et al. PKC-alpha regulates cardiac contractility and propensity toward heart failure. *Nat Med.* 2004;10(3):248-254.

33. Libby P, Lee RT. Matrix matters. *Circulation.* 2000;102(16):1874-1876.

34. Borbely A, Falcao-Pires I, van Heerebeek L, et al. Hypophosphorylation of the Stiff N2B titin isoform raises cardiomyocyte resting tension in failing human myocardium. *Circ Res.* 2009;104(6):780-786.

35. Borbely A, van Heerebeek L, Paulus WJ. Transcriptional and posttranslational modifications of titin: implications for diastole. *Circ Res.* 2009;104(1):12-14.

36. Pureza V, and Florea VG. Mechanisms for cachexia in heart failure. *Curr Heart Fail Rep.* 2013;10(4):307-314.

37. Onesti JK, Guttridge DC. Inflammation based regulation of cancer cachexia. *Biomed Res Int.* 2014; 2014:168407.

38. Anker SD, Ponikowski P, Varney S, et al. Wasting as independent risk factor for mortality in chronic heart failure. *Lancet.* 1997;349(9058):1050-1053.

39. Tisdale MJ. Biology of cachexia. *J Natl Cancer Inst.* 1997;89(23):1763-1773.

40. Levine B, Kalman J, Mayer L, Fillit HM, Packer M. Elevated circulating levels of tumor necrosis factor in severe chronic heart failure. *N Engl J Med.* 1990;323(4):236-241.

41. Kistorp C, Faber J, Galatius S, et al. Plasma adiponectin, body mass index, and mortality in patients with chronic heart failure. *Circulation.* 2005;112(12):1756-1762.

42. Florea VG, Moon J, Pennell DJ, et al. Wasting of the left ventricle in patients with cardiac cachexia: a cardiovascular magnetic resonance study. *Int J Cardiol.* 2004;97(1):15-20.

43. Ronco C, Haapio M, House AA, Anavekar N, Bellomo R. Cardiorenal syndrome. *J Am Coll Cardiol.* 2008;52(19):1527-1539.

44. Nohria A, Hasselblad V, Stebbins A, et al. Cardiorenal interactions: insights from the ESCAPE trial. *J Am Coll Cardiol.* 2008;51(13):1268-1274.

45. Bock JS, Gottlieb SS. Cardiorenal syndrome: new perspectives. *Circulation.* 2010;121(23):2592-2600.

46. Bradley SE, Bradley GP. The effect of increased intra-abdominal pressure on renal function in man. *J Clin Invest.* 1947;26(5):1010-1022.

47. Dilley JR, Corradi A, Arendshorst WJ. Glomerular ultrafiltration dynamics during increased renal venous pressure. *Am J Physiol.* 1983;244(6):F650-658.

48. Mullens W, Abrahams Z, Francis GS, et al. Importance of venous congestion for worsening of renal function in advanced decompensated heart failure. *J Am Coll Cardiol.* 2009;53(7):589-596.

49. Mullens W, Abrahams Z, Skouri HN, et al. Elevated intra-abdominal pressure in acute decompensated heart failure: a potential contributor to worsening renal function? *J Am Coll Cardiol.* 2008;51(3):300-306.

50. Marcus JT, Vonk Noordegraaf A, Roeleveld RJ, et al. Impaired left ventricular filling due to right ventricular pressure overload in primary pulmonary hypertension: noninvasive monitoring using MRI. *Chest.* 2001;119(6):1761-1765.

CHAPTER 69

The Epidemiology of Heart Failure

Ravi Karra

QUESTIONS

DIRECTIONS: Choose the one best response to each question.

69-1. A 56-year-old man presents to your clinic to follow up a recent hospitalization for acute decompensated heart failure (HF). During his hospitalization, he was noted to have an ischemic cardiomyopathy with a left ventricular (LV) ejection fraction (EF) of 30%. He is currently able to do his activities of daily living, and he denies exertional dyspnea or functional limitation. What is his American Heart Association heart failure stage?

A. A
B. B
C. C
D. D
E. Indeterminate

69-2. A 53-year-old man is transferred to your hospital for acute decompensated heart failure. He is currently stable on inotrope therapy but remains orthopneic at rest, continues to be volume overloaded, and has a rising serum creatinine. What is his INTERMACS profile?

A. 1
B. 2
C. 3
D. 4
E. 7

69-3. Which of the following is *not true* regarding the epidemiology of heart failure (HF)?

A. HF is equally prevalent in men and women
B. The incidence of HF increases with aging

C. The proportion of patients with heart failure with preserved ejection fraction (HFpEF) is increasing
D. In the United States, HF is more common in white people than in black people
E. HF is the leading cause for hospitalization among Medicare beneficiaries

69-4. Which of the following is a modifiable risk factor for heart failure?

A. Blood pressure
B. Body mass
C. Physical activity
D. Smoking
E. All of the above

69-5. Which of the following risk factors is more strongly associated with the risk of HFpEF than with the risk of HFrEF?

A. Lower ratio of forced expiratory volume in 1 second (FEV1) to forced vital capacity (FVC)
B. Prior myocardial infarction (MI)
C. Left bundle branch block (LBBB)
D. Lower hemoglobin
E. All of the above

69-6. Which of the following does *not* increase the lifetime risk for heart failure?

A. Age
B. Serum CRP levels
C. Systolic blood pressure
D. BMI
E. Heart rate

69-7. Which of the following is *true* about the prognosis of heart failure?

A. Quality of life is similar between patients with HFrEF and HFpEF
B. Fewer than 50% of symptomatic patients are alive within 5 years of initial diagnosis
C. The risk for mortality is highest immediately after hospitalization for acute decompensated heart failure
D. Obese patients are at higher risk for death after a diagnosis of heart failure
E. A, B, and C

69-8. Which of the following predict survival after a diagnosis of heart failure?

A. Right bundle branch block (RBBB)
B. The use of digoxin
C. Serum potassium
D. A diagnosis of heart failure within the prior 18 months
E. A narrow QRS duration

69-9. Which of the following is *true* about the etiology of heart failure (HF)?

A. The most common cause of HF is coronary artery disease
B. In black persons, coronary artery disease is the most common cause of HF
C. Chagas disease is an important cause of HF in Africa
D. A and B are both correct
E. B and C are both correct

69-10. Which of the following treatments for diabetes is associated with a reduced risk of heart failure?

A. Thiazolidinediones
B. Saxagliptin
C. Empagliflozin
D. B and C
E. None of the above

69-1. The answer is C. (*Hurst's The Heart, 14th Edition, Chap. 69*). Heart failure is typically a progressive syndrome resulting from risk factors (stage A) that lead to asymptomatic abnormalities of cardiac structure and function (stage B), then eventually transitioning to symptomatic HF (stage C) and decompensations/refractory symptoms (stage D) (Figure 69-1).[1] This staging system formulated by the AHA and the ACC highlights the potential importance of risk factor modification through lifestyle and pharmacologic means to prevent progression to symptomatic HF. The patient in question has a history of symptomatic heart failure, with a prior hospitalization, and has evidence for structural heart disease, with a reduced ejection fraction. Thus, he is stage C.

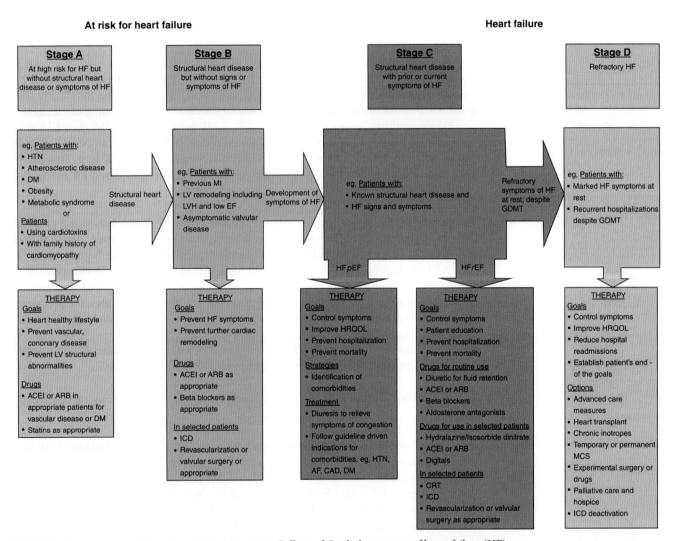

FIGURE 69-1 American Heart Association/American College of Cardiology stages of heart failure (HF).

Abbreviations: ACEI = angiotensin-converting enzyme inhibitor; AF = atrial fibrillation; ARB = angiotensin receptor blocker; CAD = coronary artery disease; CRT = cardiac resynchronization therapy; DM = diabetes mellitus; EF = ejection fraction; GDMT = guideline-directed medical therapy; HFpEF = heart failure with preserved ejection fraction; HFrEF = heart failure with reduced ejection fraction; HRQOL = health-related quality of life; HTN = hypertension; ICD = implantable cardioverter-defibrillator; LV = left ventricular; LVH = left ventricular hypertrophy; MCS = mechanical circulatory support. MI = myocardial infarction.

(Reproduced with permission from Yancy CW, Jessup M, Bozkurt B, et al. 2013 ACCF/AHA guideline for the management of heart failure: a report of the American College of Cardiology Foundation/American Heart Association Task Force on Practice Guidelines, *J Am Coll Cardiol*. 2013 Oct 15;62(16):e147-e239.)

TABLE 69-1 The INTERMACS Classification of Heart Failure

		Possible Profile Modifiers		
Profile	Description	Temporary Circulatory Support (TCS)	Arrhythmia (A)	Frequent Flyer (FF)
1.	Critical cardiogenic shock	X	X	
2.	Progressive decline on inotropic support	X	X	
3.	Stable but inotrope dependent	X (in hosp)	X	X (if home)
4.	Resting symptoms home on oral therapy		X	X
5.	Exertion intolerant		X	X
6.	Exertion limited		X	X
7.	Advanced NYHA Class III symptoms		X	

NYHA, New York Heart Association Classification. INTERMACS scores of 5 to 7 apply to New York Heart Association class III, whereas scores of 1 to 4 apply to NYHA class IV.

Reproduced with permission from Stevenson LW, Pagani FD, Young JB, et al. INTERMACS profiles of advanced heart failure: the current picture, *J Heart Lung Transplant*. 2009 Jun;28(6):535-541.

69-2. The answer is B. (*Hurst's The Heart, 14th Edition, Chap. 69*) The Interagency Registry of Mechanically Assisted Circulatory Support (INTERMACS) profile refines the classification of disease severity to inform risk assessment and the choice and the timing of mechanical circulatory support (Table 69-1).[2] For example, a HF patient with NYHA class III limitations may be further categorized as INTERMACS 5, 6, or 7, whereas an NYHA class IV patient could be further classified into INTERMACS categories 1, 2, 3, or 4. This patient continues to decline despite inotropic support and should be considered for mechanical circulatory support (option B).

69-3. The answer is D. (*Hurst's The Heart, 14th Edition, Chap. 69*) Heart failure is a common disease. In general, incidence rates increase with age and are higher in men than in women and in blacks compared to whites.[3] Older people consistently have the highest incidence rates, with an approximate two- to threefold higher incidence for each decade after age 55 (option B).[4-7] The proportion of incident HF cases with preserved compared with reduced LVEF appears to be increasing over time (option C).[8,9] In the United States, the prevalence of HF is similar between men and women at 2.3% and 2.2%, respectively, but it is more common in black (about 3.0%) than in white (about 2.2%) people (options A and D).[10] HF remains the leading cause for hospitalization among Medicare beneficiaries, although the primary hospitalization rate for HF declined from 1998 to 2008 (option E).[11]

69-4. The answer is E. (*Hurst's The Heart, 14th Edition, Chap. 69*) The AHA recognized the importance of modifiable risk factors to cardiovascular risk and developed a concept known as the Simple 7 (blood pressure, body mass, cholesterol, diet, glucose, physical activity, and smoking) (options A through D). In the ARIC study, individuals with high Simple 7 scores (indicating more healthy behaviors) were at lower lifetime risk for incident HF (14%), compared with individuals with average (27%) or poor (49%) scores.[12] These findings were corroborated by recent observations from the Framingham Heart Study.[13] Data from the Physicians' Health Study suggest that optimal modifiable risk factor profiles can lower the lifetime risk of HF by as much as 50%.[14]

69-5. The answer is A. (*Hurst's The Heart, 14th Edition, Chap. 69*) In the Framingham Heart Study, a history of hypertension, diastolic dysfunction, atrial fibrillation, female sex, and a lower ratio of FEV in 1 second to FVC were associated with a greater risk for symptomatic HFpEF compared with HFrEF (option A).[15,16] Patients with HFpEF often demonstrate exaggerated blood pressure responses to exercise, increased vascular stiffness, chronotropic incompetence, and increased baroreceptor sensitivity, and they are exquisitely sensitive to excess preload reduction. In this context, atrial fibrillation appears to be a particularly strong risk factor for HFpEF.[17] In the Framingham Heart Study, prior myocardial infarction, left bundle branch block, asymptomatic left ventricular systolic dysfunction, higher serum creatinine, and lower total blood hemoglobin concentration were significantly associated with a greater risk for HFrEF (options B, C, and D).[15,16]

69-6. The answer is B. (*Hurst's The Heart, 14th Edition, Chap. 69*) Many heart failure risk prediction models from community cohorts have been developed. Factors included in the risk prediction models vary by study, but they typically include age, sex, heart rate, systolic blood pressure, body mass index, and diabetes mellitus (options A, C, D, and E). Other factors, such as smoking status, serum creatinine, coronary heart disease, antihypertensive medication use, left ventricular hypertrophy, and valvular disease, are included to varying extents. The c-statistics for model performance are good, ranging from 0.73 to 0.87.[18-22]

69-7. The answer is E. (*Hurst's The Heart, 14th Edition, Chap. 69*) Quality of life is similar between patients with HFrEF and HFpEF, and it declines with worse NYHA classification (option A).[23-25] Survival among those with symptomatic HF (AHA/ACC stages C and D) is generally poor, with approximately 50% alive at 5 years following diagnosis (option B).[26,27] The highest-risk period appears to follow a hospitalization for HF, with 28-day and 1-year case fatality rates of 10% and 30%, respectively (option C).[28-30] Obesity, a prominent risk factor for the development of HF, paradoxically appears to be related to better outcomes among those with prevalent HF (option D).[31-36]

69-8. The answer is D. (*Hurst's The Heart, 14th Edition, Chap. 69*) To aid in prognostication, risk prediction models for mortality in HF, such as the Seattle Heart Failure Model and the Heart Failure Survival Score, have been derived and validated largely from cohorts of individuals with reduced ejection fraction and advanced HF (Table 69-2).[37,38] In a recent meta-analysis, these scores were found to be fair to modest in their discriminatory capacity for predicting death in HF, with c-statistics ranging from 0.56 to 0.81.[39] More recently, another model for predicting mortality in chronic ambulatory HF was developed by the Meta-Analysis Global Group in Chronic Heart Failure (MAGGIC) using data from 39,372 patients largely enrolled in clinical trials.[40] Factors that drive the Seattle Heart Failure Model and Heart Failure Survival Score and the MAGGIC model are given in Table 69-2 (options A–E).

TABLE 69-2 Factors Included in the Meta-Analysis Global Group in Chronic Heart Failure (MAGGIC) and Seattle Heart Failure Models for Predicting Survival in Heart Failure[38,40]

MAGGIC	Seattle Heart Failure Model
Left ventricular ejection fraction, %	Age, years
Age, years	Sex
Systolic blood pressure, mm Hg	NYHA Class
Body mass index, kg/m²	Weight, kg
Creatinine, μmol/L	Left ventricular ejection fraction, %
NYHA class	Systolic blood pressure, mm Hg
Sex	Ischemic etiology
Current smoker	ACEI, yes or no
Diabetes mellitus	β-Blocker, yes or no
Chronic obstructive pulmonary disease	ARB, yes or no
First diagnosis of HF in past 18 months	Statin, yes or no
β-Blocker, yes or no	Allopurinol, yes or no
ACEI/ARB use, yes or no	Aldosterone antagonist, yes or no
	Furosemide, yes (dose, route) or no
	Bumetanide, yes (dose, route) or no
	Torsemide, yes (dose, route) or no
	Metolazone, yes (and dose) or no
	Hydrochlorothiazide, yes (and dose) or no
	Chlorothiazide, yes (dose, route) or no
	Hemoglobin, g/dL
	Lymphocyte, %
	Uric acid, mg/dL
	Total cholesterol, mg/dL
	Sodium, mmol/L
	Biventricular pacemaker, yes or no
	Implantable cardioverter-defibrillator, yes or no
	Biventricular pacemaker with implantable cardioverter-defibrillator, yes or no
	Left bundle branch block, yes or no
	QRS duration > 150 ms, yes or no
	IABP, ventilator, or ultrafiltration, yes or no
	Number of pressors or inotropes

69-9. The answer is A. (*Hurst's The Heart, 14th Edition, Chap. 69*) Coronary artery disease is often cited as the most common cause of HF (option A).[41] Among black persons, hypertension accounted for 30.1% of incident HF, whereas coronary artery disease accounted for 29.5% (option B).[42] Chagas disease is also an important cause of HF in South America (option C).[43]

69-10. The answer is C. (*Hurst's The Heart, 14th Edition, Chap. 69*) A number of medications for the treatment of diabetes mellitus have been associated with an increased risk of HF, such as the thiazolidinediones (rosiglitazone and pioglitazone) and the dipeptidyl peptidase-4 inhibitor (saxagliptin) (options A and B).[44-46] In contrast, glucose lowering with the sodium-glucose cotransporter 2 inhibitor empagliflozin was recently demonstrated to reduce the risk of HF among individuals with prevalent diabetes mellitus (option C).[45] Higher amounts of physical activity have been associated with a reduced risk of incident HF.[47,48] Further, among middle-aged to elderly people, smoking is an established risk factor for incident HF.[19,20]

References

1. Yancy CW, Jessup M, Bozkurt B, et al. 2013 ACCF/AHA guideline for the management of heart failure: a report of the American College of Cardiology Foundation/American Heart Association Task Force on Practice Guidelines. *J Am Coll Cardiol.* 2013;62(16):e147-e239.

2. Stevenson LW, Pagani FD, Young JB, et al. INTERMACS profiles of advanced heart failure: the current picture. *J Heart Lung Transplant.* 2009;28(6):535-541.

3. Roger VL. Epidemiology of heart failure. *Circ Res.* 2013;113(6):646-659.

4. Writing Group Members, Mozaffarian D, Benjamin EJ, et al. Heart disease and stroke statistics—2016 update: a report from the American Heart Association. *Circulation.* 2016;133(4):e38-e360.

5. Croft JB, Giles WH, Pollard RA, et al. National trends in the initial hospitalization for heart failure. *J Am Geriatr Soc.* 1997;45(3):270-275.

6. Curtis LH, Whellan DJ, Hammill BG, et al. Incidence and prevalence of heart failure in elderly persons, 1994-2003. *Arch Intern Med.* 2008;168(4):418-424.

7. Gottdiener JS, Arnold AM, Aurigemma GP, et al. Predictors of congestive heart failure in the elderly: the Cardiovascular Health Study. *J Am Coll Cardiol.* 2000;35(6):1628-1637.

8. Owan TE, Hodge DO, Herges RM, et al. Trends in prevalence and outcome of heart failure with preserved ejection fraction. *N Engl J Med.* 2006;355(3):251-259.

9. Steinberg BA, Zhao X, Heidenreich PA, et al. Trends in patients hospitalized with heart failure and preserved left ventricular ejection fraction: prevalence, therapies, and outcomes. *Circulation.* 2012;126(1):65-75.

10. Writing Group Members, Mozaffarian D, Benjamin EJ, et al. Executive summary: heart disease and stroke statistics—2016 update: a report from the American Heart Association. *Circulation.* 2016;133(4):447-454.

11. Chen J, Normand SL, Wang Y, and Krumholz HM. National and regional trends in heart failure hospitalization and mortality rates for Medicare beneficiaries, 1998-2008. *JAMA.* 2011;306(15):1669-1678.

12. Folsom AR, Shah AM, Lutsey PL, et al. American Heart Association's life's Simple 7: avoiding heart failure and preserving cardiac structure and function. *Am J Med.* 2015;128(9):970-976 e2.

13. Nayor M, Enserro DM, Vasan RS, Xanthakis V. Cardiovascular health status and incidence of heart failure in the Framingham Offspring Study. *Circ Heart Fail.* 2016;9(1):e002416.

14. Djousse L, Driver JA, Gaziano JM. Relation between modifiable lifestyle factors and lifetime risk of heart failure. *JAMA.* 2009;302(4):394-400.

15. Lee DS, Gona P, Vasan RS, et al. Relation of disease pathogenesis and risk factors to heart failure with preserved or reduced ejection fraction: insights from the Framingham Heart Study of the National Heart, Lung, and Blood Institute. *Circulation.* 2009;119(24):3070-3077.

16. Lam CS, Lyass A, Kraigher-Krainer E, et al. Cardiac dysfunction and noncardiac dysfunction as precursors of heart failure with reduced and preserved ejection fraction in the community. *Circulation.* 2011;124(1):24-30.

17. Santhanakrishnan R, Wang N, Larson MG, et al. Atrial fibrillation begets heart failure and vice versa: temporal associations and differences in preserved versus reduced ejection fraction. *Circulation.* 2016;133(5):484-492.

18. Butler J, Kalogeropoulos A, Georgiopoulou V, et al. Incident heart failure prediction in the elderly: the health ABC heart failure score. *Circ Heart Fail.* 2008;1(2):125-133.

19. Agarwal SK, Chambless LE, Ballantyne CM, et al. Prediction of incident heart failure in general practice: the Atherosclerosis Risk in Communities (ARIC) Study. *Circ Heart Fail.* 2012;5(4):422-429.

20. Chahal H, Bluemke DA, Wu CO, et al. Heart failure risk prediction in the Multi-Ethnic Study of Atherosclerosis. *Heart.* 2015;101(1):58-64.

21. Ho JE, Gona P, Pencina MJ, et al. Discriminating clinical features of heart failure with preserved vs. reduced ejection fraction in the community. *Eur Heart J.* 2012;33(14):1734-1741.

22. Ho JE, Lyass A, Lee DS, et al. Predictors of new-onset heart failure: differences in preserved versus reduced ejection fraction. *Circ Heart Fail.* 2013;6(2):279-286.

23. Hobbs FD, Kenkre JE, Roalfe AK, et al. Impact of heart failure and left ventricular systolic dysfunction on quality of life: a cross-sectional study comparing common chronic cardiac and medical disorders and a representative adult population. *Eur Heart J.* 2002;23(23):1867-1876.

24. Juenger J, Schellberg D, Kraemer S, et al. Health related quality of life in patients with congestive heart failure: comparison with other chronic diseases and relation to functional variables. *Heart.* 2002;87(3):235-241.

25. Lewis EF, Lamas GA, O'Meara E, et al. Characterization of health-related quality of life in heart failure patients with preserved versus low ejection fraction in CHARM. *Eur J Heart Fail.* 2007;9(1):83-91.

26. Gerber Y, Weston SA, Redfield MM, et al. A contemporary appraisal of the heart failure epidemic in Olmsted County, Minnesota, 2000 to 2010. *JAMA Intern Med.* 2015;175(6):996-1004.

27. Roger VL, Weston SA, Redfield MM, et al. Trends in heart failure incidence and survival in a community-based population. *JAMA.* 2004;292(3):344-350.

28. Solomon SD, Dobson J, Pocock S, et al. Influence of nonfatal hospitalization for heart failure on subsequent mortality in patients with chronic heart failure. *Circulation.* 2007;116(13):1482-1487.

29. Chang PP, Chambless LE, Shahar E, et al. Incidence and survival of hospitalized acute decompensated heart failure in four US communities (from the Atherosclerosis Risk in Communities study). *Am J Cardiol.* 2014;113(3):504-510.

30. Nichols GA, Reynolds K, Kimes TM, Rosales AG, Chan WW. Comparison of risk of re-hospitalization, all-cause mortality, and medical care resource utilization in patients with heart failure and preserved versus reduced ejection fraction. *Am J Cardiol.* 2015;116(7):1088-1092.

31. Horwich TB, Fonarow GC, Hamilton MA, et al. The relationship between obesity and mortality in patients with heart failure. *J Am Coll Cardiol.* 2001;38(3):789-795.

32. Fonarow GC, Srikanthan P, Costanzo MR, et al. An obesity paradox in acute heart failure: analysis of body mass index and in-hospital mortality for 108,927 patients in the Acute Decompensated Heart Failure National Registry. *Am Heart J.* 2007;153(1):74-81.

33. Kenchaiah S, Pocock SJ, Wang D, et al. Body mass index and prognosis in patients with chronic heart failure: insights from the Candesartan in Heart failure: Assessment of Reduction in Mortality and morbidity (CHARM) program. *Circulation.* 2007;116(6):627-36.

34. Shah R, Gayat E, Januzzi JL, Jr., et al. Body mass index and mortality in acutely decompensated heart failure across the world: a global obesity paradox. *J Am Coll Cardiol.* 2014;63(8):778-785.

35. Khalid U, Ather S, Bavishi C, et al. Pre-morbid body mass index and mortality after incident heart failure: the ARIC study. *J Am Coll Cardiol.* 2014;64(25):2743-2749.

36. Sharma A, Lavie CJ, Borer JS, et al. Meta-analysis of the relation of body mass index to all-cause and cardiovascular mortality and hospitalization in patients with chronic heart failure. *Am J Cardiol.* 2015;115(10):1428-1434.

37. Aaronson KD, Schwartz JS, Chen TM, et al. Development and prospective validation of a clinical index to predict survival in ambulatory patients referred for cardiac transplant evaluation. *Circulation.* 1997;95(12):2660-2667.

38. Levy WC, Mozaffarian D, Linker DT, et al. The Seattle Heart Failure Model: prediction of survival in heart failure. *Circulation.* 2006;113(11):1424-1433.

39. Alba AC, Agoritsas T, Jankowski M, et al. Risk prediction models for mortality in ambulatory patients with heart failure: a systematic review. *Circ Heart Fail.* 2013;6(5):881-889.

40. Pocock SJ, Ariti CA, McMurray JJ, et al. Predicting survival in heart failure: a risk score based on 39 372 patients from 30 studies. *Eur Heart J.* 2013;34(19):1404-1413.

41. Gheorghiade M, Sopko G, De Luca L, et al. Navigating the crossroads of coronary artery disease and heart failure. *Circulation.* 2006;114(11):1202-1213.

42. Kalogeropoulos A, Georgiopoulou V, Kritchevsky SB, et al. Epidemiology of incident heart failure in a contemporary elderly cohort: the health, aging, and body composition study. *Arch Intern Med.* 2009;169(7):708-715.

43. Bocchi EA, Arias A, Verdejo H, et al. The reality of heart failure in Latin America. *J Am Coll Cardiol.* 2013;62(11):949-958.

44. Scirica BM, Bhatt DL, Braunwald E, et al. Saxagliptin and cardiovascular outcomes in patients with type 2 diabetes mellitus. *N Engl J Med.* 2013;369(14):1317-1326.

45. Zinman B, Wanner C, Lachin JM, et al. Empagliflozin, cardiovascular outcomes, and mortality in type 2 diabetes. *N Engl J Med.* 2015;373(22):2117-2128.

46. Singh S, Loke YK, Furberg CD. Thiazolidinediones and heart failure: a teleo-analysis. *Diabetes Care.* 2007;30(8):2148-2153.

47. Pandey A, Garg S, Khunger M, et al. Dose-response relationship between physical activity and risk of heart failure: a meta-analysis. *Circulation.* 2015;132(19):1786-1794.

48. Echouffo-Tcheugui JB, Butler J, Yancy CW, Fonarow GC. Association of physical activity or fitness with incident heart failure: a systematic review and meta-analysis. *Circ Heart Fail.* 2015;8(5):853-861.

CHAPTER 70

The Diagnosis and Management of Chronic Heart Failure

Ravi Karra

QUESTIONS

DIRECTIONS: Choose the one best response to each question.

70-1. Which of the following physical examination signs is associated with a low cardiac index?

A. Elevated jugular venous pressure
B. Peripheral edema
C. Proportional pulse pressure < 25%
D. Third heart sound
E. Square root sign

70-2. Which of the following biomarkers is predictive of outcomes from heart failure?

A. B-type natriuretic peptide (BNP)
B. Cardiac troponin
C. Soluble ST2
D. Galectin-3
E. All of the above

Questions 70-3 through 70-6 refer to the following vignette:

A 43-year-old white woman presents for a second opinion regarding her heart failure with reduced ejection fraction (HFrEF) of five years. Her evaluation is notable for a left ventricular ejection fraction (LVEF) of 30% with no significant valvular heart disease, coronary angiography without obstructive coronary artery disease (CAD), and cardiopulmonary exercise testing (CPET) with a VO_2 max of 18 mL·kg^{-1}·min^{-1} and normal VE/VCO$_2$ slope. She has NYHA class I symptoms at the moment and has never been hospitalized for acute heart failure.

70-3. Which of the following is the next best step in her management?

A. Referral for advanced heart failure therapies
B. Right heart catheterization
C. Continued titration of guideline-directed medical therapy
D. Encouragement to exercise
E. C and D are both correct

70-4. The patient now presents to your office with worsening dyspnea on exertion and a 3-pound weight gain. Her physical examination suggests adequate perfusion but congestion. Her renal function is normal. A review of her medical history reveals a sulfa allergy resulting in systemic anaphylaxis that required an ICU hospitalization. Which loop diuretic would be appropriate to use?

A. Furosemide
B. Torsemide
C. Bumetanide
D. Ethacrynic acid
E. Metolazone

70-5. After starting a diuretic, the patient's symptoms are much improved. She is feeling much better and is interested in what else she can do to prevent the progression of her heart failure. At this time, she endorses exertional dyspnea with moderate exertion. Her medical therapy includes linsiopril 10 mg daily, spironolactone 12.5 mg daily, and metoprolol tartrate 25 mg twice daily in addition to her diuretic. Her blood pressure is 115/78 mm Hg, and her heart rate is 85 bpm. Which of the following would be reasonable next steps for the management of her heart failure?

A. Change metoprolol tartrate to carvedilol
B. Change spironolactone to eplerenone
C. Change lisinopril to LCZ696
D. A and C are both correct
E. B and C are both correct

70-6. You see the patient in follow-up, and she is tolerating her medication changes. Her blood pressure is 98/65 mm Hg, and her heart rate is 92 bpm. She continues to have NYHA class II symptoms. Which of the following medication changes would be reasonable?

A. Start digitalis
B. Start warfarin
C. Start ivabradine
D. Start isosorbide
E. Start hydralazine

70-7. A 53-year-old man presents for follow-up of his ischemic cardiomyopathy. He was previously healthy until an ST-elevation myocardial infarction (MI) 2 weeks ago. He presented late and was managed medically without revascularization. A post-discharge echocardiogram showed an LVEF of 30%. Hi EKG: shows sinus rhythm with a QRS duration of 106 ms. He is tolerating maximal doses of guideline-directed medical therapy for heart failure. Which of the following is *true* of device therapy for this patient?

A. He should be evaluated for an ICD at this time
B. He should be evaluated for CRT-D at this time
C. He should undergo an echocardiogram more than 40 days after his infarct, and he should undergo evaluation for an ICD if his LVEF remains depressed
D. He should undergo an invasive EP study with ICD implantation if ventricular tachycardia is inducible
E. None of the above

70-8. You are asked to consult on a 62-year-old man with a nonischemic cardiomyopathy (LVEF of 30% for the past 8 years) and permanent atrial fibrillation. His heart failure decompensated with rapid atrial fibrillation. He has previously tried amiodarone and dofetilide but was unable to tolerate either. He is unable to tolerate higher doses of rate control. He is now interested in AV nodal ablation. He currently has a single-lead ICD. Which type of device change should he undergo at the time of nodal ablation?

A. No change to his current system
B. Upgrade to a biventricular pacing system
C. Addition of an atrial pacing lead
D. B and C are both correct
E. None of the above

70-9. Which of the following medications are recommended for the treatment of HFpEF?

A. Metoprolol
B. Carvedilol
C. Enalapril
D. Sildenafil
E. None of the above

70-10. A 54-year-old woman with which of the following conditions is most likely to benefit from cardiac resynchronization therapy?

A. LBBB, QRS duration of 160 ms, and LVEF of 25%
B. RBBB, QRS duration of 140 ms, and LVEF of 30%
C. LBBB, QRS duration of 160 ms, and LVEF of 45%
D. LBBB, QRS duration of 100 ms, and LVEF of 25%
E. None of the above

70-1. The answer is C. *(Hurst's The Heart, 14th Edition, Chap. 70)* Many findings are attributed to heart failure. However, many findings such as peripheral edema are nonspecific (option B). By contrast, findings such as elevations in jugular venous pressure and third heart sound are strongly specific for heart failure but difficult to detect, and they suffer from a lack of reproducibility (options A and D).[1,2] Furthermore, they are dependent on the patient's body habitus and can be misleading in the presence of right ventricular dysfunction and/or tricuspid regurgitation. A proportional pulse pressure [(systolic – diastolic)/systolic] of < 25% suggests a cardiac index < 2.2 $L \cdot min^{-1} \cdot m^{-2}$ (option C).[3] The cardiovascular response to the Valsalva maneuver is a simple and highly sensitive bedside test for the estimation of volume status and the detection of LV systolic dysfunction, but it is not specifically associated with a low cardiac output (option E).

70-2. The answer is E. *(Hurst's The Heart, 14th Edition, Chap. 70)* Natriuretic peptides have an AHA/ACC Class I recommendation for the diagnosis of acute heart failure and establishment of prognosis in chronic heart failure.[4] Cardiac troponin elevations in heart failure are associated with more severe disease and prognosis, but how treatments might be adjusted based on serum elevations remains unclear.[5,6] It is reasonable currently to measure levels in the hospital setting to rule out an ischemic trigger and establish prognosis. Soluble ST2 and galectin-3 are predictive of adverse outcomes in chronic heart failure and are additive in their value to natriuretic peptides.[7] Along with other prognostic factors, they can provide unique and objective information about the patient and are likely be included in future multimarker approaches to heart failure care.[8] In chronic heart failure, the measurement of cardiac troponins, ST2, and galectin-3 has an AHA/ACC Class IIb recommendation for risk stratification.[9]

70-3. The answer is E. *(Hurst's The Heart, 14th Edition, Chap. 70).* This patient has chronic stable heart failure. In the absence of decompensation or progressive symptoms, additional evaluation is not required at this time (option B). Treatment should be aimed at helping her feel better, live longer, and stay out of the hospital. Therefore, optimal medical therapy and encouragement to exercise are indicated (options C and D). A $VO_{2max} \leq 14$ $mL \cdot kg^{-1} \cdot min^{-1}$ had been suggested to prompt referral for advanced therapies, but in the current era of improved therapies, a lower threshold of 10 to 12 $mL \cdot kg^{-1} \cdot min^{-1}$ has been suggested. Some studies have suggested that the VE/VCO$_2$ slope is a better predictor of outcome than peak VO$_2$, LVEF, and NYHA class.[10] This patient is stable, and her CPET testing does not suggest advanced disease (option A).

70-4. The answer is D. *(Hurst's The Heart, 14th Edition, Chap. 70)* Loop diuretics are the backbone for the treatment of volume overload, and most patients are on maintenance doses to preserve a euvolemic state. Their dosing is usually adjusted in response to disease progression, dietary changes, and concurrent therapies.[11] Although furosemide is by far the most common oral loop diuretic, patients with resistance to oral furosemide therapy may benefit from bumetanide or torsemide, which may offer greater efficacy due to increased bioavailability and potency. All the available loop diuretics share similar toxicity, including the risk of ototoxicity in high doses (options A–C). Ethacrynic acid may be used in patients with sulfa allergy because it is the only loop diuretic that does not contain sulfa (option D). Metolazone and chlorothiazide can be used in conjunction with loop diuretics to overcome diuretic resistance (option E).

70-5. The answer is D. *(Hurst's The Heart, 14th Edition, Chap. 70)* Beta-blockers should be initiated in all stable heart failure patients except those who have a clear contraindication to their use. In clinical trials, beta-blockers reduce mortality (including sudden cardiac death) and hospitalization by approximately 30%.[12-14] Another randomized controlled trial, the Carvedilol or Metoprolol European Trial (COMET), showed that carvedilol increased survival compared with short-acting metoprolol (option A).[15] It is recommended that spironolactone or eplerenone be used in all patients with HFrEF who are already on an ACE inhibitor (or ARB) and beta-blocker but have suboptimal response to therapy and still have NYHA class II symptoms.[9,16] For a patient who is stable on spironolactone, a change to eplerenone would be indicated with side effects related to spironolactone (option B). A first-in-class drug that involves dual inhibition of neprilysin and the angiotensin II receptor (angiotensin receptor-neprilysin inhibitor [ARNI]; LCZ696) was approved for use in HFrEF and NYHA class II to IV heart failure based on a trial that randomized 8442 patients to LCZ696 versus enalapril (Prospective Comparison of ARNI with ARB Global Outcomes in Heart Failure with Preserved Ejection Fraction [PARADIGM-HF] trial).[17] The trial was stopped early due to significant reductions in the primary end point after a median duration of follow-up of 27 months. LCZ696 reduced the primary composite end point of cardiovascular death or heart failure hospitalization by 20%. Thus, a change from lisinopril to LCZ696 would be indicated (option C).

70-6. **The answer is C.** *(Hurst's The Heart, 14th Edition, Chap. 70)* The Digitalis Investigators Group (DIG) trial included a cohort of 988 patients with heart failure and relatively preserved ejection fraction (> 45%) in sinus rhythm.[18] Treatment with digoxin did not reduce all-cause or heart failure mortality but led to a 28% reduction in heart failure admissions. Clinicians can consider adding digoxin if patients have persistent symptoms on guideline-recommended therapy. This patient's symptoms are stable, so digoxin would not be indicated (option A). The results of the A-HEFT study led the US FDA to approve BiDil for African American patients with NYHA class III or IV heart failure and reduced ejection fraction. This patient is white, has stable symptoms, and does not have much blood pressure room, so isosorbide and hydralazine are not indicated (options D and E).[19] Ivabradine involves the inhibition of the I_f current node. It slows down the sinus node rate in patients who are in sinus rhythm. It is approved for stable patients with HFrEF who have a resting heart rate of at least 70 bpm on maximally tolerated beta-blockers (option C). Derangements in the clotting cascade are common in heart failure. However, large trials testing vitamin K antagonism in HFrEF without atrial fibrillation yielded no evidence of improvement in outcomes (option B).[20,21]

70-7. **The answer is C.** *(Hurst's The Heart, 14th Edition, Chap. 70)* The following are Class I recommendations for ICD use in primary prevention, according to the ACC/AHA 2013 guidelines: (1) for the primary prevention of SCD to reduce mortality in patients with both ischemic and nonischemic cardiomyopathy and LVEF ≤ 35% with NYHA class II or III symptoms on guideline-recommended medical therapy for at least 3 months, and (2) for the primary prevention of SCD in patients who are at least 40 days post–myocardial infarction and with LVEF ≤ 30% and NYHA class I symptoms or more while receiving guideline-recommended medical therapy.[9] For secondary prevention, ICDs are indicated for survivors of cardiac arrest and in patients with sustained ventricular arrhythmias, irrespective of LVEF. ICD therapy should only be offered to patients who have a reasonable expectation of survival beyond a year and lack of frailty or advanced comorbid conditions.

70-8. **The answer is B.** *(Hurst's The Heart, 14th Edition, Chap. 70)* Cardiac synchronization therapy (CRT) is indicated in heart failure patients who have an indication for conventional right ventricular pacing that alters cardiac activation in a manner similar to a native LBBB. Finally, because effective CRT requires high rates of biventricular pacing, the benefit to patients with underlying atrial fibrillation is greatest in patients who have undergone concomitant atrioventricular node ablation (options A and B).[22,23] An atrial pacing lead would not be useful since this patient has permanent atrial fibrillation (option C).

70-9. **The answer is E.** *(Hurst's The Heart, 14th Edition, Chap. 70).* There is no proven effective treatment that improves mortality in HFpEF (option E). Beta-blockers are commonly prescribed for patients with diastolic dysfunction based on the notion that slowing the sinus rate will prolong diastole and promote ventricular filling.[24] Despite this theoretical benefit, there is little to no evidence that beta-blockers improve exercise capacity or clinical outcomes, although data are quite limited in this regard (options A and B).[25-29] The available data do not support the use of ACE inhibitors/ARBs as a disease-modifying therapy in HFpEF, although they are clearly safe and still may be effective as antihypertensives in this population (option C).[30-32] In animal models of pressure-overload hypertrophy, sildenafil improves ventricular structure and function dramatically.[33] However, in the Phosphodiesterase-5 Inhibition to Improve Clinical Status and Exercise Capacity in Diastolic Heart Failure (RELAX) trial, sildenafil did not improve exercise capacity, neurohormones, ventricular function, or quality of life (option D).[34]

70-10. **The answer is A.** *(Hurst's The Heart, 14th Edition, Chap. 70)* Approximately a third of patients with HFrEF have prolongation of the QRS interval on ECG, inferring a degree of mechanical dyssynchrony of the failing heart, which is associated with worse clinical outcomes.[35] CRT or biventricular pacing is accomplished through simultaneous pacing of both the left and the right ventricles and can lead to improvements in echocardiographic and hemodynamic parameters, functional status (average of 1–2 mL/kg/min increase in peak VO$_2$), and clinical outcomes (reduction in hospitalizations and all-cause mortality). CRT is recommended for patients in normal sinus rhythm with LVEF ≤ 35% and a left bundle branch block (LBBB) with QRS of ≥ 120 ms (option A). Less clarity exists for patients with non-LBBB patterns on ECG, those who are not in normal sinus rhythm, or those with wide QRS but ≤ 150 ms (options B, C, and D).

References

1. Drazner MH, Rame JE, Stevenson LW, Dries DL. Prognostic importance of elevated jugular venous pressure and a third heart sound in patients with heart failure. *N Engl J Med.* 2001;345(8):574-581.

2. Ishmail AA, Wing S, Ferguson J, et al. Interobserver agreement by auscultation in the presence of a third heart sound in patients with congestive heart failure. *Chest.* 1987;91(6):870-873.

3. Stevenson LW, Perloff JK. The limited reliability of physical signs for estimating hemodynamics in chronic heart failure. *JAMA.* 1989;261(6):884-888.

4. Yancy CW, Jessup M, Bozkurt B, et al. 2013 ACCF/AHA guideline for the management of heart failure: executive summary: a report of the American College of Cardiology Foundation/American Heart Association Task Force on practice guidelines. *Circulation.* 2013;128(16):1810-1852.

5. Januzzi JL, Jr., Filippatos G, Nieminen M, Gheorghiade M. Troponin elevation in patients with heart failure: on behalf of the third Universal Definition of Myocardial Infarction Global Task Force: Heart Failure Section. *Eur Heart J.* 2012;33(18):2265-2271.

6. O'Connor CM, Fiuzat M, Lombardi C, et al. Impact of serial troponin release on outcomes in patients with acute heart failure: analysis from the PROTECT pilot study. *Circ Heart Fail.* 2011;4(6):724-732.

7. Ahmad T, Fiuzat M, Neely B, et al. Biomarkers of myocardial stress and fibrosis as predictors of mode of death in patients with chronic heart failure. *JACC Heart Fail.* 2014;2(3):260-268.

8. Ky B, French B, Levy WC, et al. Multiple biomarkers for risk prediction in chronic heart failure. *Circ Heart Fail.* 2012;5(2):183-190.

9. Yancy CW, Jessup M, Bozkurt B, et al. 2013 ACCF/AHA guideline for the management of heart failure: a report of the American College of Cardiology Foundation/American Heart Association Task Force on Practice Guidelines. *J Am Coll Cardiol.* 2013;62(16):e147-e239.

10. Arena R, Myers J, Abella J, et al. Development of a ventilatory classification system in patients with heart failure. *Circulation.* 2007;115(18):2410-2417.

11. Michael Felker G. Diuretic management in heart failure. *Congest Heart Fail.* 2010;16 Suppl 1:S68-S72.

12. Bohm M, Maack C, Wehrlen-Grandjean M, Erdmann E. Effect of bisoprolol on perioperative complications in chronic heart failure after surgery (Cardiac Insufficiency Bisoprolol Study II (CIBIS II)). *Z Kardiol.* 2003;92(8):668-676.

13. The Cardiac Insufficiency Bisoprolol Study II (CIBIS-II): a randomised trial. *Lancet.* 1999;353(9146):9-13.

14. Effect of metoprolol CR/XL in chronic heart failure: Metoprolol CR/XL Randomised Intervention Trial in Congestive Heart Failure (MERIT-HF). *Lancet.* 1999;353(9169):2001-2007.

15. Poole-Wilson PA, Swedberg K, Cleland JG, et al. Comparison of carvedilol and metoprolol on clinical outcomes in patients with chronic heart failure in the Carvedilol Or Metoprolol European Trial (COMET): randomised controlled trial. *Lancet.* 2003;362(9377):7-13.

16. McMurray JJ, Adamopoulos S, Anker SD, et al. ESC guidelines for the diagnosis and treatment of acute and chronic heart failure 2012: The Task Force for the Diagnosis and Treatment of Acute and Chronic Heart Failure 2012 of the European Society of Cardiology. Developed in collaboration with the Heart Failure Association (HFA) of the ESC. *Eur J Heart Fail.* 2012;14(8):803-869.

17. McMurray JJ, Packer M, Desai AS, et al. Angiotensin-neprilysin inhibition versus enalapril in heart failure. *N Engl J Med.* 2014;371(11):993-1004.

18. Ahmed A, Rich MW, Fleg JL, et al. Effects of digoxin on morbidity and mortality in diastolic heart failure: the ancillary digitalis investigation group trial. *Circulation*. 2006;114(5):397-403.

19. Taylor AL, Ziesche S, Yancy C, et al. Combination of isosorbide dinitrate and hydralazine in blacks with heart failure. *N Engl J Med*. 2004;351(20):2049-2057.

20. Cleland JG, Findlay I, Jafri S, et al. The Warfarin/Aspirin Study in Heart failure (WASH): a randomized trial comparing antithrombotic strategies for patients with heart failure. *Am Heart J*. 2004;148(1):157-164.

21. Cokkinos DV, Haralabopoulos GC, Kostis JB, Toutouzas PK, HELAS investigators. Efficacy of antithrombotic therapy in chronic heart failure: the HELAS study. *Eur J Heart Fail*. 2006;8(4):428-432.

22. Brignole M, Botto G, Mont L, et al. Cardiac resynchronization therapy in patients undergoing atrioventricular junction ablation for permanent atrial fibrillation: a randomized trial. *Eur Heart J*. 2011;32(19): 2420-2429.

23. Upadhyay GA, Choudhry NK, Auricchio A, Ruskin J, Singh JP. Cardiac resynchronization in patients with atrial fibrillation: a meta-analysis of prospective cohort studies. *J Am Coll Cardiol*. 2008;52(15):1239-1246.

24. Bergstrom A, Andersson B, Edner M, et al. Effect of carvedilol on diastolic function in patients with diastolic heart failure and preserved systolic function. Results of the Swedish Doppler-echocardiographic study (SWEDIC). *Eur J Heart Fail*. 2004;6(4):453-461.

25. Conraads VM, Metra M, Kamp O, et al. Effects of the long-term administration of nebivolol on the clinical symptoms, exercise capacity, and left ventricular function of patients with diastolic dysfunction: results of the ELANDD study. *Eur J Heart Fail*. 2012;14(2):219-225.

26. Ambrosio G, Flather MD, Bohm M, et al. Beta-blockade with nebivolol for prevention of acute ischaemic events in elderly patients with heart failure. *Heart*. 2011;97(3):209-214.

27. Yamamoto K, Origasa H, Hori M, J-DHF Investigators. Effects of carvedilol on heart failure with preserved ejection fraction: the Japanese Diastolic Heart Failure Study (J-DHF). *Eur J Heart Fail*. 2013;15(1):110-118.

28. Hernandez AF, Hammill BG, O'Connor CM, et al. Clinical effectiveness of beta-blockers in heart failure: findings from the OPTIMIZE-HF (Organized Program to Initiate Lifesaving Treatment in Hospitalized Patients with Heart Failure) registry. *J Am Coll Cardiol*. 2009;53(2):184-192.

29. Farasat SM, Bolger DT, Shetty V, et al. Effect of beta-blocker therapy on rehospitalization rates in women versus men with heart failure and preserved ejection fraction. *Am J Cardiol*. 2010;105(2):229-234.

30. Yusuf S, Pfeffer MA, Swedberg K, et al. Effects of candesartan in patients with chronic heart failure and preserved left-ventricular ejection fraction: the CHARM-Preserved Trial. *Lancet*. 2003;362(9386):777-781.

31. Cleland JG, Tendera M, Adamus J, et al. The perindopril in elderly people with chronic heart failure (PEP-CHF) study. *Eur Heart J*. 2006;27(19):2338-2345.

32. Massie BM, Carson PE, McMurray JJ, et al. Irbesartan in patients with heart failure and preserved ejection fraction. *N Engl J Med*. 2008;359(23):2456-2467.

33. Takimoto E, Champion HC, Li M, et al. Chronic inhibition of cyclic GMP phosphodiesterase 5A prevents and reverses cardiac hypertrophy. *Nat Med*. 2005;11(2):214-222.

34. Redfield MM, Chen HH, Borlaug BA, et al. Effect of phosphodiesterase-5 inhibition on exercise capacity and clinical status in heart failure with preserved ejection fraction: a randomized clinical trial. *JAMA*. 2013;309(12):1268-1277.

35. Saxon LA, Ellenbogen KA. Resynchronization therapy for the treatment of heart failure. *Circulation*. 2003;108(9):1044-1048.

CHAPTER 71

Evaluation and Management of Acute Heart Failure

Ravi Karra

QUESTIONS

DIRECTIONS: Choose the one best response to each question.

71-1. Which of the following is *true* about outcomes of acute heart failure (AHF)?

A. In-hospital mortality is greater for patients with heart failure with reduced ejection fraction (HFrEF) than for patients with heart failure with preserved ejection fraction (HFpEF)

B. About 25% of patients are readmitted within 30 days of hospital discharge

C. About 30% of patients die within 6 months of hospitalization

D. After an initial hospitalization, subsequent hospitalizations tend to be shorter

E. None of the above

71-2. Which of the following contributes to renal dysfunction in AHF?

A. Elevated right-sided pressures

B. Diminished cardiac output

C. Renin-angiotensin-aldosterone system (RAAS) activation

D. Sympathetic nervous system (SNS) activation

E. All of the above

71-3. An 85-year-old black woman with HFpEF is admitted for AHF and is administered intravenous diuretics. Her course is complicated by hypotension and acute renal failure (as determined by an increase in her BUN and Cr) despite elevated filling pressures. She has been persistently hyponatremic. Which of the following features is associated with an adverse prognosis?

A. Hypotension

B. Older age

C. Increase in BUN

D. Black race

E. All of the above

71-4. Which of the following physical examination signs are associated with congestion?

A. Orthopnea

B. Square wave blood pressure response to Valsalva

C. Dyspnea

D. Both A and B are correct

E. None of the above

71-5. A 57-year-old man with HFrEF is admitted with AHF. On your assessment, you note that he is "warm" and "wet." Which of the following is correct regarding management of his volume?

A. Continuous infusion of furosemide is not superior to bolus dosing for relieving congestion

B. The addition of a thiazide to a loop diuretic can help to spare potassium losses

C. The use of tolvaptan improves mortality related to AHF

D. Ultrafiltration should be a first-line treatment strategy

E. Nesiritide relieves congestion better than standard loop diuretics

71-6. A 62-year-old man with an ischemic cardiomyopathy with LVEF of 25% is admitted with AHF. His extremities are cool, and his renal function has worsened over his baseline. His blood pressure is 96/76 mm Hg, and his heart rate is 110 bpm. Which of the following is *true* of inotrope therapy in patients with AHF?

A. Milrinone's effect is dependent on β-receptors
B. Milrinone can be used independently of renal function
C. Dobutamine is renally cleared
D. Dobutamine and milrinone are both proarrhythmic
E. Levosimendan is approved for AHF in the United States

71-7. Which of the following *is not* among the performance measures for coordinating transitions of care after HF hospitalizations?

A. Written materials explaining discharge medications
B. Educational materials detailing activity level, diet, and weight monitoring
C. Documented discussion of code status
D. Written materials with follow-up visit instructions
E. Written materials explaining what to do if symptoms worsen

71-8. Which of the following *are not* risk factors for readmission after a hospitalization for AHF?

A. Older age
B. Nonischemic cardiomyopathy
C. Low systolic blood pressure
D. Increased BUN
E. Increased heart rate

71-9. Which of the following is *not* a part of the definition of cardiogenic shock?

A. LVEF < 25%
B. Systolic blood pressure < 90 mm Hg for > 30 minutes
C. A drop in mean arterial pressure > 30 mm Hg below baseline
D. Cardiac index < 1.8 L/min/m^2 without hemodynamic support
E. Pulmonary capillary wedge pressure (PCWP) > 15 mm Hg

71-10. Which of the following is *true* regarding the use pulmonary artery catheters (PACs) for tailored therapy in patients with AHF?

A. PACs should be used to guide the management of AHF
B. PAC use during hospitalization improves the number of days alive out of the hospital
C. PAC use for ADHF is associated with fewer adverse events
D. PACs can play a role in carefully selected patients for whom hemodynamics are unclear or AHF symptoms are persistent
E. None of the above

71-1. The answer is B. *(Hurst's The Heart, 14th Edition, Chap. 71)* AHF is a harbinger of poor outcomes and is associated with significant mortality after discharge. Recent trends suggest in-hospital mortality rates range from 2% to 5% and are similar when comparing HFpEF to HFrEF (option A).[1,2] Postdischarge mortality for these two groups approaches 10% at 90-day follow-up,[3] whereas approximately 30% of patients die within 1 year of hospitalization (option C).[2,4] Despite concerted efforts to reduce rehospitalizations for AHF, nearly 25% of patients are readmitted within 30 days of discharge, and 50% are readmitted by 6 months (option B).[5,6] Each subsequent hospitalization following the index stay is associated with increasing risk of death (option D).

71-2. The answer is E. *(Hurst's The Heart, 14th Edition, Chap. 71)* While historically worsening renal function (WRF) in AHF was considered a consequence of reduced cardiac output ("underperfusion"), it has become increasingly apparent that right-sided congestion (eg, right atrial pressure) plays an important role. Multiple studies have failed to show a correlation between cardiac output and WRF in AHF, with the exception of extreme reductions in output (option B).[7-10] In contrast, several studies show a correlation between elevated right atrial pressure and intra-abdominal pressure with WRF (option A).[7-9,11] Neurohormonal activation plays a critical role in WRF in the setting of decompensation. The downstream effects of RAAS and SNS activation include angiotensin II and catecholamine-induced renal efferent arteriolar constriction, which increases glomerular filtration at the expense of renal blood flow (options C and D). Additionally, the stimulation of aldosterone secretion increases sodium resorption and exacerbates volume overload and congestion, which in turn promotes WRF. Chronic RAAS and SNS activation may lead to renal interstitial fibrosis and inflammation, resulting in chronic kidney disease.[12]

71-3. The answer is E. *(Hurst's The Heart, 14th Edition, Chap. 71)* The Acute Decompensated Heart Failure National Registry (ADHERE) "risk tree" was derived from an analysis of 39 admission variables in over 60,000 AHF patients.[13] Investigators found that the best predictors of in-patient mortality were markers of renal dysfunction (elevated blood urea nitrogen and creatinine) and lower blood pressure (options A and C). Additionally, the Get With the Guidelines–Heart Failure (GWTG-HF) risk score was derived from a cohort of over 39,000 patients admitted with AHF between 2007 and 2009.[13] This score incorporates a number of admission variables associated with mortality risk in a multivariable analysis: age, systolic blood pressure, blood urea nitrogen, heart rate, sodium, COPD, and nonblack race (options B and D). This model has been validated for use across a wide spectrum of AHF patients and is effective in both HFpEF and HFrEF patients.[13] These scores represent just a few of the many AHF risk scores available for clinical use.

71-4. The answer is D. *(Hurst's The Heart, 14th Edition, Chap. 71)* The conventional approach to therapy in AHF begins with bedside determination of the hemodynamic profile. Nohria et al described four patient profiles based on volume and perfusion status.[14] This simple classification has proven to be very useful in clinical practice:

Profile A: Patients without evidence of congestion with adequate perfusion ("dry-warm")
Profile B: Patients with congestion but adequate perfusion ("wet-warm")
Profile C: Patients with congestion and hypoperfusion ("wet-cold")
Profile L: Patients without congestion, with hypoperfusion ("dry-cold")[13]

Survival analysis revealed that clinical profiles predicted outcomes in HF, with profiles B and C portending increased risk of death or urgent transplantation, adding prognostic value even when limited to patients with New York Heart Association (NYHA) class III and IV symptoms. The presence of congestion was determined by orthopnea and/or physical exam evidence of jugular venous distention, pulmonary rales, hepatojugular reflux, ascites, peripheral edema, leftward radiation of the pulmonic heart sound, or a square wave blood pressure response to the Valsalva maneuver (options A–C). Perfusion status was determined by the presence of narrow pulse pressure ([systolic − diastolic]/systolic blood pressure < 25%), pulsus alternans, symptomatic hypotension, cool extremities, and/or impairment in mentation.[14]

71-5. The answer is A. (*Hurst's The Heart, 14th Edition, Chap. 71*) The mainstay of diuretic therapy is loop diuretics (furosemide, torsemide, bumetanide, and ethacrynic acid). The Diuretic Optimization Strategies Evaluation (DOSE) trial randomized AHF patients to low-dose (equal to daily diuretic dose) or high-dose (2.5 times total daily dose) furosemide, administered as either an intravenous bolus every 12 hours or as a continuous infusion. The study found no significant difference between strategies in the patient-reported global assessment of symptoms and no change in serum creatinine from baseline to 72 hours (option A).[15] Thiazides may be useful as an addition in patients on chronic loop diuretics because they may overcome loop diuretic resistance, but they should be used with caution because they can cause severe electrolyte disturbances such as profound hypokalemia (option B). The Efficacy of Vasopressin Antagonism in Heart Failure Outcome Study with Tolvaptan (EVEREST) trial revealed a clinical benefit with vasopressin, with significant weight reduction and dyspnea scores at 24 hours and decreased volume retention at day 7. Despite this, there were no observed differences in hospitalization or mortality at 10-month follow-up (option C).[16] The ACC/AHA guidelines currently state that UF is reasonable in certain patients with refractory congestion once other strategies have failed (option D).[17] Nesiritide reduces LV filling pressures and relieves dyspnea but may lead to hypotension. However, the Acute Study of Clinical Effectiveness of Nesiritide in Decompensated Heart Failure Subsequent trial failed to reach statistical significance for either relief of dyspnea or HF readmission or death at 30 days compared with placebo (option E).[18]

71-6. The answer is D. (*Hurst's The Heart, 14th Edition, Chap. 71*) Milrinone, a phosphodiesterase-3 inhibitor, decreases the degradation of cyclic adenosine monophosphate, thus increasing protein kinase A, leading to phosphorylation of multiple myocardial targets downstream, augmenting contractility. The mechanism of action of milrinone is independent of β-adrenergic receptors, which are downregulated in HF (option A). Milrinone has a half-life of roughly 2.4 hours and is renally cleared (option B). In clinical trials, milrinone use did not result in decreased duration of hospitalization and was associated with a nonsignificant higher mortality both in hospital and after discharge, as well as higher rates of new-onset atrial arrhythmias and sustained hypotension requiring intervention.[19] Dobutamine is a sympathomimetic agent whose mechanism of action is through the stimulation of β₁ receptors. Dobutamine has a half-life of 2 minutes with largely hepatic clearance (option C). Both milrinone and dobutamine can cause a tachycardic response and are often arrhythmogenic, portending a higher risk of mortality (option D). The Randomized Multicenter Evaluation of Intravenous Levosimendan Efficacy trial and Survival of Patients with Acute Heart Failure in Need of Intravenous Inotrope Support trial failed to show an overall mortality benefit in levosimendan compared with placebo or dobutamine, respectively, and currently the drug is not approved for use in AHF in the United States (option E).[20,21]

71-7. The answer is C. (*Hurst's The Heart, 14th Edition, Chap. 71*) To optimize post-hospitalization outcomes, clinicians should follow published guidelines.[17] A critical performance measure set forth for HF hospitalization involves care coordination and transition of care, which includes written discharge instructions or educational materials provided to patients explaining discharge medications (option A), activity level, diet, weight monitoring (option B), follow-up visit instructions (option D), and what to do if symptoms worsen (option E).[22]

71-8. The answer is B. (*Hurst's The Heart, 14th Edition, Chap. 71*) Several risk factors for rehospitalization have been identified, including but not limited to advanced age (option A); ischemic etiology (option B); low systolic blood pressure (option C); increased heart rate; higher NYHA class at discharge; laboratory abnormalities such as low admission hemoglobin, admission and discharge creatinine, and increased blood urea nitrogen (option D);

other testing abnormalities such as prolonged QRS on electrocardiogram; echocardiographic parameters such as lower ejection fraction; higher systolic pulmonary artery pressure; and right ventricular tissue Doppler imaging.[5] Similarly, natriuretic peptide levels at admission and on discharge predict readmission risk, and post-discharge measurement also guides further risk stratification.[5]

71-9. The answer is A. (*Hurst's The Heart, 14th Edition, Chap. 71*) Cardiogenic shock is defined as systemic tissue hypoperfusion caused by inadequate cardiac output despite adequate circulatory volume and filling pressure. Hemodynamic criteria include systolic blood pressure < 90 mm Hg for > 30 minutes (option B), a drop in mean arterial pressure > 30 mm Hg below baseline with cardiac index < 1.8 L/min/m^2 without hemodynamic support (options C and D), and a PCWP > 15 mm Hg (option E).[23,24]

71-10. The answer is D. (*Hurst's The Heart, 14th Edition, Chap. 71*) Pulmonary artery catheters (PACs) have historically been used as part of a "tailored therapy" approach in AHF. More recently, the routine use of PAC-guided management has been discouraged.[25] The Evaluation Study of Congestive Heart Failure and Pulmonary Artery Catheterization and Effectiveness (ESCAPE) trial evaluated the use of PACs in patients hospitalized with HF in whom the use of a PAC was deemed to be of potential benefit but not essential.[26] The use of PACs was compared to clinical assessment alone in 433 patients with comparable baseline characteristics, including severe elevation in PCWP, diminished LV ejection fraction, and cardiac index 1.9 ± 0.6 L/min/m^2. The ESCAPE trial reported no differences between groups in the primary end point of days alive out of the hospital (option B). Subgroup analysis showed a trend toward improved outcomes in the PAC group in the highest enrollment centers and a trend in favor of the PAC group for functional assessment (6-minute walk, Minnesota Living With Heart Failure testing), but also a trend toward more adverse events (option C). It is important to note that the ESCAPE trial excluded patients whom physicians felt clearly required PAC for optimal management and involved physician investigators who were highly experienced in the evaluation and treatment of HF. With the bedside availability of astute physical exam skills, serum biomarkers and laboratory results, and point-of-care and advanced imaging techniques, PAC should be reserved for selective situations.[27] The ACC/AHA guidelines state that invasive hemodynamic monitoring should not be routinely used, but it can play a role in carefully selected patients for whom hemodynamics are unclear or AHF symptoms are persistent (option D).[17]

References

1. Steinberg BA, Zhao X, Heidenreich PA, et al. Trends in patients hospitalized with heart failure and preserved left ventricular ejection fraction: prevalence, therapies, and outcomes. *Circulation.* 2012;126(1):65-75.

2. Kociol RD, Hammill BG, Fonarow GC, et al. Generalizability and longitudinal outcomes of a national heart failure clinical registry: Comparison of Acute Decompensated Heart Failure National Registry (ADHERE) and non-ADHERE Medicare beneficiaries. *Am Heart J.* 2010;160(5):885-892.

3. Fonarow GC, Stough WG, Abraham WT, et al. Characteristics, treatments, and outcomes of patients with preserved systolic function hospitalized for heart failure: a report from the OPTIMIZE-HF Registry. *J Am Coll Cardiol.* 2007;50(8):768-777.

4. Shahar E, Lee S, Kim J, et al. Hospitalized heart failure: rates and long-term mortality. *J Card Fail.* 2004;10(5):374-379.

5. Giamouzis G, Kalogeropoulos A, Georgiopoulou V, et al. Hospitalization epidemic in patients with heart failure: risk factors, risk prediction, knowledge gaps, and future directions. *J Card Fail.* 2011;17(1):54-75.

6. Ross JS, Chen J, Lin Z, et al. Recent national trends in readmission rates after heart failure hospitalization. *Circ Heart Fail.* 2010;3(1):97-103.

7. Damman K, van Deursen VM, Navis G, et al. Increased central venous pressure is associated with impaired renal function and mortality in a broad spectrum of patients with cardiovascular disease. *J Am Coll Cardiol.* 2009;53(7):582-588.

8. Guglin M, Rivero A, Matar F, Garcia M. Renal dysfunction in heart failure is due to congestion but not low output. *Clin Cardiol.* 2011;34(2):113-116.

9. Mullens W, Abrahams Z, Francis GS, et al. Importance of venous congestion for worsening of renal function in advanced decompensated heart failure. *J Am Coll Cardiol.* 2009;53(7):589-596.

10. Ljungman S, Laragh JH, Cody RJ. Role of the kidney in congestive heart failure. Relationship of cardiac index to kidney function. *Drugs.* 1990;39 Suppl 4:10-21; discussion 2-4.

11. Mullens W, Abrahams Z, Skouri HN, et al. Elevated intra-abdominal pressure in acute decompensated heart failure: a potential contributor to worsening renal function? *J Am Coll Cardiol.* 2008;51(3):300-306.

12. Mezzano SA, Ruiz-Ortega M, Egido J. Angiotensin II and renal fibrosis. *Hypertension.* 2001;38(3 Pt 2): 635-638.

13. Fonarow GC, Adams KF, Jr., Abraham WT, et al. Risk stratification for in-hospital mortality in acutely decompensated heart failure: classification and regression tree analysis. *JAMA.* 2005;293(5):572-580.

14. Nohria A, Tsang SW, Fang JC, et al. Clinical assessment identifies hemodynamic profiles that predict outcomes in patients admitted with heart failure. *J Am Coll Cardiol.* 2003;41(10):1797-1804.

15. Felker GM, Lee KL, Bull DA, et al. Diuretic strategies in patients with acute decompensated heart failure. *N Engl J Med.* 2011;364(9):797-805.

16. Konstam MA, Gheorghiade M, Burnett JC, Jr., et al. Effects of oral tolvaptan in patients hospitalized for worsening heart failure: the EVEREST Outcome Trial. *JAMA.* 2007;297(12):1319-1331.

17. Yancy CW, Jessup M, Bozkurt B, et al. 2013 ACCF/AHA guideline for the management of heart failure: a report of the American College of Cardiology Foundation/American Heart Association Task Force on Practice Guidelines. *J Am Coll Cardiol.* 2013;62(16):e147-e239.

18. O'Connor CM, Starling RC, Hernandez AF, et al. Effect of nesiritide in patients with acute decompensated heart failure. *N Engl J Med.* 2011;365(1):32-43.

19. Klein L, O'Connor CM, Leimberger JD, et al. Lower serum sodium is associated with increased short-term mortality in hospitalized patients with worsening heart failure: results from the Outcomes of a Prospective Trial of Intravenous Milrinone for Exacerbations of Chronic Heart Failure (OPTIME-CHF) study. *Circulation.* 2005;111(19):2454-2460.

20. Packer M, Colucci W, Fisher L, et al. Effect of levosimendan on the short-term clinical course of patients with acutely decompensated heart failure. *JACC Heart Fail.* 2013;1(2):103-111.

21. Mebazaa A, Nieminen MS, Filippatos GS, et al. Levosimendan vs. dobutamine: outcomes for acute heart failure patients on beta-blockers in SURVIVE. *Eur J Heart Fail.* 2009;11(3):304-311.

22. Bonow RO, Bennett S, Casey DE, Jr., et al. ACC/AHA clinical performance measures for adults with chronic heart failure: a report of the American College of Cardiology/American Heart Association Task Force on Performance Measures (Writing Committee to Develop Heart Failure Clinical Performance Measures) endorsed by the Heart Failure Society of America. *J Am Coll Cardiol.* 2005;46(6):1144-1178.

23. Antonelli M, Levy M, Andrews PJ, et al. Hemodynamic monitoring in shock and implications for management. International Consensus Conference, Paris, France, 27-28 April 2006. *Intensive Care Med.* 2007;33(4):575-590.

24. Reynolds HR, Hochman JS. Cardiogenic shock: current concepts and improving outcomes. *Circulation.* 2008;117(5):686-697.

25. Kahwash R, Leier CV, Miller L. Role of the pulmonary artery catheter in diagnosis and management of heart failure. *Cardiol Clin.* 2011;29(2):281-288.

26. Binanay C, Califf RM, Hasselblad V, et al. Evaluation study of congestive heart failure and pulmonary artery catheterization effectiveness: the ESCAPE trial. *JAMA.* 2005;294(13):1625-1633.

27. Shah MR, Miller L. Use of pulmonary artery catheters in advanced heart failure. *Curr Opin Cardiol.* 2007;22(3):220-224.

CHAPTER 72

Cardiac Transplantation

Ravi Karra

QUESTIONS

DIRECTIONS: Choose the one best response to each question.

72-1. Which of the following is *not an indication* for heart transplantation?

A. NYHA functional class IIIb–IV symptoms despite optimal medical and device therapy
B. VO_2 max of ≤ 12 to 14 mL/kg/min and/or VO_2 max < 50% predicted and/or VE/VCO_2 slope > 35 on cardiopulmonary exercise stress testing (CPET)
C. Cardiogenic shock not expected to recover
D. Intractable ventricular arrhythmias, uncontrolled with standard antiarrhythmic, device, or ablative therapy
E. Congenital heart disease with severe, fixed pulmonary hypertension

72-2. You are contacted to evaluate a potential heart as a donor for transplantation. Which of the following are favorable donor characteristics?

A. Cardiac index > 2.4 L/min·m²
B. Left ventricular (LV) wall thickness > 13 mm
C. Donor-recipient body size match (usually within 20% to 30% of height and weight)
D. All of the above
E. Both A and C are correct

72-3. A 44-year-old man is admitted for acute cardiogenic shock. He is transferred to your center with an intra-aortic balloon pump (IABP) and dobutamine infusion. After stabilization, he is able to be weaned successfully from the IABP. He is listed for heart transplantation and discharged home with home dobutamine. What is his UNOS status?

A. 1A
B. 1B

C. 2
D. 7
E. None of the above

72-4. Which of the following is a consequence of denervation of the transplanted heart?

A. Coronary ischemia continues to result in chest pain
B. Resting heart rate is low
C. Exercise intolerance
D. Digoxin is an effective agent for rate control
E. Atropine can increase heart rate

72-5. Which of the following is associated with a better prognosis following heart transplantation?

A. Retransplantation
B. Older age of donor organs
C. Higher transplant center volume
D. Both B and C are correct
E. None of the above

72-6. A 43-year-old woman has recently received an orthotopic heart transplant. She is being counseled about the requirement for immunosuppression and has several questions about the side effects of her medications. Which of the following is appropriate to tell her?

A. Tacrolimus is thought to result in fewer episodes of acute rejection compared to cyclosporine
B. Calcineurin inhibitors are not associated with renal dysfunction
C. Mycophenolate mofetil (MMF) is not associated with gastrointestinal intolerance
D. Sirolimus may cause coronary artery vasculopathy (CAV)
E. High-risk steroids are *not* associated with an increased infection risk

72-7. A 43-year-old woman who has recently received an orthotopic heart transplant presents with generalized malaise. She ran out of her immunosuppressive medications 1 week ago. An echocardiogram shows an LVEF of 25%. Her endomyocardial biopsy is shown in Figure 72-1. Which of the following is the most appropriate next step in her management?

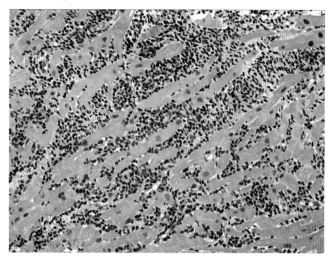

FIGURE 72-1 Endomyocardial biopsy for the patient in question 72-7.

A. An increase in her oral steroid dosing as an outpatient
B. Change from tacrolimus to cyclosporine
C. Anti-thymocyte globulin
D. Both A and C are correct
E. None of the above

72-8. A 57-year-old man underwent orthotopic heart transplantation 20 years ago and presents with progressive exertional dyspnea. He is found to have a normal LVEF, but coronary angiography suggests CAV. Which of the following is *true* of CAV?

A. Coronary angiography typically shows discrete, focal stenosis
B. CAV results from concentric, intimal thinning
C. Proliferation signal inhibitors (PSIs) can reduce the progression of CAV
D. Prognosis with therapy is good
E. None of the above

72-9. Which of the following pathogens warrants antimicrobial prophylaxis for the first year after heart transplantation?

A. HIV
B. Pneumocystis
C. HCV
D. MRSA
E. None of the above

72-10. Which of the following is *true* regarding risk for malignancy following heart transplantation?

A. Malignancy is a rare cause of late mortality in heart transplant recipients
B. The most common type of malignancy after heart transplantation is colorectal cancer
C. Post-transplant lymphoproliferative disorder (PTLD) is related to EBV infection and the degree of immunosuppression
D. Immunosuppression should be increased when PTLD is identified
E. Routine preventive screening for malignancy should be avoided in patients who have undergone cardiac transplantation

72-1. **The answer is E.** (*Hurst's The Heart, 14th Edition, Chap. 72*) The goal of a heart transplant evaluation is to determine if (1) the patient's cardiac status is limited enough, on optimal medical therapy, to benefit from heart transplantation (ie, "sick enough") (options A, B, and C); (2) the patient does not have comorbidities that would preclude heart transplantation (ie, "well enough"); and (3) the patient demonstrates compliance and possesses adequate social support ("can adapt to new transplant lifestyle"). The cardiopulmonary exercise stress test measures maximal oxygen consumption (VO_2 max), which is proportional to cardiac output. Patients with a peak VO_2 of more than 14 mL/kg/min have 1- and 2-year survival rates that are comparable or better than those achieved with transplantation, and these patients should be managed medically and should undergo serial exercise testing.[1,2] In the early years of heart transplantation, it was discovered that a normal donor right ventricle (RV) cannot increase its external workload acutely to overcome elevated pulmonary vascular resistance (PVR), resulting in acute RV failure and cardiogenic shock postoperatively.[3] Elevated PVR remains a strong risk factor for RV failure and early postoperative mortality. A pulmonary artery systolic pressure above 50 to 60 mm Hg, a PVR value above 5 Wood units, or a transpulmonary gradient above 15 to 20 mm Hg is usually considered prohibitive of successful heart transplantation (option E).

72-2. **The answer is E.** (*Hurst's The Heart, 14th Edition, Chap. 72*) To be considered suitable donors for cardiac transplantation, brain-dead individuals must meet certain minimum criteria. Most cardiac donors are younger than 55 years, although older donors may be used selectively in critically ill or older recipients. There should be no evidence of severe cardiothoracic trauma or cardiac puncture. An initial echocardiogram is performed to identify significant structural heart disease such as left ventricular hypertrophy or dysfunction, occlusive coronary artery disease, valvular dysfunction, and congenital lesions (options A and B). Donors with these conditions are typically excluded, although selected marginal organs may be allocated to higher risk recipients. Donors should also be size-matched to recipients (option C) Angiography is performed to exclude significant coronary artery disease in male donors older than age 45 and in female donors older than age 50 but may also be performed in younger patients with multiple risk factors for coronary artery disease. Patients with active malignancy (excluding nonmelanocytic skin cancers and certain isolated brain tumors) or severe systemic infections are typically excluded.

72-3. **The answer is B.** (*Hurst's The Heart, 14th Edition, Chap. 72*) The UNOS status helps to preferentially allocate organs to those patients with the highest risk for mortality in the absence of transplantation. Criteria for 1A listing include temporary mechanical circulatory support, left ventricular assist device (LVAD) complication, or continuous infusion of single high-dose inotrope or multiple inotropes in addition to continuous hemodynamic monitoring of LV filling pressures (option A). Status 1B patients are stable patients with an LVAD for more than 30 days or who require continuous inotropes but do not meet 1A criteria (option B). Status 2 patients are patients meeting criteria for heart transplantation but who do not meet 1A or 1B criteria (option C). Status 7 patients are temporarily inactive due to a change in condition (option D).

72-4. **The answer is C.** (*Hurst's The Heart, 14th Edition, Chap. 72*) When the donor heart is placed into the recipient, both afferent (from the heart to the central nervous system) and efferent (from the central nervous system to the heart) nerve supply is lost. The loss of afferent nerve supply means that the recipient will not experience angina with the exception of a small subgroup that may have reinnervation (option A).[4] The consequences of the loss of efferent nerves are related to the loss of vagal tone and the postganglionic direct release of norepinephrine stores in response to exercise. With the loss of vagal tone, heart transplant recipients have a higher than normal resting heart rate, usually around 90 to 110 bpm (option B). The lack of efferent nerves also means that the transplant recipient must rely on circulating catecholamines to respond to exercise, so there is a blunting of the heart rate's response to exercise (option C). Similarly, after exercise, the heart rate returns to baseline more slowly because of the gradual decline of circulating catecholamine concentrations to baseline. Some cardiac drugs are not effective in the denervated heart. As a result of the lack of vagal tone, digoxin will have little effect on sinoatrial and atrioventricular conduction velocity and will not achieve rate control if the transplanted heart develops atrial fibrillation (option D). However, the inotropic effects of digoxin persist after transplantation. Similarly, the parasympatholytic effect of atropine will not increase heart rate in transplanted hearts (option E).

72-5. The answer is C. *(Hurst's The Heart, 14th Edition, Chap. 72)* An in-depth analysis of risk factors for survival at 1, 5, 10, 15, and 20 years after transplantation is provided in the ISHLT registry report.[5] The strongest risk factors for 1-year mortality, associated with a 50% or more increase, are mainly related to technical issues and the underlying disease responsible for transplantation, including the use of temporary circulatory support, congenital cardiomyopathy versus nonischemic cardiomyopathy, prior transplant, and pretransplant ventilatory support or dialysis. Risk factors for 5- and 10-year mortality, on the other hand, are mostly related to immunologic issues and toxicity related to immunosuppression, including dialysis or infection after transplant, rejection during the first posttransplant year, and lack of immunosuppression therapy with a combination of at least two of the following classes: cell cycle inhibitors, calcineurin inhibitors, and PSIs. Other factors affecting 20-year survival include etiology for transplantation, sex, age, ischemic time, and center volume. Patients receiving retransplant and those receiving transplant for ischemic heart disease or valvular heart disease have a lower likelihood of survival past 20 years after transplant compared with patients who receive an allograft for nonischemic cardiomyopathy (option A). Younger donor age, younger recipient age, lower allograft ischemic time, and higher center volume are additional factors associated with long-term survival, and these risk factors appear consistent across countries (options B and C).

72-6. The answer is A. *(Hurst's The Heart, 14th Edition, Chap. 72)* Since the introduction of cyclosporine in the early 1980s, the calcineurin inhibitors have remained the cornerstone of maintenance immunosuppressive therapy in patients undergoing solid organ transplantation.[6] Tacrolimus is favored over cyclosporine based on evidence from clinical trials suggesting that tacrolimus-based immunosuppression is associated with decreased rates of acute rejection (option A).[7,8] Although nephrotoxicity is seen with both agents, there is more hypertension and dyslipidemia observed with cyclosporine and a higher incidence of new-onset insulin-requiring diabetes observed with tacrolimus (option B).[9,10] MMF has replaced azathioprine as the preferred antimetabolite agent in recent years based on a clinical trial demonstrating a significant reduction in both mortality and in the incidence of treatable rejection at 1 year with MMF versus azathioprine.[11] MMF is classically associated with GI intolerance (option C). Mycophenolate sodium is an enteric-coated, delayed-release formulation developed to improve the upper gastrointestinal tolerability of MMF. It is therapeutically similar to MMF with respect to the prevention of both biopsy-proven and treated acute rejection episodes, graft loss, or death.[12] Sirolimus and everolimus are often used in place of MMF in patients with rejection, allograft vasculopathy, malignancy, and viral infections such as cytomegalovirus to prevent recurrence or progression (option D).[13] Although steroids are highly effective for the prevention and treatment of acute rejection, their long-term use is associated with a number of adverse effects, including new-onset or worsening diabetes mellitus, hyperlipidemia, hypertension, fluid retention, myopathy, osteoporosis, and a predisposition toward opportunistic infections (option E).

72-7. The answer is D. *(Hurst's The Heart, 14th Edition, Chap. 72)* This patient has severe acute cellular rejection (ACR) with dense infiltrates and myocyte damage. The management of rejection proceeds in a stepwise fashion based on the severity of rejection detected on biopsy and the patient's presentation. If the patient is asymptomatic (no HF symptoms and normal left ventricular ejection fraction), treatment options include oral pulse steroids, targeting higher levels of immunosuppressive medications, switching from cyclosporine to tacrolimus, or switching from MMF to a PSI (option B).[8,14-17] Given the equivalent success of intravenous and oral corticosteroid therapy for the treatment of asymptomatic ACR, an outpatient course of oral corticosteroids is often the first-line treatment (option A).[18] For patients with HF symptoms or reduced ejection fraction, treatment is more aggressive, with intravenous corticosteroids and cytolytic therapy with antithymocyte globulin (option C).

72-8. The answer is C. *(Hurst's The Heart, 14th Edition, Chap. 72)* Despite improvements in immunosuppression over the past three decades, the incidence of CAV has not significantly decreased, and its development continues to limit long-term survival in patients undergoing cardiac transplantation. In CAV, the major epicardial vessels, their branches, and often the intramyocardial divisions display uniform, diffuse involvement extending along their entire length. The asymmetric and calcified plaques or lesions composed of cholesterol that are characteristic of conventional atherosclerosis are not found in uncomplicated lesions of vessels affected by CAV (option A). Histopathologic sections show a concentrically thickened intimal layer composed of modified smooth muscle cells, foamy macrophages, and variable numbers of histiocytes and lymphocytes within a connective tissue matrix that ranges from loose, edematous, and myxoid in early lesions to densely hyalinized and fibrotic in older lesions (option B).[19] Intraluminal thrombosis is uncommon. Clinically apparent CAV is associated with a poor prognosis, and therefore, prevention is an important strategy (option D). The PSIs also show significant promise in reducing the progression of intimal thickening by IVUS (option C).[14,15,20,21] Retransplantation may be considered for patients with advanced CAV.

72-9. The answer is B. *(Hurst's The Heart, 14th Edition, Chap. 72)* Given the degree of immunosuppression, all transplant recipients receive antimicrobial prophylaxis for oral candidiasis, toxoplasmosis and pneumocystis, and cytomegalovirus over the first post-transplant year (options A, B, C, and D). The use of vaccines in heart transplant recipients remains controversial. Live vaccines are definitely contraindicated because of the patients' immunosuppressed states. Even dead vaccines may pose a risk because they can promote activation of the immune system and cause rejection.[22]

72-10. The answer is C. *(Hurst's The Heart, 14th Edition, Chap. 72)* Malignancy is one of the most common causes of late mortality in heart transplant recipients (option A).[23] Cutaneous malignancies are the most common type after heart transplantation, mainly squamous cell and basal cell carcinomas (option B).[24] Post-transplant lymphoproliferative disorder (PTLD), most commonly a B-cell lymphoma related to EBV infection, may occur after transplantation (option C).[25,26] Risk factors for the development of PTLD include the use of cytolytic therapy for induction and EBV serostatus (with EBV-seronegative recipients of EBV-seropositive donors being at the highest risk).[26,27] The most critical point of treatment of malignancies is prevention. Heart transplant recipients should undergo routine health maintenance screenings with their primary care physicians, including mammograms, pap smears, prostate exams, and colonoscopies as indicated for nontransplant patients. In addition, patients are instructed to use sun protection and to establish care with a dermatologist for routine skin exams (option E). The initial approach to malignancy is reduction of immunosuppression, and this may be the only treatment required for some forms of PTLD (option D).

References

1. Mancini DM, Eisen H, Kussmaul W, et al. Value of peak exercise oxygen consumption for optimal timing of cardiac transplantation in ambulatory patients with heart failure. *Circulation.* 1991;83(3):778-786.
2. Mehra MR, Canter CE, Hannan MM, et al. The 2016 International Society for Heart Lung Transplantation listing criteria for heart transplantation: a 10-year update. *J Heart Lung Transplant.* 2016;35(1):1-23.
3. Costard-Jackle A, Fowler MB. Influence of preoperative pulmonary artery pressure on mortality after heart transplantation: testing of potential reversibility of pulmonary hypertension with nitroprusside is useful in defining a high risk group. *J Am Coll Cardiol.* 1992;19(1):48-54.
4. Stark RP, McGinn AL, Wilson RF. Chest pain in cardiac-transplant recipients. Evidence of sensory reinnervation after cardiac transplantation. *N Engl J Med.* 1991;324(25):1791-1794.

5. Lund LH, Edwards LB, Kucheryavaya AY, et al. The Registry of the International Society for Heart and Lung Transplantation: thirty-second official adult heart transplantation report—2015; focus theme: early graft failure. *J Heart Lung Transplant*. 2015;34(10):1244-1254.

6. Reitz BA, Bieber CP, Raney AA, et al. Orthotopic heart and combined heart and lung transplantation with cyclosporin-A immune suppression. *Transplant Proc*. 1981;13(1 Pt 1):393-396.

7. Grimm M, Rinaldi M, Yonan NA, et al. Superior prevention of acute rejection by tacrolimus vs. cyclosporine in heart transplant recipients—a large European trial. *Am J Transplant*. 2006;6(6):1387-1397.

8. Kobashigawa JA, Miller LW, Russell SD, et al. Tacrolimus with mycophenolate mofetil (MMF) or sirolimus vs. cyclosporine with MMF in cardiac transplant patients: 1-year report. *Am J Transplant*. 2006;6(6):1377-1386.

9. Taylor DO, Barr ML, Radovancevic B, et al. A randomized, multicenter comparison of tacrolimus and cyclosporine immunosuppressive regimens in cardiac transplantation: decreased hyperlipidemia and hypertension with tacrolimus. *J Heart Lung Transplant*. 1999;18(4):336-345.

10. Ye F, Ying-Bin X, Yu-Guo W, Hetzer R. Tacrolimus versus cyclosporine microemulsion for heart transplant recipients: a meta-analysis. *J Heart Lung Transplant*. 2009;28(1):58-66.

11. Kobashigawa J, Miller L, Renlund D, et al. A randomized active-controlled trial of mycophenolate mofetil in heart transplant recipients. Mycophenolate Mofetil Investigators. *Transplantation*. 1998;66(4):507-515.

12. Kobashigawa JA, Renlund DG, Gerosa G, et al. Similar efficacy and safety of enteric-coated mycophenolate sodium (EC-MPS, myfortic) compared with mycophenolate mofetil (MMF) in de novo heart transplant recipients: results of a 12-month, single-blind, randomized, parallel-group, multicenter study. *J Heart Lung Transplant*. 2006;25(8):935-941.

13. Kobashigawa J, Ross H, Bara C, et al. Everolimus is associated with a reduced incidence of cytomegalovirus infection following de novo cardiac transplantation. *Transpl Infect Dis*. 2013;15(2):150-162.

14. Keogh A, Richardson M, Ruygrok P, et al. Sirolimus in de novo heart transplant recipients reduces acute rejection and prevents coronary artery disease at 2 years: a randomized clinical trial. *Circulation*. 2004;110(17):2694-2700.

15. Eisen HJ, Tuzcu EM, Dorent R, et al. Everolimus for the prevention of allograft rejection and vasculopathy in cardiac-transplant recipients. *N Engl J Med*. 2003;349(9):847-858.

16. Mancini D, Pinney S, Burkhoff D, et al. Use of rapamycin slows progression of cardiac transplantation vasculopathy. *Circulation*. 2003;108(1):48-53.

17. Kobashigawa JA, Patel J, Furukawa H, et al. Five-year results of a randomized, single-center study of tacrolimus vs microemulsion cyclosporine in heart transplant patients. *J Heart Lung Transplant*. 2006;25(4):434-439.

18. Kobashigawa JA, Stevenson LW, Moriguchi JD, et al. Is intravenous glucocorticoid therapy better than an oral regimen for asymptomatic cardiac rejection? A randomized trial. *J Am Coll Cardiol*. 1993;21(5):1142-1144.

19. Pucci AM, Forbes RD, Billingham ME. Pathologic features in long-term cardiac allografts. *J Heart Transplant*. 1990;9(4):339-345.

20. Eisen HJ, Kobashigawa J, Starling RC, et al. Everolimus versus mycophenolate mofetil in heart transplantation: a randomized, multicenter trial. *Am J Transplant*. 2013;13(5):1203-1216.

21. Kobashigawa JA, Pauly DF, Starling RC, et al. Cardiac allograft vasculopathy by intravascular ultrasound in heart transplant patients: substudy from the Everolimus versus mycophenolate mofetil randomized, multicenter trial. *JACC Heart Fail*. 2013;1(5):389-399.

22. Schaffer SA, Husain S, Delgado DH, Kavanaugh L, Ross HJ. Impact of adjuvanted H1N1 vaccine on cell-mediated rejection in heart transplant recipients. *Am J Transplant*. 2011;11(12):2751-2754.

23. Stehlik J, Edwards LB, Kucheryavaya AY, et al. The Registry of the International Society for Heart and Lung Transplantation: twenty-seventh official adult heart transplant report—2010. *J Heart Lung Transplant*. 2010;29(10):1089-1103.

24. Vajdic CM, van Leeuwen MT. Cancer incidence and risk factors after solid organ transplantation. *Int J Cancer*. 2009;125(8):1747-1754.

25. Opelz G, Henderson R. Incidence of non-Hodgkin lymphoma in kidney and heart transplant recipients. *Lancet*. 1993;342(8886-8887):1514-1516.

26. Swinnen LJ, Costanzo-Nordin MR, Fisher SG, et al. Increased incidence of lymphoproliferative disorder after immunosuppression with the monoclonal antibody OKT3 in cardiac-transplant recipients. *N Engl J Med*. 1990;323(25):1723-1728.

27. Walker RC. Pretransplant assessment of the risk for posttransplant lymphoproliferative disorder. *Transplant Proc*. 1995;27(5 Suppl 1):41.

CHAPTER 73

Mechanically Assisted Circulation

Ravi Karra

DIRECTIONS: Choose the one best response to each question.

73-1. Which of the following is *not* among the indications for destination therapy (DT) left ventricular assist device (LVAD) implantation?

A. Continuous infusion of inotropic medications for at least 7 days
B. NYHA class IIIb or IV functional limitations on maximally tolerated medical therapy
C. Left ventricular (LV) ejection fraction < 25%
D. Peak oxygen consumption of < 14 mL/kg/min
E. Need for acute mechanical circulatory support (MCS) for at least 7 days

73-2. A 43-year-old man develops cardiogenic shock after an acute myocardial infarction (MI). An intra-aortic balloon pump (IABP) is inserted. Which of the following is *not true* about the IABP tracing in Figure 73-1?

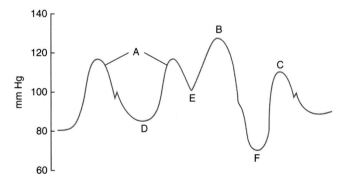

FIGURE 73-1 IABP tracing for question 73-2.

(Adapted with permission from Trost JC, Hillis LD. Intra-aortic balloon counterpulsation, *Am J Cardiol.* 2006 May 1;97(9):1391-1398.)

A. A reflects unassisted systole
B. B is an augmented diastolic beat
C. C and F are a part of an assisted beat
D. D is an unassisted end diastolic pressure
E. E indicates balloon deflation

73-3. A 67-year-old woman received an orthotopic heart transplant 6 months ago. She presents with generalized malaise and new onset heart failure. Echocardiography confirms allograft dysfunction, and serum PCR demonstrates HCMV viremia. Which of the following is *true* about HCMV myocarditis?

A. Myocardial infection with HCMV is usually observed in immunocompetent hosts
B. Myocardial pathology is notable for an infiltrate by eosinophils
C. Viral infection is restricted to myocytes
D. In immunosuppressed patients, infection often occurs by reactivation of a latent infection
E. First-line treatment is with acyclovir

73-4. Which of the following is *not true* of short-term mechanical support devices?

A. The Impella devices are axial flow LVADs that are mounted on a catheter designed to rest in the left ventricle (LV)
B. In the traditional configuration, the TandemHeart pump draws blood from the left atrium
C. The PVAD and AB5000 are pneumatic extracorporeal pumps
D. The CentriMag system and the Rotaflow systems are pulsatile pumps
E. The Impella RP and the Protek Duo Cannula system provide right ventricular (RV) support by draining blood from the right atrium (RA) and ejecting blood into the pulmonary artery (PA)

73-5. Which of the following is *true* of cardiac MRI (CMR) findings of acute myocarditis?

A. CMR findings are diagnostic but not prognostic
B. Late gadolinium enhancement (LGE) is present in a noncoronary distribution
C. CMR would show decreased myocardial edema
D. Early gadolinium enhancement (EGE) is normal
E. The presence of a pericardial effusion increases the diagnostic accuracy of CMR for myocarditis

73-6. Which of the following is *not* a complication of venoarterial extracorporeal membrane oxygenation (VA ECMO) used for cardiogenic shock?

A. Bleeding at the cannulation site
B. Ipsilateral limb ischemia when the femoral artery is cannulated
C. Pulmonary edema without an LV vent
D. Thrombocytosis
E. Inflammation

73-7. Which of the following is *true* about durable mechanical circulatory support?

A. The HeartMate II device is a pulsatile flow LVAD
B. The HeartMate II device is approved for bridge to transplantation (BTT) and DT use
C. The HeartWare device is approved for DT use only
D. The Syncardia Total Artificial Heart (Syncardia, Tucson, AZ) is approved for DT use in patients with severe biventricular heart failure
E. The Excor LVAD is approved as a DT device for children in the United States.

73-8. A 53-year-old woman with an implanted continuous flow LVAD presents with worsening exertional dyspnea, edema, and abdominal distension. Her LVAD pump parameters indicated decreased flows and several suction events. An echocardiogram shows a decompressed LV and dilated RV. Which of the following is *true* of right heart failure (RHF) associated with LVAD support?

A. Isolated late-onset RV failure after LVAD implantation is unlikely
B. A ratio of central venous pressure to pulmonary capillary wedge pressure < 0.63 is a risk factor for early RV failure
C. Preoperative elevation of bilirubin, the need for inotropic support, and hemodynamic instability are predictors of early RHF after LVAD implantation
D. LVAD speed adjustment is unlikely to be helpful
E. Inotropic therapy is not needed with an LVAD in place

73-9. A 47-year-old woman with an axial flow LVAD presents with fatigue and dark stools. Which of the following is *true* of gastrointestinal bleeding (GI) with LVAD support?

A. The use of systemic anticoagulation increases the risk for GI bleeding
B. An acquired deficiency of von Willebrand factor may increase the risk for GI bleeding
C. AVMs in the small bowel are a major cause of bleeding in patients supported with an LVAD
D. All of the above are correct
E. None of the above is correct

73-10. A 48-year-old man supported by an axial flow LVAD develops tea-colored urine, increased pump powers, and heart failure symptoms. An echocardiographic ramp study shows that the LV does *not* decompress with increased pump speeds. Which of the following lab abnormalities would be expected in this patient?

A. An elevated serum creatinine
B. Increased lactate dehydrogenase (LDH)
C. Decreased plasma free hemoglobin
D. Increased bilirubin
E. B and C

73-1. The answer is A. (*Hurst's The Heart, 14th Edition, Chap. 73*) The DT LVAD population continues to grow. Eligible patients have NYHA class IIIb or IV functional limitations on maximally tolerated medical therapy (option B), an LV ejection fraction < 25% (option C), and a peak oxygen consumption of < 14 mL/kg/min (option D). In less stable patients, treatment with continuous infusion of inotropic medications for at least 14 days (option A) or the need for acute circulatory support for at least 7 days are also indications for durable LVAD therapy (option E).

73-2. The answer is E. (*Hurst's The Heart, 14th Edition, Chap. 73*) Option A reflects unassisted systole. Option B is an augmented diastolic beat. Options C and F are assisted systole and diastole respectively. Option D is an unassisted end diastolic pressure. Option E indicates balloon inflation, and it is an important landmark to assess the timing of balloon inflation.

73-3. The answer is D. (*Hurst's The Heart, 14th Edition, Chap. 73*) Myocardial infection with HCMV is more commonly observed in immunocompromised hosts (option A). The myocardial pathology is characterized by T-cell inflammatory infiltrate and by the presence of typical intranuclear amphophilic inclusion bodies that specifically immune-stain with anti-HCMV antibodies (option B). The virus infects both myocytes and endothelial cells (option C). Children become infected early in life in developing countries, whereas up to 80% of the adult population is infected in developed nations. The course of primary infection is usually mild or asymptomatic in immunocompetent hosts as HCMV establishes a latent but persistent infection reflecting the inability of the immune system to clear the infection; immune evasion mechanisms allow infected cells to escape both innate and adaptive effector immunity.[1] In immunosuppressed patients (eg, solid organ or bone marrow transplantation recipients), the infection can be reactivated to result in systemic and organ infection; the heart is a possible target for tissue infection, especially in heart transplant recipients (option D). For herpes simplex virus types 1 and 2 and for varicella zoster virus, acyclovir (or its prodrug valacyclovir) and famciclovir have greatly reduced the burden of disease and have demonstrated a remarkable safety record. Ganciclovir and valganciclovir remain the drugs of choice for HCMV infection in immunocompromised hosts (option E).[2,3]

73-4. The answer is D. (*Hurst's The Heart, 14th Edition, Chap. 73*) The Impella (Abiomed, Danvers, MA) is a catheter-mounted, axial flow VAD demonstrated to provide more hemodynamic support than IABP. The catheter is inserted into the LV using an over-the-wire technique. The device draws blood from the LV and ejects it into the aortic root (option A). The TandemHeart Pump and Cannula System (CardiacAssist, Pittsburgh, PA) is another percutaneous device for LV support. The left heart drainage cannula is inserted from the femoral vein into the left atrium across the intra-atrial septum. Outflow from the pump is into the femoral artery and descending aorta (option B). The paracorporeal ventricular assist device (PVAD; St. Jude Medical, St. Paul, MN) and the AB5000 pump (Abiomed, Danvers, MA) are older, pulsatile devices that can be used for right, left, or biventricular support. Right heart drainage is achieved with a surgically attached right atrial or RV cannula, whereas the left heart is drained with a surgically attached LV apical cannula. Outflow from the right heart pump consists of a graft cannula sewn to the main pulmonary artery, whereas outflow from the left heart consists of a graft cannula attached to the ascending aorta. The cannulas exit the body below the sternotomy incision and are attached to pneumatic pumps that rest on the anterior abdominal wall (option C). Two examples of continuous flow devices are the CentriMag pump (St. Jude Medical, St. Paul, MN) and the Rotaflow pump (Maquet, Wayne, NJ). Like the pulsatile devices, rotary flow systems provide right heart and/or left heart support and use surgically attached cannulas tunneled out of chest onto the upper abdomen (option D). The Impella RP and the Protek Duo Cannula system are newer devices meant to support the right ventricle. They provide RV support by draining blood from the RA and ejecting blood into the PA (option E).

The Impella RP and the Protek Duo Cannula system provide RV support by draining blood from the RA and ejecting blood into the PA.

73-5. **The answer is B.** *(Hurst's The Heart, 14th Edition, Chap. 73)* CMR provides a detailed morphofunctional description of ventricular involvement and offers important prognostic information.[4] There is a substantially lower risk of events in patients with suspected myocarditis but normal CMR findings (option A).[5] According to the Lake Louise CMR criteria, acute myocarditis is associated with (1) increased regional or global myocardial signal intensity in T2-weighted images (indicating myocardial edema); (2) increased global myocardial early gadolinium enhancement (EGE) ratio between myocardium and skeletal muscle in T1-weighted images (supporting hyperemia/capillary leakage); and (3) at least one focal lesion with nonischemic distribution in LGE T1-weighted images (suggestive of cell injury/necrosis) (options B, C, and D).[4] The diagnostic accuracy does not increase with the addition of pericardial effusion (option E).[6]

73-6. **The answer is D.** *(Hurst's The Heart, 14th Edition, Chap. 73)* ECMO is another temporary MCS strategy capable of supporting the cardiovascular and respiratory systems. VA ECMO consists of a circuit in which blood is drawn from the venous circulation, oxygenated, and returned to the arterial system. Adverse events associated with VA ECMO are related to the cannulation and artificial blood circuit as well as the underlying shock state that prompted treatment (option A). Peripheral arterial complications associated with VA ECMO include bleeding, arterial obstruction, and distal extremity ischemia. When femoral arterial cannulation is used, ipsilateral lower extremity perfusion must be monitored (option B). VA ECMO does not directly unload the LV, and blood return from an incompetent aortic valve or from pulmonary venous return may cause LV distention resulting in progressive ventricular distention and hydrostatic pulmonary circulatory injury. The placement of an LV vent via the apex or right superior pulmonary vein with return of blood to the ECMO circuit can prevent this complication (option C). ECMO support is associated with blood component abnormality coagulopathies. Hemolysis related to blood contact with the ECMO tubing is usually not clinically significant as long as appropriate cannulas and pump speeds are used. Thrombocytopenia may result from platelet consumption or clumping. Exposure of the blood volume to the artificial surfaces may trigger inflammatory responses manifested as fever, leukocytosis, or peripheral arterial vasodilation requiring vasopressors (options D and E).

73-7. **The answer is B.** *(Hurst's The Heart, 14th Edition, Chap. 73)* The HeartMate II LVAD (St. Jude Medical, Minneapolis, MN) is a continuous flow LVAD implanted in the left upper quadrant of the abdomen (option A). HeartMate II has US approval for BTT and DT (option B).[7,8] The HeartWare HVAD (HeartWare, Framingham, MA) is a continuous, centrifugal flow device that is smaller than HeartMate II and is implanted in the pericardial space. The HVAD has US approval for BTT based on a 140-patient trial that compared HVAD outcomes to a contemporaneously enrolled INTERMACS cohort that received an approved LVAD (option C).[9] The Syncardia Total Artificial Heart (Syncardia, Tucson, AZ) is the only commercially available TAH that has achieved BTT approval in patients with severe biventricular heart failure (option D).[10] The Excor Pediatric VAD (Berlin Heart, Woodlands, TX) is a miniaturized, pneumatically driven, extracorporeal LVAD manufactured with stroke volumes from 10 to 60 mL to fulfill the hemodynamic needs of children from newborn through adolescence. The Excor device is approved as a BTT for children in the United States.[11]

73-8. **The answer is C.** *(Hurst's The Heart, 14th Edition, Chap. 73)* RV failure is an important cause of morbidity and mortality in LVAD-supported patients. Preimplant prediction is best accomplished by integrating multiple data elements. A ratio of central venous pressure to pulmonary capillary wedge pressure > 0.63 is a risk factor for early RV failure (option B).[12] Many other clinical variables have been identified in multivariate analyses as associated with the development of early RV failure. These include a lack of hemodynamic stability, the use of inotropic or vasopressor support, and markers of liver injury (option C).[13] Furthermore, although the focus of many analyses has been on early RV failure, there is increasing evidence that a syndrome of late RV failure can develop months to years after LVAD implantation (option A). This may be in part a result of residual RV dysfunction that manifests later in the clinical course, ongoing myocyte injury leading to declining contractility of the unsupported RV, or a new insult to the RV myocardium. Similar to early RV failure, management of this clinical syndrome requires careful consideration of relative right- and left-sided filling pressures, which can be concordant or discordant. In patients with concordant elevation in left- and right-sided filling pressures, diuretic therapy and LVAD speed adjustment may be key therapeutic interventions (option D). However, elevated right-sided pressures in the setting of low or normal left-sided pressures may require consideration of inotropic support to improve RV contractility (option E).

73-9. The answer is D. *(Hurst's The Heart, 14th Edition, Chap. 73)* Both surgical and nonsurgical bleeding are common adverse events associated with LVAD therapy. Bleeding in LVAD recipients results from hematologic alterations, including acquired von Willebrand disease, impaired platelet aggregation, and the requisite use of antiplatelet agents and anticoagulation (options A and B).[14,15] Acquired von Willebrand disease, a consequence of high shear stress generated in the LVAD, exposes enzymatic cleavage sites on the von Willebrand protein with resultant proteolysis to smaller molecular weight fragments that are less effective at platelet binding.[16,17] LVAD patients have measurable reductions of large-molecular-weight von Willebrand factor multimers within 30 days after implantation but restoration following heart transplantation, suggesting a primary role of the device.[18-20] Reduced pulse pressure leads to alterations in microcirculatory flow, promoting the proliferation of arteriovenous malformations (AVMs) in the GI tract.[15] AVMs have been identified as the bleeding source in up to one-third of GI bleeding events and are most commonly identified in the small bowel (option C).[21]

73-10. The answer is B. *(Hurst's The Heart, 14th Edition, Chap. 73)* This patient has a classic presentation for LVAD pump thrombosis. Elevated levels of lactate dehydrogenase, plasma free hemoglobin, and hemoglobinuria associated with alterations in consumed pump power help confirm the diagnosis (options B and C). The other options are possible but are more indirectly related to hemolysis (options A and D). Medical management strategies include hemodynamic stabilization, enhanced anticoagulation, and systemic or intraventricular thrombolysis.[22,23] Most patients, however, will require LVAD exchange; this recommendation is based largely on the observation of improved survival for the patient cohort managed with device removal versus noninvasive management.[23]

References

1. Poole E, Sinclair J. Sleepless latency of human cytomegalovirus. *Med Microbiol Immunol.* 2015;204(3):421-429.
2. Field HJ, Vere Hodge RA. Recent developments in anti-herpesvirus drugs. *Br Med Bull.* 2013;106:213-249.
3. Owers DS, Webster AC, Strippoli GF, Kable K, Hodson EM. Pre-emptive treatment for cytomegalovirus viraemia to prevent cytomegalovirus disease in solid organ transplant recipients. *Cochrane Database Syst Rev.* 2013(2):CD005133.
4. Friedrich MG, Sechtem U, Schulz-Menger J, et al. Cardiovascular magnetic resonance in myocarditis: A JACC White Paper. *J Am Coll Cardiol.* 2009;53(17):1475-1487.
5. Schumm J, Greulich S, Wagner A, et al. Cardiovascular magnetic resonance risk stratification in patients with clinically suspected myocarditis. *J Cardiovasc Magn Reson.* 2014;16:14.
6. Lurz P, Eitel I, Klieme B, et al. The potential additional diagnostic value of assessing for pericardial effusion on cardiac magnetic resonance imaging in patients with suspected myocarditis. *Eur Heart J Cardiovasc Imaging.* 2014;15(6):643-650.
7. Miller LW, Pagani FD, Russell SD, et al. Use of a continuous-flow device in patients awaiting heart transplantation. *N Engl J Med.* 2007;357(9):885-896.
8. Slaughter MS, Rogers JG, Milano CA, et al. Advanced heart failure treated with continuous-flow left ventricular assist device. *N Engl J Med.* 2009;361(23):2241-2251.
9. Aaronson KD, Slaughter MS, Miller LW, et al. Use of an intrapericardial, continuous-flow, centrifugal pump in patients awaiting heart transplantation. *Circulation.* 2012;125(25):3191-3200.
10. Copeland JG, Smith RG, Arabia FA, et al. Cardiac replacement with a total artificial heart as a bridge to transplantation. *N Engl J Med.* 2004;351(9):859-867.

11. Fraser CD, Jr., Jaquiss RD, Rosenthal DN, et al. Prospective trial of a pediatric ventricular assist device. *N Engl J Med.* 2012;367(6):532-541.

12. Kormos RL, Teuteberg JJ, Pagani FD, et al. Right ventricular failure in patients with the HeartMate II continuous-flow left ventricular assist device: incidence, risk factors, and effect on outcomes. *J Thorac Cardiovasc Surg.* 2010;139(5):1316-1324.

13. Matthews JC, Koelling TM, Pagani FD, Aaronson KD. The right ventricular failure risk score: a pre-operative tool for assessing the risk of right ventricular failure in left ventricular assist device candidates. *J Am Coll Cardiol.* 2008;51(22):2163-2172.

14. John R, Boyle A, Pagani F, Miller L. Physiologic and pathologic changes in patients with continuous-flow ventricular assist devices. *J Cardiovasc Transl Res.* 2009;2(2):154-158.

15. Suarez J, Patel CB, Felker GM, et al. Mechanisms of bleeding and approach to patients with axial-flow left ventricular assist devices. *Circ Heart Fail.* 2011;4(6):779-784.

16. Tsai HM, Sussman, II, Nagel RL. Shear stress enhances the proteolysis of von Willebrand factor in normal plasma. *Blood.* 1994;83(8):2171-2179.

17. Baldauf C, Schneppenheim R, Stacklies W, et al. Shear-induced unfolding activates von Willebrand factor A2 domain for proteolysis. *J Thromb Haemost.* 2009;7(12):2096-2105.

18. Crow S, Chen D, Milano C, et al. Acquired von Willebrand syndrome in continuous-flow ventricular assist device recipients. *Ann Thorac Surg.* 2010;90(4):1263-1269; discussion 9.

19. Crow S, Milano C, Joyce L, et al. Comparative analysis of von Willebrand factor profiles in pulsatile and continuous left ventricular assist device recipients. *ASAIO J.* 2010;56(5):441-445.

20. Uriel N, Pak SW, Jorde UP, et al. Acquired von Willebrand syndrome after continuous-flow mechanical device support contributes to a high prevalence of bleeding during long-term support and at the time of transplantation. *J Am Coll Cardiol.* 2010;56(15):1207-1213.

21. Demirozu ZT, Radovancevic R, Hochman LF, et al. Arteriovenous malformation and gastrointestinal bleeding in patients with the HeartMate II left ventricular assist device. *J Heart Lung Transplant.* 2011;30(8):849-853.

22. Slaughter MS, Pagani FD, Rogers JG, et al. Clinical management of continuous-flow left ventricular assist devices in advanced heart failure. *J Heart Lung Transplant.* 2010;29(4 Suppl):S1-S39.

23. Goldstein DJ, John R, Salerno C, et al. Algorithm for the diagnosis and management of suspected pump thrombus. *J Heart Lung Transplant.* 2013;32(7):667-670.

SECTION 12

Cardiopulmonary Disease

CHAPTER 74

Pulmonary Hypertension

Patrick R. Lawler

QUESTIONS

DIRECTIONS: Choose the one best response to each question.

74-1. What physiologic characteristic of the pulmonary circulation makes it highly adaptable in the face of increased blood flow?

A. Large amount of smooth muscle cells in the vessels
B. Large vascular flow reserve
C. Small cross-sectional surface area
D. High pulmonary vascular resistance to flow
E. All of the above

74-2. A mother brings her 9-week-old infant to clinic for a regular checkup. She notes that he has not been feeding well and gets tired easily. On physical examination, a continuous murmur is auscultated consistent with a patent ductus arteriosus (PDA). What pathophysiologic mechanism is responsible for this disease manifestation?

A. Pulmonary pressure drops significantly lower than systemic blood pressure after birth
B. Pulmonary pressure fails to rise above systemic blood pressure after birth
C. Pulmonary pressure is nearly equal to systemic blood pressure at birth
D. Pulmonary pressure fails to drop below systemic blood pressure after birth
E. None of the above

74-3. A 57-year-old man was diagnosed with pulmonary arterial hypertension (PAH) 6 months ago, and he was started on a calcium channel blocker. Follow-up Doppler echocardiography reveals a decreased pulmonary artery systolic blood pressure. Is this finding anticipated to portend a good prognosis?

A. No, the decreased pressure could be due to hemodynamic deterioration

B. Yes, Doppler echocardiography is sufficient to monitor PH
C. No, Doppler echocardiography does not assess RV function
D. Yes, the decreased pulmonary pressure is indicative of treatment efficacy
E. None of the above are correct

74-4. Which of the following statements about pulmonary hypertension (PH) and left heart failure is *correct*?

A. Diastolic heart failure has a better prognosis than heart failure with decreased systolic function
B. The degree of PH and the RV ejection fraction are prognostic for LV failure
C. Elevated PVR is a contraindication to surgical elimination of an obstruction causing pulmonary venous hypertension
D. Patients with heart failure with preserved ejection fraction tend to be older males with a history of hypertension
E. PH that accompanies LV failure is sufficient to cause RV failure

74-5. A 64-year-old woman presents to your clinic with shortness of breath, episodes of dizziness, and recurrent chest pain. Following a thorough history and a physical examination, idiopathic PAH is suspected. Which of the following is consistent with this diagnosis?

A. Patient is a female over the age of 60
B. Pathology indicates injury to the vascular walls of the large pulmonary arteries
C. The obliterative lesion affects more than one layer of the vessel wall
D. High pulmonary arterial pressure and elevated LA filling pressures
E. All of the above

74-6. A 35-year-old woman recently diagnosed with PAH is evaluated in clinic. Which of the following is *not* contraindicated for this patient?

A. Pregnancy
B. Phlebotomy in patients with pulmonary vascular disease and cyanotic congenital heart disease
C. Appetite suppressants
D. Oral contraceptives
E. High altitudes

74-7. Which of the following statements about available PAH therapies is *correct*?

A. The development of bronchiolitis obliterans is unlikely following lung transplantation in PAH patients
B. Epoprostenol is an oral prostacyclin analogue
C. Endothelin receptor antagonists are highly effective vasodilators without adverse effects
D. Phosphodiesterase inhibitors relax pulmonary vessels without affecting systemic arterial pressure
E. Atrial septostomy is a first-line therapy for patients with severe RV pressure and volume overload

74-8. Which of the following signs and symptoms is consistent with pulmonary veno-occlusive disease (PVOD)?

A. Patients experience worsening of pulmonary edema after administration of epoprostenol
B. High pulmonary arterial pressure and high LV end-diastolic pressure
C. Pathology reveals unilateral lung edema and focal fibrosis
D. Oral PAH medications are the treatment of choice
E. None of the above

74-9. Regarding prognostic assessment in a 66-year-old male patient diagnosed with PAH, which of the following determinants predicts a more *favorable* prognosis?

A. 6-minute walk distance is 250 meters
B. Brain natriuretic peptide levels are significantly increased (> 180 pg/mL)
C. Right heart catheterization (RHC) measures right atrial pressure (RAP) < 10 mm Hg
D. Resting heart rate is > 100 bpm
E. Resting systolic blood pressure is < 100 mm Hg

74-10. Which of the following statements about the pathways regulating the proliferation and contraction of pulmonary arteriole smooth muscle cells is *correct*?

A. PDE-5 inhibitors prevent the synthesis of nitric oxide from L-arginine
B. Prostacyclin is an endothelium-derived vasoconstrictor with a short half-life
C. Dysfunctional endothelium in PAH produces decreased levels of endothelin (ET-1)
D. Endothelin (ET-1) is an endothelium-derived mitogen and vasoconstrictor of smooth muscle cells
E. All of the above

74-1. The answer is B. *(Hurst's The Heart, 14th Edition, Chap. 74)* Because of its large capacity, its great distensibility, its low resistance to blood flow, and the modest amounts of smooth muscle in the small arteries and arterioles (option A), the pulmonary circulation is not predisposed to become hypertensive. In normal individuals lying supine, the mean driving pressure (ie, the difference between the mean blood pressure in the pulmonary artery and in the left atrium, the transpulmonary gradient) is usually < 10 mm Hg. Because blood flow (cardiac output) is the same in both circulations in the absence of any systemic to pulmonary communications, the pulmonary vascular resistance (PVR) is approximately one-eighth of systemic vascular resistance (option D). The large cross-sectional surface area of the pulmonary circulation (option C), coupled with the distensibility of its thin-walled vessels and the large recruitable vascular reserve, account for these unique characteristics. During exercise, as pulmonary blood flow increases, new regions of the pulmonary vascular bed are open, and existing vasculature dilates (option B); accordingly, the pulmonary circulation is capable of accommodating a fourfold or greater increase in resting blood flow with virtually no change in pulmonary artery pressure, with a concomitant decrease in PVR.

74-2. The answer is D. *(Hurst's The Heart, 14th Edition, Chap. 74)* Immediately before birth, pulmonary and systemic arterial blood pressures are near equal (option C) and approximately 70/40 mm Hg, with a mean of 50 mm Hg. Immediately after birth, with closure of the ductus arteriosus and initiation of ventilation, pulmonary arterial pressure falls rapidly to approximately one-half of systemic levels. Thereafter, pulmonary arterial pressures gradually decrease over several weeks to reach adult levels. In some neonates, the normal PH of the fetus fails to recede normally (option D), generally as a result of either a developmental anomaly, such as a patent ductus arteriosus, or a relentless increase in pulmonary vascular tone. In such infants, the persistent PH and RV failure may become life threatening.

74-3. The answer is A. *(Hurst's The Heart, 14th Edition, Chap. 74)* In general, echocardiographic techniques have proved useful in providing a measure of RV thickness as an index of RV hypertension (option C). Estimates of RV systolic pressure can be obtained by determining regurgitant flows across the tricuspid valves using continuous-wave Doppler echocardiography. However, the diagnosis of PH should not be made without confirmatory RHC (option B) because echocardiography sometimes inaccurately estimates RV systolic pressure because of poor visualization of the tricuspid regurgitant jet. Although echocardiography is an attractive alternative to repeated cardiac catheterization in following the course of the disease and assessing the effects of therapeutic interventions in some patients, the optimal parameters to monitor have not been well characterized (option D). Furthermore, a reduction in estimated or directly measured pulmonary artery systolic pressure may be caused by either hemodynamic improvement or deterioration (option A), since the pressure may decrease as pulmonary blood flow decreases as a result of progressive right heart failure.

74-4. The answer is B. *(Hurst's The Heart, 14th Edition, Chap. 74)* LV failure is one of the most common causes of PH. When the PH is caused by pulmonary venous hypertension, relief of the pulmonary venous hypertension will reverse the pulmonary vascular disease in virtually all cases. An elevated PVR should not be a contraindication to surgery or an interventional procedure to eliminate a discrete site of obstruction causing pulmonary venous hypertension (option C). LV failure is the most common cause of RV failure; the level of PH that accompanies LV failure is infrequently sufficient to account for RV failure (option E). It turns out, for reasons that remain unclear, that it is the degree of RV hypertension (ie, PH) and the RV ejection fraction that are prognostic for LV failure and not the degree of LV failure (option B). Patients with heart failure with preserved ejection fraction tend to be older females and to have a history of systemic hypertension (option D). Although the prognosis for these patients was previously considered better than for patients with a decreased LV ejection fraction, recent data suggest otherwise (option A). Pulmonary venous hypertension caused by diastolic dysfunction is often more severe than expected.

74-5.   **The answer is C.** *(Hurst's The Heart, 14th Edition, Chap. 74)* Idiopathic pulmonary arterial hypertension (IPAH) is a disorder intrinsic to the pulmonary vascular bed that is characterized by sustained elevations in pulmonary arterial pressure and vascular resistance that generally lead to RV failure and death. The hemodynamic hallmarks of IPAH in the resting patient include a combination of high pulmonary arterial pressure, a normal or low cardiac output, and normal LA or left-sided filling pressures (option D). The disease process occurs in the small pulmonary arteries (option B) and arterioles, and the obliterative lesions can affect one or more layers of these vessels (option C). The typical picture of a patient with IPAH is that of a woman who develops one or more of the symptoms of PH. Females predominate, regardless of age, with an overall ratio of approximately 3:1 (option A).

74-6.   **The answer is B.** *(Hurst's The Heart, 14th Edition, Chap. 74)* General measures for patients with all forms of PAH include the avoidance of circumstances or substances that may aggravate the disease state. Exercise should be guided by symptoms, and exposure to high altitude (option E) may worsen PAH by producing hypoxia-induced pulmonary vasoconstriction. Pregnancy (option A), oral contraceptives (option D), and appetite suppressants (option C) should be avoided. Because anesthesia and surgery of any type pose an increased risk of hemodynamic instability and death, elective procedures should be carefully considered. Phlebotomy (option B) with replacement of fluid (eg, plasma or albumin) is helpful in patients with pulmonary vascular disease and cyanotic congenital heart disease in whom severe hypoxemia has evoked substantial polycythemia. Phlebotomy is recommended for symptoms of hyperviscosity as a result of severe polycythemia, such as headache or blurry vision, or if the hematocrit is > 65% to 70%.

74-7.   **The answer is D.** *(Hurst's The Heart, 14th Edition, Chap. 74)* Patients with PAH have several therapeutic options. Atrial septostomy has been performed in patients with severe RV pressure and volume overload refractory to maximal medical therapy (option E), but its utility is uncertain because although systemic cardiac output is increased, shunting of deoxygenated blood occurs. Phosphodiesterase (PDE-5) inhibitors, thereby enhancing NO activity, which is an endothelium-derived relaxing factor that contributes to the low initial tone of the pulmonary circulation. It has the advantage over other vasodilators of selectively relaxing pulmonary vessels without affecting systemic arterial pressure (option D). Epoprostenol is a prostacyclin analogue that works as a pulmonary vasodilator. Unfortunately, it requires continuous intravenous infusion, which is accomplished using portable pumps (option B). None of these modalities are free of complications. Although endothelin receptor antagonists are generally well tolerated, liver function must be monitored monthly because they can cause hepatic injury (option C). While hemodynamic improvement is often dramatic, transplant for PAH poses both a considerable surgical risk and the prospect of opportunistic infections that accompany lifelong immunosuppression. Rejection phenomena, notably bronchiolitis obliterans (option A), are the major limiting factors to prolonged survival.

74-8.   **The answer is A.** *(Hurst's The Heart, 14th Edition, Chap. 74)* Pulmonary veno-occlusive disease (PVOD) is thought to begin as an inflammatory-thrombotic process in the small pulmonary veins and venules and end in fibrous obliteration of the venous and venular lumens. Cardiac catheterization discloses a high pulmonary arterial pressure with a normal pulmonary wedge and LV end-diastolic pressure (option B). When epoprostenol is administered to a patient with PVOD, a pulmonary edema pattern may ensue (option A), most often acutely (although it may not occur for several days in some patients), resulting from increasing pulmonary blood flow in the face of downstream vascular obstruction. This response, when present, is usually diagnostic of PVOD. At autopsy, both lungs are involved (option C). The lungs are the seat of congestion, edema, and focal fibrosis, which may become extensive. Most experienced clinicians consider PVOD to be a contraindication to the use of oral PAH medications or intravenous epoprostenol (option D). The treatment of choice is probably lung transplant.

74-9. The answer is C. (*Hurst's The Heart, 14th Edition, Chap. 74*) The diagnosis of PAH carries with it a poor prognosis unless medical or surgical therapy succeeds in decreasing PVR. The assessment of disease severity has been evaluated using noninvasive studies and invasive tests. These include the assessment of functional classification and exercise capacity using either the 6-minute walk test to assess exercise endurance or cardiopulmonary exercise testing to evaluate exercise tolerance. A 6-minute walking distance > 400 m is associated with a better outcome, while a 6-minute walking distance < 320 m is associated with a worse outcome (option A). Assessment of RAP by right heart catheterization reveals that RAP < 10 mm Hg is considered normal and is associated with a better prognosis (option C). Brain natriuretic peptide appears to be a reasonable biomarker for disease severity (option B). Likewise, a resting heart rate > 100 bpm (option D) and resting systolic blood pressure > 100 mm Hg (option E) are associated with worse outcomes. The prognosis is largely determined by the severity of right heart dysfunction and the hemodynamic and clinical response to therapy. Table 74-1 shows a detailed list of determinants of prognosis in PAH.

TABLE 74-1 Pulmonary Arterial Hypertension: Determinants of Prognosis

Risk Factors	Better Outcome	Worse Outcome
PAH group I classification	PAH-CHD, IPAH	PAH-CTD, PoPH, HPAH, PCH, PVOD
Rate of disease progression	Gradual	Rapid deterioration over several months
Syncope	Without	Recurrent
Right heart failure	No	Yes
WHO functional class[b]	I, II	IV
Resting systolic blood pressure		< 100 mm Hg
Resting heart rate		> 100 bpm
Chest radiograph		Pleural effusions
Echocardiography	Normal RV function to minimal RV dysfunction; no effusion	Pericardial effusion (any size); significant RV dilation/dysfunction; right atrial enlargement; IVS encroachment into the LVOT; IAS encroachment into LA; decreased right-sided clearance with cavitation study
6-Minute walk distance[c]	> 400 m	< 320 m
CPET	Peak VO_2 > 10.4 mL/kg/min; peak systolic blood pressure > 120 mm Hg	Peak VO_2 < 10.4 mL/kg/min; peak systolic blood pressure < 120 mm Hg
Platelet count	> 150,000	< 50,000
Uric acid	< 7 mg/dL	> 11 mg/dL
Renal insufficiency	No	Yes
BNP	Normal to minimal increase, ie, < 180 pg/mL	Significantly increased, ie, > 180 pg/mL
Troponin	Negative	Positive
RHC	Normal/near normal RAP and CI, ie, RAP < 10 mm Hg, CI > 2.5 L/min/m²; PVR < 10 Wood units	High RAP, low CI, ie, RAP > 20 mm Hg, CI < 1.8 L/min/m²; severe elevation in PVR, ie, PVR > 24 Wood units

Abbreviations: BNP, brain natriuretic peptide; CI, cardiac index; CPET, cardiopulmonary exercise testing; IAS, interatrial septum; IVS, interventricular septum; LA, left atrium; LVOT, left ventricular outflow tract; PAH, pulmonary arterial hypertension; PCH, pulmonary capillary hemangiomatosis; peak VO2, peak oxygen uptake during exercise; PoPH, portal pulmonary hypertension; PVOD, pulmonary veno-occlusive disease; RAP, right atrial pressure; RHC, right heart catheterization; RV, right ventricle; WHO, World Health Organization.

Data from McLaughlin V, McGoon M. Pulmonary arterial hypertension, *Circulation*. 2006 Sep 26;114(13):1417-1431.

74-10. The answer is D. *(Hurst's The Heart, 14th Edition, Chap. 74)* Three major pathways (endothelin, nitric oxide, and prostacyclin) are involved in abnormal proliferation and contraction of the smooth muscle cells of the pulmonary artery in patients with PAH. These pathways correspond to important therapeutic targets in this condition and play a role in determining which of four classes of drugs—endothelin receptor antagonists, nitric oxide, phosphodiesterase type 5 inhibitors, and prostacyclin derivatives—will be used. Epoprostenol (prostacyclin, prostaglandin I_2), a metabolite of arachidonic acid, and its analogues continue to be a major focus of attention as treatments for a variety of forms of PAH. The pulmonary endothelium elaborates prostacyclin into the bloodstream, where it has a short biologic half-life and serves important functions as a vasodilator and inhibitor of smooth muscle cell proliferation (option B). Endothelin (ET-1) is a potent mitogen and vasoconstrictor that is produced in excess by the hypertensive pulmonary endothelium (option D). Circulating levels of endothelin are increased in patients with PAH (option C), and the magnitude of elevation correlates with survival. NO is synthesized in endothelial cells from one of the guanidine nitrogens of L-arginine by the enzyme NO synthase. Sildenafil and tadalafil are both PDE-5 inhibitors that enhance NO activity by inhibiting PDE-5 (option A), the enzyme responsible for catabolism of cyclic guanosine monophosphate, and are approved for the treatment of PAH. Figure 74-1 demonstrates a schematic representation of these three pathways.

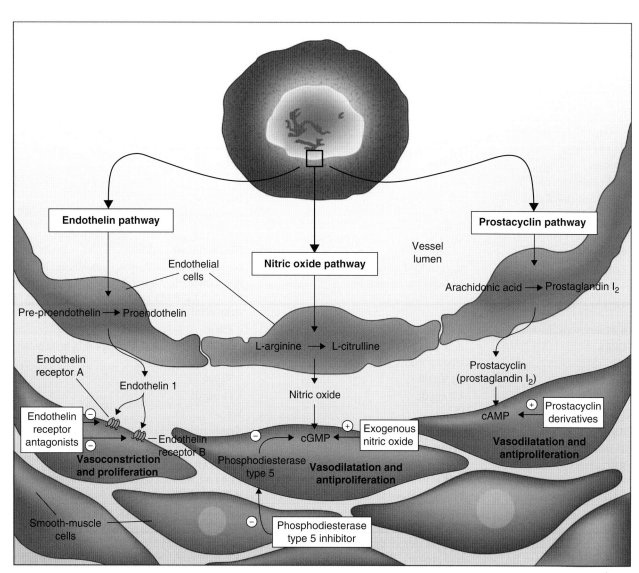

FIGURE 74-1 Three major pathways involved in abnormal proliferation and contraction of the smooth muscle cells of the pulmonary artery in patients with pulmonary arterial hypertension.

CHAPTER 75

Pulmonary Embolism

Patrick R. Lawler

QUESTIONS

DIRECTIONS: Choose the one best response to each question.

75-1. The most common origin for pulmonary emboli related to venous thromboembolic disease is from which vascular territory?

A. Deep veins of the lower extremities in the thighs
B. Deep veins of the lower extremities in the calves
C. Deep veins of the lower extremities in the foot
D. Deep veins of the upper extremities, especially the arms
E. Deep veins of the upper extremities, especially the hands

75-2. Which of the following is *not* a risk factor for venous thromboembolism?

A. Oral contraceptive use
B. Myocardial infarction and heart failure
C. Body mass index of 20 kg/m^2
D. Malignancy
E. Antithrombin III deficiency

75-3. A patient is admitted with hypoxemia due to a pulmonary embolism (PE). Which of the following is *not* a mechanism by which hypoxemia can develop in PE?

A. Intrapulmonary right-to-left shunting
B. Decreased workload of the right ventricle
C. Intracardiac right-to-left shunting
D. Decreased mixed venous oxygen level
E. Ventilation-perfusion inequality

75-4. Which of the following is a sign or symptom that suggests a massive and life-threatening PE?

A. Pleural rub
B. Tachypnea
C. Pleuritic pain
D. Syncope
E. Anxiety

75-5. Which of the following diagnostic imaging tools has become the most useful test in patients with clinically suspected acute PE?

A. Chest radiography
B. Magnetic resonance angiography (MRA)
C. Contrast-enhanced computed tomography
D. Ventilation-perfusion scanning
E. Echocardiography

75-6. An 86-year-old woman who is 3 hours post-op following open reduction and internal fixation of a femoral bone fracture is seen in the post-anesthetic care unit (PACU) for transient syncope and hypotension. She has not been receiving antithrombotic prophylaxis due to a prior history of heparin allergy. Which of the following statements regarding diagnostic approaches to this patient with suspected PE and hypotension is *correct*, provided the patient continues to remain stable?

A. She should undergo CT angiography as the initial diagnostic modality of choice
B. She should undergo D-dimer testing as the initial diagnostic modality of choice
C. She should undergo transthoracic echocardiography (TTE) as the initial diagnostic modality of choice
D. She should undergo V/Q testing as the initial diagnostic modality of choice
E. She should receive empiric thrombolytic therapy

75-7. Thrombolytic therapy of acute PE restores pulmonary perfusion more rapidly than anticoagulation alone. Which of the following is *not* considered an absolute contraindication for thrombolytic therapy?

A. Known intracranial malignancy
B. Ischemic stroke 6 months prior
C. Hemorrhagic stroke eight years prior
D. Active gastrointestinal hemorrhage
E. Suspected aortic dissection

75-8. Anticoagulation treatment is recommended for a patient with acute PE. Which of the following is *not* an appropriate therapy?

A. Intravenous unfractionated heparin
B. Subcutaneous unfractionated heparin
C. Subcutaneous fondaparinux
D. Subcutaneous low-molecular-weight heparin
E. Oral rivaroxaban

75-9. A patient with recurrent pulmonary emboli progresses to chronic thromboembolic pulmonary hypertension (CTEPH). Which of the following findings would *not* be expected in a patient with CTEPH?

A. Pulmonary microvascular disease
B. Pulmonary vascular remodeling
C. Right heart failure
D. Left heart failure
E. Inflammation

75-10. Which of the following is *not* considered a standard therapy to prevent venous thromboembolism?

A. Unfractionated heparin
B. Low-molecular-weight heparin
C. Warfarin
D. Aspirin
E. Fondaparinux

75-1. The answer is B. *(Hurst's The Heart, 14th Edition, Chap. 75)* The overwhelming majority of emboli originate from the deep veins of the lower extremities, although any venous bed can be involved. Although thrombi may form at any point along the vein wall, most originate in valve pockets. The veins of the calf are the most common site of origin, with subsequent extension of the clot proximally prior to embolization (option B). Eventually, the thrombus may expand to fill the vessel entirely, with both retrograde and proximal extension. If embolization does not occur, the thrombosis can partially or completely resolve via three mechanisms: recanalization, organization, and lysis. Upper extremity DVT has become an increasingly important clinical problem because of the increasing use of pacemakers; implantable defibrillators; and long-term, indwelling, central venous catheters. Symptomatic PE may originate from upper extremity thrombi, although it is much less common than embolization from lower extremity DVT (options D and E).

75-2. The answer is C. *(Hurst's The Heart, 14th Edition, Chap. 75)* Recent studies implicate obesity as a risk factor for VTE, particularly in developed countries. The Nurses' Health Study found that a body mass index of 29 kg/m² or greater was an independent risk factor for PE (option C).[1] Observational studies suggest that patients with myocardial infarction and heart failure are at higher risk for VTE (option B).[2] Malignancy clearly increases the risk of VTE (option D). Oral contraception, pregnancy, and the postpartum period are the most common settings in which women younger than age 40 acquire thromboembolic disease. Venous thrombosis develops in these settings three to six times more often than in age-matched women who are not on oral contraceptives (option A). Inherited thrombophilias including antithrombin III deficiency (option E), antiphospholipid antibody syndrome, the presence of factor V Lieden, and the presence of prothrombin gene mutation G20210A, increase the risk for VTE.

75-3. The answer is answer B. *(Hurst's The Heart, 14th Edition, Chap. 75)* Hypoxemia develops in the preponderance of patients with PE and has been attributed to various mechanisms, including intrapulmonary or intracardiac right-to-left shunting (option A), ventilation-perfusion (V/Q) mismatch (option E), and decreases in the mixed venous oxygen level (option D), thereby magnifying the effect of the normal venous admixture. Obstruction of the pulmonary vascular bed by embolism acutely increases the workload on the RV, a chamber ill-equipped to deal with a high-pressure load (option B). In patients with an acute increase in right ventricular afterload and a resultant increase in right heart pressures, the direction of blood flow across an incidental intracardiac shunt (such as a patent foramen ovalae or an atrial septal defect) may reverse, and a new right-to-left shunt may develop, which may worsen hypoxemia (option C). In patients without preexisting cardiopulmonary disease, obstruction of < 20% of the pulmonary vascular bed usually results in a number of compensatory events that minimize adverse hemodynamic consequences.

75-4. The answer is D. *(Hurst's The Heart, 14th Edition, Chap. 75)* Severe dyspnea and syncope are the principal symptoms that may suggest massive, life-threatening PE (option D). The mechanism is presumably obstruction to blood flow and resultant hypotension and decreased cerebral perfusion. Pleuritic chest pain and hemoptysis are common in patients with PE, but their presence is not supportive of the clinical severity (option C). Anxiety and lightheadedness are symptoms that may be caused by PE but are nonspecific (option E). Tachypnea and tachycardia are the most common signs of PE, but they are also nonspecific (option B). A pleural rub may suggest pulmonary infarction, and an accentuated pulmonic component of the second heart sound may suggest pulmonary hypertension but can also be explained by other disorders (option A). With PE of sufficient magnitude to cause RV dysfunction, a murmur of tricuspid regurgitation, systemic hypotension, or jugular venous distension might be present.

75-5. The answer is C. *(Hurst's The Heart, 14th Edition, Chap. 75)* V/Q scanning was the pivotal diagnostic test for suspected PE for many years. Although clinical indications for the study remain, chest CT has now virtually replaced lung scanning. When the chest radiograph is normal or near normal, a V/Q scan can be reliably used to diagnose PE in the presence of an unmatched perfusion defect (option D). Since the introduction of multidetector computed tomographic (MDCT) angiography, however, contrast-enhanced CT of the chest has become the most useful imaging test in patients with clinically suspected acute PE (option C). It allows rapid and comprehensive visualization of the pulmonary arteries, usually through the subsegmental level. It has the added advantage of also identifying alternate causes of dyspnea (such as pneumonia). An enlarged right ventricle on CT can also suggest right ventricular strain, supportive of a diagnosis of submassive PE. While the chest radiograph may be abnormal in patients with PE, the findings are often nonspecific and subtle (option A). Gadolinium-enhanced MRA can evaluate for PE, but it not routinely used (option B). Transthoracic echocardiography (TTE) can provide important information on right ventricular function and estimated pulmonary artery systolic pressure in the setting of PE, which can aid in risk stratification and treatment decisions (option E). Rarely, TTE can identify a clot in transit.

75-6. **The answer is A**. *(Hurst's The Heart, 14th Edition, Chap. 75)* Figure 75-1 illustrates a diagnostic approach to patients with suspected PE with shock or hypotension (massive PE). Generally, if the patient is stable for CT scan this is favored to confirm the diagnosis and define the extent of disease (option A). However, if instability precludes safely performing a CT scan, TTE can be used to support the diagnosis (option C), although the finding of acute right heart dysfunction is non-specific. V/Q scanning in such settings would be unlikely to be performed in a sufficiently timely manner (option D). D-dimer testing is not useful in a patient with high pretest probability of PE (option B). Empiric thrombolytic therapy (option E) may be considered if instability develops and TTE is suggestive of the diagnosis. The risks and benefits of thrombolytic therapy, particularly given that the patient is post-op, need to be individualized. The presence of an epidural catheter precludes thrombolysis. If contraindications are present, urgent surgical embolectomy may be considered. In contrast to this patient with suspected massive PE, a diagnostic algorithm for approaching patients presenting with suspected PE but *without* shock or persistent hypotension is summarized in Figure 75-2.

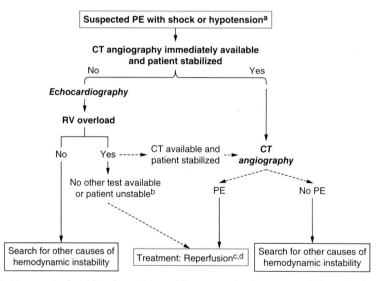

FIGURE 75-1 Diagnostic algorithm for patients with suspected pulmonary embolism (PE) with shock or hypotension.
[a]Hypotension defined as systolic blood pressure < 90 mm Hg (or needing vasopressor drugs to maintain a systolic blood pressure ≥ 90 mm Hg) or a systolic pressure drop by ≥ 40 mm Hg, for > 15 minutes, if not caused by new-onset arrhythmia, hypovolemia, or sepsis. [b]If available, consider the possibility of using a portable ventilation-perfusion scan in the setting of hemodynamic instability to confirm diagnosis. [c]Thrombolysis; alternatively catheter-based therapies or surgical embolectomy. [d]If PE is highly suspected in a critically ill patient, and a firm diagnosis cannot be established, empiric aggressive therapy may be considered. CT, computed tomography; RV, right ventricle.
(Adapted with permission from Konstantinides SV, Torbicki A, Agnelli G, et al. 2014 ESC guidelines on the diagnosis and management of acute pulmonary embolism, *Eur Heart J*. 2014 Nov 14;35(43):3033-3069.)

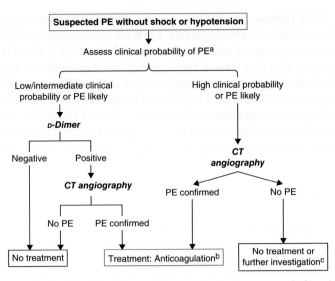

FIGURE 75-2 Diagnostic algorithm for patients with suspected pulmonary embolism (PE) without shock or hypotension.
[a]Clinical judgment or prediction rule. [b]Close monitoring for intermediate-/high-risk patients; in case of hemodynamic instability, reperfusion therapy should be considered. [c]In patients with high clinical probability of PE and negative computed tomography (CT) angiography, further testing may be considered as shown in Figure 75-8 of Fuster V et al, eds. *Hurst's The Heart.* 14th ed. 2019.
(Adapted with permission from Konstantinides SV, Torbicki A, Agnelli G, et al. 2014 ESC guidelines on the diagnosis and management of acute pulmonary embolism, *Eur Heart J.* 2014 Nov 14;35(43):3033-3069.)

75-7. **The answer is B.** Absolute contraindications for thrombolytic therapy include medical conditions that increase the possible risk of bleeding complications, such as known intracranial lesions (option A), ischemic stroke within the past 3 months (beyond 3 months, this is considered only a *relative* contraindication; option B), hemorrhagic stroke at any time (option C), active gastrointestinal hemorrhage (options D), and suspected aortic dissection.

75-8. **The answer is B.** *(Hurst's The Heart, 14th Edition, Chap. 75)* Unfractionated heparin (UFH) can be administered as an intravenous bolus followed by a maintenance dose via continuous infusion (option A); subcutaneous UFH is only used as prophylaxis and not treatment against VTE (option B). Weight-based dosing of subcutaneous LMWH is an acceptable treatment for PE (option D). Fondaparinux is administered subcutaneously on a once-daily basis in fixed doses of 5 mg for patients weighing < 50 kg, 7.5 mg for those weighing 50 to 100 kg, and 10 mg for those weighing > 100 kg (option C). Like LMWH, fondaparinux is administered in a fixed dose and does not require dose adjustment with laboratory coagulation tests. Treatment with LMWHs is more convenient for the patient and the nursing staff. Rivaroxaban is also an acceptable alternative for the treatment of VTE (option E).

75-9. **The answer is D.** *(Hurst's The Heart, 14th Edition, Chap. 75)* Approximately 30% of patients who develop CTEPH have no documented history of acute DVT or PE, and this feature greatly impedes the diagnosis. Anticardiolipin antibodies or a lupus anticoagulant has been detected in approximately 10% of patients, and elevated factor VIII levels have been detected in 40%. Apart from major pulmonary vascular obstruction, the pathophysiology of CTEPH includes pulmonary microvascular disease (option A), pulmonary vascular remodeling (option B), immune phenomena, and inflammation (option E). The median age of patients at diagnosis of CTEPH is 63 years, and both genders are equally affected. Clinical symptoms and signs are nonspecific or absent in early CTEPH, with signs of right heart failure resulting from pulmonary hypertension (group 4) only becoming evident in advanced disease (option C).

75-10. **The answer is D.** *(Hurst's The Heart, 14th Edition, Chap. 75)* Prophylaxis against VTE can be pharmacologic or nonpharmacologic. Pharmacologic prophylaxis options include low-dose UFH (option A), LMWH (option B), fondaparinux (option E), warfarin (option C), and new oral anticoagulants. LMWHs are increasingly used in clinical practice for both the prevention and treatment of established VTE. LMWH preparations are advantageous in that they have a more predictable dose-response relationship and are administered subcutaneously only once or twice daily (without monitoring), depending on the preparation. While some have advised long-term use of aspirin following discontinuation of anticoagulation therapy for the treatment of VTE, there is no documented role for aspirin in the primary prevention of VTE (option D). Early ambulation and sequential pneumatic compression devices represent nonpharmacologic prophylaxis.

References

1. Goldhaber SZ, Grodstein F, Stampfer MJ, et al. A prospective study of risk factors for pulmonary embolism in women. *JAMA*. 1997;277(8):642-645.
2. Sorensen HT, Horvath-Puho E, Lash TL, et al. Heart disease may be a risk factor for pulmonary embolism without peripheral deep venous thrombosis. *Circulation*. 2011;124(13):1435-1441.

CHAPTER 76

Cor Pulmonale: The Heart in Parenchymal Lung Disease

Patrick R. Lawler

QUESTIONS

DIRECTIONS: Choose the one best response to each question.

76-1. The pulmonary circulation is characterized by all of the following *except*:

A. It carries venous deoxygenated blood
B. Low resistance
C. Low capacitance
D. Normal mean pulmonary pressure is < 20 mm Hg at rest
E. Pulmonary vascular resistance (PVR) decreases with increased cardiac output

76-2. Which of the following lung diseases *does not* manifest as a typical cor pulmonale syndrome?

A. Acute pulmonary embolism
B. Chronic obstructive pulmonary disease (COPD)
C. Bronchiectasis
D. Sarcoidosis
E. Obstructive sleep apnea (OSA)

76-3. Which of the following statements about the pathophysiology of cor pulmonale is *correct*?

A. Pulmonary vascular remodeling is characterized by intimal wall thinning
B. Endothelial cells in the lungs respond to hypoxia with vasodilation
C. Inflammatory processes in pulmonary hypertension (PH) result in decreased vessel cross-sectional area and a decrease in PVR
D. Lung diseases associated with PH have an impairment in nitric oxide synthesis
E. All of the above

76-4. A 40-year-old woman working on a base camp on Mount Kilimanjaro for the past 5 years begins to experience headaches, dizziness, and shortness of breath. On physical examination, you notice that she also has peripheral edema. Which of the following is most likely in this situation?

A. Her arterial partial pressure of oxygen (PaO_2) is < 55 mm Hg
B. She has right ventricular hypertrophy (RVH)
C. She has polycythemia
D. She has PH
E. All of the above

76-5. A 76-year-old man with long-standing COPD comes to your office with new onset of peripheral edema. On physical examination you also note the presence of a third heart sound and jugular venous distention. You perform further tests and order an echocardiography. Which of the following echocardiographic findings is expected in this patient with suspected cor pulmonale?

A. Diminished tricuspid regurgitation velocity
B. Increased right ventricular/left ventricular ratio to > 1
C. Decreased right ventricle wall thickness
D. Increased tricuspid annular plane systolic excursion (TAPSE)
E. Decreased eccentricity index

76-6. You decide to do more testing on your 76-year-old male patient with COPD to assess his respiratory function and degree of PH. Which result is consistent with a diagnosis of cor pulmonale?

A. Reduced mean pulmonary artery pressure (mPAP)
B. Increased maximum oxygen uptake during exercise
C. Increased pulmonary arterial compliance
D. Emphysema with decreased right ventricular end-diastolic volumes (RVEDV)
E. None of the above

76-7. Obstructive sleep apnea is common in the general population but is often underdiagnosed. Which of the following characteristics associated with cor pulmonale has *not* been documented in OSA patients?

A. Right ventricular dilatation
B. Decreased ejection fraction
C. Increased dyssynchrony
D. Hypertrophy of the interventricular septum
E. Increased systolic and diastolic velocities

76-8. For the following underlying disease and treatment pairs, which is an *incorrect* treatment strategy for cor pulmonale?

A. COPD: smoking cessation, bronchodilators, steroids
B. Sarcoidosis: NSAIDs
C. Sleep apnea: continuous positive airway pressure, weight loss
D. Pulmonary fibrosis: anti-inflammatory medications, tyrosine kinase inhibitors, lung transplantation
E. Oxygen therapy when arterial PO_2 < 60 mm Hg

76-9. Which of the following electrocardiographic findings is *not* commonly associated with cor pulmonale?

A. Left axis deviation
B. Atrial fibrillation
C. P pulmonale
D. Right ventricular hypertrophy
E. None of the above

76-10. Which of the following major lung diseases is associated with cor pulmonale?

A. Kyphoscoliosis
B. Cystic fibrosis
C. Obesity-hypoventilation syndrome
D. Idiopathic interstitial pulmonary fibrosis
E. All of the above

76-1. The answer is C. *(Hurst's The Heart, 14th Edition, Chap. 76)* The pulmonary circulation (with the exception of the bronchial arteries that deliver oxygenated blood from the left heart) is characterized not only by the delivery of venous deoxygenated blood to the alveoli for oxygen uptake (option A is incorrect), but also by low resistance (option B is incorrect) and large capacitance (option C is correct). This capacitance allows the lungs to accommodate a wide range of blood flows with little increase in pulmonary arterial pressure.[1] Normal mean pulmonary pressure is < 20 mm Hg at rest (option D is incorrect), with a mean level > 25 mm Hg diagnostic of PH.[2] Although pulmonary pressures do rise with exercise, PVR normally drops further with exercise to accommodate the marked increase in cardiac output (option E is incorrect).

76-2. The answer is A. *(Hurst's The Heart, 14th Edition, Chap. 76)* Cor pulmonale describes the pathological changes and associated signs and symptoms of right ventricular failure resulting from PH.[3] Chronic cor pulmonale is typically a manifestation of various lung diseases, such as COPD (option B is incorrect), bronchiectasis (option C is incorrect), sarcoidosis (option D is incorrect) and OSA (option E is incorrect). Acute pulmonary embolism can lead to acute right heart failure, which has been termed *acute cor pulmonale*. The cardiac response to "acute cor pulmonale" differs from the typical cor pulmonale syndrome, which is characterized by early RVH and subsequent late right ventricular dilatation. In contrast, in acute pulmonary embolism, the right ventricle dilates acutely without intervening hypertrophy, leading to a volume overload rather than pressure overload right ventricular failure (option A is correct).

76-3. The answer is D. *(Hurst's The Heart, 14th Edition, Chap. 76)* Various mechanisms contribute to increased pulmonary vascular disease in parenchymal lung disease, including inflammation, destruction of lung parenchyma, obliteration as a result of fibrosis, endothelial dysfunction, and hypoxemia.[4] The severity of pulmonary vascular remodeling correlates with the severity of inflammation,[5] with intimal thickening being the most pronounced pathologic abnormality (option A is incorrect). The resultant decrease in cross-sectional area and vasodilatory capacity leads to an increase in PVR (option C is incorrect). As in the systemic circulation, the endothelium plays a key role in mediating vascular dilation. Unlike the systemic circulation, endothelial cells in the pulmonary circulation respond to hypoxia with signaling leading to vasoconstriction ("hypoxic vasoconstriction"—designed to optimize ventilation and perfusion matching to facilitate optimal gas exchange) as opposed to vasodilation (option B is incorrect). COPD and other lung diseases associated with PH have been shown to have impairment in the three major pathways that regulate pulmonary vascular tone, including an impairment of nitric oxide synthesis (option D is correct).

76-4. The answer is E. *(Hurst's The Heart, 14th Edition, Chap. 76)* Chronic mountain sickness is a disease that develops after many years of living at high altitude and in some cases can progress to cor pulmonale. It is characterized by polycythaemia (high hemoglobin concentration in the blood) (option C is correct) and hypoxemia (low levels of oxygen in the blood), which usually becomes evident with arterial partial pressure of oxygen (PO_2) < 55 mm Hg (option A is also correct). Hypoxia has been considered a key mediator in PH associated with various parenchymal lung diseases, and it can indeed be a cause of PH as seen in chronic mountain sickness (option D is also correct). The clinical manifestations of cor pulmonale are usually nonspecific and reflect the signs and symptoms of right heart failure, including RVH (option B is also correct). Thus, cor pulmonale that developed in this patient with chronic mountain sickness could manifest with all of the symptoms above (option E is the correct answer).

76-5. The answer is B. *(Hurst's The Heart, 14th Edition, Chap. 76)* Transthoracic echocardiography is very useful for the detection of cor pulmonale and its antecedent PH. Its salient features include the detection of RVH, right ventricular enlargement, and elevated tricuspid regurgitation velocity (used to estimate the pulmonary artery systolic pressure from the modified Bernoulli question: $PASP = 4v_{TR}^2$), which is indicative of increased gradient between the right ventricle and right atrium (option A is incorrect). Echocardiography can also measure the decrease in TAPSE, which reflects the longitudinal myocardial shortening of the right ventricle and reflects global right ventricular function (option D is incorrect). Right ventricular dimensions are increased in cor pulmonale and are accompanied by increases in wall thickness (option C is incorrect). Normally the right ventricle appears to be smaller than the left ventricle on the four-chamber view, with the apex being formed by the left ventricle. With the development of cor pulmonale, the right ventricle enlarges, and the right ventricular/left ventricular ratio increases to > 1 (option B is incorrect). When pressure and volume overload of the right ventricle develop, the left ventricle assumes a D shape as the intraventricular septum flattens (in systole and in diastole, respectively). This leads to an abnormally high ratio (> 1) between the left ventricular anteroposterior and septolateral dimensions (eccentricity index) (option E is incorrect).

76-6. The answer is D. *(Hurst's The Heart, 14th Edition, Chap. 76)* COPD is an inflammatory disease characterized by a combination of small airway disease (obstructive bronchiolitis) and destruction of the parenchyma (emphysema), with the contribution of each component varying between patients.[6] Patients with COPD ofen have abnormally high mPAP (option A is incorrect).[7] Patients with PH also have decreased exercise capacity with significantly lower maximum oxygen uptake during exercise (option B is incorrect). The "blue bloater" (chronic bronchitis) phenotype, in contrast to the "pink puffer" (emphysema), has traditionally been associated with cor pulmonale. A recent analysis from the Multi-Ethnic Study of Atherosclerosis (MESA)[8] investigating COPD surprisingly found lower RVEDV with no change in right ventricular mass in COPD patients compared with controls (option D is correct). The findings may have been mediated partly by more emphysema rather than chronic bronchitis in the population. Finally, increased pulmonary artery stiffness (decreased compliance) is not only a characteristic and relatively early sign of PH, but it may also play a role in the progression of the disease (option C is incorrect).[9,10]

76-7. The answer is E. *(Hurst's The Heart, 14th Edition, Chap. 76)* Both OSA and central sleep apnea have been associated with cor pulmonale. OSA is common and underdiagnosed, with moderate to severe OSA affecting up to 10% of the adult population in the United States.[11] Abnormalities in right ventricular function, decreased strain and ejection fraction (option B is incorrect), increased dyssynchrony[12] (option C is incorrect), right ventricular dilatation (option A is incorrect), hypertrophy of the interventricular septum (option D is incorrect), and reduced tissue Doppler–determined systolic and diastolic velocities[13] (option E is correct) have been documented in patients with OSA.

76-8. The answer is B. *(Hurst's The Heart, 14th Edition, Chap. 76)* Treatment of cor pulmonale is mostly aimed at the underlying lung disease, with oxygen therapy when arterial oxygen is below 60 mm Hg (option E is incorrect) (Table 76-1). The treatment of cor pulmonale in COPD is geared to treating the underlying inflammatory process that may exacerbate arterial thickening and PH. It also focuses on the risk factors for COPD, with smoking being the most important (option A is incorrect). OSA is characterized by hypoventilation during sleep and is associated with obesity. The mainstays of therapy are therefore weight loss, continuous positive airway pressure treatment, and bariatric surgery (option C is incorrect). In fact, improvements in all symptoms of cor pulmonale have been observed with treatment of the OSA with continuous positive airway pressure during sleep.[14] Sarcoidosis is characterized by the presence of noncaseating granulomas in multiple organs, with the lungs being most commonly affected. Therapy for sarcoidosis is mainly anti-inflammatory with steroids (option B is correct). There is no specific treatment for PH in idiopathic pulmonary fibrosis (IPF), however recently both pirfenidone, a small-molecule anti-inflammatory drug, and nintedanib, a tyrosine kinase inhibitor, were approved for the treatment of IPF. IPF is also the leading cause for lung transplantation (option D is incorrect).[15]

TABLE 76-1 Treatment Principles of Cor Pulmonale

Treat underlying disease
Chronic obstructive pulmonary disease: smoking cessation, bronchodilators, steroids (inhaled for maintenance therapy/systemic for exacerbations)
Sarcoidosis: steroids
Sleep apnea: continuous positive airway pressure, weight loss, corrective surgery
Pulmonary fibrosis: perfinidone, nintedanib, lung transplantation
Oxygen supplementation if arterial PO_2 < 60 mm Hg
Loop diuretics for volume overload
Consider torsemide if gut edema suspected/diuretic resistance
PH-specific therapies: unproven
Endothelin receptor antagonists contraindicated in pulmonary fibrosis

Abbreviations: PH, pulmonary hypertension; PO_2, partial pressure of oxygen.

76-9. **The answer is A.** (Hurst's The Heart, 14th Edition, Chap. 76) The clinical manifestations of cor pulmonale are nonspecific and reflect the signs and symptoms of right heart failure. Electrocardiographic findings in cor pulmonale include evidence of right axis deviation (option A is correct) and not left axis deviation, RVH (option D is incorrect), right ventricular strain, P pulmonale secondary to right atrial enlargement (option C is incorrect), and hypertrophy. Common accompanying arrhythmias include atrial fibrillation (option B is incorrect), atrial flutter, and multifocal atrial tachycardia in addition to premature atrial and ventricular contractions.[16]

76-10. **The answer is E.** (Hurst's The Heart, 14th Edition, Chap. 76) A listing of lung diseases that have been associated with cor pulmonale is provided in Table 76-2. All of these have chronic hypoxemia in common, and indeed without significant hypoxemia, cor pulmonale does not typically develop. In IPF, PH is found in a third of patients and is associated with worse prognosis (option D is correct).[17] The obesity-hypoventilation syndrome involves a complex interaction between impaired respiratory mechanics, decreased ventilatory drive, and obstructive sleep apnea and is associated with significant mortality and morbidity (option C is also correct). As mentioned previously, any lung condition that causes low oxygen level in the blood over a long time can lead to cor pulmonale, including cystic fibrosis (option B is also correct) and severe curving of the upper part of the spine (kyphoscoliosis) (option A is also correct).

TABLE 76-2 Major Lung Diseases Associated with Cor Pulmonale

Obstructive lung diseases
Chronic obstructive pulmonary disease
Cystic fibrosis
Bronchiectasis
Bronchiolitis obliterans
Restrictive lung diseases
Sarcoidosis
Neuromuscular diseases
Kyphoscoliosis
Sequelae of pulmonary tuberculosis
Pneumoconiosis
Drug-related lung diseases
Extrinsic allergic alveolitis
Connective tissue diseases
Idiopathic interstitial pulmonary fibrosis
Interstitial pulmonary fibrosis of known origin
Hypoventilation syndromes
Obstructive sleep apnea
Obesity-hypoventilation syndrome (formerly Pickwickian syndrome)
Central sleep apnea
Hypoxic vasoconstriction
Mountain sickness

References

1. Chemla D, Castelain V, Hervé P, Lecarpentier Y, Brimioulle S. Haemodynamic evaluation of pulmonary hypertension. *Eur Respir J.* 2002 Nov; 20(5):1314-1331.

2. Hoeper MM, Bogaard HJ, Condliffe R, et al. Definitions and diagnosis of pulmonary hypertension. *J Am Coll Cardiol.* 2013;62(25 Suppl):D42-D50.

3. Weitzenblum E, Chaouat A. Cor pulmonale. *Chron Resp Dis.* 2009;6(3):177-185.

4. Rowan SC, Keane MP, Gaine S, McLoughlin P. Hypoxic pulmonary hypertension in chronic lung diseases: novel vasoconstrictor pathways. *Lancet Respir Med.* 2016;4(3):225-236.

5. Peinado VI, Barbera JA, Ramirez J, et al. Endothelial dysfunction in pulmonary arteries of patients with mild COPD. *Am J Physiol.* 1998;274(6 Pt 1):L908-L913.

6. Global Initiative for Chronic Obstructive Lung Disease. Global strategy for diagnosis, management and prevention of COPD. http://goldcopd.org/guidelines-global-strategy-for-diagnosis-management.html. Accessed July 24, 2016.

7. Vonbank K, Funk GC, Marzluf B, et al. Abnormal pulmonary arterial pressure limits exercise capacity in patients with COPD. *Wien Klin Wochenschr.* 2008;120(23-24):749-755.

8. Kawut SM, Poor HD, Parikh MA, et al. Cor pulmonale parvus in chronic obstructive pulmonary disease and emphysema: the MESA COPD study. *J Am Coll Cardiol.* 2014;64(19):2000-2009.

9. Sanz J, Kariisa M, Dellegrottaglie S, et al. Evaluation of pulmonary artery stiffness in pulmonary hypertension with cardiac magnetic resonance. *JACC Cardiovasc Imaging.* 2009;2(3):286-295.

10. Ben-Yehuda O, Barnett C. Magnetic resonance assessment of pulmonary artery compliance: a promising diagnostic and prognostic tool in pulmonary hypertension? *JACC Cardiovasc Imaging.* 2009;2(3):296-298.

11. Peppard PE, Young T, Barnet JH, Palta M, Hagen EW, Hla KM. Increased prevalence of sleep-disordered breathing in adults. *Am J Epidemiol.* 2013;177(9):1006-1014.

12. Vitarelli A, Terzano C, Saponara M, et al. Assessment of right ventricular function in obstructive sleep apnea syndrome and effects of continuous positive airway pressure therapy: a pilot study. *Can J Cardiol.* 2015;31(7):823-831.

13. Shivalkar B, Van de Heyning C, Kerremans M, et al. Obstructive sleep apnea syndrome: more insights on structural and functional cardiac alterations, and the effects of treatment with continuous positive airway pressure. *J Am Coll Cardiol.* 2006;47(7):1433-1439.

14. Colish J, Walker JR, Elmayergi N, et al. Obstructive sleep apnea: effects of continuous positive airway pressure on cardiac remodeling as assessed by cardiac biomarkers, echocardiography, and cardiac MRI. *Chest.* 2012;141(3):674-681.

15. Kistler KD, Nalysnyk L, Rotella P, Esser D. Lung transplantation in idiopathic pulmonary fibrosis: a systematic review of the literature. *BMC Pulm Med.* 2014;14:139.

16. Goudis CA, Konstantinidis AK, Ntalas IV, Korantzopoulos P. Electrocardiographic abnormalities and cardiac arrhythmias in chronic obstructive pulmonary disease. *Int J Cardiol.* 2015;199:264-273.

17. Lettieri CJ, Nathan SD, Barnett SD, Ahmad S, Shorr AF. Prevalence and outcomes of pulmonary arterial hypertension in advanced idiopathic pulmonary fibrosis. *Chest.* 2006;129(3):746-752.

CHAPTER 77

Sleep-Disordered Breathing and Cardiac Disease

Patrick R. Lawler

QUESTIONS

DIRECTIONS: Choose the one best response to each question.

77-1. Which of the following characteristics is associated with central sleep apnea (CSA)?

A. Retrognathism
B. Obesity
C. Ongoing respiratory effort
D. Cheyne–Stokes respiration (CSR)
E. Upper airway obstruction

77-2. Which of the following techniques is considered the gold standard for diagnosing sleep-disordered breathing (SDB)?

A. Multichannel sleep polygraphy
B. Polysomnography (PSG)
C. Transthoracic impedance sensor
D. Nocturnal heart rate monitor
E. Epworth Sleepiness Scale

77-3. A 33-year-old woman presents to your clinic with symptoms of fatigue, morning headaches, and daytime sleepiness. She is worried that she may have obstructive sleep apnea (OSA) as did her father. Which of the following factors predisposes this patient the *most* to SDB?

A. She is a regular smoker
B. She has a a normal BMI
C. She is Asian
D. She is a premenopausal female
E. All of the above

77-4. Which laboratory finding suggests a diagnosis of SDB?

A. Elevated urinary norepinephrine
B. Decreased cortisol levels
C. Decreased levels of plasminogen activator inhibitor-1 (PAI-1)
D. Increased insulin sensitivity
E. All of the above

77-5. Which of the following statements about SDB and cardiac disease is *not correct*?

A. Apnea-hypopnea index (AHI) > 20/h is a significant risk factor for sudden cardiac death
B. SDB is associated with a decreased risk of ventricular cardiac arrhythmias
C. SDB is characterized by a nondipping blood pressure pattern
D. Negative thoracic pressure can initiate episodes of atrial fibrillation
E. SDB patients have a higher frequency of ST-segment depression episodes

77-6. A 68-year-old woman with a history of heart failure with preserved ejection fraction (HFpEF) is evaluated for possible SDB. Given her condition, which of the following is *correct*?

A. Patients with heart failure often do not present with classic symptoms of SDB
B. HFpEF patients predominantly have CSA
C. There is a positive correlation between daytime sleepiness and daytime muscle sympathetic nervous system activity
D. Beta-blockers increase daytime sleepiness in HF patients
E. The prevalence of OSA increases with the severity of HF syndrome

77-7. A 44-year-old obese man with long-standing untreated SDB has a new onset of shortness of breath. His mean pulmonary arterial pressure is 35 mm Hg at rest. Which of the following statements is *correct*?

A. The patient developed pulmonary hypertension as a result of hypoxemia
B. The patient will likely benefit from continuous positive airway pressure (CPAP) treatment
C. Right ventricular failure is uncommon in his case
D. SDB can result in pulmonary arteriolar remodeling
E. All of the above

77-8. A patient with newly diagnosed SDB is counseled on treatment options, and a recommendation is made for lifestyle modifications. Which of the following is *not* appropriate for the treatment of SDB?

A. Bariatric surgery
B. PAP therapy
C. Oral appliances
D. Carbon dioxide therapy
E. Positional therapy

77-9. What is *complex sleep apnea*?

A. Untreated sleep apnea
B. CSA/CSR that develops in OSA patients receiving PAP therapy
C. OSA that progresses to HF
D. SDB in patients with more than one comorbidity
E. None of the above

77-10. What is the main advantage of adaptive servo-ventilation (ASV) over other positive airway treatment modalities?

A. It is set to a single pressure that remains constant thoughout the night
B. It has two pressure settings, one for inhalation and one for exhalation
C. It adapts to the patient's breathing pattern and can suppress complex sleep apnea
D. Its use is associated with lower overall mortality and lower cardiovascular mortality
E. None of the above

77-1. **The answer is D.** *(Hurst's The Heart, 14th Edition, Chap. 77)* Sleep-disordered breathing can present as either OSA, CSA, or a combination of both. In OSA, there is collapse of the pharynx during sleep with consequent upper airway obstruction (option E). Predisposing factors include obesity (option B), a short neck, and retrognathism (option A). In OSA, there is evidence of ongoing respiratory effort throughout the apneic-hypopneic event (option C), often with paradoxical movement of the chest and abdomen as breathing against a closed airway is attempted. In contrast, apneas and hypopneas in CSA are accompanied by a marked reduction or cessation of respiratory effort. In CSA, the underlying abnormality is in the regulation of breathing in the respiratory centers of the brainstem. In normal physiology, minute ventilation during sleep is primarily regulated by chemoreceptors in the brainstem and carotid bodies, which trigger an increase in respiratory drive in response to a rise in partial pressure of arterial carbon dioxide ($PaCO_2$), thus maintaining $PaCO_2$ within a narrow range. Patients with HF and CSA tend to have an exaggerated respiratory response to carbon dioxide, so that modest rises in $PaCO_2$ that may occur during sleep result in inappropriate hyperventilation. One of the hallmarks of CSA is CSR (option D), characterized by a periodic pattern of hyperventilation followed by hypoventilation.

77-2. **The answer is B.** *(Hurst's The Heart, 14th Edition, Chap. 77)* More than 50% of patients with OSA and cardiovascular disease (CVD) do not report symptoms of unrestful sleep, but rather present with symptoms of CVD.[1] In addition, patients with HF and SDB do not tend to complain of daytime sleepiness, possibly because of the high sympathetic tone found in HF. Screening questionnaires that include questions about daytime sleepiness, such as the Epworth Sleepiness Scale, can thus be insensitive (option E).[2] Attended in-hospital PSG, including the assessment of respiratory movement, oxygen saturation, nasal and oral airflow, snoring, electroencephalography, electrocardiography, electromyography, and ocular movement, has long been considered the gold standard test for sleep disorders (option B). While multichannel sleep polygraphy (option A) with oxygen saturation, nasal airflow, and chest and abdominal movement recorded is more widely available, an advantage of PSG over polygraphy is that periods of wakefulness are easily identified, and therefore, the AHI can be recorded during sleep only, increasing its accuracy of diagnosis. Nocturnal heart rate variability (option D), whether on a 24-hour tape or from an implanted device, reflects autonomic tone but does not appear to be a useful approach to screening. A recent study has reported a high sensitivity and specificity for the diagnosis of moderate to severe SDB by a pacemaker algorithm using transthoracic impedance minute ventilation sensors[3] (option C), but further research is required.

77-3. **The answer is C.** *(Hurst's The Heart, 14th Edition, Chap. 77)* The prevalence of SDB is two- to threefold higher in men than in women, although sex differences decrease after women reach menopause (option D).[4] Differences in the prevalence of SDB among individuals of varied racial and ethnic backgrounds likely reflect genetic factors that influence craniofacial shape, body fat distribution, and physiologic risk factors for SDB, as well as the influence of environmental factors. Several studies of Asian populations, with lower rates of obesity than in many Western societies, have identified a relatively high prevalence of SDB, which is likely attributable to race-based differences in craniofacial morphology (option C). Although exposure to tobacco smoke may increase upper airway inflammation and snoring, smoking is not a firmly established risk factor for SDB (option A). Approximately 40% to 60% of cases of SDB are attributable to being overweight. It is estimated that a 1% increase in body mass index is associated with a 3% increase in AHI. Excess body weight increases susceptibility to upper airway collapsibility by increased mechanical loading of the upper airway (option B).

77-4. The answer is A. *(Hurst's The Heart, 14th Edition, Chap. 77)* The physiologic consequences of SDB are many and affect multiple systems. Sympathetic nervous system activity is heightened in SDB, with increased muscle sympathetic nervous system activity and elevated urinary norepinephrine concentrations (option A). Furthermore, urinary norepinephrine increases in parallel with the severity of SDB, the number of arousals, and the degree of oxygen desaturation. Studies have suggested associations between sleep apnea and insulin resistance that are independent of obesity.[5] SDB was found to be associated with a reduction in insulin sensitivity (option D), glucose effectiveness, and pancreatic β-cell function.[6] Further predisposition toward metabolic dysfunction may occur through the effects of SDB on the hypothalamic-pituitary-adrenal axis. Experimental partial or total sleep deprivation has been shown to increase levels of plasma cortisol on the following evening at a time when the circadian rhythm of the hypothalamic-pituitary-adrenal axis is at its nadir (option B). There is some evidence for a hypercoagulable state in sleep apnea, which may contribute to the increased risk of vascular events. For example, sleep apnea has been associated with increased levels of plasminogen activator inhibitor-1 (PAI-1)[7] (option C), a molecule that inhibits fibrinolysis and has been shown to contribute to atherothrombotic events and an increased risk of recurrent myocardial infarction.

77-5. The answer is B. *(Hurst's The Heart, 14th Edition, Chap. 77)* The hemodynamic profile of blood pressure patterns in SDB is characterized by a nondipping blood pressure pattern (option C). Repetitive upper airway obstructions associated intermittent negative intrathoracic pressure swings, sleep deprivation, and recurrent episodes of hypoxemia and hypercapnia individually and interactively contribute to sympathetic activation and elevated blood pressure even during nonsleep periods. The negative thoracic pressure during obstructive respiratory events was identified as the most relevant factor for the perpetuation and initiation of atrial fibrillation (option D). Negative thoracic pressure changes result in the increased occurrence of atrial premature contractions, potentially triggering AF episodes. Furthermore, individuals with SDB have a threefold increase in their odds of having nonsustained ventricular tachycardia and almost twice the odds of having complex ventricular ectopy (option B).[8] An AHI of > 20/h was a significant and independent risk factor for incident sudden cardiac death, including in patients with heart failure (option A). Finally, studies have reported a high prevalence of ST-segment depression in patients with SDB during sleep (option E), adding that these ST-segment changes were related to heightened sympathetic tone and sleep fragmentation.[9]

77-6. The answer is A. *(Hurst's The Heart, 14th Edition, Chap. 77)* SDB is common in patients with both HF with reduced ejection fraction and HF with preserved ejection fraction (HFpEF), with no difference in prevalence between the two groups. The prevalence of CSA/CSR appears to increase as the symptomatic severity of the HF syndrome increases, while the prevalence of OSA decreases[10,11] (Figure 77-1) (option E). The predominant type of SDB in HFpEF appears to be OSA (70% to 80%) (option B). One of the interesting features of SDB in patients with HF compared to general SDB patients is a relative lack of symptoms, especially of daytime somnolence, which could contribute to the lack of recognition and detection of SDB in HF patients (option A). One possible explanation for a lack of daytime sleepiness in HF patients with SDB is the increased sympathetic nervous system activity in HF patients compared with healthy subjects, which is increased even further in the presence of OSA. In fact, a significant inverse correlation between the degree of subjective daytime sleepiness and daytime muscle sympathetic nervous system activity has been documented in patients with HF and OSA (option C). Furthermore, patients with HF are often taking medications that can cross the blood-brain barrier and affect sleep, such as certain beta-blockers (including metoprolol) (option D).

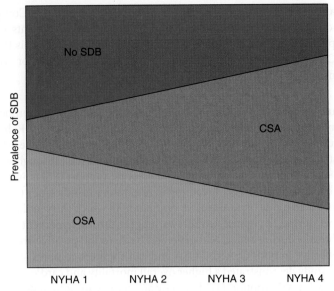

FIGURE 77-1 Prevalence of sleep-disordered breathing (SDB) by symptomatic severity of heart failure.
CSA, central sleep apnea; NYHA, New York Heart Association; OSA, obstructive sleep apnea.
(Modified with permission from Jing J, Huang T, Cui W, et al. Effect on quality of life of continuous positive airway pressure in patients with obstructive sleep apnea syndrome: a meta-analysis, *Lung.* 2008 May-Jun;186(3):131-144.)

77-7. **The answer is E.** *(Hurst's The Heart, 14th Edition, Chap. 77)* Pulmonary hypertension is defined as a mean pulmonary arterial pressure of > 25 mm Hg at rest or > 30 mm Hg during exercise. Acute changes in pulmonary arterial pressures have been observed to occur during apneas. The primary mechanism likely to be involved with the development of pulmonary hypertension in SDB is hypoxemia (option A), which reflexively increases pulmonary arterial pressures. The pulmonary hypertension associated with SDB is thought to be a result of a combination of precapillary and postcapillary factors, including pulmonary arteriolar remodeling (option D) and hyperreactivity to hypoxia, left ventricular diastolic dysfunction, and left atrial enlargement. Although measurable changes in the structure and function of the right ventricle have been reported in association with SDB, the clinical significance of these changes is uncertain. Right ventricular failure in SDB appears to be uncommon (option C) and is more likely if there is coexisting left-sided heart disease or chronic hypoxic respiratory disease. CPAP treatment results in a significant decrease in pulmonary artery pressure and a significant decrease in total pulmonary vascular resistance (option B).

77-8. **The answer is D.** *(Hurst's The Heart, 14th Edition, Chap. 77)* Lifestyle modifications to improve activity and diet are important in the management of SDB. Weight loss and bariatric surgery highly benefit patients with OSA (option A). Patients in whom SDB occurs either exclusively or predominantly in a supine sleep position should be counseled regarding positional therapy, using techniques that discourage sleep in the supine position (option E). PAP therapy delivered through a nasal or nasal-oral mask stabilizes the airway and thus prevents collapse and is the standard treatment for SDB (option B). Oral appliances, worn during sleep and usually fitted by a dentist, may be used to extend the dimensions of the airway and may be effective in select patients, such as those with mild SDB, with positional SDB, or without marked obesity (option C). Finally, carbon dioxide therapy reduces AHI in CSA but at the expense of hyperventilation and poor sleep quality, and thus it is not used clinically (option D).

77-9. The answer is B. *(Hurst's The Heart, 14th Edition, Chap. 77)* Complex sleep apnea is a type of CSA characterized by the emergence of CSR in patients receiving positive airway pressure therapy (option B). This treatment-induced CSR is thought to arise in HF and OSA patients with heightened chemoreceptor sensitivity, or with pronounced sleep fragmentation.

77-10. The answer is C. *(Hurst's The Heart, 14th Edition, Chap. 77)* A number of different positive airway treatment modalities exist for CSA/CSR, namely CPAP, bilevel positive airway pressure (BiPAP), and ASV (Figure 77-2). CPAP machines have a fixed or automatically adjusted expiratory pressure (EPAP) that remains constant throughout the night (option A). BiPAP monitors have a fixed EPAP and pressure support (PS) at inspiration, usually with a fixed backup rate to trigger breathing in respiratory insufficiency (option B). ASV is a more sophisticated mode of noninvasive ventilation in which the ventilator increases inspiratory support during hypopnea, withdraws support during hyperventilation, provides mandatory breaths during apnea, and generates background positive airway pressure. Therefore, it is effective in both CSA and OSA and can suppress complex sleep apnea. Nevertheless, a recent study demonstrated a higher overall mortality and cardiovascular mortality in those treated with ASV (option D), driven by an increase in sudden death.

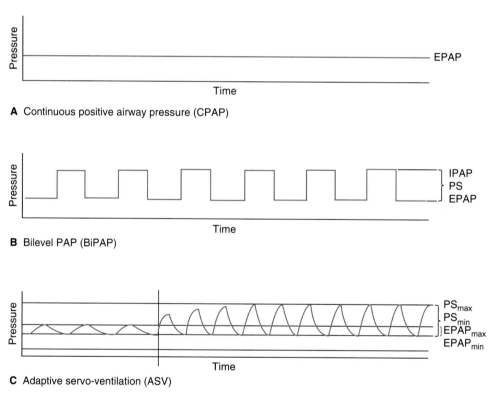

A Continuous positive airway pressure (CPAP)

B Bilevel PAP (BiPAP)

C Adaptive servo-ventilation (ASV)

FIGURE 77-2 Different positive airway treatment modalities.
(Reproduced with permission from Linz D, Woehrle H, Bitter T, et al. The importance of sleep-disordered breathing in cardiovascular disease, *Clin Res Cardiol.* 2015 Sep;104(9):705-718.)

References

1. Somers VK, White DP, Amin R, et al. Sleep apnea and cardiovascular disease: an American Heart Association/American College of Cardiology Foundation Scientific Statement from the American Heart Association Council for High Blood Pressure Research Professional Education Committee, Council on Clinical Cardiology, Stroke Council, and Council on Cardiovascular Nursing. *J Am Coll Cardiol.* 2008;52:686-717.
2. Taranto Montemurro L, Floras JS, Millar PJ, et al. Inverse relationship of subjective daytime sleepiness to sympathetic activity in patients with heart failure and obstructive sleep apnea. *Chest.* 2012;142:1222-1228.
3. Defaye P, de la Cruz I, Martí-Almor J, et al. A pacemaker transthoracic impedance sensor with an advanced algorithm to identify severe sleep apnea: the DREAM European study. *Heart Rhythm.* 2014;11:842-848.

4. Won C, Guilleminault C. Gender differences in sleep disordered breathing: implications for therapy. *Exp Rev Respir Med.* 2015;9:221-231.

5. Punjabi NM, Polotsky VY. Disorders of glucose metabolism in sleep apnea. *J Appl Physiol.* 2005;99:1998-2007.

6. Punjabi NM, Beamer BA. Alterations in glucose disposal in sleep-disordered breathing. *Am J Respir Crit Care Med.* 2009;179:235-240.

7. von Kanel R, Loredo JS, Ancoli-Israel S, et al. Association between polysomnographic measures of disrupted sleep and prothrombotic factors. *Chest.* 2007;131:733-739.

8. Mehra R, Benjamin EJ, Shahar E, et al. Association of nocturnal arrhythmias with sleep-disordered breathing: the Sleep Heart Health Study. *Am J Respir Crit Care Med.* 2006;173:910-916.

9. Alonso-Fernandez A, Garcia-Rio F, Racionero MA, et al. Cardiac rhythm disturbances and ST-segment depression episodes in patients with obstructive sleep apnea–hypopnea syndrome and its mechanisms. *Chest.* 2005;127:15-22.

10. Oldenburg O, Lamp B, Faber L, Teschler H, Horstkotte D, Topfer V. Sleep-disordered breathing in patients with symptomatic heart failure: a contemporary study of prevalence in and characteristics of 700 patients. *Eur J Heart Fail.* 2007;9:251-257.

11. Bitter T, Faber L, Hering D, Langer C, Horstkotte D, Oldenburg O. Sleep-disordered breathing in heart failure with normal left ventricular ejection fraction. *Eur J Heart Fail.* 2009;11:602-608.

SECTION 13

Rhythm and Conduction Disorders

CHAPTER 78

Electrophysiologic Anatomy

Jacqueline Joza

QUESTIONS

DIRECTIONS: Choose the one best response to each question.

78-1. Which of the following is *false* regarding the the heart borders and surrounding structures?

A. The right border of the heart is formed exclusively by the right atrium
B. The inferior border is marked by the right ventricle
C. The left border is formed by the aortic arch, the pulmonary veins, and the left ventricle
D. The left atrium forms most of the posterior border
E. The pulmonary trunk crosses over the root of the aorta anteriorly such that the aorta ascends behind

78-2. Regarding the right atrium, which of the following is *true*?

A. The right atrium is rightward and anterior when compared to the left atrium, which is leftward and posterior
B. The right atrium is more superior (cephalad) than the left atrium
C. During embryonic development, the eustachian valve separates the sinus venosus from the heart
D. The sinus node is a subepicardial structure that is found at the posteroseptal aspect of the superior vena cava–right atrial junction
E. The tendon of Todaro guards the orifice of the coronary sinus

78-3. Which of the following regarding the left atrium is *false*?

A. The remnant of the vein of Marshall or ligament of Marshall runs on the lateral epicardial aspect of the neck of the appendage, anterior to the left pulmonary veins
B. The orifices of the left pulmonary veins are more superiorly located than those of the right pulmonary veins
C. Triggered activity from the pulmonary vein muscle sleeves can initiate atrial fibrillation
D. Unlike the right atrium, virtually all the pectinate muscles in the left atrium are confined to the appendage
E. In approximately 5% of normal hearts, the fossa ovalis is patent

78-4. Which of the following statements is *false?*

A. Each ventricle has three components: the inlet, the outlet, and the apex
B. The right ventricular outflow tract is posterior and slightly leftward to that of the left ventricle
C. The right ventricle is the most anteriorly situated cardiac chamber in the normal heart
D. The moderator band is characteristic of the right ventricle
E. When the heart is viewed from the front, most of the left ventricle is behind the right ventricle

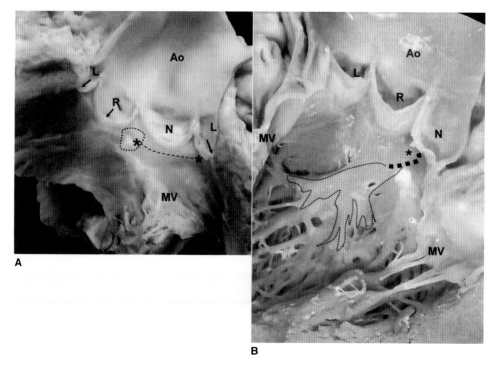

FIGURE 78-1 (A) The left ventricular outflow tract incised through the left coronary aortic sinus. (B) The aortic root is displayed by cutting through the anterior leaflet of the mitral valve.

78-5. Figure 78-1 displays the left ventricular outflow tract incised through the left coronary aortic sinus (Figure 78-1A), and the aortic root displayed by cutting through the "anterior" leaflet of the mitral valve (Figure 78-1B). What two different structures do the straight broken lines represent?

A. His bundle; chordae tendinae
B. Aortic-mitral fibrous continuity; atrioventricular conduction bundle
C. aortic-mitral fibrous continuity; left anterior fascicle
D. ligament of marshall; atrioventricular conduction bundle
E. coronary sinus; crista terminalis

78-6. Which of the following statements regarding the coronary veins is *incorrect*?

A. The greater coronary venous system drains 85% of the venous flow
B. The main coronary veins in the greater coronary venous system include the great, middle, and small cardiac veins
C. The anterior interventricular vein runs parallel to the circumflex artery
D. The coronary sinus ostium is usually between 5 and 15 mm in diameter
E. The valve of Vieussens is a flimsy valve that can provide some resistance to coronary sinus catheter placement

78-7. Regarding the sinus node, which of the following is *correct*?

A. The inferior aspect of the sinus nodal tissue can extend down > 50% of the length of the crista terminalis toward the inferior vena cava
B. Nodal tissues are penetrated by the septal artery
C. The tissue surrounding the sinus node is dominated by Na^+ channels
D. Bachmann's bundle is a prominent interatrial muscle bridge that extends across the floor of the right atrium, through the coronary sinus, and into the left atrium
E. Conduction over Bachmann's bundle is slow, and it leads to late endocardial activation of the left atrium

78-8. Which of the following statements regarding the atrioventricular conduction system is *incorrect*?

A. In the normal heart, the atrioventricular conduction system provides the only pathway of muscular continuity between the atrial and ventricular myocardium
B. The compact atrioventricular node is located near the apex of the triangle of Koch
C. The atrioventricular node receives its blood supply from the sinoatrial nodal artery
D. The compact atrioventricular node is approximately 5 mm long and 5 mm wide in the adult
E. Most of the time, extensions from the compact node pass to the right and left sides of the artery

78-9. Which of the following statements is *correct*?

A. Compared to that of the tricuspid valve, the mitral valve annulus is closer to the apex and has a septal leaflet

B. The aortomitral continuity is a site from which triggered idiopathic ventricular arrhythmias can originate

C. The papillary muscles are relatively thin structures, making them easy targets for ablation of ventricular arrhythmias originating within

D. The apex of the left ventricle is very thick, measuring approximately 15 to 20 mm in normal hearts

E. Fine muscular strands within the left ventricle are called intermediary bands

78-10. Which of the following statements is *incorrect*?

A. The right aortic sinus may be used to map and ablate focal atrial tachycardias that have their earliest activation in the vicinity of the His bundle area

B. Superiorly, at the apex of the triangle of Koch, the penetrating bundle of His passes through the central fibrous body, coursing leftward

C. The landmark for the atrioventricular conduction bundle is immediately inferior to the fibrous area, between the right and noncoronary aortic sinuses

D. The left bundle branch fans out as it descends in the subepicardium of the septal surface of the left ventricle

E. Both bundle branches are insulated as they descend toward the apical parts of the ventricles

78-1. **The answer is C.** *(Hurst's The Heart, 14th Edition, Chap. 78)* The sloping left border is often described as having three to four "moguls" on the chest x-ray, which correspond to the aortic arch, pulmonary artery (not pulmonary veins), and left ventricle (superior to inferior). Occasionally, the left atrial appendage is visible between the pulmonary artery and the left ventricle. The aortic knob appears above the pulmonary trunk. The right border of the heart is formed exclusively by the right atrium (option A), with the superior and inferior caval veins joining at its upper and lower margins. The inferior border lying horizontally on the diaphragm is marked by the right ventricle (option B). The left atrium is the most posterior cardiac chamber (closest to the spine), and the esophagus is immediately behind the left atrium (option D). In the hilum, the aortic knob is superior and rightward and the main pulmonary artery (or pulmonary trunk) is inferior and leftward (option E). The pulmonary trunk crosses over the root of the aorta anteriorly such that the aorta ascends behind or posterior to it.

78-2. **The answer is A.** *(Hurst's The Heart, 14th Edition, Chap. 78)* The right atrium is rightward and anterior, whereas the left atrium is leftward and posterior. The *left atrium* is also more superior (cephalad) than the right atrium (option B). During embryonic development, the crista terminalis (not the eustachian valve) separates the sinus venosus from the heart: it separates the smooth-walled posterior or venous atrium from the anterior trabeculated atrium (option C). The eustachian valve, guarding the entrance of the inferior vena cava, is a fibrous extension from the inferior margin of the crista terminalis. Sometimes the valve is perforated or netlike and is often described as a Chiari network. The sinus node (option D) is a subepicardial structure in the cephalad aspect of the sulcus terminalis (a fat-filled groove that corresponds internally to the crista terminalis) at the *anterolateral aspect* of the superior vena cava–right atrial junction. The thebesian valve (not the tendon of Todaro) often guards the orifice of the coronary sinus, and it is often fenestrated (option E). A complete and imperforate thebesian valve is rare, but it can cause an inability to cannulate the coronary sinus. The fibrous tendon of Todaro is a continuation of the free border of the eustachian ridge. The tendon of Todaro penetrates the musculature of the sinus septum, which separates the fossa ovalis from the os of the coronary sinus.[1]

78-3. **The answer is E.** *(Hurst's The Heart, 14th Edition, Chap. 78)* In approximately 20% to 25% (*not 5%*) of normal hearts, the fossa is patent, even though on the left atrial side the valve is large enough to overlap the rim. This is because the adhesion of the valve to the rim is incomplete, leaving a gap usually in the anterosuperior margin corresponding to a C-shaped mark in the left atrial side just behind the anterior atrial wall (Option E). The oblique vein of Marshall is obliterated in a majority of individuals, and the remnant of this vein (the ligament of Marshall) enters the coronary sinus and passes superiorly to inferiorly, between the left atrial appendage and the left superior pulmonary vein (this region is termed the Coumadin ridge) (Option A). The orifices of the left pulmonary veins are more superiorly located than those of the right pulmonary veins (option B). Typically, there are four pulmonary veins (left superior, left inferior, right superior, and right inferior). Sometimes there is a fifth pulmonary vein (usually a right middle pulmonary vein), and sometimes two of the veins will share a common antrum (eg, a left common antrum). Triggered activity from the pulmonary vein muscle sleeves can initiate atrial fibrillation (option C). These sources of ectopic activity are targeted during pulmonary vein isolation for the treatment of drug-refractory atrial fibrillation.[2,3] Unlike the right atrium, virtually all of the pectinate muscles in the left atrium are confined to the appendage (option D).

78-4. **The answer is B.** *(Hurst's The Heart, 14th Edition, Chap. 78)* The curvature places the right ventricular outflow tract *anteriorly* and slightly leftward to that of the left ventricle, resulting in a characteristic "crossover" relationship between right and left ventricular outflow tracts. Each ventricle has three components: the inlet containing the atrioventricular valve, the outlet leading to the arterial valve, and the apical trabecular component (option A). The right ventricle is the most anteriorly situated cardiac chamber in the normal heart. It is located immediately behind the sternum (option C). Coarse muscular trabeculations crisscross the apical portion of the right ventricle, and one of them (the moderator band) is characteristic of the right ventricle (option D). The moderator band bridges the ventricular cavity between the body of the septomarginal trabeculation and the parietal wall, giving rise to the anterior papillary muscle along the way. When the heart is viewed from the front, most of the left ventricle is behind the right ventricle (option E).

78-5. **The answer is B.** (*Hurst's The Heart, 14th Edition, Chap. 78*) The broken line in Figure 78-1A represents the aortic-mitral fibrous continuity with the fibrous trigones (asterisks) at each end. The aortic leaflets have been removed to show the muscular components (arrows) in the right (R) and left (L) coronary aortic sinuses that may be the source of aortic cusp ventricular tachycardia. In Figure 78-1B, the aortic root is displayed by cutting through the "anterior" leaflet of the mitral valve. The broken line represents the atrioventriular conduction bundle, which passes between the membranous septum (asterisk) and the muscular septum. The irregularly drawn shape represents the left bundle branch and its three fascicles.

78-6. **The answer is C.** (*Hurst's The Heart, 14th Edition, Chap. 78*) The great cardiac vein is a continuation of the coronary sinus and is also continuous with the anterior interventricular vein, which runs parallel to the left anterior descending artery (*not* the circumflex artery). (Option A) The venous return from the myocardium either is channeled via small thebesian veins that open directly into the cardiac chambers or, more significantly, is collected by the greater coronary venous system, which drains 85% of the venous flow.[4,5] The main coronary veins in the greater system are the great, middle, and small cardiac veins (option B). The middle cardiac vein runs alongside the posterior descending coronary artery. The great cardiac vein and middle cardiac vein (usually) drain into the coronary sinus. The coronary sinus is a critical structure in electrophysiology. Its ostium is usually between 5 and 15 mm in diameter (option D). Its transition to the great cardiac vein is marked by several structures, including the valve of Vieussens and the vein of Marshall. The valve of Vieussens marks the transition from the coronary sinus to the great cardiac vein. Found in 80% to 90% of hearts, this flimsy valve can provide some resistance to potential catheter placement (option E).

78-7. **The answer is A.** (*Hurst's The Heart, 14th Edition, Chap. 78*) The "tail" of the sinus nodal tissue can extend down more than 50% of the length of the crista terminalis toward the inferior vena cava. The node is richly supplied with nerves from both the sympathetic chains and the vagus nerve. Nodal tissues are penetrated by the sinoatrial nodal artery, which arises from the right coronary artery in 65% of individuals (option B).[6] The tissue surrounding the sinus node is dominated by calcium channel activation (as opposed to Na^+) (option C), and therefore, sinus node exit conduction is slow and decremental, similar to the atrioventricular node.[6] (Option D) Bachmann's bundle is a prominent interatrial muscle bridge that extends across the roof (*not floor*) of the atria anterosuperior to the fossa ovalis. Conduction over Bachmann's bundle leads to early (*not late*) endocardial activation in the anterior left atrium in order to help facilitate interatrial synchrony[6] (option E).

78-8. **The answer is C.** (*Hurst's The Heart, 14th Edition, Chap. 78*) The atrioventricular node receives its blood supply from the *atrioventricular nodal artery*, which arises from the right coronary artery in 80%, the left circumflex artery in 10%, and both in 10% of hearts. In the normal heart (without accessory pathway connections), the atrioventricular conduction system provides the only pathway of muscular continuity between atrial and ventricular myocardium (option A). There is an interface of transitional cells between ordinary atrial myocardium and the histologically specialized cells that make up the atrioventricular node. The compact atrioventricular node was described by Tawara in 1906 and is located near the apex of the triangle of Koch (option B).[7] In the adult, the compact atrioventricular node is approximately 5 mm in length and width (option D). Most of the time, extensions from the compact node pass to the right and left sides of the artery[8] (option E). The right extension courses parallel and adjacent to the tricuspid annulus, whereas the left extension projects toward the mitral vestibule.

78-9. The answer is B. *(Hurst's The Heart, 14th Edition, Chap. 78)* The aortomitral continuity is a structure of particular importance and is another site from which triggered idiopathic ventricular arrhythmias can originate.[9] Compared to that of the tricuspid valve, the mitral valve annulus is *farther* away from the apex and does *not* have a septal leaflet (option A). The mitral leaflets are attached via tendinous cords exclusively to two groups of papillary muscles: anterolateral and posteromedial papillary muscles. The papillary muscles can be sources for ventricular arrhythmias that are often *difficult* to ablate given their location and motion within the left ventricular cavity as well as the *thick* nature of the papillary muscles (option C). At the apex, the muscular wall tapers to a thickness of 1 to 2 mm in normal hearts (*not 15 to 20 mm*), and the trabeculations are finer than those found in the right ventricle (Option D). Fine muscular strands, or so-called *false tendons* (*not intermediary bands*), extend between the septum and the papillary muscles or the parietal wall. They often carry the distal ramifications of the left bundle branch and have been implicated in idiopathic left ventricular tachycardia.

78-10. The answer is A. *(Hurst's The Heart, 14th Edition, Chap. 78)* The *noncoronary* aortic sinus (not the *right aortic sinus*), being immediately adjacent to the paraseptal region of the left and right atria and close to the superior atrioventricular junction, may be used to map and ablate focal atrial tachycardias that have their earliest activation in the vicinity of the His bundle area—so-called parahisian atrial tachycardiac. Superiorly, at the apex of the triangle of Koch, the penetrating bundle of His passes through the central fibrous body, coursing leftward (option B). This short bundle of specialized myocardium encased in a fibrous sheath is a direct extension of the compact atrioventricular node, enabling atrial activity to be conveyed to the ventricles. In relationship to the aortic valve, the landmark for the atrioventricular conduction bundle is immediately inferior to the fibrous area between the right and noncoronary aortic sinuses (option C). The bundle is sandwiched between the membranous septum and the crest of the ventricular septum. After a short distance, the bundle bifurcates into the left and right bundle branches. The left bundle branch fans out as it descends in the subepicardium of the septal surface of the left ventricle (option D). In contrast, the right bundle branch is cordlike and descends through the musculature of the ventricular septum to emerge in the subendocardium at the base of the medial papillary muscle to run in the septomarginal trabeculation. Along its descent, a prominent branch crosses to the parietal wall within the moderator band. Both bundle branches are insulated as they descend toward the apical parts of the ventricles (option E). The branches then ramify as the Purkinje fibers, running in the subendocardium and into the myocardium in a netlike fashion.

References

1. Ho SY, Anderson RH. How constant anatomically is the tendon of Todaro as a marker for the triangle of Koch? *J Cardiovasc Electrophysiol.* 2000;11:83-89.
2. Zipes DP, Knope RF. Electrical properties of the thoracic veins. *Am J Cardiol.* 1972;29:372-376.
3. Haissaguerre M, Jais P, Shah DC, et al. Spontaneous initiation of atrial fibrillation by ectopic beats originating in the pulmonary veins. *N Engl J Med.* 1998;339:659-666.
4. Gensini GG, Digiorgi S, Coskun O, Palacio A, Kelly AE. Anatomy of the coronary circulation in living man; coronary venography. *Circulation.* 1965;31:778-784.
5. Habib A, Lachman N, Christensen KN, Asirvatham SJ. The anatomy of the coronary sinus venous system for the cardiac electrophysiologist. *Europace.* 2009;11(suppl 5):v15-v21.
6. Dobrzynski H, Anderson RH, Atkinson A, et al. Structure, function and clinical relevance of the cardiac conduction system, including the atrioventricular ring and outflow tract tissues. *Pharmacol Ther.* 2013;139:260-288.
7. Tawara S. *Das Reizleitungssystem des Saugetierherzens: Eine Anatomisch-Histologische Studie Uber Das Atrioventrikularbundel Und Die Purkinjeschen Faden.* Jena, Germany: Verlag von Gustav Fischer; 1906.
8. Inoue S, Becker AE. Posterior extensions of the human compact atrioventricular node: a neglected anatomic feature of potential clinical significance. *Circulation.* 1998;97:188-193.
9. Hai JJ, Chahal AA, Friedman PA, et al. Electrophysiologic characteristics of ventricular arrhythmias arising from the aortic mitral continuity-potential role of the conduction system. *J Cardiovasc Electrophysiol.* 2015;26:158-163.

CHAPTER 79

Mechanisms of Cardiac Arrhythmias and Conduction Disturbances

Jacqueline Joza

QUESTIONS

DIRECTIONS: Choose the one best response to each question.

79-1. A 45-year-old woman presents to the emergency department after experiencing frequent and intermittent regular palpitations over the last several days. Her presenting electrocardiogram reveals ventricular bigeminy, and monitoring demonstrates rapid runs of ventricular tachycardia of the same morphology as her premature ventricular contractions (PVCs). The consultant cardiologist diagnoses her with right ventricular outflow tract ventricular tachycardia. Which of the following tachycardias shares the same arrhythmia mechanism?

A. Bundle branch reentry tachycardia
B. AV reentry using an accessory bypass tract
C. Atrial flutter
D. Atrial tachycardia
E. AV nodal reentry tachycardia

79-2. A 79-year-old man is admitted overnight to the coronary care unit for symptomatic severe sinus bradycardia. You have held his beta-blocker and have tentatively scheduled the implantation of a permanent dual-chamber pacemaker for the following day. Due to his persistent heart rate of 35 bpm associated with weakness, you decide to start isoproterenol. Which of the following regarding the I_f current is *incorrect*?

A. The I_f current is referred to as a "funny" current because, unlike most voltage-sensitive currents, it is activated by hyperpolarization

B. The I_f is a mixed Na-K inward current modulated by the autonomic nervous system through cyclic adenosine monophosphate
C. I_f is responsible for heart rate control by the autonomic nervous system
D. The contributions of the I_f and the potassium channel (I_K) are equal in the SA node, AV node, and Purkinje fibers
E. The depolarization of I_f activates L-type Ca ($I_{Ca,L}$) current, which provides Ca to activate the type 2 cardiac ryanodine receptor (RyR2)

79-3. An 85-year-old woman is sent to the emergency department after significant sinus node dysfunction with > 5 second sinus pauses noted on her recent holter monitor. Her resting ECG today demonstrates severe sinus bradycardia with a junctional escape at 50 bpm. Regarding the sinus node and the subsidiary pacemakers, which of the following is *correct*?

A. The potential range of the pacemaker cells in the SA/AV nodes and the Purkinje fibers is –90 to –65mV and –70 to –35mV, respectively
B. Cells in the AV node have the fastest intrinsic rates
C. Subsidiary atrial pacemakers with more negative diastolic potentials (–75 to –70 mV) than SA nodal cells are located at the junction of the inferior right atrium
D. Acetylcholine can significantly reduce Purkinje automaticity by inhibiting the parasympathetic influence, a phenomenon termed *accentuated antagonism*
E. Adenosine has important effects on His-Purkinje system activation rate at baseline

79-4. Which of the following statements concerning automaticity is *correct*?

A. Heart failure and atrial fibrillation (AF) may only be associated with significant AV node dysfunction

B. Mutation of HCN4 may cause changes in HCN4 channel expression and kinetics, leading to long QT syndrome type 2

C. Depolarization-induced automaticity refers to the phenomenon whereby atrial and ventricular myocardial cells display spontaneous diastolic depolarization or automaticity under resting conditions

D. Abnormal automaticity is enhanced by β-adrenergic agonists and by the reduction of external potassium

E. *Overdrive suppression* refers to the intrinsic ability of the His-Purkinje system to suppress spontaneous junctional tachycardia

79-5. A 22-year-old male patient is resuscitated following an out-of-hospital cardiac arrest that occurred while he was playing soccer. While he is being monitored in the intensive care unit, he develops frequent runs of bidirectional VT. The patient's father and paternal grandfather both died suddenly in their 20s. Which of the following statements is *false*?

A. Delayed afterdepolarizations (DADs) occur because of the spontaneous release of Ca from the sarcoplasmic reticulum

B. The patient has a likely diagnosis of catecholaminergic polymorphic VT

C. Flecainide may suppress exercise-induced arrhythmias in this patient

D. The term *diastolic Ca-voltage coupling gain* is used to describe membrane potential (V_m) responses to elevated Ca during diastole

E. A critical prolongation of repolarization accompanies most, but not all, DADs.

79-6. A 29-year-old man is sent to you in consultation for syncope. Your tentative diagnosis is early repolarization syndrome (ERS). Which of the following might *not* be noted on his ECG?

A. Low voltage in the inferior leads

B. ST-segment or J_t elevation in the inferolateral plus anterior or right ventricular leads

C. Notch or slur of the terminal part of the QRS

D. ST-segment or J_t elevation in the lateral leads

E. J_p exceeding 0.1 mV in two or more contiguous inferior and/or lateral leads

79-7. The main differences between Brugada syndrome (BrS) and ERS include all of the following *except*:

A. The RVOT is affected in BrS as opposed to the inferior left ventricle in ERS

B. Greater inducibility of VF during electrophysiologic study in BrS than in ERS

C. Greater elevation of J_o, J_p, or J_t (ST-segment elevation) in response to sodium channel blockers in BrS than in ERS

D. Patients may be totally asymptomatic in ERS until presenting with sudden cardiac arrest, as opposed to BrS where symptoms are typically present early on

E. A higher prevalence of AF in BrS than in ERS

79-8. Which of the following statements regarding extracardiac arrhythmogenicity is *incorrect*?

A. The pulmonary veins are important sources of atrial fibrillation (AF)

B. Rapid activations from other thoracic veins, such as the superior vena cava and the vein of Marshall, are important for AF to occur and sustain

C. The embryologic development of the pulmonary veins is closely related to the development of the sinus venosus segment of the heart, which are known to be structures that can generate automaticity

D. Because of the short action potential duration, the pulmonary veins are also prone to the development of late phase 3 early afterdepolarizations (EADs) and triggered arrhythmias

E. The myocardial fiber orientation within the pulmonary veins is organized in a parallel fashion

79-9. A 70-year-old woman presents to the emergency department following a syncopal episode. She was standing in her kitchen and suffered a sudden loss of consciousness. She awoke on the floor with a large laceration to her forehead. Her medications include sotalol and hydrochlorothiazide. Her EKG reveals a prolongation in her QT interval, with isolated premature ventricular contractions (PVCs) occurring on the T wave. Which of the following statements regarding the PVCs is *incorrect*?

A. A critical prolongation of repolarization accompanies most, but not all EADs

B. Drugs that block Ca currents may reduce repolarization reserve and predispose the cells to EADs

C. Antiarrhythmic drugs with class III action generally induce EAD activity at slow stimulation rates and totally suppress EADs at rapid rates

D. An EAD occurs when the balance of current active during phase 2 or 3 of the action potential shifts in the inward direction

E. EADs develop more in midmyocardial M cells and Purkinje fibers than in epicardial or endocardial cells when exposed to action potential duration-prolonging agents

79-10. You are consulted on a 55-year-old woman who presents after three episodes of sustained rapid palpitations of sudden onset. Each episode required an emergency department visit, where a narrow QRS tachycardia was noted with an Rsr' noted in lead V1. The tachycardia was always promptly terminated with adenosine. Which of the following statements regarding the patient's presumed arrhythmia is *correct*?

A. Two functionally or anatomically distinct potential pathways exist that do not join proximally or distally

B. Unidirectional block must occur for initiation and maintenance of the arrhythmia

C. Interruption of the arrhythmia circuit along its path should result in a change in the rate of the arrhythmia

D. Reentry can be classified as functional but not anatomical

E. The ring model is the prototypical example of reentry around an anatomical obstacle: it first emerged as a concept when Mayer reported the results of experiments in pigs

79-1. The answer is D. *(Hurst's The Heart, 14th Edition, chap. 79).* The arrhythmic mechanism of right ventricular outflow tract ventricular tachycardia is enhanced or abnormal impulse formation (either triggered or automatic activity). Atrial tachycardia occurs as a result of enhanced pacemaker activity of ectopic sites within the atria. The arrhythmic mechanism of atrial tachycardia is either enhanced or abnormal impulse formation (from enhanced automaticity or triggered activity) as well as reentry. Bundle branch reentry tachycardia (option A), AV reentry using an accessory bypass tract (WPW or concealed accessory AV connection) (option B), atrial flutter (option C), and AV nodal reentry tachycardia (option E) are all reentrant tachycardias.

79-2. The answer is D. *(Hurst's The Heart, 14th Edition, chap. 79).* The contributions of the I_f and the potassium channel (I_K) *differ* in the SA node/AV nodes and Purkinje fibers because of the different potential ranges of these two pacemaker types (ie, –70 to –35 mV and –90 to –65 mV, respectively). The I_f current is referred to as a "funny" current because, unlike most voltage-sensitive currents, it is activated by hyperpolarization (from –40/–50 mV to –100/–110 mV) rather than depolarization (option A). At the end of the action potential, the I_f is activated and is responsible for early diastolic depolarization that gradually depolarizes the sarcolemmal membrane.[1,2] The I_f is a mixed Na-K inward current modulated by the autonomic nervous system through cyclic adenosine monophosphate[3] (option B). Sympathetic stimulation (isoproterenol) increases the I_f, whereas parasympathetic stimulation (acetylcholine) reduces it. These findings suggest that I_f is responsible for heart rate control by the autonomic nervous system (option C). The depolarization activates L-type Ca current ($I_{Ca,L}$), which provides Ca to activate the type 2 (cardiac) ryanodine receptor (RyR2) (option E). The activation of RyR2 initiates sarcoplasmic reticulum Ca release (Ca-induced Ca release), leading to contraction of the heart, a process known as excitation–contraction coupling.

79-3. The answer is C. *(Hurst's The Heart, 14th Edition, chap.79).* Subsidiary atrial pacemakers with more negative diastolic potentials (–75 to –70 mV) than SA nodal cells are located at the junction of the inferior right atrium and the inferior vena cava, near or on the eustachian ridge.[4,5] Other atrial pacemakers have been identified in the crista terminalis[6] as well as at the orifice of the coronary sinus[7] and in the atrial muscle that extends into the tricuspid and mitral valves.[5,6] The contribution of the hyperpolarization-activated pacemaker current (I_f) and potassium channel (I_K) differs in SA node/AV nodes (–70 to –35 mV) and Purkinje fiber (–90 to –65 mV) because of the different potential ranges of these two pacemaker types (option A). Cells in the SA node (*not* the AV node, option B) have the fastest intrinsic rates, therefore the SA node is the primary pacemaker in the normal heart. In the His-Purkinje system, parasympathetic effects are less apparent than those of the sympathetic system. (Option D) Although acetylcholine produces little in the way of a direct effect, it can significantly reduce Purkinje automaticity by inhibiting the sympathetic (*not* parasympathetic) influence, a phenomenon termed *accentuated antagonism*.[8-10] Adenosine has *no* effects on His-Purkinje system activation rate at baseline, but it reduces its activation rate during isoproterenol infusion (option E). These findings suggest that adenosine's effects on the human His-Purkinje system are primarily antiadrenergic and are thus consistent with the concept of accentuated antagonism.

79-4. The answer is D. *(Hurst's The Heart, 14th Edition, chap. 79).* Similar to normal automaticity, abnormal automaticity is enhanced by β-adrenergic agonists and by the reduction of external potassium. Because the conductance of I_{K1} channels is sensitive to extracellular potassium concentration, hypokalemia can lead to a major reduction in I_{K1}, leading to depolarization and the development of enhanced or abnormal automaticity, particularly in Purkinje pacemakers. Common diseases, such as heart failure and AF, may be associated with significant SA node dysfunction[11,12] (option A). Malfunction of membrane voltage clocks and Ca clocks might both be present in these common diseases. A mutation of *HCN4*, which makes up part of the channels that carry I_f, can lead to familial bradycardia,[13-15] which can be associated with a variant of noncompaction syndrome, *not* long QT syndrome (option B). Depolarization-induced automaticity refers to the development of spontaneous diastolic depolarization or automaticity of the atrial and ventricular myocytes *only* when they are depolarized[16] (option C). This results in the development of repetitive impulse initiation. The membrane potential at which abnormal automaticity develops ranges between –70 and –30 mV. *Overdrive suppression* refers to the ability to inhibit the automaticity of all pacemakers within the heart by overdrive pacing (option E). Under normal conditions, all subsidiary pacemakers are overdrive-suppressed by SA nodal activity. The mechanisms of overdrive suppression are thought to be related to pacing-induced intracellular accumulation of Ca and Na.[17,18]

79-5. **The answer is E.** *(Hurst's The Heart, 14th Edition, chap. 79).* A critical prolongation of repolarization accompanies most, but not all, EADs (*not* DADs). The patient in the question has a likely diagnosis of catecholaminergic polymorphic VT (CPVT) based on the classic finding of bidirectional VT as a result of alternans in Ca caused by a "leaky" ryanodine receptor (option B). DADs occur because of the spontaneous release of Ca from the sarcoplasmic reticulum (option A), which activates the I_{NCX} and results in oscillations of transmembrane potentials that occur after full repolarization of the action potential.[19] Knollmann's laboratory[20] discovered that flecainide prevented adrenergic stress-induced arrhythias in a mouse model of CPVT and in humans with calsequestrin (CASQ2) and ryanodine receptor (RYR2) mutations (option C). *Diastolic Ca-voltage coupling gain* is a term used to describe membrane potential (V_m) responses to elevated Ca during diastole (option D). This concept is based on the finding that the same magnitude of sarcoplasmic reticulum Ca release may induce DADs in the Purkinje fibers but not in the epicardial cells.

79-6. **The answer is A.** *(Hurst's The Heart, 14th Edition, chap. 79).* Low voltage is not specifically seen in ERS. ERS is characterized by J waves, J_o elevation, notch or slur of the terminal part of the QRS (option C), and ST-segment or J_t elevation in the lateral (type I) (option D), inferolateral (type II), or inferolateral plus anterior or right ventricular leads (type III) (option B). The J_p should exceed 0.1 mV in two or more contiguous inferior and/or lateral leads as per the taskforce recommendations for measurement and reporting of ER and J waves[21] (option E). It was further recommended that the start of the end QRS notch or J wave be designated as J_o and the termination as J_t. An ER pattern is often encountered in healthy individuals, particularly in young black individuals and athletes, and can be observed in acquired conditions, including hypothermia and ischemia.

79-7. **The answer is D.** *(Hurst's The Heart, 14th Edition, chap. 79).* Patients with either BrS or ERS may be totally asymptomatic until their initial presentation with sudden cardiac arrest. Differences between the two syndromes include: (1) the region of the heart most affected (RVOT vs inferior left ventricle) (option A); (2) greater incidence of late potentials in signal-averaged ECGs in BrS (60%) versus ERS (7%)[22]; (3) greater inducibility of VF during electrophysiologic study in BrS than in ERS (option B); (4) greater elevation of J_o, J_p, or J_t (ST-segment elevation) in response to sodium channel blockers in BrS versus ERS (option C); and (5) higher prevalence of AF in BrS versus ERS (option E).[23]

79-8. **The answer is E.** *(Hurst's The Heart, 14th Edition, chap. 79)* The *complex* myocardial fiber orientation in the pulmonary veins and at the pulmonary vein–left atrial junction can cause conduction blocks and facilitate reentrant excitations in that region.[24] Rapid activations in the pulmonary veins are responsible for triggering AF (option A). Rapid activations from other thoracic veins, such as the superior vena cava and the vein of Marshall,[25,26] are also important for AF to occur and sustain (option B). The embryologic development of the pulmonary veins is closely related to the development of the sinus venosus segment of the heart, which are known to be structures that can generate automaticity[27-29] (option C). Because of the short APD, the pulmonary veins are also prone to the development of late phase 3 EADs and triggered arrhythmias[30-32] (option D).

79-9. The answer is B. *(Hurst's The Heart, 14th Edition, chap. 79)* Drugs that block potassium channels (*not* Ca) may reduce repolarization reserve and predispose the cells to EADs (eg, class Ia and III antiarrhythmic agents). Although specific mechanisms of EAD induction can differ, a critical prolongation of repolarization accompanies most, but not all EADs (option A). Antiarrhythmic drugs with class III action generally induce EAD activity at slow stimulation rates and totally suppress EADs at rapid rates[33-34] (option C). An EAD occurs when the balance of current active during phase 2 or 3 of the action potential shifts in the inward direction (option D). If the change in the current-voltage relation results in a region of net inward current during the plateau range of membrane potentials, it leads to a depolarization or EAD. EADs develop more in midmyocardial M cells and Purkinje fibers than in epicardial or endocardial cells when exposed to action potential duration-prolonging agents (option E). This is in part a result of the presence of a weaker I_{Ks} in M cells.[35]

79-10. The answer is B. *(Hurst's The Heart, 14th Edition, chap. 79)* The patient likely has a diagnosis of typical atrioventricular nodal reentry tachycardia for which the underlying arrhythmia mechanism is reentry. Three criteria were developed by Mines to identify circus movement reentry: (1) an area of unidirectional block must exist (option B); (2) the excitatory wave progresses along a distinct pathway, returning to its point of origin and then following the same path again (ie, the circuit pathway *connects* at the proximal and distal ends) (option A); (3) interruption of the reentrant circuit at any point along its path should terminate the circus movement (option C). Reentry can be classified as anatomic *and* functional, although there is a gray zone in which both functional and anatomical factors are important in determining the characteristics of reentral excitation (option D). The ring model is the prototypical example of reentry around an anatomical obstacle. It first emerged as a concept shortly after the turn of the last century when Mayer reported the results of experiments involving the subumbrella tissue of a jellyfish (*Sychomedusa cassiopeia*)[36] (option E). The muscular disk did not contract until ringlike cuts were made and pressure and a stimulus applied. This caused the disk to "spring into rapid rhythmical pulsation so regular and sustained as to recall the movement of clockwork."

References

1. Bucchi A, Baruscotti M, Robinson RB, DiFrancesco D. Modulation of rate by autonomic agonists in SAN cells involves changes in diastolic depolarization and the pacemaker current. *J Mol Cell Cardiol.* 2007;43:39.
2. Difrancesco D. The role of the funny current in pacemaker activity. *Circ Res.* 2010;106:434-446.
3. Accili EA, Robinson RB, DiFrancesco D. Properties and modulation of I_f in newborn versus adult cardiac SA node. *Am J Physiol.* 1997;272:H1549-H1552.
4. Jones SB, Euler DE, Hardie E, Randall WC, Brynjolfsson G. Comparison of SA nodal and subsidiary atrial pacemaker function and location in the dog. *Am J Physiol.* 1978;234:H471-H476.
5. Rozanski GJ, Lipsius SL. Electrophysiology of functional subsidiary pacemakers in canine right atrium. *Am J Physiol.* 1985;249:H594-H603.
6. Hogan PM, Davis LD. Evidence for specialized fibers in the canine right atrium. *Circ Res.* 1968;23:387-396.
7. Wit AL, Cranefield PF. Triggered activity in cardiac muscle fibers of the simian mitral valve. *Circ Res.* 1976;38:85-98.
8. Levy MN, Martin P, Zieske H. Sympathetic and parasympathetic interactions upon the left ventricle of the dog. *Circ Res.* 1966;19:5-10.
9. Levy MN, Zieske H. Effect of enhanced contractility on the left ventricular response to vagus nerve stimulation in dogs. *Circ Res.* 1969;24:303-311.
10. Levy MN. Sympathetic-parasympathetic interactions in the heart. *Circ Res.* 1971;29:437-445.
11. Sanders P, Kistler PM, Morton JB, Spence SJ, Kalman JM. Remodeling of sinus node function in patients with congestive heart failure: reduction in sinus node reserve. *Circulation.* 2004;110:897-903.
12. Elvan A, Wylie K, Zipes DP. Pacing-induced chronic atrial fibrillation impairs sinus node function in dogs: electrophysiological remodeling. *Circulation.* 1996;94:2953-2960.
13. Milanesi R, Baruscotti M, Gnecchi-Ruscone T, DiFrancesco D. Familial sinus bradycardia associated with a mutation in the cardiac pacemaker channel. *N Engl J Med.* 2006;354:151-157.
14. Schulze-Bahr E, Neu A, Friederich P, et al. Pacemaker channel dysfunction in a patient with sinus node disease. *J Clin Invest.* 2003;111:1537-1545.

15. Nof E, Luria D, Brass D, et al. Point mutation in the HCN4 cardiac ion channel pore affecting synthesis, trafficking, and functional expression is associated with familial asymptomatic sinus bradycardia. *Circulation.* 2007;116:463-470.

16. Mohabir R, Ferrier GR. Effects of ischemic conditions and reperfusion on depolarization-induced automaticity. *Am J Physiol.* 1988;255:H992-H999.

17. Greenberg YJ, Vassalle M. On the mechanism of overdrive suppression in the guinea pig sinoatrial node. *J Electrocardiol.* 1990;23:53-67.

18. Gadsby DC, Cranefield PF. Electrogenic sodium extrusion in cardiac Purkinje fibers. *J Gen Physiol.* 1979;73:819-837.

19. Bers DM, Ginsburg KS. Na:Ca stoichiometry and cytosolic Ca-dependent activation of NCX in intact cardiomyocytes. *Ann N Y Acad Sci.* 2007;1099:326-338.

20. Watanabe H, Chopra N, Laver D, et al. Flecainide prevents catecholaminergic polymorphic ventricular tachycardia in mice and humans. *Nat Med.* 2009;15:380-383.

21. Macfarlane P, Antzelevitch C, Haissaguerre M, et al. Consensus paper: early repolarization pattern. *J Am Coll Cardiol.* 2015;66:470-477.

22. Kawata H, Noda T, Yamada Y, et al. Effect of sodium-channel blockade on early repolarization in inferior/lateral leads in patients with idiopathic ventricular fibrillation and Brugada syndrome. *Heart Rhythm.* 2012;9:77-83.

23. Junttila MJ, Tikkanen JT, Kentta T, et al. Early repolarization as a predictor of arrhythmic and nonarrhythmic cardiac events in middle-aged subjects. *Heart Rhythm.* 2014;11:1701-1706.

24. Chou CC, Nihei M, Zhou S, et al. Intracellular calcium dynamics and anisotropic reentry in isolated canine pulmonary veins and left atrium. *Circulation.* 2005;111:2889-2297.

25. Hwang C, Wu TJ, Doshi RN, Peter CT, Chen PS. Vein of Marshall cannulation for the analysis of electrical activity in patients with focal atrial fibrillation. *Circulation.* 2000;101:1503-1505.

26. Tsai CF, Tai CT, Hsieh MH, et al. Initiation of atrial fibrillation by ectopic beats originating from the superior vena cava: electrophysiological characteristics and results of radiofrequency ablation. *Circulation.* 2000;102:67-74.

27. Bliss DF, Hutchins GM. The dorsal mesocardium and development of the pulmonary veins in human embryos. *Am J Cardiovasc Pathol.* 1995;5:55-67.

28. Webb S, Brown NA, Wessels A, Anderson RH. Development of the murine pulmonary vein and its relationship to the embryonic venous sinus. *Anat Rec.* 1998;250:325-334.

29. DeRuiter MC, Gittenberger-de Groot AC, Wenink AC, Poelmann RE, Mentink MM. In normal development pulmonary veins are connected to the sinus venosus segment in the left atrium. *Anat Rec.* 1995;243:84-92.

30. Patterson E, Lazzara R, Szabo B, et al. Sodium-calcium exchange initiated by the Ca^{2+} transient: an arrhythmia trigger within pulmonary veins. *J Am Coll Cardiol.* 2006;47:1196-1206.

31. Patterson E, Po SS, Scherlag BJ, Lazzara R. Triggered firing in pulmonary veins initiated by in vitro autonomic nerve stimulation. *Heart Rhythm.* 2005;2:624-631.

32. Patterson E, Jackman WM, Beckman KJ, et al. Spontaneous pulmonary vein firing in man: relationship to tachycardia-pause early afterdepolarizations and triggered arrhythmia in canine pulmonary veins in vitro. *J Cardiovasc Electrophysiol.* 2007;18:1067-1075.

33. Davidenko JM, Cohen L, Goodrow R, Antzelevitch C. Quinidine-induced action potential prolongation, early afterdepolarizations, and triggered activity in canine Purkinje fibers. Effects of stimulation rate, potassium, and magnesium. *Circulation.* 1989;79:674-686.

34. Roden DM, Hoffman BF. Action potential prolongation and induction of abnormal automaticity by low quinidine concentrations in canine Purkinje fibers: relationship to potassium and cycle length. *Circ Res.* 1986;56:857-867.

35. Liu DW, Antzelevitch C. Characteristics of the delayed rectifier current (IKr and IKs) in canine ventricular epicardial, midmyocardial, and endocardial myocytes. *Circ Res.* 1995;76:351-365.

36. Mayer AG. Rhythmical pulsations in scyphomedusae. *Publication 47 of the Carnegie Institute.* 1906:1-62.

CHAPTER 80

Genetics of Channelopathies and Clinical Implications

Jacqueline Joza

QUESTIONS

DIRECTIONS: Choose the one best response to each question.

80-1. A 28-year-old woman is seen in consult after a near drowning episode. Both her presenting EKG and her baseline EKG today reveal a QTc of 490 ms. Which of the following genetic mutations paired with its responsible ion channel is most likely responsible for this patient's channelopathy?

A. $KCNH2$ / I_{Kr}
B. $KCNQ1$ / I_{Ks}
C. $KCNQ1$ / I_{Na}
D. $KCNH2$ / I_{Ks}
E. $KCNJ2$ / I_{K1}

80-2. Based on current guidelines, all of the following patients may be given a presumptive diagnosis of long QT syndrome *except*:

A. An asymptomatic 22-year-old female, on no medications, with a QTc of 485 ms in repeated ECGs
B. An asymptomatic 10-year-old female with a normal ECG and a positive mutation in the $KCNH2$ gene discovered on cascade screening
C. A 25-year-old female drug user on methadone, with resuscitated cardiac arrest and a QTc of 490 ms
D. A 22-year-old female, on no medications, with one episode of unexplained syncope and a QTc of 465 ms on several ECGs
E. A 22-year-old female with a prior syncope, QTc of 465 ms, and T wave notching

80-3. Which of the following represents a Class III recommendation for the management of long QT syndrome (LQTS)?

A. ICD implant in addition to beta-blocker therapy in asymptomatic carriers of a pathogenic mutation in $KCNH2$ or $SCN5A$ when the QTc is > 500 ms
B. Electrophysiology study for sudden cardiac death risk stratification
C. Beta-blocker use in carriers of a causative LQTS mutation and normal QT interval
D. ICD implantation in LQTS patients who experienced syncope and/or VT while receiving an adequate dose of beta-blockers
E. Sodium channel blocker use to shorten the QT interval in LQTS3 patients with a QTc > 500 ms

80-4. Two rhythm strips of a 19-year-old male patient being worked up for syncope are shown in Figure 80-1. The *upper panel* is during an exercise stress test, and the *lower panel* is during Holter monitoring. Which of the following is the most likely diagnosis?

A. Arrhythmogenic right ventricular dysplasia
B. Long QT syndrome
C. Short QT syndrome
D. Catecholaminergic polymorphic VT
E. Brugada syndrome

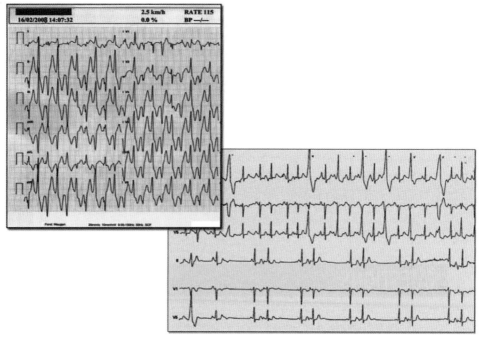

FIGURE 80-1 Arrhythmias in catecholaminergic polymorphic ventricular tachycardia (CPVT). The *upper panel* shows bidirectional ventricular tachycardia during an exercise stress test at low workload and arising at a sinus heart rate of 115 bpm. An example of supraventricular arrhythmias is shown in the *lower panel*.

80-5. A 40-year-old man presents to the emergency department for acute right knee pain. He denies any chest pain, nausea, dyspnea, or palpitations. His presenting ECG demonstrates ST elevations in leads V_1-V_2 (J point elevation ≥ 2 mm with coved ST segments), and he is taken to the cath lab emergently. Normal coronary arteries are demonstrated on coronary angiogram. He denies any history of syncope. Which of the following is *not* recommended at this time?

A. ICD implantation
B. Electrophysiology study
C. Extended monitoring
D. Counseling about avoiding large meals
E. Genetic testing

80-6. A 35-year-old woman with known Brugada syndrome undergoes urgent appendectomy. A code blue is called to the OR. When you arrive, you note that the patient is in electrical storm. What specific therapy should the patient receive at this point?

A. Flecainide IV
B. Epinephrine
C. Amiodarone IV
D. Esmolol infusion
E. Isoproterenol infusion

80-7. Which of the following genes have *not* been implicated in Brugada syndrome?

A. SCN5A
B. CASQ2
C. CACNB2
D. KCNE3
E. CACNA1c

80-8. You are assessing a 25-year-old man with evidence of a QTc interval of 350 ms. Which of the following additional pieces of history would be the *least* suggestive of a diagnosis of short QT syndrome (SQTS)?

A. Confirmed gain-of-function mutation in KCNH2
B. Confirmed loss-of-function mutation in KCNH2
C. Sudden cardiac death history in a 30-year-old brother
D. Survival from a VT episode in a structurally normal heart
E. Family history of SQTS

80-9. You are counseling a 25-year-old male patient regarding his diagnosis of long QT syndrome type 1 (LQTS1). He was incidentally discovered to have a loss-of-function mutation in the *KCNQ1* gene based on cascade screening after his mother suffered a resuscitated sudden cardiac arrest. Which of the following statements is *incorrect*?

A. Penetrance is defined as the ratio between the number of individuals showing the disease phenotype and the number of carriers of a given mutation

B. Penetrance is a common finding in all inherited arrhythmogenic diseases

C. Population studies have demonstrated that the heritable component of various ECG parameters is negligible

D. Variable penetrance can be the result of the presence of modulatory genetic factors, known as genetic modifiers

E. The QT interval and risk of events in LQTS patients are modulated by single nucleotide polymorphisms (SNPs)

80-10. A newborn boy is diagnosed with failure to thrive. His ECG reveals a markedly prolonged QTc, and a hearing test reveals sensorineural deafness. Which of the following syndromes is most consistent with the patient's findings?

A. Andersen–Tawil syndrome
B. Timothy syndrome
C. Jervell and Lange-Nielsen syndrome
D. Romano–Ward syndrome
E. Brugada syndrome

80-1. **The answer is B.** *(Hurst's The Heart, 14th Edition, Chap. 80)* The patient most likely has long QT syndrome type 1 (LQTS1), for which the classic trigger is strenuous swimming. The gene mutation associated with LQTS1 is *KCNQ1*, which is the gene of the I_{Ks} current (slow component of the delayed rectifier current) (option B). I_{Ks} is mostly active during phase 3 of the action potential, but its role in the control of repolarization becomes more evident during adrenergic stimulation since the current is mainly activated by catecholamines. Thus, the consequences of *KCNQ1* mutations, leading to reduced I_{Ks}, become more evident during increased sympathetic tone (eg, exercise, acute emotions) with a failure to shorten the action potential (ie, QT interval). LQTS2 is due to loss of function mutations in the *KCNH2* gene, which encodes for the α-subunit (pore-forming protein) of the I_{Kr} (rapid component of the delayed rectifier) channel, which participates in the control of cardiac repolarization during phase 3 (option A). Exposure to loud noises in LQTS2 patients should be avoided. LQTS3 is due to gain of function mutations in *SCN5A* that induce an increase of the late component of I_{Na}, leaving the peak (fast) component of the current unaffected or only mildly altered (option C: *SCN5A* / I_{Na} is the correct pairing). Option D: *KCNH2* / I_{Kr} is the correct pairing. A mutation in *KCNJ2* would lead to LQTS7, also known as Andersen–Tawil syndrome (option E).[1] The gene encodes for the cardiac inward rectifier I_{K1} current gene that participates in the control of the late repolarization phase and resting membrane potential. LQTS7 is a rare variant (< 1%) that can sometimes include extracardiac manifestations (periodic paralysis and dysmorphic features).

80-2. **The answer is C.** *(Hurst's The Heart, 14th Edition, Chap. 80)* The patient has a prolonged QT measured at 490 ms and was resuscitated from cardiac arrest. However, the patient is on methadone, which is well known to cause QT prolongation, and therefore a diagnosis of long QT syndrome cannot be made at the present time. Current guidelines indicate that long QT syndrome (LQTS) can be diagnosed under the following conditions: (1) either QTc ≥ 480 ms in repeated 12-lead ECGs (option A) or LQTS risk score > 3 (option E); (2) confirmed pathogenic LQTS mutation, irrespective of the QT duration (option B); or (3) a QTc ≥ 460 ms in repeated 12-lead ECGs in patients with unexplained syncope in the absence of secondary causes for QT prolongation (option D). These new diagnostic criteria substantially facilitate the clinical diagnosis since they permit the exclusion of patients with isolated (ie, with no family history, symptoms, or genetic mutation) and borderline QTc (440 to 460 ms).

80-3. **The answer is B.** *(Hurst's The Heart, 14th Edition, Chap. 80)* An invasive electrophysiology study is considered a Class III recommendation, and it should *not* be performed for sudden cardiac death risk stratification. Implantation of an ICD may be considered in addition to beta-blocker therapy in asymptomatic carriers of a pathogenic mutation in *KCNH2* or *SCN5A* when the QTc is > 500 ms (option A, Class IIb recommendation). Beta-blockers should be considered in carriers of a causative LQTS mutation who have a normal QT interval (option C, Class IIa recommendation). ICD implantation in addition to beta-blockers should be considered in LQTS patients who experienced syncope and/or VT while receiving an adequate dose of beta-blockers (option D, Class IIa recommendation). Sodium channel blockers (mexiletine, flecainide, or ranolazine) may be considered as add-on therapy to shorten the QT interval in LQTS3 patients with a QTc > 500 ms (option E, Class IIb recommendation). Because the response to this approach is not invariably positive (nonresponders), acute oral drug testing in the hospital setting may be advisable before chronic administration.[2]

80-4. **The answer is D.** *(Hurst's The Heart, 14th Edition, Chap. 80).* Arrhythmias in catecholaminergic polymorphic ventricular tachycardia (CPVT) are shown in Figure 80-1. The *upper panel* shows bidirectional ventricular tachycardia during an exercise stress test at low workload and arising at a sinus heart rate of 115 bpm. This distinctive pattern that appears during exercise is an alternating 180-degree QRS axis on a beat-to-beat basis.

The *lower panel* is an example of a supraventricular arrhythmia that can also be observed in patients with CPVT. Bidirectional ventricular tachycardia would not specifically be seen in arrhythmogenic right ventricular dysplasia (option A), short QT syndrome (option B), LQTS (option C), or Brugada syndrome (option E).

80-5. **The answer is A.** *(Hurst's The Heart, 14th Edition, Chap. 80)* The patient most likely has a spontaneous type 1 Brugada pattern on his ECG. An ICD should *not* be implanted in a patient with a spontaneous type 1 ECG without a history of syncope. Of concern is that the risk of life-threatening events in a patient with a spontaneous type 1 ECG pattern is double that of patients without spontaneous ST-segment elevation.[3] The inducibility of ventricular tachycardia (VT) or ventricular fibrillation (VF) at programmed electrical stimulation (PES) has been proposed for these patients, but there are conflicting results, and the approach remains controversial (option E). Overall, the most recent meta-analysis shows that the inducibility of VT/VF at PES with up to two extra stimuli is associated with an approximately threefold increased risk of cardiac arrest during follow-up.[4] However, patients with a negative PES still have a significant burden of events (approximately 1% per year).[4] Extended monitoring with either a Holter monitor or an implantable monitor should be considered (option C). Patients with Brugada syndrome should be counseled for lifestyle changes, including avoidance of drugs that may induce ST-segment elevation in the right precordial leads (http://www.brugadadrugs.org), avoidance of excessive alcohol intake and large meals (option D), and prompt treatment of any fever with antipyretic drugs. A referral to a specialized center for consideration for genetic testing should be made (option E).

80-6. **The answer is E.** *(Hurst's The Heart, 14th Edition, Chap. 80)* Isoproterenol or quinidine should be considered in patients with Brugada syndrome to treat electrical storms. Local anesthetics (bupivicaine) and other agents used for general anesthesia (eg, propofol) may exacerbate the ECG pattern in Brugada syndrome and potentially trigger arrhythmias, as seen in this patient. Flecainide is a sodium channel blocker that is used to uncover a type 1 brugada ECG pattern in suspected patients (option A). It is not used to acutely treat ventricular arrhythmias. Epinephrine (option B) is incorrect. Amiodarone (option C) and esmolol infusion (option D) are not specific therapies to treat electrical storm in the Brugada patient.

80-7. **The answer is B.** *(Hurst's The Heart, 14th Edition, Chap. 80)* Calsequestrin 2 (*CASQ2*) is the gene responsible for the autosomal recessive variant of CPVT.[5] Calsequestrin is a calcium-buffering protein located in the sarcoplasmic reticulum (SR) that controls the SR Ca^{2+} concentration, and it modulates the ryanodine receptor open probability. Mutations in the *SCN5A* gene account for 20% of cases of Brugada syndrome (option A). Cardiac calcium channel mutations have been reported in a few Brugada syndrome patients, and three genes have been involved: *CACNA1c* (option E), *CACNB2* (option C), and *CACNA2D1*. They all encode for subunits that cooperate to form the multimeric structure of the channel. A common feature of Brugada syndrome associated with calcium channel mutations is the presence of a short QT interval, which is reported to be constantly in the lower range of normal or even below normal in some patients. *KCNE3* (option D), is implicated in mutations leading to an increase in the cardiac transient outward potassium (I_{to}) current. Overall, potassium-related Brugada syndrome is considered a rare occurrence.

80-8. **The answer is B.** *(Hurst's The Heart, 14th Edition, Chap. 80)* A loss-of-function mutation in *KCNH2* would result in a *prolonged* QT interval, and it is considered a causative mutation in long QT syndrome type 2. Three short QT syndrome (SQTS) variants manifest with "isolated" short ventricular repolarization. These variants are found in association with gain-of-function mutations in *KCNH2* (SQTS1) (option A), *KCNQ1* (SQTS2), and *KCNJ2* (SQTS3). SQTS can be diagnosed in the presence of QTc < 340 ms (Class Ic)[6] and can also be considered (Class IIa) in the presence of a QTc ≤ 360 ms and one or more of the following: (1) confirmed pathogenic mutation (option A); (2) family history of SQTS (option E); (3) family history of sudden death at age < 40 years (option C); or (4) survival from a VT/VF episode in the absence of heart disease (option D).

80-9. **The answer is C.** *(Hurst's The Heart, 14th Edition, Chap. 80)* Population studies have demonstrated that the heritable component of various ECG parameters is between 25% and 45% of the total variance, and it includes the QT, RR, and PR intervals and RR variability.[7] Penetrance is defined as the ratio between the number of individuals showing the disease phenotype and the number of carriers of a given mutation (option A). Penetrance is a common finding in all inherited arrhythmogenic diseases (option B). Variable penetrance should always be considered when assessing families with suspected inherited arrhythmias, and it should prompt the use of genetic testing in all available family members whenever a mutation is identified in the proband (option D). Specific data have been observed for few SNPs on the *NOS1AP* gene that are associated with a twofold increased risk of events in LQTS with QTc < 500 ms[8] (option E).

80-10. **The answer is C.** *(Hurst's The Heart, 14th Edition, Chap. 80)* QT prolongation and arrhythmic risk may be observed in Jervell and Lange-Nielsen syndrome where patients are known to have associated sensorineural deafness. *KCNQ1* and *KCNE1* mutations, when present in "double dose" (homozygosity) and inherited as a recessive trait, cause the Jervell and Lange-Nielsen syndrome. *KCNJ2* causes the LQTS7 variant,[1] also known as Andersen–Tawil syndrome (option A), and it is characterized by hypokalemic periodic paralysis, facial dimorphism, and autosomal dominant inheritance. Timothy syndrome (option B) is characterized by a prolonged QT interval with associated syndactyly, autism spectrum disorders, congenital cardiac defects, and metabolic abnormalities, with sporadic presentation or parental mosaicism. Two clinical signs (QT prolongation with or without syncope) define the most common LQTS presentation, the so-called Romano–Ward syndrome, which has autosomal dominant inheritance (option D). Brugada syndrome (option E) is characterized by a particular ECG pattern of ST-segment elevation in leads V_1 to V_3 and incomplete or complete right bundle branch block in the absence of signs of acute myocardial ischemia.

References

1. Priori SG, Wilde AA, Horie M, et al. HRS/EHRA/APHRS expert consensus statement on the diagnosis and management of patients with inherited primary arrhythmia syndromes: document endorsed by HRS, EHRA, and APHRS in May 2013 and by ACCF, AHA, PACES, and AEPC in June 2013. *Heart Rhythm.* 2013;10:1932-1963.
2. Priori SG, Ruan Y, O'Rourke B, Liu N, Napolitano C. Sodium current disorders: geneticist's view, in Abriel H (ed): *Cardiac Sodium Channel Disorders.* Philadelphia: Elsevier; 2014:825-833.
3. Priori SG, Napolitano C, Gasparini M, et al. Natural history of Brugada syndrome. Insights for risk stratification and management. *Circulation.* 2002;105:1342-1347.
4. Sroubek J, Probst V, Mazzanti A, et al. Programmed ventricular stimulation for risk stratification in the Brugada syndrome: a pooled analysis. *Circulation.* 2016;133:622-630.
5. Priori SG, Napolitano C, Tiso N, et al. Mutations in the cardiac ryanodine receptor gene (*hRyR2*) underlie catecholaminergic polymorphic ventricular tachycardia. *Circulation.* 2001;103:196-200.
6. Priori SG, Blomstrom-Lundqvist C, Mazzanti A, et al. 2015 ESC guidelines for the management of patients with ventricular arrhythmias and the prevention of sudden cardiac death: the Task Force for the Management of Patients with Ventricular Arrhythmias and the Prevention of Sudden Cardiac Death of the European Society of Cardiology (ESC). Endorsed by: Association for European Paediatric and Congenital Cardiology (AEPC). *Eur Heart J.* 2015;36:2793-2867.
7. Marsman RF, Tan HL, Bezzina CR. Genetics of sudden cardiac death caused by ventricular arrhythmias. *Nat Rev Cardiol.* 2014;11:96-111.
8. Napolitano C, Novelli V, Francis MD, Priori SG. Genetic modulators of the phenotype in the long QT syndrome: state of the art and clinical impact. *Curr Opin Genet Dev.* 2015;33:17-24.

CHAPTER 81

Approach to the Patient with Cardiac Arrhythmias

Jacqueline Joza

QUESTIONS

DIRECTIONS: Choose the one best response to each question.

81-1. A 40-year-old woman presents to your clinic complaining of palpitations that have become more frequent in the last few years, having occurred three times in the last year. They are described as rapid, regular, of sudden onset and sudden offset, with no clear precipitant. Three years ago, a supraventricular tachycardia was noted on EKG, which terminated abruptly with adenosine administration in the emergency department. Her transthoracic echo at that time revealed a structurally normal heart. She regularly drinks 1 to 2 cups of coffee per day, and she does *not* ingest other caffeinated products. With regard to caffeine intake, what advice do you give her?

A. She should limit her caffeine intake to 1 cup of coffee per day
B. She should stop all caffeine consumption
C. Caffeine is not clearly linked with paroxysmal SVT
D. She should increase her intake to assess whether caffeine is a precipitant for her palpitations
E. She should drink tea instead

81-2. Which of the following is most in favor with cardiac syncope as opposed to a seizure?

A. Waking with a cut tongue
B. Loss of consciousness with emotional stress
C. Head turning to one side during loss of consciousness
D. Prolonged standing prior to event
E. Abnormal behavior noted

81-3. A subset of patients with manifest preexcitation (delta wave) should undergo ablation. All of the following patients with a preexcitation pattern on their baseline ECG should undergo ablation *except*:

A. 35-year-old male, asymptomatic with a pathway refractory period of < 250 ms
B. 35-year-old male with recurrent palpitations and documented narrow-QRS supraventricular tachycardia
C. 35-year-old male, asymptomatic with a pathway refractory period < 450 ms
D. 25-year-old male with resuscitated cardiac arrest
E. 35-year-old male with recurrent palpitations and documented wide-complex tachycardia

81-4. A 65-year-old man is referred for pacemaker implantation based on bradycardia that is documented on a resting ECG. The patient is asymptomatic. His ECG reveals 2:1 AV block. Which of the following statements is *correct*?

A. Exercise will improve Mobitz II AV block
B. Exercise will improve Mobitz I AV block
C. Exercise will improve complete AV block
D. Atropine will worsen Mobitz II AV block
E. Atropine will improve Mobitz I AV block

81-5. All of the following clinical tools may be used for improved risk stratification for the development of ventricular arrhythmias *except*:

A. Signal-averaged electrocardiogram
B. Head-up tilt table testing
C. T-wave alternans
D. Transthoracic echocardiography
E. Autonomic evaluation including heart rate variability

81-6. T-wave alternans (TWA) may be used in risk stratification for patients at risk for ventricular arrhythmias. Which of the following statements is *incorrect*?

A. TWA reflects dispersion of repolarization in animal models and human hearts
B. Subtle oscillations can be revealed as microvolt-level TWA, which has a high negative predictive value for ventricular arrhythmias
C. In patients with a left ventricular ejection fraction < 35%, patients with negative TWA have a < 5% risk of sudden cardiac arrest in a 1-year period
D. The use of TWA has a class II indication in managing patients at risk for ventricular arrhythmias
E. TWA predicted ICD therapy in the MUSTT trial, but it is currently of adjunctive value

81-7. A 75-year-old woman recently suffered a mild stroke. She is otherwise healthy. As part of her workup for cryptogenic stroke, an implantable loop recorder (ILR) is implanted. What are the potential advantages of ILR?

A. The ability to detect rare events that may be missed by other monitoring modalities
B. The ability to record events that are patient-triggered
C. The ability to record events that are auto-triggered
D. Lack of need for patient compliance
E. All of the above

81-8. Limitations of modern-day ECG recordings include all of the following *except*:

A. Battery or motor failure slowing the tape speed
B. Patient-related artifacts such as during tooth brushing
C. Data-recording artifacts from loose skin-electrode contact
D. ECG noise from medical equipment such as infusion pumps
E. Patient-related artifacts such as the Parkinson tremor

81-9. You are consulted on a 20-year-old woman with recurrent syncope in the emergency department. You suspect recurrent vasovagal syncope and refer her for head-up tilt table testing. Which of the following statements concerning head-up tilt table testing is *correct*?

A. It may be used to discriminate postural orthostatic tachycardia syndrome (POTS) from inappropriate sinus tachycardia
B. It consists of footrest-supported head-up tilting to 85 to 95 degrees for 30 to 45 minutes
C. In patients with vasovagal syncope, this position may lead to venous pooling and loss of consciousness
D. Infusions of isoproterenol or nitroglycerin may be used to increase the study specificity
E. The test itself has very good reproducibility

81-10. Cardiac magnetic resonance (CMR) has an increasing role in arrhythmia management. In which of the following scenarios would a CMR prove to be the *least* useful for a 55-year-old male patient?

A. Sustained ventricular tachycardia within 72 hours of an acute myocardial infarction
B. Newly diagnosed hypertrophic cardiomyopathy, for presence of scar
C. Planned epicardial VT ablation, for localization of the coronary arteries
D. Planned pulmonary vein isolation, for left atrial and pulmonary vein anatomy
E. T-wave inversions V_1 to V_4 and a family history of SCD, for presence of cardiomyopathy

81-1. The answer is C. (*Hurst's The Heart, 14th Edition, Chap. 81*). Neither alcohol nor caffeine is clearly linked with paroxysmal SVT or sustained ventricular tachycardias. The link between caffeine and arrhythmias is unclear, and perhaps more clear for sinus tachycardia than supraventricular tachycardias (SVT).[1] Options A and B suggest reducing or discontinuing caffeine intake, but there are no data to suggest that this will reduce her symptoms or arrhythmia burden.

81-2. The answer is D. (*Hurst's The Heart, 14th Edition, Chap. 81*). Scoring systems exist to separate cardiac syncope from seizures (see Table 81-1 in *Hurst's The Heart*, 14th Edition).[2] It is essential to document neurological prodromes or sequelae that may suggest the aura or postictal state of seizures or focal neurological abnormalities that may point to a nonarrhythmic etiology, including waking with a cut tongue (option A), loss of consciousness with emotional stress (option B), head turning to one side during the loss of consciousness (option C), the presence of abnormal behavior (option E), postictal confusion, and prodromal deja vu. Criteria more in favor of a syncopal episode include any presyncope, loss of consciousness with prolonged standing or sitting, and diaphoresis before a spell (option D).

81-3. The answer is C. (*Hurst's The Heart, 14th Edition, Chap. 81*). Ablation of pathways with a short refractory period (< 250 ms) is recommended (option A).[3] Any patient with Wolff-Parkinson-White (WPW) syndrome (characterized by documented SVT or symptoms consistent with SVT in a patient with ventricular preexcitation during sinus rhythm) should be referred for electrophysiology study and ablation (options B and E). Rapid anterograde accessory pathway conduction during atrial fibrillation can result in sudden cardiac death in patients with a manifest accessory pathway, with a 10-year risk ranging from 0.15% to 0.24% (option D).[4]

81-4. The answer is B. (*Hurst's The Heart, 14th Edition, Chap. 81*) Exercise or isoproterenol will improve Mobitz I or Wenckebach block (option B), but it will worsen (not improve) Mobitz II A block (option A) and complete AV block (option C). Atropine may improve (not worsen) Mobitz II block (option D) and worsen (not improve) Wenckebach block (option E). A diagnosis of Mobitz II or complete heart block typically warrants pacemaker therapy.[5] Patients with newly diagnosed high-grade AV block should also be evaluated for sarcoid, amyloid, and Lyme disease in endemic areas.

81-5. The answer is B. (*Hurst's The Heart, 14th Edition, Chap. 81*) There is increasing general interest in the science and practice of improving risk stratification for ventricular arrhythmias. Indices such as abnormal conduction (signal-averaged ECG [SAECG])(option A), indices of abnormal repolarization (microvolt changes in the T wave) (option C), and measures of unfavorable autonomic balance, specifically heart rate variability (which measures variability in sinus cycle length) (option E) may be used. Reduced heart rate variability < 100 ms is associated with increased mortality.[6] The SAECG detects low-amplitude signals occurring late in the QRS complex that may reflect slow conduction near diseased myocardium, which may predispose to reentry.[7] Transthoracic echo (option D) is used to measure the left-ventricular ejection fraction (LVEF), which may alone be sufficient to proceed with ICD therapy. Head-up tilt table testing (option B) is used in the evaluation of syncope and may be useful in patients with a suspected diagnosis of vasovagal syncope.

81-6. The answer is E (*Hurst's The Heart, 14th Edition, Chap. 81*). T-wave alternans (TWA) is an ECG measure of beat-to-beat oscillations in the T wave and reflects dispersion of repolarization and increased risk for ventricular arrhythmias (option A).[8,9] Subtle oscillations have a high negative predictive value for ventricular arrhythmias (option B). In patients with implantable cardioverter-defibrillator (ICD) indications (ie, left-ventricular ejection fraction [LVEF] < 35%), individuals with a negative TWA have a low (< 5%) risk of sudden cardiac arrest in a 1-year period (option C).[10] Patients with relatively preserved LVEF (35% to 45%) with a positive TWA test may also be at higher risk for ventricular arrhythmias.[10] Signal-averaged ECG (not TWA) predicted ICD therapy in the MUSTT trial (option E).[6]

81-7. **The answer is E.** *(Hurst's The Heart, 14th Edition, Chap. 81)* Implantable loop recorders (ILR) provide long-term outpatient ECG recordings for periods of years, and they are ideal for detecting rare events missed by other modalities (option A). Specifically, the devices store summary trend data, including heart rates, and record events that are patient-triggered but also auto-triggered based on heart rate and other threshold criteria (options B and C). Current ILRs are injected through millimeter-sized incisions, and risks such as infection or bleeding are uncommon.

81-8. **The answer is A.** *(Hurst's The Heart, 14th Edition, Chap. 81)* Battery or motor failure could be seen in earlier analog tape systems, which could slow the tape speed which, when played back, mimicked tachycardia. Present-day recordings do not use analog systems. Patient-related artifacts may result from involuntary muscle contractions, such as the Parkinsonian tremor of 4 to 5 Hz that can be mistaken for atrial flutter (option E), or movements such as brushing teeth that can be confused with ventricular tachycardia (option B).[11] Data recording artifacts are mostly from loose skin-electrode contact (option C), myopotentials, electrical noise, or mechanical stimulation of the electrode.[12] ECG noise can result from various devices as a 60 Hz signal, including digital ECG amplifiers or medical equipment such as infusion pumps and transcutaneous or implanted nerve stimulators.

81-9. **The answer is C.** *(Hurst's The Heart, 14th Edition, Chap. 81)* In patients with vasovagal syncope, this position may lead to venous pooling and loss of consciousness, helping to establish the diagnosis. Tilt table testing is not used to discriminate postural orthostatic tachycardia syndrome (POTS) from inappropriate sinus tachycardia (option A). Holter monitoring is essential to aid in the diagnosis of inappropriate sinus tachycardia, of which the definition is a sinus heart rate > 100 bpm at rest, with a mean 24-h heart rate > 90 bpm not due to appropriate physiological responses or primary causes such as hyperthyroidism or anemia. Tilt table testing, however, may be useful in the evaluation of younger patients with a suspected diagnosis of vasovagal syncope, in the evaluation of postural orthostatic tachycardia syndrome (POTS), and to discriminate between reflex and orthostatic hypotension syncope.[13] It consists of footrest-supported head-up tilting to 60 to 70 degrees (not 85 to 95 degrees) for 30 to 45 minutes (option B).[14] Infusions of isoproterenol or nitroglycerin are used to increase the study sensitivity (not the specificity) at the cost of decreasing specificity (option D). Although an important diagnostic tool, the test has limited specificity, sensitivity, and reproducibility (option E).

81-10. **The answer is C.** *(Hurst's The Heart, 14th Edition, Chap. 81)*. Although CMR is important to guide certain electrophysiologic procedures, including pulmonary vein isolation (atrial fibrillation ablation) (option D), computed tomography (CT) (and not CMR) is specifically more helpful than CMR in localizing the coronary arteries in patients having an epicardial VT ablation (option C). In addition to detailed information about cardiac structure and function, CMR can quantify and localize myocardial scar. For patients with coronary disease, the presence of extensive ventricular scar may indicate increased risk for ventricular arrhythmias (option A).[15] In patients with hypertrophic cardiomyopathy, CMR identification of ventricular scar may help determine eligibility for ICD therapy[16] (option B). CMR may assist in conditions such as arrhythmogenic right ventricular cardiomyopathy (ARVC) (option E).

References

1. Frost L, Vestergaard P. Caffeine and risk of atrial fibrillation or flutter: The Danish Diet, Cancer, and Health Study. *Am J Clin Nutr.* 2005;81:578-582.
2. Sheldon R, Rose S, Ritchie D, et al. Historical criteria that distinguish syncope from seizures. *J Am Coll Cardiol.* 2002;40:142-148.

3. Al-Khatib SM, Arshad A, Balk EM, et al. Risk stratification for arrhythmic events in patients with asymptomatic pre-excitation: A systematic review for the 2015 ACC/AHA/HRS guideline for the management of adult patients with supraventricular tachycardia: a report of the American College of Cardiology/ American Heart Association Task Force on Clinical Practice Guidelines and the Heart Rhythm Society. *J Am Coll Cardiol.* 2016 Apr 5;67(13):1624-1638.

4. Brembilla-Perrot B, Moulin-Zinsch A, Sellal JM, et al. Impact of transesophageal electrophysiologic study to elucidate the mechanism of arrhythmia on children with supraventricular tachycardia and no preexcitation. *Pediatr Cardiol.* 2013;34:1695-1702.

5. Epstein AE, DiMarco JP, Ellenbogen KA, et al. 2012 ACCF/AHA/HRS focused update incorporated into the ACCF/AHA/HRS 2008 guidelines for device-based therapy of cardiac rhythm abnormalities: a report of the American College of Cardiology Foundation/American Heart Association Task Force on Practice Guidelines and the Heart Rhythm Society. *J Am Coll Cardiol.* 2013;61:e6-e75.

6. Goldberger JJ, Basu A, Boineau R, et al. Risk stratification for sudden cardiac death: a plan for the future. *Circulation.* 2014;129:516-526.

7. Narayan SM, Cain ME. The signal-averaged ECG: an overview. *UpToDate Cardiol.* 2015. Epub ahead of print.

8. Narayan SM. T-wave alternans and the susceptibility to ventricular arrhythmias. *J Am Coll Cardiol.* 2006;47:269-281.

9. Narayan SM, Bayer JD, Lalani G, Trayanova NA. Action potential dynamics explain arrhythmic vulnerability in human heart failure: a clinical and modeling study implicating abnormal calcium handling. *J Am Coll Cardiol.* 2008;52:1782-1792.

10. Verrier RL, Klingenheben T, Malik M, et al. Microvolt T-wave alternans physiological basis, methods of measurement, and clinical utility: consensus guideline by International Society for Holter and Noninvasive Electrocardiology. *J Am Coll Cardiol.* 2011;58:1309-1324.

11. Knight BP, Pelosi F, Michaud GF, Strickberger SA, Morady F. Clinical consequences of electrocardiographic artifact mimicking ventricular tachycardia. *N Engl J Med.* 1999;341:1270-1274.

12. Prystowsky EN, Fogel R. Evaluating the patient with arrhythmias. In: Fuster V, Walsh R, Harrington R, eds. *Hurst's The Heart,* 13th ed. New York: McGraw-Hill; 2011:949-962.

13. Sheldon RS, Grubb BP 2nd, Olshansky B, et al. 2015 Heart Rhythm Society expert consensus statement on the diagnosis and treatment of postural tachycardia syndrome, inappropriate sinus tachycardia, and vasovagal syncope. *Heart Rhythm.* 2015;12:e41-e63.

14. Moya A, Sutton R, Ammirati F, et al. Task force for the diagnosis and management of syncope of the European Society of Cardiology, European Heart Rhythm Association, Heart Failure Association, and Heart Rhythm Society. Guidelines for the diagnosis and management of syncope (version 2009). *Eur Heart J.* 2009;30:2631-2671.

15. Kwong RY, Chan AK, Brown KA, et al. Impact of unrecognized myocardial scar detected by cardiac magnetic resonance imaging on event-free survival in patients presenting with signs or symptoms of coronary artery disease. *Circulation.* 2006;113:2733-2743.

16. O'Hanlon R, Grasso A, Roughton M, et al. Prognostic significance of myocardial fibrosis in hypertrophic cardiomyopathy. *J Am Coll Cardiol.* 2010;56:867-874.

CHAPTER 82

Invasive Diagnostic Electrophysiology

Jacqueline Joza

QUESTIONS

DIRECTIONS: Choose the one best response to each question.

82-1. All of the following are reasonable indications for a diagnostic electrophysiology study (EPS) *except*:

A. Evaluation of sinus node function in patients with suspected sick sinus syndrome
B. Delineation of the mechanism of wide-complex tachycardia
C. Evaluation of syncope in an airline pilot
D. Patient with coronary artery disease with a preserved left ventricular ejection fraction and a 5-beat run of non-sustained ventricular tachycardia
E. Wolff-Parkinson-White (WPW) syndrome when pre-excitation persists with exercise on stress testing

82-2. After a complete workup is performed in a 55-year-old woman with syncope, the etiology remains unclear. You decide to send her for an EPS. She wants to know the possible complications of EPS. All of the following are complications of EPS alone, without catheter ablation, *except*:

A. Pneumothorax (0.2%)
B. Cardiac perforation (0.2%)
C. Vascular access complications (0.4%)
D. Thromboembolic events (≈0.5%)
E. Mortality (0.1%)

82-3. During EPS, intracardiac electrograms from various locations in the heart, along with the 12-lead surface electrocardiogram (ECG), are recorded and displayed. Which of the following is *correct* regarding intracardiac electrogram measurements?

A. The AH interval is measured between the atrial and ventricular electrograms on the His catheter
B. The AH interval varies with autonomic tone
C. The HV interval is affected by autonomic tone
D. The normal range of the HV interval is 55 to 75 ms
E. In manifested preexcitation, WPW syndrome, the HV interval is often > 35 ms.

82-4. (See Figure 82-1.) A 55-year-old woman is referred for an EPS after having been diagnosed with a supraventricular tachycardia on ECG. She has recurrent palpitations lasting longer than 30 minutes at a time. What arrhythmia is present in the intracardiac tracing in Figure 82-1?

A. Atrioventricular reentrant tachycardia (AVRT)
B. Atrial tachycardia (AT)
C. Ventricular tachycardia (VT)
D. Wolff–Parkinson–White (WPW)
E. Junctional tachycardia (JT)

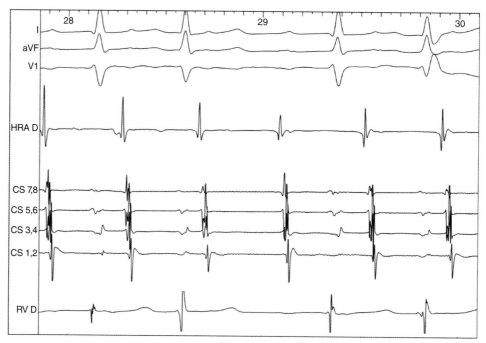

FIGURE 82-1 Intracardiac electrogram (question 82-4).

Abbreviations: surface electrocardiographic leads I, aVF, and V₁ are present; HRA D = high right atrium distal catheter tip; CS = coronary sinus, with CS 1, 2 at the distal coronary sinus; RV D = right ventricle distal catheter tip.

82-5. In which of the following cases does an asymptomatic 55-year-old male patient have an indication for permanent pacing?

A. Type II second-degree AV block that occurs during night-time hours on Holter monitoring and that is present with concomitant sinus rate slowing

B. Resting type I second-degree AV nodal block in a patient taking metoprolol

C. Second-degree AV block at the intra-Hisian level noted on EPS

D. Wide right bundle branch block and left anterior fascicular block

E. Pauses of 3 s during atrial fibrillation

82-6. A 66-year-old woman presents to the emergency department with highly symptomatic palpitations. Her ECG demonstrates cavotricuspid isthmus dependent (typical) atrial flutter. With regard to the mechanism of this tachycardia, which of the following is *incorrect*?

A. The mechanism requires unidirectional block in one pathway

B. The mechanism requires two functionally or anatomically separate pathways

C. The mechanism requires recovery of excitability in the blocked pathway in order to initiate or maintain the tachycardia

D. The mechanism includes triggered activity for its initiation

E. The mechanism is shared among other arrhythmias, including atrioventricular reentrant tachycardia (AVRT)

82-7. A 65-year-old man presents to the emergency department with sudden-onset palpitations that are associated with lightheadedness. While being monitored, the patient has recurrent symptoms, and the rhythm strip reveals a wide-complex tachycardia at 130 bpm. Which of the following is *least* likely to be part of your differential diagnosis?

A. Ventricular pacing

B. Fascicular ventricular tachycardia

C. Atrial tachycardia with aberrancy

D. Antidromic tachycardia (WPW syndrome)

E. Artifact

82-8. All of the following are findings suggestive of an arrhythmic etiology of syncope *except*:

A. Sinus bradycardia at 56 bpm

B. Left bundle branch block

C. Type 1 Brugada pattern

D. Pre-excitation pattern (WPW syndrome)

E. T-wave inversions V₁ through V₄

82-9. An EPS for the induction of ventricular arrhythmias is indicated for a 65-year-old man in all of the following situations *except*:

A. Syncope and a prior myocardial infarction
B. Asymptomatic with coronary artery disease, left ventricular ejection fraction 38%, and nonsustained ventricular tachycardia
C. Wide-complex tachycardia of unclear etiology
D. Recurrent ventricular tachycardia, to guide catheter ablation
E. Asymptomatic with long QT syndrome type 1

82-10. An 80-year-old man presents to the emergency department with a syncopal episode. The ECG recording taken by the EMS reveals a narrow-complex tachycardia at 180 bpm with evidence of an r' in lead V_1. Regarding this arrhythmia, which of the following statements is *incorrect*?

A. Atrioventricular nodal reentrant tachycardia (AVNRT) is a reentry arrhythmia involving the two pathways of the AV node
B. In typical AVNRT, antegrade conduction is via the slow pathway and retrograde conduction is via the fast pathway
C. Dual AV node physiology is demonstrated during an EPS
D. In typical AVNRT, the AV node excites the ventricle and atrium in parallel; hence the VA relationship is 2:1
E. Rarely AVNRT may demonstrate 2:1 AV block resulting from functional infranodal block

ANSWERS

82-1. **The answer is D.** *(Hurst's The Heart, 14th Edition, Chap. 82).* Electrophysiology study may be indicated in patients with coronary artery disease, depressed left ventricular ejection fraction (< 40%), and nonsustained ventricular tachycardia, where the induction of sustained VT or VF is an indication for an implantable cardioverted defibrillator (ICD). Evaluation of sinus node function in patients with suspected sick sinus syndrome is an indication for testing. A diseased sinus node is suggested by the presence of a prolonged sinus node recovery time (SNRT) > 1500 ms and inappropriate sinus bradycardia (option A). EPS is indicated for the evaluation of tachyarrhythmias, including the delineation of narrow- and wide-complex tachycardias, for diagnosis and/or for tachycardia mechanism prior to ablation (option B). EPS may be performed for the evaluation of syncope, including evaluation in high-risk occupations (airline pilots, bus drivers, etc.) (option C) as well as for syncope of unclear etiology and in patients with structural heart disease. Risk stratification for WPW syndrome may be performed when pre-excitation persists with exercise on stress testing (option E).

82-2. **The answer is A.** *(Hurst's The Heart, 14th Edition, Chap. 82).* Pneumothorax is not a complication of an EPS. Options B through E represent possible complications and their present-day rates of occurrence. Thrombophlebitis (0.6%) is an additional potential complication. Patients should not be exposed even to this minimal risk if there is no benefit expected from EPS.

82-3. **The answer is B.** *(Hurst's The Heart, 14th Edition, Chap. 82).* The AH interval is measured between the atrial and His (not ventricular) electrograms on the His catheter and corresponds to conduction time from the low interatrial septum to the His, which is an indirect measure of the AV node conduction (option A). The AH interval does vary with autonomic tone: increased vagal tone would increase the AH interval, whereas increased sympathetic or decreased vagal tone would shorten it (option B).[1,2] The normal AH interval during sinus rhythm is approximately 55 to 130 ms.[3] The HV interval is not affected by autonomic tone (option C), and the normal range is 35 to 55 ms (option D).[3] In manifested preexcitation, WPW syndrome, the HV interval is often < 35 ms.

82-4. **The answer is B.** *(Hurst's The Heart, 14th Edition, Chap. 82).* Atrial tachycardia is seen in this tracing of a patient undergoing EPS for supraventricular tachycardia. The intracardiac electrograms demonstrate that there are more atrial electrograms than ventricular electrograms, which is consistent here with a diagnosis of atrial tachycardia. In atrioventricular reentrant tachycardia (AVRT) or orthodromic reciprocating tachycardia, the ventricular-to-atrial (VA) relationship is 1:1 with a long VA time (VA > 70 ms) (option A). Pacing maneuvers are required to differentiate AVRT from atypical AVNRT and atrial tachycardia. This is not ventricular tachycardia (option C) because there are not more ventricular electrograms than atrial electrograms. This is not WPW because there is no preexcitation present on the surface leads, the QRS is narrow (except for the fourth QRS complex, which is of RBBB morphology), and an arrhythmia using a concealed retrograde accessory pathway (such as AVRT) is not present (option D). Junctional tachycardia would have simultaneous ventricular and atrial electrograms, for which maneuvers would need to be performed to distinguish it from typical atrioventricular nodal reentry tachycardia (AVNRT) (option E).

82-5. **The answer is C.** *(Hurst's The Heart, 14th Edition, Chap. 82).* A second-degree AV block at the intra- or infra-Hisian level, which is most commonly associated with type II block, is pathological and indicates a need for permanent pacing. Rarely, type II second-degree AV block can occur in the AV node during periods of high vagal tone and is seen with concomitant sinus rate slowing, which confirms that the mechanism of block is caused by increased vagal tone (option A). Resting type I second-degree AV block can be seen with high vagal tone in young athletes and with medications such as beta-blockers, calcium channel blockers, and digoxin (option B).[4] A right bundle branch block and left anterior fascicular block alone are not enough to warrant permanent pacing (option D). During atrial fibrillation, pauses > 5 s (not 3 s) are suggestive of high-degree AV block (option E).

82-6. **The answer is D.** *(Hurst's The Heart, 14th Edition, Chap. 82).* The mechanism of all tachyarrhythmias is either macro-reentry or focal. Macro-reentrant arrhythmias are most common. Focal arrhythmias may be caused by automaticity, microreentry, or triggered activity (option D).[5] Cavotricuspid isthmus dependent (typical) atrial flutter is a macro-reentrant tachycardia that shares its mechanism with atrioventricular reentrant tachycardia (option E). Reentry requires (1) two functionally or anatomically separate pathways (option A), (2) unidirectional block in one pathway (option B), and (3) recovery of excitability in the blocked pathway to initiate or maintain reentry (option C).[6]

82-7. **The answer is B.** *(Hurst's The Heart, 14th Edition, Chap. 82).* Fascicular ventricular tachycardia (VT) is typically a VT of *narrow* complex that originates from one of the fascicles. Ventricular pacing (option A), supraventricular tachycardias with aberrancy (option C), antidromic tachycardia associated with WPW syndrome (option D), artifact (option E), and scar-mediated ventricular tachycardia or bundle-branch reentry tachycardia are all important diagnostic considerations when a wide-complex tachycardia is present.

82-8. **The answer is A.** *(Hurst's The Heart, 14th Edition, Chap. 82).* Sinus bradycardia alone does not necessarily suggest an arrhythmic etiology for syncope. *Severe* sinus bradycardia may be suggestive of the cause for syncope, however, or if the sinus bradycardia is clearly correlated with symptoms. Bundle branch block (in particular left bundle branch or bifascicular block) (option B), type 1 Brugada ECG pattern (option C), pre-excitation pattern (option D), and T-wave inversions V_1 through V_4 (suggestive of ischemia versus arrhythmogenic right ventricular cardiomyopathy) (option E) are other findings suggestive of an arrhythmic etiology of syncope.

82-9. **The answer is E.** *(Hurst's The Heart, 14th Edition, Chap. 82).* There is no role for EPS specifically as it relates to long QT syndrome. Options A through D are all indications for EPS.

82-10. **The answer is D.** *(Hurst's The Heart, 14th Edition, Chap. 82).* In typical AVNRT, the AV node excites the ventricle and atrium in parallel; hence the VA relationship is 1:1 (not 2:1) and often simultaneous (VA time ≤ 60 ms). Atrioventricular nodal reentrant tachycardia (AVNRT) is a reentry arrhythmia involving the two pathways of the AV node (option A). In typical AVNRT, antegrade conduction is via the slow pathway and retrograde conduction is via the fast pathway (option B). During EPS, atrial pacing demonstrates evidence of dual AV node pathways (option C). Rarely, AVNRT may demonstrate 2:1 AV block resulting from functional infranodal block.[7]

References

1. Seides SF, Josephson ME, Batsford WP, Weisfogel GM, Lau SH, Damato AN. The electrophysiology of propranolol in man. *Am Heart J.* 1974;88:733-741.
2. Cannom DS, Rider AK, Stinson EB, Harrison DC. Electrophysiologic studies in the denervated transplanted human heart. II. Response to norepinephrine, isoproterenol and propranolol. *Am J Cardiol.* 1975;36:859-866.
3. Dhingra RC, Rosen KM, Rahimtoola SH. Normal conduction intervals and responses in sixty-one patients using His bundle recording and atrial pacing. *Chest.* 1973;64:55-59.
4. Corino VD, Sandberg F, Platonov PG, et al. Non-invasive evaluation of the effect of metoprolol on the atrioventricular node during permanent atrial fibrillation. *Europace.* 2014;16 suppl 4:iv129-iv134. doi: 10.1093/europace/euu246.

5. Del Carpio Munoz F, Buescher TL, Asirvatham SJ. Teaching points with 3-dimensional mapping of cardiac arrhythmia: how to overcome potential pitfalls during substrate mapping? *Circ Arrhythm Electrophysiol.* 2011;4:e72-e75.

6. Tse G. Mechanisms of cardiac arrhythmias. *J Arrhythm.* 2016;32:75-71.

7. Man KC, Brinkman K, Bogun F, et al. 2:1 Atrioventricular block during atrioventricular node reentrant tachycardia. *J Am Coll Cardiol.* 1996;28:1770-1774.

CHAPTER 83

Atrial Fibrillation, Atrial Flutter, and Atrial Tachycardia

Jacqueline Joza

QUESTIONS

DIRECTIONS: Choose the one best response to each question.

83-1. A 60-year-old man presents to you in consult after his second episode of atrial fibrillation (AF) in 2 years. Regarding the classification of AF, which is *incorrect*?

A. Paroxysmal AF is characterized by self-terminating episodes that generally last < 7 days
B. AF that lasts > 7 days is generally termed *persistent*
C. Long-standing AF may be diagnosed when AF has been continuous for at least 1 year
D. Permanent AF is diagnosed once a patient has failed cardioversion or when further attempts to terminate AF is deemed futile
E. AF may be labeled *chronic* when a diagnosis of AF has been present for at least 5 years

83-2. The mechanism of AF may be multifactorial. Which one of the following statements regarding the pathophysiology of AF is *correct*?

A. Rapidly firing ectopic foci in the pulmonary arteries have been shown to be the underlying mechanism of most paroxysmal AF
B. The pulmonary vein musculature of patients with paroxysmal AF may demonstrate an *increased* effective refractory period and conduction delay
C. In patients with paroxysmal AF, most triggering foci that are mapped during electrophysiologic study occur within the inferior vena cava, the right atrial appendage, and the anterior interventricular vein

D. Rotors or spiral wave reentry has shown importance as a perpetuating mechanism for AF
E. The greater the amount of atrial fibrosis, the more likely is the success of catheter ablation using standard ablation approaches

83-3. Regarding the hemodynamic effects of AF on the heart, which of the following statements is *false*?

A. The LV end-diastolic pressure decreases
B. There is a loss of mechanical AV synchrony
C. There is a paradoxical increase in the LV contractility
D. The stroke volume is reduced
E. There is an increase in the left atrial mean diastolic pressure

83-4. A 50-year-old man was admitted to the CCU with an NSTEMI. A coronary angiogram revealed an 80% lesion in the left anterior descending artery, for which a drug-eluting stent was placed. A transthoracic echo revealed an LVEF of 50% to 55% without significant valvular disease. On auscultation, the patient's lungs are clear, and there is no S3. Forty-eight hours after percutaneous coronary intervention, the patient develops AF. Which antiarrhythmic medication would be *contraindicated* as a rhythm-control agent?

A. Amiodarone
B. Dofetilide
C. Dronedarone
D. Propafenone
E. Sotalol

83-5. Which of the following statements regarding oral anticoagulation is *correct* for a 75-year-old woman with hypertension and AF?

A. She should only continue lifelong oral anticoagulation if she develops persistent or permanent AF

B. Her CHA$_2$DS$_2$-VASc score is 3

C. Her transthoracic echocardiogram reveals mitral stenosis, and as such, oral anticoagulation with a novel oral anticoagulant (NOAC) is indicated

D. Oral anticoagulation is specifically recommended for patients with a prior stroke, TIA, or CHA$_2$DS$_2$-VASc score of 3 or more

E. Meta-analysis of studies comparing aspirin with placebo suggests a relative risk reduction in stroke of approximately 22% with aspirin.

83-6. You are counseling a patient prior to initiating an NOAC. Which one of the following answers is *incorrect*?

A. Dabigatran is a direct competitive inhibitor of thrombin

B. Rivaroxaban inhibits coagulation factor X

C. NOACs have not been proven safe and effective in patients with AF and rheumatic mitral stenosis

D. Edoxaban inhibits coagulation factor IIa

E. NOACs have not been proven safe to use in patients with a mechanical valve

83-7. You decide to start a 50-year-old man on an anti-arrhythmic medication for his AF. Which one of the following statements is *incorrect*?

A. Class Ic drugs should be combined with a beta-blocker or calcium channel blocker to decrease the risk of atrial flutter with a 1:1 ventricular response

B. Monitoring the QRS duration and the PR interval is important during class Ic therapy

C. Sotalol prolongs the ventricular refractoriness and the QT interval

D. Efforts to avoid hypokalemia and hypomagnesemia are important in patients receiving antiarrhythmic drugs

E. Class III drugs should be combined with a beta-blocker or calcium channel blocker to decrease the risk of QT prolongation

83-8. Which of the following is *not* a reasonable oral anticoagulation strategy surrounding cardioversion?

A. Oral warfarin with a therapeutic INR for 3 to 4 weeks before cardioversion, followed by continued warfarin therapy for a minimum of 4 weeks

B. Oral anticoagulation is unnecessary if the transesophageal echo is negative for intracardiac clot, and the patient is cardioverted with ibutilide

C. NOAC for 3 weeks before cardioversion followed by a NOAC for a minimum of 4 weeks

D. In patients without high risk factors for stroke, anticoagulation can be discontinued approximately 4 weeks after cardioversion

E. Transesophageal echocardiography (TEE) and intravenous heparin immediately before cardioversion followed by oral warfarin for a minimum of 4 weeks

83-9. You decide to start your patient on dronedarone after electrical cardioversion. Which of the following statements is *incorrect*?

A. Dronedarone is a noniodinated benzofuran derivative of amiodarone

B. Dronedarone blocks multiple channels, including sodium, potassium, and calcium

C. Dronedarone is indicated in patients with permanent AF

D. Dronedarone has noncompetitive antiadrenergic effects

E. Dronedarone is contraindicated in patients with class II to IV heart failure

83-10. Your patient, an 84-year-old woman with a normal LV ejection fraction and dual-chamber pacemaker, continues to have significant palpitations from her AF, despite drug therapy. You decide to refer her for an AV node ablation. Which of the following statements is *incorrect*?

A. Rhythm control with antiarrhythmic medications is more successful after AV node ablation

B. AV node ablation does not change the long-term need for anticoagulation

C. Patients may become pacemaker dependent after AV node ablation as a result of an inadequate escape rhythm

D. Right ventricular pacing produces an abnormal LV contraction sequence, and acute worsening of hemodynamics has been observed in some patients

E. The development of right ventricular pacing-induced cardiomyopathy can occur

83-1. The answer is E. (*Hurst's The Heart, 14th Edition, Chap. 83*). Atrial fibrillation is classified into four categories: *paroxysmal*, *persistent*, *long-standing persistent*, and *permanent*.[1] The definition of *chronic* AF (option E) varies greatly in the literature, and the term is best avoided. Paroxysmal AF is characterized by self-terminating episodes that generally last < 7 days (most < 24 hours) (option A), whereas persistent AF generally lasts > 7 days (option B) and often requires electrical or pharmacologic cardioversion. Long-standing AF has been continuous for at least a year (option C). Many patients have both paroxysmal and persistent episodes of AF, and in general, we characterize such patients by their more typical form of AF. AF is classified as permanent when a patient has failed cardioversion or when further attempts to terminate the arrhythmia are deemed futile (option D).

83-2. The answer is D. (*Hurst's The Heart, 14th Edition, Chap. 83*) A variety of electrophysiologic and structural factors promote the perpetuation of AF. Recently, rotors or spiral wave reentry has shown importance as a perpetuating mechanism for AF in humans.[2-6] Ablation of these rotors can lead to the termination of AF in some patients. Spontaneous ectopy from the muscular sleeves of pulmonary veins can serve as triggers of AF. Rapidly firing ectopic foci in *pulmonary veins* have been shown to be the underlying mechanism of most paroxysmal AF[7,8] (option A). The pulmonary vein musculature of patients with paroxysmal AF demonstrates a markedly *reduced* effective refractory period and conduction delay (option B).[9] Although most triggering foci that are mapped during electrophysiologic studies occur in the pulmonary veins in patients with paroxysmal AF, foci within the superior vena cava,[10] the ligament of Marshall,[11] and the musculature of the coronary sinus[12] have been identified (option C). AF itself seems to produce a variety of alterations of atrial architecture that further contribute to atrial remodeling, mechanical dysfunction, and perpetuation of fibrillation, a concept of AF begetting more AF. Of note, recent data suggest the greater the atrial fibrosis, the less likely is the success of catheter ablation using standard ablation approaches[13] (option E).

83-3. The answer is C. (*Hurst's The Heart, 14th Edition, Chap. 83*) LV contractility is reduced in AF. Atrial fibrillation produces several adverse hemodynamic effects, including loss of atrial contraction, a rapid ventricular rate, and an irregular ventricular rhythm. The loss of mechanical AV synchrony (option B) may have a dramatic impact on ventricular filling and cardiac output when there is reduced ventricular compliance, as with LV hypertrophy from hypertension, restrictive cardiomyopathy, hypertrophic cardiomyopathy, or the increased ventricular stiffness associated with aging. The loss of AV synchrony results in a decrease in LV end-diastolic pressure (LVEDP) (option A) as the loading effect of atrial contraction is lost, thereby reducing stroke volume (option D) and LV contractility (option C) by the Frank-Starling mechanism. Although there is a reduction in the LVEDP, there is an increase in the left atrial mean diastolic pressure (option E).

83-4. The answer is D. (*Hurst's The Heart, 14th Edition, Chap. 83*) Class Ic medications, including propafenone and flecainide, are contraindicated in the setting of coronary artery disease. In this patient, with the presence of structural heart disease from coronary artery disease, without heart failure present, initial pharmacological therapy for a rhythm control strategy includes dofetilide (option B), dronedarone (option C), and sotalol (option E). Alternative pharmacological options include amiodarone (option A).

83-5. The answer is E. (*Hurst's The Heart, 14th Edition, Chap. 83*). True: the relative risk reduction of aspirin as compared to placebo is approximately 22%. The 2012 ESC guidelines and 2014 ACC/AHA/HRS guidelines recommend the use of the CHA_2DS_2-VASc risk score, which recognizes that stroke risk in patients with AF is related to age as a continuous variable, acknowledges the higher, albeit unequal, risk of stroke faced by women, and incorporates the less validated risk associated with vascular disease, prior MI, complex aortic plaque, and peripheral arterial disease, although these may contribute unequally. Oral anticoagulants are recommended for patients with a prior stroke, TIA, or CHA_2DS_2-VASc score of 2 or more (option D); either oral anticoagulants, aspirin, or no antithrombotic therapy can be considered for a CHA_2DS_2-VASc of 1; and antithrombotic therapy may be omitted for a CHA_2DS_2-VASc score of 0.[1] There is no difference in the indications for antithrombotic therapy between paroxysmal, persistent, and permanent AF (option A). The patient's CHA_2DS_2-VASc score is 4 (1 point for female sex, 2 points for age ≥ 75, and 1 point for hypertension) (option B). Mitral stenosis is well known to be associated with a high risk for stroke in AF patients, and *warfarin* (not NOAC) anticoagulation is indicated in all such patients (option C).

83-6. **The answer is D.** *(Hurst's The Heart, 14th Edition, Chap. 83).* Rivaroxaban (option B), apixaban, and edoxaban (option D) inhibit coagulation factor Xa, whereas dabigatran (option A) is a direct competitive inhibitor of thrombin (coagulation factor IIa). NOACs have been shown to be noninferior or of superior efficacy against all stroke (ischemic plus hemorrhagic) and systemic embolism with rates of major bleeding comparable to or lower than warfarin. Considered collectively, the NOACs have been associated with significantly lower risks of intracerebral hemorrhage than even well-adjusted warfarin in the trials leading to their approval for clinical use, generally better outcomes even in cases when major bleeding occurred, and lower rates of all-cause mortality when used for thromboembolism prevention in patients with nonvalvular AF. These agents have not been proven safe or effective in patients with AF associated with rheumatic mitral stenosis (option C) or mechanical heart valves (option E), and experience in patients with AF who have undergone bioprosthetic heart valve replacement or valve repair is limited.

83-7. **The answer is E.** *(Hurst's The Heart, 14th Edition, Chap. 83)* Many agents are effective for maintaining sinus rhythm in patients with AF.[1] Because class Ic drugs may suppress AF but promote atrial flutter, they are combined with a beta-blocker or calcium channel blocker to decrease the risk of atrial flutter with 1:1 ventricular response, a potentially life-threatening situation (option A). Monitoring the QRS duration and PR interval is important during class Ic therapy (option B). Sotalol, dofetilide, and amiodarone prolong ventricular refractoriness and the QT interval (option C). Monitoring the QT interval during the initiation of therapy is important. If possible, avoid corrected QT intervals of > 500 to 520 ms with sotalol and dofetilide, but longer QT intervals may occur without a risk of proarrhythmia in patients receiving amiodarone. Periodic ECGs should be obtained on an outpatient basis in patients receiving antiarrhythmic drugs, and efforts to avoid hypokalemia and hypomagnesemia are important (option D).

83-8. **The answer is B.** *(Hurst's The Heart, 14th Edition, Chap. 83)* Oral anticoagulation management is identical for both chemical and electrical cardioversion. There are two basic anticoagulation strategies before cardioversion: (1) oral warfarin with a therapeutic INR (2-3) for 3 to 4 weeks before cardioversion followed by continued warfarin therapy for a minimum of 4 weeks (option A), or (2) TEE and intravenous heparin immediately before cardioversion followed by oral warfarin thereafter (option E).[14] The recent AHA/ACC/HRS guidelines suggest the use of a NOAC for 3 weeks before cardioversion is reasonable,[1] but there are few prospective data supporting this. The left atrial mechanical function may be significantly impaired for up to several weeks after cardioversion from AF to sinus rhythm. This *stunning* effect on the atria may occur after either electrical or pharmacologic cardioversion[15-17] and is more marked with a longer duration of AF. In patients without high risk factors for stroke, anticoagulation can be discontinued approximately 4 weeks after cardioversion (option D). If the patient has a standard indication for warfarin before cardioversion, anticoagulation should be continued indefinitely after cardioversion unless a clear reversible cause of AF has been corrected.

83-9. **The answer is C.** *(Hurst's The Heart, 14th Edition, Chap. 83)* Dronedarone is the most recent oral antiarrhythmic drug approved for the treatment of patients with AF and atrial flutter.[18] It is a noniodinated benzofuran derivative of amiodarone (option A).[19] Like amiodarone, it blocks multiple channels (option B), including sodium, potassium, and calcium, and has noncompetitive antiadrenergic effects (option D). Compared with placebo in two randomized controlled trials, dronedarone prolonged the median times to recurrence of arrhythmia.[20] In a multicenter randomized controlled trial of > 4600 patients, dronedarone reduced the incidence of hospitalization from cardiovascular events or death in patients who had AF.[21] A follow-up study, PALLAS, failed to demonstrate a benefit on a similar end point when dronedarone was administered to patients with heart disease and permanent AF. Based on this study and ANDROMEDA, which enrolled recently hospitalized patients with heart failure,[22] dronedarone is contraindicated in patients with permanent AF (option C), those with class II to IV heart failure (option E), and those with recent decompensation requiring hospitalization or referral to a specialized heart failure clinic.

83-10. **The answer is A.** (Hurst's The Heart, 14th Edition, Chap. 83) Catheter ablation of the AV conduction system and permanent pacemaker implantation is a highly effective means of establishing permanent rate control (not rhythm control) during AF in selected patients.[22-24] Despite the many favorable effects of this procedure, there are several limitations. First, AV nodal ablation does not change the long-term need for anticoagulation (option B). Second, although an adequate junctional escape rhythm may be present after ablation, patients may become pacemaker dependent as a result of an inadequate escape rhythm (option C). Third, right ventricular pacing produces an abnormal LV contraction sequence, and acute worsening of hemodynamics has been observed in some patients (option D). The development of a right-ventricular pacing-induced cardiomyopathy can occur (option E). In the post AV node ablation evaluation (PAVE) trial, patients who received biventricular versus right ventricular apical pacing, especially those with abnormal LV ejection fractions before ablation, had longer 6-minute walking distances and higher LV ejection fractions after ablation.[25]

References

1. January CT, Wann L S, Alpert JS, et al. 2014 AHA/ACC/HRS Guideline for the management of patients with atrial fibrillation: a report of the American College of Cardiology/American Heart Association Task Force on Practice Guidelines and the Heart Rhythm Society. Circulation. 2014; online ISSN:1524-1539.

2. Prystowsky EN, Padanilam BJ, Fogel RI. Treatment of atrial fibrillation. JAMA. 2015;314(3):278-288.

3. Davidenko JM, Pertsov AV, Salomonsz R, et al. Stationary and drifting spiral waves of excitation in isolated cardiac muscle. Nature. 1992;355:349-351.

4. Nishida K, Datino T, Macle L, Nattel S. The present and future state-of-the-art review, atrial fibrillation ablation: translating basic mechanistic insights to the patient. J Am Coll Cardiol. 2014;64:823-831.

5. Narayan SM, Krummen DE, Rappel WJ. Clinical mapping approach to diagnose electrical rotors and focal impulse sources for human atrial fibrillation. J Cardiovasc Electrophysiol. 2012;23:447-454.

6. Narayan SM, Krummen DE, Shivkuman K, et al. Treatment of atrial fibrillation by the ablation of localized sources: CONFIRM (Conventional Ablation for Atrial Fibrillation With or Without Focal Impulse and Rotor Modulation) trial. J Am Coll Cardiol. 2012;60:628-636.

7. Haissaguerre M, Jais P, Shah DC, et al. Spontaneous initiation of atrial fibrillation by ectopic beats originating in the pulmonary veins. N Engl J Med. 1998;339:659-666.

8. Chen SA, Hsieh MH, Tai CT, et al. Initiation of atrial fibrillation by ectopic beats originating from the pulmonary veins: electrophysiologic characteristics, pharmacologic responses and effects of radiofrequency ablation. Circulation. 1999;100:1879-1886.

9. Tse HF, Lau CP, Kou W, et al. Prevalence and significance of exit block during arrhythmias arising in pulmonary veins. J Cardiovasc Electrophysiol. 2000;11:379-386.

10. Tsai CF, Tai CT, Hsieh MH, et al. Initiation of atrial fibrillation by ectopic beats originating from the superior vena cava: Electrophysiological characteristics and results of radiofrequency ablation. Circulation. 2000;102:67-74.

11. Doshi RN, Wu TJ, Yashima M, et al. Relation between ligament of Marshall and adrenergic atrial tachyarrhythmia. Circulation. 1999;100:876-883.

12. Chen PS, Chou CC. Coronary sinus as an arrhythmogenic structure. J Cardiovasc Electrophysiol. 2002;13:863-864.

13. Marrouche NF, Wilber D, Hindricks G, et al. Association of atrial tissue fibrosis identified by delayed enhancement MRI and atrial fibrillation catheter ablation: the DECAAF study. JAMA. 2014;311(5): 498-506.

14. Klein EA. Assessment of cardioversion using transesophageal echocardiography (TEE) multicenter study (ACUTE I): clinical outcomes at eight weeks. *J Am Coll Cardiol.* 2000;36:324.

15. Antonielli E, Pizzuti A, Bassignana A, et al. Transesophageal echocardiographic evidence of more pronounced left atrial stunning after chemical (propafenone) rather than electrical attempts at cardioversion from atrial fibrillation. *Am J Cardiol.* 1999;84:1092-1110.

16. Bellotti P, Spirito P, Lupi G, Vecchio C. Left atrial appendage function assessed by transesophageal echocardiography before and on the day after elective cardioversion for nonvalvular atrial fibrillation. *Am J Cardiol.* 1998;81:1199-1202.

17. Mitusch R, Garbe M, Schmucker G, et al. Relation of left atrial appendage function to the duration and reversibility of nonvalvular atrial fibrillation. *Am J Cardiol.* 1995;75:944-947.

18. Connolly SJ, Camm AJ, Halperin JL, et al. Dronedarone in high-risk permanent atrial fibrillation. *N Engl J Med.* 2011;365:2268-2276. doi: 10.1056/NEJMoa1109867.

19. Laughlin JC, Kowey PR. Dronedarone: a new treatment for atrial fibrillation. *J Cardiovasc Electrophysiol.* 2008;19:1220-1226.

20. Singh BN, Connolly SJ, Crijns HJ, et al. Dronedarone for maintenance of sinus rhythm in atrial fibrillation or flutter. *N Engl J Med.* 2007;357:987-999.

21. Hohnloser SH, Crijns HJ, van Eickels M, et al; for the ATHENA Investigators. Effect of dronedarone on cardiovascular events in atrial fibrillation. *N Engl J Med.* 2009;360:668-678.

22. Marshall HJ, Harris ZI, Griffith MJ, et al. Prospective randomized study of ablation and pacing versus medical therapy for paroxysmal atrial fibrillation: effects of pacing mode and mode-switch algorithm. *Circulation.* 1999;99:1587-1592.

23. Kay GN, Ellenbogen KA, Giudici M, et al. The Ablate and Pace Trial: a prospective study of catheter ablation of the AV conduction system and permanent pacemaker implantation for treatment of atrial fibrillation: APT Investigators. *J Interv Card Electrophysiol.* 1998;2:121-135.

24. Brignole M, Gianfranchi L, Menozzi C, et al. Assessment of atrioventricular junction ablation and DDDR mode-switching pacemaker versus pharmacological treatment in patients with severely symptomatic paroxysmal atrial fibrillation: a randomized controlled study. *Circulation.* 1997;96:2617-2624.

25. Doshi RN, Daoud EG, Fellows C, et al. Left ventricular-based cardiac stimulation post AV nodal ablation evaluation (the PAVE study). *J Cardiovasc Electrophysiol.* 2005;16:1160-1165.

CHAPTER 84

Supraventricular Tachycardia: Atrial Tachycardia, Atrioventricular Nodal Reentry, and Wolff–Parkinson–White Syndrome

Jacqueline Joza

QUESTIONS

DIRECTIONS: Choose the one best response to each question.

84-1. You are called by the anesthesiologist to see a 75-year-old woman who is post-op a left hip replacement. Intra-operative monitoring revealed a sudden-onset narrow QRS tachycardia, which abruptly terminated after several minutes. All of the following statements are correct regarding atrioventricular nodal reentrant tachycardia (AVNRT) *except*:

A. AVNRT occurs in approximately 10% of the general population
B. AVNRT accounts for up to two-thirds of all cases of paroxysmal supraventricular tachycardia (PSVT)
C. The usual age of onset is beyond the fourth decade of life
D. Men are twice as commonly affected as women
E. AVNRT can result in significant debility and decreased quality of life

84-2. Regarding AVNRT, which of the following statements is *correct*?

A. Five types of AVNRT have been described
B. The most prevalent type of AVNRT is called "typical" or "slow/fast" AVNRT
C. Atypical AVNRT may be differentiated into fast/slow, slow/slow, and fast/fast AVNRT
D. Only typical or atypical AVNRT may be induced in any one patient
E. Autopsy studies have reported that the site of successful slow pathway ablation is approximately 5 cm superior to the compact AV node

84-3. You are shown an ECG of a narrow-complex tachycardia by the emergency room physician. After the administration of one dose of 6 mg IV of adenosine, the tachycardia persists at a rate of 140 bpm. The ECG reveals a long-RP tachycardia. The differential diagnosis of this rhythm includes all of the following *except*:

A. Atypical AVNRT
B. Sinus tachycardia
C. Atrioventricular reciprocating tachycardia (AVRT) with a slowly conducting pathway
D. Typical AVNRT
E. Atrial tachycardia

84-4. The electrocardiographic characteristics of AVNRT are unique. Which of the following statements is *incorrect*?

A. Regular ventricular rates of 120 to 200 bpm are typically seen, but the rate may exceed 200 bpm
B. In typical AVNRT, the P wave is usually obscured by the QRS or may be seen slightly before or after the QRS complex
C. ST-segment depressions observed during tachycardia are predictive of ischemia
D. Functional bundle branch block (BBB) may develop during AVNRT, producing a wide QRS tachycardia, but the BBB should not affect the rate of the tachycardia
E. QRS alternans is observed more often in association with accessory pathway-mediated tachycardias than during AVNRT

84-5. A 65-year-old man is taken by ambulance to the emergency department. His ECG reveals a narrow-complex tachycardia with a short RP interval. Which of the following is *not* an AHA/ACC/HRS class I recommendation for the acute treatment of AVNRT?

A. Intravenous beta-blockers, diltiazem, or verapamil
B. Adenosine
C. Synchronized cardioversion in hemodynamically *stable* AVNRT when pharmacologic therapy does not terminate the tachycardia or is contraindicated
D. Synchronized cardioversion if hemodynamically *unstable* AVNRT when initial measures do not terminate the tachycardia or are not feasible
E. Vagal maneuvers

84-6. A 25-year-old man is referred to your clinic after an episode of palpitations. His baseline ECG reveals sinus rhythm with pre-excitation. All of the following are features of accessory pathways (AP) *except*:

A. Patients with tetralogy of Fallot who also have WPW syndrome often have more than one AP
B. APs capable of antegrade conduction are referred to as *manifest*
C. Most antegrade-conducting APs exhibit rapid, non-decremental conduction
D. APs are present in 0.15% to 0.25% of the general population
E. There is a higher prevalence of APs in first-degree relatives of patients with WPW syndrome

84-7. A 40-year-old man is referred to you after a routine ECG reveals pre-excitation. The patient describes a recent episode of irregular, rapid palpitations lasting several minutes that occurred after a workout at the gym. Which of the following statements is *correct*?

A. If an accessory pathway (AP) has a very long antegrade refractory period, atrial fibrillation may result in a rapid ventricular response with subsequent degeneration to ventricular fibrillation
B. The risk of sudden death has been shown to be higher if the shortest R-R interval during atrial fibrillation is < 450 ms
C. 50% of patients with WPW syndrome also have atrial fibrillation
D. The incidence of sudden cardiac death from WPW syndrome has been estimated at 3.5% to 5%
E. In the context of atrial fibrillation and the presence of an accessory pathway, surgical or catheter ablation of accessory pathways can result in the elimination of atrial fibrillation as well

84-8. A 20-year-old woman presents to you in follow-up concerning her intermittent palpitations. Her baseline ECG reveals pre-excitation. Her past medical history is significant for a structurally abnormal heart diagnosed by echocardiogram that has been present since birth. Which congenital abnormality does this patient most likely have?

A. Tetralogy of Fallot
B. Arrhythmogenic right ventricular dysplasia
C. Bicuspid aortic valve
D. Corrected transposition of the great vessels
E. Pulmonary atresia

84-9. A 45-year-old woman presents to the emergency department with sudden-onset rapid palpitations that have been sustained for the last two hours. You are shown two of her ECGs taken several minutes apart. The first reveals a narrow-complex tachycardia at 170 bpm and the second reveals a wide-complex tachycardia (LBBB morphology) at 140 bpm. Which of the following is the most likely diagnosis?

A. Atrioventricular reentrant tachycardia (AVRT) involving a right-sided pathway
B. AVRT involving a left-sided pathway
C. AVNRT
D. Atrial tachycardia
E. Ventricular tachycardia

84-10. Routine screening of a 28-year-old pilot reveals the presence of pre-excitation. Concerning the management of asymptomatic pre-excitation in this patient, which of the following is most *correct*?

A. The ACC/AHA/HRS Guidelines for the Management of Patients with Supraventricular Arrhythmias gives electrophysiologic testing and catheter ablation a class III classification for the treatment of patients with asymptomatic pre-excitation
B. Catheter ablation is strongly suggested in patients < 25 years old
C. The loss of pre-excitation after the administration of procainamide or ajmaline is the gold standard for diagnosing a low-risk accessory pathway
D. Catheter ablation of the accessory pathway is reasonable in asymptomatic patients if the presence of pre-excitation precludes specific employment
E. An electrophysiologic study in risk stratification of the accessory pathway has not been shown to add any further information

84-1. The answer is D. *(Hurst's The Heart, 14th Edition, Chap. 84)* Women are affected twice as often as men. Atrioventricular nodal reentrant tachycardia (AVNRT) is an important arrhythmia for several reasons. First, AVNRT is extremely common and occurs in approximately 10% of the general population (option A); it accounts for up to two-thirds of all cases of PSVT (option B). Although AVNRT can occur at any age, it is extremely uncommon before age 5. The usual age of onset is beyond the fourth decade of life and is later than the usual age of onset of accessory pathway-mediated tachycardias (option C). A second reason for the importance of AVNRT is the fact that it can result in significant debility and decreased quality of life (option E).

84-2. The answer is B. *(Hurst's The Heart, 14th Edition, Chap. 84)* Three types of AVNRT have been described (option B) (Figure 84-1).[1] Typical or slow/fast AVNRT is the most prevalent type, accounting for 85% to 90% of cases (option B). Representing the other 10% to 15% of cases, atypical AVNRT can be further differentiated into fast/slow and slow/slow (or intermediate) AVNRT (option C). Induction of typical and atypical AVNRT in the same patient is possible but unusual (option D). The typical or slow/fast AVNRT is thought to use the slow pathway for antegrade conduction and the fast pathway for retrograde conduction. When an atrial premature complex blocks the fast pathway and proceeds slowly along the slow pathway, the fast pathway has enough time to recover from its refractoriness. This allows the impulse to activate the fast pathway retrogradely and return to the atrium, giving rise to an AV nodal reentrant echo beat. The impulse then travels down along the

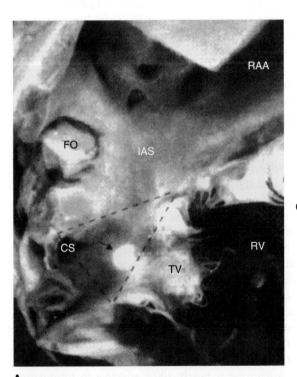

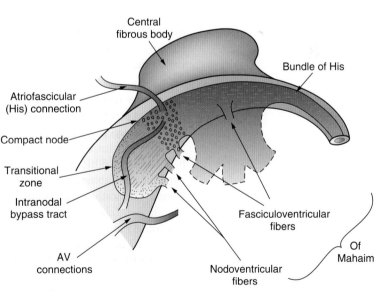

FIGURE 84-1 Structure of the atrioventricular (AV) node. (A) Heart specimen from patient with atrioventricular nodal reentrant tachycardia (AVNRT). Koch triangle is formed by tendon of Todaro, coronary sinus (CS), ostium, and septal attachment of tricuspid valve (TV). Arrow represents site of successful ablation. (B) Schematic drawing depicting the three zones of the AV node and various types of perinodal and atrioventricular bypass tracts. FO, fossa ovalis; IAS, interatrial septum; RAA, right atrial appendage; RV, right ventricle. (Part A reproduced with permission from Olgin JE, Ursell P, Kao AK, et al. Pathological findings following slow pathway ablation for AV nodal reentrant tachycardia, *J Cardiovasc Electrophysiol* 1996 Jul;7(7):625-631. Part B reproduced with permission from Singer I. *Interventional Electrophysiology*, 2nd ed. New York: Lippincott Williams & Wilkins; 2001.)

slow pathway again, continuation giving rise to AVNRT. Systematic anatomic investigation of the AV node in patients with AVNRT is lacking. No obvious histologic abnormalities have been identified among patients with AVNRT versus patients without AVNRT. Several recent autopsy studies have reported that the sites of successful slow pathway ablation were clearly away from the histologic compact AV node, approximately 1 or 2 cm *inferior* and *posterior* to it (option E) (Figure 84-1).

84-3. The answer is D. (*Hurst's The Heart, 14th Edition, Chap. 84*) The differential diagnosis for a long-RP tachycardia (where the RP interval ≥ PR interval) includes atypical AVNRT (option A), sinus tachycardia (option B), atrioventricular reciprocating tachycardia (AVRT) with a slowly conducting pathway (eg, permanent junctional reciprocating tachycardia [PJRT]) (option C), atrial tachycardia (option E), and sinus node reentry. Typical AVNRT is an example of a short-RP tachycardia (where the RP interval < PR interval).

84-4. The answer is C. (*Hurst's The Heart, 14th Edition, Chap. 84*) Significant ST-segment depressions can be observed during tachycardia in nearly 25% to 50% of patients with AVNRT, and this is *not* predictive of ischemia. AVNRT is characterized by a tachycardia with a narrow QRS complex with sudden onset and termination generally at regular rates between 120 and 200 bpm (option A). Uncommonly, the rate can be lower; occasionally, especially in children, it may exceed 200 bpm. The rate of tachycardia may vary from episode to episode. In typical or slow/fast AVNRT, anterograde AV node conduction usually exceeds 200 ms. Because the retrograde conduction is through the fast pathway, the VA interval is short, resulting in superimposition of the P wave onto the QRS complex on the surface electrocardiogram (ECG) (option B). Usually, the P wave is obscured by the QRS or may be seen slightly before or after the QRS complex. The presence of a pseudo r wave in lead V_1 or a pseudo S wave in leads II, III, and aVF suggests typical AVNRT. Functional BBB may develop, producing a wide QRS tachycardia. However, functional BBB should not affect the rate of tachycardia (option D). Studies have reported that QRS alternans is observed more often in association with AP-mediated tachycardias than during AVNRT (option E). Newly acquired T-wave inversions after termination of AVNRT, commonly in anterior or inferior leads, can be seen in nearly 40% of patients. They may be seen immediately after termination of tachycardia, or they may develop within 6 hours, and they can persist for a variable duration. This occurrence is also not related to the rate or duration of tachycardia. This is also not the result of coronary artery disease but is caused by repolarization abnormalities, probably because of ionic current alterations resulting from the rapid rate.

84-5. The answer is A. (*Hurst's The Heart, 14th Edition, Chap. 84*) The American College of Cardiology, American Heart Association, and the Heart Rhythm Society (ACC/AHA/HRS) have recently published updated guidelines on the management of supraventricular arrhythmias.[2] Intravenous (class IIa recommendation) or oral (class IIb recommendation) beta-blockers, diltiazem, or verapamil may be reasonable for acute treatment in hemodynamically stable patients with AVNRT. Intravenous amiodarone may be considered in hemodynamically stable patients with AVNRT when other therapies are ineffective or contraindicated (class IIb recommendation). Because of the known influence of autonomic tone on AV nodal conduction, maneuvers that increase vagal tone, such as the Valsalva (option E) and Mueller maneuvers, gagging, carotid sinus massage, and occasionally exposing the face to ice water, can be used to terminate the tachycardia. The effect of vagal maneuvers is most pronounced on the slow pathway. Adenosine, a purinergic blocking agent that causes acute and transient AV nodal blockade, is the drug of choice for acute termination of AVNRT (option B). Adenosine is nearly 100% effective in terminating AVNRT. Synchronized cardioversion in stable or unstable patients with AVNRT are both class I recommendations when other measures are unsuccessful (options C and D).

84-6. The answer is A. (*Hurst's The Heart, 14th Edition, Chap. 84*) Accessory pathways (AP) are anomalous, typically extranodal connections that connect the epicardial surfaces of the atrium and ventricle along the AV groove. Accessory bypass tracts, which conduct antegrade from the atrium to the ventricle and therefore are detectable on an ECG, are reportedly present in 0.15% to 0.25% of the general population (option D). A higher prevalence of 0.55% has been reported in first-degree relatives of patients with WPW syndrome (option E). APs can be classified based on their site of origin and insertion, location along the mitral or tricuspid annulus, type of conduction, and properties of conduction (decremental or nondecremental). APs usually exhibit rapid, nondecremental conduction, similar to that which is present in normal His-Purkinje tissue and atrial or ventricular myocardium (option C). Approximately 8% of APs display decremental antegrade or retrograde conduction. Whereas APs that are capable only of retrograde conduction are referred to as concealed, those capable of antegrade conduction are referred to as manifest, demonstrating pre-excitation on a standard ECG (option B). Patients with Ebstein anomaly (*not* tetralogy of Fallot) who also have WPW syndrome often have more than one AP (option A).

84-7. **The answer is E.** (*Hurst's the Heart, 14th Edition, Chap. 84*) Atrial fibrillation is an uncommon but potentially serious arrhythmia in patients with the WPW syndrome. If an accessory pathway (AP) has a *short* antegrade refractory period, atrial fibrillation may result in a rapid ventricular response with subsequent degeneration to ventricular fibrillation[3-5] (option A). The risk of sudden death has been shown to be higher if the shortest R-R interval is < 250 ms during spontaneous or induced atrial fibrillation[3] (option B). It has been estimated that one-third of patients with WPW syndrome also have atrial fibrillation (option C). The incidence of sudden cardiac death in patients with WPW syndrome has been estimated to range from 0.15% to 0.39%[3-5] (option D). APs appear to play a pathophysiologic role in the development of atrial fibrillation in these patients because most are young and do not have structural heart disease. Furthermore, surgical or catheter ablation of APs usually results in the elimination of atrial fibrillation as well (option E). Given the high prevalence of atrial fibrillation among patients with WPW syndrome and the concern for sudden cardiac death resulting from rapid preexcited atrial fibrillation, the low annual incidence of sudden death among patients with WPW syndrome is reassuring.

84-8. **The answer is D.** (*Hurst's The Heart, 14th Edition, Chap. 84*) Accessory pathways (AP) can more commonly occur in patients with corrected transposition of the great vessels (l-transposition) where a "double-reversal" of the ventricles and the great arteries is present. In this case, the anomaly of the left (tricuspid) valve is associated with APs to the functioning systemic ventricle (anatomic right ventricle). Nearly 10% of patients with Ebstein anomaly have pre-excitation. Options A through C and E are not associated with an increased risk of WPW syndrome.

84-9. **The answer is B.** (*Hurst's The Heart, 14th Edition, Chap. 84*) The development of BBB aberration during tachycardia can be useful in determining both the presence of and the participation of an AP in tachycardia. An increase in tachycardia cycle length caused by an increase in VA conduction time with functional BBB is consistent with the presence of an accessory pathway ipsilateral to the BBB. In this example, an increase in the tachycardia cycle length from 170 bpm/350 ms to 140 bpm/430 ms with the development of a left BBB strongly suggests an AVRT involving a left-sided pathway.

84-10. **The answer is D.** (*Hurst's The Heart, 14th Edition, Chap. 84*) Catheter ablation of the accessory pathway (AP) is reasonable in asymptomatic patients if the presence of pre-excitation precludes specific employment, such as pilots. Most patients with asymptomatic pre-excitation have a good prognosis. Because of the small but real risks associated with invasive procedures, electrophysiology study (EPS) is not mandated for risk stratification or ablative therapy. The ACC/AHA/HRS Guidelines for the Management of Patients with Supraventricular Arrhythmias gives electrophysiologic testing and catheter ablation when indicated a IIA classification for the treatment of patients with asymptomatic pre-excitation[2] (options A and B), meaning that it is reasonable to offer EPS with or without ablation in selected patients after a thorough discussion of the risks and benefits of the procedure. The detection of intermittent pre-excitation—which is characterized by an abrupt loss of the delta wave, normalization of the QRS complex, and an increase in the PR interval during a continuous ECG recording—is evidence that an AP has a relatively long refractory period and is unlikely to precipitate ventricular fibrillation. The loss of pre-excitation after the administration of antiarrhythmic drugs such as procainamide or ajmaline has also been used to indicate a low-risk subgroup. These noninvasive tests are generally considered inferior to EPS in the assessment of the risk of sudden cardiac death. Because of this, *they play little role in patient management at present* (option C). Based on the results of multiple studies, as well as the well-established safety and efficacy of catheter ablation of APs, an increasing proportion of electrophysiologists, particularly pediatric electrophysiologists, now advocate screening EPS and prophylactic catheter ablation when a high-risk AP is uncovered (option E).

References

1. Katritsis DG, Josephson ME. Classification of electrophysiological types of atrioventricular nodal re-entrant tachycardia: a reappraisal. *Europace.* 2013;15(9):1231-1240. Epub 2013 Apr 23.
2. Page RL, Joglar JA, Caldwell MA, et al. 2015 ACC/AHA/HRS guideline for the management of adult patients with supraventricular tachycardia: a report of the American College of Cardiology/American Heart Association Task Force on Clinical Practice Guidelines and the Heart Rhythm Society. *J Am Coll Cardiol.* 2016 Apr 5; 67(13):e27-e115. doi: 10.1016/j.jacc.2015.08.856. Epub 2015 Sep 24.
3. Klein GJ, Bashore TM, Sellers TD, et al. Ventricular fibrillation in the Wolff-Parkinson-White syndrome. *N Engl J Med.* 1979;301:1080-1085.
4. Timmermans C, Smeets JL, Rodriguez LM, et al. Aborted sudden death in the Wolff-Parkinson-White syndrome. *Am J Cardiol.* 1995;76:492-494.
5. Pappone C, Santinelli V, Rosanio S, et al. Usefulness of invasive electrophysiologic testing to stratify the risk of arrhythmic events in asymptomatic patients with Wolff-Parkinson-White pattern: results from a large prospective long-term follow-up study. *J Am Coll Cardiol.* 2003;41(2):239-244.

CHAPTER 85

Ventricular Arrhythmias

Jacqueline Joza

QUESTIONS

DIRECTIONS: Choose the one best response to each question.

85-1. You are seeing a 45-year-old man in consult for very frequent premature ventricular contractions (PVCs). You counsel the patient regarding his risk of developing a PVC-induced cardiomyopathy (CM). What is the lowest percentage of PVCs over a 24-hour period that is associated with a higher risk of developing CM?

A. 2%
B. 5%
C. 10%
D. 15%
E. 20%

85-2. A 48-year-old perimenopausal woman presents to the emergency department with incessant palpitations that have been occurring over the last month. Transthoracic echocardiogram is normal. An electrocardiogram reveals ventricular bigeminy and short runs of nonsustained ventricular tachycardia (VT). The morphology of the ventricular ectopy is as follows: LBBB morphology in V_1 with a precordial transition at V_5, an inferior axis, negative in aVL and aVR, and slight negativity in lead I. Regarding this type of VT, which of the following is *false*?

A. This arrhythmia is often provoked by exercise and emotional stress
B. In women, these occur more often during premenstrual, perimenopausal, and gestational periods
C. When RV dysfunction is present on transthoracic echo, a cardiac-MRI should be considered

D. The success rate for medical therapy is excellent
E. The proposed cellular mechanism is cyclic adenosine monophosphate–mediated (cAMP) triggered activity from delayed afterdepolarizations

85-3. Fascicular VT is a specific subtype of idiopathic VT. All of the following are clinical features of this VT *except*:

A. Structurally normal heart
B. VT with a relatively narrow QRS (< 140 ms) characterized by a right bundle branch block (RBBB) pattern in V_1 and a superior axis
C. Induction with atrial pacing
D. Sensitivity to diltiazem
E. Typical presentation is in patients between 15 and 40 years of age

85-4. A 75-year-old patient presents to the emergency department with sustained VT requiring external defibrillation. His past medical history is significant for a previous myocardial infarction that required acute percutaneous coronary intervention to the distal left anterior descending artery. His transthoracic echocardiogram reveals akinesis of the entire anterior and anterolateral wall and apex. Which of the following ECG features of the VT would be *least* likely to be observed?

A. LBBB pattern in V_1 with positive R waves in lead I
B. Inferior axis (positive leads in II, III, aVF)
C. Dominant S waves in V_3, V_4
D. Dominant R waves in V_3, V_4
E. RBBB pattern with dominant R waves in V_1

85-5. Monitoring of a 55-year-old woman in the coronary care unit reveals approximately 20 to 30 PVCs per hour. She is 24 hours post stenting of her proximal right coronary artery after presenting with an inferior STEMI. Which of the following is *false* regarding her PVCs?

A. Improved survival has been demonstrated when PVCs are treated with an antiarrhythmic agent

B. Lidocaine may be considered temporarily when recurrent hemodynamically significant ventricular arrhythmias occur in the setting of an acute myocardial infarction

C. Her electrolytes and acid-base imbalance should be corrected

D. β-adrenergic blocking agents or amiodarone are the preferred pharmacologic interventions in the setting of frequent and persistent ventricular ectopy that results in hemodynamic instability

E. Prophylactic use of an antiarrhythmic agent is not recommended

85-6. A 75-year-old man presents to the emergency room with sustained monomorphic VT at 160 bpm. He was seated at the dinner table when he describes sudden-onset dizziness and palpitations. His chest x-ray demonstrates clear lungs, and electrolytes are all within normal limits. A transthoracic echocardiogram reveals a left ventricular ejection fraction (LVEF) of 45% to 50% with akinesis of the inferior wall. At baseline, he can walk up several flights of stairs without difficulty, and he had joined a running club a few years ago, where he trains several times per week. His past medical history is significant for diet-controlled diabetes mellitus type II, prior myocardial infarction 15 years ago, and dyslipidemia. As part of his treatment with amiodarone, he will also receive an implantable cardioverter defibrillator (ICD). Which of the following statements is *false?*

A. All patients with VT should be treated with a beta-blocker unless prohibited

B. Acute ischemia is a less likely cause of his presentation

C. The ICD should be programmed with a longer VT detection time

D. Amiodarone in combination with a beta-blocker is a reasonable option

E. The VT zone on the ICD should be programmed to 158 bpm so as to avoid inappropriate shocks

85-7. For a 65-year-old woman, in which of the following cases is an ICD *not* indicated?

A. Survivor of cardiac arrest due to ventricular fibrillation where a completely reversible cause has been excluded

B. With structural heart disease and hemodynamically stable sustained VT

C. With nonsustained VT due to a prior myocardial infarction with an LV ejection fraction of < 40% and inducible VF at electrophysiology study

D. With an LV ejection fraction of 35%, remote myocardial infarction, and NYHA functional class I

E. Syncope of undetermined origin with hemodynamically significant sustained VT induced at electrophysiology study

85-8. A 70-year-old man presents with an anterior STEMI and undergoes percutaneous coronary intervention to his proximal left anterior descending artery. While he is being monitored in the coronary care unit overnight, the nurse notices 1 minute of a wide-complex tachycardia at 90 bpm. The patient is sleeping. Which of the following statements concerning this arrhythmia is *false?*

A. Typical rates of this rhythm are between 40 and 120 bpm

B. Its presence is associated with an increase in long-term mortality

C. Fusion beats may be seen at the onset and termination of the arrhythmia

D. This rhythm may be also associated with dilated CM

E. The incidence is not affected by the location of myocardial infarction or the infarct size

85-9. Concerning the Sudden Cardiac Death in Heart Failure Trial (SCD-HeFT), which of the following statements is *false?*

A. The patients included in the study were all primary prevention patients

B. The study compared ICD versus amiodarone versus optimal medical therapy

C. Patients were required to have an LVEF < 35% for enrollment

D. After a 5-year follow-up, the annual mortality of patients on optimal medical therapy was 7% to 8% per year

E. The addition of an ICD decreases mortality by 8% compared with optimal medical therapy alone

85-10. All of the following statements are *true* regarding Chagas disease *except:*

A. Chagas disease is a major cause of CM and VT in Central and South America, and it is a growing problem in the United States as a result of immigration patterns

B. *Trypanosoma cruzi* is transmitted to humans via triatome insect vectors

C. Recurrent monomorphic VT is common in chronic Chagas CM

D. Histologic examination of patients with Chagas disease reveals focal and diffuse fibrosis of the myocardium, predominantly in the endocardium

E. The ACC/AHA/HRS 2008 guidelines recommend an ICD for primary prevention of sudden death in patients with Chagas disease

85-1. **The answer is C.** *(Hurst's The Heart, 14th Edition, Chap. 84)* Clinical evidence of an association between frequent PVCs and a dilated CM has been demonstrated.[1-5] A higher burden of PVCs over a 24-hour period is associated with higher risk, but the development of CM associated with a burden as low as 10% has been described.[1] Current studies regarding the role of PVCs in the development of a CM demonstrate the following: (1) left ventricular dysfunction can occur when PVCs are present for a prolonged period of time; (2) LV dysfunction occurs among patients with a high frequency of PVCs; and (3) among patients with a PVC-induced CM, LVEF improves in most patients when the PVCs can be eliminated with radiofrequency catheter ablation. A number of electrocardiographic and other factors have been associated with an increased risk of PVC-induced CM, but further assessment is ongoing. A higher burden, retrograde ventriculoatrial (VA) conduction,[2] PVC QRS duration,[3,7] site of origin,[7] interpolation,[5] male gender,[4] PVCs throughout the day,[4] epicardial origin,[8] and coupling interval dispersion[9] have been described as potential contributing factors.

85-2. **The answer is D.** *(Hurst's The Heart, 14th Edition, Chap. 84)* The ventricular tachycardia that is suggested is an "outflow tract" VT. With a LBBB morphology in V_1, late transition at V_5, and an inferior axis, the most likely origin is from the right ventricular outflow tract (RVOT). "Outflow tract" VT occurs in young to middle-aged patients without structural heart disease. This arrhythmia is often provoked by exercise and emotional stress (option A). Recurrence may be associated with exercise, stress, or caffeine, and in women, it occurs more often during premenstrual, perimenopausal, and gestational periods (option B). For RVOT PVCs, while further imaging studies are often not required, patients with PVCs from the right ventricle (RV), with RV dysfunction or enlargement on echocardiogram or multiform RV-origin PVCs, should be considered for further evaluation to exclude arrhythmogenic RV cardiomyopathy (ARVC) or cardiac sarcoidosis. This workup should include a cardiac MRI (option C)[10] and possibly a positron emission tomography–computed tomography (PET-CT) scan.[11] The proposed cellular mechanism of outflow tract PVCs is cyclic adenosine monophosphate–mediated (cAMP) triggered activity from delayed afterdepolarizations.[12] This mechanism is supported by the sensitivity of the arrhythmia to adenosine infusion, which often terminates the arrhythmia. Initial treatment of RVOT PVCs should be the avoidance of potential exogenous stimulants (such as caffeine, excess alcohol, recreational drugs) or a trial of β-adrenergic blocking or calcium channel–blocking agents. However, the success rate for medical therapy is low (< 50%) in this population (option D).[13-14]

85-3. **The answer is D.** *(Hurst's The Heart, 14th Edition, Chap. 84)* Fascicular VT is characterized by an RBBB pattern with a left superior axis on a 12-lead ECG (option B). Belhassen and Laniado[15] were the first to describe the sensitivity of this tachycardia to verapamil (option D) in 1981. The arrhythmia usually presents in patients between 15 and 40 years of age (option E). Patients typically have a structurally normal heart (option A), but they may present with an incessant VT, and a reversible tachycardia-mediated CM can develop. The site of origin of the tachycardia is usually in the region of the left posterior fascicle (inferior posterior LV septum),[16] but other regions have been described, although they are less common. At electrophysiology study, fascicular VT is typically induced with atrial pacing (option C).[17] Patients with fascicular VT have a good prognosis, responding well to verapamil for acute termination of VT as well as for long-term arrhythmia control. Catheter ablation is an excellent option for those patients who are unresponsive to verapamil or prefer not to take medications long-term.

85-4. **The answer is A.** *(Hurst's The Heart, 14th Edition, Chap. 84)* The anatomic substrate from which ischemic VT originates usually involves a healed scar after an acute myocardial infarction (MI). The interplay of healthy, damaged (border zone), and scarred (fibrotic) myocardium serves as a setting for slowed conduction and reentry.[18-19] A 12-lead ECG should be obtained whenever possible to help localize the origin of the VT. The patient in the question has suffered a previous large anterior myocardial infarction with akinesis of his entire anterior and anterolateral walls and apex. On 12-lead ECG of the VT, options B through E may all be consistent with this patient's presenting VT: (option B) an inferior axis suggests an exit site at the anterior wall; (option C) dominant S waves in V_3, V_4 suggest an apical exit site; (option D) dominant R waves in V_3, V_4 suggest a basal exit site; (option E) an RBBB pattern with a dominant R wave in V_1 indicates a left ventricular exit site of the VT. An LBBB pattern in V_1 suggests exit in the right ventricle or interventricular septum, which is *least* likely to be observed in this patient (option A).

85-5. **The answer is A.** (*Hurst's The Heart, 14th Edition, Chap. 84*) While the association between PVCs after myocardial infarction (MI) and adverse events has been established, there is no clear benefit to routinely treating PVCs with antiarrhythmics in this setting. The association of PVCs with sudden cardiac death previously led to the routine use of intravenous lidocaine in patients following MIs.[20] Subsequent randomized controlled studies (CAST trial) demonstrated poorer survival when PVCs were treated with antiarrhythmic agents (option A).[21] Based on these findings, the routine prophylactic use of antiarrhythmic agents for patients after an MI is not recommended (option E). In patients with frequent ventricular ectopy, electrolyte and acid-base imbalance should be corrected (option C). If frequent and persistent ventricular ectopy results in hemodynamic instability (which is rare), a β-adrenergic blocking agent or amiodarone are the preferred pharmacologic interventions (option D). Lidocaine may be considered temporarily when recurrent hemodynamically significant ventricular arrhythmias occur in the setting of acute MI (option B).[22]

85-6. **The answer is E.** (*Hurst's The Heart, 14th Edition, Chap. 84*) When antiarrhythmic agents are initiated in patients with an ICD, care must be taken in programming the device because antiarrhythmic medications can have varying effects on defibrillation thresholds, and they *may slow the rate of the VT below a programmed detection zone* (option E). The VT zone of this patient on amiodarone should therefore be programmed to a much lower zone than his initial presenting VT. All patients with VT with an ischemic etiology should be treated with a beta-blocker unless prohibited by hypotension, bradycardia, or other clinical factors (ie, reactive airway disease, vasospastic coronary disease) (option A). Reversible factors contributing to VT, such as congestive heart failure exacerbation, acute ischemia, or electrolyte abnormalities, should be diagnosed rapidly and treated. However, while concerning in the setting of polymorphic VT, acute ischemia is rarely a cause of monomorphic VT (option B). Monomorphic VT in the setting of structural heart disease suggests underlying myocardial fibrosis/scar. In a randomized study of patients with ICDs implanted for inducible or spontaneously occurring VT or VF, patients randomized to β-adrenergic blockers alone, sotalol alone, or amiodarone plus beta-blocker, amiodarone plus beta-blocker resulted in significantly fewer shocks compared with beta-blocker or sotalol alone (option D).[23] ICD programming with longer VT detection times (option C) and more ATP therapies can help minimize shocks for nonsustained episodes of VT or inappropriate shocks from supraventricular arrhythmias.[24-26]

85-7. **The answer is D.** (*Hurst's The Heart, 14th Edition, Chap. 84*) ICD therapy is recommended in patients with an LVEF < 35% due to prior myocardial infarction who are at least 40 days post-myocardial infarction and are in NYHA functional class II or III. If the patient is NYHA class I with a remote myocardial infarction, the LVEF must be < 30% to be considered for ICD implantation. Options A through C and E are all class I indications for ICD implant. Class I indications include: (1) primary or secondary prevention of SCD in patients who are survivors of cardiac arrest due to ventricular fibrillation or hemodynamically unstable sustained VT after evaluation to define the cause of the event and to exclude any completely reversible causes (level of evidence [LOE] A); (2) patients with structural heart disease and spontaneous sustained VT whether hemodynamically stable or unstable (LOE B); (3) patients with syncope of undetermined origin with clinically relevant, hemodynamically significant sustained VT or ventricular fibrillation induced at electrophysiologic study (LOE B); (4) ICD therapy is recommended in patients with an LVEF < 35% due to prior myocardial infarction who are at least 40 days post–myocardial infarction and are in NYHA functional class II or III (LOE A); (5) ICD therapy is recommended in patients with nonischemic dilated CM who have an LVEF ≤ 35% and who are in NYHA functional class II or III (LOE B); (6) ICD therapy is indicated in patients with LV dysfunction due to prior myocardial infarction who are at least 40 days post-myocardial infarction, have an LVEF < 30%, and are in NYHA functional class I (LOE A); (7) ICD therapy is indicated in patients with nonsustained VT due to prior myocardial infarction, LVEF < 40% and inducible ventricular fibrillation or sustained VT at electrophysiologic study (LOE B).

85-8. **The answer is B.** *(Hurst's The Heart, 14th Edition, Chap. 84)* Accelerated idioventricular rhythm (AIVR) is typically an automatic rhythm originating in the ventricle with rates between 40 and 120 bpm (option A). It is often seen gradually accelerating beyond the sinus rate, resulting in isorhythmic atrioventricular dissociation.[29] Fusion beats may be seen at the onset and termination of the arrhythmia (option C). AIVR may be associated with ischemic CM, acute coronary syndromes, rheumatic heart disease, dilated CM (option D), and acute myocarditis.[30] Furthermore, AIVR has been described in patients with no apparent heart disease.[31] In the setting of acute coronary syndromes, AIVR is considered to be a noninvasive, albeit nonspecific, marker for successful reperfusion after thrombolytic therapy. The incidence of AIVR is not affected by the location of MI or the infarct size (option E). The presence of AIVR after an MI is not associated with an increase in mortality (opton B).[32] The mechanism of AIVR is thought to be increased automaticity in a region of the ventricle; however, in some instances, such as in myocardial ischemia and digitalis toxicity, the mechanism may be caused by triggered activity.[33]

85-9. **The answer is E.** *(Hurst's The Heart, 14th Edition, Chap. 84)* The Sudden Cardiac Death in Heart Failure Trial (SCD-HeFT)[34] is the largest randomized primary prevention trial (2521 patients) comparing ICD versus amiodarone versus optimal medical therapy in patients with LVEF < 35% (options A, B, and C). This study did not require the presence of NSVT for enrollment. Patients enrolled in SCD-HeFT also had New York Heart Association functional class II to III heart failure symptoms. After a 5-year follow-up period, this study demonstrated that (1) the annual mortality of patients on optimal medical therapy was 7% to 8% per year (option D); (2) amiodarone, when used as a primary preventative agent, does *not* improve survival over optimal medical therapy for heart failure; and (3) the addition of an ICD decreases mortality by 23% compared with optimal medical therapy alone (HR = 0.77; 95% CI, 0.62–0.96; *P* = .007)(option E).[34]

85-10. **The answer is D.** *(Hurst's The Heart, 14th Edition, Chap. 84)* Chagas disease is the major cause of CM and VT in Central and South America and is a growing problem in the United States[35] as a result of immigration patterns (option A). The protozoan *Trypanosoma cruzi* is transmitted to humans via triatome insect vectors (option B). The etiology of chronic Chagas CM and associated VT is likely a combined effect of direct parasitism, autoimmune reaction, inflammatory effects, microvascular destruction, and autonomic dysregulation. Recurrent monomorphic VT is common in chronic Chagas CM (option C). Most VTs can be induced with programmed stimulation and entrained during VT, favoring reentry as the predominant mechanism. Histologic examination of patients with Chagas disease reveals focal and diffuse fibrosis of the myocardium, predominantly in the *subepicardium* and interspersed with surviving myocardial fibers (option D). Classically, ablation for VT is performed in the epicardium for this reason. Sudden death is the most common cause of death in Chagas disease, accounting for 55% to 65% of deaths.[36] Therefore the ACC/AHA/HRS 2008 guidelines recommend an ICD for primary prevention of sudden death in patients with Chagas disease (option E).

References

1. Baman TS, Lange DC, Ilg KJ, et al. Relationship between burden of premature ventricular complexes and left ventricular function. *Heart Rhythm*. 2010;7:865-869.

2. Ban JE, Park HC, Park JS, et al. Electrocardiographic and electrophysiological characteristics of premature ventricular complexes associated with left ventricular dysfunction in patients without structural heart disease. *Europace*. 2013;15:735-741.

3. Deyell MW, Park KM, Han Y, et al. Predictors of recovery of left ventricular dysfunction after ablation of frequent ventricular premature depolarizations. *Heart Rhythm*. 2012;9:1465-1472.

4. Hasdemir C, Ulucan C, Yavuzgil O, et al. Tachycardia-induced cardiomyopathy in patients with idiopathic ventricular arrhythmias: the incidence, clinical and electrophysiologic characteristics, and the predictors. *J Cardiovasc Electrophysiol*. 2011;22: 663-668.

5. Olgun H, Yokokawa M, Baman T, et al. The role of interpolation in PVC-induced cardiomyopathy. *Heart Rhythm*. 2011;8:1046-1049.

6. Bogun F, Crawford T, Reich S, et al. Radiofrequency ablation of frequent, idiopathic premature ventricular complexes: comparison with a control group without intervention. *Heart Rhythm*. 2007;4:863-867.

7. Del Carpio Munoz F, Syed FF, Noheria A, et al. Characteristics of premature ventricular complexes as correlates of reduced left ventricular systolic function: study of the burden, duration, coupling interval, morphology and site of origin of PVCs. *J Cardiovasc Electrophysiol*. 2011;22:791-798.

8. Sadron Blaye-Felice M, Hamon D, Sacher F, et al. Premature ventricular contraction-induced cardiomyopathy: related clinical and electrophysiologic parameters. *Heart Rhythm*. 2016 Jan;13(1):103-110. doi: 10.1016/j.hrthm.2015.08.025. Epub 2015 Aug 18.

9. Kawamura M, Badhwar N, Vedantham V, et al. Coupling interval dispersion and body mass index are independent predictors of idiopathic premature ventricular complex-induced cardiomyopathy. *J Cardiovasc Electrophysiol*. 2014;25:756-762.

10. Aquaro GD, Pingitore A, Strata E, et al. Cardiac magnetic resonance predicts outcome in patients with premature ventricular complexes of left bundle branch block morphology. *J Am Coll Cardiol*. 2010;56:1235-1243.

11. Marchlinski FE, Deely MP, Zado ES. Sex-specific triggers for right ventricular outflow tract tachycardia. *Am Heart J*. 2000;139:1009-1013.

12. Lerman BB, Ip JE, Shah BK, et al. Mechanism-specific effects of adenosine on ventricular tachycardia. *J Cardiovasc Electrophysiol*. 2014;25:1350-1358.

13. Stec S, Sikorska A, Zaborska B, et al. Benign symptomatic premature ventricular complexes: short- and long-term efficacy of antiarrhythmic drugs and radiofrequency ablation. *Kardiol Pol*. 2012;70:351-358.

14. Krittayaphong R, Bhuripanyo K, Punlee K, et al. Effect of atenolol on symptomatic ventricular arrhythmia without structural heart disease: a randomized placebo-controlled study. *Am Heart J*. 2002;144:e10.

15. Belhassen B, Rotmensch HH, Laniado S. Response of recurrent sustained ventricular tachycardia to verapamil. *Br Heart J*. 1981;46:679-682.

16. Nogami A, Naito S, Tada H, et al. Demonstration of diastolic and presystolic Purkinje potentials as critical potentials in a macroreentry circuit of verapamil-sensitive idiopathic left ventricular tachycardia. *J Am Coll Cardiol*. 2000;36:811-823.

17. Zipes DP, Foster PR, Troup PJ, Pedersen DH. Atrial induction of ventricular tachycardia: reentry versus triggered automaticity. *Am J Cardiol*. 1979;44:1-8.

18. de Bakker JM, van Capelle FJ, Janse MJ, et al. Reentry as a cause of ventricular tachycardia in patients with chronic ischemic heart disease: electrophysiologic and anatomic correlation. *Circulation*. 1988;77:589-606.

19. Josephson ME, Horowitz LN, Farshidi A. Continuous local electrical activity. A mechanism of recurrent ventricular tachycardia. *Circulation*. 1978;57:659-665.

20. MacMahon S, Collins R, Peto R, et al. Effects of prophylactic lidocaine in suspected acute myocardial infarction. An overview of results from the randomized, controlled trials. *JAMA*. 1988;260:1910-1916.

21. Echt DS, Liebson PR, Mitchell LB, et al. Mortality and morbidity in patients receiving encainide, flecainide, or placebo. The Cardiac Arrhythmia Suppression Trial. *N Engl J Med*. 1991;324:781-788.

22. Tosaki A, Balint S, Szekeres L. Protective effect of lidocaine against ischemia and reperfusion-induced arrhythmias and shifts of myocardial sodium, potassium, and calcium content. *J Cardiovasc Pharmacol*. 1988;12:621-628.

23. Connolly SJ, Dorian P, Roberts RS, et al. Comparison of beta-blockers, amiodarone plus beta-blockers, or sotalol for prevention of shocks from implantable cardioverter defibrillators: the OPTIC Study: a randomized trial. *JAMA*. 2006;295:165-171.

24. Moss AJ, Schuger C, Beck CA, et al. Reduction in inappropriate therapy and mortality through ICD programming. *N Engl J Med*. 2012;367:2275-2283.

25. Wathen MS, DeGroot PJ, Sweeney MO, et al. Prospective randomized multicenter trial of empirical antitachycardia pacing versus shocks for spontaneous rapid ventricular tachycardia in patients with implantable cardioverter-defibrillators: Pacing Fast Ventricular Tachycardia Reduces Shock Therapies (PainFREE Rx II) trial results. *Circulation*. 2004;110:2591-2596.

26. Wathen MS, Sweeney MO, DeGroot PJ, et al. Shock reduction using antitachycardia pacing for spontaneous rapid ventricular tachycardia in patients with coronary artery disease. *Circulation*. 2001;104:796-801.

27. Epstein AE, DiMarco JP, Ellenbogen KA, et al. ACC/AHA/HRS 2008 guidelines for device-based therapy of cardiac rhythm abnormalities: a report of the American College of Cardiology/American Heart Association Task Force on Practice Guidelines (Writing Committee to Revise the ACC/AHA/NASPE 2002 Guideline Update for Implantation of Cardiac Pacemakers and Antiarrhythmia Devices) developed in collaboration with the American Association for Thoracic Surgery and Society of Thoracic Surgeons. *J Am Coll Cardiol*. 2008;51:e1-e62.

28. Epstein AE, DiMarco JP, Ellenbogen KA, et al. 2012 ACCF/AHA/HRS focused update incorporated into the ACCF/AHA/HRS 2008 guidelines for device-based therapy of cardiac rhythm abnormalities: a report of the American College of Cardiology Foundation/American Heart Association Task Force on Practice Guidelines and the Heart Rhythm Society. *J Am Coll Cardiol*. 2013;61:e6-e75.

29. Gallagher JJ, Damato AN, Lau SH. Electrophysiologic studies during accelerated idioventricular rhythms. *Circulation*. 1971;44:671-677.

30. Gressin V, Louvard Y, Pezzano M, Lardoux H. Holter recording of ventricular arrhythmias during intravenous thrombolysis for acute myocardial infarction. *Am J Cardiol*. 1992;69:152-159.

31. Nakagawa M, Hamaoka K, Okano S, et al. Multiform accelerated idioventricular rhythm (AIVR) in a child with acute myocarditis. *Clin Cardiol*. 1988;11:853-855.

32. Norris RM, Mercer CJ. Significance of idioventricular rhythms in acute myocardial infarction. *Prog Cardiovasc Dis*. 1974;16:455-468.

33. Sclarovsky S, Strasberg B, Fuchs J, et al. Multiform accelerated idioventricular rhythm in acute myocardial infarction: electrocardiographic characteristics and response to verapamil. *Am J Cardiol*. 1983;52:43-47.

34. Bardy GH, Lee KL, Mark DB, et al. Amiodarone or an implantable cardioverter-defibrillator for congestive heart failure. *N Engl J Med*. 2005;352:225-237.

35. Traina MI, Sanchez DR, Hernandez S, et al. Prevalence and impact of Chagas disease among Latin American immigrants with nonischemic cardiomyopathy in Los Angeles, California. *Circ Heart Fail*. 2015;8:938-943.

36. Rassi A Jr., Rassi SG, Rassi A. Sudden death in Chagas' disease. *Arq Bras Cardiol*. 2001;76:75-96.

CHAPTER 86

Bradyarrhythmias

Jacqueline Joza

QUESTIONS

DIRECTIONS: Choose the one best response to each question.

86-1. Which of the following statements concerning the blood supply of the electrical conduction system is *false*?

A. The left bundle receives its blood supply from the AV nodal artery, posterior descending artery, and branches of the left anterior descending artery
B. The sinus node receives its blood supply from the sinoatrial nodal artery arising from the right coronary artery in 60% of patients
C. The sinus node receives its blood supply from the sinoatrial nodal artery arising from the circumflex artery in 40% of patients
D. The AV node is supplied by the AV nodal artery arising from the right coronary artery in 10% of patients and from the left circumflex artery in the remaining 90%
E. The His bundle is supplied by the AV nodal artery as well as branches of the left anterior descending artery

86-2. A 25-year-old woman presents to your office in consultation for severe sinus bradycardia. Her resting ECG reveals a heart rate at 28 bpm. She is entirely asymptomatic from her bradycardia. All of the following represent possible etiologies of her sinus node dysfunction *except*:

A. Hormonal fluctuations during premenstrual, perimenopausal, and gestational periods
B. Mutation in the hyperpolarization-activated cyclic nucleotide-gated (HCN) channel
C. Previous closure of an atrial septal defect of the sinus-venosus type
D. Collagen vascular disease
E. Mutation in the cardiac sodium channel gene, *SCN5A*

86-3. A 70-year-old woman is sent to the emergency department after her primary care physician notices her to be bradycardic at 50 bpm. The resting ECG reveals sinus bradycardia at 50 bpm, without intracardiac conduction delay. The patient denies any significant dyspnea, palpitations, lightheadedness or chest pain at rest or with exertion. She takes no medications. You decide to perform an exercise treadmill test. Which of the following concerning chronotropic incompetence (CI) is *false*?

A. CI is defined as the inability of the sinus node to achieve at least 50% of the age-predicted maximal heart rate
B. CI may be secondary to drugs with negative chronotropic effects
C. CI is present in 20% to 60% of patients with sinus node dysfunction
D. CI is common in patients with heart failure
E. CI may be diagnosed when there is a failure to attain > 80% of the HR reserve measured during a graded exercise test

86-4. A 69-year-old man recently underwent implantation of a dual-chamber pacemaker for sinus node dysfunction. His baseline ECG prior to the pacemaker was consistent with sinus bradycardia at 48 bpm without intracardiac conduction delay (PR 170 ms; QRS 64 ms), and Holter monitoring had demonstrated frequent daytime sinus pauses of > 5 seconds. The pacemaker is programmed DDDR 50 to 120 bpm. His ECG today demonstrates atrial and ventricular pacing. Which of the following pacemaker programming settings would be *least* likely to increase his incidence of atrial fibrillation and congestive heart failure?

A. DDD 50 bpm; sensed AV delay 150 ms; paced AV delay 180 ms
B. AAIR 50 to 120 bpm
C. VVI 50 bpm
D. DDDR 50 to 120 bpm; sensed AV delay 150 ms; paced AV delay 180 ms
E. VVIR 50 to 120 bpm

86-5. Implantation of a dual-chamber pacemaker is indicated in the setting of hypersensitive carotid sinus syndrome and neurocardiogenic syncope in which of the following patients?

A. A 35-year-old woman with minimally symptomatic neurocardiogenic syncope that is associated with bradycardia documented spontaneously or at the time of tilt-table testing

B. A 25-year-old woman with recurrent syncope without clear provocative events and with a hypersensitive cardioinhibitory response of 2 seconds

C. A 25-year-old woman with recurrent syncope caused by spontaneously occurring carotid sinus stimulation and carotid sinus pressure that induces ventricular asystole of > 3 seconds

D. A 35-year-old woman with a hyperactive cardioinhibitory response to carotid stimulation in the absence of symptoms or in the presence of vague symptoms

E. A 25-year-old woman with situational vasovagal syncope in which avoidance behavior is effective

86-6. A 40-year-old man presents to the emergency department with increased dyspnea on exertion. His ECG reveals sinus rhythm with complete heart block. Which of the following statements is *incorrect*?

A. If the patient is taking lithium, this medication should be held first before consideration of pacemaker implantation

B. This patient may harbor a mutation in the *SCN5A* gene

C. This patient should undergo further evaluation with a high-resolution chest CT and/or cardiac MRI

D. His presentation may be explained by the presence of a Lamin A/C mutation

E. If the patient has a diagnosis of myotonic dystrophy, a pacemaker should be deferred until immune modulatory therapy is initiated

86-7. The monitoring of an 80-year-old man, post-op hip replacement, reveals sinus rhythm with 2:1 atrioventricular block. Which of the following statements is *false*?

A. A 2:1 AV block with normal QRS duration or with a very long PR interval generally suggests block in the AV node

B. A 2:1 AV block in the presence of bundle branch block, especially in the setting of a normal PR interval, favors block below the AV node but is not diagnostic

C. Carotid sinus stimulation may worsen the degree of block if it is in the AV node

D. Carotid sinus stimulation may worsen the ratio of AV conduction and decrease the ventricular rate if the block is located in the His–Purkinje system

E. Both A and C are false

86-8. For a 70-year-old woman, in which of the following cases should cardiac resynchronization be considered?

A. LVEF 45%, NYHA class I, and complete heart block

B. LVEF 30%, NYHA class I, and complete heart block

C. LVEF 35%, NYHA class II, and high-degree AV block

D. LVEF 60%, NYHA class II, and complete heart block

E. LVEF 60%, NYHA class III, and complete heart block

86-9. You are seeing a 75-year-old woman in consult for an abnormal electrocardiogram. She is asymptomatic. Her electrocardiogram reveals a right bundle branch block and left anterior fascicular block. Which of the following circumstances would persuade you to implant a pacemaker?

A. If at electrophysiology study, a prolonged HV interval of ≥ 60 ms was observed

B. If a first-degree AV block was also noted on ECG

C. No other circumstances: just implant a dual-chamber pacemaker to prevent syncope

D. Alternating bundle branch block

E. Both B and D are correct

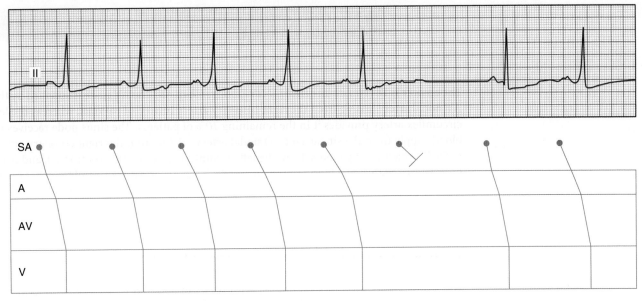

FIGURE 86-1 Telemetry strip and Ladder diagram demonstrating a sinus pause.

86-10. Refer to the telemetry strip with accompanying ladder diagram (Figure 86-1). The diagnosis is most consistent with:

A. Tachycardia-bradycardia syndrome
B. Sinoatrial exit block
C. Sinus arrest
D. Chronotropic incompetence
E. Persistent atrial standstill

86-1. **The answer is D.** *(Hurst's The Heart, 14th Edition, Chap. 86)* The AV node is supplied by the AV nodal artery arising from the right coronary artery in *90%* of patients, whereas the left circumflex artery provides it in the remaining *10%* of patients. The sinus node receives its blood supply from the sinoatrial (SA) nodal artery arising from the right coronary artery in 59% (option B) of patients, from the left circumflex artery in 38% (option C), and from both arteries with a dual blood supply in 3%. Both the AV nodal artery and branches of the left anterior descending artery supply the bundle of His (option E). The left bundle has a rich blood supply from the AV nodal artery, posterior descending artery, and branches of the left anterior descending artery (option A).

86-2. **The answer is A.** *(Hurst's The Heart, 14th Edition, Chap. 86)* Hormonal changes have not been shown to be associated with sinus node dysfunction (SND). SND can occur in children and young adults without structural heart disease. In addition to autosomal inheritance, polygenetic susceptibility to SND has been described. Mutations in the hyperpolarization-activated cyclic nucleotide-gated channel (HCN), specifically HCN4 (option B), result in a lack of channel responsiveness to cyclic AMP or reduction in the funny current (I_f), leading to sinus bradycardia, chronotropic incompetence, and atrial fibrillation.[1] Mutations in calcium (Ca^{2+}) channels and Ca^{2+} handling proteins (ryanodine receptor [RYR2] or calsequestrin 2[CASQ2]) are also associated with SND.[2] Mutations in the cardiac sodium channel gene, *SCN5A* (option E), have been reported in families to result in primary cardiac conduction disease. The spectrum of conduction diseases associated with *SCN5A* varies widely, but it includes sinus node dysfunction, atrial standstill, AV block, and progressive cardiac conduction disease (PCCD). An inherited form of Lev-Lenégre disease is associated with loss-of-function mutations in *SCN5A* and can exist alone or as overlap syndromes with Brugada or long QT syndrome. Mutations in ankyrinB (ANKB) are associated with long QT type 4 and familial sinus node dysfunction by disrupting the membrane and Ca^{2+} clocks.[3-4] Rare cases of sinus node dysfunction requiring pacemaker therapy have been reported with Lyme disease (*Borrelia burgdorferi* infection).[5] In children and young adults, damage to the sinus node during atrial surgery (closure of atrial septal defects of the sinus-venosus type, Mustard procedure for transposition of great arteries) has been commonly associated with sinus node dysfunction (option C). An idiopathic degenerative disorder of the sinus node is the most common cause for intrinsic SND, but ischemic heart disease is responsible in a significant number of patients. Other potential causes of SND include long-standing hypertension, cardiomyopathy (especially infiltrative disorders such as amyloidosis and sarcoidosis), inflammation (collagen vascular disease [option D], rheumatic fever or pericarditis), viral myocarditis, valvular heart disease or heart transplant, atrial arrhythmias, and inherited neuromuscular disorders. Finally, drugs and autonomic nervous system influences are also important causes of SND in patients without structural abnormalities.

86-3. **The answer is A.** *(Hurst's The Heart, 14th Edition, Chap. 86)* Chronotropic incompetence (CI) is most commonly defined as the inability of the sinus node to achieve at least 85%, 80%, or less commonly 70% of the age-predicted maximal heart rate (APMHR, 220 – age) obtained during an incremental dynamic exercise test (option A). CI has also been determined from change in HR from rest to peak exercise during an exercise test, commonly referred to as the HR reserve. Adjusted (percent) HR reserve is determined from the change in HR from rest to peak exercise divided by the difference of the resting HR and the APMHR. Most studies in the literature have used failure to attain >80% of the HR reserve, measured during a graded exercise test, as the primary criterion for CI (option E).[6] It is present in approximately 20% to 60% of patients with sinus node dysfunction (option C). Although the resting heart rates may be normal, these patients may have either the inability to increase their heart rate during exercise or unpredictable fluctuations in heart rate during activity. Some patients may initially experience a normal increase in heart rate with exercise, which then plateaus or decreases inappropriately.

Chronotropic incompetence may be secondary to intrinsic sinus node dysfunction or secondary to drugs with negative chronotropic effects (option B). Chronotropic incompetence is also common in patients with heart failure (option D).[7]

86-4. **The answer is B.** *(Hurst's The Heart, 14th Edition, Chap. 86)* It is now well accepted that long-term right ventricular (RV) pacing causes a deterioration of left ventricular (LV) function through complex effects on regional ventricular wall strain and loading conditions. This deterioration is thought to result from intraventricular dyssynchrony between different regions of the left ventricle induced by RV apical pacing. Sweeney and coworkers demonstrated, by careful review of data from MOST, that an increase in the frequency of ventricular pacing in patients with sick sinus syndrome who had a narrow native QRS complex was associated with an increased incidence of atrial fibrillation and congestive heart failure.[8] These observations were confirmed by Wilkoff and colleagues in the Dual Chamber and VVI Implantable Defibrillator (DAVID) study, in which backup ventricular pacing and dual-chamber pacing were prospectively compared in patients with dual-chamber defibrillators.[9] A composite of congestive heart failure, hospitalization, and death was increased by a factor of 1.6 in patients with an increased frequency of ventricular pacing. In patients with sinus node dysfunction, it is recommended to have the pacemaker programmed to either AAI(R) or DDD(R) with an algorithm that minimizes unnecessary ventricular pacing. Only option B would prevent unnecessary ventricular pacing. DDD pacing (with or without rate-response on) (options A and D) with a paced AV delay of 180 ms would result in unnecessary ventricular pacing in this patient with a baseline PR of 170 ms. Options C and E would result in unnecessary ventricular pacing with AV dyssynchrony.

86-5. **The answer is C.** *(Hurst's The Heart, 14th Edition, Chap. 86)* A hypersensitive response to carotid sinus stimulation of 5 to 10 seconds is defined as asystole caused by sinus arrest or AV block of > 3 seconds (cardioinhibitory), a substantial symptomatic decrease in systolic blood pressure of 50 mm Hg or more (vasodepressor), or both (mixed). Option C is the only correct answer. In option A, neurocardiogenic syncope must be significantly symptomatic and associated with documented bradycardia before a pacemaker is indicated. In option B, recurrent syncope in the presence of a hypersensitive cardioinhibitory response of 3 or more seconds is necessary. Options D and E represent class III indications for pacemaker implantation.

86-6. **The answer is E.** *(Hurst's The Heart, 14th Edition, Chap. 86)* Mutations in the cardiac-specific sodium channel gene (*SCN5A*) have been associated with progressive cardiac conduction system disease (PCCD) (option B).[10] A variety of inherited heart diseases has been reported to be associated with dilated cardiomyopathy and conduction system disease, including disorders of the nuclear envelope proteins lamin A and C (option D).[11] Lamin A/C is necessary for the structural integrity of the nucleus. This patient may well harbor a lamin A/C mutation. Many common drugs, including β-adrenergic blockers, calcium channel antagonists, digoxin, class I and III antiarrhythmic drugs, tricyclic antidepressants, phenothiazines, lithium (option A), and donepezil (a cholinesterase inhibitor used to treat Alzheimer disease), can cause AV conduction disturbances. Cardiac sarcoidosis should be considered in the differential diagnosis in a young patient presenting with CHB.[12] The current expert consensus on arrhythmias associated with cardiac sarcoidosis is that in patients aged < 60 years presenting with unexplained Mobitz II second-degree AV block or complete heart block, further evaluation with high-resolution chest CT and/or cardiac MRI may be necessary for diagnosis.[13] Certain neuromuscular disorders (myotonic dystrophy, Kearns–Sayre syndrome, peroneal muscular atrophy, Erb limb-girdle dystrophy, Emory–Dreifuss muscular dystrophy, and X-linked muscular dystrophies) may give rise to progressive and insidiously developing conduction disorders of the His–Purkinje system. Myotonic dystrophy (option E) and Kearns–Sayre syndrome are associated with a high incidence of unpredictable and rapidly progressive conduction system disease[14] for which therapy for myotonic dystrophy has *not* been shown to reverse the presence of AV block.

86-7. **The answer is D.** *(Hurst's The Heart, 14th Edition, Chap. 86)* In patients with a 2:1 AV block, vagal maneuvers are helpful in diagnosing the level of AV block. Carotid sinus stimulation may worsen the degree of block if it is in the AV node (option C), whereas slowing of the sinus rate may paradoxically *improve* the ratio of AV conduction and *increase* ventricular rate if the block is located in the His–Purkinje system (option D). A 2:1 AV block pattern with normal QRS duration or with a very long PR interval generally suggests block in the AV node (option A). A 2:1 AV block pattern in the presence of bundle branch block, especially in the setting of a normal PR interval, favors block below the AV node, but it is not diagnostic (option B). A prolonged electrocardiographic recording may sometimes reveal a transition to varying degrees of AV block (3:2 or 4:3), with type I or type II features that aid in the diagnosis. Rarely, Wenckebach conduction may be noted in the His–Purkinje system.

86-8. **The answer is C.** *(Hurst's The Heart, 14th Edition, Chap. 86)* Current guidelines indicate that cardiac resynchronization therapy (CRT) can be useful for patients with symptomatic heart failure (HF) and LVEF ≤ 35% who are expected to require frequent ventricular pacing (> 40%) after device implantation. The only answer option with these criteria is option C. The role of biventricular (BiV) pacing in patients with AV block and a *normal* LVEF or *only modest* depression of LV function remains unsettled. The Biventricular Versus RV Pacing in Heart Failure Patients with Atrioventricular Block (BLOCK HF) study was a prospective trial that randomized 691 patients with mild to moderate heart failure (NYHA class I, II, or III), LV dysfunction (LVEF ≤ 0.50), and AV block to RV pacing versus BiV pacing with an average follow-up of 37 months.[15] Patients randomly assigned to biventricular pacing had a significantly lower incidence of the primary outcome (time to death from any cause, an urgent care visit for heart failure that required intravenous therapy, or a 15% or more increase in the left ventricular end-systolic volume index) over time than did those assigned to RV pacing (hazard ratio, 0.74; 95% credible interval, 0.60 to 0.90).

86-9. **The answer is D.** *(Hurst's The Heart, 14th Edition, Chap. 86)* Alternating bundle branch block in the setting of chronic bifascicular and trifascicular block, even in asymptomatic patients, is a sign of advanced conduction disturbance, and it is an indication for implantation of a pacemaker (class I indication, level of evidence: B). Patients with bifascicular block (right bundle branch block and left anterior or posterior fascicular block) or left bundle branch block and left axis deviation have a 6% annual incidence of progression to complete heart block.[16] In patients with acute MI, the development of new bifascicular block and first-degree AV block is associated with a very high risk (42%) for progression to high-grade AV block. It is generally recommended that these patients undergo prophylactic temporary pacing. The patient in the question did not have an acute MI, and asymptomatic bifascicular block with a first degree AV block is not an indication to proceed with pacing. In patients with bundle branch block, His-bundle recordings can occasionally be helpful in identifying patients at high risk for progression to high-grade AV block. The incidental findings of markedly prolonged H-V interval (> 100 ms) (*not* ≥ 60ms – option A) or atrial-pacing–induced infra-Hisian block[17] that is not physiologic during an electrophysiology study is believed to indicate a high risk for progression to advanced AV block, and prophylactic permanent pacing is recommended.

86-10. **The answer is B.** *(Hurst's The Heart, 14th Edition, Chap. 86)* The telemetry strip demonstrates a sinus pause that is twice the length of the preceding P-P interval, suggesting sinoatrial exit block. The ladder diagram depicts sinoatrial (SA) nodal type I exit block. In SA exit block, the impulse is formed in the sinus node but fails to conduct to the atria. In sinus arrest (option C), there is a failure of the sinus node to discharge with lack of atrial activation of sinus origin. This results in the absence of P waves and periods of ventricular asystole if lower pacemakers (junctional or ventricular) do not initiate escape beats. Tachycardia-bradycardia syndrome (option A) is defined as sinus bradycardia interspersed with periods of atrial tachyarrhythmias; it is a common manifestation of sinus node dysfunction. Chronotropic incompetence (option D) is defined as the inability of the sinus node to achieve at least 80% to 85% of the age-predicted maximal heart rate (220 – age) during an incremental dynamic exercise test. Persistent atrial standstill (option E) is a rare clinical syndrome in which there is no spontaneous atrial activity, and the atria cannot be electrically stimulated. The surface ECG usually reveals junctional bradycardia without atrial activity. This must be distinguished from fine atrial fibrillation with complete heart block. Atria are generally fibrotic and without any functional myocardium.

References

1. Duhme N, Schweizer PA, Thomas D, et al. Altered HCN4 channel C-linker interaction is associated with familial tachycardia-bradycardia syndrome and atrial fibrillation. *Eur Heart J*. 2013;34:2768-2775.

2. Venetucci L, Denegri M, Napolitano C, Priori SG. Inherited calcium channelopathies in the pathophysiology of arrhythmias. *Nat Rev Cardiol*. 2012;9:561-575.

3. Butters TD, Aslanidi OV, Inada S, et al. Mechanistic links between Na⁺ channel (*SCN5A*) mutations and impaired cardiac pacemaking in sick sinus syndrome. *Circ Res*. 2010;107:126-137.

4. Le Scouarnec S, Bhasin N, Vieyres C, et al. Dysfunction in ankyrin-B-dependent ion channel and transporter targeting causes human sinus node disease. *Proc Natl Acad Sci USA*. 2008;105:15617-15622.

5. Robinson ML, Kobayashi T, Higgins Y, et al. Lyme carditis. *Infect Dis Clinic North Am*. 2015;29:255-268.

6. Okin PM, Lauer MS, Kligfield P. Chronotropic response to exercise: improved performance of ST-depression criteria after adjustment for heart rate reserve. *Circulation*. 1996;94:3226-3231.

7. Brubaker PH, Kitzman DW. Chronotropic incompetence: causes, consequences and management. *Circulation*. 2011;123:1010-1020.

8. Sweeney MO, Helkamp AS, Ellenbogen KA, et al. Adverse effect of ventricular pacing on heart failure and atrial fibrillation among patients with a normal QRS duration in a clinical trial of pacemaker therapy for sinus node dysfunction. *Circulation*. 2003;107:2932-2937.

9. Wilkoff BL, Cook JR, Epstein AE, et al. Dual chamber pacing or ventricular backup pacing in patients with an implantable defibrillator: the Dual Chamber and VVI Implantable Defibrillator (DAVID) trial. *JAMA*. 2002;288:3115-3123.

10. Kovach JR, Benson DW. Conduction disorders and Na$_v$1.5. *Card Electrophysiol Clin*. 2014;6:723-731.

11. Lamas GA, Lee KL, Sweeney M, et al. Ventricular pacing or dual chamber pacing for sinus node dysfunction. *N Engl J Med*. 2002;346:1854-1862.

12. Doughan AR, Williams BR. Cardiac sarcoidosis. *Heart*. 2006;92:282-288.

13. Birnie DH, Sauer DH, Bogan F, et al. HRS expert consensus statement on the diagnosis and management of arrhythmias associated with cardiac sarcoidosis. *Heart Rhythm*. 2014;11:1304-1323.

14. Kabunga P, Lau AK, Phan K, et al. Systematic review of cardiac electrical disease in Kearns-Sayre syndrome and mitochondrial cytopathy. *Int J Cardiol*. 2015;181:303-310.

15. Curtis AB, Worley SJ, Adamson PB, et al. Biventricular pacing for atrioventricular block and systolic dysfunction. *N Eng J Med*. 2013;368:1585-1593.

16. Dhingra RC, Amat-Y-Leon F, Wyndham C, et al. Significance of left axis deviation in patients with left bundle branch block. *Am J Cardiol*. 1978;42:551-556.

17. Scheinman MM, Peters RW, Suave MJ, et al. Value of the H-Q interval in patients with bundle branch block and the role of prophylactic permanent pacing. *Am J Cardiol*. 1982;50:1316-1322.

CHAPTER 87

Antiarrhythmic Drugs

Jacqueline Joza

DIRECTIONS: Choose the one best response to each question.

87-1. All of the following are sodium channel blockers *except*:

A. Flecainide
B. Procainamide
C. Disopyramide
D. Sotalol
E. Quinidine

87-2. You are seeing a 50-year-old man in the emergency department for new-onset atrial fibrillation (AF). The patient's palpitations started 2 hours ago. The emergency room doctor has already given a dose of intravenous metoprolol, which has resulted in minimal slowing of the ventricular rate. You decide to give oral propafenone due to its marked increase in sodium channel blockade during tachycardia. This specific characteristic of class Ic antiarrhythmics is known as:

A. Reverse use dependence
B. Use dependence
C. Reentry
D. Triggered activity
E. Abnormal automaticity

87-3. Which of the following medications or risk factors is *least* likely to concern you for the development of torsades de pointes?

A. Quinidine
B. Procainamide
C. Congenital long QT syndrome
D. Female gender
E. Amiodarone

87-4. Why are the class Ia antiarrhythmic drugs relatively contraindicated in structural heart disease?

A. They inhibit the sodium current (I_{Na}) at higher doses leading to conduction slowing and a decrease in myocardial contractility
B. They inhibit the rapidly activating delayed rectifier potassium current (I_{Kr}) at higher doses leading to conduction slowing and a decrease in myocardial contractility
C. They decrease myocardial contractility primarily through an α-blocking effect that can produce hypotension
D. They inhibit the L-type calcium current ($I_{Ca,L}$) in the sinoatrial and AV nodes, causing bradycardia and decreased myocardial contractility
E. They exert a strong α-adrenergic blocking effect that may decrease myocardial contractility

87-5. Which one of the following pairs of medications and their responsible metabolic enzymes is matched *incorrectly*?

A. Metoprolol/CYP2D6
B. Amiodarone/CYP3A4
C. Flecainide/CYP2D6
D. Diltiazem/CYP2D6
E. Lidocaine/CYP3A4

87-6. A 21-year-old man is brought to the hospital by ambulance after a syncopal episode. He has been followed for asymptomatic preexcitation (delta wave) on his baseline electrocardiogram. In the emergency department he develops an irregular wide-complex tachycardia consistent with preexcited AF. You decide to give intravenous procainamide. All are potential adverse effects of procainamide *except*:

A. Hypotension
B. Photosensitivity
C. Systemic lupus erythematosus–like reaction
D. Granulocytosis
E. QT prolongation

87-7. A 70-year-old woman known for ischemic cardiomyopathy presents to the emergency department with palpitations and dizziness. She is found to be in ventricular tachycardia (VT) at a rate of 180 bpm. Her current medications include carvedilol 3.125 mg twice daily, ramipril 5 mg once daily, digoxin 0.125 mg once daily, and warfarin. You start intravenous amiodarone. Which of the following statements is *incorrect*?

A. Amiodarone has properties of all four classes of the Vaughan-Williams classification
B. Amiodarone may raise the plasma concentration of digoxin
C. If continuing amiodarone long-term, hepatic, thyroid, and pulmonary functions need to be assessed on a regular basis
D. The dose of warfarin should be decreased to prevent a supratherapeutic international normalized ratio
E. Intravenous amiodarone, as compared to oral dosing, exhibits an acute inhibitory effect on I_{Kr}, I_{Ks}, I_{K1}, and I_{to}

87-8. A 30-year-old woman is brought by ambulance to the hospital after a syncopal episode. In the ambulance she develops a wide complex tachycardia with a stable blood pressure. Electrocardiogram confirms VT. She is given a small dose of an intravenous beta-blocker without change in the rhythm. At arrival, the patient states that she may be pregnant. Which of the following medications would be *most* suitable to convert her VT?

A. Lidocaine
B. Dronedarone
C. Amiodarone
D. Flecainide
E. Mexiletine

87-9. You are seeing a 60-year-old man with AF. He has failed both flecainide and sotalol for rhythm control managment, but the patient is not interested in catheter ablation for his AF at this time. You consider starting dronedarone. Which of the following scenarios should dronedarone *not* be started in?

A. First-degree AV block
B. Permanent AF
C. Mitral valve prolapse
D. Hypothyroidism
E. Chronic obstructive pulmonary disease

87-10. Digoxin is eliminated by a single pathway that uses P-glycoprotein. Coadministration with which of the following would *not* result in digoxin toxicity?

A. Amiodarone
B. Quinidine
C. Verapamil
D. Azithromycin
E. Dabigatran

ANSWERS

87-1. **The answer is D.** *(Hurst's The Heart, 14th Edition, Chap. 87)* d,l-Sotalol is a racemate of *d* and *l* isomers, and it is a Vaughan-Williams class III antiarrhythmic drug that blocks potassium channels, specifically the rapidly activated component of the delayed rectifier outward potassium current (I_{Kr}).[1] In addition, the *l* isomer also exhibits nonselective beta-blocking activity. Electrophysiologic effects of sotalol include an increase in action potential duration in both the atria and ventricles and a decrease in sinus rate and AV conduction. Flecainide (option A) is a sodium channel blocker (class Ic antiarrhythmic drug), which specifically blocks the channel in its open state with slow recovery from block. Procainamide (option B), disopyramide (option C), and quinidine (option E) are all Vaughan-Williams class Ia antiarrhythmic drugs. These block the sodium channel in its open state, with an intermediate recovery from block. They also inhibit I_{Kr} at relatively lower concentrations. There is moderate phase 0 depression and conduction slowing with prolongation of the action potential. Lidocaine and mexiletine are both examples of class Ib antiarrhythmic drugs that block the sodium channel in its inactivated state.

87-2. **The answer is B.** *(Hurst's The Heart, 14th Edition, Chap. 87)* The class Ic drugs (flecainide and propafenone) dissociate from the sodium channels in the resting state very slowly, exhibiting strong use dependence that manifests as a marked increase in sodium channel blockade during tachycardia. This is thought to be responsible for the increased efficacy of the class Ic antiarrhythmic drugs in slowing and converting tachycardia with minimal effects at normal sinus rates. However, strong use dependence of a drug on I_{Na} may be proarrhythmic (eg, flecainide-induced atrial flutter or VT) when the effect of the drug on conduction slowing is stronger than its effect on the effective refractory period. Reverse use dependence (option A) is observed during inhibition of I_{Kr}, which is enhanced during *bradycardia* when the channel is "not frequently used," leading to more significant action potential prolongation at slow heart rates. Most of the class III drugs, such as sotalol, demonstrate reverse use dependence. Reentry (option C), triggered activity (option D), and abnormal automaticity (option E) are all mechanisms of arrhythmia initiation.

87-3. **The answer is E.** *(Hurst's The Heart, 14th Edition, Chap. 87)* Torsades de pointes (TdP) requires QT prolongation.[2] It is widely accepted that TdP is initiated by early afterdepolarization (EAD)–dependent triggered activity and maintains itself via functional reentry.[3] Class Ia and class III antiarrhythmic drugs that block I_{Kr} and/or increase late I_{Na} may facilitate the development of TdP. Quinidine (option A) and procainamide (option B) are class Ia antiarrhythmics that may cause a prolongation in the QT interval. Interestingly, amiodarone (option E), a commonly used class III antiarrhythmic drug, significantly prolongs the QT interval but rarely causes TdP. Amiodarone prolongs the action potential duration without producing EADs and reduces transmural dispersion of repolarization, probably as a consequence of its effects on multiple ionic channels and receptors.[4] Marked QT prolongation and resultant TdP are more likely to occur in patients with reduced repolarization reserve. Clinical diseases or factors that are associated with reduced repolarization reserve include congenital long QT syndrome (option C), bradycardia, female sex (option D), ventricular hypertrophy, electrolyte disturbances such as hypokalemia and hypomagnesemia, and coadministration of other QT-prolonging agents or drugs that delay the clearance of the drugs from the body.

87-4. **The answer is A.** *(Hurst's The Heart, 14th Edition, Chap. 87)* The class Ia antiarrhythmic drugs include quinidine, procainamide, and disopyramide. The common electrophysiologic feature of class Ia drugs is that the drugs block the rapidly activating delayed rectifier potassium current (I_{Kr}) at relatively lower concentrations than their effect on I_{Na}. This is the reason they may cause QT prolongation that may lead to torsades de pointes. However, at higher doses, they inhibit I_{Na}, with an intermediate time constant of dissociation from the sodium channel, leading to conduction slowing and a decrease in myocardial contractility (option A). Consequently, the class Ia agents are relatively contraindicated in structural heart disease. Quinidine also has α-blocking effect that can produce hypotension (option C) but is not the mechanism through which it causes decreased myocardial contractility. Class IV antiarrhythmic drugs (the nondihydropyridine calcium channel blockers) such as verapamil and diltiazem specifically inhibit calcium-dependent ($I_{Ca,L}$) slow action potentials in the sinoatrial and AV nodes and should be avoided in patients with advanced heart failure or hypotension (option D). In addition to inhibiting sympathetic activity through β-adrenergic blockade, carvedilol and labetalol (class II antiarrhythmics) also have strong α-adrenergic blocking effect (option E). Although β-adrenergic blockers, when used in patients with compensated heart failure, reduce symptoms of heart failure and improve survival, their use in patients with decompensated heart failure who need inotropic support of intravenous agents should be avoided.

87-5. **The answer is D.** *(Hurst's The Heart, 14th Edition, Chap. 87)* CYP3A4 is the most prevalent enzyme in the liver and plays a role in the metabolism of many drugs, including amiodarone (option B), quinidine, lidocaine (option E), and many calcium channel blockers including diltiazem (option D). This enzyme is inhibited by multiple agents, which include cimetidine, erythromycin, fluconazole, and grapefruit juice. Use of these agents causes the accumulation of higher concentrations of the parent compound and thus an exaggerated electrophysiologic effect. CYP2D6 is the enzyme responsible for the metabolism of propafenone, flecainide (option C), acebutolol, metoprolol (option A), and propranolol. Most patients are *extensive metabolizers*, which means that a large percentage of the parent compound is transformed into a metabolite with activity that is identical to, similar to, or dissimilar from the parent. However, 5% to 10% are *poor metabolizers*, producing poor clearance with increased drug concentration, for which significant beta blockade can occur with an increased risk of asthma.

87-6. **The answer is B.** *(Hurst's The Heart, 14th Edition, Chap. 87)* In Wolff-Parkinson-White syndrome (preexcitation of the ventricles via accessory pathway(s) between the atria and ventricles), AF with rapid ventricular response may mimic VT, in which AV-blocking agents are relatively contraindicated. Intravenous procainamide inhibits conduction in the accessory pathway(s) and therefore effectively slows the ventricular response to AF. Procainamide can cause nausea, anorexia, vomiting, rash, and granulocytosis (option D). Intravenous administration of procainamide may result in hypotension (option A). A systemic lupus erythematosus–like reaction (option C) is fairly common (10%–20%), particularly in slow acetylators who have a higher procainamide concentration and a lower NAPA level. Procainamide can cause QT prolongation (option E), likely via its active metabolite NAPA. However, the incidence of TdP is lower than with quinidine, and it typically only occurs at high plasma concentrations (> 30 µg/mL). Photosensitivity is an adverse effect of *amiodarone*.

87-7. **The answer is E.** *(Hurst's The Heart, 14th Edition, Chap. 87)* While amiodarone is designated as a class III agent, it has properties of all four classes of the Vaughan-Williams classification (option A). The electrophysiologic effects of intravenous amiodarone differ from oral amiodarone; when given intravenously, amiodarone exhibits acute inhibitory effects on I_{Na} and $I_{Ca,L}$ (option E), whereas oral amiodarone has a delayed onset of action, which takes at least 2 to 3 days, that mainly targets outward currents. Chronic administration of amiodarone inhibits multiple outward potassium currents, including I_{Kr}, I_{Ks}, I_{K1}, and I_{to}. Amiodarone exerts its antiadrenergic effects by noncompetitive binding to β-adrenergic receptors and inhibition of agonist-induced increases in adenylate cyclase activity. These combined effects may lead to QT prolongation, a slight increase in QRS duration, and a profound inhibitory effect on sinus node and AV conduction. Amiodarone may raise the plasma concentration of digoxin (option B) and warfarin (option D), leading to serious toxicities. Therefore, doses of these two drugs often need to be adjusted when amiodarone is started. Because amiodarone may cause significant extracardiac adverse effects, hepatic, thyroid, and pulmonary functions need to be assessed on a regular basis (option C).

87-8. **The answer is A.** *(Hurst's The Heart, 14th Edition, Chap. 87)* The strong majority of antiarrhythmic drugs are US Food and Drug Administration (FDA) Category C, meaning

TABLE 87-1 Antiarrhythmic Drugs and Pregnancy

Drug	FDA Class[a]	Indications	Possible Adverse Effects	Comments
Quinidine	C	SVT/CBT and VT	Maternal and fetal thrombocytopenia, eighth nerve toxicity, and TdP	Long record of safety
Procainamide	C	SVT/CBT, VT, or undiagnosed WCT	Lupus-like syndrome with long-term use and TdP	Long record of safety
Disopyramide	C	Limited experience Induction of labor	Uterine contractions, premature labor, and TdP	Limited experience
Lidocaine	B	VT	CNS adverse effects and bradycardia	Long record of safety
Mexiletine	C	VT	CNS adverse effects and fetal bradycardia	Limited usage
Flecainide	C	SVT/CBT and selected VT	?	Used in fetal SVT with hydrops fetalis; more recent evidence of safety
Propafenone	C	SVT/CBT and selected VT	?	Used in fetal SVT with hydrops fetalis
β-Blockers	B-D	SVT, AF/AFL, selected VT, and LQTS	Intrauterine growth retardation, fetal bradycardia, hypoglycemia, and apnea	Generally safe; avoid during first trimester
Sotalol	B	SVT and VT	Bradycardia and TdP	Limited experience
Amiodarone	D	Life-threatening VT	Fetal hyper- or hypothyroidism, growth retardation, prematurity, bradycardia, and malformation	Avoid during first trimester
Dronedarone	X	–	Fetal vascular and skeletal malformations	Absolutely contraindicated in pregnancy
Ibutilide	C	Acute termination of AF/AFL	TdP	Limited record of safety
Verapamil	C	SVT, AF/AFL, and selected VT	Maternal hypotension, fetal bradycardia, and AV block	Relatively safe
Diltiazem	C	SVT and AF/AFL	Maternal hypotension, fetal bradycardia, and AV block	Verapamil preferred
Digoxin	C	SVT and AF/AFL	Low birth weight and premature labor	Long record of safety
Adenosine	C	Acute termination of SVT	Transient dyspnea and fetal bradycardia	Short duration of effect

aFDA pregnancy categories: A, no risk demonstrated in well-controlled studies in humans; B, no evidence of risk in humans; C, risk cannot be ruled out; D, positive evidence of risk; X, contraindicated in pregnancy. Abbreviations: AF/AFL, atrial fibrillation/flutter; AV, atrioventricular; CNS, central nervous system; FDA, Food and Drug Administration; LQTS, long QT syndrome; SVT, supraventricular tachycardia; SVT/CBT, supraventricular tachycardia using concealed bypass tract; TdP, torsade de pointes; VT, ventricular tachycardia; WCT, wide complex tachycardia; ?, unknown.
Modified with permission from Joglar JA, Page RL. Antiarrhythmic drugs in pregnancy. *Curr Opin Cardiol.* 2001 Jan;16(1):40-45.

that risk to the fetus cannot be ruled out (see Table 87-1). This is because of the paucity of randomized control trials (animal or human) necessary to demonstrate a higher level of evidence-based safety. Lidocaine (option A) is well tolerated and widely used in pregnancy, and it is classified as FDA pregnancy Category B (no evidence of risk in humans). Intravenous lidocaine is administrated primarily for the acute management of life-threatening ventricular arrhythmias. Flecainide (option D) appears to be a well-tolerated option for maternal arrhythmias, particularly AF, and it has evidence of safety in data with its use in treating fetal tachyarrhythmias.[5] Because propafenone (FDA pregnancy Category C, but more limited experience in pregnancy) and flecainide (FDA pregnancy Category C) have good transplacental passage, both have been used as second-line therapy for sustained fetal supraventricular arrhythmias, particularly in the presence of hydrops fetalis, that are refractory to digoxin.[5-6] Experience with mexiletine (FDA pregnancy Category C) (option E) in pregnancy is more limited.[6-7] Mexiletine may cause adverse CNS effects and fetal bradycardia. Dronedarone (option B) is an FDA Category X and is absolutely contraindicated because it has animal data showing teratogenic effects, specifically vascular and skeletal malformations. Amiodarone (option C) should be totally avoided or used with extreme caution for arrhythmias that are refractory to other drugs and are life threatening. Amiodarone causes hypothyroidism or hyperthyroidism, congenital abnormalities, bradycardia, premature labor, low birth weight, and prematurity.[8-9] Amiodarone is excreted in breast milk and can cause hypothyroidism or hyperthyroidism, but not significant bradycardia, in breast-fed infants.

87-9. The answer is B. *(Hurst's The Heart, 14th Edition, Chap. 87)* Dronedarone was approved for the treatment of atrial fibrillation and flutter by the US Food and Drug Administration (FDA) in 2009. It is an analog of amiodarone but is a noniodinated benzofuran derivative with the most significant molecular modification being removal of iodine and the addition of a methane sulfonyl group. Based on an adverse effect on mortality in ANDROMEDA (Antiarrhythmic Trial with Dronedarone in Moderate-to-Severe Congestive Heart Failure Evaluating Morbidity Decrease), dronedarone should be avoided in patients with advanced heart failure.[10-11] In addition, dronedarone should not be used in patients with permanent AF (option B) because of an increased risk for heart failure, stroke, and death with use in this population. This recommendation is based upon data from the PALLAS (Permanent Atrial Fibrillation Outcome Study Using Dronedarone on Top of Standard Therapy) trial, which was terminated early as a result of excess mortality and morbidity in patients in the dronedarone treatment group versus control.[12] Dronedarone is *not* associated with thyroid, neurologic, ocular, or pulmonary toxicity. Dronedarone leads to dose-dependent prolongation of the QT interval, but no TdP has been reported. Like amiodarone, it has a very low proarrhythmic risk, differentiating it from most other antiarrhythmics. The most common adverse effects of dronedarone are gastrointestinal, including nausea, vomiting, and diarrhea. Options A, C, D, and E do not represent contraindications to dronedarone use.

87-10. The answer is E. *(Hurst's The Heart, 14th Edition, Chap. 87)* Drug interactions resulting from interference with elimination also may occur. For example, digoxin is eliminated by a single pathway that uses P-glycoprotein. P-glycoprotein activity is inhibited by many drugs, including amiodarone (option A), quinidine (option B), verapamil (option C), and azithromycin (option D).[13] Thus, the coadministration of these agents with digoxin can result in digoxin toxicity. No potential interaction is noted between dabigatran and digoxin.

References

1. Hohnloser SH, Woosley RL. Sotalol. *N Engl J Med.* 1994;331:31-38.
2. Yan GX, Lankipalli RS, Burke JF, et al. Ventricular repolarization components on the electrocardiogram: cellular basis and clinical significance. *J Am Coll Cardiol.* 2003;42:401-409.
3. Yan GX, Wu Y, Liu T, et al. Phase 2 early after depolarization as a trigger of polymorphic ventricular tachycardia in acquired long-QT syndrome: direct evidence from intracellular recordings in the intact left ventricular wall. *Circulation.* 2001;103:2851-2856.
4. Van Opstal JM, Schoenmakers M, Verduyn SC, et al. Chronic amiodarone evokes no torsade de pointes arrhythmias despite QT lengthening in an animal model of acquired long-QT syndrome. *Circulation.* 2001;104:2722-2727.
5. Jaeggi ET, Carvalho JS, De Groot E, et al. Comparison of transplacental treatment of fetal supraventricular tachyarrhythmias with digoxin, flecainide, and sotalol: results of a nonrandomized multicenter study. *Circulation.* 2011;124:1747-1754.
6. Vergani P, Mariani E, Ciriello E, et al. Fetal arrhythmias: natural history and management. *Ultrasound Med Biol.* 2005;31:1-6.
7. Gregg AR, Tomich PG. Mexiletine use in pregnancy. *J Perinatol.* 1988;8:33-35.
8. Magee LA, Downar E, Sermer M, et al. Pregnancy outcome after gestational exposure to amiodarone in Canada. *Am J Obstet Gynecol.* 1995;172:1307-1311.
9. Bartalena L, Bogazzi F, Braverman LE, et al. Effects of amiodarone administration during pregnancy on neonatal thyroid function and subsequent neurodevelopment. *J Endocrinol Invest.* 2001;24:116-130.
10. Patel C, Yan GX, Kowey PR. Dronedarone. *Circulation.* 2009;120:636-644.
11. Kober L, Torp-Pedersen C, McMurray JJ, et al. Increased mortality after dronedarone therapy for severe heart failure. *N Engl J Med.* 2008;358:2678-2687.
12. Connolly SJ, Camm AJ, Halperin JL, et al. Dronedarone in high-risk permanent atrial fibrillation. *N Engl J Med.* 2011; 365:2268-2276.
13. Fromm MF, Kim RB, Stein CM, et al. Inhibition of P-glycoprotein-mediated drug transport: a unifying mechanism to explain the interaction between digoxin and quinidine. *Circulation.* 1999;99:552-557.

CHAPTER 88

Catheter-Ablative Techniques

Jacqueline Joza

QUESTIONS

DIRECTIONS: Choose the one best response to each question.

88-1. During the introduction of diagnostic catheters into the coronary sinus, right ventricle, and His regions, a right anterior oblique (RAO) fluoroscopy view is used. Which of the following cardiac structures can be differentiated with an RAO view?

A. Right atrium and left atrium
B. Atria and ventricles
C. Right ventricle and left ventricle
D. Medial and lateral cardiac silhouette
E. Septal and free wall

88-2. A 65-year-old woman is undergoing an electrophysiology study and ablation for atrial tachycardia. During the tachycardia, a map of the right atrium is created through the annotation of the local activation time (electrogram) compared to a fixed reference point (eg, the proximal coronary sinus catheter). What is this type of mapping called?

A. Entrainment mapping
B. Substrate mapping
C. Activation mapping
D. Pace mapping
E. Fluoroscopic mapping

88-3. During radiofrequency ablation for typical AV nodal reentrant tachycardia, the slow pathway is modified. The ablation catheter is positioned at the low posterior septum. At what temperature does cell death begin to occur?

A. 43°C to 49°C
B. ≥ 72°C

C. ≥ 50°C
D. ≥ 25°C
E. 90°C to 100°C

88-4. A 75-year-old woman is considering ablation of her recurrent and highly symptomatic supraventricular tachycardia. Electrocardiograms during the tachycardia reveal a narrow complex tachycardia with a short RP, consistent with probable typical AV nodal reentrant tachycardia (AVNRT). What is the success rate and approximate risk of permanent pacemaker implantation, respectively, of AVNRT ablation?

A. ≥ 95%/1%
B. ≥ 85%/1%
C. ≥ 95%/0.1%
D. ≥ 98%/0.01%
E. ≥ 85%/1%

88-5. A 25-year-old woman is being followed for persistent palpitations associated with dyspnea on minimal exertion. After some time, a diagnosis of inappropriate sinus tachycardia (IST) has been given. The long-term success of sinus node modification is limited, with frequent recurrences and persistent symptoms, and thus the role of ablation for IST is controversial. If she were to undergo IST ablation, which of the following complications would be *least* likely to occur?

A. Superior vena cava obstruction
B. Phrenic nerve paralysis
C. Sinus node dysfunction
D. Myocardial perforation
E. Pulmonary vein stenosis

88-6. You are having difficulty controlling the ventricular response rate of an 88-year-old woman with permanent atrial fibrillation (AF). Despite high doses of a beta-blocker and a calcium channel blocker, her ventricular rate persists at 110 to 130 bpm at rest. She underwent implantation of a dual-chamber pacemaker several years earlier for tachy-brady syndrome. Which of the following statements concerning atrioventricular node (AVN) ablation for this patient is *correct*?

A. Post-AVN ablation, she may discontinue oral anticoagulation

B. Post-AVN ablation, her risk of sudden cardiac death from polymorphic VT is high

C. Post-AVN ablation, she will no longer be in AF

D. Post-AVN ablation, an appropriate pacemaker setting is VVI 60 bpm

E. If she has poor left ventricular function before the procedure, her left ventricular function will definitely improve with AVN ablation

88-7. You are seeing a 42-year-old man in consult for premature ventricular contractions (PVCs). His baseline electrocardiogram reveals ventricular bigeminy. Which of the following is *not* an indication to pursue PVC ablation?

A. Symptoms that do not improve with medical therapy

B. PVC burden > 4000 / 24 hours, asymptomatic

C. Nonischemic cardiomyopathy, asymptomatic

D. PVC-triggered ventricular fibrillation episode

E. Medical therapy not desired

88-8. A 35-year-old woman presents to the emergency department with frequent symptomatic premature ventricular contractions (PVCs). Which of the following is *not* a characteristic of right ventricular outflow tract (RVOT) PVCs?

A. Left bundle branch block configuration in V_1

B. Inferiorly directed axis

C. Early precordial transition

D. May be suppressed with anesthesia

E. Negativity in leads aVR and aVL

88-9. The risk of complete heart block is small, but it is present during radiofrequency ablation of specific arrhythmias. Which of the following ablations is *least* likely to result in complete heart block?

A. PVC ablation at the interventricular septum

B. Anteroseptal WPW ablation

C. PVC ablation at the left coronary cusp of the aortic valve

D. Atrial tachycardia ablation at the noncoronary cusp of the aortic valve

E. Atypical atrioventricular nodal reentrant tachycardia ablation

88-10. Focal atrial tachycardias (ATs) represent approximately 10% of supraventricular tachycardias referred for ablation. Which of the following statements regarding focal ATs is *incorrect*?

A. Ablation for focal ATs is successful in $\geq$ 80% of patients

B. Foci in the left atrium often have a P wave that is positive in leads I and aVL

C. ATs may be paroxysmal, may occur in repetitive bursts, or may be incessant

D. Foci in the right atrium tend to have a negative terminal component in V_1

E. AT foci may originate at the crista terminalis, coronary sinus, and mitral valve annulus, among other regions

88-1. The answer is B. *(Hurst's The Heart, 14th Edition, Chap. 88)* Fluoroscopy provides a two-dimensional projection of the cardiac anatomy and catheter orientation, yet it is operator dependent, using either a single plane of view or two orthogonal views to create a three-dimensional location of catheters. The right anterior oblique (RAO) and the left anterior oblique (LAO) are common views. The RAO is a profile view of the heart. This differentiates the atrial and the ventricular components (option B); however, there is overlap of the left- and right-sided structures. The LAO view is an end-on view from the apex to base with foreshortening of the long axis of the heart. The LAO projection facilitates differentiating the left from the right side chambers (options A and C), the left and right heart borders (option D), and the septal from the free wall aspect within a chamber (option E).

88-2. The answer is C. *(Hurst's The Heart, 14th Edition, Chap. 88)* Cardiac mapping is performed with the acquisition of data during an arrhythmia; it can be achieved in a point-by-point manner or by the use of multielectrode mapping of multiple points simultaneously.[1] In *activation mapping* (option C), the local activation time (electrogram) can be annotated compared to a fiducial reference point (surface electrocardiogram [ECG] or fixed intracardiac electrode). Compilation of the activation times at all sites within a chamber depicts the spread of the activation wavefront. Macroreentrant arrhythmias occur as a result of continuous repetitive activation around a reentry circuit, and they are usually amenable to continuous resetting by pacing at a slightly faster mechanism and location of the reentry circuit (*entrainment mapping*) (option A).[2] *Substrate mapping* (option B) can be performed during sinus rhythm or during an arrhythmia (along with activation mapping) to identify diseased myocardial sites. Arrhythmogenic sites may have low-voltage, fractionated, or late activated electrograms that are targets for ablation.[3] *Pace mapping* (option D) is performed by pacing from various sites and comparing the generated surface ECG morphology to the template arrhythmia.[4] A pace match may identify regions close to the site of origin of a focal arrhythmia or the exit site of a reentrant tachycardia.[5]

88-3. The answer is C. *(Hurst's The Heart, 14th Edition, Chap. 88)* Initial attempts at catheter ablation of the AV node for supraventricular tachycardias were with high-energy direct current (DC) shocks. These were painful and resulted in uncontrolled lesions with a risk of life-threatening complications. The advent of radiofrequency (RF) energy in the ~500 kHz range has permitted more controlled and effective ablation by thermal injury. Reversible loss of myocardial excitability occurs between 43°C and 50°C (option A), and cell death occurs at tissue temperatures above 50°C (option C).[6] When the temperature reaches 100°C, plasma proteins denature to form a coagulum. The coagulum causes a sharp rise in the impedance and a corresponding fall in the current density, thereby limiting further lesion growth. The RF current density is highest at the electrode-tissue interface, and a 1- to 2-mm rim of tissue in contact with the electrode is resistively heated (ohmic heating). Passive conductive heating of the surrounding tissue results in a larger lesion.[7]

88-4. The answer is A. *(Hurst's The Heart, 14th Edition, Chap. 88)* AV nodal reentrant tachycardia (AVNRT) ablation is acutely successful in > 95% of cases, and it has a 5% recurrence rate.[8,9] The major risk is inadvertent damage to the compact AV node producing heart block that requires permanent pacemaker implantation (~1%).[8,9] Cryoablation has a lower risk of heart block but also has lower long-term efficacy.[10,11] Slow pathway ablation in the inferoseptal region may result in elevation of sinus heart rates for up to 6 months, possibly related to ablation of adjacent autonomic nerve fibers.[12]

88-5. The answer is E. *(Hurst's The Heart, 14th Edition, Chap. 88)* Inappropriate sinus tachycardia (IST) is an unccomon disorder characterized by sinus tachycardia out of proportion to physiologic demand. IST is often associated with fatigue and palpitations that respond poorly to pharmacologic therapy.[13] Catheter ablation is feasible to target sinus node tissue along the crista terminalis. The septal portion of the crista has the most rapid automaticity and is initially targeted, often reducing the sinus rate.[14] Ablation can be difficult because of the epicardial location of the sinus node, and epicardial ablation can be considered. The long-term success is limited, with frequent recurrences and persistent symptoms despite rate control in some patients.[14] Complications include superior vena cava obstruction, phrenic nerve paralysis, and sinus node dysfunction.[13,14] The role of ablation for IST is controversial, and it is not often recommended—even as a measure of last resort, with nonablative therapy being the accepted approach.

88-6. **The answer is B.** *(Hurst's The Heart, 14th Edition, Chap. 88)* Catheter ablation of the atrioventricular node (AVN) to create complete heart block with implantation of a permanent pacemaker is an option for controlling the heart rate in patients with AF and difficult-to-control ventricular rates.[15] This is typically a low-risk, relatively quick procedure with high efficacy. The heart rate is controlled without medications, and the ventricular rate in AF is regularized (option C). This leads to improvements in quality of life, exercise tolerance, and ejection fraction.[16] Several potential disadvantages require careful consideration before using this strategy. The atria usually continue to fibrillate, so patients remain at risk for thromboembolic complications (option A), and as a result, patients should remain on oral anticoagulation as determined by their stroke risk. The abrupt restoration of a slower rate with ventricular pacing has been associated with occasional cases of sudden death possibly caused by polymorphic VT (torsades de pointes) (option B). This risk appears to be largely mitigated by setting the pacemaker lower rate to 90 bpm for the first several weeks and then gradually reducing the rate over time (option D).[17] Further, chronic right ventricular (RV) apical pacing has important adverse hemodynamic consequences in some patients. Patients with poor left ventricular function and mitral regurgitation are at greatest risk for aggravation of heart failure with RV pacing, and biventricular pacemaker for cardiac resynchronization therapy may be warranted (option E).[16]

88-7. **The answer is B.** *(Hurst's The Heart, 14th Edition, Chap. 88)* Premature ventricular complexes (PVCs) can arise from any ventricular tissue, yet the outflow tracts and adjacent epicardial regions, papillary muscles, tricuspid and mitral valve annuli, and the fascicular conduction system are more common as sources of this form of arrhythmia.[4] Frequent PVCs can cause symptoms of palpitations, dyspnea, chest pain, lightheadedness, and anxiety. A very high burden of PVCs, typically > 10,000 or 20,000 per 24 hours (option B), can depress the left ventricular systolic function in a subset of patients. Analogous to tachycardia-mediated cardiomyopathy, suppression of PVCs can result in the resolution of ventricular dysfunction (option C).[4,18] PVC suppression may also be indicated when a consistent PVC triggers sustained ventricular fibrillation (option D) or tachycardia and results in syncope or implanted cardioverter-defibrillator (ICD) shocks.[4,19]

PVCs occasionally respond to beta-blockers or calcium channel blockers, and antiarrhythmic drugs like flecainide, sotalol, or amiodarone may be effective. When one or two PVC morphologies predominate, PVC ablation can be performed when drug therapy is ineffective (option A), not tolerated, or not desired (option E).[4,20]

88-8. **The answer is C.** *(Hurst's The Heart, 14th Edition, Chap. 88)* Most commonly, premature ventricular contractions (PVCs) arise from the right ventricular outflow tract (RVOT), and they have a left bundle branch block configuration in lead V_1 (option A) with an inferiorly directed axis (option B) and tall positive QRS complexes in leads II, III, and aVF. Leads aVR and aVL are negative, suggesting an origin at the left or right outflow tract (option E), and a *late* precordial transition (as compared to the native QRS) is seen in RVOT PVCs (option C). PVCs may be suppressed with anesthesia (option D), but they are sometimes inducible with isoproterenol or rapid ventricular pacing, resulting in calcium loading of cells and triggering of PVCs.[21] Activation mapping is critical to identify the earliest site of activation, and often a prepotential at the earliest site is the target of ablation.

88-9. **The answer is C.** *(Hurst's The Heart, 14th Edition, Chap. 88)* Ablation in proximity to the atrioventricular (AV) node, the fast pathway, and the His bundle in the mid and anterior septal region presents a risk of complete heart block. AV block can occur during ablation for typical or atypical AV nodal reentrant tachycardia (AVNRT) (option E), septal atrial tachycardias, mid and anteroseptal accessory pathways (option B), junctional tachycardia, and para-Hisian or septal PVCs (option A) or VT. Focal atrial tachcyardias arising from the peri-AV nodal region can be ablated from the noncoronary cusp (aortic sinus of Valsalva) because of its anatomic apposition with the anteroseptum (option D).[22] Injury to the essential AV conduction system can occur from the right heart chambers, aortic root, left ventricle, and left atrium. Ablation at the left coronary cusp should not result in heart block due to the distance from the AV node (option C). Because there is no distinct electrogram signature for the AV node, safety depends on an understanding of the critical anatomic relationships of the conduction system and on close monitoring of AV conduction during ablation. Early recognition of rapid junctional beats is crucial, and cryoablation may be considered when the risk of irreversible AV block with radiofrequency ablation is high.

88-10. **The answer is B.** *(Hurst's The Heart, 14th Edition, Chap. 88)* Focal atrial tachycardia (AT) represents approximately 10% of SVTs referred for ablation. AT may be paroxysmal, may occur in repetitive bursts, or may be incessant (option C). It may respond to beta-blockers, calcium channel blockers, and membrane-active antiarrhythmic drugs. Catheter ablation is an alternative to pharmacologic therapy.[8] AT foci tend to occur in specific anatomic locations, including the crista terminalis, tricuspid or mitral annulus, coronary sinus, atrial appendages, and the pulmonary veins (option E). Foci in the left atrium often have a P wave that is negative in leads I and aVL and positive in lead V_1 (option B); those from the right atrium tend to have a negative terminal component in V_1 (option D). AT originating from the septum has narrow P waves, whereas foci in the free walls have wider P waves, on account of simultaneous or sequential activation of the two atria.[8,23] The wide range of possible locations requires accurate mapping to identify the earliest site of activation to target ablation. Paroxysmal AT can, however, be difficult to induce in the electrophysiology lab, especially when sedation or anesthesia is used. Ablation is successful in > 80% of patients, with reported recurrence rates after successful ablation ranging from 4% to 27% (option A).[8]

References

1. Thajudeen A, Jackman WM, Stewart B, et al. Correlation of scar in cardiac MRI and high-resolution contact mapping of left ventricle in a chronic infarct model. *PACE.* 2015;38:663-674.

2. Stevenson WG, Sager PT, Friedman PL. Entrainment techniques for mapping atrial and ventricular tachycardias. *J Cardiovasc Electrophysiol* 1995;6:201-216.

3. Komatsu Y, Daly M, Sacher F, et al. Endocardial ablation to eliminate epicardial arrhythmia substrate in scar-related ventricular tachycardia. *J Am Coll Cardiol.* 2014;63:1416-1426.

4. Noheria A, Deshmukh A, Asirvatham SJ. Ablating premature ventricular complexes: justification, techniques, and outcomes. *Methodist DeBakey Cardiovasc J.* 2015;11:109-120.

5. de Chillou C, Groben L, Magnin-Poull I, et al. Localizing the critical isthmus of postinfarct ventricular tachycardia: the value of pace-mapping during sinus rhythm. *Heart Rhythm.* 2014;11:175-181.

6. Nath S, Lynch C 3rd, Whayne JG, Haines DE. Cellular electrophysiological effects of hyperthermia on isolated guinea pig papillary muscle. Implications for catheter ablation. *Circulation.* 1993;88:1826-1831.

7. Wittkampf FH, Nakagawa H. RF catheter ablation: lessons on lesions. *PACE.* 2006;29:1285-1297.

8. Wu J, Wu J, Olgin J, et al. Mechanisms underlying the reentrant circuit of atrioventricular nodal reentrant tachycardia in isolated canine atrioventricular nodal preparation using optical mapping. *Circ Res.* 2001;88:1189-1195.

9. Calkins H, Yong P, Miller JM, et al. Catheter ablation of accessory pathways, atrioventricular nodal reentrant tachycardia, and the atrioventricular junction: final results of a prospective, multicenter clinical trial. The Atakr Multicenter Investigators Group. *Circulation.* 1999;99:262-270.

10. Andrade JG, Khairy P, Dubuc M. Catheter cryoablation: biology and clinical uses. *Circ Arrhythm Electrophysiol.* 2013;6:218-227.

11. Jackman WM, Beckman KJ, McClelland JH, et al. Treatment of supraventricular tachycardia due to atrioventricular nodal reentry, by radiofrequency catheter ablation of slow-pathway conduction. *N Engl J Med.* 1992;327:313-318.

12. Becker AE, Anderson RH, Durrer D, Wellens HJ. The anatomical substrates of Wolff-Parkinson-White syndrome. A clinicopathologic correlation in seven patients. *Circulation.* 1978;57:870-879.

13. Marrouche NF, Beheiry S, Tomassoni G, et al. Three-dimensional nonfluoroscopic mapping and ablation of inappropriate sinus tachycardia. Procedural strategies and long-term outcome. *J Am Coll Cardiol.* 2002;39:1046-1054.

14. Perez FJ, Schubert CM, Parvez B, et al. Long-term outcomes after catheter ablation of cavo-tricuspid isthmus dependent atrial flutter: a meta-analysis. *Circ Arrhythm Electrophysiol.* 2009;2:393-401.

15. Curtis AB, Worley SJ, Adamson PB, et al. Biventricular pacing for atrioventricular block and systolic dysfunction. *N Engl J Med.* 2013;368:1585-1593.

16. Ozcan C, Jahangir A, Friedman PA, et al. Sudden death after radiofrequency ablation of the atrioventricular node in patients with atrial fibrillation. *J Am Coll Cardiol.* 2002;40:105-110.

17. January CT, Wann LS, Alpert JS, et al. 2014 AHA/ACC/HRS guideline for the management of patients with atrial fibrillation: a report of the American College of Cardiology/American Heart Association task force on practice guidelines and the Heart Rhythm Society. *Circulation.* 2014;130:e199-e267.

18. Haissaguerre M, Shoda M, Jais P, et al. Mapping and ablation of idiopathic ventricular fibrillation. *Circulation.* 2002;106:962-967.

19. Aliot EM, Stevenson WG, Almendral-Garrote JM, et al. EHRA/HRS expert consensus on catheter ablation of ventricular arrhythmias: developed in a partnership with the European Heart Rhythm Association (EHRA), a registered branch of the European Society of Cardiology (ESC), and the Heart Rhythm Society (HRS); in collaboration with the American College of Cardiology (ACC) and the American Heart Association (AHA). *Heart Rhythm.* 2009;6:886-933.

20. Lerman BB. Mechanism, diagnosis, and treatment of outflow tract tachycardia. *Nat Rev Cardiol.* 2015;12:597-608.

21. Nogami A, Naito S, Tada H, et al. Demonstration of diastolic and presystolic Purkinje potentials as critical potentials in a macroreentry circuit of verapamil-sensitive idiopathic left ventricular tachycardia. *J Am Coll Cardiol.* 2000;36:811-823.

22. Olshansky B, Sullivan RM. Inappropriate sinus tachycardia. *J Am Coll Cardiol.* 2013;61:793-801.

23. Park J, Wi J, Joung B, et al. Prevalence, risk, and benefits of radiofrequency catheter ablation at the aortic cusp for the treatment of mid- to anteroseptal supra-ventricular tachyarrhythmias. *Int J Cardiol.* 2013;167:981-986.

CHAPTER 89

Pacemakers and Defibrillators

Jacqueline Joza

DIRECTIONS: Choose the one best response to each question.

89-1. A 74-year-old man presents to the emergency department with shoulder pain. His past medical history is significant for a prior anterior wall myocardial infarction 3 years ago. Serial troponins are negative, and the shoulder pain is deemed to be musculosketal. An echocardiogram reveals an ejection fraction of 55%. However, his serial ECGs reveal sinus rhythm with alternating bundle branch blocks. His medications include aspirin 80 mg once daily and amlodipine 5 mg once daily. Which of the following statements is *correct*?

A. Proceed with dual-chamber pacemaker
B. Proceed with dual-chamber implantable cardioverter defibrillator (ICD)
C. Do not implant a device
D. Proceed with single-chamber pacemaker
E. Proceed with biventricular pacemaker

89-2. A 70-year-old woman with remote implantation of a dual-chamber pacemaker for symptomatic sinus bradycardia is hospitalized for several days with an episode of new-onset atrial fibrillation. During her hospitalization, her pacemaker was reprogrammed to VVI 60 bpm. You are seeing her in follow-up and note that she is now back in sinus rhythm. Which of the following is a *known* effect of single-chamber (ventricular-only) pacing in the presence of sinus rhythm?

A. Increased incidence of ventricular tachycardia
B. Increased mortality
C. Improved quality of life
D. Increased incidence of pacemaker syndrome
E. Decreased incidence of atrial fibrillation

89-3. In which of the following patients would the implantation of a pacemaker *not* be indicated?

A. 65-year-old woman, asymptomatic, permanent atrial fibrillation and one 5-second pause while awake
B. 35-year-old woman, asymptomatic sinus bradycardia at 35 bpm while awake
C. 65-year-old man, asymptomatic third-degree AV block during exercise stress testing in the absence of myocardial ischemia
D. 35-year-old man, asymptomatic, limb-girdle muscular dystrophy and type II second-degree AV block
E. 65-year-old man, asymptomatic, episodes of third-degree AV block with an escape rate of 35 bpm while awake

89-4. A 50-year-old man with a history of myocardial infarction 1 year ago presents with intermittent dizziness. He denies any chest pain, dyspnea, or syncope. In the emergency department, a 10-beat run of nonsustained VT is seen on the monitor. A transthoracic echocardiogram reveals a left ventricular ejection fraction (LVEF) of 35% to 40%, slightly decreased from an echo performed 2 years ago. Active coronary disease is ruled out with a stress-MIBI. Which of the following constitutes the next *best* course of action?

A. Implantation of an implantable cardioverter-defibrillator
B. Initiation of amiodarone
C. Referral for electrophysiology study
D. Referal for outpatient Holter monitoring
E. Organize for a wearable cardioverter-defibrillator

89-5. Which of the following patients represents a class III indication for cardiac resynchronization therapy (CRT) (assuming that all are on guideline-directed medical therapy)?

A. NYHA class II, LVEF ≤ 35%, atrial fibrillation, complete heart block

B. NYHA ambulatory class IV, LVEF ≤ 35%, sinus rhythm, RBBB 135 ms

C. NYHA class II, LVEF ≤ 35%, sinus rhythm, RBBB 135 ms

D. NYHA class II, LVEF ≤ 35%, sinus rhythm, LBBB > 150 ms

E. NYHA class II, LVEF ≤ 35%, sinus rhythm, LBBB 120 ms

89-6. An 80-year-old woman with a dual-chamber pacemaker presents with intermittent ventricular undersensing. Her ventricular lead is programmed to a unipolar configuration for improved sensing. When compared to a bipolar configuration, which of the following regarding a unipolar configuration is *incorrect*?

A. May lead to myopotential oversensing

B. Far-field sensing may be decreased

C. Cross-talk may be increased

D. May lead to skeletal muscle stimulation

E. Unipolar leads have one electrode in contact with the myocardium

89-7. A 70-year-old man is in a motor vehicle accident, with crush injury sustained to his upper torso. You decide to interrogate his implantable cardioverter-defibrillator because you suspect a lead fracture based on the CT scan. Which of the following statements is *incorrect*?

A. The lead impedance may be high

B. The lead impedance may be within normal limits

C. The lead impedance may be low

D. Both A and B are correct

E. Both B and C are correct

89-8. Regarding pacemaker nomenclature, which of the following is *false*?

A. The first letter represents the chamber being paced

B. The second letter represents the chamber being sensed

C. The third position describes the response of the device to a paced event

D. The device can either inhibit pacing output from one or both of its leads or it can trigger pacing after the sensed event

E. The fourth position refers to the programmability of the device: R for rate-responsive pacing

89-9. An 85-year-old woman presents with symptomatic sinus pauses of 5 seconds during waking hours. You refer her for pacemaker implantation. She wants to know the potential risks associated with the implant. Specifically, she would like to know about the possibility of pacemaker infection. Which of the following statements is *correct*?

A. The rate of acute infection after initial pacemaker implantation is approximately 3.5%

B. Early infections are generally caused by coagulase-negative staphylococci

C. Transthoracic echocardiography is the gold standard to determine whether vegetations are present on the pacemaker leads

D. The presence of hematoma after pacemaker implantation does not increase the risk for infection

E. Incisional or superficial infection with no bacteremia or involvement of the device can usually be managed with oral antibiotic therapy

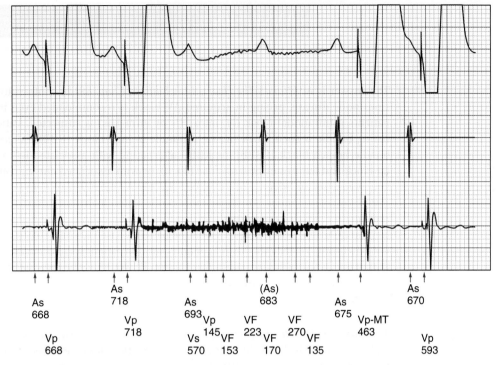

FIGURE 89-1 Surface electrocardiogram and atrial and ventricular electrograms with event markers are shown. As, atrial sensed; VF, ventricular fibrillation; Vp, ventricular paced; Vs, ventricular sensed.

89-10. Refer to Figure 89-1. For a 55-year-old man with a dual-chamber defibrillator, which of the following represents the most likely diagnosis?

A. Pacemaker-mediated tachycardia
B. Atrial fibrillation leading to mode switch
C. Ventricular capture failure
D. Atrial lead undersensing
E. Oversensing of diaphragmatic myopotentials

89-1. The answer is A. *(Hurst's The Heart, 14th Edition, Chap. 89)* In contrast to indications for sinus node disease, pacing in acquired AV block is recommended even in *asymptomatic* patients if infranodal block (ie, intra-His or infra-His) is suspected. Patients with alternating bundle branch block (ie, right bundle branch block [RBBB] alternating with left bundle branch block [LBBB], or RBBB alternating with associated left anterior fascicular block and left posterior fascicular block), or with associated chronic bifascicular block and type 2 second-degree or advanced AV block, meet a class I indication for pacing, *irrespective of symptoms.* An implantable cardioverter defibrillator (option B) would not be indicated because of the normal cardiac function on echo. A single-chamber pacemaker (option D) would not be correct given the patient's baseline sinus rhythm and the need for AV synchrony. Despite the likely scenario that this patient will be ventricular pacing most of the time, a biventricular pacemaker (option E) would not be indicated at this time given the normal cardiac function and the absence of New York Heart Association class II and greater.

89-2. The answer is D. *(Hurst's The Heart, 14th Edition, Chap. 89)* The largest randomized pacemaker study for isolated sinus node disease was the Mode Selection Trial (MOST).[1] The trial randomized a total of 2010 patients to either dual-chamber (atrial and ventricular) or single-chamber (ventricular-only) pacing. Neither the primary end point of death (option B) from any cause or nonfatal stroke, nor the secondary end point—a composite of death, stroke, or heart failure hospitalization—differed between patients assigned to either dual-chamber or ventricular-only pacing. The incidence of atrial fibrillation was less common with dual-chamber pacing (HR 0.79, $P = .008$) (option E), and heart failure scores were better ($P < .0001$), as were quality of life metrics (option C). Importantly, close to one-third of patients assigned to ventricular pacing crossed over to dual-chamber pacing. This was driven by the incidence of the pacemaker syndrome in half of all crossovers (option D). Notable here is that MOST had a strict definition for pacemaker syndrome, requiring the documentation of both symptoms of dyspnea or syncope and demonstration of ventriculoatrial (VA) conduction or blood pressure reduction of 20 mm Hg or more during ventricular-only pacing.

89-3. The answer is B. *(Hurst's The Heart, 14th Edition, Chap. 89)* Options A and C through E are all class I indications for permanent pacing. Class I recommendations for pacing for sinus node disease hinge primarily on the presence of symptoms. The indication for pacing exists when the heart rate is < 40 bpm and a *clear association between significant symptoms* consistent with bradycardia and the actual presence of bradycardia has not been documented (class IIa) or when patients are *minimally symptomatic* with chronic heart rates < 40 bpm while awake (class IIb).

89-4. The answer is C. *(Hurst's The Heart, 14th Edition, Chap. 89)* An implantable cardioverter-defibrillator (ICD) would be indicated in this patient if sustained ventricular tachycardia (VT) or ventricular fibrillation (VF) were induced with programmed electrical stimulation during electrophysiology (EP) study. The Multicenter Unsustained Tachycardia Trial (MUSTT) included 704 patients with coronary artery disease (> 4 days from the most recent myocardial infarction or revascularization procedure), left ventricular ejection fraction (LVEF) ≤ 40%, and asymptomatic nonsustained VT (NSVT) (lasting for ≥ 3 beats) who underwent EP study.[2] Patients with sustained VT or VF at the EP study were then randomized, either to antiarrhythmic therapy with ICD or EP-guided antiarrhythmic therapy, or to no antiarrhythmic therapy. The trial showed that, although patients with EP-guided therapy demonstrated a lower risk of arrhythmia, the risk of arrhythmic death was lowered only in patients assigned to ICD (RR 0.24 versus those who received EP-guided antiarrhythmic therapy, $P < .001$). Perhaps more than any other secondary-prevention trial, MUSTT makes a compelling argument for ICD among patients with CAD and inducible VT or VF, above and beyond medical therapy. A single-chamber ICD (option A) would not be indicated at this time without an LVEF of ≤ 35% with NYHA functional class II or III, or an LVEF of ≤ 30% with NYHA functional class I. Options B, D, and E would not be indicated at this time.

89-5. **The answer is C.** (*Hurst's The Heart, 14th Edition, Chap. 89*) CRT is *not* recommended for patients with NYHA class I or II symptoms and non-LBBB pattern with QRS duration < 150 ms (level of evidence: B): class III recommendation. However, CRT may be considered in patients with *NYHA class III or ambulatory class IV* symptoms (option B) with an LVEF of ≤ 35% with sinus rhythm, a non-LBBB pattern, and a QRS duration 120 to 149 ms on guideline-directed medical therapy (GDMT). CRT can be useful in patients with an LVEF ≤ 35%, sinus rhythm LBBB with a QRS duration of 120 to 149 ms, with NYHA class II, III, or ambulatory IV symptoms on GDMT (option E), and in patients with an LVEF ≤ 35% and atrial fibrillation on GDMT if (a) the patient requires ventricular pacing or otherwise meets CRT criteria (option A), and (b) AV nodal ablation or pharmacologic rate control will allow near 100% ventricular pacing with CRT. Finally, a class I indication is met for patients with an LVEF ≤ 35%, sinus rhythm, LBBB with a QRS duration ≥ 150 ms, and NYHA class II, III, or ambulatory IV symptoms on GDMT (option D).

89-6. **The answer is B.** (*Hurst's The Heart, 14th Edition, Chap. 89*) Pacing leads are identified as unipolar or bipolar based on the number of electrodes in contact with the myocardium, although all leads use a circuit with cathodal and anodal terminals. For example, unipolar leads carry a single conductor to a single electrode present at the lead tip (cathode), which is in contact with the myocardial tissue, and the surface of the pacemaker acts as the anodal terminal (option E). Bipolar lead systems, on the other hand, house two conductors in the lead body leading to a cathodal tip electrode and an anodal ring electrode, 10 to 20 mm proximal to the tip electrode. Most modern pacing systems allow for bipolar leads to be "programmed unipolar" based on the clinical scenario—for example, to increase the field of view for sensing or possibly to reduce the pacing output needed to capture the myocardium at a particular location. Downsides to the unipolar configuration are greater susceptibility than the bipolar configuration to myopotential oversensing (option A), far-field sensing (option B), cross-talk (atrial stimulus sensed by ventricular channel or vice-versa) (option C), and skeletal muscle stimulation (option D).

89-7. **The answer is D.** (*Hurst's The Heart, 14th Edition, Chap. 89*) Lead impedance is the resistance to the flow of current from the generator to the myocardial tissue through the lead. Although there is a wide variability of normal lead impedances (250 to 1200 Ω), chronic lead impedances should not vary widely between outpatient follow-up visits. A fractured lead exhibits markedly elevated lead impedance (option A). Insulation breaks are indicated by reduced lead impedances (option C). Lead fractures or insulation breaks often are intermittent problems. Therefore, normal lead impedances and pacing and sensing thresholds do not rule out these problems (option B). The leads can be stressed by having the patient change position and do various provocative arm movements (eg, isometric exercise) to facilitate the diagnosis of lead-related problems that are not otherwise observed. Many pacemakers intermittently monitor lead impedance and alert the physician to measured impedances that are out of the typical range.

89-8. **The answer is C.** (*Hurst's The Heart, 14th Edition, Chap. 89*) The North American Society of Pacing and Electrophysiology and the British Pacing and Electrophysiology Group established a five-letter pacemaker code to describe basic pacemaker mode and function.[3,4] The first letter represents the chamber being paced (option A) and the second the chamber being sensed (option B): A for atrium, V for ventricle, and D for both atrium and ventricle. The third position describes the response of the device to a *sensed* event (option C): I for inhibition, T for triggered, and D for both inhibition and triggering. The device can either inhibit (I) pacing output from one or both of its leads, or it can trigger (T) pacing after the sensed event (option D). In a DDD pacemaker, a sensed atrial event inhibits the atrial pacing channel and triggers ventricular pacing after a programmable AV delay. The fourth position refers to the programmability of the device: R for rate-responsive pacing (option E). The fifth position refers to antitachycardia function for pacemakers only; with the evolution of implantable defibrillators, this position is rarely used.

89-9. The answer is E. *(Hurst's The Heart, 14th Edition, Chap. 89)* The use of prophylactic antibiotics and pocket irrigation with antibiotic solutions has decreased the rate of acute infections after pacemaker implantations to < 1% to 2% in most series (option A). Periprocedural antibiotics have been validated in double-blinded clinical trials, and cefazolin is a commonly used agent.[5] Ongoing trials (PADIT) are being run to determine whether periprocedural antibiotics truly mitigate the infection risk.[6] Although early infections are generally caused by *Staphylococcus aureus* (option B) and may be aggressive, late infections associated with CIEDs may be associated with coagulase-negative staphylococci, and their course tends to be indolent.[7] The signs of infection include local inflammation and abscess formation, erosion of the pacer, and fever with positive blood cultures without an identifiable focus of infection. Post-procedural hematomas have been associated with an increased risk of infection.[8] Transesophageal echocardiography (*not transthoracic*) helps determine whether vegetations are present on the pacemaker leads (option C). Incisional or superficial infection with no bacteremia or involvement of the CIED can usually be managed with oral antibiotic therapy (option E). With that said, complete system removal is advocated for source control in patients with definite evidence of CIED system involvement (subcutaneous, transvenous, or epicardial) or lead-associated vegetation or valvular endocarditis without definite involvement of the leads (class I indication).[7] Patients with bacteremia but no localizing evidence of generator-site or clear lead involvement are a challenging group. In patients with relapsing or occult staphylococcal bacteremia, system explant is recommended (class I), and it may also be reasonable for gram-negative bacteremia (class IIa).

89-10. The answer is E. *(Hurst's The Heart, 14th Edition, Chap. 89)* Figure 89-1 reveals oversensing of diaphragmatic myopotentials causing inhibition of ventricular output. The surface electrocardiogram and atrial and ventricular electrograms with event markers are shown. The patient developed dizzy spells caused by underlying complete heart block and inhibition of pacing because of oversensing. The ventricular lead was repositioned in the right ventricular outflow tract, eliminating the diaphragmatic oversensing. In a single-chamber pacemaker or defibrillator, oversensing leads to the inhibition of the pacing channel and causes inappropriate pauses. However, in dual-chamber devices, oversensing elicits either inappropriate inhibition or triggering, depending on the channel in which oversensing occurs and the programmed pacing mode. Oversensing in the ventricular channel in the DDD or DDI mode results in the inhibition of both atrial and ventricular outputs and resetting of timing cycles. In patients with complete heart block, this may result in ventricular asystole (Figure 89-1). The artifact is noted in the lower (ventricular) channel and is too rapid (nonphysiologic) to represent atrial fibrillation; therefore option B is incorrect. Evidence for ventricular capture is present in the first and last two QRS complexes in the tracing (option C). There is no evidence of atrial undersensing (option D) or pacemaker-mediated tachycardia (option A).

References

1. Lamas GA, Lee KL, Sweeney MO, et al. Ventricular pacing or dual-chamber pacing for sinus-node dysfunction. *N Engl J Med.* 2002;346(24):1854-1862.
2. Buxton AE, Lee KL, Fisher JD, Josephson ME, Prystowsky EN, Hafley G. A randomized study of the prevention of sudden death in patients with coronary artery disease. Multicenter Unsustained Tachycardia Trial Investigators. *N Engl J Med.* 1999;341(25):1882-1890.
3. Singh JP, Klein HU, Huang DT, et al. Left ventricular lead position and clinical outcome in the multicenter automatic defibrillator implantation trial–cardiac resynchronization therapy (MADIT-CRT) trial. *Circulation.* 2011;123(11):1159-1166.
4. Bernstein AD, Camm AJ, Fletcher RD, et al. The NASPE/BPEG generic pacemaker code for antibradyarrhythmia and adaptive-rate pacing and antitachyarrhythmia devices. *Pacing Clin Electrophysiol.* 1987;10(4 Pt 1):794-799.

5. de Oliveira JC, Martinelli M, Nishioka SA, et al. Efficacy of antibiotic prophylaxis before the implantation of pacemakers and cardioverter-defibrillators: results of a large, prospective, randomized, double-blinded, placebo-controlled trial. *Circ Arrhythm Electrophysiol.* 2009;2(1):29-34.

6. Krahn AD, Philippon F, Exner DV, et al. Prevention of arrhythmia device infection trial (PADIT): pilot study results. *Canadian Journal of Cardiology.* 2012;28(5):S394.

7. Baddour LM, Epstein AE, Erickson CC, et al. Update on cardiovascular implantable electronic device infections and their management: a scientific statement from the American Heart Association. *Circulation.* 2010;121(3):458-477.

8. Birnie DH, Healey JS, Wells GA, et al. Pacemaker or defibrillator surgery without interruption of anticoagulation. *N Engl J Med.* 2013;368(22):2084-2093.

CHAPTER 90

Diagnosis and Management of Syncope

Jacqueline Joza

QUESTIONS

DIRECTIONS: Choose the one best response to each question.

90-1. Obstructive cardiac disorders associated with syncope include all of the following *except*:

A. Pulmonary embolism
B. Hypertrophic cardiomyopathy
C. Atrial myxoma
D. Cardiac tamponade
E. Supraventricular tachycardia

90-2. A 70-year-old woman presents after experiencing her third syncopal episode in the last year. The syncopal events always occur upon standing from a seated position. Which of the following does *not* occur immediately upon standing from a supine position?

A. Approximately 300 to 800 mL of blood is displaced to the lower limbs and the inferior mesenteric area
B. There is a mean decrease in stroke volume of approximately 40% within the first few seconds of standing
C. The discharge rate of the aortic arch and carotid sinus baroreceptors is increased
D. A decrease in efferent vagal activity is observed, with an increase in efferent sympathetic activity
E. A 10 to 15 bpm increase in heart rate is observed, with an approximately 10 mm Hg increase in diastolic blood pressure

90-3. A 60-year-old man presents to your office in consultation for syncope. He describes several episodes that occurred in the summertime. Which of the following aspects of his medical and medication history would convince you of a diagnosis of pure autonomic failure?

A. Use of a monoamine oxidase inhibitor
B. A history of constipation
C. A history of diabetes
D. A new diagnosis of sarcoidosis
E. Construction worker as an occupation

90-4. A 75-year-old man suffers a syncopal episode while shaving. Which of the following statements concerning the etiology of the syncope is *incorrect*?

A. A vasodepressor response may result
B. A cardioinhibitory response may result
C. Impulses to the medulla oblongata will activate efferent sympathetic and vagal efferent nerve fibers
D. Aortic arch baroreceptors are activated
E. This cause of syncope is most common in men ≥ 50 years old

90-5. You have followed a 52-year-old man in your clinic for frequent orthostatic syncope. In addition to a profound drop in the systolic pressure upon standing, he exhibited rigidity with a mild intention tremor. With time, he developed severe slurring of his speech, urinary and rectal incontinence, gait disturbance, and truncal ataxia. The patient died 5 years after his diagnosis. Which of the following represents the *correct* diagnosis?

A. Postural orthostatic tachycardia syndrome (POTS)
B. Neurocardiogenic syncope
C. Carotid sinus hypersensitivity
D. Multiple system atrophy
E. Acute autonomic failure

90-6. A 60-year-old man who complains of frequent dizziness has a sudden syncopal episode while painting his ceiling. Which of the following is *consistent* with an etiology of subclavian steal syndrome?

A. Increased brachial arterial pressure in one arm
B. Femoral bruit
C. Retrograde shunting to the distal subclavian artery
D. Adduction of the shoulder is a common precipitant
E. Vasospasm occurs at the level of the proximal subclavian artery

90-7. You decide to send your 25-year-old female patient for tilt-table testing. Which of the following is *false*?

A. The specificity of tilt-table testing is near 90%
B. The sensitivity of tilt-table testing is between 20% and 74%
C. The specificity of tilt-table testing increases with pharmacologic provocation
D. The reproducibility of the test (in a time frame ranging from several hours to weeks) is 80% to 90% for an initially positive response
E. The reproducibility of the test (in a time frame ranging from several hours to weeks) is 30% to 90% for an initially negative response

90-8. In which of the following scenarios would tilt-table testing be *least* useful?

A. 45-year-old man with unclear history of syncope versus epilepsy
B. 35-year-old woman with syncope at the sight of blood

C. 55-year-old man with syncope with longstanding diagnosis of diabetes
D. 45-year-old man with recurrent unexplained falls
E. 35-year-old man with recurrent syncope with injury in the absence of organic heart disease

90-9. You are counseling your 30-year-old female patient on treatment for her neurocardiogenic syncope. Which of the following is *not* a recommended treatment?

A. Tilt training
B. Isometric countermaneuvers
C. Sleeping with the head of the bed elevated 6 inches above the feet
D. Knee-high elastic support stockings, 10 to 15 mm Hg compression.
E. Salt and water loading

90-10. Abnormal tilt-table responses can be classified into five groups. Which of the following is *not* an example of a tilt-table response?

A. Epileptic response
B. Dysautonomic response
C. Postural tachycardic response
D. Classic neurocardiogenic response
E. Cerebral syncope

ANSWERS

90-1. **The answer is E.** (*Hurst's The Heart, 14th Edition, Chap. 90*) Obstruction to cardiac output in the left or right side of the heart may cause syncope. The relationship of syncope to exertion may provide clues to the etiology. Loss of consciousness during or immediately after exertion can occur with any of the cardiac causes of syncope, but it is particularly common and may be the presenting symptom in patients with certain obstructive lesions, including aortic stenosis and hypertrophic cardiomyopathy (option B). Studies suggest that in such patients, the failure of cardiac output to increase adequately during exercise together with a reflex decrease in peripheral vascular resistance may play a role.[1] Nonexertional syncope related to acute decreases in preload or afterload or to inotropic stimulation may also occur in either aortic stenosis or hypertrophic cardiomyopathy. Other cardiac disorders associated with syncope include mitral stenosis, typically in the setting of tachycardia or other arrhythmia, atrial myxoma (option C), obstruction in the pulmonary vasculature as a result of pulmonary artery hypertension, pulmonary stenosis, or pulmonary embolism (option A), cardiac tamponade (option D) which affects both the right and left sides of the heart, tetralogy of Fallot, and prosthetic mitral or aortic valve malfunction.

90-2. **The answer is C.** (*Hurst's The Heart, 14th Edition, Chap. 90*) In the normal supine individual, approximately one-quarter of the blood volume is in the thorax. On standing, there is a gravity-mediated displacement of between 300 and 800 mL of blood to both the dependent extremities and the inferior mesenteric area (option A).[2] Approximately 50% of this displacement occurs within the first few seconds of standing, resulting in a drop in venous return to the heart and a mean fall in stroke volume of approximately 40% (option B).[2] In the normal subject, accommodation to this change in posture occurs in < 1 minute. Immediately on standing, muscle contractions in the legs, abdomen, and arms, in concert with the venous valvular system, support blood pressure by facilitating venous return.[2-3] The reduction in venous return with upright posture is followed by a slow progressive fall in arterial pressure and cardiac filling that produces less stretch and *reduces* the discharge rate of aortic arch and carotid sinus baroreceptors (option C). Fibers from these mechanoreceptors travel with unmyelinated vagal fibers from the atria and the ventricles to the nucleus tractus solitarii and other areas of the medulla that modulate vascular tone. In the resting supine position, impulses from these fibers increase efferent parasympathetic activity and have an inhibitory effect on efferent sympathetic activity to the heart. After standing, the drop in arterial pressure receptor firing in the carotid sinuses decreases efferent vagal activity and increases efferent sympathetic activity (option D), producing a reflex increase in heart rate and peripheral vasoconstriction. As a result, the assumption of an upright posture results in a 10 to 15 bpm increase in heart rate, minimal change in systolic blood pressure, and an approximately 10 mm Hg increase in diastolic blood pressure (option E).[4]

90-3. **The answer is B.** (*Hurst's The Heart, 14th Edition, Chap. 90*) *Pure autonomic failure* (PAF) refers to the diffuse state of autonomic failure present as evidenced by impaired bladder, bowel, thermoregulatory, motor, and sexual function (all in the absence of somatic nerve involvement).[5] The onset of symptoms in PAF is usually between ages 50 and 75 years, and it affects twice as many men as women.[6] PAF is manifested by orthostatic hypotension, syncope, and near syncope, neurocardiogenic bladder, constipation (option B), heat intolerance, an inability to sweat, and erectile dysfunction. Typically, the onset of symptoms is gradual and insidious, often with sensations of positional weakness, lightheadedness, and dizziness.[7] Male patients often report that the earliest signs of PAF were erectile dysfunction and diminished libido; women often report that their earliest symptoms were urinary retention and incontinence.[8] Although not the initial symptom, syncope may be the event that prompts the patient to seek medical attention. Whereas PAF may result in severe functional impairment, it sometimes leads to death.[8] In contrast, secondary forms of autonomic failure may occur in conjunction with another illness (such as amyloidosis, sarcoidosis [option D] or diabetes [option C]), in the setting of a known biochemical or structural alteration, or following exposure to various drugs or toxins (heavy metals such as lead [option E], alcohol, or some chemotherapeutic agents). Various pharmacologic agents, such as monoamine oxidase inhibitors (option A) among others, may cause or worsen orthostatic intolerance.

90-4. The answer is D. *(Hurst's The Heart, 14th Edition, Chap. 90)* Syncope caused by carotid sinus hypersensitivity is most common in men ≥ 50 years old (option E) and is precipitated by pressure on the *carotid sinus* baroreceptors, *not the aortic arch* (option D), typically in the setting of shaving, a tight collar, or turning the head to one side. Activation of carotid sinus baroreceptors gives rise to impulses to the medulla oblongata that, in turn, activate efferent sympathetic nerve fibers to the heart and blood vessels, cardiac vagal efferent nerve fibers, or both (option C). In patients with carotid sinus hypersensitivity, these responses may cause sinus arrest or AV block (a cardioinhibitory response—option B), vasodilatation (a vasodepressor response—option A), or both (a mixed response). The underlying mechanisms responsible for the syndrome are not clear, and validated diagnostic criteria do not exist.

90-5. The answer is D. *(Hurst's The Heart, 14th Edition, Chap. 90)* Multiple system atrophy (MSA) is a more severe form of autonomic failure, first reported by Shy and Drager in 1960.[9] In contrast to pure autonomic failure (PAF), these patients display not only significant orthostatic hypotension but also urinary and rectal incontinence, anhidrosis, iris atrophy, external ocular palsy, erectile dysfunction, rigidity, and tremor. As with PAF, the condition is twice as common in men as in women and usually starts in the fifth and sixth decades of life.[6] Although MSA may initially be indistinguishable from PAF, patients with MSA eventually experience somatic nervous system involvement.[10] Postural orthostatic tachycardia syndrome (POTS) (option A) is a somewhat less severe autonomic insufficiency in which heart rate increases excessively in response to upright posture.[11] Neurocardiogenic syncope (option B) is a type of reflex syncope referring to vasodepressor or vasovagal syncope. Carotid sinus hypersensitivity (option C) is precipitated by pressure on the carotid sinus baroreceptors, typically in the setting of shaving, a tight collar, or turning the head to one side. Acute autonomic failure (option E) is dramatic in presentation.[12] The onset is surprisingly rapid and is characterized by severe widespread failure of both parasympathetic and sympathetic components of the autonomic nervous system, while the somatic system is unaffected. Patients may have such profound orthostatic hypotension that merely trying to sit up in bed causes syncope.[13] Many suffer from complete anhidrosis and disturbances in bowel and bladder function that result in abdominal pain, cramping, bloating, nausea, and vomiting. Cardiac denervation is common, resulting in a fixed heart rate of 45 to 50 bpm and chronotropic incompetence.[14]

90-6. The answer is C. *(Hurst's The Heart, 14th Edition, Chap. 90)* Syncope in the *subclavian steal syndrome* is caused by major occlusive disease (*not vasospasm*) of the subclavian artery proximal to the origin of the vertebral artery. During upper extremity exercise, blood flow is shunted retrograde, by the circle of Willis, to the distal subclavian artery (option C). The consequent decrease in cerebral circulation induces cerebral ischemia.[15] This syndrome is suggested by the findings of *diminished* brachial arterial pressure on the affected side (option A), a bruit that is maximal over the *supraclavicular area* (not the femoral area—option B) adjacent to the origin of the vertebral artery, and the induction of symptoms by exercise of the involved extremity. Hyperextension and lateral rotation of the neck may cause syncope through the mechanical narrowing of the vertebral arteries by skeletal deformities of the cervical spine (option D). Such symptoms have been observed in patients with Klippel–Feil deformity, cervical spondylosis, and severe cervical osteoarthritis.

90-7. The answer is C. *(Hurst's The Heart, 14th Edition, Chap. 90)* The specificity of tilt-table testing is reported to be near 90% (option A), but lower when pharmacologic provocation is used (option C). The sensitivity of the test is reported to be between 20% and 74% (option B), the variability a result of differences in study populations, protocols, and the absence of a true "gold standard" to which the results of the test can be compared.[16,17] The reproducibility of the test (in a time frame ranging from several hours to weeks) is

80% to 90% for an initially positive response (option D), but less for an initially negative response (ranging from 30% to 90%) (option E).

90-8. The answer is B. *(Hurst's The Heart, 14th Edition, Chap. 90)* A young, otherwise healthy person with a history that strongly suggests neurocardiogenic syncope and no evidence of life-threatening condition may not require tilt-table testing after an initial episode of syncope (option B).[18] Indications for head-up tilt-table testing include: (1) unexplained recurrent (or single) syncope that is associated with injury or significant risk of injury in the absence of organic heart disease (option E) or (2) in the setting of organic heart disease after a cardiac cause is excluded; (3) recurrent syncope in which the determination of an increased predisposition to neurocardiogenic syncope could alter treatment; (4) differentiating conclusive syncope from epilepsy (option A); (5) evaluation of recurrent near syncope or dizziness; (6) evaluation of syncope in autonomic failure syndromes (option C); (7) exercise- or postexercise-induced syncope in the absence of organic heart disease for patients in whom exercise stress testing cannot reproduce an episode; and (8) evaluation of recurrent unexplained falls (option D).

90-9. The answer is D. *(Hurst's The Heart, 14th Edition, Chap. 90)* A variety of physical maneuvers have been used to treat the syndromes of orthostatic intolerance. Tilt training (option A) has been advocated; for neurocardiogenic syncope, however, long-term compliance is often poor.[19-21] Isometric countermaneuvers (option B), such as tensing of the arm and leg muscles, can sometimes prevent neurocardiogenic syncope if used at the first onset of symptoms.[22,23] Sleeping with the head of the bed elevated 6 inches above the feet is reported to be useful in neurocardiogenic syncope and the autonomic failure syndromes (option C). Elastic support stockings can be helpful in some patients; to be truly effective, however, they must be *waist high* and provide a *minimum of 30 mm Hg* of ankle counterpressure (option D). In some patients, salt and water loading increase intravascular volume and are effective in controlling syncope (option E). See Table 90-1 for therapies for orthostatic intolerance syndromes.

TABLE 90-1 Orthostatic Intolerance Syndrome Therapies

Treatment	Application	NCS	PD	HA	OH	Problems
Reconditioning	Aerobic exercise 20 min 3 times/wk	X	X	X	X	If done too vigorously may worsen symptoms
Physical maneuvers (tilt training, etc.)	30 min 3 times/d	X				Noncompliance is common
Sleeping with head tilted upright	During sleep	X		X	X	
Hydration	2 L PO/d	X	X		X	Edema
Salt	2-4 g/d	X	X		X	Edema
Fludrocortisone	0.1-0.2 mg PO qd	X	X		X	Hypokalemia, hypomagnesemia, edema
Metoprolol	25-100 mg bid	X				Fatigue
Labetalol	100-200 mg PO bid			X		Fatigue
Midodrine	5-10 mg PO tid	X	X		X	Nausea, scalp itching, supine hypertension
Methylphenidate	5-10 mg PO tid	X	X	X		Anorexia, insomnia, dependency
Bupropion	150-300 mg XL/qd		X	X	X	Tremor, agitation, insomnia
Clonidine	0.1-0.3 mg PO bid / 0.1-0.3 mg patch qwk			X		Dry mouth, blurred vision
Pyridostigmine	30-60 mg PO/d		X		X	Nausea, diarrhea
SSRI-escitalopram	10 mg PO/d	X	X		X	Tremor, agitation, sexual problems
Erythropoietin	10,000-20,000 µg SC qwk	X	X		X	Pain at injection site, expensive
Octreotide	50-200 µg SC tid		X	X	X	Nausea, diarrhea, gallstone
Permanent pacing		X				
Ivabradine	5-7.5 mg PO BID	X	X			Nausea, flashing lights
Droxidopa	100-600 mg PO TID				X	Nausea, supine hypertension

Abbreviations: HA, hyperadrenergic postural orthostatic tachycardia syndrome; NCS, neurocardiogenic syncope; OH, orthostatic hypotension; PD, partial dysautonomia; SSRI, selective serotonin reuptake inhibitor.

90-10. The answer is A. *(Hurst's The Heart, 14th Edition, Chap. 90)* Abnormal tilt-table responses can be classified into five groups.[16] The first is referred to as a *classic neurocardiogenic response* (option D), which is characterized by an abrupt drop in blood pressure. When accompanied by a significant drop in heart rate, this is referred to as a *vasovagal response*; in the absence of a decrease in heart rate, a *vasodepressor response*. A second pattern referred to as *dysautonomic* (or *delayed orthostatic*) (option B), is characterized by a gradual progressive fall in blood pressure with relatively little change in heart rate. This pattern is often noted in the autonomic failure syndromes. The third pattern, termed a *postural tachycardic response* (option C), is associated with a > 30 bpm increase in heart rate (or a heart rate of > 120 bpm) during the first 10 minutes of the baseline tilt. The fourth pattern is called *cerebral syncope* (option E). These patients experience syncope in the absence of systematic hypotension concomitant with intense cerebral vasoconstriction (as determined by transcranial Doppler), as well as cerebral hypoxia (as determined by electroencephalogram). The fifth response pattern is *psychogenic*. These patients experience loss of consciousness in the absence of systemic hypotension or any observable change in electroencephalogram or transcranial Doppler recording.[24] They are often found to suffer from psychiatric disorders that range from conversion reactions to severe depression.[25] Patients suffering from conversion reactions are not consciously aware of these events.[26] Many patients with psychogenic syncope are young women who have been victims of sexual abuse.[25]

References

1. Marian A. Hypertrophic cardiomyopathy: from genetics to treatment. *Eur J Clic Invest.* 2010;40(4):360-369.
2. Streeten D. Physiology of the microcirculation. In: Streeten D, ed. *Orthostatic Disorders of the Circulation.* New York: Plenum; 1987:1-12.
3. Thompson WO, Thompson PK, Daily ME. The effect of upright posture on the composition and volume of the blood in man. *J Clin Invest.* 1988;5:573-609.
4. Wieling W, van Lieshout JJ. Maintenance of postural normotension in humans. In: Low P, Benarroch E, eds. *Clinical Autonomic Disorders.* 3rd ed. Philadelphia, PA: Lippincott Williams & Wilkins; 2008:57-67.
5. Freeman R. Pure autonomic failure. In: Robertson D, Biaggiona I, eds. *Disorders of the Autonomic Nervous System.* Luxembourg: Harwood Academic; 1995:83-106.
6. Low PA, Banister R. Multiple system atrophy and pure autonomic failure. In: Low P, ed. *Clinical Autonomic Disorders,* 2nd ed. Philadelphia, PA: Lippincott-Raven; 1997:555-575.
7. Bannister R, Iodice V, Vichayanrat E, Mathias C. Clinical features and evaluation of the primary chromic autonomic failure syndromes. In: Mathias C, Bannister R, eds. *Autonomic Failure: A Textbook of Clinical Disorders of the Autonomic Nervous System.* 5th ed. Oxford, UK: Oxford University Press; 2013:485-497.
8. Kaufmann H, Schatz IT. Pure autonomic failure. In: Robertson D, Biaggioni I, Burnstock G, Low P, Paton J, eds. *Primer on the Autonomic Nervous System.* 3rd ed. San Diego, CA: Academic Press; 2012:467-468.
9. Shy GM, Drager GA. A neurologic syndrome associated with orthostatic hypotension. *Arch Neurol.* 1960;3:511-527.
10. Robertson D, Gilman S. Multiple system atrophy. In: Robertson D, Biaggioni I, Burnstock G, Low P, Paton J, eds. *Primer on the Autonomic Nervous System.* 3rd ed. San Diego, CA: Academic Press; 2012:453-454.
11. Grubb BP. The postural tachycardia syndrome. *Circulation* 2008;117(21):2814-2817.
12. Grubb BP, Kosinski DJ. Acute pandysautonomic syncope. *Eur J Cardiac Pacing Electrophysiol.* 1997;7:10-14.
13. Low P, Sandroni P. Autonomic neuropathies. In: Low P, Benarroch E., eds. *Clinical Autonomic Disorders.* 3rd ed. Philadelphia, PA: Lippincott Williams & Wilkins; 2008:400-422.
14. Yaki MD, Fronera AT. Acute autonomic neuropathy. *Arch Neurol.* 1975;32:132-133.
15. Bousser MG, Dubois B, Castaigne P. Transient loss of consciousness in ischemic cerebral events: a study of 557 ischemic strokes and transient ischemic attacks. *Ann Intern Med.* 1980;132:300-307.
16. Grubb BP, Kosinski D. Tilt table testing: concepts and limitations. *Pacing Clin Electrophysiol.* 1997;20:781-787.
17. Benditt D, Ferguson D, Grubb BP, Kapoor WN, Kugler L, Lerman BB. Tilt table testing for accessing syncope and its treatment: an American College of Cardiology Consensus Document. *J. Am Coll Cardiol.* 1996;28:263-267.
18. Strickberger SA, Benson DW, Biaggioni I, et al. AHA/ACCF scientific statement on the evaluation of syncope: from the American Heart Association Councils on Clinical Cardiology, Cardiovascular Nursing, Cardiovascular Disease in the Young, and Stroke, and the Quality of Care and Outcomes Research Interdisciplinary Working Group; and the American College of Cardiology Foundation; in collaboration with the Heart Rhythm Society; endorsed by the American Autonomic Society. *Circulation.* 2006;113(2):316-327.
19. Ector H, Reybrouck T, Heidbuchel H, Gewillig M, Van de Weif F. Tilt training: a new treatment for recurrent neurocardiogenic syncope or severe orthostatic intolerance. *Pacing Clin Electrophysiol.* 1998;21:193-196.

20. Di Girolamo E, Di Iorio C, Leonzio L, Sabatini P, Barsotti A. Usefulness of tilt training program for the prevention of refractory neurocardiogenic syncope in adolescents: a controlled study. *Circulation.* 1999;100:1798-1801.

21. Abe H, Kondo S, Kohshi K, Nakashima Y. Usefulness of orthostatic self training for the prevention of neurocardiogenic syncope. *Pacing Clin Electrophysiol.* 2002;25:1454-1458.

22. Brignole M, Croci F, Menozzi C, et al. Isometric arm counter-pressure maneuvers to abort impending vasovagal syncope. *J Am Coll Cardiol.* 2002;40:2054-2060.

23. Krediet P, van Dijk N, Linzer M, Liehout J, Wieling W. Management of vasovagal syncope: controlling or aborting faints by leg crossing and muscle tensing. *Circulation.* 2002;106:1684-1689.

24. Grubb BP, Samoil D, Kosinski D, et al. Cerebral syncope: loss of consciousness associated with cerebral vasoconstriction in the absence of systematic hypotension. *Pacing Clin Electrophysiol.* 1988;21:652-658.

25. Grubb BP, Gerald G, Wolfe DA, Samoil D, Davenport CW, Homan RW. Syncope and seizure of psychogenic origin: identification with head upright tilt table testing. *Clin Cardiol.* 1992;15:839-842.

26. Kouakam C, Lacriox D, Klug D, Baux P, Marquie C, Kacet S. Prevalence and significance of psychiatric disorders in patients evaluated for recurrent neurocardiogenic syncope. *Am J Cardiol.* 2002;89:530-535.

CHAPTER 91

Sudden Cardiac Death

Jacqueline Joza

QUESTIONS

DIRECTIONS: Choose the one best response to each question.

91-1. Which of the following statements is *correct* regarding the incidence of sudden cardiac death (SCD)?

A. The annual incidence of SCD is higher in whites than in African Americans in the United States

B. SCD accounts for approximately 50% of all sudden deaths in patients younger than age 20

C. The majority of cardiac arrest victims are women

D. The average age for SCD is under the age of 60

E. The incidence of SCD in the United States, Europe, and Asia is approximately 40 to 100 SCDs per 100,000 persons

91-2. A 60-year-old man presents to your clinic for his yearly visit. You are counseling him on lifestyle factors and their correlation with the risk for SCD. Which of the following statements is *incorrect*?

A. The Physicians' Health Study demonstrated a decreased risk of SCD in men who consumed light to moderate amounts of alcohol (two to six drinks per week) compared with those who drank rarely or never

B. Smoking decreases the ventricular fibrillation (VF) threshold

C. Those that stop smoking have a prompt reduction in coronary heart disease mortality rate irrespective of the duration of previous tobacco use

D. In a substudy of the Physicians' Health Study, increased levels of omega-3 fatty acids were associated with a reduced risk of SCD, but fish consumption and omega-3 fatty acid levels had no association with myocardial infarction or total cardiovascular mortality

E. No link has been observed between emotional stress and SCD

91-3. Acute myocardial ischemia leads to intracellular and extracellular acidosis and loss of myocellular membrane integrity with efflux of potassium and influx of calcium. Among the electrophysiologic effects of ischemia, which of the following statements is *incorrect*?

A. In late phases after myocardial infarction, when the infarction is healed, automaticity is the principal mechanism of ventricular arrhythmias

B. Fast sodium and slow calcium channels in partially depolarized fibers may remain inactive

C. Rapid polymorphic ventricular tachycardia (VT) and VF are characteristic arrhythmias during the early stages of ischemia

D. Within the first 3 days of myocardial infarction, SCD may occur as a result of VF initiated by frequent, early premature ventricular complexes

E. Accelerated idioventricular rhythms associated with reperfusion have no prognostic significance for the development of late arrhythmias, and they usually subside after 2 to 3 days

91-4. A 55-year-old woman is seeing you in consult for idiopathic/nonischemic dilated cardiomopathy (DCM). Which statement is *correct*?

A. The total mortality rate for idiopathic DCM is 2% to 5% annually

B. The proportion of sudden to nonsudden cardiac deaths is increased in idiopathic DCM

C. SCD in idiopathic DCM is mainly attributable to pulseless electrical activity

D. The only clinical variable that identifies patients with a higher risk of SCD is unexplained syncope

E. The electrophysiology study is considered a useful screening tool in patients with idiopathic DCM

91-5. A 35-year-old woman presents after an episode of syncope. Her transthoracic echocardiogram reveals bileaflet mitral valve prolapse with moderate regurgitation and a left ventricular ejection fraction (LVEF) of 50%. All of the following are prognostic indicators for sudden death in mitral valve prolapse *except*:

A. A history of syncope
B. A family history of sudden death at a young age
C. A short QT interval
D. An abnormal LVEF
E. Frequent complex ventricular ectopy

91-6. A 75-year-old man with ischemic cardiomyopathy has developed worsening renal failure over the last couple of years. He is about to start his first session of hemodialysis. Which of the following is *false* concerning his risk of SCD?

A. Chronic kidney disease is an independent risk factor for cardiovascular disease and coronary heart disease
B. Statins do not have any effect on cardiovascular mortality or SCD in patients with diabetes and ESRD
C. The SCD risk is elevated at 1.7-fold in the first 12 hours after the initiation of chronic dialysis
D. Despite primary prevention ICDs, patients with chronic kidney disease have a two- to five-fold elevated risk of total mortality compared to those with normal renal function
E. ICD implantation for the primary prevention of SCD was associated with a 42% reduction in total mortality

91-7. Which of the following pairings of medications and their pro-arrhythmic mechanisms is *incorrectly* matched?

A. Procainamide / QT prolongation from blockade of repolarizing potassium currents
B. Flecainide / promotion of reentrant VT
C. Sildenafil / increasing intracellular calcium levels
D. Methadone / coronary vasoconstriction and increased sympathetic tone
E. Flecainide / enhancement of AV nodal conduction

91-8. Electrocardiographic parameters reported to be associated independently with an increased risk of SCD include all of the following *except*:

A. Biatrial enlargement
B. Atrial fibrillation
C. Left bundle branch block
D. Left ventricular hypertrophy
E. QT interval prolongation

91-9. A 60-year-old woman presents for urgent follow-up after describing several brief episodes of dizziness. She denies any true syncope. Her past medical history is significant for a prior myocardial infarction 1 year ago. A recent Holter monitor revealed a short run of nonsustained VT, 10 beats at 178 bpm. Transthoracic echocardiogram demonstrates a LVEF of 40%. You decide to refer her for electrophysiology study (EPS). Which of the following statements is *incorrect*?

A. In patients who present with sustained monomorphic VT, the clinical rhythm is reproducibly inducible in most patients
B. Induction of nonsustained ventricular arrhythmias, polymorphic VT, or VF is specific and should prompt the implantation of a defibrillator
C. EPS has a poor negative predictive value in patients with severely compromised EF (< 30%)
D. EPS does predict future arrhythmic events independent of LVEF
E. The MUSTT trial included post–myocardial infarction patients with LVEF fractions below 40%, with a history of nonsustained VT

91-10. A 78-year-old man presents to your office with worsening dyspnea over the last year. He is now unable to climb a flight of stairs without shortness of breath and mild lightheadedness. His past medical history is significant for myocardial infarction 15 years ago. A transthoracic echo reveals a LVEF of 20%, despite optimal medical therapy. He is reluctant to implant an ICD because he is concerned about the up-front risks involved in the implantation. Which of the following trials compared amiodarone versus ICD in this patient population?

A. CIDS
B. CABG-Patch
C. SCD-HeFT
D. DINAMIT
E. MADIT-II

91-1. The answer is E. *(Hurst's The Heart, 14th Edition, Chap. 91)* Recent data from the United States, Europe, and Asia have demonstrated an incidence of approximately 40 to 100 SCDs per 100,000 persons[1-6] (option E), with significant geographical variation. The majority of cardiac arrest victims are *men* (option C), and the average age is *more than* 60 years (option D).[1,2,7] The incidence of SCD increases along with the prevalence of ischemic heart disease at older ages.[8,9] This trend is independent of gender or race. SCD accounts for approximately 20% of all sudden deaths in patients younger than age 20 (option B).[10] Structural cardiac abnormalities can be identified in the majority of young victims of SCD[11]; however, autopsy-based studies suggest that 20% to 35% of sudden deaths in young adults occur in the absence of identifiable structural abnormalities.[12,13] Many of these deaths are likely caused by genetically based arrhythmogenic disorders. The annual incidence of SCD has been shown to be higher in African Americans than in whites in numerous studies.[8,14-16]

91-2. The answer is E. *(Hurst's The Heart, 14th Edition, Chap. 91)* There are many reports linking stress, particularly emotional stress, to SCD (option E). Patients experiencing intense anger tend to have higher rates of ICD discharges,[17] and an estimated sevenfold greater relative risk of appropriate ICD discharge occurs during mental and physical stress.[18] ICD discharge rates in New York City remained elevated for up to 30 days after the 2001 terrorist attack.[19] Observations suggest that lifestyle factors such as alcohol consumption, cigarette smoking, diet, exercise, and stress are significantly correlated with the risk of sudden death.[9,17,20] Individuals who consume large amounts of alcohol (more than five drinks per day) have increased risks of ventricular arrhythmia and SCD.[21] However, a prospective analysis of 21,537 subjects in the Physicians' Health Study demonstrated a decreased risk of SCD in men who consumed light to moderate amounts of alcohol (two to six drinks per week) compared with those who drank rarely or never (option A).[20] Cigarette smoking is one of the few coronary risk factors associated with a disproportionate increase in the risk of SCD. In the Framingham Study, the annual incidence of SCD increased from 13 per 1000 persons in nonsmokers to 31 per 1000 persons in those smoking > 20 cigarettes per day.[22] Smoking has been shown to induce physiologic changes that predispose to SCD, such as increased platelet adhesiveness and catecholamine release, decreased VF threshold (option B), acceleration of heart rate, increased blood pressure, coronary spasm, reduced oxygen-carrying capacity by the accumulation of carboxyhemoglobin, and impairment of myoglobin utilization.[22] Those who stop smoking have a prompt reduction in CHD mortality rate irrespective of the duration of previous tobacco use (option C).[23] Omega-3 fatty acids (such as those found in fish) have been shown to have antiarrhythmic properties in experimental animal models,[24] and the administration of omega-3 fatty acids has been associated with reduced inducibility for monomorphic VT in patients with CAD undergoing ICD implantation.[25] In a substudy of the Physicians' Health Study, increased levels of omega-3 fatty acids were associated with a reduced risk of SCD,[26] and men who consumed fish at least once per week also had a significant reduction in SCD risk. Fish intake and omega-3 fatty acid levels had no association with myocardial infarction or total cardiovascular mortality (option D).[27]

91-3. The answer is A. *(Hurst's The Heart, 14th Edition, Chap. 91)* In the late phases after myocardial infarction (MI), when the infarction is healed, *reentrant* excitation (not automaticity—option A) is the principal mechanism of ventricular arrhythmias. Critical areas of the reentrant circuit are formed by surviving myocardial cells in the epicardial and endocardial border zone of a healed infarction, as well as surviving intramural fibers within the infarct zone.[28] Fast sodium and slow calcium channels in partially depolarized fibers may remain inactive, thereby prolonging refractoriness even after the completion of repolarization (option B). This may further contribute to electrical inhomogeneities within and around the ischemic zone, causing conduction delays, unidirectional block, and reentrant arrhythmias.[29] Rapid polymorphic VT and VF are the characteristic arrhythmias during the early stages of ischemia (option C).[30] Within the first 3 days of myocardial infarction, SCD may occur as a result of VF initiated by frequent, early, premature ventricular complexes (PVCs) (option D). Such PVCs have been shown in experimental models to be predominantly the result of impulse formation consistent with abnormal automaticity. Other manifestations of abnormal automaticity are accelerated idioventricular rhythms associated with reperfusion. These arrhythmias appear to arise, for the most part, from surviving Purkinje fibers in the subendocardial border zone of a transmural infarction. They have no prognostic significance for the development of late arrhythmias, and they usually subside after 2 to 3 days at approximately the same time that the resting membrane potential and action potential duration of Purkinje fibers normalize (option E).[31]

91-4.   **The answer is D.** *(Hurst's The Heart, 14th Edition, Chap. 91)* Idiopathic dilated cardiomyopathy (DCM) is the substrate for approximately 10% of SCDs in the adult population. The total mortality rate for idiopathic DCM is high, reaching 10% to 50% annually (*not 2–5%*—option A), and is most closely tied to the severity of left ventricular dysfunction.[32] Mortality rates are higher among patients with advanced heart failure, but the proportion of sudden to nonsudden cardiac deaths in these patients is *not* increased (option B).[33] SCD in idiopathic DCM is usually attributed to both polymorphic and monomorphic ventricular tachyarrhythmias (*not pulseless electrical activity*—option C) occurring in the setting of a high frequency of complex ventricular ectopy.[34] However, the terminal event may also be caused by pump failure with asystole or electromechanical dissociation, especially in patients with advanced left ventricular dysfunction.[35] The only clinical variable that identifies patients with a higher risk of SCD is unexplained syncope (option D), and these patients should undergo further electrophysiologic (EP) evaluation. The induction of polymorphic VT or VF during EP testing is nonspecific, and the probability of inducing sustained monomorphic VT in this population is less than 10% (option E).[36] Therefore, an EP study is not considered a useful screening tool in patients with idiopathic DCM. However, when sustained monomorphic VT does occur in patients with nonischemic dilated cardiomyopathy, the mechanism is usually reentry.

91-5.   **The answer is C.** *(Hurst's The Heart, 14th Edition, Chap. 91)* The most important prognostic indicators for sudden death in mitral valve prolapse (MVP) are a history of syncope (option A), and family history of sudden death at a young age (option B), as well as significant mitral regurgitation, abnormal left ventricular function (option D), and a *prolonged* QT interval (*not short*—option C)[37] Women with significant bileaflet MVP and frequent complex ventricular ectopy may also be at increased risk for SCD (option E).[38] Late gadolinium enhancement of the papillary muscles and inferobasal left ventricle by cardiac MRI in patients with MVP has been associated with complex ventricular arrhythmias,[39,40] and fibrosis in similar areas has been detected in patients with MVP and without any other structural heart disease who died suddenly.[40] It remains unclear if this fibrosis is directly related to abnormal leaflet motion.

91-6.   **The answer is E.** *(Hurst's The Heart, 14th Edition, Chap. 91)* Sudden cardiac death is a common cause of mortality in patients with end-stage renal disease (ESRD). Chronic kidney disease is an independent risk factor for cardiovascular disease and CHD (option A).[41] Factors beyond worsening coronary artery disease likely contribute to this elevated risk, however, because the risk of SCD remains significantly elevated in patients on dialysis even after surgical revascularization with coronary artery bypass grafting,[42] and the treatment of patients with diabetes and ESRD on hemodialysis with statins had no effect on cardiovascular mortality or SCD, despite approximately 40% reductions in median low-density lipoprotein cholesterol (option B).[43,44]

   Shifts in electrolytes and the dialysis procedure itself may also contribute to SCD risk. SCD risk is elevated 1.7-fold in the first 12 hours after the initiation of chronic dialysis (option C), and it is elevated threefold in the 12 hours prior to the initiation of chronic dialysis after a 72-hour intradialytic interval.[45] Patients with severe renal dysfunction and patients on dialysis have been excluded from most ICD trials. In a meta-analysis of patients in the MADIT-I, MADIT-II, and SCD-HeFT studies, primary prevention ICD implantation was not associated with survival benefit in patients with an estimated glomerular filtration rate < 60 mL/min/1.73 m^2 (stage 3 chronic kidney disease).[46] However, in a retrospective study of 6042 dialysis patients, ICD implantation for the *secondary* prevention of SCD was associated with a 42% reduction in total mortality (*not primary prevention*—option E).[47]

91-7. **The answer is D.** *(Hurst's The Heart, 14th Edition, Chap. 91)* The most common form of proarrhythmia, seen with Vaughan-Williams class IA and class III antiarrhythmics, stems from QT interval prolongation resulting from the blockade of repolarizing potassium currents (primarily I_{Kr}) and is accordingly sometimes referred to as the "acquired" long QT syndrome (option A). Proarrhythmia with different underlying mechanisms has been seen with other drugs that do not prolong the QT interval. For example, the Cardiac Arrhythmia Suppression Trial (CAST) showed an increase in mortality in postinfarction patients treated with the class IC antiarrhythmic drugs encainide or flecainide compared with placebo, despite the documented suppression of PVCs.[48] It is believed that these potent sodium channel blockers exacerbate ischemia-induced myocardial conduction delays and promote reentrant VTs (option B).[49] Class IC antiarrhythmic agents can also lead to proarrhythmia by converting atrial fibrillation to atrial flutter at slower than usual atrial rates, allowing one-to-one conduction of the flutter waves (referred to as "enhanced atrioventricular [AV] nodal conduction") (option E). For this reason, AV nodal blocking agents should be administered concomitantly with these medications in atrial fibrillation patients. Phosphodiesterase inhibitors, such as sildenafil and other positive inotropic agents, may promote arrhythmias by increasing intracellular calcium levels. These medications have been shown to be proarrhythmic and to increase the risk of SCD, despite their beneficial effects on hemodynamic parameters.[50] Methadone produces toxicity by *prolonging repolarization* and QTc, leading to torsade de pointes (option D).

91-8. **The answer is A.** *(Hurst's The Heart, 14th Edition, Chap. 91)* In survivors of out-of-hospital cardiac arrest, the presence of AV block or intraventricular conduction defects on ambulatory ECG (72 hours) is associated with a higher recurrence rate of cardiac arrest.[51] Other ECG parameters reported to be associated independently with an increased risk of SCD are prolongation of the QT interval (option E),[52] increased dispersion of the QT interval,[53] atrial fibrillation (option B), left bundle branch block (option C), and left ventricular hypertrophy (option D).[54] Biatrial enlargement, independently, has not been demonstrated to increase the risk of SCD. The detection of nonsustained ventricular tachycardia (NSVT) by ambulatory ECG monitoring has been reported to be of value in the risk stratification of patients for SCD, particularly after myocardial infarction.[55-56] The incidence of SCD in the 2 years after myocardial infarction in 766 patients enrolled in a prospective multicenter study increased with the frequency of PVCs detected during 24-hour ECG monitoring from 3% for < 1 per hour to 14% for > 30 per hour; similarly, patients with NSVT had a higher (17%) incidence of SCD than did those with single PVCs (6%).[56]

91-9. **The answer is B.** *(Hurst's The Heart, 14th Edition, Chap. 91)* Induction of sustained monomorphic VT at electrophysiology study (EPS) is the generally accepted end point for programmed ventricular stimulation, whereas the induction of nonsustained ventricular arrhythmias, polymorphic VT, or VF may be nonspecific findings (option B), depending on the aggressiveness of the stimulation protocol.[57,58] Information obtained during EPS, such as VT rate, morphology, origin, mechanism, and hemodynamic stability, is valuable in planning appropriate therapy. In patients who present with sustained monomorphic VT, the clinical rhythm is reproducibly inducible in most patients, especially in those with prior myocardial infarction (option A).[57] Although EP testing does predict future arrhythmic events independent of LVEF (option D) in the presence of prior myocardial infarction, concern has been raised regarding the poor negative predictive value of electrophysiolgic studies in patients with severely compromised ejection fraction (< 30%) (option C).[59] EPS inducibility (as well as nonsustained VT on ambulatory monitoring) was an entry criterion for the Multicenter Unsustained Tachycardia Trial (MUSTT) and the Multicenter Automatic Defibrillator Implantation Trial (MADIT), the first major clinical trials to demonstrate a survival benefit for ICDs over drug therapy in the primary prevention of SCD.[60,61]

MUSTT and MADIT included post–myocardial infarction patients with LVEFs below 40% and 35%, respectively (option E).

91-10. **The answer is C.** *(Hurst's The Heart, 14th Edition, Chap. 91)* The SCD-HeFT trial enrolled > 2500 patients with class II (70%) and III heart failure and LVEF ≤ 35% as a result of either ischemic or nonischemic cardiomyopathy and randomized them to ICD, amiodarone, or placebo, in addition to standard medical therapy.[62] After a median of 45 months, all-cause mortality in the ICD, amiodarone, and placebo arms was 22%, 28%, and 29%, respectively. The benefit of ICDs in the trial was highly statistically significant and appeared similar between ischemic and nonischemic subgroups, but it was greater for patients with class II than for those with class III heart failure—an observation not seen in other ICD trials.[62] The Canadian Implantable Defibrillator Study (CIDS)[63] randomized 659 patients with resuscitated VF or VT or with unmonitored syncope to ICD or amiodarone. After 3 years of follow-up, ICDs were associated with a 33% reduction in arrhythmic death and a 20% reduction in total mortality that did not reach statistical significance (option A). The Coronary Artery Bypass Graft (CABG) Patch Trial found no significant difference in the primary end point of total mortality in patients with ejection fractions of < 30% and an abnormal signal-averaged ECG (SAECG) randomized to ICD or no ICD at the time of CABG (option B).[64] These negative findings were attributed to the benefit of complete revascularization and possibly to the poor positive predictive value of the SAECG. ICDs do not appear to be of benefit immediately after large myocardial infarctions. The Defibrillator in Acute Myocardial Infarction Trial (DINAMIT) randomized 674 patients with recent (6 to 40 days) myocardial infarction LVEF < 35%, and depressed heart rate variability on 24-hour monitoring to ICD or no ICD (option D). In contrast to other trials that excluded patients with very recent infarcts, DINAMIT found no benefit from prophylactic ICD implantation.[65] MADIT-II compared ICD implantation to conventional therapy in 1232 patients with ischemic cardiomyopathy (average 3 years post-infarction) (option E).[66] After 20 months of follow-up, a risk reduction of 31% was observed in patients who underwent ICD implantation.[66]

References

1. de Vreede-Swagemakers JJ, Gorgels AP, Dubois-Arbouw WI, et al. Out-of-hospital cardiac arrest in the 1990's: a population-based study in the Maastricht area on incidence, characteristics and survival. *J Am Coll Cardiol.* 1997;30(6):1500-1505.

2. Chugh SS, Jui J, Gunson K, et al. Current burden of sudden cardiac death: multiple source surveillance versus retrospective death certificate-based review in a large U.S. community. *J Am Coll Cardiol.* 2004;44(6):1268-1275.

3. Stecker EC, Reinier K, Marijon E, et al. Public health burden of sudden cardiac death in the United States. *Circ Arrhyth Electrophysiol.* 2014;7(2):212-217.

4. Byrne R, Constant O, Smyth Y, et al. Multiple source surveillance incidence and aetiology of out-of-hospital sudden cardiac death in a rural population in the west of Ireland. *Eur Heart J.* 2008;29(11):1418-1423.

5. Hua W, Zhang LF, Wu YF, et al. Incidence of sudden cardiac death in China: analysis of 4 regional populations. *J Am Coll Cardiol.* 2009;54(12):1110-1118.

6. Nichol G, Thomas E, Callaway CW, et al. Regional variation in out-of-hospital cardiac arrest incidence and outcome. *JAMA.* 2008;300(12):1423-1431.

7. Eisenberg MS, Horwood BT, Cummins RO, Reynolds-Haertle R, Hearne TR. Cardiac arrest and resuscitation: a tale of 29 cities. *Ann Emerg Med.* 1990;19(2):179-186.

8. Zheng ZJ, Croft JB, Giles WH, Mensah GA. Sudden cardiac death in the United States, 1989 to 1998. *Circulation.* 2001;104(18):2158-2163.

9. Kannel WB, Cupples LA, D'Agostino RB. Sudden death risk in overt coronary heart disease: the Framingham Study. *Am Heart J.* 1987;113(3):799-804.

10. Wren C, O'Sullivan JJ, Wright C. Sudden death in children and adolescents. *Heart.* 2000;83(4):410-413.

11. Maron BJ, Gohman TE, Aeppli D. Prevalence of sudden cardiac death during competitive sports activities in Minnesota high school athletes. *J Am Coll Cardiol.* 1998;32(7):1881-1884.

12. Eckart RE, Scoville SL, Campbell CL, et al. Sudden death in young adults: a 25-year review of autopsies in military recruits. *Ann Intern Med.* 2004;141(11):829-834.

13. di Gioia CR, Autore C, Romeo DM, et al. Sudden cardiac death in younger adults: autopsy diagnosis as a tool for preventive medicine. *Hum Pathol.* 2006;37(7):794-801.

14. Becker LB, Han BH, Meyer PM, et al. Racial differences in the incidence of cardiac arrest and subsequent survival. The CPR Chicago Project. *N Engl J Med.* 1993;329(9):600-606.

15. Reinier K, Nichols GA, Huertas-Vazquez A, et al. Distinctive clinical profile of blacks versus whites presenting with sudden cardiac arrest. *Circulation*. 2015;132(5):380-387.

16. Cowie MR, Fahrenbruch CE, Cobb LA, Hallstrom AP. Out-of-hospital cardiac arrest: racial differences in outcome in Seattle. *Am J Pub Health*. 1993;83(7):955-959.

17. Lampert R, Joska T, Burg MM, Batsford WP, McPherson CA, Jain D. Emotional and physical precipitants of ventricular arrhythmia. *Circulation*. 2002;106(14):1800-1805.

18. Fries R, Konig J, Schafers HJ, Bohm M. Triggering effect of physical and mental stress on spontaneous ventricular tachyarrhythmias in patients with implantable cardioverter-defibrillators. *Clin Cardiol*. 2002;25(10):474-478.

19. Steinberg JS, Arshad A, Kowalski M, et al. Increased incidence of life-threatening ventricular arrhythmias in implantable defibrillator patients after the World Trade Center attack. *J Am Coll Cardiol*. 2004;44(6):1261-1264.

20. Albert CM, Manson JE, Cook NR, Ajani UA, Gaziano JM, Hennekens CH. Moderate alcohol consumption and the risk of sudden cardiac death among US male physicians. *Circulation*. 1999;100(9):944-950.

21. McElduff P, Dobson AJ. Case fatality after an acute cardiac event: the effect of smoking and alcohol consumption. *J Clin Epidemiol*. 2001;54(1):58-67.

22. Kannel WB. Update on the role of cigarette smoking in coronary artery disease. *Am Heart J*. 1981;101(3): 319-328.

23. Hallstrom AP, Cobb LA, Ray R. Smoking as a risk factor for recurrence of sudden cardiac arrest. *N Engl J Med*. 1986;314(5):271-275.

24. Billman GE, Kang JX, Leaf A. Prevention of sudden cardiac death by dietary pure omega-3 polyunsaturated fatty acids in dogs. *Circulation*. 1999;99(18):2452-2457.

25. Metcalf RG, Sanders P, James MJ, Cleland LG, Young GD. Effect of dietary n-3 polyunsaturated fatty acids on the inducibility of ventricular tachycardia in patients with ischemic cardiomyopathy. *J Am Coll Cardiol*. 2008;101(6):758-761.

26. Albert CM, Campos H, Stampfer MJ, et al. Blood levels of long-chain n-3 fatty acids and the risk of sudden death. *N Engl J Med*. 2002;346(15):1113-1118.

27. Albert CM, Hennekens CH, O'Donnell CJ, et al. Fish consumption and risk of sudden cardiac death. *JAMA*. 1998;279(1):23-28.

28. Josephson ME, Horowitz LN, Farshidi A, Kastor JA. Recurrent sustained ventricular tachycardia. 1. Mechanisms. *Circulation*. 1978;57(3):431-440.

29. Dillon SM, Allessie MA, Ursell PC, Wit AL. Influences of anisotropic tissue structure on reentrant circuits in the epicardial border zone of subacute canine infarcts. *Circ Res*. 1988;63(1):182-206.

30. Pogwizd SM, Corr PB. Mechanisms underlying the development of ventricular fibrillation during early myocardial ischemia. *Circ Res*. 1990;66(3):672-695.

31. Janse MJ, Wit AL. Electrophysiological mechanisms of ventricular arrhythmias resulting from myocardial ischemia and infarction. *Physiol Rev*. 1989;69(4):1049-1169.

32. Tamburro P, Wilber D. Sudden death in idiopathic dilated cardiomyopathy. *Am Heart J*. 1992;124(4): 1035-1045.

33. Packer M. Lack of relation between ventricular arrhythmias and sudden death in patients with chronic heart failure. *Circulation*. 1992;85(1 Suppl):I50-I56.

34. Larsen L, Markham J, Haffajee CI. Sudden death in idiopathic dilated cardiomyopathy: role of ventricular arrhythmias. *Pacing Clin Electrophysiol*. 1993;16(5 Pt 1): 1051-1059.

35. Luu M, Stevenson WG, Stevenson LW, Baron K, Walden J. Diverse mechanisms of unexpected cardiac arrest in advanced heart failure. *Circulation*. 1989;80(6):1675-1680.

36. Grimm W, Hoffmann J, Menz V, Luck K, Maisch B. Programmed ventricular stimulation for arrhythmia risk prediction in patients with idiopathic dilated cardiomyopathy and nonsustained ventricular tachycardia. *J Am Coll Cardiol*. 1998;32(3):739-745.

37. Puddu PE, Pasternac A, Tubau JF, Krol R, Farley L, de Champlain J. QT interval prolongation and increased plasma catecholamine levels in patients with mitral valve prolapse. *Am Heart J*. 1983;105(3):422-428.

38. Sriram CS, Syed FF, Ferguson ME, et al. Malignant bileaflet mitral valve prolapse syndrome in patients with otherwise idiopathic out-of-hospital cardiac arrest. *J Am Coll Cardiol*. 2013;62(3):222-230.

39. Han Y, Peters DC, Salton CJ, et al. Cardiovascular magnetic resonance characterization of mitral valve prolapse. *JACC Cardiovasc Imaging*. 2008;1(3):294-303.

40. Basso C, Perazzolo Marra M, Rizzo S, et al. Arrhythmic mitral valve prolapse and sudden cardiac death. *Circulation*. 2015;132(7):556-566.

41. Sarnak MJ, Levey AS, Schoolwerth AC, et al. Kidney disease as a risk factor for development of cardiovascular disease: a statement from the American Heart Association Councils on Kidney in Cardiovascular Disease, High Blood Pressure Research, Clinical Cardiology, and Epidemiology and Prevention. *Circulation*. 2003;108(17):2154-2169.

42. Herzog CA, Strief JW, Collins AJ, Gilbertson DT. Cause-specific mortality of dialysis patients after coronary revascularization: why don't dialysis patients have better survival after coronary intervention? *Nephrol Dial Transplant*. 2008;23(8):2629-2633.

43. Wanner C, Krane V, Marz W, et al. Atorvastatin in patients with type 2 diabetes mellitus undergoing hemodialysis. *N Engl J Med*. 2005;353(3):238-248.

44. Fellstrom BC, Jardine AG, Schmieder RE, et al. Rosuvastatin and cardiovascular events in patients undergoing hemodialysis. *N Engl J Med.* 2009;360(14):1395-1407.

45. Bleyer AJ, Hartman J, Brannon PC, Reeves-Daniel A, Satko SG, Russell G. Characteristics of sudden death in hemodialysis patients. *Kidney Int.* 2006;69(12):2268-2273.

46. Pun PH, Al-Khatib SM, Han JY, et al. Implantable cardioverter-defibrillators for primary prevention of sudden cardiac death in CKD: a meta-analysis of patient-level data from 3 randomized trials. *Am J Kid Dis.* 2014;64(1):32-39.

47. Herzog CA, Li S, Weinhandl ED, Streif JW, Collins AJ, Gilbertson DT. Survival of dialysis patients after cardiac arrest and the impact of implantable cardioverter defibrillators. *Kidney Int.* 2005;68(2):818-825.

48. Echt DS, Liebson PR, Mitchell LB, et al. Mortality and morbidity in patients receiving encainide, flecainide, or placebo. The Cardiac Arrhythmia Suppression Trial. *N Engl J Med.* 1991;324(12):781-788.

49. Nattel S, Pedersen DH, Zipes DP. Alterations in regional myocardial distribution and arrhythmogenic effects of aprindine produced by coronary artery occlusion in the dog. *Cardiovasc Res.* 1981;15(2):80-85.

50. Packer M, Medina N, Yushak M. Hemodynamic and clinical limitations of long-term inotropic therapy with amrinone in patients with severe chronic heart failure. *Circulation.* 1984;70(6):1038-1047.

51. Myerburg RJ, Conde CA, Sung RJ, et al. Clinical, electrophysiologic and hemodynamic profile of patients resuscitated from prehospital cardiac arrest. *Am J Med.* 1980;68(4):568-576.

52. Algra A, Tijssen JG, Roelandt JR, Pool J, Lubsen J. QTc prolongation measured by standard 12-lead electrocardiography is an independent risk factor for sudden death due to cardiac arrest. *Circulation.* 1991;83(6):1888-1894.

53. Barr CS, Naas A, Freeman M, Lang CC, Struthers AD. QT dispersion and sudden unexpected death in chronic heart failure. *Lancet.* 1994;343(8893):327-329.

54. Zimetbaum PJ, Buxton AE, Batsford W, et al. Electrocardiographic predictors of arrhythmic death and total mortality in the multicenter unsustained tachycardia trial. *Circulation.* 2004;110(7):766-769.

55. Risk stratification and survival after myocardial infarction. *N Engl J Med.* 1983;309(6):331-336.

56. Bigger JT, Jr., Fleiss JL, Kleiger R, Miller JP, Rolnitzky LM. The relationships among ventricular arrhythmias, left ventricular dysfunction, and mortality in the 2 years after myocardial infarction. *Circulation.* 1984;69(2):250-258.

57. Ruskin JN. Role of invasive electrophysiological testing in the evaluation and treatment of patients at high risk for sudden cardiac death. *Circulation.* 1992;85(1 Suppl):I152-I159.

58. DiCarlo LA, Jr., Morady F, Schwartz AB, et al. Clinical significance of ventricular fibrillation-flutter induced by ventricular programmed stimulation. *Am Heart J.* 1985;109(5 Pt 1):959-963.

59. Buxton AE, Lee KL, DiCarlo L, et al. Electrophysiologic testing to identify patients with coronary artery disease who are at risk for sudden death. Multicenter Unsustained Tachycardia Trial Investigators. *N Engl J Med.* 2000;342(26):1937-1945.

60. Buxton AE, Lee KL, Fisher JD, Josephson ME, Prystowsky EN, Hafley G. A randomized study of the prevention of sudden death in patients with coronary artery disease. Multicenter Unsustained Tachycardia Trial Investigators. *N Engl J Med.* 1999;341(25):1882-1890.

61. Moss AJ, Hall WJ, Cannom DS, et al. Improved survival with an implanted defibrillator in patients with coronary disease at high risk for ventricular arrhythmia. Multicenter Automatic Defibrillator Implantation Trial Investigators. *N Engl J Med.* 1996;335(26):1933-1940.

62. Bardy GH, Lee KL, Mark DB, et al. Amiodarone or an implantable cardioverter-defibrillator for congestive heart failure. *N Engl J Med.* 2005;352(3):225-237.

63. Connolly SJ, Gent M, Roberts RS, et al. Canadian implantable defibrillator study (CIDS): a randomized trial of the implantable cardioverter defibrillator against amiodarone. *Circulation.* 2000;101(11):1297-1302.

64. Bigger JT, Jr. Prophylactic use of implanted cardiac defibrillators in patients at high risk for ventricular arrhythmias after coronary-artery bypass graft surgery. Coronary Artery Bypass Graft (CABG) Patch Trial Investigators. *N Engl J Med.* 1997;337(2):1569-1575.

65. Hohnloser SH, Kuck KH, Dorian P, et al. Prophylactic use of an implantable cardioverter-defibrillator after acute myocardial infarction. *N Engl J Med.* 2004;351(24):2481-2488.

66. Moss AJ, Zareba W, Hall WJ, et al. Prophylactic implantation of a defibrillator in patients with myocardial infarction and reduced ejection fraction. *N Engl J Med.* 2002;346(12):877-883.

CHAPTER 92

Cardiopulmonary and Cardiocerebral Resuscitation

Jacqueline Joza

QUESTIONS

DIRECTIONS: Choose the one best response to each question.

92-1. Which of the following statements concerning out-of-hospital cardiac arrests is *incorrect*?

A. A family history of cardiac arrest in a first-degree relative is associated with a twofold increase in the risk of cardiac arrest
B. The majority of out-of-hospital cardiac arrests occur at a home or residence
C. The median age for out-of-hospital cardiac arrest is 66 years
D. The incidence of cardiac arrest with an initial rhythm of VF is decreasing over time
E. The incidence of cardiac arrest is decreasing

92-2. You are speaking with your patient and his family in the coronary care unit after he underwent coronary percutaneous intervention for an anterior ST elevation myocardial infarction. The patient's wife asks about the utility of learning cardiopulmonary resuscitation (CPR) in the event that her husband has an arrhythmic event. Which of the following statements is *incorrect*?

A. Untrained lay rescuers should provide compression-only (hands-only) CPR, with or without dispatcher guidance, for adult victims of cardiac arrest
B. The rescuer should continue compression-only CPR until the arrival of an AED or rescuers with additional training
C. All lay rescuers should, at a minimum, provide chest compressions for victims of cardiac arrest
D. If the trained lay rescuer can perform rescue breaths, he or she should add rescue breaths in a ratio of 15 compressions to 2 breaths

E. The rescuer should continue CPR until an AED arrives and is ready for use, EMS providers take over care of the victim, or the victim starts to move

92-3. You are teaching a course on advanced life support to medical students. One student asks you about the recommended chest compression rate and chest compression depth during CPR. Your answer is:

A. Rate of 100 to 120/min; compression to a depth of 2 inches (5 cm)
B. Rate of 80 to 100/min; compression to a depth of 2.7 inches (7 cm)
C. Rate of 120 to 150/min; compression to a depth of 2.7 inches (7 cm)
D. Rate of 100 to 120/min; compression to a depth of 2.7 inches (7 cm)
E. Rate of 120 to 150/min; compression to a depth of 2 inches (5 cm)

92-4. A code blue is called for an in-hospital cardiac arrest. Which of the following statements about medications during cardiopulmonary resuscitation is *correct*?

A. Amiodarone should be used in the event of failure to terminate VF/polymorphic VT with three stacked shocks or with the first shock
B. Lidocaine q3-5 min should be used in the setting of an initial nonshockable rhythm
C. Vasopressin q3-5 min should be used in the setting of asystole as the initial presenting rhythm
D. High-dose epinephrine q3-5 min should be used for VF as the initial presenting rhythm
E. Epinephrine in combination with vasopressin should be used during asystolic arrest

92-5. A 50-year-old man suffers a witnessed cardiac arrest while at a busy restaurant. The presenting rhythm is ventricular fibrillation requiring several shocks for the return of spontaneous circulation. He is brought into the emergency department, and you wish to initiate an induced hypothermia protocol. Which of the following statements is *incorrect*?

A. The three phases of the hypothermia protocol are (1) the cooling phase for the first 24 hours, (2) the rewarming phase, and (3) the maintenance phase

B. A head CT scan should be performed on every patient before initiating the hypothermia protocol

C. One of the exclusion criteria includes a patient with multiorgan failure

D. During the invasive cooling phase, the goal temperature is 33°C (although targeted temperature management of 36°C can be considered)

E. Normothermia maintenance takes effect when the patient reaches 37°C

92-6. Cooling technologies for the induction of hypothermia following cardiac arrest can be divided into invasive (core cooling) and noninvasive (surface cooling) methods. The advantages of invasive cooling over surface cooling include all of the following *except*:

A. No risk of surface cooling–induced skin lesions

B. Ease of accessibility to patient, that is, no need to cover large areas of the skin to achieve cooling

C. Fewer and smaller temperature fluctuations in the maintenance phase

D. Continuous central temperature measurement in some types of endovascular catheter is possible

E. Ease of use; can be applied by nurses without a physician being present

92-7. A 65-year-old man is resuscitated from cardiac arrest that occurred while he was exercising. With the return of spontaneous circulation, which of the following hemodynamic goals should be instituted?

A. Correct hypotension for a systolic blood pressure > 80 mm Hg

B. Correct hypotension for a systolic blood pressure > 90 mm Hg

C. Correct hypotension for a systolic blood pressure > 120 mm Hg

D. Correct hypotension for a mean arterial pressure of 50 mm Hg

E. Correct hypotension for a mean arterial pressure of 80 mm Hg

92-8. Possible side effects of the cooling phase of the induced hypothermia protocol include all of the following *except*:

A. Coagulopathy

B. Hyperglycemia

C. Infection

D. Shivering

E. Junctional tachycardia

92-9. You are reviewing the protocol for out-of-hospital cardiac arrests. Which of the following statements is *incorrect*?

A. 1.5 minutes to 3 minutes of chest compressions should be given prior to shock delivery

B. Naloxone should be administered if opioid overdose is suspected

C. During cardiopulmonary resuscitation, 1 breath every 6 seconds (10 breaths per minute) while continuous chest compressions are being performed is reasonable

D. Rescuers should avoid leaning on the chest between compressions

E. The routine use of automated mechanical chest compression devices should be avoided

92-10. Public-access defibrillation (PAD) programs for patients with out-of-hospital cardiac arrests constitute an important prevention measure. Which of the following is *not* an essential component of the implementation of the PAD program?

A. Creation of a community of cardiac arrest survivors

B. A planned and practiced response, which ideally includes identification of locations and neighborhoods where there is a high risk of cardiac arrest and ensuring that bystanders are aware of the location of the automatic external defibrillators

C. Training of anticipated rescuers in cardiopulmonary resuscitation and in the use of the automatic external defibrillator

D. An integrated link with the local EMS system

E. A program of ongoing quality improvement

ANSWERS

92-1. The answer is E. (*Hurst's The Heart, 14th Edition, Chap. 92*) The American Heart Association (AHA) statistical data from 2015[1] reveal that the incidence of cardiac arrest is *not* decreasing, but the incidence of cardiac arrest with an initial rhythm of VF is decreasing over time (option D).[2] The median age for out-of-hospital cardiac arrest is 66 years (option C). According to the CARES registry, in 2013 most out-of-hospital cardiac arrests occurred at a home or residence (69.5%).[3] A family history of cardiac arrest in a first-degree relative is associated with a twofold increase in the risk of cardiac arrest.[4-5]

92-2. The answer is D. (*Hurst's The Heart, 14th Edition, Chap. 92*) Favorable neurologic outcome at discharge was observed in patients who were treated under the 2005 guidelines with a compression-ventilation ratio of 30:2, with a slightly higher survival than those patients treated under the 2000 guidelines with a compression-ventilation ratio of 15:2 (8.9% vs 6.5%; RR 1.37 [95% CI, 0.98–1.91]).[6-7] Options A through C and E are correct.

92-3. The answer is A. (*Hurst's The Heart, 14th Edition, Chap. 92*) For the critical outcome of survival to hospital discharge according to chest compression rates, evidence exists from two observational studies[8-9] representing 13,469 adult patients. They compared chest compression rates of > 140/min, 120 to 139/min, < 80/min, and 80 to 99/min with the control rate of 100 to 119/min. When compared with the control chest compression rate of 100 to 119/min, there was a 4%, 2%, 2%, and 1% decrease in survival to hospital discharge with compression rates of > 140/min, 120 to 139/min, 80 to 90/min, and < 80/min, respectively.

During manual CPR, rescuers should perform chest compressions to a depth of at least 2 inches (5 cm) for an average adult, while avoiding excessive chest compression depths (> 2.4 inches [6 cm]). Compressions create blood flow primarily by increasing intrathoracic pressure and directly compressing the heart, which in turn results in critical blood flow and oxygen delivery to the heart and brain. Rescuers often do not compress the chest deeply enough despite the recommendation to "push hard." Although a compression depth of at least 2 inches (5 cm) is recommended, as noted above the 2015 guidelines update incorporates new evidence about the potential for an upper threshold of compression depth (> 2.4 inches [6 cm]) beyond which complications may occur.

92-4. The answer is A. (*Hurst's The Heart, 14th Edition, Chap. 92*) Antiarrhythmic drugs can be used during cardiac arrest for refractory ventricular dysrhythmias. The 2015 guideline recommendations for antiarrhythmic drugs for cardiac arrest suggest the use of amiodarone in adult patients with refractory VF/polymorphic VT to improve rates of return of spontaneous circulation, where lidocaine (option B) or nifekalant may be used as alternatives. The 2015 guidelines recommend against the routine use of magnesium in adult patients. The 2015 guidelines suggest vasopressin should not be used instead of epinephrine in cardiac arrest (option C).[10] A single randomized controlled trial with 336 patients comparing multiple doses of single-dose epinephrine with multiple doses of standard-dose vasopressin in the emergency department for out-of-hospital cardiac arrest did not show any advantage for survival to discharge with favorable neurologic outcome, or return of spontaneous circulation with vasopressin.[11] High-dose epinephrine (at least 0.2 mg/kg or 5 mg bolus dose) was compared with single-dose epinephrine (1 mg bolus dose). Two randomized controlled studies including 1920 patients did not show an advantage of the high dose over the low dose for survival to hospital discharge (option D).[12,13] Randomized studies comparing epinephrine with vasopressin + epinephrine combination therapy showed no advantage with combination therapy (option E).[14-16]

92-5. The answer is B. (*Hurst's The Heart, 14th Edition, Chap. 92*) The hypothermia protocol is recommended for patients > 18 years of age who sustained a cardiac arrest and remain in a coma. The patient must be comatose, not following commands or demonstrating purposeful movements. The three phases include (1) cooling phase for the first 24 hours, (2) rewarming phase, which begins after 24 hours at the target temperature and begins rewarming by increasing 0.25°C per hour to 37°C, and (3) maintenance phase, where normothermia maintenance takes effect when the patient reaches 37°C (options A and E). A head CT without contrast is recommended only if it is clinically indicated and will not delay transfer to the cardiac catheterization laboratory (option B). Twenty-four hours of cooling therapy at a temperature goal of 33°C is recommended (option D). The dose of temperature management is controversial, and some centers cool patients to 36°C; this is based on a large study comparing temperature management at 33°C to maintaining a core temperature of 36.0°C which concluded that each core temperature had equally good outcomes.[17] Patients excluded from the hypothermia protocol include patients who are awake, suffered prolonged ischemic times, experience refractory shock, demonstrate multiorgan failure (option C), or have severe underlying illnesses, including terminal illnesses and do-not-resuscitate (DNR) status.

92-6. **The answer is E.** (*Hurst's The Heart, 14th Edition, Chap. 92*) Endovascular catheters are an effective method of inducing therapeutic hypothermia. Continuous core temperature monitoring is required and is generally accomplished using a temperature probe in the bladder (urinary catheter) or the rectum. The catheters are usually inserted into the inferior vena cava through the femoral vein. There is no evidence for a difference in outcome based on cooling method. All of the options represent advantages of invasive cooling over surface cooling *except* option E. The advantages of surface cooling over invasive cooling include its ease of use and its ability to be applied by nurses without a physician being present; the lack of invasive procedures required and therefore the avoidance of mechanical complications; the ability for surface cooling to be started immediately; the lack of risk for catheter-induced thrombus formation; and its applicability for use outside the intensive care unit setting.

92-7. **The answer is B.** (*Hurst's The Heart, 14th Edition, Chap. 92*) It may be reasonable to avoid and immediately correct hypotension (systolic blood pressure < 90 mm Hg, mean arterial pressure < 65 mm Hg) during post–cardiac arrest care.[10]

Studies of patients after cardiac arrest have found that a systolic blood pressure < 90 mm Hg or a mean arterial pressure of < 65 mm Hg is associated with higher mortality and diminished functional recovery, while systolic arterial pressures of > 100 mm Hg are associated with better recovery. Although higher pressures appear superior, specific systolic or mean arterial pressure targets could not be identified because trials typically studied a bundle of many interventions, including hemodynamic control. Also, because baseline blood pressure varies from patient to patient, different patients may have different requirements to maintain optimal organ perfusion.

92-8. **The answer is E.** (*Hurst's The Heart, 14th Edition, Chap. 92*) Typically sinus bradycardia, or a slow junctional rhythm (*not tachycardia*) may be observed during the cooling phase. In addition to serum electrolyte imbalance during the cooling phase, with resultant low levels of potassium, magnesium, calcium, and phosphate, other side effects include: (1) Coagulopathy (option A) for which if active bleeding does occur, an evaluation of coagulation factors and platelets should be performed and deficiencies corrected. (2) Hyperglycemia (option B), which suppresses insulin release and causes insulin resistance. (3) Infection (option C), which is usually multifactorial and can be caused by emergency intubation and intravenous catheter insertion and aspiration pneumonia at the time of arrest. Furthermore, the hypothermia itself can suppress white blood cell production and impair neutrophil and macrophage function. All measures to reduce ventilator-associated pneumonia are employed, including elevating the head of the bed. (4) Shivering (option D), which must be prevented by the administration of sedation and neuromuscular blocking agents upon the induction of hypothermia.

92-9. **The answer is A.** (*Hurst's The Heart, 14th Edition, Chap. 92*) Numerous studies have addressed the question of whether a benefit is conferred by providing a specified period (typically 1.5 to 3 minutes) of chest compressions before shock delivery, as compared to delivering a shock as soon as the AED can be readied. No difference in outcome has been shown. For witnessed adult cardiac arrest when an AED is immediately available, it is reasonable that the defibrillator be used as soon as possible. For patients with known or suspected opioid addiction who are unresponsive with no normal breathing but a pulse, it is reasonable for appropriately trained lay rescuers and BLS providers to administer intramuscular (IM) or intranasal (IN) naloxone in addition to providing standard BLS care (option B). The 2015 guidelines suggest that it may be reasonable for the provider to deliver one breath every 6 seconds (10 breaths per minute) while continuous chest compressions are being performed (ie, during CPR with an advanced airway) (option C).[18] Rescuers should avoid leaning on the chest between compressions, to allow full chest wall recoil for adults in cardiac arrest (option D). Automated mechanical chest compression devices should not be used in the place of manual chest compressions because no benefit or harm was shown when automated and manual chest compressions were compared.[10]

92-10. The answer is A. *(Hurst's The Heart, 14th Edition, Chap. 92)* It is recommended that public-access defibrillation (PAD) programs for patients with out-of-hospital cardiac arrests be implemented in public locations where there is a relatively high likelihood of witnessed cardiac arrest (ie, airports, casinos, sports facilities). There is clear and consistent evidence of improved survival from cardiac arrest when a bystander performs CPR and rapidly uses an AED. Options B through E are all essential components of the PAD programs.

References

1. Mozaffarian D, Benjamin EJ, et al. Heart disease and stroke statistics: 2015 update. A report from the American Heart Association. *Circulation*. 2015;17:e205-e214.

2. Cobb LA, Fahrenbruch CE, Olsufka M, Copass MK. Changing incidence of out-of-hospital ventricular fibrillation, 1980-2000. *JAMA*. 2002;288:3008-3013.

3. Centers for Disease Control and Prevention. 2013 Cardiac Arrest Registry to Enhance Survival (CARES) nationalsummaryreport.https://mycares.net/sitepages/uploads/2014/2013CARESNationalSummaryReport .pdf. Accessed July 15, 2014.

4. Maron BJ, Doerer JJ, Haas TS, Tierney DM, Mueller FO. Sudden deaths in young competitive athletes: analysis of 1866 deaths in the United States, 1980-2006. *Circulation*. 2009;119:1085-1092.

5. Harmon KG, Asif IM, Klossner D, Drezner JA. Incidence of sudden cardiac death in National Collegiate Athletic Association athletes. *Circulation*. 2011;123:1594-1600.

6. Hinchey PR, Myers JB, Lewis R, et al.; Capital County Research Consortium. Improved out-of-hospital cardiac arrest survival after the sequential implementation of 2005 AHA guidelines for compressions, ventilations, and induced hypothermia: the Wake County experience. *Ann Emerg Med*. 2010;56:348-357.

7. Olasveengen TM, Vik E, Kuzovlev A, Sunde K. Effect of implementation of new resuscitation guidelines on quality of cardiopulmonary resuscitation and survival. *Resuscitation*. 2009;80:407-411.

8. Idris AH, Guffey D, Aufderheide TP, et al. Resuscitation Outcomes Consortium Investigators. Chest compression rates and survival following out-of-hospital cardiac arrest. *Crit Care Med*. 2015;45:840-848.

9. Idris AH, Guffey D, Aufderheide TP, et al. Resuscitation Outcomes Consortium (ROC) Investigators. Relationship between chest compression rates and outcomes from cardiac arrest. *Circulation*. 2012;125: 3004-3012.

10. Callaway CW, Soar J, et al. Part 4: Advanced life support: 2015 international consensus on cardiopulmonary resuscitation and emergency cardiovascular care science with treatment recommendations. *Circulation*. 2015;132(16 suppl 1):S84-S145.

11. Mukoyama T, Kinoshita K, Nagao K, Tanjoh K. Reduced effectiveness of vasopressin in repeated doses for patients undergoing prolonged cardiopulmonary resuscitation. *Resuscitation*. 2009;80:755-761.

12. Callaham M, Madsen CD, Barton CW, et al. A randomized clinical trial of high-dose epinephrine and nonepinephrine vs standard-dose epinephrine in prehospital cardiac arrest. *JAMA*. 1992;268:2667-2672.

13. Gueugniaud PY, Mols P, Goldstein P, et al. A comparison of repeated high doses and repeated standard does of epinephrine for cardiac arrest outside the hospital. European Epinephrine Study Group. *N Engl J Med*. 1998;339:1595-1601.

14. Gueugniaud PY, David JS, Chanzy E, et al. Vasopressin and epinephrine vs. epinephrine alone in cardiopulmonary resuscitation. *N Engl J Med*. 2008;359:21-30.

15. Ong ME, Tiah L, Leong BS, et al. A randomized, double-blind, multi-centre trial comparing vasopressin and adrenaline in patients with cardiac arrest presenting to or in the emergency department. *Resuscitation*. 2012;83:953-960.

16. Wenzel V, Krismer AC, Arntz HR, et al.; European Resuscitation Council Vasopressor During Cardio-pulmonary Resuscitation Study Group. A comparison of vasopressin and epinephrine for out-of-hospital cardiopulmonary resuscitation. *N Engl J Med.* 2004;350(2):105-113.

17. Nielsen N, Wetterslev J, Cronberg T, et al.; TTM Trial Investigators. Targeted temperature management at 33 °C versus 36 °C after cardiac arrest. *N Engl J Med.* 2013;369:2197-2206.

18. Travers AH, Perkins GD, Berg RA, et al. Part 3: Adult basic life support and automated external defibrilla-tion. 2015 international consensus on cardiopulmonary resuscitation and emergency cardiovascular care science with treatment recommendations. *Circulation.* 2015;132(suppl 1):S51-S83.

SECTION 14

Diseases of the Great Vessels and Peripheral Vessels

CHAPTER 93

Diseases of the Aorta

Jacqueline Joza

QUESTIONS

DIRECTIONS: Choose the one best response to each question.

93-1. The aorta is an elastic artery with a trilaminar wall. Which of the following statements is *incorrect* regarding the layers that make up the aorta?

A. The innermost lining of the tunica intima is the endothelium
B. An internal elastic membrane forms the outer lining of the tunica intima
C. Within the tunica adventitia lie the nervi vasorum and vasa vasorum
D. The vasa vasorum develops into a capillary network supplying the adventitia and media of the abdominal aorta
E. The tunica media is comprised of elastin, smooth muscle cells, collagen, and ground substance

93-2. A 75-year-old man who smokes and is known for hypertension presents to the emergency department with chest pain. Troponins are mildly positive, but the electrocardiogram does not demonstrate acute ischemia. CT angiography of the aorta is performed, which reveals a contrast-filled pouch-like protrusion in the thoracic aorta, in the absence of an intimal flap or false lumen. A transesophageal echocardiogram confirms a localized, crater-like protrusion of the aortic lumen into the aortic wall. Which of the following *best* represents the diagnosis?

A. Fusiform aneurysm
B. Saccular aneurysm
C. Intramural hematoma
D. Penetrating aortic ulcer
E. Aortic transection

93-3. A middle-aged woman who is followed for a remote myocardial infarction, hypertension, and dyslipidemia is seen in follow-up in your clinic. Which of the following clinical characteristics is *not* associated with an increased likelihood of the presence of a thoracic aortic aneurysm?

A. The presence of liver cysts
B. Past medical history of an intracranial aneurysm
C. Past medical history of temporal arteritis
D. Bovine aortic arch configuration
E. A positive thumb-palm sign

93-4. Which of the following pairs of thoracic aortic aneurysm syndromes with their genetic mutation correlates is *incorrect*?

A. Marfan syndrome / Fibrillin 1 mutation
B. Ehlers–Danlos syndrome / *COL3A1* mutation
C. Loeys–Dietz syndrome / *TGFBR1* and *TGFBR2* mutations
D. Bicuspid aortic valve / *NOTCH1* mutation
E. Familial thoracic aortic aneurysm / *KCNH2* mutation

93-5. A 65-year-old man has a past medical history significant for an abdominal aortic aneurysm (AAA). He complains of intermittent chest pain, and the referring physician suspects an aneurysm of the thoracic aorta. Due to the presence of chronic renal failure, an echocardiogram (as opposed to a CT scan) is requested by the referring physician. Which of the following is *incorrect* regarding the potential limitations of echo for imaging the aorta?

A. A transesophageal echo will be limited by the tracheal air column in imaging the upper portion of the ascending aorta
B. Adequate sedation for transesophageal echo is required to avoid hypertension, which could extend an aortic dissection or instigate a potential rupture
C. A transthoracic echo can mainly visualize the proximal several centimeters of the ascending aorta
D. A transthoracic echo will miss an aneurysm of the mid-portion of the ascending aorta
E. A transeophageal echo will only visualize the beginning of an aneurysm in the proximal aorta and will therefore underestimate its size

93-6. You are asked to see a patient with chest pain in the emergency department. The patient is a 65-year-old man with a 20 pack-year history of cigarette smoking. The internal medicine resident tells you that the D-dimer is elevated. Which of the following is *true* regarding a D-dimer in the setting of an acute aortic dissection?

A. The D-dimer is useful as a predictor for aortic dissection
B. The D-dimer is poorly sensitive in the detection of acute aortic dissection
C. The D-dimer is highly specific in the detection of acute aortic dissection
D. The D-dimer elevation reflects the longitudinal extent of aortic dissection
E. The D-dimer does not predict the mortality of a patient with aortic dissection

93-7. A 45-year-old woman with Marfan's syndrome undergoes a regular imaging evaluation of her aorta. At what absolute size (cm) of her ascending and descending thoracic aorta respectively should she undergo surgical intervention?

A. 5.0 cm (ascending) / 6.0 cm (descending)
B. 5.5 cm (ascending) / 6.0 cm (descending)
C. 5.0 cm (ascending) / 6.5 cm (descending)
D. 4.5 cm (ascending) / 5.0 cm (descending)
E. 5.0 cm (ascending) / 5.0 cm (descending)

93-8. Pathologic and histologic examination of an aorta and its branches is performed during autopsy of a 40-year-old woman who died suddenly. On gross examination, the left subclavian artery is substantially narrowed, and she demonstrates evidence of healed pericarditis. Molecular autopsy reveals a positive mutation in the *IL12B* gene. Which of the following aortopathies did this patient have?

A. Giant cell arteritis
B. Takayasu disease
C. Infectious aortitis
D. HLA-B27-associated spondyloarthorpathy
E. Syphilitic aortitis

93-9. A 55-year-old man was incidentally found to have an AAA while having an ultrasound as part of a work-up for renal stones. Which of the following statements regarding asymptomatic AAAs is *incorrect*?

A. AAAs between 4 and 5 cm in diameter are associated with a 1% per year risk of rupture
B. AAAs 5.5 cm in diameter or larger should be repaired
C. Patients with an infrarenal AAA measuring 4.0 to 5.4 cm should be monitored by ultrasound or CT scan every 2 years
D. Infrarenal AAAs < 4.0 cm in diameter pose a very low risk of rupture, and monitoring by ultrasound yearly is reasonable
E. Similar size indications for intervention should apply to both endovascular and surgical therapy for AAA

93-10. Regarding the medical management of aortic aneurysms, which of the following statements is *incorrect*?

A. Beta-blockers have been shown to delay aortic dissection and death in patients with Marfan syndrome
B. The data regarding angiotensin receptor blocking drugs for the attenuation of progression of aortic disease remain inconclusive
C. Doxycycline has shown promise in large-scale clinical trials in patients with AAAs
D. Statins have been shown to have a substantial benefit for thoracic aortic aneurysms, most pronounced for descending and thoracoabdominal aneurysms
E. Cyclooxygenase 2 inhibitory anti-inflammatory agents have not been associated with consistent clinical benefit

93-1. **The answer is D.** *(Hurst's The Heart, 14th Edition, Chap. 93)* The vasa vasorum supplies the adventitia and media of the *thoracic* aorta (the vasa vasorum do *not* supply the media of the abdominal aorta). The major conductance vessel of the body, the aorta is an elastic artery with a trilaminar wall: the tunica intima, tunica media, and tunica adventitia.[1,2] The innermost lining of the tunica intima is the endothelium, resting on a thin basal lamina (option A). An internal elastic membrane forms the outer lining of the tunica intima (option B). The tunica media is approximately 1 mm thick, comprised of elastin, smooth muscle cells, collagen, and ground substance (option E). The predominance of elastic fibers in the aortic wall and their arrangement as circumferential lamellae distinguish it from the smaller muscular arteries. Surrounding the tunica media is the tunica adventitia, which is composed of loose connective tissue, including fibroblasts, relatively small amounts of collagen fibers, elastin, and ground substance. The adventitia strengthens the aorta and is essential to aortic surgeons for secure suturing of tissues. Within the tunica adventitia lie the nervi vasorum and vasa vasorum. Unlike the elastic fibers of the arterial wall, which are highly distensible, collagen is inelastic and provides the tensile strength required to prevent deformation and rupture of the aortic wall.

93-2. **The answer is C.** *(Hurst's The Heart, 14th Edition, Chap. 93)* An intramural hematoma represents a concentric, circumferentially oriented collection of thrombus in the aortic wall, without the discrete transluminal flap typical of aortic dissection. A gross morphologic classification distinguishes true aneurysms as fusiform (most common) or saccular. A fusiform aneurysm (option A) is roughly cylindrical and affects the entire circumference of the aorta; a saccular aneurysm is an outpouching of only a portion of the aortic circumference (option B). Frequently, a small neck provides continuity between the aortic lumen and the saccular aneurysm. Aortic dissection refers to a splitting of the medial layer of the aortic wall, permitting longitudinal propagation of blood between the components of the aortic wall. Aortic dissection is the most common cause of death due to human aortic disease.[3] Acute aortic transection, a consequence of trauma, involves localized disruption of an intrinsically normal aortic wall, which is resistant to propagating dissection (option E). A penetrating aortic ulcer involves localized perforation of the medial layer of the aortic wall beneath an atherosclerotic plaque (option D).

93-3. **The answer is A.** *(Hurst's The Heart, 14th Edition, Chap. 93)* Renal cysts, *not liver cysts*, have been associated with an increased likelihood for the presence of a thoracic aortic aneurysm. Aneurysms are often clinically silent until rupture or dissection occurs, and these catastrophes are most often fatal. Thus the detection of asymptomatic aneurysms is paramount. "Guilt by association" has been proposed as a strategic approach to aneurysm detection[4] capitalizing on eight clinical correlates of thoracic aortic aneurysm: (1) Intracranial (option B) or (2) abdominal aneurysm that illustrates the coincidence of aneurysms in multiple vascular beds. Patients with thoracic aneurysms have an approximately 10% likelihood of concurrent intracranial aneurysms.[5] (3) Bovine aortic arch configuration (option D) and other arch anomalies, like the direct origin of the left vertebral artery from the aortic arch or aberrant right subclavian artery, occur more often in patients with thoracic aortic aneurysm than in the general population.[6,7] (4) Bicuspid aortic valve, which is associated with structural abnormalities of the ascending aorta, including aortic coarctation. (5) Renal cysts (*not* liver cysts), which may reflect excess MMP activity.[8] (6) Family history. (7) A positive thumb-palm sign, which echoes the importance of a family history of aortic aneurysmal disease. (8) Temporal arteritis.

93-4. **The answer is E.** *(Hurst's The Heart, 14th Edition, Chap. 93)* The *KCNH2* gene mutation is found in long QT syndrome type 2, *not* familial thoracic aortic aneurysms.

To date, as many as 21 genes have been linked with familial or syndromic thoracic aortic aneurysms and dissection (see Fig. 93-12 in *Hurst's The Heart*, 14th edition),[9] and the discovery of additional candidate genes is likely. These encode molecules that regulate extracellular matrix (*FBN1, FBN2, COL1A1, COL1A2, COL3A1*), the cytoskeleton of smooth muscle cells (*ACTA2, MYH11, MYLK*), and the TGF-β signaling pathway (*TGFβ2, TGFBR1, TGFBR2, SMAD3, SLC2A10*). Most known mutations predispose to aortic aneurysm formation. Marfan syndrome (option A) is linked to an autosomal dominant anomaly in the gene regulating the synthesis of fibrillin type 1, a large glycoprotein that directs and orients elastin in the developing aorta.[10] Marfan syndrome was widely attributed to structural abnormalities and weaknesses of the aortic wall until dysregulation of TGF-β signaling was identified as a more reliable correlate.[11-13] TGF-β controls a panoply of cell functions. As fibrillin 1 binds TGF-β in an inactive complex, increased TGF-β signaling develops as a compensatory mechanism and plays a role in the pathogenesis of the degeneration of elastic fibers, the accumulation of mucoid material within the medial layer of the aortic wall, and accelerated cystic medial necrosis that characterize this disease. Ehlers–Danlos syndrome (option B) is an inherited connective tissue disorder less common than Marfan syndrome but also associated with aneurysm formation.[14-15] Although aneurysm formation and aortic dissection may occur in most types of Ehlers–Danlos syndrome, they are more frequent in the vascular type (type IV), which results from a mutation of the *COL3A1* gene.[16] Loeys–Dietz syndrome (option C), which is caused by mutations in the *TGFBR1* and *TGFBR2* genes, is associated with aortic and arterial aneurysms that enlarge rapidly and are prone to rupture; in one series, the mean age at death was 26 years.[17,18] The specific genetic mutations in humans with bicuspid valve (option D) have proven complex and multifactorial; abnormalities in the *NOTCH1* gene have been documented, but only in some bicuspid patients.[19] Evidence shows that excess MMP activity characterizes both the valve tissue and the aortic wall in bicuspid patients.

93-5. **The answer is E.** *(Hurst's The Heart, 14th Edition, Chap. 93)* A transesophageal echo (TEE) will be able to easily see an aneurysm involving the *proximal* aorta, but it will have difficulty in visualizing an aneurysm that is predominantly in the *mid-ascending aorta*. The TEE will also underestimate the size of an aneurysm in the mid-ascending aorta. A transthoracic echocardiogram (TTE) can only visualize the proximal several centimeters of the ascending aorta (option C), perhaps to just above the sinotubular junction in a patient with good echo windows. Thus a TTE will miss an aneurysm of the mid-portion of the ascending aorta (option D). Even TEE is limited by the interposed tracheal air column and can be "blinded" to the upper portion of the ascending aorta (option A).

93-6. **The answer is D.** *(Hurst's The Heart, 14th Edition, Chap. 93)* D-dimer is a byproduct of fibrin degradation. D-dimer is a useful biomarker in acute aortic dissection. It is 99% sensitive (option B) in the detection of acute aortic dissection.[20] If the D-dimer is not elevated, the patient does not have aortic dissection. However, D-dimer is extremely nonspecific (option C), being elevated in patients with pulmonary embolism and coronary thrombosis, essentially in any state in which thrombosis and thrombolysis proceed. The extent of D-dimer elevation reflects the longitudinal extent of aortic dissection (option D), predicts the mortality of patients with aortic dissection (option E), and differentiates dissection from MI. However, because D-dimer elevation occurs *after* the dissection, it is not useful as a predictor (option A).

93-7. **The answer is A.** *(Hurst's The Heart, 14th Edition, Chap. 93)* In non-Marfan patients, when viewed in terms of cumulative lifetime risk, the natural history of thoracic aortic aneurysms is characterized by an abrupt increment in the incidence of dissection or rupture at a maximum diameter of 6 cm for the ascending aorta; these events tend to occur at a larger dimension at the level of the descending aorta. Yearly risks of rupture, dissection, or death reflect a stepwise increment in risk as the aorta expands, rising most dramatically to 14.1% at a dimension of 6 cm.[21-23] Based on this observation, patients without overwhelming comorbidities should undergo resection of thoracic aortic aneurysm before the maximum diameter reaches 5.5 to 6.0 cm. The descending aorta enlarges somewhat more rapidly than the ascending aorta. For patients with Marfan syndrome or a family history of this disease, a criterion of 5 cm is usually applied because these patients are more prone to rupture or dissection.[21-23] Lacking evidence from prospective trials, surgical repair of aortic root or ascending aortic aneurysms in patients with bicuspid aortic valves is generally recommended at diameters ≥ 5.5 cm.[24] Surgical intervention may be considered when the aortic diameter reaches ≥ 5.0 cm, when aortic expansion occurs at a rate in excess of 0.5 cm annually, or in those with a family history of aortic dissection.[24,25] As for aortic aneurysms confined to the chest or abdomen, the dimensional criteria for surgical intervention apply only to asymptomatic aneurysms. *Symptomatic aortic aneurysms at any level should be resected regardless of size.* The development of symptoms frequently portends rupture and mandates surgical or endovascular repair.

93-8. The answer is B. *(Hurst's The Heart, 14th Edition, Chap. 93)* Because of its predilection for the brachiocephalic vessels, this arteritis has been labeled *pulseless disease* and *aortic arch syndrome*. Recently, a genetic underpinning for Takayasu disease has been discovered, with mutations in the *HLA-B* and *IL12B* genes.[26,27] Histologic examination during active stages of the disease discloses a granulomatous arteritis similar to giant-cell arteritis and to the aortitis associated with the seronegative spondyloarthropathies and Cogan syndrome. In later stages, medial degeneration, fibrous scarring, intimal proliferation, and thrombosis result in narrowing of the vessel. Aneurysm formation is less common than stenosis, but aneurysm rupture is an important cause of death in patients with Takayasu arteritis. Angiographically, the left subclavian artery is narrowed in approximately 90% of patients. The right subclavian artery, left carotid artery, and brachiocephalic trunk follow closely in frequency of stenosis. Clinical pericarditis has been observed infrequently, but healed pericarditis is often encountered at necropsy. The American College of Rheumatology has identified six major criteria for the diagnosis of Takayasu arteritis.[28] Onset of illness by age 40 years avoids overlap with giant-cell arteritis. Other criteria include upper-extremity claudication; diminished brachial pulses; > 10 mm Hg difference between systolic blood pressure in the arms; subclavian or aortic bruit; and narrowing of the aorta or a major branch. The presence of three of these six criteria carries high diagnostic accuracy. Giant-cell arteritis (option A) involves extracranial arteries, including the aorta, but the peak incidence is later in life. Infectious aortitis (option C) is a primary infection of the aortic wall that causes aortic aneurysms, more often saccular than fusiform. *Staphylococcus*, *Salmonella*, and *Pseudomonas* species are the most frequent pathogens causing primary aortic infections.[29] Aortitis is present in a substantial portion of patients with ankylosing spondylitis and Reiter syndrome; > 90% have the histocompatibility antigen HLA-B27 (option D). Treponemal infection produces chronic aortitis in approximately 10% of patients with untreated tertiary syphilis (option E) and is the primary cause of death in about the same proportion of cases, but there is evidence of the process at autopsy in about half of patients who have had untreated syphilis for > 10 years.[30]

93-9. The answer is C. *(Hurst's The Heart, 14th Edition, Chap. 93)* In general, patients with infrarenal or juxtarenal AAAs measuring 4.0 to 5.4 cm in diameter should be monitored by ultrasonography or CT scans every *6 months (not every 2 years)* to detect expansion. Repair may be beneficial in selected patients with aneurysms. Abdominal aortic aneurysms between 4 and 5 cm in diameter are associated with a 1% per year risk of rupture, and decisions regarding surveillance or surgery should be individualized based on age, familial features, and an assessment of surgical risk (option A). Aneurysms 5.5 cm in diameter or larger carry a substantial risk of rupture and should be repaired (option B). For patients with aneurysms smaller than 4.0 cm in diameter, monitoring by ultrasonography examination yearly is reasonable (option D). Intervention is not recommended for patients with asymptomatic infrarenal or juxtarenal aneurysms smaller than 5.0 cm in diameter in men or 4.5 cm in women. A meta-analysis found that these criteria should be employed as well for *endovascular* treatment of AAAs, and that similar size indications for intervention should apply to both endovascular and surgical therapy (option E).[31]

93-10. The answer is A. *(Hurst's The Heart, 14th Edition, Chap. 93)* Patients with aortic aneurysms are commonly treated with β-adrenergic antagonist drugs to decrease systolic arterial wall stress, but the effectiveness of this strategy has been validated only in one long-term study of 70 patients with clinical features of Marfan syndrome.[32,33] The value of β-adrenergic antagonist drugs in patients with and without Marfan syndrome is controversial.[34-38]

Among the concerns, in addition to the potential for side effects, is evidence that beta-blockers decrease the elasticity of the aortic wall. The evidence that beta-blockers delay aortic dilatation in Marfan patients is quite equivocal, and there is, further, simply no evidence of effectiveness in preventing the vital clinical end points of aortic dissection and death.[38] Angiotensin receptor blocking drugs (ARBs) (option B) represent a potential alternative to beta-blockers in patients with Marfan syndrome,[39-41] based on groundbreaking work by Dietz and colleagues, which showed the benefit of losartan in a mouse model and in infants with Marfan disease.[39-41] The concept was developed that ARBs (acting on the TGF-β pathway) can attenuate the progression of aortic disease in Marfan patients. However, a randomized clinical trial comparing the losartan to atenolol showed no difference in rates of progressive aortic root dilation among children and young adults with Marfan syndrome,[42] but the issue remains unresolved in part because of concerns about dose selection. The antibiotic agent doxycycline (option C), an MMP inhibitor, has shown promise in large-scale clinical trials in patients with AAAs.[43] Cyclooxygenase (COX) 2 inhibitory anti-inflammatory agents have not been associated with consistent clinical benefit (option D).[44] A retrospective study in large numbers of patients with thoracic aortic aneurysm suggested substantial benefit in meaningful clinical end points from statin therapy for thoracic aortic aneurysm, most pronounced for descending and thoracoabdominal aneurysms (option E).[45]

References

1. The circulatory system. In: Junqueira LC, Carneiro J, eds. *Basic Histology: Text and Atlas*. 11th ed. New York: McGraw-Hill Access Medicine (electronic format); 2005.
2. Sanz J, Einstein AJ, Fuster V. Acute aortic dissection: Anti-impulse therapy. In: Elefteriades JA, ed. *Acute Aortic Disease*. New York: Informa Healthcare USA; 2007:229-248.
3. Anagnostopoulos CE. *Acute Aortic Dissections*. Baltimore, MD: University Park Press; 1975.
4. Elefteriades JA, Sang A, Kuzmik G, Hornick M. Guilt by association: paradigm for detecting a silent killer (thoracic aortic aneurysm). *Open Heart*. 2015;2:e000169.
5. Kuzmik GA, Feldman M, Tranquilli M, Rizzo JA, Johnson M, Elefteriades JA. Concurrent intracranial and thoracic aortic aneurysms. *Am J Cardiol*. 2010;105:417-420.
6. Hornick M, Moomiaie R, Mojibian H, et al. "Bovine" aortic arch: a marker for thoracic aortic disease. *Cardiology*. 2012;123:116-124.
7. Dumfarth J, Chou AS, Ziganshin BA, et al. Atypical aortic arch branching variants: A novel marker for thoracic aortic disease. *J Thorac Cardiovasc Surg*. 2015;149:1586-1592.
8. Ziganshin BA, Theodoropoulos P, Salloum MN, et al. Simple renal cysts as markers of thoracic aortic disease. *J Am Heart Assoc*. 2016;5:e002248.
9. Ziganshin BA, Bailey AE, Coons C, et al. Routine genetic testing for thoracic aortic aneurysm and dissection in a clinical setting. *Ann Thorac Surg*. 2015;100:1604-1611.
10. Jondeau G, Delorme G, Guiti C. [Marfan syndrome]. *Rev Prat*. 2002;52:1089-1093.
11. Franken R, Radonic T, den Hartog AW, et al. The revised role of TGF-beta in aortic aneurysms in Marfan syndrome. *Neth Heart J*. 2015;23:116-121.
12. Loeys BL. Angiotensin receptor blockers: a panacea for Marfan syndrome and related disorders? *Drug Discov Today*. 2015;20:262-266.
13. Yuan SM, Ma HH, Zhang RS, Jing H. Transforming growth factor-beta signaling pathway in Marfan's syndrome: a preliminary histopathological study. *VASA*. 2011;40:369-374.
14. Callewaert B, Malfait F, Loeys B, De Paepe A. Ehlers-Danlos syndromes and Marfan syndrome. *Best Pract Res Clin Rheumatol*. 2008;22:165-189.
15. De Paepe A, Malfait F. The Ehlers-Danlos syndrome, a disorder with many faces. *Clin Genet*. 2012;82:1-11.
16. Pepin M, Schwarze U, Superti-Furga A, Byers PH. Clinical and genetic features of Ehlers-Danlos syndrome type IV, the vascular type. *N Engl J Med*. 2000;342:673-680.
17. Loeys BL, Schwarze U, Holm T, et al. Aneurysm syndromes caused by mutations in the TGF-beta receptor. *N Engl J Med*. 2006;355:788-798.
18. Loeys BL, Chen J, Neptune ER, et al. A syndrome of altered cardiovascular, craniofacial, neurocognitive and skeletal development caused by mutations in *TGFBR1* or *TGFBR2*. *Nat Genet*. 2005;37:275-281.
19. McKellar SH, Tester DJ, Yagubyan M, Majumdar R, Ackerman MJ, Sundt TM 3rd. Novel *NOTCH1* mutations in patients with bicuspid aortic valve disease and thoracic aortic aneurysms. *J Thorac Cardiovasc Surg*. 2007;134:290-296.
20. Ohlmann P, Faure A, Morel O, et al. Diagnostic and prognostic value of circulating D-dimers in patients with acute aortic dissection. *Crit Care Med*. 2006;34:1358-1364.

21. Davies RR, Goldstein LJ, Coady MA, et al. Yearly rupture or dissection rates for thoracic aortic aneurysms: simple prediction based on size. *Ann Thorac Surg.* 2002;73:17-27.

22. Davies RR, Gallo A, Coady MA, et al. Novel measurement of relative aortic size predicts rupture of thoracic aortic aneurysms. *Ann Thorac Surg.* 2006;81:169-177.

23. Elefteriades JA, Ziganshin BA, Rizzo JA, et al. Indications and imaging for aortic surgery: size and other matters. *J Thorac Cardiovasc Surg.* 2015;149:S10-S13.

24. Hiratzka LF, Creager MA, Isselbacher EM, et al. Surgery for aortic dilatation in patients with bicuspid aortic valves: a statement of clarification from the American College of Cardiology/American Heart Association Task Force on Clinical Practice Guidelines. *J Am Coll Cardiol.* 2016;67:724-731.

25. Wojnarski CM, Svensson LG, Roselli EE, et al. Aortic dissection in patients with bicuspid aortic valve-associated aneurysms. *Ann Thorac Surg.* 2015;100:1666-1674.

26. Terao C. Revisited HLA and non-HLA genetics of Takayasu arteritis: where are we? *J Hum Genet* 2016;61:27-32.

27. Alibaz-Oner F, Direskeneli H. Update on Takayasu's arteritis. *Presse Med.* 2015;44:e259-e265.

28. Arend WP, Michel BA, Bloch DA, et al. The American College of Rheumatology 1990 criteria for the classification of Takayasu arteritis. *Arthritis Rheum.* 1990;33:1129-1134.

29. Takagi H, Kato T, Matsuno Y, et al. Aortic dissection without Marfan's syndrome in ankylosing spondylitis. *J Thorac Cardiovasc Surg.* 2004;127:600-602.

30. Jackman JD, Jr., Radolf JD. Cardiovascular syphilis. *Am J Med.* 1989;87:425-433.

31. Filardo G, Powell JT, Martinez MA, Ballard DJ. Surgery for small asymptomatic abdominal aortic aneurysms. *Cochrane Database Syst Rev.* 2015;2:CD001835.

32. Shores J, Berger KR, Murphy EA, Pyeritz RE. Progression of aortic dilatation and the benefit of long-term beta-adrenergic blockade in Marfan's syndrome. *N Engl J Med.* 1994;330:1335-1341.

33. Yin FC, Brin KP, Ting CT, Pyeritz RE. Arterial hemodynamic indexes in Marfan's syndrome. *Circulation.* 1989;79:854-862.

34. Gersony DR, McClaughlin MA, Jin Z, Gersony WM. The effect of beta-blocker therapy on clinical outcome in patients with Marfan's syndrome: a meta-analysis. *Int J Cardiol.* 2007;114:303-308.

35. Gao L, Mao Q, Wen D, Zhang L, Zhou X, Hui R. The effect of beta-blocker therapy on progressive aortic dilatation in children and adolescents with Marfan's syndrome: a meta-analysis. *Acta Paediatr.* 2011;100:e101-e105.

36. Chun AS, Elefteriades JA, Mukherjee SK. Medical treatment for thoracic aortic aneurysm: much more work to be done. *Prog Cardiovasc Dis.* 2013;56:103-108.

37. Chun AS, Elefteraides JA, Mukherjee SK. Do beta-blockers really work for prevention of aortic aneurysms? Time for reassessment. *Aorta (Stamford).* 2013;1:45-51.

38. Ziganshin BA, Mukherjee SK, Elefteriades JA. Atenolol versus losartan in Marfan's syndrome. *N Engl J Med.* 2015;372:977-978.

39. Brooke BS, Habashi JP, Judge DP, Patel N, Loeys B, Dietz HC 3rd. Angiotensin II blockade and aortic-root dilation in Marfan's syndrome. *N Engl J Med.* 2008;358:2787-2795.

40. Matt P, Schoenhoff F, Habashi J, et al. Circulating transforming growth factor-beta in Marfan syndrome. *Circulation.* 2009;120:526-532.

41. Habashi JP, Judge DP, Holm TM, et al. Losartan, an AT1 antagonist, prevents aortic aneurysm in a mouse model of Marfan syndrome. *Science.* 2006;312:117-121.

42. Lacro RV, Dietz HC, Sleeper LA, et al. Atenolol versus losartan in children and young adults with Marfan's syndrome. *N Engl J Med.* 2014;371:2061-2071.

43. Hackmann AE, Thompson RW, LeMaire SA. Long-term suppressive therapy: clinical reality and future prospects. In: Elefteriades JA, ed. *Acute Aortic Disease.* New York: Informa Healthcare; 2007:309-330.

44. Cipollone F, Prontera C, Pini B, et al. Overexpression of functionally coupled cyclooxygenase-2 and prostaglandin E synthase in symptomatic atherosclerotic plaques as a basis of prostaglandin E(2)-dependent plaque instability. *Circulation.* 2001;104:921-927.

45. Stein LH, Berger J, Tranquilli M, Elefteriades JA. Effect of statin drugs on thoracic aortic aneurysms. *Am J Cardiol.* 2013;112:1240-1245.

CHAPTER 94

Cerebrovascular Disease and Neurologic Manifestations of Heart Disease

Jacqueline Joza

QUESTIONS

DIRECTIONS: Choose the one best response to each question.

94-1. A 50-year-old woman with mitral valve prolapse (MVP) presents to the hospital with three days of fever. Blood cultures are positive for a *Candida* species, and transesophageal echo confirms the presence of a possible vegetation on the posterior mitral valve leaflet. Which of the following statements is *correct*?

A. Warfarin should be given to prevent embolization
B. Embolic complications are unusual in patients with infective endocarditis
C. Myotic aneurysms can cause fatal subarachnoid bleeding
D. Libman–Sacks endocarditis refers to valve lesions occurring in patients with rheumatoid arthritis
E. MVP is a relatively common source of embolic stroke

94-2. A 75-year-old woman awakes from sleep with new left-sided weakness. Which of the following statements regarding cerebral infarction is *incorrect*?

A. MRI is more sensitive for the detection of acute brain infarcts than CT
B. MRI can image hemosiderin
C. The presence of superficial wedge-shaped infarcts in multiple different vascular territories is highly suggestive of a cardioembolic origin
D. The mechanism of hemorrhagic infarction is reperfusion of ischemic zones after iatrogenic opening of an occluded artery or after restoration of the circulation after a period of systemic hypoperfusion
E. Hemorrhagic cerebral infarction is considered characteristic of a thrombotic mechanism

94-3. Which of the following would be *least* likely to suggest the presence of a paradoxical embolism?

A. Prolonged airplane flight
B. Presence of factor V Leiden
C. Pulmonary embolism within a short time after a neurologic ischemic event
D. The sudden onset of stroke during straining
E. Increased brain natriuretic peptide (BNP) level

94-4. Different brain regions have selective vulnerability to hypoxic-ischemic damage. Which of the following regions are particularly vulnerable to injury?

A. The basal ganglia
B. The cerebral cortex
C. The hippocampus
D. The thalamus
E. Both B and C are correct

94-5. A 65-year-old woman is diagnosed with a subarachnoid hemorrhage (SAH). Which of the following findings would be *least* likely to be observed on electrocardiogram?

A. QT prolongation
B. QRS widening
C. U waves
D. Tall, peaked T waves
E. Large T-wave inversions

94-6. A 70-year-old man presents at the insistence of his wife. She has noticed her husband neglecting his left space, with a lack of awareness of his deficit. Which of the following effected arteries is responsible for this patient's findings?

A. Right middle cerebral artery
B. Internal carotid artery
C. Anterior cerebral artery
D. Left middle cerebral artery
E. Left posterior cerebral artery

94-7. You would like to initiate intravenous heparin in a patient with a moderate-sized middle cerebral infarct. The patient was found to have atrial fibrillation, and a transesophageal echo revealed a thrombus in the left atrial appendage. All of the following would delay or be contraindications to the use of intravenous heparin *except*:

A. The presence of a large cerebral infarct
B. Uncontrolled hypertension
C. Less than 48 hours from time of infarct
D. Bacterial endocarditis
E. Sepsis

94-8. A 55-year-old man presents to the hospital with left arm and leg weakness. The time is 3.5 hours after the onset of symptoms. Which of the following regarding t-PA is *incorrect* in this setting?

A. This patient has a 6% to 12% chance of intracranial bleeding
B. Patients with distal intracranial arterial embolic occlusions do well with thrombolysis
C. Patients with internal carotid artery occlusions in the neck are typically good responders to intravenous thrombolysis
D. Where possible, vascular imaging should precede the administration of thrombolysis
E. Intra-arterially administered prourokinase thrombolysis has also been proven to be very effective in opening arteries within the anterior circulation

94-9. Hypertension especially damages the deep arteries that penetrate perpendicularly from the major intracranial arteries. Which of the following constitutes a major pattern of brain ischemia in patients with hypertension?

A. Discrete lacunar infarcts
B. Diffuse, patchy, white and gray matter degeneration with gliosis
C. Arterial vasoconstriction
D. Both A and B are correct
E. Both A and C are correct

94-10. A 48-year-old man is brought to the hospital by ambulance with right arm weakness. A CT scan demonstrates the presence of an intracerebral hemorrhage. The patient has no known history of hypertension. All of the following are possible etiologies for an acute elevation of blood pressure resulting in an intracerebral hemorrhage *except*:

A. Amyloid angiopathy
B. Intracranial operations on the fifth cranial nerve
C. Pheochromocytoma
D. Recent onset of arterial hypertension
E. Cocaine use

94-1. **The answer is C.** *(Hurst's The Heart, 14th Edition, Chap. 94)* Embolic complications are *common* in patients who have infective endocarditis (option B).[1,2] Mycotic aneurysms can cause fatal subarachnoid bleeding (option C). Bleeding can also result from vascular necrosis as a result of an infected embolus.[2] Embolization usually stops when the infection is controlled.[3] Warfarin does *not* prevent embolization and is contraindicated in patients with endocarditis and known cerebral embolism (option A) unless there are other important lesions such as prosthetic valves or pulmonary embolism. In children and young adults with congenital heart defects, especially those with right-to-left shunts and polycythemia, brain abscess is an important complication. Valve lesions occur in patients with systemic lupus erythematosus (Libman–Sacks endocarditis)[4] (*not rheumatoid arthritis*), antiphospholipid antibody syndrome,[5] cancer, and other debilitating diseases (nonbacterial thrombotic endocarditis). Mitral valve prolapse (MVP) as a source of embolic stroke continues to be controversial.[1,6] Several small clinical series have reported cerebral embolism in MVP patients who lacked other possible embolic sources.[6-9] In the absence of atrial fibrillation, MVP/mitral regurgitation is probably *not* associated with a significant increase in the risk of first or recurrent stroke.[8-10]

94-2. **The answer is E.** *(Hurst's The Heart, 14th Edition, Chap. 94)* Hemorrhagic infarction has long been considered characteristic of *embolic* (*not a thrombotic mechanism*), especially when the artery leading to the infarct is patent.[11] MRI, particularly with the use of MR diffusion-weighted and MR gradient recall echo (GRE) imaging, is much more sensitive for the detection of acute brain infarcts than is CT (option A). MR is also superior in detecting hemorrhagic infarction by imaging hemosiderin (option B). The mechanism of hemorrhagic infarction is reperfusion of ischemic zones after iatrogenic opening of an occluded artery (eg, endarterectomy, fibrinolytic treatment) or after the restoration of the circulation after a period of systemic hypoperfusion (option D). Hemorrhage then occurs into proximal reperfused regions of brain infarcts.[1,12,13] Emboli usually cause the occlusion of distal branches and produce surface infarcts that are roughly triangular, with the apex of the triangle pointing inward. CT and MRI findings can suggest that an ischemic stroke was cardioembolic by the location and shape of the lesions on imaging;[14] for example, finding the presence of superficial wedge-shaped infarcts in multiple different vascular territories (option C), hemorrhagic infarction, and visualization of thrombi within arteries.

94-3. **The answer is E.** *(Hurst's The Heart, 14th Edition, Chap. 94)* Elevated BNP level does not increase the possibility of diagnosis of a paradoxical embolism from a patent foramen ovale. When four of the following five criteria are met, the presence of paradoxical embolism may be established with a high degree of certainty[1,15-17]: (1) situations that promote thrombosis of the deep veins of the leg or pelvis (eg, long sitting in one position, such as prolonged airplane flight, or recent surgery)(option A), (2) increased coagulability (eg, the use of oral contraceptives, the presence of factor V Leiden (option B), dehydration, and other inherited or acquired thrombophilia), (3) the sudden onset of stroke during Valsalva or other maneuvers that promote right-to-left shunting of blood (eg, sexual intercourse, straining at stool) (option C), (4) pulmonary embolism within a short time before or after the neurologic ischemic event (option D), and (5) the absence of other putative causes of stroke after thorough evaluation.

94-4. **The answer is E.** *(Hurst's The Heart, 14th Edition, Chap. 94)* Different brain regions have selective vulnerability to hypoxic-ischemic damage. Regions that are most remote and at the edges of major vascular supply are more liable to sustain hypoperfusion injury. These zones are usually referred to as border zones or watersheds. The cerebral cortex and hippocampus are particularly vulnerable to injury.[18-21] In the cerebral cortex, the border zone regions are between the anterior cerebral artery and middle cerebral artery (MCA), and between the MCA and posterior cerebral artery. The basal ganglia (option A) and thalamus (option D) are most involved if hypoxia is severe but some circulation is preserved. This situation applies most to hanging, strangulation, drowning, and carbon monoxide exposure.[22] Cerebellar neurons may also be selectively injured.[23]

94-5. The answer is B. *(Hurst's The Heart, 14th Edition, Chap. 94)* In stroke patients, especially those with SAH, QRS widening on ECG is not typically demonstrated. However, the ECG may show a prolonged QT interval (option A); giant, wide, roller coaster–inverted T waves (option D); and U waves (option C).[24] These changes are often called *cerebral T waves*. Patients with stroke undergoing continuous ECG monitoring have a high incidence of T-wave and ST-segment changes, various arrhythmias, and cardiac enzyme abnormalities. ECG changes may include a prolonged QT interval, depressed ST segments, flat or inverted T waves, and U waves.[24-28] Less often, tall, peaked T waves (option D) and elevated ST segments are noted. Myocardial enzyme release and echocardiographic regional wall motion abnormalities are associated with impaired left ventricular performance after SAH.

94-6. The answer is A. *(Hurst's The Heart, 14th Edition, Chap. 94)* Neurologic symptoms and signs depend on the region of the brain that is ischemic. Table 94-1 describes the most common signs in cerebrovascular occlusive disease at various sites.[12,29] Contralateral motor, sensory, and visual loss is present in a middle cerebral artery (MCA) occlusion. A right MCA occlusion will result in neglect of the left space, lack of awareness of deficit, apathy, and impersistence, whereas a left MCA occlusion will result in aphasia.

TABLE 94-1 **Common Signs in Cerebrovascular Occlusive Disease at Various Sites**

ICA origin	Ipsilateral transient monocular blindness; MCA and ACA signs
ICA siphon (proximal to ophthalmic artery)	Same as ICA origin
ICA siphon (distal to ophthalmic artery)	MCA and ACA signs
ACA	Contralateral weakness of the lower limb and shoulder shrug
MCA	Contralateral motor, sensory, and visual loss Left: Aphasia Right: Neglect of left space, lack of awareness of deficit apathy, impersistence
AChA	Contralateral motor, sensory, and visual loss, usually without cognitive changes
Subclavian artery (proximal to VA)	Lack of arm stamina, cool hand, transient dizziness, veering, diplopia
VA origin	Same as subclavian, but no ipsilateral arm or hand findings
VA intracranially	Lateral medullary syndrome; staggering and veering (cerebellar infarction)
BA	Bilateral motor weakness; ophthalmoplegia and diplopia
PCA	Contralateral hemianopia and hemisensory loss Left: Alexia with agraphia Right: Neglect of left visual space

Abbreviations: ACA, anterior cerebral artery; AChA, anterior choroidal artery; BA, basilar artery; ICA, internal carotid artery; MCA, middle cerebral artery; PCA, posterior cerebral artery; VA, vertebral artery.

94-7. The answer is C. *(Hurst's The Heart, 14th Edition, Chap. 94)* If there is considerable residual at-risk brain tissue, the direct treatment relies on the location and severity of the causative vascular lesion. Standard dose heparin is usually given by intravenous infusion, keeping the APTT between 60 and 100s (1.5–2 x control APTT). It is given as *immediate* therapy for definite cardiac-origin cerebral embolism. However, a large cerebral infarct (option A), hypertension (option B), bacterial endocarditis (option D), or sepsis (option E) would delay or contraindicate its use. Intravenous heparin should also be used in the setting of a severe stenosis or occlusion of the internal carotid artery (ICA) origin, ICA siphon, middle cerebral artery, vertebral artery, or basilar artery with less than a large clinical deficit. Subsequent treatment could consist of warfarin or surgery in these patients.

94-8. **The answer is C.** (*Hurst's The Heart, 14th Edition, Chap. 94*) Patients with internal carotid artery occlusions in the neck and intracranially *rarely* reperfuse after intravenous thrombolytic therapy, especially if collateral circulation is poor. Thrombolytic drugs, especially recombinant tissue-type plasminogen activator (rt-PA) and streptokinase, have been given intravenously and intra-arterially in patients with acute brain ischemia. In a study in which the arterial lesions were undefined, intravenous therapy with rt-PA given within 90 minutes and 3 hours of ischemia onset, in the aggregate, provided a statistically significant benefit.[30] Additionally, in a more recent study, intravenous t-PA was found to be of overall benefit even when given 3 to 4.5 hours after ischemic stroke symptom onset.[31] Unfortunately, in these and other studies, approximately 6% to 12% of patients treated with thrombolytic agents developed important intracranial bleeding (option A). Uncontrolled studies show that patients with distal intracranial arterial embolic occlusions do well with intravenous thrombolytic therapy (option B).[32-37] Intra-arterially administered prourokinase thrombolysis has also been proven to be very effective in opening blocked intracranial arteries within the anterior circulation (option E).[38] The dose, timing, mode of delivery, and target group for therapy remain unsettled. Vascular imaging should precede the administration of thrombolytic agents (option D). Brain and vascular imaging can guide physicians as to who should receive thrombolytics and by what route.[39]

94-9. **The answer is D.** (*Hurst's The Heart, 14th Edition, Chap. 94*) The two major patterns of brain ischemia in patients with hypertension are *discrete lacunar infarcts* and a more *diffuse, patchy, white, and gray matter degeneration with gliosis*. Both are caused by sclerotic changes in deep intracerebral arteries and arterioles. The term *lacune* (hole) refers to a small, deep infarct caused by lipohyalinosis of the penetrating artery feeding the ischemic brain tissue.[40,41] Vasoconstriction and symptoms of diffuse brain swelling can be seen in aneurysmal SAH. The two most important neurologic complications of aneurysmal SAH are rebleeding and brain ischemia caused by vasoconstriction (so-called vasospasm). Vasoconstriction of arteries is thought to be caused by blood or blood products that bathe the adventitia of arteries.[42-45]

94-10. **The answer is A.** (*Hurst's The Heart, 14th Edition, Chap. 94*) Intracerebral hemorrhage (ICH) accounts for approximately 10% of all strokes.[12,46] Head trauma, vascular malformations, bleeding diatheses, drugs (especially anticoagulants, amphetamines, and cocaine), amyloid angiopathy, and intracranial aneurysms account for some cases.[47,48] Although amyloid angiopathy does cause ICH, it is *not* through a mechanism of causing an acute elevation of blood pressure. Traditionally, spontaneous ICH has usually been equated with hypertensive hemorrhage. Many patients, however, have no history of hypertension or associated changes of hypertensive vasculopathy at necropsy.[49-51] Acute elevations of blood pressure and/or blood flow to the brain can cause ICH by the sudden increase in blood pressure, causing vessel breakage.[52] Causes of acute changes in blood pressure or blood flow that can result in ICH include: drugs (especially cocaine and amphetamines) (option E), recent onset of arterial hypertension (option D), pheochromocytoma (option C), cold hemorrhages (exposure to freezing ambient temperatures), dental chair hemorrhages, intracranial operations on the fifth cranial nerve (option B), stereotactic treatment of the fifth cranial nerve for trigeminal neuralgia, carotid endarterectomy (reflex hypertension and reperfusion), cardiac transplantation, especially in children, surgical repair of congenital heart disease in children, and migraines.

References

1. Caplan LR. Brain embolism. In: Caplan LR, Hurst JW, Chimowitz MI, eds. *Clinical Neurocardiology*. New York: Marcel Dekker; 1999:35-185.
2. Kanter MC, Hart RG. Neurologic complications of infective endocarditis. *Neurology*. 1991;41:1015-1020.

3. Nighoghossian N, Derex L, Loire R, et al. Giant lambl excrescences: an unusual source of cerebral embolism. *Arch Neurol.* 1997;54:41-44.

4. Galve E, Candell-Riera J, Pigrau C, et al. Prevalence, morphology, types and evaluation of cardiac valvular disease in systemic lupus erythematosus. *N Engl J Med.* 1988;319:817-823.

5. Barbut D, Borer JS, Wallerson D, et al. Anticardiolipin antibody and stroke: possible relation of valvular heart disease and embolic events. *Cardiology.* 1991;79:99-109.

6. Barnett HJM, Jones MW, Boughner DR, et al. Cerebral ischemic events associated with prolapsing mitral valve. *Arch Neurol.* 1976;33:777-782.

7. Barnett HJM, Boughner DR, Taylor DW, et al. Further evidence relating mitral valve prolapse to cerebral ischemic events. *N Engl J Med.* 1980;302:139-144.

8. Sandok BA, Giuliani ER. Cerebral ischemic events in patients with mitral valve prolapse. *Stroke.* 1982;13:448-450.

9. Lauzier S, Barnett HJM. Cerebral ischemia with mitral valve prolapse and mitral annulus calcification. In: Furlan AJ, ed. *The Heart and Stroke.* London, UK: Springer-Verlag; 1987:63-100.

10. Kernan WN, Ovbiagele B, Black HR, et al. Guidelines for the prevention of stroke in patients with stroke and transient ischemic attack. *Stroke.* 2014;45(7):2160-2236.

11. Fisher CM, Adams RD. Observations on brain embolism. *J Neuropathol Exp Neurol.* 1951;10:92-94.

12. Caplan LR. *Stroke: A Clinical Approach.* 3rd ed. Boston, MA: Butterworth-Heinemann; 2000.

13. Fisher CM, Adams RD. Observations on brain embolism with special reference to hemorrhagic infarction. In: Furlan AJ, ed. *The Heart and Stroke.* London, UK: Springer-Verlag; 1987:17-36.

14. Ringlestein EB, Koschorke S, Holling A, et al. Computed tomographic patterns of proven embolic brain infarcts. *Ann Neurol.* 1989;26:759-765.

15. Jones HR, Caplan LR, Come PC, et al. Cerebral emboli of paradoxical origin. *Ann Neurol.* 1983;13:314-319.

16. Biller J, Adams HP, Johnson MR, et al. Paradoxical cerebral embolism: eight cases. *Neurology.* 1986;36:1356-1360.

17. Gautier JC, Durr A, Koussa S, et al. Paradoxical cerebral embolism with a patent foramen ovale: A report of 29 patients. *Cerebrovasc Dis.* 1991;1:193-202.

18. Brierley J, Meldrum B, Brown A. The threshold and neuropathology of cerebral "anoxic-ischemic" cell change. *Arch Neurol.* 1973;29:367-373.

19. Brierley JB, Adams JH, Graham DI, et al. Neocortical death after cardiac arrest: a clinical, neurophysiological report of two cases. *Lancet.* 1971;2:560-565.

20. Dougherty JH, Rawlinson DG, Levy DE, et al. Hypoxic-ischemic brain injury and the vegetative state: clinical and neuropathologic correlation. *Neurology.* 1981;31:991-997.

21. Cummings JL, Tomiyasu U, Read S, et al. Amnesia with hippocampal lesions after cardiopulmonary arrest. *Neurology.* 1984;34:679-681.

22. Dooling E, Richardson EP. Delayed encephalopathy after strangling. *Arch Neurol.* 1976;33:196-199.

23. Lance J, Adams RD. The syndrome of intention and action myoclonus as a sequel to hypoxic encephalopathy. *Brain.* 1963;86:111-133.

24. Burch GE, Myers R, Abildskov JA. A new electrocardiographic pattern observed in cerebrovascular accidents. *Circulation.* 1954;9:719-723.

25. Caplan LR, Hurst JW. Cardiac and cardiovascular findings in patients with nervous system disease: strokes. In: Caplan LR, Hurst JW, Chimowitz MI, eds. *Clinical Neurocardiology.* New York: Marcel Dekker; 1999:303-312.

26. Dimant J, Grob D. Electrocardiographic changes and myocardial damage in patients with acute cerebrovascular accidents. *Stroke.* 1977;8:448-455.

27. Rolak LA, Rokey R. Electrocardiographic features. In: Rolak LA, Rokey R, eds. *Coronary and Cerebral Vascular Disease.* Mt. Kisco, NY: Futura; 1990:139-197.

28. Goldstein DS. The electrocardiogram in stroke: relationship to pathophysiological type and comparison with prior tracings. *Stroke.* 1979;10:253-259.

29. Caplan LR. Cerebrovascular disease: large artery occlusive disease. In: Appel S, ed. *Current Neurology.* Vol. 87. Chicago, IL: Year Book; 1988:179-226.

30. National Institute of Neurological Disorders and Stroke rt-PA Study Group. Tissue plasminogen activator for acute ischemic stroke. *N Engl J Med.* 1995;333:1581-1587.

31. Hacke W, Kaste M, Bluhmki E, et al. Thrombolysis with alteplase 3 to 4.5 hours after acute ischemic stroke. *N Engl J Med.* 2008;359:1317-1329.

32. del Zoppo GJ, Poeck K, Pessin MS, et al. Recombinant tissue plasminogen activator in acute thrombotic and embolic stroke. *Ann Neurol.* 1992;32:78-86.

33. Wolpert SM, Bruckmann H, Greenlee R, et al. Neuroradiologic evaluation of patients with acute stroke treated with recombinant tissue plasminogen activator. *AJNR Am J Neuroradiol.* 1993;14:3-13.

34. Pessin MS, del Zoppo GJ, Furlan AJ. Thrombolytic treatment in acute stroke: review and update of selected topics. In: Moskowitz MA, Caplan LR, eds. *Cerebrovascular Diseases: Nineteenth Princeton Stroke Conference.* Boston, MA: Butterworth-Heinemann; 1995:409-418.

35. Furlan A, Higashida R, Wechsler L, et al. Intra-arterial prourokinase for acute ischemic stroke. The PROACT II study: a randomized controlled trial—prolyse in acute cerebral thromboembolism. *JAMA.* 1999;282:2003-2011.

36. Caplan LR, Mohr JP, Kistler JP, et al. Should thrombolytic therapy be the first-line treatment for acute ischemic stroke? *N Engl J Med*. 1997;337:1309-1313.

37. Caplan LR. Intracranial branch atheromatous disease. *Neurology*. 1989;39:1246-1250.

38. Caplan LR. Lacunar infarction: A neglected concept. *Geriatrics*. 1976;31:71-75.

39. Caplan LR. Binswanger's disease revisited. *Neurology*. 1995;45:626-633.

40. Fisher CM, Caplan LR. Basilar artery branch occlusion: a cause of pontine infarction. *Neurology*. 1971;21:900-905.

41. Fisher CM. Bilateral occlusion of basilar artery branches. *J Neurol Neurosurg Psychiatry*. 1977;40:1182-1189.

42. Heros R, Zervas NT, Varsos V. Cerebral vasospasm after subarachnoid hemorrhage: an update. *Ann Neurol*. 1983;14:599-608.

43. Kassell N, Sasaki T, Colohan A, et al. Cerebral vasospasm following aneurysmal subarachnoid hemorrhage. *Stroke*. 1985;16:562-572.

44. MacDonald RL, Weir BK. A review of hemoglobin and the pathogenesis of cerebral vasospasm. *Stroke*. 1991;22:971-982.

45. Ostergaard JR. Warning leaks in subarachnoid hemorrhage. *BMJ*. 1990;301:190-191.

46. Mohr J, Caplan LR, Melski J, et al. The Harvard cooperative stroke registry: a prospective study. *Neurology*. 1978;28:754-762.

47. Edelman RR, Mattle HP, Atkinson DJ, et al. MR angiography. *AJR Am J Roentgenol*. 1990;154:937-946.

48. Eckstein HH, Ringleb P, Allenberg JR, et al. Results of the Stent-Protected Angioplasty versus Carotid Endarterectomy (SPACE) study to treat symptomatic stenosis at 2 years: a multinational, prospective, randomised trial. *Lancet Neurol*. 2008;7:893-902.

49. Schlesinger MJ, Reiner L. Focal myocytolysis of heart. *Am J Pathol*. 1955;31:443-459.

50. Bahemuka M. Primary intracerebral hemorrhage and heart weight: a clinicopathological case-control review of 218 patients. *Stroke*. 1987;18:531-536.

51. Brott T, Thalinger K, Hertzberg V. Hypertension as a risk factor for spontaneous intracerebral hemorrhage. *Stroke*. 1986;17:1078-1083.

52. Caplan LR. Intracerebral hemorrhage revisited. *Neurology*. 1988;38:624-627.

CHAPTER 95

Carotid Artery Stenting

Patrick R. Lawler

QUESTIONS

DIRECTIONS: Choose the one best response to each question.

95-1. Which of the following is *incorrect* regarding asymptomatic carotid stenosis?

A. The severity of the carotid bruit correlates with the severity of the stenosis
B. Patients are likely to have collaterals to the affected hemisphere
C. Stroke risk in these patients is mainly from embolism plaque
D. Revascularization can be considered for patients with > 80% asymptomatic stenosis
E. None of the above are incorrect

95-2. During a routine physical examination, a carotid bruit is auscultated in a 46-year-old obese man. The results from a duplex ultrasound and angiography confirm asymptomatic carotid stenosis. Regarding treatment options, which of the following arguments in favor of interventional therapy is *incorrect*?

A. Statin therapy is not effective in decreasing the total number of fatal strokes
B. Compliance with medical treatment may be diminished due to the lack of symptoms
C. Response to medical treatment of an established stroke is unpredictable
D. Revascularization subjects the patient to small risks that are spread out over time
E. All of the above are incorrect

95-3. A 50-year-old man presents to your clinic with complaints of dizziness and frequent headaches. Duplex ultrasound of the carotid arteries reveal a severe stenosis in the left internal carotid artery. Which of the following factors is *not* generally considered a contraindication to carotid artery stenting (CAS)?

A. Dementia
B. A 90° angle between the ICA and the ECA
C. Severe stenosis with TIMI grade III flow in the vessel
D. Severe ICA stenosis with "string sign"
E. Extensive circumferential calcification of the ICA

95-4. Which of the following is *correct* regarding the evaluation of patients for CAS?

A. Antihypertensive agents and beta-blockers should be withheld the day of the procedure
B. A neurological exam is *not* mandatory when evaluating a patient for a possible carotid intervention
C. CT angiography is the standard noninvasive method for the evaluation of carotid artery stenosis
D. It is advantageous to perform the carotid intervention during a coronary angiography
E. All of the above are correct

95-5. Your patient is scheduled to undergo CAS. Which of the following is *incorrect* about the use of embolic protection devices (EPDs) during this procedure?

A. The use of occlusive EPDs is restricted to patients with robust collateral circulation to the affected hemisphere
B. With EPDs, all steps of the carotid intervention are completely protected from emboli
C. Nonocclusive EPDs function like filters that preserve antegrade flow
D. Proximal occlusive EPDs function by the interruption of antegrade flow and flow reversal
E. None of the above are incorrect

95-6. Which of the following is *correct* regarding the procedure of CAS?

A. The procedure is performed under general anesthesia
B. An EPD is placed cephalad to the area of stenosis
C. Following stent deployment, the balloon should be deflated as quickly as possible
D. The use of glycoprotein IIb/IIIa inhibitors is recommended
E. Hypotension in the postprocedure period is normal and never worrisome

95-7. Which of the following scenarios is of concern during the intraprocedural management of a patient undergoing CAS?

A. The use of glycoprotein IIb/IIIa inhibitors during the procedure
B. Frequent yawning by the patient during the procedure
C. Increased blood pressure in the postprocedure period
D. Persistent hypotension in the postprocedure period
E. All of the above

95-8. Cerebral hyperperfusion syndrome (CHS) is an infrequent but devastating outcome of CAS. Which of the following regarding CHS is *correct*?

A. The most common clinical symptom is confusion
B. Calcium antagonists and nitrates are indicated in the treatment of CHS
C. CHS is usually symptomatic and thus easy to detect
D. Antihypertensives and anticonvulsant therapy are the mainstay of treatment
E. CHS is defined as an increase in blood flow of > 80% from baseline associated with a neurological deficit

95-9. What was the main conclusion of the CREST study regarding the management of patients with symptomatic carotid disease?

A. Myocardial infarcts occurred more often in the CAS cohort
B. The risk of restenosis was greater for the CEA group
C. The primary composite end point of stroke, MI, or death was similar between CEA and CAS
D. There were significant differences in outcomes in men versus women
E. The incidence of major disabling strokes was greater in the CAS group

95-10. Which of the following is *incorrect* regarding the evaluation of carotid stenting and carotid endarterectomy in different subgroups?

A. CEA is safer and more effective in patients who have undergone prior radiotherapy
B. Patients with carotid artery stenosis who need CABG may benefit from CAS prior to CABG
C. In case of restenosis, CAS following prior CEA is associated with low complication rates
D. CAS shows greater efficacy at younger ages, CEA at older ages
E. None of the above are incorrect

95-1. **The answer is A.** *(Hurst's The Heart, 14th Edition, Chap. 95)* The detection of a carotid bruit during a clinical exam often leads to the diagnosis of asymptomatic carotid stenosis. However, neither the presence nor the severity of the bruit correlates with the severity of the stenosis (option A). The absence of symptoms in patients with severe, hemodynamically significant stenosis signals the presence of robust collaterals to the culprit hemisphere (option B) — most often from the contralateral carotid artery via a patent anterior communicating artery or from the VB circulation via a posterior communicating artery. The stroke risk in these patients is mainly from embolization from the stenotic plaque in the extracranial ICA to the intracranial vessel(s) rather than from complete occlusion of the carotid artery in the neck (option C). Per current guidelines, it is reasonable to consider revascularization for patients with > 80% asymptomatic stenosis and low periprocedural risk (option D).[1]

95-2. **The answer is D.** *(Hurst's The Heart, 14th Edition, Chap. 95)* Proponents of medical treatment for asymptomatic disease argue that revascularization treatment for asymptomatic carotid stenosis subjects the patient to periprocedural risks that are immediate as opposed to the small risks with medical therapy that are spread out over time (option D).[2] On the other hand, there are important considerations supporting the case for an interventional approach in asymptomatic patients. Because the first presentation in a patient with asymptomatic disease can be a major devastating stroke, there is no active treatment that will predictably reverse the neurological deficit of a stroke, and response to treatment of an established stroke is unpredictable (option C), significant efforts have been directed at primary stroke prevention. Furthermore, a meta-analysis[3] of randomized trials in asymptomatic patients found that statins were effective in decreasing the total number of strokes but not fatal strokes (option A). In addition, medical treatment requires a lifelong patient commitment, and hence its value and impact on outcomes depend on patient compliance. Medication cost, side effects, and a perceived lack of any immediate benefit (because patients are asymptomatic) all compromise patient compliance (option B).

95-3. **The answer is C.** *(Hurst's The Heart, 14th Edition, Chap. 95)* A patient who is high risk for CEA does not automatically become suitable (ie, standard risk) for CAS. Patients with poor "brain reserve" and brain function are more likely to clinically manifest neurological events related to periprocedural embolization. Examples of patients with poor brain reserve include those who have experienced a prior large stroke, multiple small strokes or lacunar infarcts, and those with dementia (option A). Lesion and vessel features that are ideal for stenting include a narrow, acute angle between the ICA and the ECA. The wider this bifurcation (ie, approaching or exceeding 90°), the greater is the anticipated technical difficulty in advancing a distal embolic protection filter device with a fixed-wire system (option B). The degree of stenosis severity and eccentricity/concentricity are not problems as long as the flow in the vessel is normal (TIMI grade III) (option C). A severe stenosis in association with less than TIMI III flow ("string sign") (option D) and an occluded carotid artery are contraindications for CAS. Likewise, extensive circumferential calcification of the internal carotid artery makes a lesion unsuitable for CAS (option E).

95-4. **The answer is A.** *(Hurst's The Heart, 14th Edition, Chap. 95)* Most if not all carotid revascularization procedures are elective and not ad hoc (ie, proceeding to perform a carotid intervention during another scheduled invasive procedure, eg, coronary angiography) (option D). A comprehensive history and physical, including a detailed neurological exam, is a mandatory first step when evaluating a patient for a possible carotid intervention (option B). The standard noninvasive method for the evaluation of carotid artery stenosis is duplex ultrasonography. CT angiography is less operator dependent, but it exposes the patient to iodinated contrast and radiation. Moreover, most carotid bifurcations are calcified, which may interfere with accurate interpretation of stenosis severity on CTA (option C). Antihypertensive agents and beta-blockers are generally withheld the day of the procedure to avoid exaggerating the bradycardia and hypotension resulting from carotid baroreceptor stimulation (option A). After the procedure, the blood pressure and heart rate need to be followed closely, and these medications can be given as soon as the clinical situation permits.

95-5. **The answer is B.** *(Hurst's The Heart, 14th Edition, Chap. 95)* Because placement of the sheath occurs before the deployment of the EPD and release of emboli occurs to some degree during all stages of the carotid intervention, no steps of the carotid intervention can ever be completely "emboli protected" (option B). A number of EPDs are available; they can be broadly categorized as flow-interrupting (occlusive) and flow-preserving devices. Although flow-interrupting, occlusive-type EPDs are intuitively appealing (no blood flow = no emboli), there have been some issues with their use. For example, it is mandatory to demonstrate a robust collateral circulation to the hemisphere that is being treated to permit occlusion and interruption of antegrade flow in the ipsilateral carotid artery (option A). The rationale for the use of the proximal occlusion devices is based on interruption of antegrade flow and "flow reversal" in the ipsilateral internal carotid artery (option D). The nonocclusive, flow-preserving devices are the filters. The underlying principle and rationale for use is the same for all filter EPDs: preserving antegrade flow while preventing the passage of the embolic debris (option C).

95-6. **The answer is B.** *(Hurst's The Heart, 14th Edition, Chap. 95)* The procedure is performed under local anesthesia; sedation is not recommended (option A). The heart rate, rhythm, blood pressure, and neurological status should be closely monitored throughout the intervention. A suitable distal EPD is placed cephalad to the stenosis (option B), and the dwell time of the EPD should be tracked. A self-expanding nitinol stent is deployed across the bifurcation. The stent is postdilated using a 5.0-mm balloon, restricting this step to a single inflation. Balloon deflations should be performed gradually, typically over 30 to 45 seconds (option C). The use of glycoprotein IIb/IIIa inhibitors is contraindicated (option D). Although "low blood pressure" is not unusual in the post-procedure period, other causes such as retroperitoneal hemorrhage related to access site bleeding should be excluded as a cause of any unexplained, persistent hypotension (option E).

95-7. **The answer is E.** *(Hurst's The Heart, 14th Edition, Chap. 95)* During the procedure, the neurological status of the patient should be monitored at frequent intervals. Any departure from baseline, including frequent yawning in a nonsedated patient, can point to a neurological event (which at times can be very subtle) that should not be ignored (option B). Close attention should be paid to the management of the blood pressure after the procedure. There are two main problems with persistent hypotension (option D): (1) patients with a periprocedural embolic event or a severe contralateral carotid stenosis can become symptomatic; and (2) patients with baseline renal insufficiency typically have an elevation of creatinine. The combination of contrast exposure and persistent postprocedure hypotension results in worsening of renal function. On the other hand, if the drop in blood pressure is less than expected and continues to be high following postdilatation (eg, in the post-endarterectomy patient with severe post-CEA restenosis), this situation increases the risk of hyperperfusion syndrome (option C). Finally, recognizing that the use of glycoprotein IIb/IIIa inhibitors during carotid stenting is contraindicated (option A), and with careful monitoring of the hemodynamics, the chances of an intracerebral bleed can be minimized.

95-8. **The answer is D.** *(Hurst's The Heart, 14th Edition, Chap. 95)* Cerebral hyperperfusion is defined as an increase in blood flow of > 100% from baseline, and cerebral hyperperfusion syndrome (CHS) is hyperperfusion associated with a neurological deficit (option E). Although CHS does not occur frequently, its consequences can be devastating. An increase in ipsilateral blood flow to the affected cerebral hemisphere may occur after carotid stenting (or endarterectomy); it is usually asymptomatic (option C). The most common clinical symptom of cerebral hyperperfusion is headache (option A). Patients with CHS can present with a variety of neurological deficits, including isolated speech disturbance.

Lowering blood pressure and anticonvulsant therapy are the most important treatments to reduce the degree of cerebral edema and seizures (option D). As vasorelaxation may further increase cerebral blood flow, calcium antagonists and nitrates are contraindicated in the treatment of CHS (option B).

95-9. **The answer is C.** *(Hurst's The Heart, 14th Edition, Chap. 95)* The results of the CREST trial showed that both CEA and CAS are excellent treatment options.[4,5] There was no difference in the outcomes in women versus men (option D). The primary composite end point of periprocedural stroke, MI, or death was similar between CEA and CAS (option C). The incidence of major disabling strokes or death was extremely low and was not different between the two treatment modalities (option E). Periprocedural minor strokes were greater in the CAS group, but by 6 months, the deficits were not different. There was no survival disadvantage in patients with minor strokes. However, MI occurred more often in the CEA cohort (option A), and this negatively affected survival. Over a follow-up period that extended to 10 years, freedom from ipsilateral stroke and the risk of restenosis were similar for the CEA and CAS groups (option B), supporting the clinical and device durability of CAS.

95-10. **The answer is A.** *(Hurst's The Heart, 14th Edition, Chap. 95)* In the CREST study,[4,5] an interaction between age and treatment efficacy was detected, leading CREST investigators to conclude that "carotid-artery stenting tended to show greater efficacy at younger ages, and carotid endarterectomy at older ages" (option D). There are no guidelines or consenus on the optimum approach to treating a patient with asymptomatic carotid artery stenosis who needs CABG. Patients with bilateral severe carotid artery disease or a contralateral occlusion may benefit from carotid revascularization prior to CABG, and CAS when feasible may be a safer alternative (option B). Because radiation-induced vascular stenosis may be associated with fibrosis and scarring of the skin and subcutaneous tissue, surgical therapy is more complicated and may lead to postoperative necrosis, infections, wound breakdown, and cranial nerve injuries. For these reasons, CAS is safer and more effective in the postradiated patient (option A). If restenosis occurs in the early years after CEA, revision CEA is technically challenging and is associated with higher complication rates than primary surgery, with increased rates of stroke, TIA, and cranial nerve injury. CAS following prior CEA is associated with low complication rates, and stent restenosis is not significantly higher than that seen with primary CAS (option C).

References

1. Brott TG, Halperin JL, Abbara S, et al. ASA/ACCF/AHA/AANN/AANS/ACR/ASNR/CNS/SAIP/SCAI/SIR/SNIS/SVM/SVS: guidelines on the management of patients with extracranial carotid and vertebral artery disease. *J Am Coll Cardiol.* 2011;57:1002-1044.
2. Spence JD, Pelz D, Veith FJ. Asymptomatic carotid stenosis: identifying patients at high enough risk to warrant endarterectomy or stenting. *Stroke.* 2014 Mar;45(3):655-657.
3. De Caterina R, Scarano M, Marfisi R, et al. Cholesterol-lowering interventions and stroke: insights from a meta-analysis of randomized controlled trials. *J Am Coll Cardiol.* 2010;55:198-211.
4. Brott TG, Hobson RW 2nd, Howard G, et al. Stenting versus endarterectomy for treatment of carotid-artery stenosis. *N Engl J Med.* 2010;363:11-23.
5. Brott TG, Howard G, Roubin GS, et al. CREST investigators long-term results of stenting versus endarterectomy for carotid-artery stenosis. *N Engl J Med.* 2016;374(11):1021-1031.

CHAPTER 96

Diagnosis and Management of Diseases of the Peripheral Arteries

Patrick R. Lawler

QUESTIONS

DIRECTIONS: Choose the one best response to each question.

96-1. A 43-year-old man presents to clinic with a dull lower limb pain that is brought on after 30 minutes of walking and is relieved by rest. He is a smoker with a blood pressure of 145/95 mm Hg, and he stopped taking his prescribed statin medication 3 months ago. Rank the following factors by their relative risk for peripheral artery disease (PAD):

A. Smoking > hypertension > hypercholesterolemia
B. Hypertension > smoking > hypercholesterolemia
C. Hypercholesterolemia > hypertension > smoking
D. Hypertension > hypercholesterolemia > smoking
E. Smoking = hypertension = hypercholesterolemia

96-2. The 43-year-old man from question 96-1 undergoes exercise testing while measuring his segmental pressures to assess the potential presence of a stenotic lesion. His ankle-brachial index (ABI) at rest and postexercise was 0.92 and 0.85, respectively. Which of the following statements about ABI values and risk of PAD is *correct*?

A. The risk of death increases with increasing ABI
B. A decrease in ABI without symptoms is associated with a better prognosis
C. This patient has the same risk of having an MI as someone with ABI > 1.40
D. ABI < 1.00 is considered normal
E. None of the above is correct

96-3. A 53-year-old woman with diabetes mellitus presents to clinic for a routine physical examination. She has no symptoms to report, her blood pressure is 120/80 mm Hg, and she affirms taking her diabetes medication consistently. What else should be assessed in this patient at risk for PAD?

A. Claudication
B. Nonhealing wounds
C. Tobacco use
D. Peripheral pulses
E. All of the above are correct

96-4. Which of the following statements about claudication is *incorrect*?

A. It occurs in a single or multiple muscle groups
B. Relief with rest is independent of position
C. Claudication worsens after a period of inactivity
D. Symptoms occur proximal to the level of stenosis or occlusion
E. Pain changes in character and/or location as the lesion progresses

96-5. A 64-year-old woman is examined for signs of lower extremity ischemia and PAD. Which of the following findings would be consistent with this?

A. Elevated surface temperature of the limb
B. Presence of livedo reticularis
C. Increased hair growth on the feet
D. A red/purplish coloration of the foot (rubor) that persists with elevation
E. All of the above are correct

96-6. A 64-year-old man with diabetes mellitus and a history of renal insufficiency presents to the emergency room with severe cramping and pain in his right leg that began at rest. Following a proper physical examination, you decide to do imaging to confirm the presence of arterial stenosis. Which of the following imaging modalities should you use?

A. Duplex ultrasound
B. Magnetic resonance angiography (MRA) with gadolinium contrast
C. CT angiography (CTA)
D. Conventional angiography
E. None of the above

96-7. A 44-year-old hypertensive man complains of muscle cramps that are brought on by walking uphill. He undergoes a lower-extremity arterial exercise treadmill test. Following exercise, what finding would be consistent with arterial stenosis?

A. Increased ABI
B. Decreased systolic blood pressure
C. Abnormal Doppler signal proximal to the stenosis
D. A larger pressure gradient across the stenosis
E. Increased peripheral resistance

96-8. Which of the following statements about behavioral modification therapy for claudication is *correct*?

A. Bicycling provides superior lower-extremity benefits to walking
B. Supervised exercise programs are superior to stent revascularization
C. Both supervised and nonsupervised programs are equally effective
D. Patients should walk until the initiation of pain, then rest for relief and start walking again
E. Walking programs likely provide benefit by preventing the formation of collateral arteries

96-9. A 66-year-old man presents to the emergency room with new-onset headache and jaw claudication. Laboratory findings reveal an elevated sedimentation rate, and angiography shows a narrowing of the vertebral arteries. The patient responds to corticosteroid therapy. What is the most likely diagnosis?

A. Giant cell (temporal) arteritis (GCA)
B. Takayasu arteritis (TA)
C. Fibromuscular dysplasia (FMD)
D. Thromboangiitis obliterans (TAO)
E. Raynaud phenomenon

96-10. What is the pathophysiologic mechanism of primary Raynaud phenomenon?

A. Unilateral ischemia of small-sized arteries of the finger
B. Exaggerated vasoconstriction reflex
C. Cold-induced vasodilation of small arteries
D. Emotional vasodilation response
E. None of the above

ANSWERS

96-1. **The answer is A.** (*Hurst's The Heart, 14th Edition, Chap. 96*) Many of the risk factors for PAD are the same as those for coronary artery disease (CAD), with tobacco and diabetes having an even greater effect.[1,2] Smoking and diabetes constitute the highest risk factors for the development of PAD (option A). Tobacco use, current and past, is associated with a two- to fourfold increase in relative risk for PAD. Diabetes mellitus has a similar increase in relative risk. Other modifiable risk factors include hyperhomocysteinemia, hyperlipidemia, and hypertension. Hypertension and homocysteinemia represent a moderate risk and are associated with a one- to threefold increase in relative risk for PAD, while hypercholesterolemia is considered the lowest risk factor and is associated with a one- to twofold increased risk for PAD. Table 96-1 demonstrates a detailed ranking of risk factors for PAD.

TABLE 96-1 **Risk Factors for Peripheral Artery Disease**

High Risk	Moderate Risk	Low Risk
Two- to fourfold increase	One- to threefold increase	One- to twofold increase
Smoking	Hypertension	Hypercholesterolemia
Diabetes mellitus	Homocysteinemia	

96-2. **The answer is C.** (*Hurst's The Heart, 14th Edition, Chap. 96*) Segmental pressures and exercise testing provide a simple and accurate method of determining the presence, severity, and approximate location of stenotic lesions. The most commonly reported segmental pressure is the ankle-brachial index (ABI). An ABI ≥ 1.0 is generally considered normal (option D). Severe disease is present when the ABI is < 0.50. The risk of death increases as the ABI decreases (option A). Lower-extremity symptoms not associated with a decrease in the ABI do not demonstrate an increase in mortality (option B). In contrast, a decrease in ABI without symptoms still portends an increase in cardiovascular morbidity and mortality. Patients with ABI > 1.40 and between 0.91 and 1.00 have a similar risk of having an MI or stroke (option C).[3]

96-3. **The answer is E.** (*Hurst's The Heart, 14th Edition, Chap. 96*) Most individuals with PAD have no lower-extremity symptoms, and the diagnosis will be missed if ABI testing is reserved exclusively for those with classic claudication symptoms. Identifying PAD in those without classic intermittent claudication symptoms remains challenging. Appropriate criteria for screening patients for suspected PAD includes a history of walking impairment, claudication (option A), ischemic rest pain, or nonhealing wounds (option B). Screening for these factors is recommended as part of a standard review of symptoms for adults 50 years and older who have atherosclerosis risk factors and for adults 70 years and older.[4] Patients in whom screening for PAD should be undertaken include those over 65 years old and those 50 years or older with a history of diabetes mellitus or tobacco abuse (option C), complaints of claudication, evidence of reduced pulses (option D), or established atherosclerotic disease. In addition, many diabetes patients are asymptomatic because of peripheral neuropathy, and they should be screened appropriately.

96-4. **The answer is D.** (*Hurst's The Heart, 14th Edition, Chap. 96*) Claudication is a stereotypical, reproducible distress in single or multiple muscle groups of the lower extremity (option A) brought on by sustained exercise and relieved by rest. The distress changes in character or location as the flow-limiting lesion(s) progress (option E). When workload is increased by rapid pace, a burden, or walking uphill or over rough terrain, the distance or time to onset will shorten. When the distance to onset or severity abruptly changes, thrombosis in situ or an embolic event should be considered. In general, symptoms occur distal to the level of stenosis or occlusion (option D). Relief with rest is independent of position (option B) and is usually complete within 5 minutes. Claudication often worsens after a period of inactivity (option C), such as hospitalization, but returns to baseline with reconditioning.

96-5. The answer is B. *(Hurst's The Heart, 14th Edition, Chap. 96)* A red or purplish color of the forefoot during dependency (dependent rubor) is common with severe ischemia. Rubor caused by ischemia will change to pallor with elevation; in contrast, rubor caused by cellulitis usually persists with elevation (option D). Loss of normal hair growth is also a marker of ischemia (option C). Livedo reticularis is a transient, bluish discoloration with a lacy pattern found on the extremities that can present as a symptom of serious vascular disease (option B). It is most apparent after exposure to cold or emotion and fades with warming or exercise. It is more common in women and fair-skinned individuals. Additionally, on palpation, one can observe that surface temperature is reduced when perfusion is compromised (option A).

96-6. The answer is A. *(Hurst's The Heart, 14th Edition, Chap. 96)* Conventional angiography (option D) provides reproducible information with high resolution not yet matched by other modalities. Drawbacks include the risk of distal embolization and arterial damage at the puncture site. Iodinated contrast is used and poses a small but real risk of anaphylactoid reaction and contrast nephropathy. CT angiography (CTA) (option C) provides detailed anatomic information without the need for arterial access, but iodinated contrast is still required. Magnetic resonance angiography (MRA) provides information similar to CTA without the need for iodinated contrast. For those at risk of contrast nephropathy or anaphylactoid reaction, it is a safe and accurate alternative to CTA and conventional angiography. However, most studies use gadolinium as a contrast agent (option B), which puts patients with a low creatinine clearance at risk of gadolinium-induced nephrogenic systemic fibrosis. Duplex ultrasound (option A) assesses not only arterial anatomy but also the hemodynamic effects of stenosis. Contrast is not required, and no ionizing radiation is used. Ultrasound is portable and captures images in real time, allowing both bedside and intraoperative monitoring of therapy.

96-7. The answer is D. *(Hurst's The Heart, 14th Edition, Chap. 96)* Lower-extremity arterial exercise testing is performed by walking on a treadmill at a standardized protocol. Select parts of the lower-extremity study (ie, ABIs or CWD at the common femoral level) are performed before and after exercise. With exercise, the systolic blood pressure increases (option B) as peripheral resistance decreases (option E), resulting in a larger pressure gradient across the stenosis (option D) and lower ABI (option A) and abnormal Doppler signals distal to the stenosis (option C). A decrease in ABI or a change in Doppler signal may be detected after exercise. Even if the resting values are normal, a decreased ABI following exercise predicts an increase in mortality.

96-8. The answer is B. *(Hurst's The Heart, 14th Edition, Chap. 96)* Walking programs should be initiated in all patients with claudication, with both typical and atypical symptoms.[5] Supervised exercise programs appear superior to stent revascularization (option B), even for those with aortoiliac PAD. Unfortunately, bicycling (option A) and other forms of exercise used for cardiovascular conditioning do not provide the same lower-extremity benefit as walking. The effectiveness of a supervised walking program is well demonstrated, and supervised programs are more effective than nonsupervised programs (option C). Patients should walk until they near their maximal pain threshold, then rest for relief before walking until they reach their pain threshold again (option D). The mechanism of improvement is unclear, but increased collateral formation or recruitment (option E), muscle training, improved oxygen uptake, and improved mechanics of walking may be involved.

96-9. The answer is A. *(Hurst's The Heart, 14th Edition, Chap. 96)* Thromboangiitis obliterans (TAO) (option D), or Buerger disease, is an inflammatory vasculopathy affecting small and medium-sized arteries and veins caused by an inflammatory, highly cellular intraluminal thrombus. The initial involvement is often in digital, pedal, and hand vessels; patients may present with ulceration of one or more digits. Episodes of recurrent superficial phlebitis are common. Fibromuscular dysplasia (FMD) (option C) most commonly affects women and has been described in almost all arteries. Although early reports described the renal arteries as being affected most often, more recent data suggest that FMD was found equally in the renal and carotid/vertebral arteries. Raynaud phenomenon (option E) is classically defined as discoloration episodes of white ischemia, then blue stasis, and then red hyperemia during the recovery phase. Takayasu arteritis (TA) (option B) and giant cell (temporal) arteritis (GCA) (option A) are similar in pathologic process but affect different age groups. TA occurs in those younger than age 40 years, and GCA usually affects those older than age 50 years. TA generally involves arteries below the neck, and GCA generally involves arteries above the diaphragm. Both GCA and TA have characteristic clinical and laboratory findings, including an elevated sedimentation rate and typical angiographic features of smooth, tapered narrowing in large and medium-sized arteries. For GCA, visual changes in the setting of an elevated sedimentation rate, jaw claudication, or a pulse deficit should be treated as a medical emergency with parenteral corticosteroids.

96-10. **The answer is B.** *(Hurst's The Heart, 14th Edition, Chap. 96)* Raynaud phenomenon is classically defined as discoloration episodes of white ischemia, then blue stasis, and then red hyperemia during the recovery phase. Primary Raynaud phenomenon is defined as episodes of bilateral color changes induced by cold or emotion without evidence of ischemia or other disease occurring for 2 years. This represents most cases and, in some sense, can be considered simply the exaggerated response of a normal reflex of vasoconstriction (option B). The pathophysiology of exaggerated vasoconstriction is complex but appears to involve both local and systemic pathways. Most patients with primary Raynaud phenomenon require no therapy and quickly learn to keep not only hands but the whole body warm.

References

1. Criqui MH, Aboyans V. Epidemiology of peripheral artery disease. *Circ Res.* 2015;116(9): 1509-1526.
2. Cimminiello C. PAD. Epidemiology and pathophysiology. *Thromb Res.* 2002;106(6): V295-V301.
3. Jones WS, Patel MR, Rockman CB, et al. Association of the ankle-brachial index with history of myocardial infarction and stroke. *Am Heart J.* 2014;167(4):499-505.
4. Rooke TW, Hirsch AT, Misra S, et al. 2011 ACCF/AHA focused update of the guideline for the management of patients with peripheral artery disease (updating the 2005 guideline): a report of the American College of Cardiology Foundation/American Heart Association Task Force on Practice Guidelines. *J Am Coll Cardiol.* 2011;58(19):2020-2045.
5. Lane R, Ellis B, Watson L, Leng GC. Exercise for intermittent claudication. *Cochrane Database Syst Rev.* 2014;7:CD000990.

CHAPTER 97

Diagnosis and Management of Diseases of the Peripheral Venous System

Patrick R. Lawler

QUESTIONS

DIRECTIONS: Choose the one best response to each question.

97-1. Which of the following is *not* characteristic of the venous system?

A. Low resting vascular tone
B. Low resistance
C. High distensibility
D. Low compliance
E. Bicuspid valves

97-2. Which of the following is *not* considered part of Virchow's Triad of risk factors for venous thrombosis?

A. Stasis of blood flow
B. Hemophilia
C. Endothelial injury
D. Hypercoagulable state
E. All of the above

97-3. A 60-year-old woman presents to the emergency room with unilateral leg pain and swelling of 4 days' duration. She has a history of hypertension and has recently returned from a trip to Australia. Which of the following findings does *not* support a diagnosis of DVT?

A. Increased respiratory variation of venous flow on ultrasound
B. Wells score of 3 points
C. Visualization of a dilated noncompressible vein on ultrasound
D. Elevated D-dimer test
E. Skin erythema

97-4. An 80-year-old man is diagnosed with distal calf vein DVT. Which of the following findings is an indication for anticoagulation therapy in this patient?

A. History of DVT
B. Thrombus is 6 cm in length
C. Thrombus is near the sapheno-popliteal junction
D. Limb swelling, erythema, and severe pain
E. All of the above

97-5. Which of the following statements about venous insufficiency is *correct*?

A. Skin hyperpigmentation is caused by hemosiderin deposition resulting from edema
B. Excessive compression can result in lipodermatosclerosis
C. Symptoms are exacerbated by prolonged elevation
D. Primary venous insufficiency is autosomal recessive with complete penetrance
E. All of the above are correct

97-6. A 63-year-old woman presents to clinic with limb swelling, erythema, and pain on compression. As part of her evaluation, she undergoes imaging and physiologic testing to define the venous anatomy and assess the presence of obstructive lesions. Which of the following is *correct*?

A. Impedance plethysmography (IPG) allows precise localization of the level of disease
B. Plethysmography measures pressure changes in the limb resulting from venous outflow or reflux disease
C. Duplex ultrasound performed during a Valsalva maneuver can assess venous reflux
D. Magnetic resonance venography is the gold standard for the direct visualization of venous flow and collaterals
E. All of the above are correct

97-7. A 56-year-old man with venous insufficiency and recurrent ulcerations undergoes treatment with end-ovenous laser ablation of affected veins after several failed attempts at conservative therapy. What is the mechanism by which this procedure improves venous insufficiency?

A. A rotational wire induces vein spasm while a chemical sclerosing agent is injected to ablate the vein

B. Injected hypertonic saline causes endothelial damage, resulting in thrombosis and fibrosis of the treated veins

C. A small scalpel is used to make incisions in the skin and physically remove the diseased vein

D. Under ultrasound guidance, a thermal source injures the vein wall, causing occlusion

E. None of the above

97-8. A 25-year-old woman with a leg ulceration presents to your clinic for evaluation. What distinguishing characteristic will allow confirmation that this is a venous (and *not* arterial) ulcer?

A. Localization at the tip of toes

B. Dark eschar

C. Granulation tissue

D. Painful

E. Dry and ischemic

97-9. A 25-year-old patient with venous insufficiency and venous ulcer treatment is evaluated in your clinic. What is the *most* important component of venous ulcer treatment?

A. Compression therapy

B. Improve arterial perfusion

C. Good skin care

D. Nonirritating dressing

E. None of the above

97-10. Which of the following is *not* appropriate to treat venous ulcers?

A. Pentoxifylline

B. Horse chestnut seed extract

C. Diuretics

D. Both A and B are not appropriate

E. None of the above are appropriate

97-1. The answer is D. *(Hurst's The Heart, 14th Edition, Chap. 97)* The lower extremity venous system includes the deep, superficial, and perforating veins, which work in concert to return blood to the heart. Unlike the arterial system, the venous system is low resistance (option B) and must overcome gravitational and hydrostatic pressure forces to achieve blood return to the heart. The venules and veins have very thin walls and low resting basal tone (option A), which allows for enormous distensibility (option C). Having thin, floppy vascular walls also means that veins tend to have very high compliances (option D). As such, large increases in blood volume are required to even slightly enhance the internal blood pressure, and small changes in hydrostatic forces, central pressure, and/or external forces result in changes of the vein diameter. Venous blood flow is reliant upon muscular leg contraction as well as bicuspid venous valves (option E) that open and close to prevent backflow. Together, muscular leg contraction and venous valves help to overcome hydrostatic forces within the vein itself.

97-2. The answer is B. *(Hurst's The Heart, 14th Edition, Chap. 97)* Venous thrombosis may occur as a result of the risks as identified in Virchow's Triad: stasis (option A), endothelial injury (option C), and the hypercoagulable state (option D), or it may occur without any known risk factors (unprovoked venous thrombosis). Stasis, or interrupted blood flow, typically occurs due to prolonged immobility (eg, on a plane), hospitalization, and varicose veins. Endothelial injury increases the risk of venous thrombosis via the activation of the coagulation cascade and recruitment of inflammatory cytokines. Lastly, any hypercoagulable state that facilitates blood clotting (eg, obesity, pregnancy, cancer) will result in changes of the constitution of blood and predispose to venous thrombosis. Hemophilia (option B) is a disorder of impaired blood clotting, resulting in increased bleeding and easy bruising; it does not typically constitute a risk factor for venous thrombosis.

97-3. The answer is A. *(Hurst's The Heart, 14th Edition, Chap. 97)* The classic clinical description of DVT includes unilateral pain, limb swelling, skin erythema (option E), and warmth, with symptoms acute to subacute in onset. The use of clinical prediction scores, like the Wells score, can be helpful in the initial evaluation of a patient with possible DVT (Table 97-1). A Wells score ≥ 3 points suggests a high probability of DVT (option B). A positive D-dimer test indicates the presence of elevated fibrin degradation products (D-dimers) in the blood and suggests an ongoing cycle of blood clot (thrombus) formation and breakdown in the body (option D). Findings that support the diagnosis of DVT on duplex ultrasonography include a dilated noncompressible vein (option C) resulting from the presence of thrombus, direct visualization of thrombus, as well as altered venous flow dynamics with a lack of respiratory variation (option A) resulting from outflow obstruction or a lack of flow augmentation with calf muscle compression, indicating distal obstruction between the calf muscle and the ultrasound transducer.

TABLE 97-1 Wells Score for Assessing Probability of Deep Vein Thrombosis

+1 Point Each:	
Active malignancy	
Paralysis, paresis, or recent plaster immobilization of lower limb	
Recently bedridden > 3 days and/or major surgery within 4 weeks	
Localized tenderness along distribution of lower extremity deep veins	
Entire lower limb swollen	
Calf swelling > 3 cm compared with the asymptomatic leg	
Strong family history of DVT (≥ 2 first-degree relatives with history of DVT)	
−2 Points if Alternative Diagnosis to DVT Is at Least as Likely	
Probability:	
High	≥ 3 points
Moderate	1-2 points
Low	≤ 0 points

97-4. **The answer is E.** *(Hurst's The Heart, 14th Edition, Chap. 97)* Incidence rates of VTE increase exponentially with age. In the case of distal calf vein DVT, it is estimated that approximately 15% to 25% will progress to the popliteal vein or result in a pulmonary embolus (PE).[1,2] For this reason, patients with distal DVT can be treated with anticoagulation (particularly if symptomatic) or an ultrasound surveillance program (ie, 1–2 week follow-up, particularly if there is a significant risk of bleeding on anticoagulation) to evaluate for thrombus propagation if anticoagulation is to be withheld. Cases in which anticoagulation should be considered over surveillance include severe associated symptoms (option D), extensive thrombus (> 5 cm in length or involving multiple veins) (option B), thrombosis in close proximity to the deep veins (5 cm from the sapheno-popliteal junction and 10 cm from the sapheno-femoral junction) (option C), lack of identifiable and reversible provoking factors, active cancer, recurrent VTE (option A), and in-patient status. All of the above are indications to start this patient on anticoagulation therapy (option E).

97-5. **The answer is A.** *(Hurst's The Heart, 14th Edition, Chap. 97)* Venous insufficiency occurs as a result of inadequate venous outflow resulting from incompetent venous valves or obstruction. It may be either primary or secondary in etiology. Primary disease is thought to be autosomal dominant with incomplete penetrance (option D). No candidate genes have been identified; however, familial studies in twins confirm a heritable influence on the development of the disease. Symptoms are exacerbated by prolonged standing and dependency, as well as during pregnancy or other volume overload states. Elevation typically relieves the symptoms (option C). The diagnosis of chronic venous insufficiency is often clinical as the characteristic skin changes and symptoms readily expose the disease. Skin hyperpigmentation is caused by hemosiderin deposition resulting from long-standing venous hypertension (option A). Venous hypertension causes edema, which leads to transudation of interstitial fluid and hemosiderin in the skin and subcutaneous space, usually above the medial malleolus, leading to stasis dermatitis. If this remains untreated (lack of compression), lipodermatosclerosis occurs (option B). In this advanced manifestation of venous insufficiency, the skin is indurated and fibrotic with more extensive pigmentation and erythema.

97-6. **The answer is C.** *(Hurst's The Heart, 14th Edition, Chap. 97)* For patients in whom therapies beyond conservative measures may be considered, such as recurrent venous ulceration or painful varicosities despite a trial of compression therapy, duplex ultrasonography is standard for evaluation. The goal of the exam is to define the anatomy and malfunctioning veins, as well as the extent of insufficiency. The duplex exam for venous insufficiency includes provocative maneuvers to unmask abnormal reversal of flow in the vein. The Valsalva maneuver is performed by asking the patient to bear down, thereby increasing intrathoracic pressure and potentially reversing the transvalvular gradient (option C). Physiologic testing with plethysmography relies on volume change in the limb as a result of venous outflow or reflux disease (option B). Unlike the duplex ultrasound assessment, plethysmography modalities do not precisely localize the level of disease (option A). MR venography shows promise in overcoming the contrast issue seen with CT, but catheter-based venography is the gold standard for the direct visualization of venous flow and collaterals (option D).

97-7. **The answer is D.** *(Hurst's The Heart, 14th Edition, Chap. 97)* For patients with lifestyle-limiting symptoms or complications related to venous insufficiency, advanced therapies to ablate the offending veins may be considered. Endovenous procedures such as laser therapy or radiofrequency ablation are most often used for the treatment of reflux in the GSV and SSV. Under ultrasound guidance, these modalities use a thermal source to cause injury to the vein wall, which leads to vein occlusion (option D). Recently, mechanochemical endovenous ablation techniques have emerged in lieu of thermal therapies of the GSV and SSV. The technique uses a rotational wire that induces vein spasm while infusing a chemical sclerosing agent to ablate the vein (option A). Chemical ablation with sclerosing agents is an alternative to thermal therapies, without the mechanical counterpart described above. A variety of agents are available, such as hypertonic saline, which cause endothelial damage and subsequent thrombosis and fibrosis of the treated veins (option B). Vein stripping and phlebectomy or microphlebectomy procedures are less often used today, but surgery may still be preferred in patients with previous failure of endovenous therapy (option C).

97-8. The answer is C. *(Hurst's The Heart, 14th Edition, Chap. 97)* Venous ulcers are the most common type of leg ulceration and the most severe manifestation of venous disease. The evaluation of a venous ulcer should include a thorough medical history and physical assessment, including area and depth measurements of the ulcer. Venous ulcers are generally wet, with good granulation tissue (option C), and they localize to the gaiter area of the leg with a predilection for the medial malleoli. The granulation tissue is new connective tissue that forms on the surface of the wound and helps during the healing process. In contrast, arterial (ischemic) ulcers are painful (option D) and often located distally (tips of toes, over pressure points) (option A). Unlike venous ulcers, they are dry (option E) and have a dark eschar (option B) due to a lack of blood supply.

97-9. The answer is A. *(Hurst's The Heart, 14th Edition, Chap. 97)* Once venous disease is confirmed, compression therapy with wound care is the foundation of venous ulcer treatment. However, four cardinal tenets (Table 97-2) promote wound healing, and in the setting of an active ulcer, each should be considered and optimized. Edema control is the most important tenet. Without adequate control of edema with compression therapy (option A), the ulcer will not heal.

Nevertheless, ensuring adequate arterial perfusion (option B), good skin care (option C), and the use of nonirritating dressings (ie, saline wet to dry, Profore four-layer wrap, Unna Boot) on the ulcer itself are also important for proper ulcer wound healing.

TABLE 97-2 **The Cardinal Tenets of Venous Ulcer Healing**

1. Edema control: this is the most important. Without adequate control of edema, the ulcer will not heal.
2. Assure adequate arterial perfusion.
3. Good skin care.
4. Put a nonirritating dressing (ie, saline wet to dry, Profore four-layer wrap, Unna Boot) on the ulcer itself.

97-10. The answer is C. *(Hurst's The Heart, 14th Edition, Chap. 97)* The main body of evidence surrounding the pharmacology of venous disease and venous ulcers includes pentoxifylline and the saposides (horse chestnut seed extracts). Horse chestnut seed (option B) is thought to inhibit enzymes, such as hyaluronidase, which are activated by accumulated leukocytes in limbs affected by chronic venous disease, thereby reducing associated leg edema and pain, although long-term safety and efficacy have not been established. Pentoxifylline (option A) has been studied in the treatment of advanced venous disease and may promote venous ulcer healing via its anti-inflammatory properties and rheolytic activities. Several trials suggest modestly improved healing rates with pentoxifylline, although the magnitude of effect is small, and its role in the treatment of venous disease is unclear. Diuretics are not useful to control limb swelling related to venous insufficiency in the absence of congestive heart failure (option C).

References

1. Stevens SM, Woller SC, Bauer KA, et al. Guidance for the evaluation and treatment of hereditary and acquired thrombophilia. *J Thromb Thrombolysis.* 2016;41(1): 154-164.
2. Hughes MJ, Stein PD, Matta F. Silent pulmonary embolism in patients with distal deep venous thrombosis: systematic review. *Thromb Res.* 2014;134(6):1182-1185.

SECTION 15

Miscellaneous Conditions and Cardiovascular Disease

CHAPTER 98

Perioperative Evaluation for Noncardiac Surgery

Jonathan Afilalo

DIRECTIONS: Choose the one best response to each question.

98-1. As with most clinical cases, the cornerstone of perioperative management is a conscientious history and physical exam. Eliciting the patient's functional status is of paramount importance in the stepwise algorithm for risk stratification; this is often quantified in terms of metabolic equivalents (METs) that the patient habitually performs. Which of the following activities falls short of the 4 MET cutoff used to define patients with acceptable functional capacity who may *not* need functional testing in the absence of acute decompensated cardiac conditions?

A. Heavy housework
B. Bicycling
C. Doubles tennis
D. Bowling
E. Walking up a hill

98-2. In patients who present with acute coronary syndromes (ACS), cardiac catheterization is generally recommended for defining coronary anatomy, stratifying risk, and devising the optimal treatment and revascularization strategy when appropriate. Which of the following statements about the perioperative management of a patient with ACS who is scheduled to undergo a noncardiac surgery is *true*?

A. If noncardiac surgery must be performed within a matter of weeks, balloon angioplasty without stenting is preferred
B. If noncardiac surgery is not essential but still time sensitive, drug-eluting stents (DESs) are preferred
C. If DESs are implanted, noncardiac surgery should ideally be delayed for 2 years

D. Noncardiac surgery may be considered at 30 days in the era of second- and third-generation DESs
E. All of the above

98-3. Atrial fibrillation is the most commonly encountered perioperative cardiac arrhythmia. Which of the following statements about the perioperative management of a patient with permanent atrial fibrillation is *false*?

A. Patients treated with a rate control strategy may continue to be treated with such a strategy throughout the perioperative period
B. Bleeding risk has generally been low in observational studies that have examined anticoagulation bridging
C. The best strategy for patients with atrial fibrillation who undergo noncardiac surgery is bridging when thromboembolic risk is low
D. In patients with atrial fibrillation and prosthetic heart valves, anticoagulation bridging should be considered
E. All of the above are false

98-4. Active cardiac disease can exist in the form of ongoing ischemia, uncontrolled arrhythmia, decompensated heart failure, and severe symptomatic valve disease. Which of the following conduction diseases is most likely to represent an active cardiac arrhythmia warranting preoperative treatment?

A. Frequent premature atrial contractions
B. Sinus arrhythmia
C. Symptomatic sinus bradycardia
D. Second-degree Mobitz type I heart block
E. All of the above

98-5. In patients with implanted cardiac rhythm devices, special attention should be paid to the use of monopolar electrocautery during surgery and its potential interaction with device programming and function. Which of the following statements about patients with implanted cardiac rhythm devices is *true*?

A. In cases where only unipolar cautery or a harmonic scalpel will be used, disruption of implanted rhythm devices is extremely unlikely

B. Bipolar electrocautery used above the umbilicus poses the highest risk of interaction with implanted rhythm devices

C. In pacemaker-dependent patients, reprogramming to the DOO or VOO setting can increase the risk of oversensing and failure to pace

D. In patients with implanted cardioverter-defibrillators (ICDs), turning off tachytherapies is recommended

E. All of the above

98-6. A propensity-matched study from a single tertiary care center of patients undergoing noncardiac surgery revealed that moderate-to-severe or severe mitral regurgitation (MR) was associated with worse outcomes driven by a higher rate of composite 30-day mortality, myocardial infarction, heart failure, and stroke.[7] Which of the following predictors was *not* associated with a poor outcome?

A. Myxomatous etiology of MR

B. Diabetes mellitus

C. Reduced LVEF < 35%

D. History of carotid endarterectomy

E. All of the above

98-7. Perioperative risk can generally be divided into two components: the inherent risk associated with the operation and the risk attributed to the patient's specific conditions. Both operation-related and patient factors are considered revised cardiac risk index (RCRI). Which of the following patient factors is *not* included in the RCRI?

A. Ischemic heart disease

B. Congestive heart failure

C. Cerebrovascular disease

D. Kidney disease

E. Pulmonary disease

98-8. Perioperative testing should be limited to circumstances that would change management independent of the surgery planned. Which of the following statements about perioperative testing is *false*?

A. Revascularization in stable coronary disease prior to surgery has not been associated with improved outcomes

B. The risk of perioperative complications is inversely proportional to the number of metabolic equivalent (METs) a patient performs on a habitual basis

C. Formal functional testing is not indicated when a patient can easily and repetitively perform over 4 METs on a habitual basis

D. A 12-lead ECG should always be obtained

E. Preoperative left ventricular function assessment is appropriate in patients with dyspnea of unknown origin

98-9. The available evidence regarding the role of preoperative stress testing is primarily derived from single center studies using dobutamine stress echocardiography (DSE) or radionuclide myocardial perfusion imaging (MPI).[11-14] Which of the following statements about the predominant findings from these studies is *true*?

A. Patients with moderate areas of ischemia are at higher perioperative risk of myocardial infarction (MI) and death

B. Functional testing has a high negative predictive value

C. Evidence of prior MI without inducible ischemia has little predictive value for perioperative events

D. The risk of an adverse event during a preoperative stress test is very low

E. All of the above are true

98-10. The use of perioperative beta-blockade continues to be debated. The Perioperative Ischemic Evaluation (POISE) trial was a multicenter trial that randomized 8351 adults scheduled to undergo noncardiac surgery to metoprolol or placebo.[15] Which of the following statements regarding the effects of beta-blocker therapy in the POISE trial is *false*?

A. Higher risk of clinically significant bradycardic episodes

B. Higher risk of clinically significant hypotensive episodes

C. Higher risk of stroke

D. Higher risk of death from noncardiovascular causes but lower risk of death from cardiovascular causes

E. All of the above are false

98-1. The answer is D. *(Hurst's the Heart, 14th Edition, Chap. 98)* Understanding a patient's functional status is key in guiding management decisions. Excellent functional status, > 10 METs, includes activities such as boxing, judo, and cross-country skiing. Good functional status, 7 to 10 METs, includes bicycling, fencing, and kayaking. Moderate functional status, 4 to 6 METs, includes golf while carrying clubs, doubles tennis (option C), walking 7 kph, walking up a hill (option E), climbing a flight of stairs, or doing heavy housework (option A). Poor functional status, < 4 METs, includes light activities limited to driving, bowling (option D), and fishing from a bank.

98-2. The answer is A. *(Hurst's the Heart, 14th Edition, Chap. 98)* If noncardiac surgery must be performed within a matter of weeks, balloon angioplasty without stenting may be considered (option A). If surgery is not essential but still time sensitive, bare metal stenting (BMS) rather than drug-eluting stents (DESs) (option B) can be used if lesion parameters permit. If DESs are implanted, surgery should also ideally be delayed for 1 year, not 2 years (option C). However, surgery may be considered at 180 days, not 30 days (option D), as the risk of stent thrombosis may have stabilized, particularly in the era of second- and third-generation DESs.[1-3]

98-3. The answer is C. *(Hurst's The Heart, 14th Edition, Chap. 98)* A known history of clinically stable atrial fibrillation does not require modified management or special evaluation other than a consideration of how to manage perioperative anticoagulation (option A). Observational data indicate that when pursued, bridging anticoagulation can be done safely (option B).[4-6] The best strategy for patients and surgeries with atrial fibrillation and low thromboembolic risk is interruption of anticoagulation (option C). In cases of high thromboembolic risk, resulting from either patient comorbidities or prosthetic heart valves, an informed discussion should take place with patients with consideration of perioperative anticoagulation bridging (option D).

98-4. The answer is C. *(Hurst's The Heart, 14th Edition, Chap. 98)* High-degree conduction disease, such as symptomatic bradycardia (option C), sick sinus syndrome, second-degree Mobitz type II heart block, and complete heart block, can significantly complicate the perioperative period and therefore warrants therapeutic consideration beforehand. Frequent supraventricular contractions (option A), sinus arrhythmia, (option B), and Mobitz type I heart block (option D) are usually benign and do not warrant preemptive therapy in most cases, unless there is a significant underlying cause, such as acute coronary ischemia, that is responsible.

98-5. The answer is D. *(Hurst's The Heart, 14th Edition, Chap. 98)* In cases where only bipolar (not monopolar [option A]) electrocautery or a harmonic scalpel will be used, disruption of implanted rhythm devices is extremely unlikely. However, in cases where monopolar (not bipolar [option B]) electrocautery will be used above the umbilicus, disruption of implanted rhythm devices is more likely. In pacemaker-dependent patients, reprogramming to the DOO or VOO setting can minimize (not maximize [option C]) oversensing and failure to pace. In patients with implanted cardioverter-defibrillators (ICDs), turning off tachytherapies is helpful to avoid unnecessary patient shocks (option D).

98-6. The answer is A. *(Hurst's The Heart, 14th Edition, Chap. 98)* Important predictors of poor postoperative outcome were: ischemic etiology of MR (not myxomatous etiology [option A]), diabetes mellitus (option B), reduced LVEF < 35% (option C), and a history of carotid endarterectomy (option D).

98-7. The answer is E. *(Hurst's The Heart, 14th Edition, Chap. 98)* The RCRI is a simple and validated tool that assesses the risk of a major cardiac perioperative event, defined as myocardial infarction, pulmonary edema, ventricular fibrillation or primary cardiac arrest, or complete heart block.[8] The RCRI consists of history of ischemic heart disease (option A), congestive heart failure (option B), cerebrovascular disease (option C), kidney disease (preoperative creatinine > 2 mg/dL or > 176 umol/L [option D]), insulin treatment, and high-risk surgical operation. Pulmonary disease (option E), while it may be important and prognostic in certain cases, is not included in the RCRI.

98-8. The answer is D. *(Hurst's The Heart, 14th Edition, Chap. 98)* Revascularization in stable coronary disease prior to surgery has not been associated with improved outcomes (option A).[9] Outcomes are improved in patients with higher functional status as approximated by the METs (option B),[10] such that formal functional testing is not indicated when a patient can easily and repetitively perform over 4 METs on a habitual basis (option C), and an even stronger argument against testing can be made above 10 METs. Obtaining a 12-lead ECG should generally be reserved for patients with known arrhythmia, coronary or peripheral arterial disease, and structural heart disease, not routinely in all patients (option D). Preoperative left ventricular function assessment is appropriate in patients with dyspnea of unknown origin and in patients with known left ventricular dysfunction and worsening or poorly controlled symptoms (option E).

98-9. The answer is E. *(Hurst's The Heart, 14th Edition, Chap. 98)* The predominant findings are summarized as follows: Moderate to large areas of ischemia are associated with a higher perioperative risk of MI and death (option A), functional testing has a high negative predictive value (option B), evidence of prior MI without inducible ischemia has little predictive value for perioperative events (option C), and both DSE and MPI have been shown to be safe when appropriately performed in this clinical context (option D).

98-10. The answer is D. *(Hurst's The Heart, 14th Edition, Chap. 98)* POISE revealed that perioperative beta-blockade improved the composite end point of perioperative cardiac events, but at the expense of more bradycardic (option A) and hypotensive (option B) episodes, strokes (option C), and most importantly, deaths. The risk of all-cause death was higher in the beta-blocker group (3.1% vs 2.3%, HR 1.33; 95% CI 1.03–1.74; $P = 0.0317$), and there was no difference in the risk of cardiovascular death (1.8% vs 1.4%, HR 1.30; 95% CI 0.92–1.83; $P = 0.1368$) (option D). Although some have criticized POISE for choices in beta-blocker dosing and frequency that may exceed those used in clinical practice, further investigations have also confirmed equivocal findings with perioperative beta-blockade.[16,17]

References

1. Wijeysundera DN WH, Yun L, Wąsowicz M, Beattie WS, Velianou JL, Ko DT. Risk of elective major noncardiac surgery after coronary stent insertion: a population-based study. *Circulation* 2012;126:1355-1362.
2. Hawn M, Graham L, Richman J, Itani K, Henderson W, Maddox T. Risk of major adverse cardiac events following noncardiac surgery in patients with coronary stents. *JAMA.* 2013;310:1462-1472.
3. Levine G, Bates E, Bittl J, et al. 2016 ACC/AHA guideline focused update on duration of dual antiplatelet therapy in patients with coronary artery disease: a report of the American College of Cardiology/American Heart Association Task Force on Clinical Practice Guidelines. *J Am Coll Cardiol.* 2016;68(10):1082-1115.
4. Douketis J, Johnson J, Turpie A. Low-molecular-weight heparin as bridging anticoagulation during interruption of warfarin: assessment of a standardized periprocedural anticoagulation regimen. *Arch Intern Med.* 2004;164:1319-1326.
5. Dunn A, Spyropoulos A, Turpie A. Bridging therapy in patients on long-term oral anticoagulants who require surgery: the Prospective Peri-operative Enoxaparin Cohort Trial (PROSPECT). *J Thromb Haemost.* 2007;5:2211-2218.
6. Spyropoulos A, Turpie A, Dunn A, et al. Clinical outcomes with unfractionated heparin or low-molecular-weight heparin as bridging therapy in patients on long-term oral anticoagulants: the REGIMEN registry. *J Thromb Haemost.* 2006;4:1246-1252.
7. Bajaj N, Agarwal S, Rajamanickam A, et al. Impact of severe mitral regurgitation on postoperative outcomes after noncardiac surgery. *Am J Med.* 2013;126:529-535.

8. Lee T, Marcantonio E, Mangione C, et al. Derivation and prospective validation of a simple index for prediction of cardiac risk of major noncardiac surgery. *Circulation*. 1999;100:1043-1049.

9. McFalls E, Ward H, Moritz T, et al. Coronary-artery revascularization before elective major vascular surgery. *N Engl J Med*. 2004;351:2795-2804.

10. Crawford R, Cambria R, Abularrage C, et al. Preoperative functional status predicts perioperative outcomes after infrainguinal bypass surgery. *J Vasc Surg*. 2010;51:351-358.

11. Lentine K, Costa S, Weir M, et al. American Heart Association Council on the Kidney in Cardiovascular Disease and Council on Peripheral Vascular Disease; American Heart Association; American College of Cardiology Foundation. Cardiac disease evaluation and management among kidney and liver transplantation candidates: a scientific statement from the American Heart Association and the American College of Cardiology Foundation. Endorsed by the American Society of Transplant Surgeons, American Society of Transplantation, and National Kidney Foundation. *Circulation*. 2012;126:617-663.

12. Douglas PS GM, Haines DE, Lai WW, et al. ACCF/ASE/AHA/ASNC/HFSA/HRS/ SCAI/SCCM/SCCT/ SCMR 2011 appropriate use criteria for echocardiography. A report of the American College of Cardiology Foundation Appropriate Use Criteria Task Force, American Society of Echocardiography, American Heart Association, American Society of Nuclear Cardiology, Heart Failure Society of America, Heart Rhythm Society, Society for Cardiovascular Angiography and Interventions, Society of Critical Care Medicine, Society of Cardiovascular Computed Tomography, and Society for Cardiovascular Magnetic Resonance. Endorsed by the American College of Chest Physicians. *J Am Coll Cardiol*. 2011;57:1126-1166.

13. Baron J, Mundler O, Bertrand M, et al. Dipyridamole-thallium scintigraphy and gated radionuclide angiography to assess cardiac risk before abdominal aortic surgery. *N Engl J Med*. 1994;330:663-669.

14. Mangano D, London M, Tubau J, et al. Dipyridamole thallium-201 scintigraphy as a preoperative screening test. A reexamination of its predictive potential. Study of Perioperative Ischemia Research Group. *Circulation*. 1991;84:493-502.

15. Devereaux P, Beattie W, Choi P, et al. How strong is the evidence for the use of perioperative beta blockers in non-cardiac surgery? Systematic review and meta-analysis of randomised controlled trials. *BMJ*. 2005;331:313-321.

16. Lindenauer P, Pekow P, Wang K, Mamidi D, Gutierrez B, Benjamin E. Perioperative beta-blocker therapy and mortality after major noncardiac surgery. *N Engl J Med*. 2005;353:349-361.

17. London M, Hur K, Schwartz G, Henderson W. Association of perioperative β-blockade with mortality and cardiovascular morbidity following major noncardiac surgery. *JAMA*. 2013;309:1704-1713.

CHAPTER 99

Anesthesia and the Patient with Cardiovascular Disease

Jonathan Afilalo

QUESTIONS

DIRECTIONS: Choose the one best response to each question.

99-1. The effects of intraoperative neuraxial block and postoperative epidural analgesia on major cardiovascular outcomes after noncardiac surgery remain controversial. In a propensity-weighted study of 10,010 high-risk noncardiac surgical patients, neuraxial block was associated with a reduction in which of the following complications?

A. Composite death, myocardial infarction, or stroke
B. Death
C. Myocardial infarction
D. Clinically important hypotension
E. None of the above

99-2. In general, there are no definite recommendations for choosing a particular anesthetic to decrease the risk of perioperative cardiac events. In which of the following surgical procedures may a neuraxial technique be advantageous to enable early recognition of complications?

A. Transurethral resection of prostate
B. Mastectomy
C. Colectomy
D. Small bowel resection
E. Nephrectomy

99-3. Although there is limited evidence to guide the safe use of neuraxial anesthesia in patients receiving novel anticoagulant drugs, this is not an absolute contraindication. Which of the following statements about best practice recommendations for the management of novel anticoagulant drugs before neuraxial manipulation is *false*?

A. The risk of spinal hematoma is significantly increased in the presence of concomitant antiplatelet drugs
B. Coagulation assays (for dabigatran) and anti-Xa assays (for apixaban, edoxaban, and rivaroxaban) should be used to determine when the anticoagulant effect is at a safe level
C. Apixaban and rivaroxaban should be discontinued for at least 1 day before neural manipulation
D. Dabigatran should be discontinued for at least 4 to 5 days before neural manipulation
E. Discontinuation times should be even longer in patients with renal insufficiency

99-4. Most intravenous anesthetics exhibit some degree of cardiovascular depression in the form of reduced cardiac output or vasodilation. Which of the following intravenous anesthetics may *not* be indicated in a patient with severely compromised cardiac function?

A. Fentanyl
B. Remifentanil
C. Propofol
D. Etomidate
E. Ketamine

99-5. Succinylcholine is a depolarizing short-acting neuromuscular blocker that is associated with a rapid onset and short duration of action. Which of the following iatrogenic effects may *not* be caused by the use of succinylcholine?

A. Hypokalemia
B. Tachycardia
C. Hypertension
D. Bradycardia
E. Hypotension

99-6. Appropriate patient selection is crucial to avoid potentially catastrophic complications (eg, paraplegia) when planning for an intraoperative central neuraxial anesthesia or postoperative neuraxial analgesia in patients receiving anticoagulation or potent antiplatelet therapy. Which of the following agents is generally contraindicated for neuraxial manipulation?

A. Glycoprotein IIb/IIIa antagonists
B. Prasugrel
C. Clopidogrel
D. Low molecular weight heparins
E. All of the above are contraindicated

99-7. Perioperative monitoring has contributed significantly to the attainment of the level of safety provided by modern anesthesia, allowing for more complex surgeries in even the highest-risk patients. The American Society of Anesthesiologists established standards for basic intraoperative monitoring in 1986.[9] Subsequently, indications for intra-arterial and central venous monitoring were established. Which of the following forms of intraoperative monitoring is *not* required based on these guidelines?

A. Basic monitoring for all patients should include blood pressure, ECG, pulse oximetry, capnometry, and body temperature
B. Intra-arterial monitoring for patients with right heart failure
C. Intra-arterial monitoring for patients undergoing major aortic surgery
D. Central venous monitoring for patients with a history of ischemic heart disease
E. Central venous monitoring for patients with a history of tricuspid stenosis

99-8. The indications for pulmonary arterial catheter (PAC) monitoring are based on a combination of patient-related and procedural factors. The American Society of Anesthesiologists published practice parameters to guide practitioners in the appropriate use of the PAC. Which of the following factors may justifiably warrant placement of a PAC for intraoperative monitoring?

A. Pulmonary arterial systolic pressure of 75 mm Hg
B. Systemic arterial pressure of 175/75 mm Hg
C. Severe tricuspid valve regurgitation
D. High-risk vascular surgery
E. All of the above

99-9. Less invasive and noninvasive methods of cardiovascular monitoring are continually being developed. Which of the following methods may *not* be used to estimate cardiac output?

A. Central venous contour analysis
B. Arterial pressure waveform analysis
C. Indicator dilution technique
D. Electrical bioimpedance
E. Esophageal Doppler ultrasound

99-10. The American Society of Anesthesiologists currently does not recommend routine brain function monitoring in patients undergoing general anesthesia.[12] Which of the following factors may *not* be associated with an increased risk of intraoperative awareness?

A. Prior history of intraoperative awareness
B. Recent history of myocardial infarction
C. Morbid obesity
D. Substance abuse
E. Chronic pain patients with opioid tolerance

99-1. The answer is E. *(Hurst's The Heart, 14th Edition, Chap. 99)* There is little scientific evidence that any particular anesthetic approach is superior to its reasonable alternatives.[1-7] In this substudy from the POISE-2 trial, neither neuraxial block nor postoperative epidural analgesia were associated with a statistically significant effect on death (option B), myocardial infarction (option C), stroke, hypotension (option D), or the composite end point (option A). In another study of 98,290 elective colectomies,[8] neuraxial technique was associated with a decreased risk of thromboembolism and cerebrovascular events, but it was associated with an increased risk of myocardial infarction, urinary tract infection, postoperative ileus, and blood transfusions.

99-2. The answer is A. *(Hurst's The Heart, 14th Edition, Chap. 99)* In certain defined surgical procedures such as transurethral resection of prostate (option A), a neuraxial technique may be advantageous in enabling early recognition of complications. This is not applicable in all circumstances (options B, C, D, E), and clinical judgment must be exercised to make the best choices in individual circumstances. Regional anesthetics and monitored anesthesia care are not infrequently converted to general anesthetics intraoperatively as a result of unexpectedly long surgery, patient discomfort, or changes in the surgical plan. No practitioner can be certain that a particular technique will be adequate for the surgical procedure, given the unpredictability of the situation, and the anesthesiologist must have flexibility to alter the technique as needed.

99-3. The answer is B. *(Hurst's The Heart, 14th Edition, Chap. 99)* There is a significantly increased risk of spinal hematoma with concomitant use of other drugs that affect hemostasis, as well as platelet inhibitors (option A). The "safe" time interval between the last dose of novel anticoagulants and safe neuraxial anesthesia not known, but there are recommended time delays that appear to be associated with an acceptably low risk. For dabigatran, the recommendation is at least 4 to 5 days (option D), and longer wait times in cases of renal insufficiency (option E). For rivaroxaban the recommended delay is at least 22 to 26 h, and for apixaban 26 to 30 h (option C). In patients taking argatroban or bivalirudin, neuraxial anesthesia is probably best avoided. Routine coagulation assays, including ecarin clotting assays and anti-factor Xa assays, are unreliable and of little value to guide neuraxial anesthesia (option B).

99-4. The answer is C. *(Hurst's The Heart, 14th Edition, Chap. 99)* The use of synthetic opioids (fentanyl [option A], sufentanil, or remifentanil [option B]), etomidate (option D), or ketamine (option E) may be preferred in patients with severely compromised cardiac function because they tend to maintain hemodynamic stability. Ketamine is unique among the intravenous anesthetic agents in that it increases blood pressure, heart rate, systemic vascular resistance, and cardiac output. Conversely, propofol decreases blood pressure, systemic vascular resistance, and cardiac output, and long-term administration can exert a negative effect on myocardial contractile function.

99-5. The answer is A. *(Hurst's The Heart, 14th Edition, Chap. 99)* Succinylcholine's cardiovascular effects depend on whether nicotinic or muscarinic receptor effects predominate in a given patient. Thus, tachycardia (option B) and hypertension (option C) or bradycardia (option D) and hypotension (option E) may occur. Vagal effects tend to predominate with repeated doses or in children. In patients with various disorders (including neuromuscular diseases, recent burns, and massive trauma), hyperkalemic (not hypokalemia [option A]) cardiac arrest may occur because of exaggerated release of intracellular potassium from myocytes.

99-6. The answer is E. *(Hurst's The Heart, 14th Edition, Chap. 99)* It is prudent to avoid neuraxial manipulation in patients who are receiving potent antiplatelet drugs that include glycoprotein IIb/IIIa antagonists (option A), adenosine diphosphate inhibitors (clopidogrel, prasugrel [options B, C]), and low molecular weight heparins (option D) at the time of the planned anesthesia. There are currently limited data on the safe use of novel oral anticoagulants such as the direct thrombin inhibitors and factor Xa inhibitors in patients considered for neuraxial anesthesia.

99-7. The answer is D. *(Hurst's The Heart, 14th Edition, Chap. 99)* Intraoperative monitoring that is required based on these guidelines include the following: (1) heart rate, (2) electrocardiogram (ECG), (3) blood pressure, (4) pulse oximetry, (5) capnometry, and (6) body temperature (option A). The indications for the use of more invasive monitors, such as intra-arterial and central venous monitoring, vary and depend on patient- and surgery-specific factors, as well as the institution and practitioner preferences; some of the recommended indications are outlined in Tables 99-5 and 99-6 of *Hurst's The Heart,* 14th edition (options B, C, E).[10] A history of ischemic heart disease, when stable and compensated, is not an indication per se for central venous line placement and monitoring during noncardiac surgery (option D).

99-8. The answer is A. *(Hurst's The Heart, 14th Edition, Chap. 99)* Many clinicians believe that patients with clinically significant pulmonary hypertension (option A), severe aortic stenosis, or severe cardiac dysfunction undergoing surgery with expected large fluid shifts or hemodynamic instability may benefit from PAC monitoring.[11] Systemic hypertension (option B) is not an indication for PAC monitoring, nor is "high-risk" surgery (option D) in the absence of large fluid shifts. PAC monitoring is less reliable in the presence of severe tricuspid valve regurgitation (option C), and this in and of itself should not constitute an indication for PAC monitoring.

99-9. The answer is A. *(Hurst's The Heart, 14th Edition, Chap. 99)* Cardiac output can be estimated using arterial pressure waveform analysis (option B), the indicator dilution technique (option C), electrical bioimpedance (option D), and esophageal Doppler ultrasound (option E). Central venous pressure and contour analysis is used to estimate cardiac filling parameters, not cardiac output (option A).

99-10. The answer is B. *(Hurst's The Heart, 14th Edition, Chap. 99)* An elevated risk of intraoperative awareness is associated with a prior history of intraoperative awareness (option A), morbid obesity (option C), substance abuse (option D), chronic pain patients with opioid tolerance (option E), and certain procedures such as trauma surgery. Brain function monitoring should thus be considered for use on a case-by-case basis. A history of myocardial infarction is not linked to a higher rate of intraoperative awareness (option B).

References

1. Tuman KJ, McCarthy RJ, March RJ, et al. Effects of epidural anesthesia and analgesia on coagulation and outcome after major vascular surgery. *Anesth Analg.* 1991;73:696-704.
2. Baron JF, Bertrand M, Barre E, et al. Combined epidural and general anesthesia versus general anesthesia for abdominal aortic surgery. *Anesthesiology.* 1991;75:611-618.
3. Bode RH Jr, Lewis KP, Zarich SW, et al. Cardiac outcome after peripheral vascular surgery: comparison of general and regional anesthesia. *Anesthesiology.* 1996;84:3-13.
4. Christopherson R, Beattie C, Frank SM, et al. Perioperative morbidity in patients randomized to epidural or general anesthesia for lower extremity vascular surgery. *Anesthesiology.* 1993;79:422-434.
5. Mofidi R, Nimmo AF, Moores C, et al. Regional versus general anaesthesia for carotid endarterectomy: impact of change in practice. *Surgeon.* 2006;4:158-162.
6. Verhoeven EL, Cina CS, Tielliu IF, et al. Local anesthesia for endovascular abdominal aortic aneurysm repair. *J Vasc Surg.* 2005;42:402-409.
7. Leslie K, McIlroy D, Kasza J, et al. Neuraxial block and postoperative epidural analgesia: effects on outcomes in the POISE-2 trial. *Br J Anaesth.* 2016;116:100-112.

8. Poeran J, Yeo H, Rasul R, Opperer M, Memtsoudis SG, Mazumdar M. Anesthesia type and perioperative outcome: open colectomies in the United States. *J Surg Res*. 2015;193:684-692.

9. American Society of Anesthesiologists. Standards for basic intraoperative monitoring. Approved by House of Delegates on October 21, 1986 and last amended on October 21, 1998. Park Ridge, IL. http://www.asahq.org/publicationsAndServices/standards/02.pdf. Accessed May 12, 2010.

10. Reich DL, Mittnacht A, Manecke G, Kaplan JA. Chapter 14: monitoring of the heart and vascular system. In: Kaplan JA, Reich DL, Savino JS, eds. *Kaplan's Cardiac Anesthesia*, 6th ed. Philadelphia, PA: Saunders Elsevier; 2011:416-451.

11. Judge O, Ji F, Fleming N, Liu H. Current use of the pulmonary artery catheter in cardiac surgery: a survey study. *J Cardiothorac Vasc Anesth*. 2015;29:69-75.

12. Practice advisory for intraoperative awareness and brain function monitoring. A report by the American Society of Anesthesiologists task force on intraoperative awareness. *Anesthesiology*. 2006;104:847-864.

CHAPTER 100

Rheumatologic Diseases and the Cardiovascular System

Jacqueline Joza

QUESTIONS

DIRECTIONS: Choose the one best response to each question.

100-1. A 55-year-old woman presents to the emergency department with positional chest pain, worse with lying flat and with inspiration. On physical exam, she is noted to have a symmetrical polyarthritis affecting the small joints of her hands and feet, including a swan-neck deformity of the fingers, ulnar deviation of the metacarpophalangeal joints, and a boutonniere deformity of the thumb. The most common cardiovascular manifestations of this systemic autoimmune disease include all of the following *except*:

A. Conduction system disease
B. Pericarditis
C. Valvular disease
D. Cardiomyopathy
E. Coronary vasculitis

100-2. A 60-year-old woman with rheumatoid arthritis (RA) is sent to you for discussion about her overall risk of developing coronary artery disease. Which of the following statements is *correct*?

A. 10% of deaths in RA are attributable to cardiovascular disease
B. The prevalence of cardiovascular disease is higher in patients with RA than in diabetics
C. When compared with controls, women with RA have a fivefold higher rate of myocardial infarction
D. Systemic inflammation in RA is hypothesized to accelerate atherosclerosis
E. The C-reactive protein normalizes in most patients with RA who are judged to be in clinical remission

100-3. A 20-year-old woman presents to your clinic after having been lost to follow-up. She had been told that she had an electrical conduction disease since birth. The patient's family history is significant for her mother having an autoimmune disorder. Her baseline electrocardiogram reveals sinus rhythm with AV dissociation and a narrow junctional escape at 50 bpm. Previously asymptomatic, she has recently noticed increased dyspnea with exertion. She has no other significant medical history. Which of the following concerning this patient is *incorrect*?

A. The patient's mother likely had positive serum anti-Ro or anti-La antibodies during her pregnancy
B. 20% to 30% of women with anti-Ro antibodies will give birth to infants with neonatal lupus syndrome or congenital heart block
C. Myocardial inflammation and fibrosis in the fetus is the mechanism by which infants of mothers who have positive serum anti-Ro or anti-La antibodies develop heart block
D. The probability that the patient's younger sister has congenital heart block is 20%
E. Treatment of dexamethasone may be helpful in converting first- and second-degree heart block in the infant

100-4. A 50-year-old man presents with pericarditis, arthralgia, and fever. He was recently started on a medication to treat a "cardiac problem." Which of the following medications is *least* likely to be the cause of his presentation?

A. Quinidine
B. Hydralazine
C. Propafenone
D. Procainamide
E. Mexiletine

100-5. A 36-year-old woman with a history of multiple miscarriages, prior lower extremity deep vein thrombosis, and resolved thrombocytopenia presents to your office after a transthoracic echocardiogram revealed mild thickening of her mitral valve. She has no cardiac complaints. Her complete blood count is within normal limits. This patient should be started on which of the following medications?

A. Warfarin
B. Low-dose aspirin daily
C. Metoprolol
D. Ramipril
E. Spironolactone

100-6. A 75-year-old woman presented 1 year ago with temporal artery tenderness, headache, jaw claudication, and mild visual loss. After treatment with steroids, she returned to her usual state of health. Today, she presents to the emergency department with severe upper back pain. Which of the following is the most likely diagnosis given her past medical history?

A. Vertebral compression fracture
B. Cauda equina syndrome
C. Nephrolithiasis
D. Aortic dissection
E. Acute pancreatitis

100-7. A 50-year-old man suffered an anterior ST elevation myocardial infarction 1 year ago and was treated with percutaneous coronary intervention with placement of a drug-eluting stent to the proximal left anterior descending artery. As part of his medication regimen, he is taking a statin. In the last several weeks, he has noticed worsening bilateral proximal leg muscle weakness. Which of the following is *more* suggestive of a statin-related myopathy than of a primary inflammatory myopathy?

A. Statin-related myopathies are typically associated with significant myalgia when compared to primary inflammatory myopathy
B. An increase in the creatinine kinase serum level is noted in most patients with a statin-related myopathy but in only a small percentage of patients with a primary inflammatory myopathy
C. Patients with a statin-related myopathy may present with skin involvement characterized by erythematous scaliness over the knuckles
D. Statin-related myopathies may suggest an underlying paraneoplastic syndrome
E. A muscle biopsy will not be able to differentiate between a statin-related myopathy and a primary inflammatory myopathy

100-8. A 23-year-old man presents to the emergency department with crushing chest pain for which he is taken directly for coronary angiogram. The angiogram reveals several coronary artery aneurysms. As a child, he was told that he was hospitalized for several days for an illness characterized by a high fever, conjunctivitis, cervical adenopathy, swollen hands and feet, and a rash around the perineum. In this disorder, aneurysms are most frequent in which of the following coronary arteries?

A. Proximal left anterior descending artery
B. Left main coronary artery
C. Circumflex coronary artery
D. Distal right coronary artery
E. Posterior descending coronary artery

100-9. Which of the following connective tissue disorders may be transmitted in an autosomal recessive manner?

A. Marfan syndrome
B. Loeys–Dietz syndrome
C. Ehlers–Danlos syndrome
D. Osteogenesis imperfecta
E. None of the above

100-10. A 35-year-old man is referred to you from his rheumatologist for a cardiac evaluation. His blood work is positive for the presence of HLA-B27, but his serum rheumatoid factor is negative. He describes symptoms of low back and buttock pain that is worse at night and improves with exercise. He also describes pain and stiffness of his ankles, with swelling at the Achilles tendon. What is the most prevalent cardiovascular manifestation of this disease?

A. Myocarditis
B. Atrial fibrillation
C. Atrioventricular block
D. Aortitis
E. C and D

100-1. The answer is A. *(Hurst's The Heart, 14th Edition, Chap. 100)* The patient has a diagnosis of RA. Extra-articular manifestations of RA include fatigue, low-grade fever, Sjögren syndrome, rheumatoid nodules, interstitial lung disease, and vasculitis. Electrical conduction disorders are *not* specifically seen as a result of RA. Other systemic autoimmune disorders, including inflammatory myopathies (characterized by proximal muscle weakness with dermatomyositis and Gottron papules) and systemic sclerosis (where the limited form is referred to as CREST), are associated with conduction system abnormalities. In RA, the most common cardiovascular manifestations are pericarditis, valvular disease, specifically mitral valve insufficiency (option C), cardiomyopathy characterized by focal necrotizing or granulomatous myocarditis (option D), coronary vasculitis (option E) where as many as 20% of patients show histologic evidence by autopsy, and accelerated coronary artery atherosclerosis and heart failure.

100-2. The answer is D. *(Hurst's The Heart, 14th Edition, Chap. 100)* The overall mortality is increased in patients with RA,[1,2] with 40% of deaths attributable to cardiovascular disease (option A).[3,4] In a recent study, the prevalence of cardiovascular disease in RA patients was *comparable* to that of patients with diabetes (option B).[5] It is known that a significant proportion of patients with RA judged to be in clinical remission using standardized disease activity scores still show an *elevated* level of C-reactive protein (> 3 mg/L) (option E), a known risk factor for future cardiovascular mortality in patients with RA.[6] Increasing evidence supports a strong link between RA and accelerated atherosclerosis, highlighting it as an important risk factor for cardiovascular disease. Atherosclerosis is an inflammatory process driven by many of the same mediators that are associated with rheumatoid inflammation, where systemic inflammation in RA is hypothesized to accelerate atherosclerosis (option D).[7] Additionally, RA appears to be an independent risk factor for multivessel coronary artery disease,[8] and as shown in the Nurses' Health Study, women with RA have a *two*-fold higher rate of myocardial infarctions compared with controls (option C).[9]

100-3. The answer is B. *(Hurst's The Heart, 14th Edition, Chap. 100)* The patient has likely had some degree of atrioventricular block since infancy. A conduction system abnormality may occur in infants of mothers with SLE whose serum contains anti-Ro and anti-La antibodies (option A). Some of these mothers may also have been previously diagnosed with primary Sjögren syndrome, whereas others may appear healthy. Fewer than 5% of women with anti-Ro and/or anti-La antibodies will give birth to infants with neonatal lupus syndrome or congenital heart block (option B). Congenital heart block develops from the transmission of maternal anti-Ro and anti-La antibodies to the fetus, causing myocardial inflammation and fibrosis (option C).[10] Additionally, the probability of congenital heart block increases to almost 20% in subsequent offspring (option D).[11] Treatment with dexamethasone may be helpful in converting first- and second-degree heart block; however, third-degree heart block appears largely irreversible (option E).[12]

100-4. The answer is E. *(Hurst's The Heart, 14th Edition, Chap. 100)* Drug-induced systemic lupus erythematosus (DIL) may be a rare complication of certain medications, including procainamide (option D), quinidine (option A), hydralazine (option B), and propafenone (option C). Other medications associated with DIL include isoniazid, minocycline, clindamycin, and phenytoin. DIL, which affects men and women equally, is associated with the development of serum anti-histone antibodies, although only a few patients will actually develop the clinical syndrome. Common signs and symptoms of DIL include pericarditis, pleuritis, arthralgia, and fever. It is rare to develop renal or neurologic complications from DIL. The syndrome will usually resolve on its own after a short course of prednisone and discontinuation of the offending medication.[13]

100-5. The answer is B. *(Hurst's The Heart, 14th Edition, Chap. 100)* This patient has antiphospholipid syndrome (APS), which is characterized by the clinical triad of recurrent arterial or venous thromboses, pregnancy loss, and thrombocytopenia. Serologically, it is defined by the presence of anticardiolipin antibodies, anti-β_2 glycoprotein antibodies, or a positive lupus anticoagulant. Because APS may produce thrombotic occlusion of many different types and sizes of blood vessels, it can produce a variety of cardiovascular manifestations. Valvular disease is the most common APS-related cardiovascular manifestation. It is seen in both primary and secondary APS and is essentially indistinguishable from Libman–Sacks endocarditis. Patients with *asymptomatic valvular thickening* should be treated with a low-dose daily aspirin (81 mg) (option B); however, those with evidence of vegetation or embolization should be treated with systemic anticoagulation (target INR 2-3).[14]

100-6. The answer is D. *(Hurst's The Heart, 14th Edition, Chap. 100)* The patient had a diagnosis of giant-cell arteritis (GCA), also known as temporal arteritis, which is the most common vasculitis among patients older than 50 years.[15] The clinical hallmarks of GCA are temporal artery tenderness, headache, jaw claudication, and visual loss.

GCA may lead to thoracic and abdominal aortic aneurysms. In one study, 16 of 41 patients with GCA and aortic aneurysm had an acute aortic dissection, with 8 deaths.[16] Given these findings, it has been recommended that patients with GCA undergo yearly screening for aortic aneurysm using transthoracic echocardiography and abdominal ultrasonography.[17] Other cardiovascular complications rarely associated with GCA are pericarditis, myocarditis, and coronary arteritis.[18]

100-7. The answer is A. *(Hurst's The Heart, 14th Edition, Chap. 100)* Both dermatomyositis (DM) and polymyositis (PM) are two inflammatory muscle diseases that are manifested by proximal muscle weakness. It is important to rule out other forms of myopathy in patients who present with muscle weakness. Patients taking statins may develop a myopathy mimicking inflammatory muscle disease. Statin-related myopathy and inflammatory myopathy may be differentiated by certain aspects of the medical history (eg, statins usually associated with significant myalgia [option A]), the results of electromyography, and findings on muscle biopsy (option E), if necessary. For statin-induced myopathy, withdrawal of the offending drug will lead to symptom resolution. Patients with DM usually present with skin involvement characterized by erythematous scaliness over the knuckles (Gottron papules) (option C), elbows, and knees, as well as periorbital swelling and a violaceous rash around the lids, known as a heliotropic rash. They may also display a photosensitive rash over the face, chest, and back in a shawl-like distribution. Increases in serum levels of muscle enzymes, such as creatine kinase and aldolase, are present in inflammatory muscle diseases (option B). In older patients, DM and PM may evolve as a paraneoplastic syndrome (option D).

100-8. The answer is A. *(Hurst's The Heart, 14th Edition, Chap. 100)* Kawasaki disease is an acute febrile illness affecting children from ages 6 months to 8 years. In the United States, its annual incidence is approximately 6 per 100,000 children younger than 5 years, occurring, in order of decreasing frequency, in children of Asian, African American, and Caucasian descent. The affected child presents with fever, desquamative rash, conjunctivitis, and lymphadenopathy. During this acute phase of Kawasaki disease, the cardiovascular system may be affected in various ways. Pericarditis, myocarditis, mitral regurgitation, aortitis, aortic regurgitation, congestive heart failure, and arrhythmias have all been described in this illness.[19] Coronary vasculitis develops in as short a time as 2 weeks after symptom onset, but usually within 4 weeks after the onset of fever. If left untreated, this process may lead to the development of coronary aneurysms, the most serious complication of this disease.[20] Coronary artery aneurysms are most common in the proximal left anterior descending (option A) and proximal right coronary arteries, followed in frequency by the left main coronary artery (option B), circumflex coronary artery (option C), distal right coronary artery (option D), and at the take-off of the posterior descending coronary artery (option E) from the right coronary artery.[21] The predilection for coronary artery aneurysms at branch points suggests a pathologic role for shear stress.

100-9. The answer is C. (*Hurst's The Heart, 14th Edition, Chap. 100*) Ehlers–Danlos syndrome is a connective tissue disease characterized by joint hypermobility, hyperelastic skin, and easy bruising associated with aortic aneurysms and mitral valve prolapse. It may be transmitted with an autosomal dominant or an autosomal recessive inheritance. Marfan syndrome (option A), Loeys–Dietz syndrome (option B), osteogenesis imperfecta (option D), and pseudoxanthoma elasticum are all connective tissue diseases with an autosomal dominant inheritance.

100-10. The answer is E. (*Hurst's The Heart, 14th Edition, Chap. 100*) The patient most likely has a diagnosis of ankylosing spondylitis, with a positive HLA-B27. Among the group of spondyloarthropathies, ankylosing spondylitis and reactive arthritis are the most frequently associated with cardiovascular manifestations. The two most prevalent cardiovascular manifestations of the spondyloarthropathies are conduction system disease and aortitis (option D), with or without aortic insufficiency. The conduction system disease presents mainly as atrioventricular block (option C), which occurs more commonly in men that are HLA-B27 positive than in women; it often requires permanent pacemaker placement. Aortic root involvement is also associated with HLA-B27 in patients with ankylosing spondylitis[22] and reactive arthritis.[23] Aortitis may lead to dilatation and stiffening of the aortic root with aortic valvular regurgitation. Aortic valvular regurgitation is usually a late complication of the spondyloarthropathies.[24] Other less common cardiac manifestations associated with spondyloarthropathies include clinically insignificant diastolic dysfunction, supraventricular tachycardias (especially atrial fibrillation [option B]),[25] myocarditis (option A), and pericarditis.

References

1. Gabriel SE. Why do people with rheumatoid arthritis still die prematurely? *Ann Rheum Dis.* 2008; 67(suppl 3):iii30-iii34.
2. Gabriel SE. The epidemiology of rheumatoid arthritis. *Rheum Dis Clin North Am.* 2001;27(2):269-281.
3. Reilly PA, Cosh JA, Maddison PJ, et al. Mortality and survival in rheumatoid arthritis: a 25 year prospective study of 100 patients. *Ann Rheum Dis.* 1990;49(6):363-369.
4. Wolfe F, Mitchel DM, Sibley JT, et al. The mortality of rheumatoid arthritis. *Arthritis Rheum.* 1994;37(4):481-494.
5. van Halm VP, Peters MJ, Voskuyl AE, et al. Rheumatoid arthritis versus diabetes as a risk factor for cardiovascular disease: a cross-sectional study, the CARRE investigation. *Ann Rheum Dis.* 2009;68(9):1395-1400.
6. Graf J, Scherzer R, Grunfeld C, et al. Levels of C-reactive protein associated with high and very high cardiovascular risk are prevalent in patients with rheumatoid arthritis. *PLoS One.* 2009;4(7):e6242.
7. Libby P. Role of inflammation in atherosclerosis associated with rheumatoid arthritis. *Am J Med.* 2008;121(10 suppl 1):S21-S31.
8. Warrington KJ, Kent PD, Frye RL, et al. Rheumatoid arthritis is an independent risk factor for multivessel coronary artery disease: a case control study. *Arthritis Res Ther.* 2005;7(5):R984-R991.
9. Solomon DH, Karlson EW, Rimm EB, et al. Cardiovascular morbidity and mortality in women diagnosed with rheumatoid arthritis. *Circulation.* 2003;107(9):1303-1307.
10. Buyon JP, Clancy RM. Neonatal lupus: basic research and clinical perspectives. *Rheum Dis Clin North Am.* 2005;31(2):299-313, vii.
11. Julkunen H, Eronen M. The rate of recurrence of isolated congenital heart block: a population-based study. *Arthritis Rheum.* 2001;44:487-488.
12. Zeller CB, Appenzeller S. Cardiovascular disease in systemic lupus erythematosus: the role of traditional and lupus related risk factors. *Curr Cardiol Rev.* 2008;4(2):116-122.
13. Price EJ, Venables PJ. Drug-induced lupus. *Drug Saf.* 1995;12(4):283-290.
14. Lockshin M, Tenedios F, Petri M, et al. Cardiac disease in the antiphospholipid syndrome: recommendations for treatment. Committee consensus report. *Lupus.* 2003;12:518.
15. Salvarani C, Cantini F, Boiardi L, et al. Polymyalgia rheumatica and giant-cell arteritis. *N Engl J Med.* 2002;347(4):261-271.
16. Evans JM, Bowles CA, Bjornsson J, et al. Thoracic aortic aneurysm and rupture in giant cell arteritis. A descriptive study of 41 cases. *Arthritis Rheum.* 1994;37(10):1539-1547.
17. Bongartz T, Matteson EL. Large-vessel involvement in giant cell arteritis. *Curr Opin Rheumatol.* 2006;18(1):10-17.
18. Sonnenblick M, Nesher G, Rosin A. Nonclassical organ involvement in temporal arteritis. *Semin Arthritis Rheum.* 1989;19(3):183-190.

19. Barron KS. Kawasaki disease: etiology, pathogenesis, and treatment. *Cleve Clin J Med.* 2002;69(suppl 2): SII69-SII78.

20. Newburger JW, Takahashi M, Gerber MA, et al. Diagnosis, treatment, and long-term management of Kawasaki disease: a statement for health professionals from the Committee on Rheumatic Fever, Endocarditis and Kawasaki Disease, Council on Cardiovascular Disease in the Young, American Heart Association. *Circulation.* 2004;110(17):2747-2771.

21. Kitamura S, Kameda Y, Seki T, et al. Long-term outcome of myocardial revascularization in patients with Kawasaki coronary artery disease. A multicenter cooperative study. *J Thorac Cardiovasc Surg.* 1994;107(3):663-673.

22. Roldan CA, Chavez J, Wiest PW, et al. Aortic root disease and valve disease associated with ankylosing spondylitis. *J Am Coll Cardiol.* 1998;32(5):1397-1404.

23. Misukiewicz P, Carlson RW, Rowan L, et al. Acute aortic insufficiency in a patient with presumed Reiter's syndrome. *Ann Rheum Dis.* 1992;51(5):686-687.

24. Badesch DB, Tapson VF, McGoon MD, et al. Continuous intravenous epoprostenol for pulmonary hypertension due to the scleroderma spectrum of disease. A randomized, controlled trial. *Ann Intern Med.* 2000;132(6):425-434.

25. Bergfeldt L. HLA-B27-associated cardiac disease. *Ann Intern Med.* 1997;127(8 pt 1):621-629.

CHAPTER 101

The Diagnosis and Management of Cardiovascular Disease in Patients with Cancer

Jonathan Afilalo

QUESTIONS

DIRECTIONS: Choose the one best response to each question.

101-1. A 55-year-old woman, with a prior history of Hodgkin lymphoma diagnosed at the age of 19 years and treated with radiation therapy, presented to the emergency department complaining of dyspnea on minimal exertion. Her physical examination revealed a 3/6 crescendo decrescendo systolic ejection murmur and a chest wall scar from prior radiation injury. Initial investigations including blood test and ECG were unremarkable. Chest radiography showed interstitial lung fibrosis. An echo was obtained and revealed severe aortic stenosis. Which of the following is *not* a predisposing factor facilitating the development of radiation-induced aortic stenosis?

A. Total radiation dose
B. Dose per fraction
C. The volume of heart irradiated
D. Female sex
E. Younger age at the time of irradiation

101-2. Radiation-induced cardiotoxicity may affect a number of different cardiac structures. Which of the following cardiac structures is the *most* sensitive to irradiation?

A. Pericardium
B. Myocardium
C. Heart valves
D. Conduction system
E. Cardiac vasculature

101-3. A 60-year-old man with a prior history of chest wall radiation therapy was referred to the cardiology clinic complaining of progressive exertional chest pain noted upon moderately vigorous physical activity. The chest pain resolves after a few minutes' rest. His physical examination and resting ECG are unremarkable. The patient is sent for a stress echocardiogram, which is positive for inducible ischemia and confirms the clinical diagnosis of stable angina. Which of the following is typically implicated in the pathophysiology of radiation-induced ischemic heart disease?

A. Reduced ratio of capillaries to myocytes
B. Arterial and capillary narrowing
C. Precocious atherosclerosis
D. A and B are correct
E. A, B, and C are all correct

101-4. A 43-year-old woman with a past history of breast cancer treated with neoadjuvant chemotherapy and modified radical mastectomy was diagnosed with recurrent disease and was treated with paclitaxel and radiotherapy. The patient was also known for hypertension, dyslipidemia, and obesity. Baseline left ventricular ejection fraction (LVEF) was 60%, but a follow-up transthoracic echocardiogram was performed and revealed a decline in LVEF to 45%. Which of the following risk factors is *not* a plausible predisposing factor for the development of cardiotoxicity in this patient?

A. Age < 65 years
B. Hypertension
C. Silent coronary artery disease
D. Radiation therapy
E. None of the above

101-5. For the patient described in question 101-4, which of the following is commonly cited as a diagnostic criterion for chemotherapy-related cardiotoxicity?

A. > 5% reduction in LVEF to < 55% with symptoms of heart failure

B. > 10% reduction in LVEF to < 55% without symptoms of heart failure

C. > 10% reduction in LVEF to < 53% with or without symptoms of heart failure

D. > 10% reduction in LVEF to < 50% with or without symptoms of heart failure

E. All of the above

101-6. For the patient described in question 101-4, which of the following would be the best next step in management following the diagnosis of chemotherapy-related cardiotoxicity?

A. Observe and order a repeat echocardiogram if heart failure symptoms develop

B. Observe and follow up with a repeat echocardiogram in 3 weeks

C. Discontinue chemotherapy and repeat an echocardiogram in 3 months

D. Discontinue chemotherapy and start ramipril

E. Discontinue chemotherapy and start carvedilol

101-7. A 48-year-old woman with a prior history of left breast cancer diagnosed 15 years ago and treated with radiotherapy after radical surgery presented to the emergency department complaining of a 6-month history of fatigue, dyspnea on exertion, edema in the lower extremities, and ascites. Physical examination was consistent with right-sided heart failure. Initial investigations included an NT-pro-BNP of 4180 pg/mL and negative cardiac troponins. ECG showed normal sinus rhythm and nonspecific ST-T changes. Chest radiography revealed bilateral pleural effusions. Which of the following statements about radiation-induced pericardial disease is *false*?

A. A normal ECG does not rule out radiation-associated pericarditis

B. In the presence of pericardial calcification on CT, further imaging is not required to diagnose constrictive pericarditis

C. Pericardial constriction occurs in 20% of patients with radiation-induced pericardial disease

D. For refractory cases, pericardiectomy is the treatment of choice to alleviate constriction

E. Post-pericardiectomy survival is < 5% at 5 years

101-8. A 27-year-old woman with a history of stage 3 cervical cancer presented to the emergency department complaining of right lower limb pain and swelling. The patient completed her third cycle of radiotherapy a few days prior. Her physical examination revealed pitting right lower limb edema, tenderness on palpation, and positive Hommans signs. A Doppler ultrasound was obtained and revealed a deep vein thrombosis (DVT). In comparison to oral anticoagulant therapy with warfarin, which of the following

statements about subcutaneous anticoagulation with low molecular weight heparin (LMWH) is *false*?

A. LMWH is equally as effective as warfarin for the prevention of recurrent DVT

B. LMWH dosing is simpler

C. The pharmacokinetic properties of LMWH are more predictable

D. There is no need for routine laboratory monitoring with LMWH

E. Fewer drug interactions occur with LMWH

101-9. A 59-year-old woman with a recent diagnosis of locally advanced breast cancer was treated with neoadjuvant chemotherapy, including doxorubicin and trastuzumab, followed by breast-conserving surgery and adjuvant radiotherapy. A pretreament echocardiogram showed a normal LVEF of 65%. Six months post-treatment, a routinely scheduled echocardiogram was obtained and showed a dilated left ventricle with global hypokinesis and an LVEF of 27%. Which of the following statements about trastuzumab cardiotoxocity is *false*?

A. Trastuzumab cardiotoxicity is dose related

B. Trastuzumab cardiotoxicity depends on whether the drug is given alone or in combination with other cardiotoxic agents

C. The incidence of cardiotoxicity is increased in patients who previously received radiation therapy

D. The incidence of cardiotoxicity is increased in patients with preexisting cardiac disease

E. The incidence of cardiotoxicity is increased in older patients

101-10. A 36-year-old man with no known past medical history is admitted to the cardiovascular intensive care unit after suffering a stroke. Upon questioning, he reports having felt fatigued and lost weight over the past few weeks. On physical examination, he is febrile and has focal neurological deficits consistent with the acute stroke episode; a cardiovascular exam is unremarkable, as is a 12-lead ECG and chest radiograph. Echocardiography was performed to rule out a cardioembolic focus, and it showed a large pedunculated mass with a friable surface adherent to the fossa ovalis on the left side of the interatrial septum. Which of the following statements about cardiac myxomas is *false*?

A. Pathologically, myxomas appear as soft, gelatinous, mucoid, gray-white masses

B. Myxomas are the most frequent benign tumor of the heart, most commonly being found in the left atrium

C. Constitutional symptoms are rare, but when present, they are helpful for differentiating myxoma from other cardiac masses

D. An early diastolic sound, the "tumor plop," may be heard 80 to 120 ms after A2

E. Surgical resection of the myxoma is the only acceptable therapy

ANSWERS

101-1. The answer is D. *(Hurst's The Heart, 14th Edition, Chap. 101)* Multiple predisposing factors facilitating the development of radiation-induced cardiotoxicity have been recognized thus far, including total radiation dose (option A) and dose per fraction (option B), the volume of heart irradiated (option C), and the concurrent administration of additional cardiotoxic agents, such as anthracyclines and trastuzumab. Younger age at the time of irradiation (option E) and the presence of other risk factors for coronary heart disease, such as hypertension, diabetes, and smoking, are patient-specific dynamics that may heighten the risk of radiation-induced cardiotoxicity.[1] Patient sex is not a predisposing factor (option D).

101-2. The answer is A. *(Hurst's The Heart, 14th Edition, Chap. 101)* The pericardium (option A) is the most sensitive cardiac structure with regard to irradiation because it consists of tissue with rapid cell turnover. The cardinal manifestation of pericardial irradition injury is constrictive pericarditis, which often presents with signs and symptoms of right heart failure. The myocardium (option B), heart valves (option C), conduction system (option D), and cardiac vasculature (option E) are all less sensitive to the effects of irradiation than the pericardium.

101-3. The answer is E. *(Hurst's The Heart, 14th Edition, Chap. 101)* Common histologic changes observed in radiation-associated cardiotoxicity include diffuse interstitial fibrosis of the myocardium with significantly reduced ratio of capillaries to myocytes (option A); arterial and capillary narrowing (option B), leading to myocyte cell death, latent ischemia, and thrombosis; endothelial cell damage, triggering precocious atherosclerosis (option C); replacement of the pericardial fat with dense connective tissue, leading to pericardial fibrosis, effusion, or even tamponade; and fibrosis and calcification of valvular leaflets/cusps, more commonly left-sided, which suggests a mechanistic role of blood pressure levels in the pathogenesis of the lesions.

101-4. The answer is A. *(Hurst's The Heart, 14th Edition, Chap. 101)* Several risk factors contribute to the development of cardiotoxicity in patients being treated for cancer. These include nonchemotherapy risk factors such as: age > 65 years (not < 65 years [option A]), preexisting hypertension (option B), coronary artery disease, which may be silent (option C), and prior radiation therapy (option D).[2-6] Advanced age was shown to be associated with a hazard ratio of 2.25 for incident anthracycline cardiomyopathy.[2]

101-5. The answer is E. *(Hurst's The Heart, 14th Edition, Chap. 101)* The Common Terminology Criteria for Adverse Events by the National Cancer Institute defines LV dysfunction as a reduction in LVEF > 5% to < 55% with symptoms of heart failure (option A) or an asymptomatic reduction in LVEF > 10% to < 55% (option B).[7] A recent document released by the American Society of Echocardiography defines chemotherapy-related cardiac dysfunction as a decrease in the LVEF of > 10 percentage points, to a value < 53% (option C), which is deemed the normal reference value for two-dimensional echocardiography, according to this society.[8] Centers such as MD Anderson and the European Society of Medical Oncology[9] define it as a reduction in LVEF of 10% or more to < 50% with or without symptoms (option D). As a consequence, at present, a consensus definition for cardiotoxicity is still lacking, and all of the aforementioned criteria are still commonly cited (option E).

101-6. The answer is B. *(Hurst's The Heart, 14th Edition, Chap. 101)* LVEF reduction ≥ 15% from baseline with normal function is not an indication to discontinue chemotherapy. LVEF decline to < 50% (but not < 40%) during chemotherapy necessitates the reassessment of LVEF after 3 weeks, and if confirmed, it should prompt the clinician to hold chemotherapy and consider heart failure therapy (option B). LVEF decline to < 40% during chemotherapy necessitates stopping chemotherapy, discussing alternatives options, and initiating heart failure therapy (option C). Heart failure therapy revolves around angiotensin-converting enzyme inhibitors (option D) and beta-blockers (option E), although there is no need to discontinue chemotherapy at this time.

101-7. The answer is B. *(Hurst's The Heart, 14th Edition, Chap. 101)* A normal ECG does not rule out acute radiation-associated pericarditis (option A). The changes appear over a period of days and then dissipate. Imaging should start with echocardiography, followed by cardiac CT or MRI if necessary to rule out constriction (option B). Even in the presence of pericardial calcification on CT, which is highly suggestive, echocardiography is critical to elicit the hemodynamic features of constrictive pericarditis. Pericardial constriction may occur in up to 20% of patients, requiring pericardiectomy. The operative mortality is high (21%), and the postoperative 5-year survival rate is very low (1%), mostly as a result of concomitant myocardial fibrosis.[10]

101-8. The answer is A. *(Hurst's The Heart, 14th Edition, Chap. 101)* Low molecular weight heparin is more effective (not equally effective [option A]) than oral anticoagulant therapy with warfarin for the prevention of recurrent VTE in patients with cancer who have had acute, symptomatic proximal DVT, pulmonary embolism, or both.[11] Further advantages of LMWH are that the doses are more easily adjusted (option B), the pharmacokinetic properties are more predictable (option C), laboratory monitoring is minimized (option D), and fewer drug interactions occur (option E).

101-9. The answer is A. *(Hurst's The Heart, 14th Edition, Chap. 101)* Trastuzumab cardiotoxicity is not dose related (option A) but depends on whether the drug is given alone or in combination with other cardiotoxic agents, especially anthracycline agents such as doxorubicin.[4] The incidence of cardiotoxicity is also increased in older patients, those with preexisting cardiac disease, and those who previously received radiation therapy. Whereas the incidence of trastuzumab cardiotoxicity was previously as high as 27%, the reported incidence has been much lower, 3% or less, in more recent trials with closer monitoring and when the simultaneous administration of trastuzumab and anthracyclines is avoided.[5]

101-10. The answer is C. *(Hurst's The Heart, 14th Edition, Chap. 101)* Intracardiac myxoma is the most frequent benign tumor of the heart (option B). Although most (75%) are located in the left atrium (LA), myxomas are also found in the RA (18%), RV (4%), and LV (3%). Cardiac myxomas usually originate from the region of the fossa ovalis but may arise from a variety of locations within the atria. A myxoma appears as a soft, gelatinous, mucoid, usually gray-white mass, often with areas of hemorrhage or thrombosis (option A). Cardiac myxomas provoke systemic manifestations in 90% of the patients (they are not rare [option C]), characterized by weight loss, fatigue, fever, anemia (often hemolytic), and elevated erythrocyte sedimentation rate. One of the classic physical examination signs is the tumor plop (option D). Surgical resection of a myxoma is the only acceptable therapy, and in view of the dangers of embolization and sudden death, it should be performed promptly (option E).

References

1. Lancellotti P, Nkomo VT, Badano LP, et al. European Society of Cardiology Working Groups on Nuclear Cardiology and Cardiac Computed Tomography and Cardiovascular Magnetic Resonance; American Society of Nuclear Cardiology; Society for Cardiovascular Magnetic Resonance; Society of Cardiovascular Computed Tomography. Expert consensus for multi-modality imaging evaluation of cardiovascular complications of radiotherapy in adults. A report from the European Association of Cardiovascular Imaging and the American Society of Echocardiography. *Eur Heart J Cardiovasc Imaging.* 2013;14(8):721-740.
2. Swain SM, Whaley FS, Ewer MS. Congestive heart failure in patients treated with doxorubicin: a retrospective analysis of three trials. *Cancer.* 2003;97:2869-2879.
3. Billingham ME, Mason JW, Bristow MR, et al. Anthracycline cardiomyopathy monitored by morphologic changes. *Cancer Treat Rep.* 1978;62(6):865-872.

4. Seidman A, Hudis C, Pierri MK, et al. Cardiac dysfunction in the trastuzumab clinical trials experience. *J Clin Oncol.* 2002;20(5):1215-1221.

5. Perez EA, Rodeheffer R. Clinical cardiac tolerability of trastuzumab. *J Clin Oncol.* 2004;22(2):322-329.

6. Zhang S, Liu X, Bawa-Khalfe T, et al. Identification of the molecular basis of doxorubicin-induced cardiotoxicity. *Nat Med.* 2012;18(11):1639-1642.

7. Common Terminology Criteria for Adverse Events v4.03 (CTCAE). http://evs.nci .nih.gov/ftp1/CTCAE. Published June 14, 2010. Accessed June 29, 2012.

8. Plana et al. Expert consensus for multimodality imaging evaluation of adult patients during and after cancer therapy: a report from the American Society of Echocardiography and the European Association of Cardiovascular Imaging. *J Am Soc Echocardiogr.* 2014;27:911-939.

9. Curigliano G, Cardinale D, Suter T, et al. ESMO Guidelines Working Group. Cardiovascular toxicity induced by chemotherapy, targeted agents and radiotherapy: ESMO clinical practice guidelines. *Ann Oncol.* 2012;23(suppl 7):vii155-vii166.

10. Wu W, Masri A, Popovic ZB, et al. Long-term survival of patients with radiation heart disease undergoing cardiac surgery. *Circulation.* 2013;127(14):1476-1484.

11. Lee AY, Levine MN, Baker RI, et al. Low-molecular-weight heparin versus a coumarin for the prevention of recurrent venous thromboembolism in patients with cancer. *N Engl J Med.* 2003;349(2):146-153.

CHAPTER 102

HIV/AIDS and the Cardiovascular System

Mark J. Eisenberg

QUESTIONS

DIRECTIONS: Choose the one best response to each question.

102-1. Which of the following is *not* one of the most common modes of HIV transmission?

A. Blood transfusion
B. Sexual transmission (heterosexual)
C. Sexual transmission (men who have sex with men)
D. Sexual transmission (women who have sex with women)
E. Vertical transmission

102-2. A 36-year-old woman, recently diagnosed with HIV, presents to your clinic after beginning a course of highly active antiretroviral therapy (HAART). Which of the following statements about HAART and cardiovascular health is *false*?

A. Both HIV-1 infection per se and HAART, particularly where non-nucleoside reverse transcriptase inhibitors (NNRTIs) are included, may have a negative impact on myocardial function
B. Zidovudine causes a dose-dependent reversible skeletal muscle myopathy by altering mitochondrial DNA replication
C. Lipodystrophy can be seen in up to 35% of HIV/AIDS patients after 12 months of protease inhibitor (PI) or NRTI therapies
D. HIV/AIDS disease markers, such as CD4$^+$ count and viral load, are as predictive of cardiovascular risk as are correlates with traditional risk factors (age, gender, diabetes mellitus, smoking, hypertension, dyslipidemia)
E. None of the above is false

102-3. Within what window of time will over 95% of HIV-infected patients have seroconverted (become serologically positive for HIV-1 infection)?

A. 2 weeks
B. 1 month
C. 3 months
D. 6 months
E. 8 months

102-4. A 33-year-old man presents to your clinic following a recent diagnosis of HIV. As a cardiologist, which of the following statements is *false* concerning the cardiovascular assessment of HIV/AIDS patients?

A. Electrocardiography should be performed routinely to confirm sinus rhythm and allow the assessment of the QT interval
B. Echocardiographic assessment of HIV/AIDS patients is extremely useful
C. Serial echocardiography should be performed every 5 to 10 years
D. Functional stress testing may be useful for the investigation of angina chest pain
E. A history of palpitations or near syncope may indicate the need for ambulatory ECG monitoring

102-5. The hallmark of cardiomyopathy associated with HIV/AIDS is:

A. Left ventricular systolic dysfunction
B. Right ventricular systolic dysfunction
C. Left ventricular diastolic dysfunction
D. Right ventricular diastolic dysfunction
E. A & D

102-6. Which of the following statements concerning cardiovascular disease in patients with HIV/AIDS is *correct*?

A. Pericardial effusion and pericarditis are the least common cardiac abnormalities found in early HIV/AIDS autopsy studies

B. Cardiac tamponade is common in patients with heart failure or malignant infiltration

C. The finding of new cardiomegaly on chest radiography should prompt early echocardiographic assessment to evaluate for pericardial effusion

D. Pericardial effusion is found in < 10% of patients

E. All of the above

102-7. Which of the following statements concerning cardiac lymphoma in HIV/AIDS is *false*?

A. Primary cardiac lymphoma is rare in HIV-1 negative individuals, accounting for < 10% of all primary malignant cardiac tumors

B. Disseminated lymphoma may involve the myocardium more often

C. In contrast to Kaposi sarcoma, lymphoma may more commonly lead to tamponade and heart failure

D. Primary cardiac lymphoma and disseminated lymphoma involving the myocardium occur less often in HIV/AIDS

E. All of the above are false

102-8. A 48-year-old man presents to your clinic to discuss concerns about his cardiovascular health. He has been living with HIV for the past 10 years, and he has read that this may increase his risk of cardiovascular disease. Which of the following statements concerning this association is *true*?

A. Coronary heart disease (CHD) in HIV/AIDS patients occurs mostly in women and at a younger age

B. The incidence of CHD in patients with his condition appears to be up to three times that of the general male population

C. The incidence of CHD among HIV/AIDS patients results in up to 20% higher rates of acute MI, hospitalization, and in-hospital deaths for acute coronary syndromes (ACS)

D. Acute myocardial infarction is an uncommon presentation of CHD among patients with HIV/AIDS

E. A high ratio of stable angina to acute myocardial infarction exists in HIV/AIDS populations

102-9. A 60-year-old woman living with HIV is in need of a heart transplant. Which of the following statements concerning this patient's clinical needs is *false*?

A. HIV/AIDS infection increases perioperative risk

B. Surgery negatively affects the clinical course of HIV/AIDS

C. Lesions seen in the hearts of patients with HIV/AIDS, like aortic stenosis, are not pathologically similar to those of patients without HIV/AIDS

D. In some cases, health care workers' fear of infection with HIV-1 may warrant precluding the HIV/AIDS patient from possible therapies should they be considered appropriate

E. All of the above are false

102-10. Which of the following statements is *false* concerning disorders of rhythm and sudden cardiac death associated with HIV/AIDS?

A. Sudden cardiac death accounts for up to 80% of cardiac-related deaths among people living with HIV

B. HIV/AIDS patients may be predisposed to QT prolongation

C. There are potential important interactions between oral anticoagulants and highly active antiretroviral therapy (HAART) drugs

D. Autonomic dysfunction is common in patients with HIV infection

E. All of the above are false

102-1. The answer is D. *(Hurst's The Heart, 14th Edition, Chap. 102)* The most common modes of spread of HIV are sexual—heterosexual (option B) or men who have sex with men (MSM) (option C)—parenteral blood (option A) or blood product recipients, injection drug users, occupational exposure to contaminated products, and vertical transmission (mother to fetus) (option E).

102-2. The answer is D. *(Hurst's The Heart, 14th Edition, Chap. 102)* Both HIV-1 infection per se and HAART, particularly where NRTIs are included, may have a negative impact on myocardial function (option A).[1,2] NRTIs are key elements of HAART, and zidovudine has been implicated in the development of some cases of HIV/AIDS cardiomyopathy (CM). In addition to inhibiting HIV-1 reverse transcriptase, the drug causes a dose-dependent, reversible skeletal muscle myopathy by altering mitochondrial DNA replication (option B).[3] The prevalence of abnormalities may be dependent on the type and duration of HAART, but lipodystrophy can be seen in up to 35% of HIV/AIDS patients after 12 months of PI or NRTI therapies (option C), particularly with older drugs.[4] Overall, controversy persists regarding the effect of HIV/AIDS on the development of atherosclerotic diseases. The D:A:D study of 23,437 patients demonstrated a risk of MI that was related to the duration of HAART treatment. This finding was refined to focus on PI therapy and the absence of such risk in patients treated with combinations that contained non-nucleosides (NNRTI).[5–7] HIV/AIDS disease markers such as CD4$^+$ count and viral load were not predictive of cardiovascular risk compared to correlates with traditional risk factors (age, gender, diabetes mellitus, smoking, hypertension, dyslipidemia) (option D).[5,8]

102-3. The answer is D. *(Hurst's The Heart, 14th Edition, Chap. 102)* Over 95% of patients seroconvert (ie, become serologically positive for HIV-1 infection) within 6 months. This usually coincides with a surge in plasma HIV-1 RNA levels to > 1 million copies/mL (peak between 4 and 8 weeks following exposure), and a fall in the CD4$^+$ count to 300 to 400 cells/mm^3.

102-4. The answer is C. *(Hurst's The Heart, 14th Edition, Chap. 102)* Heart disease may be overlooked in HIV/AIDS patients because symptoms of breathlessness, fatigue, and poor exercise tolerance are often ascribed to other conditions associated with HIV infection.[9] Therefore, electrocardiography should be performed routinely to confirm sinus rhythm and allow the assessment of the QT interval (option A). The ECG may also alert the cardiologist to the possibility of coronary artery disease (Q-waves and ST/T-wave changes) or left ventricular hypertrophy. Echocardiographic assessment of HIV/AIDS patients is extremely useful (option B) and can be used easily to identify those cardiac conditions common in HIV/AIDS patients that may be associated with a poor outcome, including pericardial effusion,[10,11] left ventricular (LV) systolic dysfunction, heart muscle disease (cardiomyopathy), and intracardiac masses.[9,12] Echocardiography may also provide useful information on the appearance of the right ventricle (RV), provide an indirect assessment of pulmonary pressures, and reveal regional wall-motion abnormalities potentially suggestive of CAD. A history of palpitation or near syncope may indicate the need for ambulatory ECG monitoring (option E), as with Holter monitoring.[13] Functional stress testing may be useful for the investigation of angina chest pain (option D), while CT coronary angiography or cardiac magnetic resonance (CMR) may be used in specific clinical circumstances.[14] It has been suggested that any HIV/AIDS patient with traditional risk factors for the development of, or who demonstrates any potential clinical manifestation of, cardiovascular disease should have a baseline echocardiogram performed. Thereafter, serial echocardiography should be performed every 1 to 2 years (option C).

102-5. **The answer is A.** *(Hurst's The Heart, 14th Edition, Chap. 102)* The hallmark of CM associated with HIV/AIDS is global left ventricular systolic dysfunction (option A). Abnormalities of mitral inflow, specifically reduced early mitral peak velocity and other indices of diastolic dysfunction, have been noted early in the course of HIV/AIDS in patients with both reduced and preserved ejection fraction.[15] The importance of these Doppler findings requires further investigation. However, the utility of echocardiography should not be underestimated, particularly because ECG and chest x-ray may be unrewarding in these patients.

102-6. **The answer is C.** *(Hurst's The Heart, 14th Edition, Chap. 102)* Pericardial effusion and pericarditis were the most common cardiac abnormalities found in early HIV/AIDS autopsy studies (option A) and remain a significant problem in Africa, where the largest number of HIV/AIDS patients are found.[16,17] Pericardial effusion is still found in up to 40% of patients (option D), particularly in association with generalized fluid retention and advanced disease, and pulmonary hypertension.[18] Small effusions are common in patients with heart failure or malignant infiltration, but cardiac tamponade is rare (option B). The finding of new cardiomegaly on chest radiography should prompt early echocardiographic assessment to evaluate for pericardial effusion (option C).[19]

102-7. **The answer is D.** *(Hurst's The Heart, 14th Edition, Chap. 102)* Primary cardiac lymphoma is rare in HIV-1 negative individuals, accounting for < 10% of all primary malignant cardiac tumors (option A). Disseminated lymphoma may involve the myocardium more often (option B) but usually only as part of widespread tumor involvement. However, both patterns of malignant cardiac involvement occur more commonly in HIV/AIDS (option D), and although primary lymphoma involving the heart alone is uncommon in HIV/AIDS, surgical resection of a right atrial lymphoma was reported in an HIV-1 positive patient with limited short-term success.[20] Non-Hodgkin's lymphoma can similarly involve the pericardium or myocardium in HIV/AIDS. Echocardiography is useful to detect any related intracavity masses or concomitant pericardial effusions. Radionuclide and MRI scans may be required to detect more diffuse cardiac involvement. In contrast to Kaposi sarcoma, lymphoma may more commonly lead to tamponade and heart failure (option C), and conduction abnormalities should be considered in HIV/AIDS patients whose cardiovascular symptoms progress rapidly.

102-8. **The answer is B.** *(Hurst's The Heart, 14th Edition, Chap. 102)* It remains likely that some HIV/AIDS patients are at risk of acute myocardial infarction (AMI) and CHD. Compared with national registries of non-HIV/AIDS patients, CHD in HIV/AIDS patients occurs mostly in men and at a younger age (option A), suggesting that the age-adjusted incidence may be significantly higher.[16-18] The incidence of CHD appears to be up to three times that of the general male population (option B) and results in up to 40% higher rates of acute MI, hospitalization, and in-hospital deaths for acute coronary syndromes (ACS) compared with non-HIV/AIDS patients (option C).[21-25] With the improvement in survival with HIV/AIDS, the therapy for cardiovascular diseases should be similar to that in the non-HIV/AIDS population. The full mechanism underlying ACS in HIV patients remains unclear. AMI appears to be a common presentation of CHD (option D), and a high ratio of AMI to stable angina exists in HIV/AIDS populations (option E).[26]

102-9. **The answer is E.** *(Hurst's The Heart, 14th Edition, Chap. 102)* HIV/AIDS survival has improved. Consideration of cardiac surgery for treatment of cardiovascular diseases unrelated directly to HIV/AIDS is now becoming increasingly common. Although studies are limited, excellent clinical outcomes were reported with 25 patients with HIV/AIDS with an in-hospital mortality of 4%.[27,28] There is neither increased perioperative risk from HIV/AIDS infection alone (option A) nor does surgery negatively affect the clinical course of HIV/AIDS (option B) or its therapy. Lesions seen in the hearts of patients with HIV/AIDS and HIV-associated non-AIDS (HANA) heart diseases, like aortic stenosis, are similar pathologically to those of patients without HIV/AIDS (option C).[29] Some advocate consideration of HIV/AIDS patients as candidates for cardiac transplantation for appropriate cardiovascular indications and in the absence of detractors, although fears remain that immunosuppressant therapies in that scenario (peri- and post-transplant) may affect viral replication and interact with HAART agents.[30] In the era of universal precautions and rapid treatment of accidental infection in the workplace, the burden of HIV/AIDS is becoming more a routine event. Fear of becoming infected with HIV-1 is understandable, but universal precautions should limit the potential risk to health care workers and as such should not preclude the HIV/AIDS patient from possible therapies should they be considered appropriate (option D).

102-10. **The answer is E.** (*Hurst's The Heart, 14th Edition, Chap.* 102*)* Sudden cardiac death (SCD) is common with HIV infection and accounts for up to 80% of cardiac-related deaths in this group (option A). SCD occurs much more commonly than expected in the general population with similar risk factors.[31] As would be expected, SCD may be secondary to other cardiac pathology, including cardiomyopathy and pulmonary hypertension, while CHD, previous arrhythmia, hypertension, and hyperlipidemia are all prevalent comorbidities in patients with SCD.[31] HIV/AIDS patients may be predisposed to QT prolongation (option B), possibly as a consequence of some forms of treatment;[12] for example, pentamidine, which was used previously in the treatment and prophylaxis of *P. carinii* infection in select patients, is structurally similar to procainamide and may cause torsades de pointes when used intravenously or intramuscularly. With increased life expectancy in HIV/AIDS, atrial fibrillation is emerging as a significant health problem. Caution is required because there are potential important interactions between oral anticoagulants, particularly some novel oral anticoagulants and HAART drugs (option C).[32] Autonomic dysfunction is common in patients with HIV infection (option D), and this may predispose to syncopal events and dysrhythmias because of excessive sympathetic tone.[33]

References

1. Kohler JJ, Hosseini SH, Lewis W. Mitochondrial DNA impairment in nucleoside reverse transcriptase inhibitor-associated cardiomyopathy. *Chem Res Toxicol.* 2008;21:990-996.

2. Dube MP, Lipshultz SE, Fichtenbaum CJ, Greenberg R, Schecter AD, Fisher SD. Effects of HIV infection and antiretroviral therapy on the heart and vasculature. *Circulation.* 2008;118:e36-e40.

3. Lewis W, Dalakas MC. Mitochondrial toxicity of antiviral drugs. *Nature Med.* 1995;1: 417-422.

4. Bogner JR, Vielhauer V, Beckmann RA, et al. Stavudine versus zidovudine and the development of lipodystrophy. *J Acquir Immune Defic Syndr.* 2001;27:237-244.

5. Friis-Moller N, Sabin CA, Weber R, et al. Combination antiretroviral therapy and the risk of myocardial infarction. *N Engl J Med.* 2003;349:1993-2003.

6. Currier JS, Lundgren JD, Carr A, et al. Epidemiological evidence for cardiovascular disease in HIV-infected patients and relationship to highly active antiretroviral therapy. *Circulation.* 2008;118:e29-e35.

7. Benson CA, Williams PL, Currier JS, et al. A prospective, randomized trial examining the efficacy and safety of clarithromycin in combination with ethambutol, rifabutin, or both for the treatment of disseminated *Mycobacterium avium* complex disease in persons with acquired immunodeficiency syndrome. *Clin Infect Dis.* 2003;37:1234-1243.

8. Currier JS. Cardiovascular risk associated with HIV therapy. *J Acquir Immune Defic Syndr.* 2002;31(suppl 1): S16-S23; discussion S24-S25.

9. Currie PF and Boon NA. Cardiac involvement in human immunodeficiency virus infection [editorial]. *Q J Med.* 1993;86:751-753.

10. Chillo, P, Bakari M, Lwakatare J. Echocardiographic diagnoses in HIV-infected patients presenting with cardiac symptoms at Muhimbili National Hospital in Dar es Salaam, Tanzania. *Cardiovasc J Africa.* 2012;23(2):90-97.

11. Sliwa K, Carrington MJ, Becker A, Thienemann F, Ntsekhe M, Stewart S. Contribution of the human immunodeficiency virus/acquired immunodeficiency syndrome epidemic to de novo presentations of heart disease in the Heart of Soweto Study Cohort. *Eur Heart J.* 2012;33:866-874.

12. Corallo S, Mutinelli MR, Moroni M, et al. Echocardiography detects myocardial damage in AIDS: prospective study in 102 patients. *Eur Heart J.* 1988;9:887-892.

13. Fiorentini A, Petrosillo N, De Stefano A, et al. QTc interval prolongation in HIV-infected patients: a case-control study by 24-h Holter ECG recording. *BMC Cardiovasc Disord.* 2012;12:124.

14. Holloway CJ, Ntusi N, Suttie J, et al. Comprehensive cardiac magnetic resonance imaging and spectroscopy reveal a high burden of myocardial disease in HIV patients. *Circulation.* 2013;128:814-822.

15. Coudray N, de Zuttere D, Force G, et al. Left ventricular diastolic function in asymptomatic and symptomatic human immunodeficiency virus carriers: an echocardiographic study. *Eur Heart J.* 1995;16:61-67.

16. D'Ascenzo F, Cerrato E, Biondi-Zoccai G, et al. Acute coronary syndromes in human immunodeficiency virus patients: A meta-analysis investigating adverse event rates and the role of antiretroviral therapy. *Eur Heart J.* 2012;33:875-880.

17. Vittecoq D, Escaut L, Chironi G, et al. Coronary heart disease in HIV-infected patients in the highly active antiretroviral treatment era. *AIDS.* 2003;17(suppl 1):S70-S76.

18. Lewden C, Salmon D, Morlat P, et al., and Mortality Study Group. Causes of death among human immunodeficiency virus (HIV)-infected adults in the era of potent antiretroviral therapy: Emerging role of hepatitis and cancers, persistent role of AIDS. *Int J Epidemiol.* 2005;34:121-130.

19. Monsuez JJ, Kinney EL, Vittecoq D, et al. Comparison among acquired immune deficiency syndrome patients with and without clinical evidence of cardiac disease. *Am J Cardiol.* 1988;62:1311-1313.

20. Horowitz MD, Cox MM, Neibart RM, Blaker AM, Interian A Jr. Resection of right atrial lymphoma in a patient with AIDS. *Int J Cardiol.* 1992;34:139-142.

21. Klein D, Hurley LB, Quesenberry CP, Jr., Sidney S. Do protease inhibitors increase the risk for coronary heart disease in patients with HIV-1 infection? *J Acquir Immune Defic Syndr.* 2002;30:471-477.

22. Vittecoq D, Escaut L, Merad M, et al. Coronary heart disease in HIV-infected individuals. *Adv Cardiol.* 2003;40:151-162.

23. Triant VA, Lee H, Hadigan C, Grinspoon SK. Increased acute myocardial infarction rates and cardiovascular risk factors among patients with human immunodeficiency virus disease. *J Clin Endocrinol Metab.* 2007;92:2506-2512.

24. Triant VA. HIV infection and coronary heart disease: an intersection of epidemics. *J Infect Dis.* 2012;205(suppl 3):S355-S361.

25. Silverberg MJ, Leyden WA, Xu L, et al. Immunodeficiency and risk of myocardial infarction among HIV-positive individuals with access to care. *J Acquir Immune Defic Syndr.* 2014;65:160-166.

26. Sliwa K, Carrington MJ, Becker A, Thienemann F, Ntsekhe M, Stewart S. Contribution of the human immunodeficiency virus/acquired immunodeficiency syndrome epidemic to de novo presentations of heart disease in the Heart of Soweto Study Cohort. *Eur Heart J.* 2012;33:866-874.

27. Namai A, Sakurai M, Akiyama M. Cardiac surgery in three patients infected with the human immunodeficiency virus. *Gen Thorac Cardiovasc Surg.* 2008;56:465-467.

28. Filsoufi F, Salzberg SP, Harbou KT, Neibart E, Adams DH. Excellent outcomes of cardiac surgery in patients infected with HIV in the current era. *Clin Infect Dis.* 2006;43:532-536.

29. Mestres CA, Chuquiure JE, Claramonte X, et al. Long-term results after cardiac surgery in patients infected with the human immunodeficiency virus type-1 (HIV-1). *Eur J Cardiothorac Surg.* 2003;23:1007-1016 [discussion, 1016].

30. Uriel N, Mahumi N, Colombo PC, et al. Advanced heart failure in patients infected with human immunodeficiency virus: is there equal access to care? *J Heart Lung Transplant.* 2014; 33:924-930.

31. Tseng ZH, Secemsky EA, Dowdy D, et al. Sudden cardiac death in patients with human immunodeficiency virus infection. *J Am Coll Cardiol.* 2012;59:891-896.

32. HIV Drug Interactions. Complete Listing of Drug Interactions by Therapeutic Class. www.hiv-druginteractions.org. Updated February 2018.

33. Bharati S, Joshi VV, Connor EM, et al. Conduction system in children with acquired immunodeficiency syndrome. *Chest.* 1989;96:406-413.

CHAPTER 103

Heart Disease in Pregnancy

Mark J. Eisenberg

QUESTIONS

DIRECTIONS: Choose the one best response to each question.

103-1. What is the most common form of cardiovascular disease (CVD) among pregnant women in the developed world?

A. Rheumatic valve disease
B. Connective tissue disease
C. Congenital heart disease (CHD)
D. Cardiomyopathies
E. Congestive heart failure

103-2. A 27-year-old woman with previously diagnosed CVD presents to your clinic for a preconception consult. Which of the following is considered a high-risk condition in which pregnancy is *not* advised?

A. Pulmonary arterial hypertension
B. Congenital cyanotic lesions
C. Severe systemic ventricular dysfunction
D. Severe mitral stenosis
E. All of the above

103-3. By what volume has a pregnant woman's circulating plasma increased at 24 weeks of gestation?

A. 20%
B. 30%
C. 40%
D. 50%
E. None of the above

103-4. A 32-year-old woman in her second trimester of gestation presents to your clinic for a prenatal cardiac consult. Which of the following would you *not* expect to be increased upon echocardiographic exam as a result of pregnancy?

A. Stroke volume
B. Left ventricular ejection fraction
C. Left ventricular cavity dimensions
D. Wall thickness
E. Aortic size

103-5. A 36-year-old woman at 25 weeks gestation complains of worsening shortness of breath (dyspnea) at rest. Which of the following is *not* an alerting symptom that should prompt further investigation in pregnant women?

A. Angina
B. Significant resting dyspnea
C. Paroxysmal nocturnal dyspnea
D. Sustained palpitations
E. Mammary souffle

103-6. Which of the following electrocardiogram (ECG) changes could be found upon examination of a 30-year-old woman in her third trimester of gestation?

A. Sinus tachycardia
B. Left axis deviation
C. Shortened PR interval
D. Increased R/S ratio in leads V_1 and V_2
E. All of the above

103-7. A 24-year-old nulliparous woman in her first trimester of gestation presents to your clinic for prenatal consult. She reports smoking fewer than 10 cigarettes per day, on average. Which of the following is considered a maternal risk factor for neonatal events (small for gestational age, prematurity and associated complications)?

A. Cyanosis
B. Use of anticoagulants during pregnancy
C. Smoking
D. Multiple gestations
E. All of the above

103-8. Which of the following statements about preeclampsia and eclampsia is *correct*?

A. Preeclampsia is a multisystem disorder that affects 15% of pregnancies
B. Among women at high risk for preeclampsia, low-dose aspirin is not recommended to decrease the risk for preeclampsia, growth restriction, and preterm delivery
C. High-risk women are those with a history of preeclampsia, chronic hypertension, diabetes, renal disease, autoimmune diseases, and those carrying multiple gestations
D. Together, preeclampsia and eclampsia account for over two-thirds of severe obstetrical complications
E. Women with mild preeclampsia are typically delivered at 30 weeks gestation

103-9. A 35-year-old woman in her second trimester of gestation complains of a rapid and irregular heart rate. Which of the following statements about cardiac arrhythmias in pregnancy is *false*?

A. Many women with structurally normal hearts experience premature atrial and ventricular ectopy during pregnancy
B. Recurrent arrhythmia is associated with an increased risk of adverse fetal and neonatal complications
C. Women with CHD are at higher risk for developing arrhythmias requiring treatment during pregnancy
D. Electrical cardioversion should not be performed in hemodynamically unstable women
E. Orthodromic atrioventricular reciprocating tachycardia is the most common arrhythmia experienced among women with pre-excitation

103-10. A 43-year-old woman recently underwent valve replacement with a mechanical valve. She has just discovered she is 7 weeks pregnant. Which of the following statements best represents the current state of the evidence regarding anticoagulation in pregnant women with mechanical valves?

A. Low molecular weight heparin (LMWH) does not cross the placenta
B. Warfarin is the preferred agent in pregnant women with mechanical prostheses
C. Anticoagulation regimens may be interrupted during pregnancy
D. LMWH is associated with a decreased risk of valve thrombosis
E. None of the above

ANSWERS

103-1. The answer is C. *(Hurst's The Heart, 14th Edition, Chap. 103)* Preexisting and acquired CVD increases maternal and fetal morbidity and mortality during pregnancy.[1-4] Cardiovascular disease complicates > 1% of pregnancies, accounts for 20% of nonobstetric maternal death,[2] and is the leading cause of indirect maternal mortality. Congenital heart disease comprises > 50% of CVD in pregnancy (option C);[5,6] other common etiologies include rheumatic valve disease (option A) (more common in developing countries), connective tissue disease (option B), and cardiomyopathies (option D). Medical care begins in the preconception period with careful planning and anticipation of the possible complications that may occur during the antepartum, intrapartum, and postpartum periods. Risk-stratification models summarizing maternal and fetal outcomes have been developed to counsel women with CVD desiring pregnancy. Optimal patient care for the pregnant woman with CVD relies on an understanding of the unique hemodynamic changes of pregnancy and the pathophysiology, signs and symptoms, and natural history specific to each heart condition that may affect pregnancy. A multidisciplinary team approach involving cardiologists, maternal fetal medicine specialists, and anesthesiologists in a center with experience is strongly advised for the care of pregnant women with heart disease.

103-2. The answer is E. *(Hurst's The Heart, 14th Edition, Chap. 103)* Women with CVD should receive counseling about both maternal and fetal risks prior to conceiving a pregnancy. In addition, women with heart disease should be cared for in institutions with experience in treating CVD during pregnancy. There are extremely high-risk conditions in which pregnancy is not advised, including pulmonary arterial hypertension (option A), congenital cyanotic lesions (option B), severe systemic ventricular dysfunction (option C) (ejection fraction < 30%, New York Heart Association [NYHA] class > II), severe mitral stenosis (option D), severe symptomatic aortic stenosis, and significantly dilated aorta in connective tissue disorders in women with Marfan syndrome and above 5 cm in women with bicuspid aortic valve (BAV).[1] Women with CVD considering pregnancy should undergo a complete workup, including a detailed medical and surgical history and a physical exam, including oxygen saturations, electrocardiogram (ECG), appropriate cardiac imaging, and consideration of cardiopulmonary stress testing for further risk stratification.[7]

103-3. The answer is C. *(Hurst's The Heart, 14th Edition, Chap. 103)* By 24 weeks of gestation, circulating plasma volume has increased by 40% (option C), resulting in a 30% to 50% increase in cardiac output, which begins to rise as early as 5 weeks after the last menstrual cycle and steadily increases until 28 to 34 weeks.[1,8-14] A greater increase in plasma volume compared to erythrocyte mass accounts for the physiologic anemia of pregnancy. In early pregnancy, the rise in cardiac output is primarily achieved through a 40% increase in stroke volume, which peaks at 28 to 31 weeks of gestation.[9,10] In the third trimester, the increase in heart rate primarily mediates cardiac output augmentation, with an average heart rate rise of 10 to 15 beats per minute.[1,13,15] Cardiac output begins to decline late in the third trimester, but it does not return to prepregnancy values until 2 to 4 weeks postpartum.[10] Systemic vascular resistance falls early in pregnancy, primarily as a result of maturation of placental circulation and the effects of endogenous hormones, with a resulting 30% to 50% fall from prepregnancy values by the end of the second trimester, followed by an increase at the end of the third trimester.[8,10,15]

103-4. The answer is B. *(Hurst's The Heart, 14th Edition, Chap. 103)* Echocardiographic studies have revealed that while left ventricular ejection fraction (option B) remains stable, in parallel with the increase in stroke volume (option A), left ventricular cavity dimensions (option C), and wall thickness (option D), aortic size (option E), and atrial dimensions all increase during pregnancy, with return to prepregnancy values in the postpartum period.[10,12,16,17,19-21] In addition, an increase in stroke work and a decrease in left ventricular longitudinal strain has been observed in the later stages of pregnancy.[20] An increase in annular diameters resulting from chamber enlargement can result in physiologic mitral, tricuspid, and pulmonic regurgitation; the development of aortic insufficiency is rare given only a small (~5%) increase in left ventricular outflow tract diameter.[18,19,22] Despite the increase in valvular regurgitation, women rarely are symptomatic from these changes.[23] In addition, pericardial effusions without hemodynamic significance develop in 40% of women and resolve by 6 weeks postpartum.[24,25]

103-5. **The answer is E.** *(Hurst's The Heart, 14th Edition, Chap. 103)* During pregnancy, it is often challenging to distinguish between common pregnancy symptoms and concerning cardiac manifestations. Women may sense dyspnea on exertion, decreased exercise capacity, hyperventilation, peripheral edema, and palpitations. When these symptoms are mild and arise prior to 20 weeks, they are often attributable to the normal hemodynamic changes of pregnancy. Alerting symptoms during pregnancy include angina (option A), significant resting dyspnea (option B), paroxysmal nocturnal dyspnea (option C), sustained palpitations (option D), and syncope. Any symptoms that arise after 20 weeks and become progressively worse, or symptoms that significantly impair a woman from performing her daily activities, should prompt further evaluation. A mammary souffle is a benign, high-pitched continuous murmur best heard over the breasts during the third trimester and lactation, representing superficial arterial flow (option E). It is not affected by a Valsalva maneuver. Abnormal findings on cardiac exam include a holosystolic systolic murmur, any diastolic murmurs, fourth heart sound, or an exaggerated second heart sound suggesting pulmonary hypertension.[26]

103-6. **The answer is E.** *(Hurst's The Heart, 14th Edition, Chap. 103)* Electrocardiogram changes found in pregnancy include sinus tachycardia (option A), left axis deviation (option B), shortened PR interval (option C), increased R/S ratio in leads V_1 and V_2 (option D), Q waves and inverted T waves in the inferior leads, and nonspecific transient ST-T changes.[1,27] Both atrial and ventricular premature beats are common in pregnant women.[28] Echocardiography is very useful to assess ventricular function and valvular pathology during pregnancy.[18] Women should be referred for echocardiography if they present with unexplained symptoms, a history of CVD, unexpected ECG changes, or a new holosystolic or diastolic murmur.[29]

103-7. **The answer is E.** *(Hurst's The Heart, 14th Edition, Chap. 103)* There is a strong association between maternal morbidity and neonatal adverse events. Rates of neonatal complications and mortality have been reported between 20% and 37%, and from 1% to 4%, respectively. Risk factors for neonatal events included cyanosis (option A), poor functional class, smoking (option C), multiple gestations (option D), the use of anticoagulants during pregnancy (option B), and mechanical valve prosthesis. Events included small for gestational age and prematurity with its associated complications, such as respiratory distress syndrome and cerebral hemorrhage.[30]

103-8. **The answer is C.** *(Hurst's The Heart, 14th Edition, Chap. 103)* Preeclampsia is a multisystem disorder that affects 2% to 5% of pregnancies (option A) and is clinically characterized by the development of new-onset hypertension after the 20th week of gestation accompanied by proteinuria exceeding 300 mg.[31] Together, preeclampsia and eclampsia account for over one-third of severe obstetrical complications (option D), 12% of maternal mortality, and double the risk of perinatal mortality.[32,33] Among women at high risk for preeclampsia, low-dose aspirin after the 12th week of gestation is recommended to decrease the risk for preeclampsia, growth restriction, and preterm delivery (option B).[32] High-risk women are those with a history of preeclampsia, chronic hypertension, diabetes, renal disease, autoimmune diseases, and those carrying multiple gestations (option C).[32] Although delivery is the mainstay of treatment for severe preeclampsia, select women who are remote from term may be expectantly managed with close monitoring until 34 weeks of gestation provided they remain clinically stable. Women with mild preeclampsia are typically delivered at 37 weeks gestation (option E).[34] Women with a history of pregnancy-related hypertensive disorders—particularly preeclampsia—are at increased risk for future CVD.[35]

The two may relate by overlapping risk profiles (including obesity, insulin resistance, hyperlipidemia, and renal disease) or through persistent endothelial dysfunction from hypertensive disorders of pregnancy increasing the risk for future CVD; the mechanism of this association is still unclear.[35-39]

103-9. The answer is D. *(Hurst's The Heart, 14th Edition, Chap. 103)* Approximately 20% to 44% of women with preexisting tachyarrhythmias experience recurrence during pregnancy, with recurrent arrhythmia associated with an increased risk of adverse fetal and neonatal complications (option B).[1,40] Nonetheless, although palpitations are a frequent complaint in pregnancy, most do not correlate with dangerous ectopy in women without structural heart disease.[41] Many women with structurally normal hearts experience premature atrial and ventricular ectopy during pregnancy (option A),[41] yet sustained arrhythmias are rare.[42] Women with CHD are at higher risk for developing arrhythmias requiring treatment during pregnancy (option C).[1,43] Those with pre-excitation are also more likely to experience arrhythmias during pregnancy, most commonly orthodromic atrioventricular reciprocating tachycardia (option E).[28,44] When treatment is indicated, consideration should be made to avoid invasive procedures when possible, though many can now be performed with minimal or no radiation, and to use antiarrhythmic therapy sparingly given a lack of safety data with these agents, particularly in the first trimester. For hemodynamically unstable women, electrical cardioversion should be performed with close fetal monitoring (option D), though the risk to the fetus has been low.[28,45-47] It is advisable to involve a cardiac electrophysiologist with expertise in caring for pregnant women when considering arrhythmia management.

103-10. The answer is A. *(Hurst's The Heart, 14th Edition, Chap. 103)* The optimal strategy for anticoagulation in pregnant women is controversial. Although mechanical prostheses have a longer durability than bioprosthetic valves, which makes them preferable for young women who do not wish to become pregnant, they pose a significant challenge for management in pregnancy mainly because of their highly thrombogenic nature, which necessitates uninterrupted anticoagulation (option C).[48] Although warfarin is often the preferred agent in nonpregnant women with mechanical prostheses (option B), the risk of embryopathy exceeds 8% with doses over 5 mg.[1,49] The use of warfarin beyond the first trimester is associated with an increased risk of adverse fetal outcomes, including miscarriage, hemorrhage, and fetal loss, an effect that in some studies appears to be dose dependent.[1,48,50-54] However, in a recent study, rates of miscarriage or fetal loss did not differ between women who took high versus low (≤ 5 mg) doses of warfarin.[48] Low-molecular-weight heparin (LMWH) does not cross the placenta (option A), and guidelines recommend switching from warfarin to LMWH in women whose warfarin dose exceeds 5 mg. Unfortunately, available data suggest that women are at high risk for valve thrombosis during the transition from warfarin to heparin products.[1,48,49] However, LMWH is associated with an increased risk of valve thrombosis (option D).[50] Although the factors responsible for this risk are incompletely understood, many authors postulate that inadequate monitoring rather than failure of the agent itself is responsible.[50] When LMWH is used during pregnancy, both peak and trough anti-Xa levels should be monitored weekly throughout to ensure consistent therapeutic anticoagulation because the therapeutic dose required may significantly change with the increasing volume of distribution.[1,50,55-58]

References

1. European Society of Cardiology. ESC guidelines on the management of cardiovascular diseases during pregnancy: The Task Force on the Management of Cardiovascular Diseases During Pregnancy of the European Society of Cardiology (ESC). *Eur Heart J.* 2011;32(24):3147-3197.
2. Berg CJ, Mackay AP, Qin C, Callaghan WM, et al. Overview of maternal morbidity during hospitalization for labor and delivery in the United States: 1993-1997 and 2001-2005. *Obstet Gynecol.* 2009;113(5): 1075-1081.
3. Cantwell R, et al. Saving mothers' lives: Reviewing maternal deaths to make motherhood safer, 2006-2008. The eighth report of the confidential enquiries into maternal deaths in the United Kingdom. *BJOG.* 2011;118(suppl 1):1-203.

4. Ouyang DW, et al. Obstetric outcomes in pregnant women with congenital heart disease. *Int J Cardiol.* 2010;144(2):195-199.

5. Kuklina E, Callaghan W. Chronic heart disease and severe obstetric morbidity among hospitalisations for pregnancy in the USA: 1995-2006. *BJOG.* 2011;118(3): 345-352.

6. Gelson E, et al. Heart disease: why is maternal mortality increasing? *BJOG.* 2009;116(5):609-611.

7. Warnes CA, et al. ACC/AHA 2008 guidelines for the management of adults with congenital heart disease: executive summary. A report of the American College of Cardiology/American Heart Association Task Force on Practice Guidelines (writing committee to develop guidelines for the management of adults with congenital heart disease). *Circulation.* 2008;118(23): 2395-2451.

8. Nanna M, Stergiopoulos K. Pregnancy complicated by valvular heart disease: an update. *J Am Heart Assoc.* 2014;3(3):e000712.

9. Easterling TR, et al. Maternal hemodynamics in normal and preeclamptic pregnancies: a longitudinal study. *Obstet Gynecol.* 1990;76(6):1061-1069.

10. Geva T, et al. Effects of physiologic load of pregnancy on left ventricular contractility and remodeling. *Am Heart J.* 1997;133(1):53-59.

11. Mabie WC, et al. A longitudinal study of cardiac output in normal human pregnancy. *Am J Obstet Gynecol.* 1994;170(3):849-856.

12. Mone SM, Sanders SP, Colan SD. Control mechanisms for physiological hypertrophy of pregnancy. *Circulation.* 1996; 94(4):667-672.

13. Robson SC, et al. Serial study of factors influencing changes in cardiac output during human pregnancy. *Am J Physiol.* 1989;256(4 pt 2):H1060-H1065.

14. Robson SC, Dunlop W, Hunter S. Haemodynamic changes during the early puerperium. *BMJ (Clin Res Ed).* 1987;294(6579):1065.

15. Hunter S, Robson SC. Adaptation of the maternal heart in pregnancy. *Br Heart J.* 1992;68(6):540-543.

16. Gilson GJ, et al. Changes in hemodynamics, ventricular remodeling, and ventricular contractility during normal pregnancy: a longitudinal study. *Obstet Gynecol.* 1997;89(6):957-962.

17. Kametas NA, et al. Maternal left ventricular mass and diastolic function during pregnancy. *Ultrasound Obstet Gynecol.* 2001;18(5):460-466.

18. Tsiaras S, Poppas A. Cardiac disease in pregnancy: Value of echocardiography. *Curr Cardiol Rep.* 2010;12(3):250-256.

19. Ducas RA, et al. Cardiovascular magnetic resonance in pregnancy: insights from the cardiac hemodynamic imaging and remodeling in pregnancy (CHIRP) study. *J Cardiovasc Magn Reson.* 2014;16:1.

20. Savu O, et al. Morphological and functional adaptation of the maternal heart during pregnancy. *Circ Cardiovasc Imaging.* 2012;5(3):289-297.

21. Easterling TR, et al. Maternal hemodynamics and aortic diameter in normal and hypertensive pregnancies. *Obstet Gynecol.* 1991;78(6):1073-1077.

22. Campos O, et al. Physiologic multivalvular regurgitation during pregnancy: a longitudinal Doppler echocardiographic study. *Int J Cardiol.* 1993;40(3):265-272.

23. Robson SC. Incidence of Doppler regurgitant flow velocities during normal pregnancy. *Eur Heart J.* 1992;13(1):84-87.

24. Abduljabbar HS, et al. Pericardial effusion in normal pregnant women. *Acta Obstet Gynecol Scand.* 1991;70(4-5):291-294.

25. Ristic AD, et al. Pericardial disease in pregnancy. *Herz.* 2003;28(3):209-215.

26. Stout KK, Otto CM. Pregnancy in women with valvular heart disease. *Heart.* 2007;93(5):552-558.

27. Carruth JE, et al. The electrocardiogram in normal pregnancy. *Am Heart J.* 1981; 102(6 pt 1):1075-1078.

28. Enriquez AD, Economy KE, Tedrow UB. Contemporary management of arrhythmias during pregnancy. *Circ Arrhythm Electrophysiol.* 2014;7(5):961-967.

29. Mishra M, Chambers JB, Jackson G. Murmurs in pregnancy: An audit of echocardiography. *BMJ.* 1992;304(6839):1413-1414.

30. Siu SC, et al. Adverse neonatal and cardiac outcomes are more common in pregnant women with cardiac disease. *Circulation.* 2002;105(18):2179-2184.

31. Ananth CV, Keyes KM, Wapner RJ. Pre-eclampsia rates in the United States, 1980-2010: age-period-cohort analysis. *BMJ.* 2013;347:f6564.

32. LeFevre ML. Low-dose aspirin use for the prevention of morbidity and mortality from preeclampsia: U.S. Preventive Services Task Force recommendation statement. *Ann Intern Med.* 2014;161(11):819-826.

33. Henderson JT, et al. Low-dose aspirin for prevention of morbidity and mortality from preeclampsia: a systematic evidence review for the U.S. Preventive Services Task Force. *Ann Intern Med.* 2014;160(10):695-703.

34. Hypertension in pregnancy. Report of the American College of Obstetricians and Gynecologists' task force on hypertension in pregnancy. *Obstet Gynecol.* 2013;122(5):1122-1131.

35. Fraser A, et al. Associations of pregnancy complications with calculated cardiovascular disease risk and cardiovascular risk factors in middle age: The Avon Longitudinal Study of Parents and Children. *Circulation.* 2012;125(11):1367-1380.

36. Garovic VD, Hayman SR. Hypertension in pregnancy: an emerging risk factor for cardiovascular disease. *Nat Clin Pract Nephrol.* 2007;3(11):613-622.

37. Sibai BM, et al. Risk factors for preeclampsia in healthy nulliparous women: a prospective multicenter study. The National Institute of Child Health and Human Development Network of Maternal-Fetal Medicine Units. *Am J Obstet Gynecol.* 1995;172(2 pt 1):642-648.

38. Sibai BM, et al. Risk factors associated with preeclampsia in healthy nulliparous women. The Calcium for Preeclampsia Prevention (CPEP) Study Group. *Am J Obstet Gynecol.* 1997;177(5):1003-1010.

39. Kaaja R. Insulin resistance syndrome in preeclampsia. *Semin Reprod Endocrinol.* 1998;16(1):41-46.

40. Silversides CK, et al. Recurrence rates of arrhythmias during pregnancy in women with previous tachyarrhythmia and impact on fetal and neonatal outcomes. *Am J Cardiol.* 2006;97(8):1206-1212.

41. Shotan A, et al. Incidence of arrhythmias in normal pregnancy and relation to palpitations, dizziness, and syncope. *Am J Cardiol.* 1997;79(8):1061-1064.

42. Li JM, et al. Frequency and outcome of arrhythmias complicating admission during pregnancy: experience from a high-volume and ethnically-diverse obstetric service. *Clin Cardiol.* 2008;31(11):538-541.

43. Drenthen W, et al. Outcome of pregnancy in women with congenital heart disease: a literature review. *J Am Coll Cardiol.* 2007;49(24):2303-2311.

44. Gleicher N, et al. Wolff-Parkinson-White syndrome in pregnancy. *Obstet Gynecol.* 1981;58(6):748-752.

45. Page RL, et al. 2015 ACC/AHA/HRS guideline for the management of adult patients with supraventricular tachycardia: a report of the American College of Cardiology/American Heart Association Task Force on Clinical Practice Guidelines and the Heart Rhythm Society. *Circulation.* 2016;133(14):e506-e574.

46. Wang YC, et al. The impact of maternal cardioversion on fetal haemodynamics. *Eur J Obstet Gynecol Reprod Biol.* 2006;126(2):268-269.

47. Barnes EJ, Eben F, Patterson D. Direct current cardioversion during pregnancy should be performed with facilities available for fetal monitoring and emergency caesarean section. *BJOG,* 2002;109(12):1406-1407.

48. van Hagen IM, et al. Pregnancy in women with a mechanical heart valve: data of the European Society of Cardiology registry of pregnancy and cardiac disease (ROPAC). *Circulation.* 2015;132(2):132-142.

49. Nishimura RA, et al. 2014 AHA/ACC guideline for the management of patients with valvular heart disease: A report of the American College of Cardiology/American Heart Association Task Force on Practice Guidelines. *Circulation.* 2014;129(23): e521-e643.

50. Sliwa K, et al. Management of valvular disease in pregnancy: a global perspective. *Eur Heart J.* 2015;36(18):1078-1089.

51. Ayad SW, et al. Maternal and fetal outcomes in pregnant women with a prosthetic mechanical heart valve. *Clin Med Insights Cardiol.* 2016;10:11-17.

52. Pieper PG, Balci A, Van Dijk AP. Pregnancy in women with prosthetic heart valves. *Neth Heart J.* 2008;16(12):406-411.

53. Vitale N, et al. Dose-dependent fetal complications of warfarin in pregnant women with mechanical heart valves. *J Am Coll Cardiol.* 1999;33(6):1637-1641.

54. Cotrufo M, et al. Risk of warfarin during pregnancy with mechanical valve prostheses. *Obstet Gynecol.* 2002;99(1):35-40.

55. Elkayam U, Goland S. The search for a safe and effective anticoagulation regimen in pregnant women with mechanical prosthetic heart valves. *J Am Coll Cardiol.* 2012;59(12):1116-1118.

56. Kaneko T, Aranki SF. Anticoagulation for prosthetic valves. *Thrombosis.* 2013:346752.

57. McLintock C, McCowan LM, North RA. Maternal complications and pregnancy outcome in women with mechanical prosthetic heart valves treated with enoxaparin. *BJOG.* 2009;116(12):1585-1592.

58. Yinon Y, et al. Use of low molecular weight heparin in pregnant women with mechanical heart valves. *Am J Cardiol.* 2009;104(9):1259-1263.

CHAPTER 104
Traumatic Heart Disease

Mark J. Eisenberg

QUESTIONS

DIRECTIONS: Choose the one best response to each question.

104-1. What percentage of traumatic cardiac penetration injuries are lethal?

A. 30% to 40%
B. 40% to 50%
C. 50% to 60%
D. 60% to 70%
E. 70% to 80%

104-2. A 30-year-old man is brought to the emergency room following a stab wound to the left upper quadrant of his anterior chest. Which region of the heart is most likely to have been penetrated?

A. Right ventricle
B. Left ventricle
C. Right atrium
D. Left atrium
E. None of the above

104-3. Which of the following statements concerning the diagnosis of a penetrating cardiac injury is *false*?

A. Echocardiography can confirm the diagnosis of cardiac injury
B. A lack of effusion on examination by echocardiography disproves cardiac injury
C. The diagnostic gold standard is a subxiphoid window with echocardiography
D. Early diagnosis is critical to survival
E. All of the above are false

104-4. A 44-year-old woman is involved in a high-velocity motor vehicle accident and suffers blunt cardiac injury resulting from the collision. Which of the following conditions *is* consistent with blunt cardiac injury?

A. Cardiac contusion
B. Valve disruption
C. Atrial or ventricular septal defects
D. Frank cardiac rupture
E. All of the above

104-5. A 65-year-old man suffered blunt trauma to his chest following a 30-foot fall from the roof of his house. Which one of the following statements concerning blunt cardiac injury is *false*?

A. Most patients with blunt cardiac trauma are asymptomatic
B. All patients who have a significant mechanism of injury should have a screening ECG
C. Findings suggestive of cardiac contusion include nonspecific ST- and T-wave changes
D. Serial cardiac enzyme measurements are specific for the diagnosis of myocardial contusion
E. Arrhythmias such as atrial fibrillation, atrial flutter, and premature ventricular complexes are common and are usually self-limiting

104-6. A 15-year-old female equestrian is brought to the emergency room following blunt chest trauma from a horse kick to the anterior chest. Which of the following statements about valvular injury secondary to blunt chest trauma is *true*?

A. The aortic valve is most frequently involved
B. Isolated injury of the mitral valve is most common
C. Tricuspid valve injury is less commonly reported than mitral injury
D. Tricuspid valve injury is more frequently fatal than mitral valve injury
E. Mitral valve injury may become evident at a time remote from the injury as right heart failure develops

104-7. Which of the following is *not* an example of possible delayed sequelae following cardiac injury?

A. Atrial or ventricular septal defects
B. Cardiac rupture
C. Aortocardiac fistulas
D. Aortopulmonary fistulas
E. Posttraumatic pericarditis

104-8. What percentage of thoracic great vessel injuries is caused by penetrating trauma?

A. 30%
B. 50%
C. 60%
D. 70%
E. > 90%

104-9. A 74-year-old woman suffered a penetrating injury to the left upper quadrant of her anterior chest after falling over wooden furniture. The trauma team managing her care quickly suspects injury to her great vessels. Which of the following statements concerning penetrating injury of the great vessels is *correct*?

A. Penetrating injuries of the great vessels have a historically low mortality rate
B. Interposition grafts are often required
C. Operative repair of thoracic aortic injuries is almost always possible by direct aortic repair with short cross-clamp times
D. Paraplegia following the successful repair of penetrating aortic injuries is common, with prolonged aortic clamping following emergency thoracotomy
E. Adjunctive measures of cardiopulmonary bypass, bypass shunts, or active aortic shunts (eg, a centrifugal pump) are usually described for penetrating injuries but are rarely used for blunt injury

104-10. A 48-year-old man involved in a multiple motor vehicle crash receives a diagnosis of aortic transection from blunt aorta trauma. Which of the following is *not* considered a treatment option in aortic transection?

A. Immediate repair through a left thoracotomy
B. Delayed repair through a left thoracotomy if the patient is multiply injured and requires ongoing resuscitation
C. Endovascular stent graft insertion
D. A and B
E. All of the above

104-1. **The answer is E.** *(Hurst's The Heart, 14th Edition, Chap. 104)* Traumatic cardiac penetration injuries are highly lethal at 70% to 80% (option E). Penetrating injury to the heart must be suspected with any missile or knife wound to the thorax or upper abdomen. The mechanism of injury may be categorized as low, medium, or high velocity. Knife wounds are low velocity, shotgun injuries are medium velocity, and high-velocity injuries include bullet wounds caused by rifles and wounds resulting from military and civilian weapons. The amount of tissue damage is directly related to the amount of energy exchange between the penetrating object and the body part.[1]

104-2. **The answer is A.** *(Hurst's The Heart, 14th Edition, Chap. 104)* The anteriorly positioned right ventricle is most frequently injured (option A), followed by the left ventricle (option B), right atrium (option C), and left atrium (option D) (see Table 104-1 of *Hurst's The Heart*, 14th Edition).[2] Other potentially injured structures include the interatrial or interventricular septum, coronary arteries, valves, subvalvular apparatus, and conduction system.[3] Low-velocity injuries, such as stab wounds, produce damage commensurate to the structure penetrated and the size of the defect. High-velocity missiles produce injury beyond the region of myocardial penetration secondary to concussive effects and are more frequently lethal.[4-7] The primary manifestations of cardiac penetration are hemorrhage and tamponade. Valve or coronary injury may, of course, produce acute valvular incompetence or myocardial infarction. Stab victims often present with tamponade when clot and surrounding pericardial fat partially seal the pericardial defect. Injuries to the left ventricle more commonly result in overt hemorrhage. Patients presenting with tamponade may have a survival advantage, with mortality rates as low as 8% in experienced trauma centers.[4] Early diagnosis is critical to survival, and this is only possible with a high index of suspicion, bearing in mind that patients with potentially fatal wounds can be stable at presentation.

104-3. **The answer is B.** *(Hurst's The Heart, 14th Edition, Chap. 104)* Early diagnosis is critical to survival (option D), and this is only possible with a high index of suspicion, bearing in mind that patients with potentially fatal wounds can be stable at presentation. Echocardiography can confirm the diagnosis of cardiac injury (option A), but the lack of an effusion does not disprove injury (option B).[8] The diagnostic gold standard, short of exploration, is a subxiphoid window (option C).

104-4. **The answer is E.** *(Hurst's The Heart, 14th Edition, Chap. 104)* Blunt cardiac injury results from either a rapid deceleration mechanism or a direct blow to the precordium; in all cases, blunt cardiac injury requires significant force, such as that which occurs in motor vehicle crashes, pedestrians struck by motor vehicles, falls from heights, and sports-related injuries. Severe sudden abdominal compression can acutely increase pressure and blood flow to the heart, resulting in right-sided rupture. The absence of a clear definition and rapid laboratory testing makes the diagnosis of blunt cardiac injury difficult. Resulting injuries include cardiac contusion (option A), valve disruption (option B), atrial or ventricular septal defects (option C), or frank cardiac rupture (option D). These injuries vary by anatomic location (see Table 104-2 of *Hurst's The Heart*, 14th Edition). Once again, because of its anterior position, the right ventricle is the chamber most often involved. Cardiac rupture is a common mechanism of death in blunt trauma, with survival after medical care being uncommon.[9,10] For patients reaching medical care with vital signs, however, a reasonable survival rate can be expected if cardiac injury is promptly recognized and operated on.[11] Those surviving cardiac rupture more frequently have injuries to the right heart.[12] Myocardial contusion encompasses a spectrum of injuries. In its mildest form, cardiac contusion results in mild epicardial ecchymosis without functional significance. More severe contusion can cause muscular injury, dysfunction, and infarction. The true incidence of myocardial contusion following blunt trauma is difficult to discern. It is important to note that severe myocardial injury can occur with little evidence of external chest trauma.

104-5. **The answer is D.** *(Hurst's The Heart, 14th Edition, Chap. 104)* A high index of suspicion along with careful evaluation of mechanism should accompany all trauma patients from these accident scenarios, as a majority of patients with blunt cardiac trauma are asymptomatic (option A). Diagnostic testing, including chest x-ray, electrocardiogram (ECG), Holter monitoring, cardiac markers, transthoracic and transesophageal echocardiography, and cardiac computed tomography (CT) and magnetic resonance imaging (MRI), may be needed to make the diagnosis. All patients who have a significant mechanism of injury should have a screening ECG (option B). Findings suggestive of cardiac contusion include nonspecific ST- and T-wave changes (option C). Arrhythmias such as atrial fibrillation, atrial flutter, and premature ventricular complexes are also common and are usually self-limiting (option E). Ventricular tachycardia and fibrillation are uncommon in patients surviving to the hospital. With a normal ECG in an otherwise uninjured patient, the risk of complications is low. Serial cardiac enzyme measurements are nonspecific for the diagnosis of myocardial contusion in the blunt injury patient (option D).[13] In the patient who remains unstable or responds poorly to standard resuscitative efforts, echocardiography is indicated to look for regional wall-motion abnormalities or structural defects.

104-6. **The answer is A.** *(Hurst's The Heart, 14th Edition, Chap. 104)* Valve injury following blunt trauma is uncommon. The aortic valve is most frequently involved (option A), and injury can result from commissural avulsion, leaflet tears, or aortic dissection, all resulting in acute aortic insufficiency.[14,15] Isolated injury of the mitral valve is less common (option B) and most often involves rupture of the papillary muscle or chordal apparatus. Tricuspid valve injury is more commonly reported than mitral injury (option C), perhaps because the latter is often fatal (option D). Tricuspid valve injury may become evident at a time remote from the injury as right heart failure develops (option E).[16-18]

104-7. **The answer is B.** *(Hurst's The Heart, 14th Edition, Chap. 104)* Patients sustaining significant blunt or penetrating cardiac injuries require long-term follow-up. Injuries may not be appreciated at the time of trauma. Possible late sequelae include evolving atrial or ventricular septal defects (option A), progressive valvular incompetence, aortocardiac or aortopulmonary fistulas (options C and D), coronary artery fistulas, ventricular aneurysms, and posttraumatic pericarditis (option E).[19-22]

104-8. **The answer is E.** *(Hurst's The Heart, 14th Edition, Chap. 104)* More than 90% of thoracic great vessel injuries are caused by penetrating trauma (option E).[1,9] The great vessels of the chest include the aorta, its major branches at the arch (innominate, carotid, subclavian), and the major pulmonary arteries. The primary venous conduits include the superior and inferior vena cavae, their main tributaries (eg, azygous vein), and the pulmonary veins. The prevalence of great vessel injuries ranges from 0.3% to 10%.

104-9. **The answer is C.** *(Hurst's The Heart, 14th Edition, Chap. 104)* Penetrating injuries of the great vessels have a historically high mortality rate (option A). The trauma surgeon must resuscitate, diagnose, and treat the patient within minutes following admission to the trauma emergency unit. Through an emergent left thoracotomy, operative repair of thoracic aortic injuries is almost always possible by direct aortic repair with short cross-clamp times (option C). Only rarely is an interposition graft required (option B), and adjunctive measures of cardiopulmonary bypass, bypass shunts, or active aortic shunts (eg, a centrifugal pump) are usually not described for penetrating injuries but are almost exclusively used for blunt injury (option E). Paraplegia following successful repair of penetrating aortic injuries is rare, even with prolonged aortic clamping following emergency thoracotomy (option D).[1]

104-10. **The answer is E.** *(Hurst's The Heart, 14th Edition, Chap. 104)* Once a diagnosis of aortic transection from blunt aortic trauma is made, several emergent/urgent treatment options are available.[1] Immediate repair through a left thoracotomy (option A) should be considered, depending on the patient's stability and other injuries. Delayed repair is appropriate in the multiply injured patient requiring ongoing resuscitation (option B), and this management strategy has grown in popularity. Nonoperative management is not risk free, however, with as many as 4% of patients thought to be candidates for delayed repair experiencing rupture within a week of injury in some series.[23] A more recent additional option is endovascular stent graft insertion (option C) in selected patients, which has yielded promising results (see Fig. 104-3 of *Hurst's The Heart*, 14th Edition) when compared with traditional repair.[24-30] The Society for Vascular Surgery database documented endovascular treatment for acute aortic transections. Ninety-seven percent were the result of a motor vehicle accident. Sixty symptomatic patients were treated with an aortic endograft, with an all-cause mortality rate of 9.1% at 30 days and a mean operative time of 125 minutes.[31] An endovascular approach may be preferred in patients who are at higher risk for open repair, such as the elderly or those with significant lung or head injuries, making thoracotomy and heparinization less appealing.

References

1. Shahani R. Penetrating chest trauma treatment and management. *Medscape*. Accessed at www.emedicine.medscape.com/article/42569. Accessed January 2, 2016.

2. Symbas PN, Harlaftis N, Waldo WJ. Penetrating wounds: a comparison of different therapeutic methods. *Ann Surg*. 1976;183:377-381.

3. Karrel R, Shaffer MA, Franaszek JB. Emergency diagnosis, resuscitation, and treatment of acute penetrating cardiac trauma. *Ann Emerg Med*. 1982;11:504-517.

4. Degiannis E, Loogna P, Doll D, et al. Penetrating cardiac injuries: recent experience in South Africa. *World J Surg*. 2006;30:1258-1264.

5. Tyburski JG, Astra L, Wilson RF, et al. Factors affecting prognosis with penetrating wounds of the heart. *J Trauma*. 2000;48:587-591.

6. Mittal V, McAleese P, Young S, et al. Penetrating cardiac injuries. *Am Surg*. 1999;65:444-448.

7. Thourani VH, Filiciano DV, Cooper WA, et al. Penetrating cardiac trauma at an urban trauma center: a 22-year experience. *Am Surg*. 1999;65:811-818.

8. Topaloglu S, Aras D, Cagli K, et al. Penetrating trauma to the mitral valve and ventricular septum. *Tex Heart Inst J*. 2006;33:392-395.

9. Ottosen J, Guo WA. Blunt cardiac injury. Accessed at www.aast.org/blunt-cardiacinjury. January 3, 2016.

10. Tanabe T, Hashimoto M, Nishibe M, et al. Statistical analysis of deaths due to cardiovascular injuries. *Kyukyuigaku*. 1984;8:361-367.

11. Namai A, Sakurai M, Fujiwara H. Five cases of blunt traumatic cardiac rupture: success and failure in surgical management. *Gen Thorac Cardiovasc Surg*. 2007;55:200-204.

12. Pevec WC, Udekwu AO, Peitzman AB. Blunt rupture of the myocardium. *Ann Thorac Surg*. 1989;48:139-142.

13. Biffl WL, Moore FA, Moore EE, et al. Cardiac enzymes are irrelevant in the patient with suspected myocardial contusion. *Am J Surg*. 1994;168:523-528.

14. Asbach S, Siegenthaler MP, Bode C, et al. Aortic valve rupture after blunt chest trauma. *Clin Res Cardiol*. 2006;95:675-679.

15. Aris A, Delgado LJ, Montiel J, et al. Multiple intracardiac lesions after blunt chest trauma. *Ann Thorac Surg*. 2000;70:1692-1694.

16. Caparrelli DJ, Cattaneo SM, Brock MV, et al. Aortic and mitral valve disruption following nonpenetrating chest trauma. *J Trauma*. 2002;52:377-379.

17. Dounis G, Matssakas E, Poularas J, et al. Traumatic tricuspid insufficiency: a case report with review of the literature. *Eur J Emerg Med*. 2002;9:258-261.

18. Kulik A, Al-Saigh M, Yelle J, et al. Subacute tricuspid valve rupture after traumatic cardiac and pulmonary contusions. *Ann Thorac Surg*. 2006;81:1111-1112.

19. Symbas PN, DiOrio DA, Tyras DH, et al. Penetrating cardiac wounds: Significant residual and delayed sequelae. *J Thorac Cardiovasc Surg*. 1973;6:526-532.

20. Demetriades D, Charalambides C, Sareli P, et al. Late sequelae of penetrating cardiac injuries. *Br J Surg*. 1990;77:813-814.

21. Jeganathan R, Irwin G, Johnston PW, Jones JM. Traumatic left anterior descending artery-to-pulmonary artery fistula with delayed pericardial tamponade. *Ann Thorac Surg*. 2007;84:276-278.

22. Mattox KL, Limacher MC, Feliciano DV, et al. Cardiac evaluation following heart injury. *J Trauma*. 1985;25:758-765.

23. Holmes JH, Bloch RD, Hall RA, et al. Natural history of traumatic rupture of the thoracic aorta managed nonoperatively: a longitudinal analysis. *Ann Thorac Surg*. 2002;73:1149-1154.

24. Jahromi AS, Kazemi K, Safar HA, et al. Traumatic rupture of the thoracic aorta: cohort study and systematic review. *J Vasc Surg*. 2001;34:1029-1034.

25. Ott MC, Stewart TC, Lawlor DK, et al. Management of blunt thoracic aortic injuries: endovascular stents versus open repair. *J Trauma*. 2004;56:565-570.

26. Peterson BG, Matsumura JS, Morasch MD, et al. Percutaneous endovascular repair of blunt thoracic aortic transection. *J Trauma*. 2005;59:1062-1065.

27. Kokitsakis J, Kaskarelis I, Misthos P, et al. Endovascular versus open repair of blunt thoracic aortic injury: short-term results. *Ann Thorac Surg*. 2007;84:1965-1970.

28. Moainie SL, Neschis DG, Gammie JS, et al. Endovascular stenting for traumatic aortic injury: an emerging new standard of care. *Ann Thorac Surg*. 2008;85:1625-1630.

29. Saratzis NA, Saratzis AN, Melas N, et al. Endovascular repair of traumatic rupture of the thoracic aorta: single-center experience. *Cardiovasc Intervent Radiol*. 2007;30:370-375.

30. Azizzadeh A, Keyhani K, Miller C, et al. Blunt traumatic aortic injury: initial experience with endovascular repair. *J Vasc Surg*. 2009;49:1403-1408.

31. Dake MD, White RA, Diethrich EB, et al. Report on endograft management of traumatic thoracic aortic transections at 30 days and 1 year from a multidisciplinary subcommittee of the Society for Vascular Surgery Outcomes Committee. *J Vasc Surg*. 2011;53(4):1091-1096.

CHAPTER 105

The Kidney in Heart Disease

Jonathan Afilalo

QUESTIONS

DIRECTIONS: Choose the one best response to each question.

105-1. A 65-year-old man with a prior history of type 2 diabetes, congestive heart failure, coronary heart disease, and end-stage chronic kidney disease was seen in the nephrology clinic to discuss starting hemodialysis. The patient refused and decided not to return for the follow-up appointments. A few weeks later, he was brought to the emergency department by his family, who observed that his mental status was "off." The family denied any recent infections or fevers. Physical examination did not reveal focal neurological deficits, although he had asterixis and a pericardial friction rub. Laboratory investigations showed a significant increase in serum creatinine with academia. Which of the following is the next best step in the management of this patient?

A. NSAIDs
B. NSAIDs and colchicine
C. Corticosteroids
D. Hemodialysis daily for at least 1 week
E. Hemodialysis 3 times per week indefinitely

The following case should be used for questions 105-2 through 105-6.

A 66-year-old woman with a prior history of coronary heart disease, arterial hypertension, and type 2 diabetes mellitus presented to the emergency department complaining of a 2-day history of increasing dyspnea, anasarca, and dry cough. Physical examination revealed diffused edema, elevated JVP, ascites, dullness to percussion over the right lung base, and bilateral crackles. Initial blood tests revealed leukocytosis, serum creatinine of 2.9 mg/dL, and metabolic acidosis. ECG showed sinus bradycardia and LVH with strain patterns. An echocardiogram was obtained and revealed a dilated left

with a globally depressed ejection fraction of 39%, mild-to-moderate mitral and tricuspid regurgitation, and pulmonary hypertension. The patient also underwent an ultrasound of the abdomen and pelvis, which showed mild ascites with a dilated IVC, and small echogenic kidneys.

105-2. The term "cardiorenal syndrome" (CRS) has been coined to describe the entity in which concomitant cardiac and renal dysfunction is present in the same patient. Which of the following types of CRS is this patient most likely to have?

A. CRS type 1
B. CRS type 2
C. CRS type 3
D. CRS type 4
E. CRS type 5

105-3. Which of the following is the most likely underlying mechanism of renal injury and damage in the patient?

A. Subclinical inflammation
B. Impaired endothelial function
C. Embolization of thrombotic material from the heart or central arteries
D. Accelerated atherosclerosis
E. All the above

105-4. An important principle in the treatment of CRS-2 is to optimize cardiac function in order to slow or reverse the pathophysiology described in Question 105-3. Which of the following treatments has *not* been shown to be beneficial for both CKD and CHF in CRS type 2?

A. Beta-blockers
B. Cardiac resynchronization therapy
C. ACEIs
D. ARBs
E. None of the above

105-5. After 2 days of parenteral furosemide, the patient exhibited persistent volume overload with minimal change in weight and urine output. Diuretic resistance was suspected. Which of the following may *not* explain oral diuretic resistance?

A. Gut edema
B. Poor intestinal perfusion
C. Organic anions
D. Hypokalemia
E. Proteinuria

105-6. Although a multitude of factors can cause diuretic resistance, intrinsic renal adaptations to loop diuretics called the "braking phenomenon" has been implicated in this process. Which of the following strategies may be the most beneficial in this regard?

A. Thiazide-type diuretics
B. Mineralocorticoid receptor antagonists
C. Acetazolamide
D. Ultrafiltration
E. All of the above

The following case should be used for questions 105-7 and 105-8.

Two days after a complex multivessel PCI, a 67-year-old man began to complain of nausea and reduced urinary output. His past medical history was significant for stage 3B CKD, type 2 diabetes, arterial hypertension, and coronary artery disease. Initial laboratory tests revealed an acute 40% rise in serum creatinine over baseline. Contrast-induced acute kidney injury (CI-AKI) was suspected.

105-7. Which of the following measures is the most effective for reducing the risk of CI-AKI?

A. Use of as little contrast material as possible during PCI
B. Use of low-osmolar contrast agents
C. Use of iso-osmolar contrast agents
D. Administration of N-acetylcysteine
E. Volume expansion combined with forced diuresis

105-8. Although no therapy exists to obviate the risk of CI-AKI for the patient described, which of the following pharmacological agents appears to reduce the risk of CI-AKI?

A. Beta-blockers
B. Ascorbic acid
C. Fenoldopam
D. Angiotensin-converting enzyme inhibitors
E. Statins

105-9. Three days after undergoing transcatheter aortic valve replacement (TAVR), a 77-year-old man started to complain of general malaise and weakness associated with reduced urinary output. His past medical history was significant for stage 4 CKD. Initial laboratory tests revealed an acute 35% rise in serum creatinine over baseline. Which of the following is a risk factor for acute kidney injury (AKI) post-TAVR?

A. Preexisting CKD
B. Advanced age
C. Blood transfusions
D. Transapical access
E. All of the above

105-10. Two days after cardiac surgery requiring cardiopulmonary bypass, an 85-year-old woman was noted to have an acute 45% rise in serum creatinine over baseline. Her past medical history was significant for stage 3A CKD, dyslipidemia, and coronary artery disease. Which of the following is *not* a mechanism of AKI following cardiac surgery?

A. Endogenous nephrotoxins
B. Exogenous nephrotoxins
C. Tissue hypoxia and ischemia-reperfusion injury
D. Acute glomerulonephritis provoked by cardiopulmonary bypass
E. The systemic inflammatory response syndrome (SIRS)

105-1. **The answer is D.** *(Hurst's The Heart, 14th Edition, Chap. 105)* Uremic pericarditis is less responsive to anti-inflammatory therapy with NSAIDs (option A), NSAIDs plus colchicine (option B), or corticosteroids (option C), and should be treated by intensive hemodialysis—that is, daily for at least 1 week (option D). The patient will require long-term dialysis (option E), but this should be performed more often than 3 times per week to treat the uremic pericarditis.

105-2. **The answer is B.** *(Hurst's The Heart, 14th Edition, Chap. 105)* As summarized in Table 105-1, CRS is subdivided according to the temporal pattern of cardiac and renal disease. In this case, chronic abnormalities in cardiac function lead to kidney injury and dysfunction. This patient therefore has CRS type 2 (option B), which is the most common CRS.

TABLE 105-1 **Cardiorenal Syndromes**

CRS type 1	Acute worsening of cardiac function leading to kidney injury and/or dysfunction
CRS type 2	Chronic abnormalities in cardiac function leads to kidney injury and/or dysfunction
CRS type 3	Acute worsening of kidney function leads to cardiac injury and/or dysfunction
CRS type 4	Chronic kidney disease leads to heart injury and/or dysfunction
CRS type 5	Systemic extrarenal and extracardiac condition leading to simultaneous injury and/or dysfunction of both the heart and kidney

Abbreviation: CRS, cardiorennal syndrome.

105-3. **The answer is E.** *(Hurst's The Heart, 14th Edition, Chap. 105)* The pathophysiology behind the development of renal dysfunction in CRS-2 is incompletely understood. There does not appear to be a strong correlation between LVEF and estimated GFR among patients with CHF.[1] All the proposed options are correct (option E). The proposed mechanisms underlying the development of kidney dysfunction in CHF are outlined in Figure 105-1.

105-4. **The answer is A.** *(Hurst's The Heart, 14th Edition, Chap. 105)* Although beta-blockers (option A) may have some positive effects, there is insufficient evidence to conclude whether people with CKD who are not known to have heart failure derive benefit from beta-blockers.[2] Cardiac resynchronization therapy (option B), when indicated, appears to improve both ejection fraction and GFR in patients with CRS-2.[3] Antagonism of the RAAS is an important component in both heart failure and CKD therapy. Both ACEIs/ARBs (options C and D) and aldosterone antagonists attenuate excessive RAAS activation and thereby prevent renal vasoconstriction and fibrosis. However, although ACEI/ARBs are beneficial in CRS-2, there is a risk of hyperkalemia as well as of inducing arterial hypotension, resulting in worsening renal function. The risk of these complications is higher for patients with CKD than for patients without renal disease.[4,5]

105-5. **The answer is D.** *(Hurst's The Heart, 14th Edition, Chap. 105)* Several characteristics of the loop diuretics, which are not related to tubular damage or dysfunction, may explain diuretic resistance. Orally administered loop diuretic absorption may be reduced in congestive heart failure due to gut edema (option A) and poor intestinal perfusion (option B). In the plasma, > 90% of the loop diuretics will be bound to plasma protein and are therefore not filtered across the glomerulus. In order to reach the tubular lumen, they must be secreted by anion transporters in the proximal tubules. Organic anions (eg, urate) compete with the loop diuretics (option C), and their transport is inhibited by acidosis. Significant proteinuria increases protein-binding of loop diuretics in the tubular lumen and prevents their pharmacological action (option E).[6,7-10]

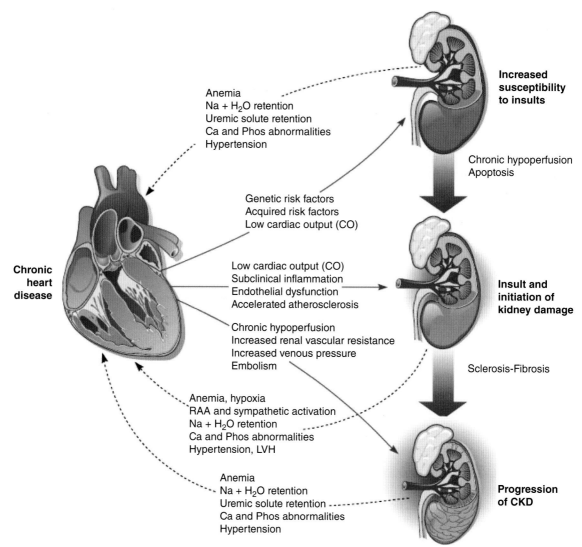

FIGURE 105-1 Proposed mechanisms of renal injury and damage in patients with congestive heart failure. Reduced cardiac function in chronic heart failure leads to a low-output state with renal hypoperfusion and congestion of the venous system (which is effectively transmitted retrograde from the great veins to the renal veins). This results in relative hypoxia of the renal parenchyma. Reduced effective circulatory volume (low-output heart failure) also leads to renin-angiotensin-aldosterone (RAA) system activation and release of vasoconstrictors (angiotensin, adrenaline, noradrenaline), which increases renal vascular resistance and further reduces renal perfusion. Chronic heart failure is associated with subclinical inflammation and impaired endothelial function, which interfere with the kidneys' autoregulatory mechanisms. Low-output heart failure also increases the risk of embolization of thrombotic material from the heart or central arteries. Microembolization may further aggravate renal hypoxia. Lastly, most risk factors for cardiovascular disease and heart failure are also risk factors for kidney disease. Accelerated atherosclerosis of the renal vessels and progression of kidney disease due to genetic or acquired risk factors likely also play a role. CKD, chronic kidney disease; LVH, left ventricular hypertrophy.

(Reproduced with permission from Ronco C, Haapio M, House AA, et al. Cardiorenal syndrome. *J Am Coll Cardiol.* 2008 Nov 4;52(19):1527-1539.)

105-6. **The answer is A.** *(Hurst's The Heart, 14th Edition, Chap. 105)* Thiazide-type diuretics (option A) are the most commonly used diuretics in patients who develop resistance to loop diuretics. Thiazide diuretics are a good choice because they act on the distal tubule NaCl symporter, which largely mediates the intrinsic renal adaptations to loop diuretics called the "braking phenomenon." In other words, with prolonged loop diuretic use, the kidney adapts by upregulating thiazide-sensitive NaCl reabsorption. Mineralocorticoid receptor antagonists (option B) and acetazolamide (option C) may also be considered, the latter being particularly useful in the setting of diuretic-induced alkalosis. Ultrafiltration (option D) may also be effective in diuretic resistance, but unfortunately the only large-scale RCT was terminated early.[11-13]

105-7. **The answer is A.** *(Hurst's The Heart, 14th Edition, Chap. 105)* The most important measures to reduce the risk of CI-AKI are to use as little contrast material as possible (option A) and to identify patients at increased risk of AKI. Whereas low-osmolar agents (option B) can be used for most patients, iso-osmolar agents (option C) are preferred for high-risk patients. The clearance of contrast can be facilitated by intravascular volume expansion by isotonic crystalloid solutions, which increase GFR and tubular flow. More aggressive volume expansion, driven either by the left ventricular end-diastolic pressure or by urine output, reduces the risk of CI-AKI.[14,15] Volume expansion may be even more effective at reducing AKI if combined with N-acetylcystein (option D) or forced diuresis (option E).[16]

105-8. **The answer is E.** *(Hurst's The Heart, 14th Edition, Chap. 105)* A number of promising substances (eg, ascorbic acid [option B] and fenoldopam [option C]) have failed to demonstrate superiority to placebo when tested in randomized trials.[17,18] However, statins (option E) appear to reduce the risk of CI-AKI, whereas renin-angiotensin-aldosterone system inhibitors (angiotensin-converting enzyme inhibitors [ACEIs; option D] and angiotensin receptor blockers [ARBs]) may increase the risk.[19-21] Statins may mediate their protective effect through several mechanisms (including the inhibition of contrast reabsorption, attenuation of inflammation, oxidative stress, endothelial dysfunction, and protection of podocytes in the glomerulus), whereas ACEIs/ARBs are thought to interfere with protective autoregulatory mechanisms, including tubuloglomerular feedback.

105-9. **The answer is E.** *(Hurst's The Heart, 14th Edition, Chap. 105)* The most important risk factors for AKI post-TAVR include: preexisting CKD (option A), hemodynamic instability or the need for circulatory support, blood transfusions (option C), transapical access (option D), amount of contrast used, diabetes, and age (option B).[22,23]

105-10. **The answer is D.** *(Hurst's The Heart, 14th Edition, Chap. 105)* The pathogenesis of AKI in the setting of cardiac surgery is incompletely understood. It is likely multifactorial, with the following factors playing a role: (1; options A and B) Nephrotoxins, both endogenous (eg, heme and iron pigments released secondary to blood trauma and hemolysis caused by blood pumps) and exogenous (eg, nonsteroidal anti-inflammatory drugs [impair autoregulation of renal blood flow] and intravenous contrast).[24-26] (2; option C) Tissue hypoxia- and ischemia-reperfusion injury secondary to intraoperative changes in systemic or local renal hemodynamics or the release of atherosclerotic emboli (eg, during aortic cross-clamping).[27,28] The renal medulla, which has a high metabolic demand and a low baseline PaO_2, is particularly susceptible to ischemia.[29] (3; option E) The systemic inflammatory response syndrome (SIRS) is triggered by major surgery and artificial conduits such as cardiopulmonary bypass machines (which do not cause acute glomerulonephritis [option D]), with activation of neutrophils, platelets, cytokines, coagulation factors, and fibrinolysis.[30]

References

1. Bhatia RS, Tu JV, Lee DS, et al. Outcome of heart failure with preserved ejection fraction in a population-based study. *N Engl J Med.* 2006;355:260-269.
2. Badve SV, Roberts MA, Hawley CM, et al. Effects of beta-adrenergic antagonists in patients with chronic kidney disease: A systematic review and meta-analysis. *J Am Coll Cardiol.* 2011;58:1152-1161.
3. Garg N, Thomas G, Jackson G, et al. Cardiac resynchronization therapy in CKD: a systematic review. *Clin J Am Soc Nephrol.* 2013;8:1293-1303.
4. Anand IS, Bishu K, Rector TS, Ishani A, Kuskowski MA, Cohn JN. Proteinuria, chronic kidney disease, and the effect of an angiotensin receptor blocker in addition to an angiotensin-converting enzyme inhibitor in patients with moderate to severe heart failure. *Circulation.* 2009;120:1577-1584.
5. Rossignol P, Cleland JG, Bhandari S, et al. Determinants and consequences of renal function variations with aldosterone blocker therapy in heart failure patients after myocardial infarction: insights from the Eplerenone Post-Acute Myocardial Infarction Heart Failure Efficacy and Survival Study. *Circulation.* 2012;125:271-279.
6. Verbrugge FH, Mullens W, Tang WH. Management of cardiorenal syndrome and diuretic resistance. *Curr Treat Options Cardiovasc Med.* 2016;18:11.

7. Kirchner KA, Voelker JR, Brater DC. Intratubular albumin blunts the response to furosemide: a mechanism for diuretic resistance in the nephrotic syndrome. *J Pharmacol Exp Ther*. 1990;252:1097-1101.

8. Vasko MR, Cartwright DB, Knochel JP, Nixon JV, Brater DC. Furosemide absorption altered in decompensated congestive heart failure. *Ann Intern Med*. 1985;102:314-318.

9. Verbrugge FH, Dupont M, Steels P et al. Abdominal contributions to cardiorenal dysfunction in congestive heart failure. *J Am Coll Cardiol*. 2013;62:485-495.

10. Uwai Y, Saito H, Hashimoto Y, Inui KI. Interaction and transport of thiazide diuretics, loop diuretics, and acetazolamide via rat renal organic anion transporter rOAT1. *J Pharmacol Exp Ther*. 2000;295:261-265.

11. Verbrugge FH, Dupont M, Steels P, et al. The kidney in congestive heart failure: "Are natriuresis, sodium, and diuretics really the good, the bad, and the ugly?" *Eur J Heart Fail*. 2014;16:133-142.

12. Costanzo MR, Negoianu D, Jaski BE, et al. Aquapheresis versus intravenous diuretics and hospitalizations for heart failure. *JACC Heart Fail*. 2016;4:95-105.

13. Kim GH. Long-term adaptation of renal ion transporters to chronic diuretic treatment. *Am J Nephrol*. 2004;24:595-605.

14. Brar SS, Aharonian V, Mansukhani P, et al. Haemodynamic-guided fluid administration for the prevention of contrast-induced acute kidney injury: the POSEIDON randomised controlled trial. *Lancet*. 2014;383:1814-2823.

15. Solomon R. Forced diuresis with the RenalGuard system: impact on contrast induced acute kidney injury. *J Cardiol*. 2014;63:9-13.

16. Kwong JS, Yu CM. Ultrafiltration for acute decompensated heart failure: a systematic review and meta-analysis of randomized controlled trials. *Int J Cardiol*. 2014;172:395-402.

17. Adolph E, Holdt-Lehmann B, Chatterjee T, et al. Renal insufficiency following radiocontrast exposure trial (REINFORCE): a randomized comparison of sodium bicarbonate versus sodium chloride hydration for the prevention of contrast-induced nephropathy. *Coronary Arterty Dis*. 2008;19:413-419.

18. Maioli M, Toso A, Leoncini M, et al. Sodium bicarbonate versus saline for the prevention of contrast-induced nephropathy in patients with renal dysfunction undergoing coronary angiography or intervention. *J Am Coll Cardiol*. 2008;52:599-604.

19. Li Y, Liu Y, Fu L, Mei C, Dai B. Efficacy of short-term high-dose statin in preventing contrast-induced nephropathy: a meta-analysis of seven randomized controlled trials. *PLoS One*. 2012;7:e34450.

20. Leoncini M, Toso A, Maioli M, Tropeano F, Villani S, Bellandi F. Early high-dose rosuvastatin for contrast-induced nephropathy prevention in acute coronary syndrome: results from the PRATO-ACS study (Protective Effect of Rosuvastatin and Antiplatelet Therapy On contrast-induced acute kidney injury and myocardial damage in patients with Acute Coronary Syndrome). *J Am Coll Cardiol*. 2014;63:71-79.

21. Han Y, Zhu G, Han L, et al. Short-term rosuvastatin therapy for prevention of contrast-induced acute kidney injury in patients with diabetes and chronic kidney disease. *J Am Coll Cardiol*. 2014;63:62-70.

22. Bagur R, Webb JG, Nietlispach F, et al. Acute kidney injury following transcatheter aortic valve implantation: predictive factors, prognostic value, and comparison with surgical aortic valve replacement. *Eur Heart J*. 2010;31:865-874.

23. Nuis RJ, Rodes-Cabau J, Sinning JM, et al. Blood transfusion and the risk of acute kidney injury after transcatheter aortic valve implantation. *Circ Cardiovasc Interv*. 2012;5:680-688.

24. Epstein M. Non-steroidal anti-inflammatory drugs and the continuum of renal dysfunction. *J Hypertens*. 2002;20:S17-S23.

25. Wright G. Haemolysis during cardiopulmonary bypass: Update. *Perfusion*. 2001;16:345-351.

26. Moat NE, Evans TE, Quinlan GJ, Gutteridge JM. Chelatable iron and copper can be released from extracorporeally circulated blood during cardiopulmonary bypass. *FEBS Lett*. 1993;328:103-106.

27. Blauth CI. Macroemboli and microemboli during cardiopulmonary bypass. *Ann Thorac Surg*. 1995;59:1300-1303.

28. Davila-Roman VG, Kouchoukos NT, Schechtman KB, Barzilai B. Atherosclerosis of the ascending aorta is a predictor of renal dysfunction after cardiac operations. *J Thorac Cardiovasc Surg*. 1999;117:111-116.

29. Brezis M, Rosen S. Hypoxia of the renal medulla: its implications for disease. *N Engl J Med*. 1995;332:647-655.

30. Paparella D, Yau TM, Young E. Cardiopulmonary bypass induced inflammation: pathophysiology and treatment. An update. *Eur J Cardiothorac Surg*. 2002;21: 232-244.

CHAPTER 106

Exercise in Health and Cardiovascular Disease

Mark J. Eisenberg

QUESTIONS

DIRECTIONS: Choose the one best response to each question.

106-1. Which of the following statements concerning the acute hemodynamics of exercise is *false*?

A. The cardiovascular control center is believed to reside in the ventrolateral medulla of the brain and to respond to both central and peripheral inputs
B. Central impulses arise from somatomotor centers of the brain
C. Peripheral impulses are generated by mechanoreceptors, found in muscles, joints, and the vascular system; chemoreceptors, found in the muscles and the vascular system; and baroreceptors, found in the vascular system
D. Central and peripheral impulses are transmitted by autonomic efferent fibers
E. The central control center regulates cardiac output (CO) and its distribution to organs and tissues according to metabolic demand

106-2. A 35-year-old triathlete presents to your clinic for a routine physical examination. Wishing to clarify his understanding of exercise physiology, he asks you to outline the physiological changes and circulatory adjustments that occur during exercise. Which of the following statements about exercise physiology is *false*?

A. Cardiac output (CO) is defined as the product of stroke volume (SV) and heart rate (HR)
B. In women, the average CO at rest is approximately 25% greater than in men

C. The magnitude of the hemodynamic response during physical activity depends on the intensity and the muscle mass involved
D. In sedentary individuals, CO during maximal exercise increases approximately four times, to an average of 20 to 22 L/min
E. In elite-class athletes, the CO can increase eightfold, to values of 35 to 40 L/min

106-3. Which of the following statements concerning the heart rate response to exercise is *correct*?

A. From rest to strenuous exercise, heart rate (HR) rapidly increases to levels of 160 to 180 bpm or higher
B. The initial rapid increase is likely the result of peripheral command influences or a slow reflex from muscle mechanoreceptors
C. The instant acceleration in HR is largely caused by vagal activation
D. Later increases result from reflex activation of the pulmonary stretch receptors, which trigger increased parasympathetic tone and more sympathetic withdrawal
E. During exercise, changes in SV account for a greater percentage of the increase in CO than does HR

106-4. Which of the following enhances diastolic ventricular filling (preload)?

A. Faster HR
B. Slower HR
C. Increased venous return
D. A or C
E. B or C

106-5. Which of the following physiological processes occurs during *intense* physical exertion?

A. Parasympathetic activity is withdrawn, and sympathetic discharge is maximal

B. A progressive decrease in blood flow to the skin occurs as the increasing cutaneous sympathetic vascular tone overcomes the thermoregulatory vasodilatory response

C. During maximal exercise, cerebral blood flow may decrease because of hyperventilation and respiratory alkalosis

D. Both A and B

E. All of the above occur

106-6. A 70-year-old woman presents to your clinic for consultation. She has recently started an exercise program at her local gym, but she expresses concern about her trainer's advice to perform resistance exercises. Which of the following statements about resistance exercise is *true*?

A. Weight training exercises have been shown to cause a significant increase in blood pressure

B. Moderate resistance training programs are safe even in subjects with cardiac disease

C. Resistance training probably contributes less significantly than does isotonic exercise to overall cardiovascular health and longevity

D. Resistance exercise should be done with care and in moderation by subjects with aortic or aortic valve disease

E. All of the above are true

106-7. Choose the *correct* statement(s):

A. At rest, CO is similar for both trained and untrained individuals

B. In untrained persons, there is only a small increase in SV during the transition from rest to exercise, and the major augmentation in CO is induced by tachycardia

C. Endurance training induces a decrease in resting parasympathetic tone and increases resting sympathetic activity

D. Both A and B are correct

E. All of the above are correct

106-8. Which of the following statements about sex-related differences in the cardiovascular effects of exercise is *correct*?

A. Adolescent females may manifest a 5% to 10% greater CO than adolescent males at any level of submaximal oxygen uptake

B. The gross maximal aerobic capacity in women is approximately 25% lower than it is in men

C. Although strength adjusted to cross-sectional muscle area is similar in men and women, men's greater muscle mass usually yields lesser isometric strength

D. During exercise, men manifest a progressive decrease in ejection fraction with little or no increase in end-diastolic volume

E. During exercise, women tend to decrease end-diastolic volume without a significant increase in ejection fraction

106-9. A 72-year-old man with no history of cardiovascular disease presents to your clinic for a routine checkup. He has read that it is important to remain physically active in old age, but he is concerned about his limited mobility. Which of the following statements concerning the overall focus for exercise training among the elderly (patients > 65 years of age) is *true*?

A. The overall focus for exercise training should be to enhance health-related fitness, reduce the risk of various chronic diseases, and improve overall quality of life

B. Only endurance-type exercise has been shown to reduce the risk of chronic disease

C. It is important to prescribe an exercise program with low-level energy expenditure, particularly during the first few weeks, with gradual increases thereafter

D. Both A and C are true

E. All of the above are true

106-10. Which of the following statements about exercise and risk factor modification is *false*?

A. Trials of exercise in both hypertensive and normotensive individuals suggest a 3- to 4-mm Hg decline in systolic blood pressure and a 2- to 3-mm Hg decline in blood pressure with both aerobic and resistive exercise training

B. Exercise is superior to metformin in the prevention of type 2 diabetes

C. While exercise in heart failure is safe and well tolerated if appropriately prescribed, it does not augment the benefits of cardiac resynchronization therapy

D. Substantial evidence supports the idea that resistance training mobilizes visceral adipose tissue in the abdominal region

E. The effects of exercise in secondary prevention are on coagulation, autonomic function, anti-ischemic and antiarrhythmic effect, and a decrease in age-related disability

106-1. The answer is D. (*Hurst's The Heart, 14th Edition, Chap. 106*) During physical activity, energy expenditure increases, and the compensatory cardiovascular response represents an integration of neural, biochemical, and physiologic factors. The cardiovascular control center is believed to reside in the ventrolateral medulla of the brain and to respond to both central and peripheral inputs (option A). Central impulses arise from somatomotor centers of the brain (option B). Peripheral impulses are generated by mechanoreceptors, found in muscles, joints, and the vascular system; chemoreceptors, found in the muscles and the vascular system; and baroreceptors, found in the vascular system (option C). These impulses are transmitted by autonomic afferent fibers (option D). The central control center regulates CO and its distribution to organs and tissues according to metabolic demand.

106-2. The answer is B. (*Hurst's The Heart, 14th Edition, Chap. 106*) The circulatory response to exercise involves a complex series of adjustments resulting in an increase in CO proportional to metabolic demands. These changes ensure that the metabolic needs of exercising muscles are met, that hyperthermia does not occur, and that blood flow to essential organs is protected. Adequate blood flow is delivered to exercising muscles through increased CO and redistribution of blood flow away from the viscera. CO is defined as the product of SV and HR (option A). The average CO at rest is approximately 5 L/min for both trained and untrained men. In women, the value is approximately 25% lower (option B). Resting CO increases immediately before the onset of physical exercise as a result of anticipatory changes in the autonomic nervous system resulting in tachycardia and increased venous return. After the onset of exercise, CO increases rapidly until steady-rate exercise is reached. CO then increases gradually until a plateau is achieved. The magnitude of the hemodynamic response during physical activity depends on the intensity and the muscle mass involved (option C). In sedentary individuals, CO during maximal exercise increases approximately four times, to an average of 20 to 22 L/min (option D). In elite-class athletes, the CO can increase eightfold, to values of 35 to 40 L/min (option E).

106-3. The answer is A. (*Hurst's The Heart, 14th Edition, Chap. 106*) From rest to strenuous exercise, HR rapidly increases to levels of 160 to 180 bpm or higher (option A). The initial rapid increase is likely the result of central command influences or a rapid reflex from muscle mechanoreceptors (option B). The instant acceleration in HR is largely caused by vagal withdrawal (option C). Later increases result from reflex activation of the pulmonary stretch receptors, which trigger increased sympathetic tone and more parasympathetic withdrawal (option D). Increased circulating catecholamines play a role as well. During exercise, changes in HR account for a greater percentage of the increase in CO than does SV (option E). Stroke volume plateaus when the CO has increased to only half of its maximum. Further increases in CO occur by increases in the HR, although HR response in older subjects can be *blunted*. Two physiologic mechanisms influence SV. Increased venous return elicits enhanced diastolic filling and more forceful systolic contraction. Neurohormonal influences also enhance contractility through direct effects.

106-4. The answer is E. (*Hurst's The Heart, 14th Edition, Chap. 106*) Diastolic ventricular filling (preload) is enhanced by slower HR or increased venous return (option E). Increased end-diastolic volume stretches myocardial fibers, enhancing the overlap of sarcomere myofilaments and improving ventricular compliance. This in turn results in enhanced contractility and greater SV. It is believed that this mechanism is responsible for increased SV during the transition from rest to exercise or from the upright to the supine position. Resting CO and SV are highest in the supine position. Supine SV is nearly maximal at rest and increases only slightly during exercise. In normal supine individuals, increased CO with exercise results predominantly from an increase in HR, with little contribution from SV. Venous return to the heart is lower in the upright position, resulting in a lower resting SV and CO. During upright exercise, however, SV can approach maximum SV observed in the recumbent position, usually without an increase in ventricular diastolic dimensions.

106-5. **The answer is E.** *(Hurst's The Heart, 14th Edition, Chap. 106)* During exertion, parasympathetic activity is withdrawn, and sympathetic discharge is maximal (option A), which results in increased release of norepinephrine from sympathetic postganglionic nerve endings. Plasma epinephrine levels are also increased. As a result, most vascular beds constrict, except those in exercising muscles, which are influenced by vasodilating metabolites. Blood flow to the skin increases during light and moderate exercise, favoring body cooling. Further increases in workload cause a progressive decrease in skin flow as the increasing cutaneous sympathetic vascular tone overcomes the thermoregulatory vasodilatory response (option B). The kidneys and splanchnic tissues extract only 10% to 25% of the oxygen available in their blood supply. Consequently, considerable reductions in blood flow to these tissues can be tolerated through increased oxygen extraction. At rest, the heart extracts approximately 75% of the oxygen in the coronary blood flow. Because of limited margin of reserve and increased myocardial demands, coronary blood flow increases fourfold during exercise. Cerebral blood flow also increases during exercise by approximately 25% to 30%.[1] During maximal exercise, however, cerebral flow may decrease because of hyperventilation and respiratory alkalosis (option C).

On cessation of exercise, there is a decrease in HR and CO secondary to withdrawal of sympathetic tone and reactivation of vagal activity. In contrast, systemic vascular resistance remains lower for some time because of persistent vasodilatation in the muscles. As a result, arterial pressure decreases, often below preexercise levels, for periods up to 12 hours into recovery.[2] Blood pressure is then stabilized at normal levels by baroreceptor reflexes.

106-6. **The answer is E.** *(Hurst's The Heart, 14th Edition, Chap. 106)* Weight lifting is considered the prototype resistance exercise and is thought to have a high isometric component. Blood pressure and HR responses during weight lifting are proportional to the relative intensity of muscle contraction, the mass of the muscle groups involved, and the duration of the contraction. Weight training exercises have been shown to cause a significant increase in blood pressure. This is thought to be the result of restricted muscle perfusion and a centrally mediated pressor response caused by enhanced muscle tension. The HR response during maximal upper body resistance exercise is lower than that seen during maximal isotonic exercise.[3] This contributes to a lower HR-blood pressure product during maximal resistance exercise compared with maximal dynamic exercise. Previous concerns regarding the safety of resistance training have been rebutted by several reports that reveal that moderate resistance training programs are safe even in subjects with cardiac disease.[4,5] At this time, it is believed that resistance training (done on a regular schedule) is useful for promoting muscle strength, flexibility, and functionality but probably contributes less significantly than does isotonic exercise to overall cardiovascular health and longevity. Resistance exercise should be done with care and in moderation by subjects with aortic or aortic valve disease.

106-7. **The answer is D.** *(Hurst's The Heart, 14th Edition, Chap. 106)* At rest, CO is similar for both trained and untrained individuals (option A). Endurance training induces an increase in resting parasympathetic tone and reduces resting sympathetic activity (option C). Heart rates below 30 bpm have been recorded for some healthy athletes. CO is maintained in such individuals by increased SV. Training-induced increase in blood volume and intrinsic myocardial factors have been cited as the source of this enhanced resting and exercise SV. During exercise, trained individuals achieve a larger maximal CO than do sedentary persons. In untrained persons, there is only a small increase in SV during the transition from rest to exercise, and the major augmentation in CO is induced by tachycardia (option B). The improved cardiac performance after conditioning is secondary to both the Frank–Starling mechanism and augmented myocardial contraction and relaxation. In previously sedentary individuals, 8 weeks of aerobic training increased SV. This change is associated with increased left ventricular end-diastolic dimension with preservation or even reduction of the end-systolic size.[6] The enhanced end-diastolic dimensions are, however, much lower than those of well-trained athletes.[7] It is not known whether this discrepancy results from prolonged training, genetic factors, or a combination of both. After cessation of training, changes largely regress within only 3 weeks, which is of great concern in adherence to exercise programs. Unfortunately, cardiovascular conditioning is more easily lost than gained, which accounts for the effort dyspnea often experienced by subjects with resumption of activity after a long absence.

106-8. **The answer is A.** *(Hurst's The Heart, 14th Edition, Chap. 106)* Available data suggest qualitatively similar responses to dynamic and static exercise in both women and men. Some quantitative differences have been demonstrated in adolescent females who manifest a 5% to 10% greater CO than adolescent males at any level of submaximal oxygen uptake (option A). This is likely related to a 10% lower hemoglobin concentration in females. To be able to deliver the same amount of oxygen, there is a proportionate increase in CO. The gross maximal aerobic capacity in women is approximately 50% lower than it is in men (option B),[8] but when adjusted to lean body mass, the difference is only 10% to 15%, a more accurate reflection of sex-related differences. The absolute number of skeletal muscle fibers and the fiber-type distribution are similar in women and men; however, for reasons that are unclear, muscle fibers in men are hypertrophied relative to those in women, resulting in greater cross-sectional muscle mass. Although strength adjusted to cross-sectional muscle area is similar in men and women, men's greater muscle mass usually yields greater isometric strength (option C).[9,10] Exercise-induced increases in SV also differ between the sexes. Men manifest a progressive increase in ejection fraction with little or no increase in end-diastolic volume (option D); in contrast, women tend to increase end-diastolic volume without a significant increase in ejection fraction (option E).[11] This results in a plateau of the ejection fraction during exercise in women compared with a progressive increase in men.

106-9. **The answer is D.** *(Hurst's The Heart, 14th Edition, Chap. 106)* Special considerations must be addressed when prescribing exercise for elderly people. A critical factor in an elderly (> 65 years of age) person's ability to function independently is mobility. The overall focus for exercise training should be to enhance health-related fitness, reduce the risk of various chronic diseases, and improve overall quality of life (option A). Considerable evidence demonstrates that physical activity, both endurance and resistance-type exercise, can significantly improve these indices (option B) and facilitate functional independence and overall well-being.[12-18] However, the exercise capacity of elderly persons, both before and after exercise training, is usually lower.[12,19,20] Furthermore, because some in this age group may have been sedentary for years, specific muscle groups are often markedly deconditioned. In addition, musculoskeletal limitations, particularly arthritis, can be severely limiting. Thus, it is important to prescribe an exercise program with low-level energy expenditure, particularly during the first few weeks (option C), with gradual increases thereafter. In these instances, however, participants can be encouraged to increase the frequency of exercise (with shorter duration), even to perhaps several times per day. Higher-intensity training must be recommended with caution in this age group because of the potential for musculoskeletal injury.

106-10. **The answer is C.** *(Hurst's The Heart, 14th Edition, Chap. 106)* Meta-analyses of randomized controlled trials of exercise in both hypertensive and normotensive individuals suggest a 3- to 4-mm Hg decline in systolic blood pressure and a 2- to 3-mm Hg decline in diastolic blood pressure with both aerobic and resistive exercise training (option A).[21,22] From a public health perspective, even such modest effects on blood pressure significantly affect CVD mortality.[23] When combined with dietary intervention, exercise lowers the incident rate of new diabetes in high-risk individuals by 42%.[24] Furthermore, it is superior to metformin in the prevention of type 2 diabetes (option B), and at least a portion of its beneficial effects appears to be independent of weight loss.[24] Exercise training can improve physiologic indices, including exercise tolerance, ventricular function, skeletal muscle function, peripheral blood flow, endothelial function, diastolic function, and quality of life.[25,26] Experience has revealed that exercise in HF is safe and well tolerated if it is appropriately prescribed and that it augments the benefits of cardiac resynchronization therapy (option C).[27,28] Resistance training has also gained favor in the treatment of obesity. Substantial evidence supports the idea that resistance training increases total fat-free mass, muscular strength, and resting metabolic rate, as well as mobilizing visceral adipose tissue in the abdominal region (option D).[29] Additional effects of exercise in secondary prevention are on coagulation, autonomic function, anti-ischemic and antiarrhythmic effects, and a decrease in age-related disability (option E).

References

1. Thomas SN, Schroeder T, Secher NH, et al. Cerebral blood flow during submaximal and maximal dynamic exercise in humans. *J Appl Physiol.* 1989;67(2):744-748.
2. Pescatello LS, Fargo AE, Leach CN Jr, et al. Short-term effect of dynamic exercise on arterial blood pressure. *Circulation.* 1991;83(5):1557-1561.
3. DeBusk RF, Valdez R, Houston N, et al. Cardiovascular responses to dynamic and static effort soon after myocardial infarction. Application to occupational work assessment. *Circulation.* 1978;58(2):368-375.
4. Ghilarducci LE, Holly RG, Amsterdam EA. Effects of high resistance training in coronary artery disease. *Am J Cardiol.* 1989;64(14):866-870.
5. Sparling PB, Cantwell JD, Dolan CM, et al. Strength training in a cardiac rehabilitation program: a six-month follow-up. *Arch Phys Med Rehabil.* 1990;71(2):148-152.
6. Ehsani AA, Hagberg JM, Hickson RC. Rapid changes in ventricular dimensions and mass in response to physical conditioning and deconditioning. *Am J Cardiol.* 1972;42:52-56.
7. Saltin B. Physiologic effects on physical conditioning. *Med Sci Sports.* 1969;1:50-56.
8. Drinkwater BL. Women and exercise: physiological aspects. *Exerc Sport Sci Rev.* 1984;12:21-51.
9. Astrand PO, Rodahl K. *Textbook of Work Physiology, Physiological Basis of Exercise.* New York: McGraw-Hill; 1986.
10. Li H, Sui X, Huang S, et al. Secular change in cardiorespiratory fitness and body composition of women: the Aerobics Center Longitudinal Study. *Mayo Clin Proc.* 2015;90(1): 43-52.
11. Higginbotham MB, Morris KG, Coleman RE, et al. Sex-related differences in the normal cardiac response to upright exercise. *Circulation.* 1984;70(3):357-366.
12. Brown M, Holloszy JO. Effects of a low-intensity exercise program on selected physical performance characteristics of 60- to 71-year olds. *Aging (Milano).* 1991;3(2):129-139.
13. Emery CF, Hauck ER, Blumenthal JA. Exercise adherence or maintenance among older adults: 1-year follow-up study. *Psychol Aging.* 1992;7(3):466-470.
14. King AC, Haskell WL, Young DR, et al. Long-term effects of varying intensities and formats of physical activity on participation rates, fitness, and lipoproteins in men and women aged 50 to 65 years. *Circulation.* 1995;91(10):2596-2604.
15. Shephard RJ. Exercise and aging: extending independence in older adults. *Geriatrics.* 1993;48(5):61-64.
16. Stewart AL, King AC, Haskell WL. Endurance exercise and health-related quality of life in 50-65-year-old adults. *Gerontologist.* 1993;33(6):782-789.
17. Doll JA, Hellkamp A, Ho PM, et al. Participation in cardiac rehabilitation programs among older patients after acute myocardial infarction. *JAMA Intern Med.* 2015;175(10):1700-1702.
18. Hupin D, Roche F, Gremeaux V, et al. Even a low-dose of moderate-to-vigorous physical activity reduces mortality by 22% in adults aged ≥60 years: a systematic review and meta-analysis. *Br J Sports Med.* 2015;49(19):1262-1267.
19. Williams MA, Maresh CM, Esterbrooks DJ, et al. Early exercise training in patients older than age 65 years compared with that in younger patients after acute myocardial infarction or coronary artery bypass grafting. *Am J Cardiol.* 1985;55(4):263-266.
20. Woo JS, Derleth C, Stratton JR, et al. The influence of age, gender, and training on exercise efficiency. *J Am Coll Cardiol.* 2006;47(5):1049-1057.
21. Suaya JA, Stason WB, Ades PA, et al. Cardiac rehabilitation and survival in older coronary patients. *J Am Coll Cardiol.* 2009;54(1):25-33.
22. Whelton SP, Chin A, Xin X, et al. Effect of aerobic exercise on blood pressure: a meta-analysis of randomized, controlled trials. *Ann Intern Med.* 2002;136(7):493-503.
23. Carlson DJ, Dieberg G, Hess NC, et al. Isometric exercise training for blood pressure management: a systematic review and meta-analysis. *Mayo Clin Proc.* 2014;89(3): 327-334.
24. Laaksonen DE, Lindstrom J, Lakka TA, et al. Physical activity in the prevention of type 2 diabetes: the Finnish diabetes prevention study. *Diabetes.* 2005;54(1):158-165.
25. Giannuzzi P, Temporelli PL, Corra U, et al. Attenuation of unfavorable remodeling by exercise training in postinfarction patients with left ventricular dysfunction: results of the exercise in left ventricular dysfunction (ELVD) trial. *Circulation.* 1997;96(6):1790-1797.

26. Flynn KE, Pina IL, Whellan DJ, et al. Effects of exercise training on health status in patients with chronic heart failure: HF-ACTION randomized controlled trial. *JAMA*. 2009;301(14):1451-1459.
27. Patwala AY, Woods PR, Sharp L, et al. Maximizing patient benefit from cardiac resyn-chronization therapy with the addition of structured exercise training: a randomized controlled study. *J Am Coll Cardiol*. 2009;53(25):2332-2339.
28. O'Connor CM, Whellan DJ, Lee KL, et al. Efficacy and safety of exercise training in patients with chronic heart failure: HF-ACTION randomized controlled trial. *JAMA*. 2009;301(14):1439-1450.
29. Tresierras MA, Balady GJ. Resistance training in the treatment of diabetes and obesity: mechanisms and outcomes. *Cardiopulm Rehabil Prev*. 2009;29(2):67-75.

SECTION 16

Populations and Social Determinants of Cardiovascular Disease

CHAPTER 107

Social Determinants of Cardiovascular Disease

Mark J. Eisenberg

QUESTIONS

DIRECTIONS: Choose the one best response to each question.

107-1. If current trends prevail, the prevalence of cardiovascular disease (CVD) in the United States is expected to rise 10% between 2010 and 2030. To what factors can this projected rise in CVD prevalence *not* be attributed?

A. An aging populace
B. An increase in major risk factors (hypertension, lack of physical activity, obesity, and diabetes)
C. Growing socioeconomic inequality
D. An increase in immigration from developing countries
E. Inequalities in the availability of clinical advances made in the diagnosis, treatment, and prevention of CVD

107-2. A 30-year-old indigenous woman presents to her local community clinic after reporting that she has been feeling unwell. Her history reveals she has type 2 diabetes and a history of alcoholism, and she suffers from major depression. Which of the following is *true* about this patient's circumstances?

A. Health disparities are likely contributors to this patient's poor health
B. Health inequalities are likely contributors to this patient's poor health
C. Health outcome disparities result from the effects of institutional barriers, provider barriers (such as cultural insensitivity, language barriers, unconscious bias, or frank racism), and patient issues (such as cultural beliefs, health literacy, adherence, and trust of the medical profession)
D. Both A and C are correct
E. All of the above are correct

107-3. Choose the *incorrect* statement:

A. Heart disease is considered a disease of affluence
B. Heart disease has emerged in both developed and developing countries
C. Evidence shows the rise and fall in the prevalence of CVD varies according to a country's stage of economic development
D. Economic globalization is a powerful mitigator of the present-day, expanding global epidemic of heart disease
E. The poorest regions of the world still see relatively low rates of CVD

107-4. Major social determinants of health include all *except* which of the following?

A. Socioeconomic status (SES)
B. Race/ethnicity
C. Sex
D. Environment
E. All of the above are social determinants of health

107-5. A 60-year-old woman presents to your clinic for a cardiac consult after reporting feeling chest pain upon physical exertion. Which of the following statements about the treatment of heart disease in women is *false*?

A. Women receive less significant treatment for CVD risk factors
B. Women are significantly more likely to be referred to cardiac rehabilitation
C. Women are more likely to experience a delay in door-to-balloon times
D. Women continue to be underrepresented in clinical trials
E. Women suffer greater in-hospital mortality before age 55 after myocardial infarction

107-6. Which of the following statements concerning morbidity and mortality among racial and ethnic minorities in the United States is *false*?

A. Hispanics have higher mortality rates than non-Hispanic whites

B. The prevalence of diabetes in Hispanic women is double that of white women

C. Almost 50% of African American women in the United States have some form of CVD

D. CVD accounts for the largest proportion of inequality in life expectancy between blacks and whites

E. Racial and ethnic minorities are less likely to have health insurance

107-7. A 41-year-old man is referred to your care from the local community clinic. He is visibly unkempt, and you learn that he has been transiently homeless for the last two years. His living circumstances have been a great source of stress in his life. You remember reading that the allostatic load (AL) heuristic model can help you understand how chronic stress may be driving this patient's ill health. Which of the following statements concerning the AL model is *false*?

A. Cumulative chronic stress is thought to lead to long-term dysregulation of allostasis

B. Evidence increasingly shows people with low SES have higher AL scores

C. Black men and women have lower AL scores than whites

D. AL burden partially explains higher mortality among blacks, independent of SES and health behaviors

E. SES adversity experience may accumulate throughout life and have a negative impact on multiple organ systems in adulthood

107-8. Over the course of your research on the social determinants of CVD, you come across an official document reporting on the occurrence of various deleterious health behaviors in the United States. Which of the following statements you have read in this report is most likely *false*?

A. Children in lower socioeconomic groups have a steeper weight gain trajectory from birth

B. Between 2003 and 2012, obesity decreased among those of higher SES but increased among those of lower SES

C. High rates of obesity are found among all racial/ethnic groups, but in particular among American Indians and Alaska Native populations

D. Differences in health behaviors account for all of the observed socioeconomic gradient in CVD

E. All of the above are correct

107-9. Which of the following does *not* constitute a strategy to mitigate disparate CVD care?

A. Performance measure-based quality improvement

B. Provider cultural competency training

C. Team-based care

D. Patient education

E. All of the above are adequate strategies

107-10. In 2011, the US Department of Health and Human Services (DHHS) published its *Action Plan to Reduce Racial and Ethnic Health Disparities*. Which of the following statements is *not* included among the five goals of this plan?

A. Transform health care

B. Strengthen the nation's health and human services infrastructure and workforce

C. Advance the health, safety, and well-being of the American people

D. Translate and disseminate research information

E. Increase the efficiency, transparency, and accountability of DHHS programs

107-1. The answer is D. (*Hurst's The Heart, 14th Edition, Chap. 107*) Cardiovascular disease is the number one cause of death around the globe, now accounting for about one in three deaths.[1] More than 80% of these CVD deaths take place in low- and middle-income countries.[2] Although mortality from CVD in the United States has been declining since the 1970s, heart disease is still the leading cause of death in America as well, accounting for approximately 31.3% of deaths in 2011.[3] The US decline in CVD mortality has been attributed to advances in prevention, diagnosis, and treatment. However, if current trends prevail, the prevalence of CVD in the United States is expected to *rise* 10% between 2010 and 2030.[4] This projected rise in CVD prevalence is attributed to a number of factors: an aging populace (option A), an increase in major risk factors (hypertension, lack of physical activity, obesity, and diabetes) (option B), and growing socioeconomic inequality (option C) that accentuate the deleterious social determinants of health. Further, the clinical advances made in the diagnosis, treatment, and prevention of CVD have not been equally available to everyone in our society (option E).[5] The United States is one of the richest nations in the world and spends more per capita on health care than any other nation, and yet America has one of the shortest life expectancies at birth of any industrialized nation, ranking 27th out of 34 Organization for Economic Cooperation and Development countries.[6]

107-2. The answer is E. (*Hurst's The Heart, 14th Edition, Chap. 107*) WHO defines *social determinants of health* as "the circumstances in which people grow, live, work, and age, and the systems put in place to deal with illness. The conditions in which people live and die are, in turn, shaped by political, social, and economic forces."[7] This broad definition recognizes that the social determinants of health are multifactorial, deeply interrelated, complex, and driven by a multitude of forces, including social, cultural, economic, and political forces. Although everyone is affected by the society in which he or she lives, some are more burdened than others by social and economic disadvantages, which in turn can result in *health disparities*. Health disparities are defined as "differences that occur by gender, race or ethnicity, education or income, disability, geographic location, or sexual orientation" (option A).[8] With respect to differences in health outcomes, the term refers to those outcomes that persist despite controlling for access to care and patient clinical factors. These outcome disparities signal the effects of institutional barriers, provider barriers (such as cultural insensitivity, language barriers, unconscious bias, or frank racism), and patient issues (such as cultural beliefs, health literacy, adherence, and trust of the medical profession) (option C).[9] The term *health disparities* not only typically connotes that the observed differences are unnecessary and avoidable, but that they are unjust as well. Some prefer to use the term *health inequalities* (option B) rather than health disparities to highlight the injustice of the observed differences in health status and health outcomes that characterize our society, while others use the two terms interchangeably.[10]

107-3. The answer is D. (*Hurst's The Heart, 14th Edition, Chap. 107*) Heart disease is considered a disease of affluence (option A). It has emerged in both developed and developing countries (option B) as industrialization and urbanization have homogenized patterns of consumption and lifestyle practices. Evidence shows that the rise and fall in the prevalence of CVD varies according to a country's stage of economic development (option C).[11] And while the poorest regions of the world still see relatively low rates of CVD (option E), regions within developing countries that are marked by increasing wealth and adoption of the Western lifestyle have seen a rapid rise in heart disease. The epidemiologic transition we are witnessing in developing countries has been compressed into a few decades, whereas the epidemic of heart disease observed in Western developed nations took place over the course of a century.[12] The swift pace of economic globalization and the rapid diffusion of the Western lifestyle are thought to be powerful drivers of the present-day, expanding global epidemic of heart disease (option D).[13]

107-4. **The answer is E.** *(Hurst's The Heart, 14th Edition, Chap. 107)* Among the major social determinants of health are SES (option A), race/ethnicity (option B), sex (option C), the environment (including social relationships, neighborhood physical and social environments, and work environment) (option D), and access to care. There is a substantial body of literature on each of these social determinants of health and also on theories of how they interact to maintain health or contribute to illness. It is beyond the scope of this chapter to explore each in detail.

107-5. **The answer is B.** *(Hurst's The Heart, 14th Edition, Chap. 107)* CVD is the leading cause of death in women in the United States, and it kills more women than the next three leading causes of death combined.[3] Significant disparities exist in cardiovascular risk factors, treatment, and outcomes based on sex.[3] Scientific evidence shows that women receive less significant treatment for CVD risk factors (option A),[14,15] are often not treated according to recommended guidelines for a number of CVD diagnoses,[16] have lower long-term adherence with statins[17] and antihypertensive medications,[18] are given significantly lower priority for emergent ambulance service than men,[19] undergo fewer invasive procedures (eg, percutaneous coronary intervention and bypass surgery),[20,21] are more likely to experience a delay in door-to-balloon times (option C),[22,23] suffer greater in-hospital mortality before age 55 after myocardial infarction (option E),[24,25] experience greater long-term mortality after myocardial infarction,[26,27] and are significantly less likely to be referred to cardiac rehabilitation (option B).[28] Further, women continue to be underrepresented in clinical trials (option D), and publications often lack sex-stratified analyses, which limits our ability to identify sex differences and provide evidence-based care that ensures safety and efficacy by sex.[29] (US legislation that requires sex-specific analysis is expected to improve these sex inequities in biomedical research.) Although biology may underlie some of these observed differences, sex bias is thought to play a substantial role in creating these health disparities.

107-6. **The answer is A.** *(Hurst's The Heart, 14th Edition, Chap. 107)* Racial and ethnic minority populations are disproportionately burdened with more illness, premature death, and disability, and they often suffer higher mortality rates than whites.[10,30] It is CVD that accounts for the largest proportion of inequality in life expectancy between blacks and whites (option D): in the United States, blacks are two to three times more likely to die of heart disease than whites.[3] Racial and ethnic minorities are less likely to have health insurance (option E),[31] face greater barriers in accessing health care, and often receive lower-quality care.[9,32] Even when minority patients have the same type of health insurance as whites, evidence reveals they tend to receive lower quality of care.[9,32] Almost 50% of African American women in the United States have some form of CVD (option C).[3] Hispanics, the largest minority in the United States, have a higher prevalence of several cardiovascular risk factors than non-Hispanic whites. Notably, Hispanic women have twice the prevalence of diabetes that white women do (about 12% vs 6%) (option B) and they often face the challenge of low SES and poor access to health care, yet Hispanics have lower mortality rates than non-Hispanic whites (option A). This has been called the "Hispanic paradox" and has been confirmed by recent cardiovascular data.[33]

107-7. **The answer is C.** *(Hurst's The Heart, 14th Edition, Chap. 107)* Allostatic load (AL) is a useful heuristic model that helps conceptualize how chronic stress drives pathophysiologic mechanisms. Cumulative chronic stress is thought to lead to long-term dysregulation of allostasis (option A) through the activation of the sympathetic nervous system and hypothalamic-pituitary axis, which promotes maladaptive wear and tear on the brain and body that, in turn, compromises resiliency.[34] Evidence is accumulating that shows people with low SES have higher AL scores (option B) (indicating greater dysregulation and increased vulnerability to disease) than those in high SES groups. One investigation studied AL scores based on 10 biomarkers and examined cardiovascular/diabetes-related mortality disparities between blacks and whites. Researchers found that black men and women had higher AL scores than whites (option C), and they concluded that AL burden partially explains higher mortality among blacks, independent of SES and health behaviors (option D).[35] This may be one of the mechanisms through which racism and discrimination exert their destructive effects. Discrimination is a source of acute and chronic stress for many oppressed group members.[36-39] SES adversity experience may accumulate throughout life and have a negative impact on multiple organ systems in adulthood, especially the cardiovascular system (option E).[40-42] Many studies in the literature now document the deleterious effects of chronic stress on the cardiovascular system, including activation of the inflammatory response, endothelial dysfunction, thrombosis, vascular hyperactivity, and metabolic disturbances.[43-47]

107-8. **The answer is D.** *(Hurst's The Heart, 14th Edition, Chap. 107)* Deleterious health behaviors (eg, smoking, inactivity, poor diet, medication nonadherence) increase the risk of CVD. According to the most recent American Heart Association statistics, between 2003 and 2012, obesity decreased among those of higher SES but increased among those of lower SES (option B).[3] Children in lower socioeconomic groups have a steeper weight gain trajectory from birth (option A), with a strong socioeconomic gradient in the prevalence of child and adult obesity.[48] It appears the die is cast early in life, as childhood SES has been shown to account for both the uptake of unhealthy behaviors and subsequent health risk in the adult years. Health behaviors vary according to race and ethnicity as well as SES. High rates of obesity are found among all racial/ethnic groups, but in particular among American Indians and Alaska Native populations (option C), of whom 39.4% are obese compared with 24.3% of non-Hispanic whites.[49] Differences in health behaviors are seen among racial and ethnic minorities. This presents the opportunity to focus interventions to promote behavioral change among high-risk populations. However, although differences in health behaviors account for some of the observed socioeconomic gradient in CVD, they do not account for all of it (option D).

107-9. **The answer is E.** *(Hurst's The Heart, 14th Edition, Chap. 107)* Comprehensively speaking, initiatives to address the CVD epidemic must entail addressing individual-level actions, health care systems, and population-wide efforts. Proximate risk factors for CVD (genomic, biologic, and behavioral) must be addressed at the individual level, and diagnosis and treatment of CVD must always receive high priority. Within this context, individual-level approaches should target high-risk individuals, especially those who are socially disadvantaged. But individual-level approaches are not enough. Public policy initiatives are needed that focus on improving access to health insurance. Further, barriers to access to care, which are multiple, need to be addressed systemically across the health care system. Evidence suggests that performance measure-based quality improvement (option A), provider cultural competency training (option B), team-based care (option C), and patient education (option D) are effective strategies for mitigating disparate CVD care and may improve outcomes.[50] The American College of Cardiology's Coalition to Reduce Racial and Ethnic Disparities in Cardiovascular Disease Outcomes (CREDO) is predicated on these strategies.

107-10. **The answer is D.** *(Hurst's The Heart, 14th Edition, Chap. 107)* In 2011 the DHHS published its *Action Plan to Reduce Racial and Ethnic Health Disparities*.[51] The goals of the plan are to (1) transform health care (option A); (2) strengthen the nation's health and human services infrastructure and workforce (option B); (3) advance the health, safety, and well-being of the American people (option C); (4) advance scientific knowledge and innovation; and (5) increase the efficiency, transparency, and accountability of DHHS programs (option E).

References

1. Lozano R, Naghavi M, Foreman K, et al. Global and regional mortality from 235 causes of death for 20 age groups in 1990 and 2010: a systematic analysis for the Global Burden of Disease Study 2010. *Lancet.* 2012;380:2095-2128.

2. World Health Organization. *Global Status Report on Noncommunicable Diseases 2014.* Geneva, Switzerland: World Health Organization; 2014.

3. Mozaffarian D, Benjamin EJ, Go AS, et al. Heart disease and stroke statistics–2015 update: a report from the American Heart Association. *Circulation.* 2015;131(4):e29-322.

4. Heidenreich PA, Albert NM, Allen LA, et al. Forecasting the impact of heart failure in the United States: a policy statement from the American Heart Association. *Circ Heart Fail.* 2013;6:606-619.

5. Pearson TA, Palaniappan LP, Artinian NT, et al. American Heart Association guide for improving cardiovascular health at the community level, 2013 update: a scientific statement for public health practitioners, healthcare providers, and health policy makers. *Circulation.* 2013;127:1730-1753.

6. Organisation for Economic Co-operation and Development. *OECD Health Statistics 2014.* http://www.oecd.org/unitedstates/Briefing-Note-UNITED-STATES-2014.pdf. Accessed November 20, 2016.

7. Commission on Social Determinants of Health. *Closing the Gap in a Generation: Health Equity through Action on the Social Determinants of Health.* Final report of the Commission on Social Determinants of Health. Geneva, Switzerland: World Health Organization; 2008. http://www.who.int/social_determinants/thecommission/final¬report/en/. Accessed December 15, 2015.

8. US Department of Health and Human Services. *Healthy People 2010.* 2nd ed. Washington, DC: US Department of Health and Human Services; 2000.

9. Institute of Medicine, Committee on Understanding and Eliminating Racial and Ethnic Disparities in Health Care. *Unequal Treatment: Confronting Racial and Ethnic Disparities in Health Care.* Washington, DC: National Academy Press; 2003.

10. Centers for Disease Control and Prevention. CDC health disparities and inequalities report—United States, 2013. *Morb Mortal Wkly Rep.* 2013;62(Suppl 3):1-189.

11. Stallones R. The rise and fall of ischemic heart disease. *Sci Am.* 1980;243:53-59.

12. Srinath K, Reddy D. Cardiovascular disease in non-Western countries. *N Engl J Med.* 2004;350:2438-2440.

13. Faergeman O. The societal context of coronary heart disease. *Eur Heart J.* 2005;7(suppl):A5-A11.

14. Jarvie JL, Foody JM. Recognizing and improving health care disparities in the prevention of cardiovascular disease in women. *Curr Cardiol Rep.* 2010;12(6):488-496.

15. Leifheit-Limson EC, D'Onofrio G, Daneshvar M, et al. Sex differences in cardiac risk factors, perceived risk, and health care provider discussion of risk and risk modification among young patients with acute myocardial infarction: the VIRGO study. *J Am Coll Cardiol.* 2015;66(18):1949-1957.

16. Hebert K, Lopez B, Horswell R, et al. The impact of a standardized disease management program on race/ethnicity and gender disparities in care and mortality. *J Health Care Poor Underserved.* 2010;21(1):264-276.

17. Lewey J, Shrank WH, Bowry AD, Kilabuk E, Brennan TA, Choudhry NK. Gender and racial disparities in adherence to statin therapy: a meta-analysis. *Am Heart J.* 2013;165(5):665-678.

18. Chapman RH, Benner JS, Petrilla AA, et al. Predictors of adherence with antihypertensive and lipid-lowering therapy. *Arch Intern Med.* 2005;165:1147-1152.

19. Melberg T, Kindervaag B, Rosland J. Gender-specific ambulance priority and delays to primary percutaneous coronary intervention: a consequence of the patients' presentation or the management at the emergency medical communications center? *Am Heart J.* 2013;166:839-845.

20. Wenger NK. Gender disparity in cardiovascular disease: bias or biology? *Expert Rev Cardiovasc Ther.* 2012;10(11):1401-1411.

21. Mumma BE, Baumann BM, Diercks DB, et al. Sex bias in cardiovascular testing: the contribution of patient preference. *Ann Emerg Med.* 2011;57(6):551-560.e4.

22. D'Onofrio G, Safdar B, Lichtman JH, et al. Sex differences in reperfusion in young patients with ST-segment-elevation myocardial infarction: results from the VIRGO study. *Circulation.* 2015;131(15):1324-1332.

23. Dreyer RP, Beltrame JF, Tavella R, et al. Evaluation of gender differences in door-to-balloon time in ST-elevation myocardial infarction. *Heart Lung Circ.* 2013;22:861-869.

24. Izadnegahdar M, Singer J, Lee MK, et al. Do younger women fare worse? Sex differences in acute myocardial infarction hospitalization and early mortality rates over ten years. *J Womens Health.* 2014;23(1):10-17.

25. Zhang Z, Fang J, Gillespie C, Wang G, Hong Y, Yoon PW. Age-specific gender differences in in-hospital mortality by type of acute myocardial infarction. *Am J Cardiol.* 2012;109(8):1097-1103.

26. Bucholz EM, Butala NM, Rathore SS, Dreyer RP, Lansky AJ, Krumholz HM. Sex differences in long-term mortality after myocardial infarction: a systematic review. *Circulation.* 2014;130(9):757-767.

27. Pancholy SB, Shantha GP, Patel T, Cheskin LJ. Sex differences in short-term and long-term all-cause mortality among patients with ST-segment elevation myocardial infarction treated by primary percutaneous intervention: a meta-analysis. *JAMA Intern Med.* 2014;174(11):1822-1830.

28. Colella TJ, Gravely S, Marzolini S, et al. Sex bias in referral of women to outpatient cardiac rehabilitation? A meta-analysis. *Eur J Prev Cardiol.* 2015;22:423-441.

29. Wenger NK. Gender disparity in cardiovascular disease: bias or biology? *Expert Rev Cardiovasc Ther.* 2012;10(11):1401-1411.

30. Foraker RE, Patel MD, Whitsel EA, Suchindran CM, Heiss G, Rose KM. Neighborhood socioeconomic disparities and 1-year case fatality after incident myocardial infarction: the Atherosclerosis Risk in Communities (ARIC) Community Surveillance (1992–2002). *Am Heart J.* 2013;165(1):102-107.

31. Kaiser Family Foundation. State health facts: uninsured rates for the nonelderly by race/ethnicity, 2012. http://kff.org/uninsured/state-indicator/rate-by-raceethnicity/. Accessed December 28, 2015.

32. Agency for Healthcare Research and Quality. *2012 National Healthcare Disparities Report.* http://archive.ahrq.gov/research/findings/nhqrdr/nhdr12/index.html. Accessed December 28, 2015.

33. Cortes-Bergoderi M, Goel K, Murad MH, et al. Cardiovascular mortality in Hispanics compared to non-Hispanic whites: a systematic review and meta-analysis of the Hispanic paradox. *Eur J Intern Med.* 2013;24(8):791-799.

34. McEwen BS, Gianaros PJ. Central role of the brain in stress and adaptation: links to socioeconomic status, health, and disease. *Ann N Y Acad Sci.* 2010;1186:190-222.

35. Duru OK, Harawa NT, Kermah D, Norris KC. Allostatic load burden and racial disparities in mortality. *J Natl Med Assoc.* 2012;104(1-2):89-95.

36. Wyatt SB, Williams DR, Calvin R, Henderson FC, Walker ER, Winters K. Racism and cardiovascular disease in African Americans. *Am J Med Sci.* 2003;325(6):315-331.

37. Clark R. Significance of perceived racism: toward understanding ethnic group disparities in health, the later years in critical perspectives on racial and ethnic differences in health in late life. In Anderson NB, Bulatao RA, Cohen B, eds. *National Research Council (US) Panel on Race, Ethnicity, and Health in Later Life.* Washington, DC: National Academies Press; 2004.

38. Brondolo E, Love EE, Pencille M, Schoenthaler A, Ogedegbe G. Racism and hypertension: a review of the empirical evidence and implications for clinical practice. *Am J Hypertens.* 2011;24(5):518-529.

39. Dolezsar CM, McGrath JJ, Herzig AJ, Miller SB. Perceived racial discrimination and hypertension: a comprehensive systematic review. *Health Psychol.* 2014;33(1):20-34.

40. Gruenewald TL, Karlamangla AS, Hu P, et al. History of socioeconomic disadvantage and allostatic load in later life. *Soc Sci Med.* 2012;74(1):75-83.

41. Seeman T, Epel E, Gruenewald T, Karlamangla A, McEwen BS. Socio-economic differ-entials in peripheral biology: cumulative allostatic load. *Ann NY Acad Sci.* 2010;1186: 223-239.

42. Whisman MA. Loneliness and the metabolic syndrome in a population-based sample of middle-aged and older adults. *Health Psychol.* 2010;29:550-554.

43. Ferdinand KC. Coronary artery disease in minority racial and ethnic groups in the United States. *Am J Cardiol.* 2006;97(2A):12A-19A.

44. Albert MA, Glynn RJ, Buring J, Ridker PM. Impact of traditional and novel risk factors on the relationship between socioeconomic status and incident cardiovascular events. *Circulation.* 2006;114:2619-2626.

45. Loucks EB, Pilote L, Lynch JW, et al. Life course socioeconomic position is associated with inflammatory markers: the Framingham Offspring Study. *Soc Sci Med.* 2010;71:187-195.

46. Liu J, Fox CS, Hickson D, et al. Fatty liver, abdominal visceral fat and cardiometabolic risk factors: the Jackson Heart Study. *Arterioscler Thromb Vasc Biol.* 2011;31(11): 2715-2722.

47. Daviglus ML, Talavera GA, Avilés-Santa ML, et al. Prevalence of major cardiovascular risk factors and cardiovascular diseases among Hispanic/Latino individuals of diverse backgrounds in the United States. *JAMA.* 2012;308:1775-1784.

48. Cameron AJ, Spence AC, Laws R, Hesketh KD, Lioret S, Campbell KJ. A review of the relationship between socioeconomic position and the early-life predictors of obesity. *Curr Obes Rep.* 2015;4(3):350-362.

49. Hutchinson RN, Shin S. Systematic review of health disparities for cardiovascular diseases and associated factors among American Indian and Alaska Native populations. *PLoS One.* 2014;9(1):e80973.

50. Yancy CW, Wang TY, Ventura HO, et al. The coalition to reduce racial and ethnic disparities in cardiovascular disease outcomes (credo): why credo matters to cardiologists. *J Am Coll Cardiol.* 2011;57(3): 245-252.

51. US Department of Health and Human Services, Office of the Secretary, Office of the Assistant Secretary for Planning and Evaluation, and Office of Minority Health. *HHS Action Plan to Reduce Racial and Ethnic Health Disparities.* Washington, DC: Office of the Assistant Secretary for Planning and Evaluation; 2011.

CHAPTER 108

Women and Ischemic Heart Disease: An Evolving Saga

Mark J. Eisenberg

QUESTIONS

DIRECTIONS: Choose the one best response to each question.

108-1. Which of the following statements about women and ischemic heart disease is *false*?

A. Women have greater CVD mortality than men
B. Despite reporting more disability, women report better quality of life than men
C. Women present later and with more comorbid conditions than men
D. Women receive fewer medical therapies and fewer interventions than men
E. The underuse of guideline-based preventive and therapeutic strategies for women is a substantial contributor to their less favorable coronary outcomes

108-2. A 60-year-old woman presents to your clinic complaining of a burning sensation in her chest at rest, which radiates down her arm. Which of the following statements concerning the development or manifestation of heart disease in women is *correct*?

A. Obstructive atherosclerotic disease of the epicardial coronary arteries remains the major cause of acute myocardial infarction (MI) for women
B. Plaque characteristics differ for women, with recent data suggesting a greater role of macrovascular disease and obstructive coronary artery disease (CAD) in the pathophysiology of coronary events in women
C. Women have more severe obstructive CAD at angiography than men
D. Both A and C are correct
E. All of the above are correct

108-3. "Sex differences" are:

A. Biologic differences, such as genetic and hormonal, increasingly acknowledged to exist even at the cellular level
B. Physiologic differences, such as a higher resting coronary blood flow
C. Another term for "gender differences"
D. Both A and B are correct
E. All of the above are correct

108-4. Approximately 15.5 million Americans live with CAD. What percentage of adult women is included within this figure?

A. 1%
B. 3%
C. 5%
D. 10%
E. 15%

108-5. A 57-year-old woman presents to your clinic for a follow-up regarding previously diagnosed CVD. Which of the following statements is *true* about the pathologic nature of this patient's atherosclerotic plaque?

A. Although plaque rupture explains half of fatal coronary events among men, 76% of events in women are due to plaque rupture
B. Plaque erosion is more common in women
C. Atherosclerotic plaque in women is defined as being less fibrous than in men
D. Both A and B are correct
E. All of the above are correct

108-6. Which of the following pregnancy complications is *not* an early indicator of increased CVD risk?

A. Preeclampsia
B. Gestational diabetes
C. Pregnancy-induced hypertension
D. Preterm delivery
E. All of the above are early indicators of increased CVD risk

108-7. A 28-year-old woman presents to your clinic for a routine check-up. She reports smoking fewer than 10 cigarettes a day, and only socially. Which of the following statements about cigarette smoking in women is *false*?

A. Although cigarette smoking rates have decreased globally, the decline is less for men than for women
B. The number of female smokers is increasing, particularly in developing countries
C. The CVD risk for female smokers is 25% higher than for male smokers
D. Smoking in association with oral contraceptive use increases the risk of acute MI, stroke, and venous thromboembolism
E. Smoking cessation is the most cost-effective risk-modifying program

108-8. Candidates for stress imaging include intermediate- or high-risk women who meet which of the following clinical criteria?

A. Functionally disabled
B. An abnormal resting ECG precluding accurate assessment of exercise-induced changes
C. High likelihood of CAD
D. Both A and B are correct
E. All of the above are correct

108-9. Which of the following statements concerning angiographic procedures in women is *false*?

A. Approximately half of women referred for angiography do not have obstructive CAD
B. Myocardial ischemia or evidence of vascular dysfunction in the setting of angiographically normal coronary arteries is a frequent occurrence in women
C. There are no diagnostic techniques that are capable of interrogating the coronary microcirculation
D. Across all female patient subsets with acute and stable ischemic heart disease, there is a lower frequency of nonobstructive CAD than in male patients
E. The adjusted hazard for major CAD events is increased approximately 90% for women and men with diffuse nonobstructive CAD

108-10. What percentage of the CABG surgical population do women constitute?

A. 10% to 20%
B. 20% to 30%
C. 30% to 40%
D. 40% to 50%
E. More than 50%

108-1. **The answer is B.** *(Hurst's The Heart, 14th Edition, Chap. 108)* Women have greater CVD mortality (option A) and report more disability and decreased quality of life (option B). They present later and with more comorbid conditions (option C) yet receive fewer medical therapies and fewer interventions than men (option D), contributing to sex-specific gaps in outcomes. These differences probably reflect both lingering diagnostic and treatment disparities and underlying biological differences. The underuse of guideline-based preventive and therapeutic strategies for women is a substantial contributor to their less favorable coronary outcomes (option E), but the spectrum of sex differences likely reflects a combination of biology and bias.

108-2. **The answer is A.** *(Hurst's The Heart, 14th Edition, Chap. 108)* The term *ischemic heart disease* (IHD) is advantageous for women because of women's lower prevalence of anatomic obstructive CAD, despite greater myocardial ischemia and associated mortality when compared to men.[1-3] Although obstructive atherosclerotic disease of the epicardial coronary arteries remains the major cause of acute MI for women (option A), symptomatic women with myocardial ischemia remain at risk even with no or minimal epicardial CAD.[4] Sex differences in nonobstructive CAD are an area of active investigation. Plaque characteristics also differ for women, with recent data suggesting a greater role of microvascular disease and nonobstructive CAD in the pathophysiology of coronary events in women (option B).[5] Other contributors to myocardial ischemia include coronary vasospasm, microvascular disease, endothelial dysfunction, and intramural coronary atherosclerosis, (ie, atherosclerotic plaque in the luminal wall with external remodeling).[6-9] The paradox of acute coronary events in women is that despite older age and a greater risk factor and anginal symptom burden with consequent morbidity and mortality, women have less severe obstructive CAD at angiography (option C).[5] A paradigm shift must occur from the consideration of anatomic obstructive CAD to IHD. Earlier risk detection must resolve the less intensive patterns of care that is more often common among women relative to men, which likely contributes to the sex-based mortality gap.[10]

108-3. **The answer is D.** *(Hurst's The Heart, 14th Edition, Chap. 108)* Sex differences are biologic differences, such as genetic and hormonal, increasingly acknowledged to exist even at the cellular level.[11-14] Sex differences are all encompassing in IHD, including anatomic (eg, smaller coronary blood vessels), physiologic (eg, higher resting coronary blood flow), age/hormonal, comorbid, and other varied risk factors uniquely affecting women. For definitional purposes, the term *gender* relates to self-identification, behavior, and its interaction with societal expectations and roles that affect all facets of IHD detection, risk, and treatment, which also uniquely influence women when compared to men.

108-4. **The answer is C.** *(Hurst's The Heart, 14th Edition, Chap. 108)* Approximately 15.5 million Americans live with CAD, a disease that affects over 5% of adult women and nearly 8% of adult men. In addition to substantial morbidity and mortality, there is a heavy economic burden associated with IHD.[15] At all ages, even among elderly people, women have a lesser prevalence of CAD. However, once clinical manifestations of IHD develop, women have a less favorable outcome than their male peers in the setting of stable IHD, acute coronary syndromes (ACS), and coronary revascularization.

108-5. **The answer is B.** *(Hurst's The Heart, 14th Edition, Chap. 108)* Pathologic data have revealed varied atherosclerotic plaque characteristics as precursors for a fatal cardiac event, including plaque rupture, erosion, and calcified nodules, findings that were also confirmed with invasive methods.[16-18] This evidence supports common mechanisms for acute events that are uniquely different for women and men. For men, plaque rupture is common and is defined within the culprit lesion as a thin, fibrous cap with a large thrombogenic lipid-rich necrotic core, expansive remodeling, and extensive plaque burden.[17-24] Although plaque rupture explains 76% of fatal coronary events among men, only half of events in women were due to plaque rupture (option A).[25] By comparison, plaque erosion is more common in women (option B) and is defined as being more fibrous (option C) ($P < 001$), with a smaller plaque burden ($P = .003$) and reduced positive remodeling ($P = .003$).[19,26-31] These data support sex-specific differences in atherosclerotic plaque, which may underlie the varying presentation and clinical outcome differences that are commonly observed in ACS registries and treatment trials. Moreover, the varying plaque features may also require future development of sex-specific targeted treatment strategies that have yet to be elucidated in current stable or acute IHD trials.

108-6. **The answer is E.** *(Hurst's The Heart, 14th Edition, Chap. 108)* Pregnancy complications, including preeclampsia (option A), gestational diabetes (option B), pregnancy-induced hypertension (option C), preterm delivery (option D), and small for gestational age at birth are early indicators of increased CVD risk. Preterm delivery (< 34 weeks of gestation) appears as an independent risk factor for subsequent long-term CVD morbidity and hospitalizations.[32] This mandates a detailed pregnancy history as an integral component of risk assessment for all women. It has been suggested that pregnancy is the first "stress test" a woman undergoes, in that the CVD and metabolic stresses of pregnancy have the potential for the early prediction of future CVD risk. It is likely that shared risk factors for preeclampsia and CVD are unmasked by the pregnancy, rather than risk being specifically caused by the preeclampsia. Preeclampsia and gestational hypertension increase by three- to sixfold the risk for subsequent hypertension and double the risk for subsequent CVD events, including stroke. Prehypertension during a normotensive pregnancy appears as an independent risk factor for predicting postpartum metabolic syndrome.[33] An increased later risk of cardiomyopathy has also been reported in women with hypertensive disorders of pregnancy.[35] Further, gestational diabetes increases by sevenfold the risk of subsequent development of type 2 diabetes.[34,36-39]

108-7. **The answer is A.** *(Hurst's The Heart, 14th Edition, Chap. 108)* Smoking is the most important preventable cause of MI in women.[40] Although cigarette smoking rates have decreased globally, the decline is less for women than men; in fact, the number of female smokers is increasing, particularly in developing countries. Nearly one in five women in the United States smoke cigarettes, with smoking among younger women more common than in younger men. The CVD risk for female smokers is 25% higher than for male smokers, with cigarette smoking tripling the MI risk for women. Moreover, smoking in association with oral contraceptive use increases the risk of acute MI, stroke, and venous thromboembolism.[41] Smoking cessation is the most cost-effective risk-modifying program.[42,43]

108-8. **The answer is E.** *(Hurst's The Heart, 14th Edition, Chap. 108)* There are decades of available evidence in women indicating that stress imaging, including stress echocardiography, myocardial perfusion SPECT or PET, and CMR imaging, has an improved diagnostic and prognostic accuracy when compared to the exercise ECG.[44-46] Candidates for stress imaging include intermediate- or high-risk women who meet the following clinical criteria: (1) functionally disabled (defined earlier) (option A); (2) an abnormal resting ECG precluding accurate assessment of exercise-induced changes (eg, left ventricular hypertrophy with repolarization changes or significant resting ST-T–wave changes) (option B); or (3) high CAD likelihood (option C).[44,47] Additional details on the appropriate candidates for stress imaging are presented in the ACC's multimodality appropriate use criteria.[48]

108-9. **The answer is D.** *(Hurst's The Heart, 14th Edition, Chap. 108)* Across all female patient subsets with acute and stable IHD, there is a higher frequency of nonobstructive CAD than in male patients (option D).[2,49,50] Included in this analysis are women with mild but obstructive CAD with < 50% stenosis. Approximately half of women referred for angiography do not have obstructive CAD (option A), including women with previously documented ischemia.[5,49,51-54] In the setting of no obstructive CAD, prognosis significantly worsens in the setting of diffuse segmental atherosclerosis (ie, more than four segments involved in the epicardial vessels).[55] The adjusted hazard for major CAD events is increased approximately 90% for women and men with diffuse nonobstructive CAD (option E).[50] Documented myocardial ischemia or evidence of vascular dysfunction in the setting of angiographically normal coronary arteries has been the focus of much research, in large part because of its frequent occurrence in women (option B). There are no diagnostic techniques that are capable of interrogating the coronary microcirculation (option C).[56,57]

108-10. **The answer is B.** *(Hurst's The Heart, 14th Edition, Chap. 108)* Women constitute 20% to 30% of the CABG surgical population (option B), about 180,000 procedures annually. Mortality is greater for women than for men, especially among younger women. Contributing factors may be an increase in nonelective surgery or late referral, reduced use of an arterial conduit, and an excess of procedural complications.

References

1. Smilowitz NR, Sampson BA, Abrecht CR, Siegfried JS, Hochman JS, Reynolds HR. Women have less severe and extensive coronary atherosclerosis in fatal cases of ischemic heart disease: an autopsy study. *Am Heart J.* 2011;161:681-688.
2. Shaw LJ, Shaw RE, Merz CN, et al. Impact of ethnicity and gender differences on angiographic coronary artery disease prevalence and in-hospital mortality in the American College of Cardiology–National Cardiovascular Data Registry. *Circulation.* 2008;117:1787-1801.
3. von Mering GO, Arant CB, Wessel TR, et al. Abnormal coronary vasomotion as a prognostic indicator of cardiovascular events in women: results from the National Heart, Lung, and Blood Institute–Sponsored Women's Ischemia Syndrome Evaluation (WISE). *Circulation.* 2004;109:722-725.
4. Hemingway H, McCallum A, Shipley M, Manderbacka K, Martikainen P, Keskimaki I. Incidence and prognostic implications of stable angina pectoris among women and men. *JAMA.* 2006;295:1404-1411.
5. Bairey Merz CN, Shaw LJ, Reis SE, et al. Insights from the NHLBI-sponsored Women's Ischemia Syndrome Evaluation (WISE) study: part II: gender differences in presentation, diagnosis, and outcome with regard to gender-based pathophysiology of atherosclerosis and macrovascular and microvascular coronary disease. *J Am Coll Cardiol.* 2006;47:S21-S29.
6. Pepine CJ, Ferdinand KC, Shaw LJ, et al. Emergence of nonobstructive coronary artery disease: a woman's problem and need for change in definition on angiography. *J Am Coll Cardiol.* 2015;66:1918-1933.
7. Ohba K, Sugiyama S, Sumida H, et al. Microvascular coronary artery spasm presents distinctive clinical features with endothelial dysfunction as nonobstructive coronary artery disease. *J Am Heart Assoc.* 2012;1:e002485.
8. Pepine CJ, Anderson RD, Sharaf BL, et al. Coronary microvascular reactivity to adenosine predicts adverse outcome in women evaluated for suspected ischemia results from the National Heart, Lung and Blood Institute WISE (Women's Ischemia Syndrome Evaluation) study. *J Am Coll Cardiol.* 2010;55:2825-2832.
9. Khuddus MA, Pepine CJ, Handberg EM, et al. An intravascular ultrasound analysis in women experiencing chest pain in the absence of obstructive coronary artery disease: a substudy from the National Heart, Lung and Blood Institute–Sponsored Women's Ischemia Syndrome Evaluation (WISE). *J Interv Cardiol.* 2010;23:511-519.
10. McSweeney JC, Rosenfeld AG, Abel WM, et al. Preventing and experiencing ischemic heart disease as a woman: state of the science: a scientific statement from the American Heart Association. *Circulation.* 2016;133:1302-1331.
11. Ouyang P, Wenger NK, Taylor D, et al. Strategies and methods to study female-specific cardiovascular health and disease: a guide for clinical scientists. *Biol Sex Diff.* 2016;7:19.
12. Miller VM, Reckelhoff JF. Sex as a biological variable: now what?! *Physiology (Bethesda).* 2016;31:78-80.
13. Miller VM, Rocca WA, Faubion SS. Sex differences research, precision medicine, and the future of women's health. *J Womens Health (Larchmt).* 2015;24:969-971.
14. Miller VM. Why are sex and gender important to basic physiology and translational and individualized medicine? *Am J Physiol Heart Circ Physiol.* 2014;306:H781-788.
15. Shaw LJ, Merz CN, Pepine CJ, et al. The economic burden of angina in women with suspected ischemic heart disease: results from the National Institutes of Health-National Heart, Lung, and Blood Institute-sponsored Women's Ischemia Syndrome Evaluation. *Circulation.* 2006;114:894-904.
16. Lansky AJ, Ng VG, Maehara A, et al. Gender and the extent of coronary atherosclerosis, plaque composition, and clinical outcomes in acute coronary syndromes. *JACC Cardiovasc Imaging.* 2012;5:S62-S72.
17. Virmani R, Burke AP, Farb A, Kolodgie FD. Pathology of the vulnerable plaque. *J Am Coll Cardiol.* 2006;47:C13-C18.
18. Hong MK, Mintz GS, Lee CW, et al. The site of plaque rupture in native coronary arteries: a three-vessel intravascular ultrasound analysis. *J Am Coll Cardiol.* 2005;46:261-265.

19. Jia H, Abtahian F, Aguirre AD, et al. In vivo diagnosis of plaque erosion and calcified nodule in patients with acute coronary syndrome by intravascular optical coherence tomography. *J Am Coll Cardiol.* 2013;62:1748-1758.

20. Narula J, Strauss HW. The popcorn plaques. *Nat Med.* 2007;13:532-534.

21. Hyafil F, Cornily JC, Feig JE, et al. Noninvasive detection of macrophages using a nanoparticulate contrast agent for computed tomography. *Nat Med.* 2007;13:636-641.

22. Osborn EA, Jaffer FA. Imaging atherosclerosis and risk of plaque rupture. *Curr Atheroscler Rep.* 2013;15:359.

23. Kolodgie FD, Gold HK, Burke AP, et al. Intraplaque hemorrhage and progression of coronary atheroma. *N Engl J Med.* 2003;349:2316-2325.

24. Burke AP, Farb A, Malcom GT, Liang YH, Smialek J, Virmani R. Coronary risk factors and plaque morphology in men with coronary disease who died suddenly. *N Engl J Med.* 1997;336:1276-1282.

25. Falk E, Nakano M, Bentzon JF, Finn AV, Virmani R. Update on acute coronary syndromes: the pathologists' view. *Eur Heart J.* 2013;34:719-278.

26. Higuma T, Soeda T, Abe N, et al. A combined optical coherence tomography and intravascular ultrasound study on plaque rupture, plaque erosion, and calcified nodule in patients with ST-segment elevation myocardial infarction: incidence, morphologic characteristics, and outcomes after percutaneous coronary intervention. *JACC Cardiovasc Interv.* 2015;8:1166-1176.

27. Lafont A. Basic aspects of plaque vulnerability. *Heart.* 2003;89:1262-1267.

28. Sheifer SE, Canos MR, Weinfurt KP, et al. Sex differences in coronary artery size assessed by intravascular ultrasound. *Am Heart J.* 2000;139:649-653.

29. Han SH, Bae JH, Holmes DR Jr, et al. Sex differences in atheroma burden and endothelial function in patients with early coronary atherosclerosis. *Eur Heart J.* 2008;29:1359-1369.

30. Vaccarino V. Ischemic heart disease in women: many questions, few facts. *Circ Cardiovasc Qual Outcomes.* 2010;3:111-115.

31. Farb A, Burke AP, Tang AL, et al. Coronary plaque erosion without rupture into a lipid core. A frequent cause of coronary thrombosis in sudden coronary death. *Circulation.* 1996;93:1354-1363.

32. Kessous R, Shoham-Vardi I, Pariente G, Holcberg G, Sheiner E. An association between preterm delivery and long-term maternal cardiovascular morbidity. *Am J Obstet Gynecol.* 2013;209:368.e1-8.

33. Lei Q, Zhou X, Zhou Y-H, et al. Prehypertension during normotensive pregnancy and postpartum clustering of cardiometabolic risk factors. *Hypertension.* 2016;68:455-463.

34. Mosca L, Benjamin EJ, Berra K, et al. Effectiveness-based guidelines for the prevention of cardiovascular disease in women—2011 update: a guideline from the American Heart Association. *Circulation.* 2011;123:1243-1262.

35. Behrens I, Basit S, Lykke JA, et al. Association between hypertensive disorders of pregnancy and later risk of cardiomyopathy. *JAMA.* 2016;315(10):1026-1033.

36. Fraser A, Nelson SM, Macdonald-Wallis C, et al. Associations of pregnancy complications with calculated cardiovascular disease risk and cardiovascular risk factors in middle age: the Avon Longitudinal Study of Parents and Children. *Circulation.* 2012;125:1367-1380.

37. Wenger NK. Recognizing pregnancy-associated cardiovascular risk factors. *Am J Cardiol.* 2014;113:406-409.

38. Bellamy L, Casas JP, Hingorani AD, Williams DJ. Pre-eclampsia and risk of cardiovascular disease and cancer in later life: systematic review and meta-analysis. *BMJ.* 2007;335:974.

39. Ahmed R, Dunford J, Mehran R, Robson S, Kunadian V. Pre-eclampsia and future cardiovascular risk among women: a review. *J Am Coll Cardiol.* 2014;63:1815-1822.

40. Njolstad I, Arnesen E, Lund-Larsen PG. Smoking, serum lipids, blood pressure, and sex differences in myocardial infarction. A 12-year follow-up of the Finnmark study. *Circulation.* 1996;93:450-456.

41. Pomp ER, Rosendaal FR, Doggen CJ. Smoking increases the risk of venous thrombosis and acts synergistically with oral contraceptive use. *Am J Hematol.* 2008;83:97-102.

42. Go AS, Mozaffarian D, Roger VL, et al. Heart disease and stroke statistics–2014 update: a report from the American Heart Association. *Circulation.* 2014;129:e28-e292.

43. Huxley RR, Woodward M. Cigarette smoking as a risk factor for coronary heart disease in women compared with men: a systematic review and meta-analysis of prospective cohort studies. *Lancet.* 2011;378:1297-1305.

44. Mieres JH, Gulati M, Bairey Merz N, et al. Role of noninvasive testing in the clinical evaluation of women with suspected ischemic heart disease: a consensus statement from the American Heart Association. *Circulation.* 2014;130:350-379.

45. Shaw LJ. Sex differences in cardiovascular imaging. *JACC Cardiovasc Imaging.* 2016;9:494-497.

46. Shaw LJ, Kohli P, Chandrashekhar Y, Narula J. Cardiovascular imaging of women: we have come a long way but still have a ways to go. *JACC Cardiovasc Imaging.* 2016;9:502-503.

47. Fihn SD, Gardin JM, Abrams J, et al. 2012 ACCF/AHA/ACP/AATS/PCNA/SCAI/ STS guideline for the diagnosis and management of patients with stable ischemic heart disease: a report of the American College of Cardiology Foundation/American Heart Association Task Force on Practice Guidelines, and the American College of Physicians, American Association for Thoracic Surgery, Preventive Cardiovascular

Nurses Association, Society for Cardiovascular Angiography and Interventions, and Society of Thoracic Surgeons. *J Am Coll Cardiol.* 2012;60:e44-e164.

48. Wolk MJ, Bailey SR, Doherty JU, et al. ACCF/AHA/ASE/ASNC/HFSA/HRS/SCAI/ SCCT/SCMR/STS 2013 multimodality appropriate use criteria for the detection and risk assessment of stable ischemic heart disease: a report of the American College of Cardiology Foundation Appropriate Use Criteria Task Force, American Heart Association, American Society of Echocardiography, American Society of Nuclear Cardiology, Heart Failure Society of America, Heart Rhythm Society, Society for Cardiovascular Angiography and Interventions, Society of Cardiovascular Computed Tomography, Society for Cardiovascular Magnetic Resonance, and Society of Thoracic Surgeons. *J Am Coll Cardiol.* 2014;63:380-406.

49. Pepine CJ, Ferdinand KC, Shaw LJ, et al. Emergence of nonobstructive coronary artery disease: a woman's problem and need for change in definition on angiography. *J Am Coll Cardiol.* 2015;66:1918-1933.

50. Jespersen L, Hvelplund A, Abildstrom SZ, et al. Stable angina pectoris with no obstructive coronary artery disease is associated with increased risks of major adverse cardiovascular events. *Eur Heart J.* 2012;33:734-744.

51. Min JK, Dunning A, Lin FY, et al. Age- and sex-related differences in all-cause mortality risk based on coronary computed tomography angiography findings results from the international multicenter CONFIRM (Coronary CT Angiography Evaluation for Clinical Outcomes: An International Multicenter Registry) of 23,854 patients without known coronary artery disease. *J Am Coll Cardiol.* 2011;58:849-860.

52. Shaw LJ, Bugiardini R, Merz CN. Women and ischemic heart disease: evolving knowledge. *J Am Coll Cardiol.* 2009;54:1561-1575.

53. Taqueti VR, Everett BM, Murthy VL, et al. Interaction of impaired coronary flow reserve and cardiomyocyte injury on adverse cardiovascular outcomes in patients without overt coronary artery disease. *Circulation.* 2015;131:528-535.

54. Lee BK, Lim HS, Fearon WF, et al. Invasive evaluation of patients with angina in the absence of obstructive coronary artery disease. *Circulation.* 2015;131:1054-1060.

55. Bittencourt MS, Hulten E, Ghoshhajra B, et al. Prognostic value of nonobstructive and obstructive coronary artery disease detected by coronary computed tomography angiography to identify cardiovascular events. *Circ Cardiovasc Imaging.* 2014;7:282-291.

56. Camici PG, Crea F. Coronary microvascular dysfunction. *N Engl J Med.* 2007;356:830-840.

57. Cecchi F, Olivotto I, Gistri R, Lorenzoni R, Chiriatti G, Camici PG. Coronary microvascular dysfunction and prognosis in hypertrophic cardiomyopathy. *N Engl J Med.* 2003;349:1027-1035.

CHAPTER 109

Race, Ethnicity, and Cardiovascular Disease

Mark J. Eisenberg

QUESTIONS

DIRECTIONS: Choose the one best response to each question.

109-1. Which of the following statements concerning race and ethnicity is *false*?

A. Race and ethnicity are precise proxies for genetic or other biological phenomena
B. Race and ethnicity are often confounded by socioeconomic status (SES)
C. Race and ethnicity are social, political, historical, and cultural constructs
D. Data on race and ethnicity can be invaluable in clinical and public health practice
E. The collection of data on race and ethnicity are crucial in the quest to advance health equity

109-2. A 21-year-old African American man presents to your clinic for a routine physical examination. Which of the following statements is *false*?

A. "Race" as an identifier lacks a clear definition
B. Culture, language, religion, and ethnicity are often strong indicators of ancestry
C. Race and ethnicity introduce provider bias about an patient's ability or willingness to accept care and may adversely affect disease management
D. Race and ethnicity are associated with differences in disease prevalence, expression, and outcome
E. All of the above

109-3. Which of the following is an example of ethnicity, as defined in the 1997 revisions to the standards for the classification of federal data on race and ethnicity?

A. Black
B. American Indian or Alaska Native

C. Asian
D. Hispanic
E. White

109-4. An 18-year-old non-Hispanic black woman presents to your clinic for a routine physical examination. You note her BMI is 32, which is classified as clinical obesity. Which of the following statements is *true* concerning the prevalence of obesity and overweight in various racial and ethnic groups, and could help you contextualize your patient's weight status?

A. In women, the prevalence of obesity and overweight is much higher in non-Hispanic blacks than in Hispanics or non-Hispanic whites
B. The prevalence of obesity and overweight among children and adolescents age 2 to 19 years is over 30%
C. Among all children age 2 to 19 years, the prevalence of overweight and obesity tends to be higher in non-Hispanic white and Hispanic children than in non-Hispanic Asian children
D. There is a greater prevalence of obesity and overweight in non-Hispanic whites and Hispanics than in non-Hispanic blacks
E. All of the above are true

109-5. Which of the following racial or ethnic groups have the highest rates of current smoking or tobacco use?

A. Non-Hispanic white men
B. Asian men
C. Non-Hispanic black men
D. Alaska native men
E. Hispanic men

109-6. Which of the following statements about racial and ethnic disparities at the provider level is *false*?

A. The race and sex of a patient have been found to independently influence how physicians manage chest pain
B. Implicit bias may operate by generating lower-quality clinical interactions and communication between (more biased) clinicians and racial and ethnic minority patients
C. There is no difference in the referral rates for black men and white men
D. Black women are approximately 60% more likely to be referred for cardiac catheterization than white men
E. Health care providers' unconscious biases may contribute to racial/ethnic disparities in the use of clinical interventions such as thrombolytic therapy for acute myocardial infarction

109-7. Rank the prevalence of hypertension-related mortality rates by race and ethnicity in the United States in 2013:

A. Non-Hispanic whites < non-Hispanic blacks < Hispanics
B. Non-Hispanic blacks < non-Hispanic whites < Hispanics
C. Hispanics < non-Hispanic blacks < non-Hispanic whites
D. Non-Hispanic whites < Hispanics < non-Hispanic blacks
E. Non-Hispanic blacks < Hispanics < non-Hispanic whites

109-8. There are racial/ethnic disparities in the risk for developing congestive heart failure (CHF). In a large cohort study of over 6000 participants of four ethnicities, which of the following groups had the highest rate of CHF?

A. Whites
B. African Americans
C. Hispanics
D. Chinese Americans
E. Alaskan Native

109-9. Which of the following is *not* among the most often cited patient-level factors and social determinants of health?

A. Behavioral and lifestyle choices
B. Cultural beliefs and practices
C. Patient preferences
D. Mistrust
E. All of the above

109-10. In an effort to help advance conceptual thinking and progress in health disparities research within the health care system, Kilbourne et al propose a framework that organizes the research agenda in three sequential phases. Choose the *correct* sequence:

A. Detection, understanding, and reduction or elimination of health disparities
B. Documentation, community outreach, and data collection
C. Advocacy, collaboration, and policy generation
D. Assessment, investment, and change implementation
E. Empowerment, activism, and community participation

109-1. The answer is A. *(Hurst's The Heart, 14th Edition, Chap. 109)* Race and ethnicity are social, political, historical, and cultural constructs (option C).[1,2] As such, they are flawed as biological concepts and inappropriate or, at best, imprecise when used as proxy for genetic or other biological phenomena (option A).[1-5] Consistent with this premise, racial and ethnic differences observed in the incidence, prevalence, morbidity, and mortality of cardiovascular diseases (CVD) should not be construed as necessarily resulting from genetic or other biological differences. Race and ethnicity are often confounded by socioeconomic status (SES) (option B). Thus, observed racial and ethnic differences that are not appropriately adjusted for SES and related factors could lead to erroneous conclusions with potentially adverse clinical and public health implications. Despite these challenges, data on race and ethnicity, when properly collected, analyzed, and interpreted, can be invaluable in clinical and public health practice (option D).[6-8] In particular, the appropriate collection and use of data on race and ethnicity are crucial in the quest to eliminate racial and ethnic disparities in cardiovascular health and to advance health equity (option E).[9,10]

109-2. The answer is B. *(Hurst's The Heart, 14th Edition, Chap. 109)* Historically, the biological concept of race has been associated with hierarchical ranking, biological determinism, eugenics, and justification for genocide, colonialism, slavery, and other social inequities.[11] It should not be a surprise that the use of racial classifications in medicine is met with skepticism and fear. A major problem with using race as an identifier is the lack of clear definition (option A).[12] Racial admixture and not knowing family ancestry further erode the utility of race classification. Race as a surrogate for biological characteristics and geographic origin is therefore imprecise. Culture, language, religion, and ethnicity have strong sociocultural components and are often poor indicators of ancestry (option B).[13] Finding better ways to measure ancestry and diversity is more likely to yield greater conceptual precision and could enable identification of useful genetic determinants of complex diseases.[13,14] Importantly, race and ethnicity have been shown to introduce provider bias about a person's ability or willingness to accept care and may adversely affect disease management (option C).[15,16] Despite these limitations, race and ethnicity are associated with differences in disease prevalence, expression, and outcome (option D).

109-3. The answer is D. *(Hurst's The Heart, 14th Edition, Chap. 109)* In October 1977, the US Government's Office of Management and Budget (OMB) announced government-wide standards for the collection of federal data on race and ethnicity. This has since been revised to account for the changing demographics of the United States.[17] These standards are required for federal data collection and are routinely used in medical and clinical research.[18,19] The revised standards contain five minimum categories for race and two categories for ethnicity, as shown in Table 109-1.

109-4. The answer is E. *(Hurst's The Heart, 14th Edition, Chap. 109)* Prominent racial and ethnic differences are seen in the prevalence of other CVD risk factors. For example, although overweight and obesity are common in US adults, with a 2011 to 2012 prevalence approaching 70% in adult men, there is a greater prevalence in non-Hispanic whites (73%) and Hispanics (80%) than in non-Hispanic blacks (69%) (option D).[20] On the other hand, in women, the prevalence of obesity and overweight is much higher in non-Hispanic blacks (82%) than in Hispanics (76%) or non-Hispanic whites (option A).[20] Among children and adolescents age 2 to 19 years, the prevalence of overweight and obesity in the 2011 to 2012 National Health and Nutrition Examination Survey (NHANES) was 31.8% (option B).[20] In general, among all children age 2 to 19 years, the prevalence of overweight and obesity tends to be higher in non-Hispanic black, non-Hispanic white, and Hispanic children than in non-Hispanic Asian children (option C).[20] Additionally, within the Hispanic population, important differences in the prevalence of overweight have been demonstrated. For example, Mexican NHANES participants have a higher mean age-adjusted prevalence of being overweight than Puerto Ricans and Cubans.[21]

TABLE 109-1 Categories of Race and Ethnicity as Defined in the 1997 Revisions to the Standards for the Classification of Federal Data on Race and Ethnicity

Race	Definition
American Indian or Alaska Native	A person having origins in any of the original peoples of North and South America (including Central America) and who maintains tribal affiliation or community attachment
Asian	A person having origins in any of the original peoples of the Far East, Southeast Asia, or the Indian subcontinent including, for example, Cambodia, China, India, Japan, Korea, Malaysia, Pakistan, the Philippine Islands, Thailand, and Vietnam
Black or African American	A person having origins in any of the black racial groups of Africa; terms such as *Haitian* and *Negro* can be used in addition to black or African American
Native Hawaiian or other Pacific Islander	A person having origins in any of original peoples of Hawaii, Guam, Samoa, or other Pacific Islands
White	A person having origins in any of the original peoples of Europe, the Middle East, or North Africa

Ethnicity	Definition
Hispanic or Latino	A person of Cuban, Mexican, Puerto Rican, South or Central American, or other Spanish culture or origin, regardless of race; the term *Spanish origin* can be used in addition to Hispanic or Latino
Not Hispanic or Latino	A person not of Cuban, Mexican, Puerto Rican, South or Central American, or other Spanish culture or origin, regardless of race; the term *not of Spanish origin* can be used in addition to not Hispanic or Latino

Reproduced with permission from Racial and Ethnic Categories and Definitions for NIH Diversity Programs and for Other Reporting Purposes; NOT-OD-089; April 8 2015. https://grants.nih.gov/grants/guide/notice-files/NOT-OD-15-089.html.

109-5. The answer is C. *(Hurst's The Heart, 14th Edition, Chap. 109)* The prevalence of current smoking or tobacco use varies significantly by race and ethnicity. Data from the 2014 NHIS in adults age 18 years and older showed a greater prevalence of current smoking in non-Hispanic black men (21.4%) (option C), non-Hispanic white men (19.9%) (option A), and Alaska Native men (18.6%) (option D) than in Asian men (13.8%) (option B) and Hispanic men (13.8%) (option E).[20] Similarly, non-Hispanic black women (13.4%), non-Hispanic white women (18.3%), and American Indian or Alaska Native women (21.6%) had a greater prevalence of current smoking than Asian women (5.5%) and Hispanic women (7.4%).[20]

109-6. The answer is D. *(Hurst's The Heart, 14th Edition, Chap. 109)* Several studies have demonstrated that health care providers' diagnostic, treatment, and referral decisions are influenced by the race/ethnicity of patients and that these influences are complex and may be modified by both patient and provider sex.[22] For example, Schulman et al[15] developed a computerized survey instrument in which actors portrayed patients with particular characteristics in scripted interviews about their symptoms in order to assess physicians' recommendations for cardiac catheterization in the evaluation of chest pain. Their findings suggested that the race and sex of a patient independently influenced how physicians managed chest pain (option A). Although the study found no difference in the referral rates for black men and white men (option C), an analysis of race–sex interactions revealed that black women were approximately 60% less likely to be referred for cardiac catheterization than white men (option D).[15] In another study assessing implicit bias, Green et al[23] also demonstrated that health care providers' unconscious biases may contribute to racial/ethnic disparities in the use of clinical interventions such as thrombolytic therapy for acute myocardial infarction (option E). The study by Schulman et al[15] is cited as an example of how providers' implicit bias, manifesting as stereotypical assumptions, may influence clinicians' decisions about referral for diagnostic or therapeutic interventions, leading to a substandard quality of care. Two other ways in which implicit bias may operate include (1) the generation of lower-quality clinical interactions and communication between (more biased) clinicians and racial and ethnic minority patients (option B) and (2) stereotype threat, wherein "individuals, often unconsciously, fear being judged negatively according to racial stereotypes."[24]

109-7. The answer is D. *(Hurst's The Heart, 14th Edition, Chap. 109)* Not surprisingly, hypertension remains a major contributor to the persisting large disparity in age-adjusted mortality rates from heart disease. The age-adjusted hypertension-related mortality rate in non-Hispanic blacks is significantly higher than the rate seen in non-Hispanic whites and Hispanics (option D).[20,25] The disparity is more dramatic when examined by sex.[20] For example, in 2013, the death rates per 100,000 population were 51.6 for non-Hispanic black men but 18.9 for non-Hispanic white men, and 20.0 for Hispanic men.[20] The corresponding rates for women were 36.5 for non-Hispanic black women, 15.8 for non-Hispanic white women, and 15.3 for Hispanic women.[20]

109-8. The answer is B. *(Hurst's The Heart, 14th Edition, Chap. 109)* In the Multi-Ethnic Study of Atherosclerosis (MESA), a cohort study of 6814 participants of four ethnicities—white (38.5%), African American (27.8%), Hispanic (21.9%), and Chinese American (11.8%)—African Americans had the highest incidence rate of CHF (option B), followed by Hispanic (option C), white (option A), and Chinese American (option D) participants (incidence rates: 4.6, 3.5, 2.4, and 1.0 per 1000 person-years, respectively).[26] In addition, African Americans had the highest proportion of incident CHF not preceded by clinical myocardial infarction (75%) compared with other ethnic groups.[26] Importantly, however, differences in the prevalence of hypertension, diabetes mellitus, and socioeconomic factors explained the higher risk of incident CHF among African Americans.[26]

109-9. The answer is E. *(Hurst's The Heart, 14th Edition, Chap. 109)* Some of the most often cited patient-level factors are behavioral and lifestyle choices, cultural beliefs and practices, patient preferences, mistrust, and nonadherence to health provider recommendations for healthful behaviors and practices. However, these factors do not exist in isolation; they are often influenced by the social determinants of health or, as defined by the World Health Organization, "the circumstances in which people are born, grow, live, work, and age, and the systems put in place to deal with illness."[27] Important within this category are conditions of residential or neighborhood environment and policies at the local, state, and national levels that also affect health and the provision of health-promoting services and resources.

109-10. The answer is A. *(Hurst's The Heart, 14th Edition, Chap. 109)* In an effort to help advance conceptual thinking and progress in health disparities research within the health care system, Kilbourne et al[29] proposed a framework that organizes the research agenda in three sequential phases: detection, understanding, and reduction or elimination of health disparities (option A). Although work in none of these phases is complete, substantial research investments have been made in the detection, documentation, and follow-up (phase 1) of racial and ethnic disparities in cardiovascular health, especially regarding non-Hispanic black and white persons in the United States.[30,31,32] Further research is needed in American Indians, Alaska Natives, and other racial/ethnic groups for whom inadequate data preclude the reliable detection of racial and ethnic disparities. In addition, we need more rigorous definitions of what constitute vulnerable populations within the concept of racial and ethnic disparities. Methodologic challenges regarding confounders and residual confounding in analyses of racial and ethnic disparities need further work.

References

1. Witzig R. The medicalization of race: scientific legitimization of a flawed social construct. *Ann Intern Med.* 1996;125(8):675-679.
2. Cooper R. A note on the biologic concept of race and its application in epidemiologic research. *Am Heart J.* 1984;108(3 Pt 2):715-722.
3. Smedley A, Smedley BD. Race as biology is fiction, racism as a social problem is real: anthropological and historical perspectives on the social construction of race. *Am Psychol.* 2005;60(1):16-26.
4. Foster MW, Sharp RR. Race, ethnicity, and genomics: social classifications as proxies of biological heterogeneity. *Genome Res.* 2002;12(6):844-850.
5. Collins FS. What we do and don't know about 'race,' 'ethnicity,' genetics and health at the dawn of the genome era. *Nat Genet.* 2004;36(11 Suppl):S13-S15.

6. Ford ME, Hill DD, Nerenz D, et al. Categorizing race and ethnicity in the HMO Cancer Research Network. *Ethn Dis*. 2002;12(1):135-140.

7. Krieger N. Refiguring "race": epidemiology, racialized biology, and biological expressions of race relations. *Int J Health Serv*. 2000;30(1):211-216.

8. Ahdieh L, Hahn RA. Use of the terms 'race,' 'ethnicity,' and 'national origins': a review of articles in the American Journal of Public Health, 1980-1989. *Ethn Health*. 1996;1(1):95-98.

9. Mensah GA, Mokdad AH, Ford ES, Greenlund KJ, Croft JB. State of disparities in cardiovascular health in the United States. *Circulation*. 2005;111(10):1233-1241.

10. Mensah GA. Eliminating disparities in cardiovascular health: six strategic imperatives and a framework for action. *Circulation*. 2005;111(10):1332-1336.

11. Tishkoff SA, Kidd KK. Implications of biogeography of human populations for 'race' and medicine. *Nat Genet*. 2004;36(11 Suppl):S21-S27.

12. Long JC, Kittles RA. Human genetic diversity and the nonexistence of biological races. *Hum Biol*. 2003;75(4):449-471.

13. Tishkoff SA, Kidd KK. Implications of biogeography of human populations for 'race' and medicine. *Nat Genet*. 2004;36(11 Suppl):S21-S27.

14. LaVeist TA. Beyond dummy variables and sample selection: what health services researchers ought to know about race as a variable. *Health Serv Res*. 1994;29(1):1-16.

15. Schulman KA, Berlin JA, Harless W, et al. The effect of race and sex on physicians' recommendations for cardiac catheterization. *N Engl J Med*. 1999;340(8):618-626.

16. Jones RG, Trivedi AN, Ayanian JZ. Factors influencing the effectiveness of interventions to reduce racial and ethnic disparities in health care. *Soc Sci Med*. 2010;70(3):337-341.

17. Office of Management and Budget. Revisions to the standards for the classification of Federal data on race and ethnicity. *Fed Reg*. 2006;62:58782-58790.

18. National Institutes of Health. *Racial and Ethnic Categories and Definitions for NIH Diversity Programs and for Other Reporting Purposes*. https://grants.nih.gov/grants/guide/notice-files/NOT-OD-15-089.html. Accessed November 21, 2016.

19. Valantine HA, Collins FS. National Institutes of Health addresses the science of diversity. *Proc Natl Acad Sci U S A*. 2015;112(40):12240-12242.

20. Mozaffarian D, Benjamin EJ, Go AS, et al. Heart disease and stroke statistics—2016 update: a report from the American Heart Association. *Circulation*. 2016;133(4):e38-e360.

21. Crespo CJ, Loria CM, Burt VL. Hypertension and other cardiovascular disease risk factors among Mexican Americans, Cuban Americans, and Puerto Ricans from the Hispanic Health and Nutrition Examination Survey. *Public Health Rep*. 1996;111(Suppl 2):7-10.

22. Institute of Medicine. *Unequal Treatment: Confronting Racial and Ethnic Disparities in Health Care*. Washington, DC: National Academies Press; 2003.

23. Green AR, Carney DR, Pallin DJ, et al. Implicit bias among physicians and its prediction of thrombolysis decisions for black and white patients. *J Gen Intern Med*. 2007;22(9):1231-1238.

24. Havranek EP, Mujahid MS, Barr DA, et al. Social determinants of risk and outcomes for cardiovascular disease: a scientific statement from the American Heart Association. *Circulation*. 2015;132(9):873-898.

25. Kung HC, Xu J. Hypertension-related mortality in the United States, 2000-2013. *NCHS Data Brief*. 2015;193:1-8.

26. Bahrami H, Kronmal R, Bluemke DA, et al. Differences in the incidence of congestive heart failure by ethnicity: the multi-ethnic study of atherosclerosis. *Arch Intern Med*. 2008;168(19):2138-2145.

27. Marmot M, Friel S, Bell R, Houweling TA, Taylor S. Closing the gap in a generation: health equity through action on the social determinants of health. *Lancet*. 2008;372(9650):1661-1669.

28. McPheeters ML, Kripalani S, Peterson NB, et al. Closing the quality gap: revisiting the state of the science (vol. 3: Quality improvement interventions to address health disparities). *Evid Rep Technol Assess (Full Rep)*. 2012;208.3:1-475.

29. Kilbourne AM, Switzer G, Hyman K, Crowley-Matoka M, Fine MJ. Advancing health disparities research within the health care system: a conceptual framework. *Am J Public Health*. 2006;96(12):2113-2121.

30. Mensah GA, Mokdad AH, Ford ES, Greenlund KJ, Croft JB. State of disparities in cardiovascular health in the United States. *Circulation*. 2005;111(10):1233-1241.

31. Agency for Health Research and Quality. *National Healthcare Quality and Disparities Report*; AHRQ Pub. No. 15-0007. Rockville, MD: Agency for Health Research and Quality; 2015.

32. Trivedi AN, Nsa W, Hausmann LR, et al. Quality and equity of care in U.S. hospitals. *N Engl J Med*. 2014;371(24):2298-2308.

CHAPTER 110

Environment and Heart Disease

Mark J. Eisenberg

QUESTIONS

DIRECTIONS: Choose the one best response to each question.

110-1. Toxic chemicals in the environment are significant causes of disease, specifically cardiovascular disease. Which of the following substances is known to be cardiotoxic?

A. Air pollution
B. Metals
C. Organophosphate insecticides
D. Nitrates
E. All of the above

110-2. Which of the following cardiovascular diseases is linked to toxic chemical exposures in the environment?

A. Hypertension
B. Arrhythmias
C. Peripheral vascular injury
D. Both A and B are correct
E. All of the above are correct

110-3. What is the most important source of atmospheric particulates in the developed, modern urban environment?

A. Household air pollution
B. Combustion of fossil fuels
C. Agricultural operations
D. Construction and demolition activities
E. Natural sources

110-4. A 48-year-old shipyard worker presents to your clinic, complaining of sluggishness, short-term memory loss, nausea, and headaches. His blood tests reveal he is anemic.

He reports some of his coworkers have been experiencing similar symptoms. You suspect lead poisoning. Which of the following statements concerning exposure to lead is *false*?

A. Inhalation is the most common route of adult exposure
B. There is a very low threshold below which lead causes no injury to the human brain
C. For children, the ingestion of lead paint chips or lead dust eroded from lead paint is the most common route of exposure
D. Ayurvedic and other nonprescription medications are sources of lead exposure
E. At high levels, lead can cause acute encephalopathy with coma, convulsions, and death

110-5. A 33-year-old woman in her first trimester of gestation presents to your clinic for a prenatal consult. She reports eating a healthy diet, particularly rich in omega-3 fatty acids derived from bluefin tuna, king mackerel, and swordfish. You recall reading that these large predatory fish at the top of the aquatic food chain may contain large bioaccumulations of methylmercury. Which of the following statements about methylmercury is *correct*?

A. Methylmercury is a mild neurotoxin
B. Methylmercury does not cross freely between maternal and fetal circulations
C. Consumption of contaminated fish is the major route of human exposure to methylmercury
D. Methylmercury is not a cardiovascular toxin
E. Mercury is transformed to methylmercury by dry land microorganisms

110-6. Polychlorinated biphenyls (PCBs), a family of chlorinated hydrocarbons, were previously used in a wide variety of industrial applications, most notably as insulating liquids in electrical generators and capacitors. Which of the following is *true* about exposure to PCBs?

A. PCBs bioaccumulate in the aquatic food chain and reach the highest levels in the predatory marine species

B. Dioxin-like PCBs have been linked to components of the metabolic syndrome, high blood pressure, elevated triglycerides, and glucose intolerance and to increased risk for obesity and diabetes

C. Because of their environmental persistence and toxicity, the manufacture and use of PCBs was banned in the United States in 1977

D. PCBs released to the environment many decades ago are still abundant in the environment

E. All of the above are true

110-7. A 6-year-old boy is brought to the emergency department showing signs and symptoms of miosis, excessive salivation, vomiting, diarrhea, and respiratory depression. You suspect acute organophosphate poisoning secondary to insecticide exposure. Which of the following is a key cardiac manifestation of acute organophosphate poisoning?

A. Bradycardia

B. ST-segment elevation

C. Atrioventricular conduction disturbances

D. Tachycardia

E. All of the above

110-8. A recent meta-analysis of 10 studies examined the cardiovascular effects of road and aircraft noise exposure conducted since the mid-1990s. What percent increase in the relative risk of ischemic heart disease was found to parallel each 10-dB increase in average noise exposure?

A. 2%

B. 5%

C. 6%

D. 8%

E. 10%

110-9. The cardiovascular consequences of global climate change will largely be the result of which contributing factor?

A. Increased surface temperatures

B. Increased oceanic temperatures

C. Increased precipitation

D. Decreased precipitation

E. Population migration

110-10. Which of the following statements is *false* concerning the health effects of the particle size of airborne particulates?

A. Larger particles (mass median airborne diameter of 10 μm and above) do not usually penetrate deeply into the lungs

B. Ultrafine particles (< 0.1 μm) may enter the systemic circulation

C. Particulate pollution is associated with hypertension

D. Most current US air regulations focus on large particles

E. All of the above

110-1. The answer is E. *(Hurst's The Heart, 14th Edition, Chap. 110)* Substances known to be cardiotoxic include air pollution (option A);[1,2] metals (option B),[3] including lead, mercury, arsenic, cobalt, and thallium; halogenated hydrocarbons, including chlorinated, brominated, and fluorinated compounds; organophosphate insecticides (option C); nitrates (option D); and carbon disulfide.

110-2. The answer is E. *(Hurst's The Heart, 14th Edition, Chap. 110)* Diseases of the heart and cardiovascular system that are linked to toxic chemical exposures in the environment include arrhythmias (option B), hypertension (option A), peripheral vascular injury (option C), cardiomyopathy, acute myocardial infarction (MI), stroke, and sudden death. Toxic chemicals that disrupt endocrine signaling can increase the risk for cardiovascular disease by causing elevated lipid levels and increasing the risk for obesity, the metabolic syndrome, and diabetes.[4,5] There is a high likelihood that beyond the known cardiotoxic chemicals, there are other chemicals in the modern environment whose toxicity to the heart and cardiovascular system has not yet been recognized.[6] These undiscovered cardiotoxins will be found hidden in plain sight among the > 80,000 new synthetic chemicals that have been invented in the past half century, which are used widely in consumer products, and which because of failure of stewardship by the chemical industry and by governments have never been tested for safety or toxicity.[6] People are widely exposed to these materials, and annual national surveys conducted by the Centers for Disease Control and Prevention find measurable levels of > 100 untested synthetic chemicals in the bodies of virtually all Americans.[7]

110-3. The answer is B. *(Hurst's The Heart, 14th Edition, Chap. 110)* Combustion of fossil fuels is the most important source of atmospheric particulates in the modern urban environment (option B). Emissions from both stationary sources—factories and coal-fired power plants—and mobile sources—cars, trucks, and buses—contribute to overall exposure, and the mix of stationary and mobile sources varies from city to city.[1,2,8] By contrast, in much of the developing world, the major source of airborne particulates is household air pollution (option A) created by the burning of biomass—wood and dried cow dung—in poorly ventilated cook stoves.[9-11]

110-4. The answer is B. *(Hurst's The Heart, 14th Edition, Chap. 110)* Patients may be exposed to lead by either inhalation or ingestion. Inhalation is the most common route of adult exposure (option A), and the most serious exposures occur among workers exposed occupationally.[12] Workers at greatest risk include smelter and foundry workers, hazardous waste workers, construction workers exposed to lead-painted steel, shipyard workers, electrical workers, and home renovators sanding or removing old lead paint.[12] For children, the ingestion of lead paint chips or, more commonly, the ingestion of the lead dust eroded from lead paint, is the most common route of exposure (option C).[13] Persons of all ages may be exposed by ingesting lead in drinking water.[13] Ayurvedic and other nonprescription medications are additional sources of exposure (option D).[14] Lead is best known as a neurotoxin. At high levels, lead can cause acute encephalopathy with coma, convulsions, and death (option E).[13] At lower levels, it can cause injury to the central and peripheral nervous systems with loss of intelligence, shortening of attention span, disruption of behavior, and slowing of nerve conduction velocity. Children are especially vulnerable to these effects.[15] There appears to be no threshold below which lead causes no injury to the human brain (option B).[15,16]

110-5. The answer is C. *(Hurst's The Heart, 14th Edition, Chap. 110)* Methylmercury is formed when airborne particles of metallic mercury emitted by industrial sources deposit in lakes, rivers, and oceans. The deposited mercury is transformed to methylmercury by marine microorganisms (option E). Methylmercury is lipophilic and highly persistent in the environment. It bioaccumulates to reach particularly high levels in predatory fish at the top of the aquatic food chain such as bluefin tuna, shark, king mackerel, and swordfish. Consumption of contaminated fish is the major route of human exposure to methylmercury (option C).[17] Methylmercury is a potent neurotoxin (option A).[18] The fetal brain is especially sensitive, and methylmercury crosses freely during pregnancy between the maternal and fetal circulations (option B). Methylmercury has been associated with major outbreaks of developmental neurotoxicity, notably Minamata disease,[19] as well as with widespread subclinical neurotoxicity.[20] Methylmercury is also a cardiovascular toxin (option D). Methylmercury exposure is associated with disturbances in cardiac rhythm, specifically decreased heart rate variability,[21] hypertension,[22,23] increased carotid arterial intima-media thickness,[24] accelerated progression of carotid atherosclerosis,[25] increased risk of MI,[24] and increased risk of coronary and cardiovascular death.[24]

110-6. **The answer is E.** *(Hurst's The Heart, 14th Edition, Chap. 110)* Because of their environmental persistence and toxicity, the manufacture and use of PCBs was banned in the United States in 1977 (option C), but PCBs released to the environment many decades ago are still abundant in the environment (option D), especially in riverine and marine sediments. PCBs bioaccumulate in the aquatic food chain and reach the highest levels in predatory marine species such as bluefin tuna, shark, king mackerel, and swordfish (option A). Consumption of contaminated fish is the major current route of exposure. The most highly cardiotoxic PCBs are congeners that most closely resemble TCDD, (eg, PCB-126). Dioxin-like PCBs have been linked to cardiovascular risk factors, specifically to components of the metabolic syndrome, high blood pressure, elevated triglycerides, and glucose intolerance[26-29] and to an increased risk for obesity and diabetes (option B).[30,31]

110-7. **The answer is E.** *(Hurst's The Heart, 14th Edition, Chap. 110)* Key cardiac manifestations of acute organophosphate poisoning are bradycardia (option A), ST-segment elevation (option B), and atrioventricular conduction disturbances (option C). Sinus tachycardia is seen in some cases (option D).[32] Longer-lasting cardiac changes include QT prolongation and polymorphic tachycardia (torsade de pointes). Complex ventricular arrhythmias are a frequently overlooked and potentially lethal aspect of acute organophosphate poisoning that can cause sudden cardiac death. Cardiac monitoring of acutely intoxicated patients for relatively long periods of time and early aggressive treatment of arrhythmias are critically important to patient survival.[32]

110-8. **The answer is C.** *(Hurst's The Heart, 14th Edition, Chap. 110)* A growing body of evidence indicates that chronic exposure to noise, especially in modern urban environments, can adversely affect health and increase the risk for ischemic heart disease. A recent meta-analysis of 10 studies examining the cardiovascular effects of road and aircraft noise exposure conducted since the mid-1990s found that the relative risk for ischemic heart disease increased by 6% with each 10-dB increase in average noise exposure (option C). The exposure-response relationship was linear and appeared to begin at an average noise level of 50 dB.[33] Concomitant exposure to air pollution does not appear to account for the association between noise exposure and heart disease.[34] Noise appears to exert its adverse effects on the cardiovascular system primarily by increasing the risk for hypertension, which in turn increases the risk for MI and stroke. Chronic nighttime noise appears to be especially hazardous and is associated with disruptions of sleep and increases in stress hormone levels and oxidative stress, which in turn may result in endothelial dysfunction and arterial hypertension.[35] Epidemiologic findings on the association between noise and cardiovascular disease are corroborated by experimental studies.[36]

110-9. **The answer is A.** *(Hurst's The Heart, 14th Edition, Chap. 110)* The cardiovascular consequences of global climate change will largely be the result of increased surface temperatures (option A). It is projected that by 2050, major US cities such as New York and Chicago may experience as many as three times their current average number of days hotter than 32°C (90°F). High temperatures are strongly associated with elevated levels of air pollution.[37] The combination of extreme heat and increased levels of air pollution will lead to increased incidence and mortality from heart disease and stroke.[38-41] The posttraumatic stress disorder and depression, which are associated with climate-related natural disasters such as extreme storms, coastal flooding, and forced migration, will further exacerbate the impacts of heat and pollution and may be expected to further increase the risk of cardiovascular disease, especially in highly vulnerable populations.[42]

110-10. **The answer is D.** (*Hurst's The Heart, 14th Edition, Chap. 110*) Particle size is a major determinant of the health impacts of airborne particulates. Larger particles with mass median airborne diameters of 10 μm and above (PM10) are usually filtered out of inhaled air in the upper airways and do not penetrate deeply into the lungs (option A), except when concentrations are so high that the normal physiologic defenses are overwhelmed, as happened in New York City after the attacks on the World Trade Center,[43] and as occurs in highly polluted indoor environments in the developing world.[11] By contrast, fine particles (< 2.5 μm in diameter) are capable of penetrating deep into the tracheobronchial tree. Ultrafine particles (< 0.1 μm) may actually translocate from inhaled air across the alveolar membranes to enter the systemic circulation (option B). Most current US air regulations focus on fine particles (option D).[44] Particulate pollution is associated with hypertension (option C),[45] increased serum lipid levels, and accelerated progression of atherosclerosis.[46-48] Toxicologic studies suggest that exposures to fine particles induce atherosclerosis and accelerate the development of atherosclerotic plaques by increasing oxidative stress, insulin resistance, endothelial dysfunction, and propensity to coagulation.[49-51] In a recent national US study, it was estimated that each 10-μg/m^3 decrease in concentration of fine particulate matter is associated with an increased life expectancy of 0.61 years.[52]

References

1. Samet J, Zeger SL, Dominici F, et al. *The National Morbidity, Mortality, and Air Pollution Study Part II: Morbidity and Mortality from Air Pollution in the United States.* Cambridge, MA: Health Effects Institute; 2000.

2. Newby DE, Mannucci PM, Tell GS, et al. Expert position paper on air pollution and cardiovascular disease. *Eur Heart J.* 2015;36(2):83-93b.

3. Solenkova NV, Newman JD, Berger JS, Thurston G, Hochman JS, Lamas GA. Metal pollutants and cardiovascular disease: mechanisms and consequences of exposure. *Am Heart J.* 2014;168:812-822.

4. Rao X, Montresor-Lopez J, Puett R, Rajagopalan S, Brook RD. Ambient air pollution: an emerging risk factor for diabetes mellitus. *Curr Diab Rep.* 2015;15(6):603.

5. Magliano DJ, Loh VH, Harding JL, Botton J, Shaw JE. Persistent organic pollutants and diabetes: a review of the epidemiological evidence. *Diabetes Metab.* 2014;40(1):1-14.

6. Landrigan PJ, Goldman L. Children's vulnerability to toxic chemicals: a challenge and opportunity to strengthen health and environmental policy. *Health Aff.* 2011;30:842-850.

7. Centers for Disease Control and Prevention. *National Report on Human Exposure to Environmental Chemicals.* Atlanta, 2015. http://www.cdc.gov/exposurereport/. Accessed November 27, 2015.

8. Global Burden of Disease 2013 Risk Factors Collaborators. Global, regional, and national comparative risk assessment of 79 behavioural, environmental and occupational, and metabolic risks or clusters of risks in 188 countries, 1990–2013: a systematic analysis for the Global Burden of Disease Study 2013. *Lancet.* 2015;386(10010):2287-2323.

9. World Health Organization. Burden of disease from household air pollution for 2012. Geneva: *World Health Organization,* 2014. http://www.who.int/phe/health_topics/outdoorair/databases/FINAL_HAP_AAP_BoD_24March2014.pdf?ua=1. Accessed July 9, 2014.

10. Laborde A, Tomasina F, Bianchi F, et al. Children's health in Latin America: the influence of environmental exposures. *Environ Health Perspect.* 2015;123:201-209.

11. Smith KR, Bruce N, Balakrishnan K, et al. Millions dead: how do we know and what does it mean? Methods used in the comparative risk assessment of household air pollution. *Annu Rev Public Health.* 2014;35:185-206.

12. Baxter PJ, Aw T-C, Cockcroft A, Durrington P, Harrington JM, eds. *Hunter's Diseases of Occupations.* 10th ed. Boca Raton, FL: CRC Press; 2010.

13. Agency for Toxic Substances and Disease Registry. *Toxicological Profile for Lead.* Atlanta, GA: Centers for Disease Control and Prevention, 2007. http://www.atsdr.cdc.gov/substances/toxsubstance.asp?toxid=22. Accessed November 28, 2015.

14. Saper RB, Philips RS, Sehgal A, et al. Lead, mercury, and arsenic in US- and Indian-manufactured Ayurvedic medicines sold via the Internet. *JAMA.* 2008;300(8):915-923.

15. Lanphear BP, Hornung R, Khoury J, et al. Low-level environmental lead exposure and children's intellectual function: an international pooled analysis. *Environ Health Perspect.* 2005;113(7):894-899.

16. World Health Organization. *Childhood Lead Poisoning.* Geneva, Switzerland: WHO; 2010.

17. Houston MC. Role of mercury toxicity in hypertension, cardiovascular disease, and stroke. *J Clin Hypertens* (Greenwich). 2011;13(8):621-627.

18. National Academy of Sciences. *Toxicological Effects of Methyl Mercury.* Washington, DC: National Academies Press; 2000.

19. Harada M. Congenital Minamata disease: intrauterine methylmercury poisoning. *Teratology.* 1978;18(2): 285-288.

20. Grandjean P, Landrigan PJ. Neurobehavioural effects of developmental toxicity. *Lancet Neurol.* 2014;13(3):330-338.

21. Choi AL, Weihe P, Budtz-Jergensen E, et al. Methylmercury exposure and adverse cardiovascular effects in Faroese whaling men. *Environ Health Perspect.* 2009;117(3):367-372.

22. Fillion M, Mergler D, Passos CJ, et al. A preliminary study of mercury exposure and blood pressure in the Brazilian Amazon. *Environ Health.* 2006;5:29-38.

23. Salonen JT, Seppanen, Nyyssonen K, et al. Intake of mercury from fish, lipid peroxidation, and risk of myocardial infarction and coronary, cardiovascular, and any death in eastern Finnish men. *Circulation.* 1995;91:645-655.

24. Salonen JT, Seppanen K, Lakka TA, et al. Mercury accumulation and accelerated progression of carotid atherosclerosis: a population-based prospective 4-year follow-up study in men in eastern Finland. *Atherosclerosis.* 2000;148:265-273.

25. Choi AL, Cordier S, Weihe P, et al. Negative confounding in the evaluation of toxicity: the case of methyl-mercury in fish and seafood. *Crit Rev Toxicol.* 2008;38(10):877-893.

26. Lee DH, Lee IK, Porta M, et al. Relationship between serum concentrations of persistent organic pollutants and the prevalence of metabolic syndrome among non-diabetic adults: results from the National Health and Nutrition Examination Survey 1999–2002. *Diabetologia.* 2007;50:1841-1851.

27. Perkins JT, Petriello MC, Newsome BJ, Hennig B. Polychlorinated biphenyls and links to cardiovascular disease. *Environ Sci Pollut Res Int.* 2016;23(3):2160-2172.

28. Arrebola JP, Fernández MF, Martin-Olmedo P, et al. Historical exposure to persistent organic pollutants and risk of incident hypertension. *Environ Res.* 2015;138:217-223.

29. Everett CJ, Mainous AG 3rd, Frithsen IL, et al. Association of polychlorinated biphenyls with hypertension in the 1999–2002 National Health and Nutrition Examination Survey. *Environ Res.* 2008;108(1):94-97.

30. Vafeiadi M, Georgiou V, Chalkiadaki G, et al. Association of prenatal exposure to persistent organic pollutants with obesity and cardiometabolic traits in early childhood: the Rhea Mother-Child Cohort (Crete, Greece). *Environ Health Perspect.* 2015;123(10):1015-1021.

31. Gore AC, Chappell VA, Fenton SE, et al. Executive summary to EDC-2: the Endocrine Society's second scientific statement on endocrine-disrupting chemicals. *Endocr Rev.* 2015;36(6):593-602.

32. Bar-Meir E, Schein O, Eisenkraft A, et al. Guidelines for treating cardiac manifestations of organo-phosphates poisoning with special emphasis on long QT and torsades de pointes. *Crit Rev Toxicol.* 2007;37(3):279-285.

33. Vienneau D, Schindler C, Perez L, et al. The relationship between transportation noise exposure and ischemic heart disease: a meta-analysis. *Environ Res.* 2015;138:372-380.

34. Tétreault LF, Perron S, Smargiassi A. Cardiovascular health, traffic-related air pollution and noise: are associations mutually confounded? A systematic review. *Int J Public Health.* 2013;58(5):649-666.

35. Münzel T, Gori T, Babisch W, Basner M. Cardiovascular effects of environmental noise exposure. *Eur Heart J.* 2014;35(13):829-836.

36. Basner M, Babisch W, Davis A, et al. Auditory and non-auditory effects of noise on health. *Lancet.* 2014;383(9925):1325-1332.

37. Kinney P. Climate change, air quality, and human health. *Am J Prev Med.* 2008; 35:459-467.

38. Krewski D, Jerrett M, Burnett RT, et al. *Extended Follow-Up and Spatial Analysis of the American Cancer Society Study Linking Particulate Air Pollution and Mortality.* Cambridge, MA: Health Effects Institute; 2009.

39. See comment in PubMed Commons below Beelen R, Stafoggia M, Raaschou-Nielsen O, et al. Long-term exposure to air pollution and cardiovascular mortality: an analysis of 22 European cohorts. *Epidemiology.* 2014;25(3):368-378.

40. Stafoggia M, Cesaroni G, Peters A, et al. Long-term exposure to ambient air pollution and incidence of cerebrovascular events: results from 11 European cohorts within the ESCAPE project. *Environ Health Perspect.* 2014;122(9):919-925.

41. Kaufman JD, Adar SD, Allen RW, et al. Prospective study of particulate air pollution exposures, subclinical atherosclerosis, and clinical cardiovascular disease: the multi-ethnic study of atherosclerosis and air pollution (MESA Air). *Am J Epidemiol.* 2012;176(9):825-837.

42. McMichael AJ, Campbell-Lendrum D, Kovats S, et al, eds. *Comparative Quantification of Health Risks, Global and Regional Burden of Disease Attributable to Selected Major Risk Factors.* Geneva, Switzerland: World Health Organization; 2004.

43. Lioy PJ, Georgopoulos P. The anatomy of the exposures that occurred around the World Trade Center site: 9/11 and beyond. *Ann NY Acad Sci.* 2006;1076:54-79.

44. US Environmental Protection Agency. *Fine Particulate (PM2.5) Designations.* http://www.epa.gov/pmdesignations. Accessed November 22, 2016.

45. Chan SH, Van Hee VC, Bergen S, et al. Long-term air pollution exposure and blood pressure in the sister study. *Environ Health Perspect.* 2015;123(10):951-958.

46. Yeatts K, Svendsen E, Creason J, et al. Coarse particulate matter (PM2.5-10) affects heart rate variability, blood lipids and circulating eosinophils in adults with asthma. *Environ Health Perspect.* 2007;115:709-714.

47. Floyd HS, Chen LC, Vallanat B, et al. Fine ambient air particulate matter exposure induces molecular alterations associated with vascular disease progression within plaques of atherosclerotic susceptible mice. *Inhal Toxicol.* 2009;21:394-403.

48. Brook RD, Rajagopalan S. Particulate matter air pollution and atherosclerosis. *Curr Atheroscler Rep.* 2010;12(5):291-300.

49. Forastiere F, Agabiti N. Assessing the link between air pollution and heart failure. *Lancet.* 2013;382(9897):1008-1010.

50. Viehmann A, Hertel S, Fuks K, et al. Long-term residential exposure to urban air pollution, and repeated measures of systemic blood markers of inflammation and coagulation. *Occup Environ Med.* 2015;72(9):656-663.

51. Hajat A, Allison M, Diez-Roux AV, et al. Long-term exposure to air pollution and markers of inflammation, coagulation, and endothelial activation: a repeat-measures analysis in the multi-ethnic study of atherosclerosis (MESA). *Epidemiology.* 2015;26(3):310-320.

52. Pope CA, Ezzati M, Dockery DW. Fine-particulate air pollution and life expectancy in the United States. *N Engl J Med.* 2009;360:376-386.

CHAPTER 111

Behavioral Cardiology: Epidemiology, Pathophysiology, and Clinical Management

Mark J. Eisenberg

QUESTIONS

DIRECTIONS: Choose the one best response to each question.

111-1. Repeatedly, studies have found that both short and long sleep, fragmented sleep, and insomnia have been linked to an increased risk for CVD. How many hours of sleep per night characterize "short" and "long" sleep, respectively?

A. ≤ 3–4 hours; > 6–7 hours
B. ≤ 4–5 hours; > 7–8 hours
C. ≤ 5–6 hours; > 8–9 hours
D. ≤ 6–7 hours; > 9–10 hours
E. ≤ 7–8 hours; > 10–11 hours

111-2. A 54-year-old woman with a recent history of major depression presents to your clinic. You remember learning about the existence of an association between depression and cardiac health. Which of the following statements about this association is *false*?

A. Major depression is found in approximately 15% of cardiac patients
B. There is a gradient relationship between the magnitude of major depressive symptoms and the occurrence of cardiac events
C. Mild levels of depression or psychological distress are not associated with an increased risk of adverse events
D. Depression is a risk factor for cardiac events among community cohorts without pre-existing CVD
E. All of the above are false

111-3. Which of the following statements concerning behavioral risk factors associated with cardiovascular disease is *true*?

A. The risk of death among those who divorce or separate, compared to married people, is highest among older men who experience divorce or separation
B. Caregiving is a stress that has not been uniformly found to be associated with an increased frequency of clinical events
C. Only dispositional pessimism has been linked to negative health outcomes
D. History of childhood abuse is associated with an approximately three fold increase in the onset of cardiovascular events by middle age
E. There is a linear relationship between the degree of life adversity and a person's sense of satisfaction

111-4. Low SES can serve as a composite chronic stressor. Which of the following mechanisms account for the increased risk associated with low SES?

A. Low SES is associated with a higher frequency of poor health habits
B. The stress associated with low SES (eg, economic hardship, job insecurity) increases the prevalence of depression
C. Pathophysiologic mechanisms that can promote CVD are also more prevalent in low-SES populations, such as more autonomic and metabolic dysfunction
D. Psychosocial stressors are potentiated when they occur among people with low SES
E. All of the above

111-5. Having a higher sense of life purpose has been associated with which of the following?

A. Reduced risk of stroke
B. Reduced risk of future physical disability
C. Reduced risk of dementia
D. Both A and C are correct
E. All of the above are correct

111-6. A 36-year-old man presents to your clinic after feeling progressively more lethargic and depressed over the last several months. You note that he has gained 15 pounds within the last year. He is not active, citing a lack of motivation and time as a challenge. Which of the following statements about the health effects of exercise is *true*?

A. Exercise training is as effective as antidepressant medication in the reduction of depressive symptoms
B. Exercise may increase the pathophysiologic risk factors associated with psychosocial risk factors
C. Exercise increases the effect of chronic stress telomere length
D. Despite its many advantages, physical fitness *cannot* buffer the relationship between depression and inflammation
E. Exercise does not protect against dementia

111-7. A 62-year-old woman who is severely overweight presents to your clinic in the company of her daughter to discuss her inability to lose weight. Although she claims to eat balanced, healthy meals, her daughter contends her mother's eating habits have not changed. In addition, the patient is a current smoker with a 25 pack-year history. You have learned that physician management of patients' health behaviors can be addressed according to a three-component model of behavior change. Which of the following is *not* included among these components?

A. Assessing patients' preparedness for behavior change
B. Promoting patients' motivation for initiating behavioral change
C. Helping patients in their execution of behavioral change
D. Helping patients sustain the long-term practice of new health behaviors
E. Both A and D are correct

111-8. Which of the following health-related New Year's resolutions is most likely to induce action?

A. "This year, I'm going to lose weight."
B. "This year, I will commit to exercising."
C. "This year, I will commit to joining a health club."
D. "This year, I will commit to exercising at the gym three times per week."
E. "This year, I really want to lose weight."

111-9. Psychosocial interventions within cardiac practice can be organized according to a tiered approach. Which of the following interventions is *not* included in a tiered system?

A. Physician management
B. Ancillary staff management
C. Behavioral specialists and programs
D. Patient empowerment
E. All of the above are included in the tiered approach

111-10. Which of the following statements concerning the management of health behaviors and psychosocial risk factors is *correct*?

A. There is increasing recognition that positive psychosocial functioning is protective of health
B. To date, there is modest translation of interventions into conventional practice
C. Practical barriers include developing more affordable interventions
D. An increasing number of techniques and tools have been developed to promote patient motivation and to assist in the execution and long-term maintenance of new health behaviors
E. All of the above

111-1. **The answer is C.** *(Hurst's The Heart, 14th Edition, Chap. 111)* Poor sleep is a newer arena that has been increasingly studied for its adverse health effects. The study of sleep has included the examination of both sleep duration and the quality of sleep. The definition of short and long sleep is arbitrary, but in most studies, short sleep has been defined as ≤ 5 to 6 hours a night and long sleep as > 8 to 9 hours a night (option C). Repeatedly, studies have found that both short and long sleep, fragmented sleep, and insomnia have been linked to an increased risk for CVD. A meta-analysis of 15 studies found short sleep to be associated with a greater risk of either developing or dying from CVD (relative risk [RR], 1.48; 95% confidence interval [CI], 1.22–1.80), and a similar risk was associated with long sleep.[1] Similarly, a meta-analysis of 13 prospective studies involving 122,501 subjects found that insomnia was associated with a risk ratio of 1.45 (95% CI, 1.29–1.63) for the development of CVD or cardiac events.[2]

111-2. **The answer is C.** *(Hurst's The Heart, 14th Edition, Chap. 111)* Major depression, which is characterized by depressed mood and/or lack of interest in nearly all activities for ≥ 2 weeks, in conjunction with at least four to five out of nine other psychological symptoms (eg, change in appetite, insomnia, fatigue, guilt), is found in approximately 15% of cardiac patients (option A), and milder depressive symptoms also occur in another 15% of cardiac patients.[3] Epidemiologic studies have consistently demonstrated the potency of depression as a risk factor for cardiac events among community cohorts without preexisting CVD (option D); it is also a risk factor for recurrent events among patients with preexisting CVD. Epidemiologic studies have also demonstrated a gradient relationship between the magnitude of depressive symptoms and the occurrence of adverse cardiac events (option B). Notably, even mild levels of depression or of overall psychological distress have been found to be associated with an increased risk of adverse events compared to patients without symptoms (option C), as demonstrated, for instance, in a recent large follow-up of 68,222 individuals who were assessed for psychological distress using the 12-item General Health Questionnaire.[4]

111-3. **The answer is B.** *(Hurst's The Heart, 14th Edition, Chap. 111)* Pessimism is commonly characterized as a general personality disposition toward expecting negative outcomes in the future. Pessimists have an explanatory style of invoking self-blame for negative events, as well as a general personality disposition toward expecting negative outcomes in the future. Both dispositional and explanatory pessimism have been linked to negative health outcomes (option C). A common stressor is marital stress. A large meta-analysis of 104 studies that examined data concerning the mortality risk associated with marital dissolution found that the risk of death among those who divorced or separated, compared to married people, was age dependent, with the risk being highest among younger men who experienced divorce or separation (option A). In addition, the meaning that is invested within a given life situation may be a potential modifier of perceived stress and clinical outcomes. For instance, caregiving is a stress that has not been uniformly found to be associated with an increased frequency of clinical events (option B). A third stressor is the enduring effects of childhood abuse or trauma. In a particularly large study, the Nurses' Health Study,[1,5] which involved a 16-year follow-up of 66,798 women, a history of childhood abuse was common, having occurred in approximately one-fifth of the women, and within this subgroup, it was associated with an approximately 1.5-fold increase in the onset of cardiovascular events by middle age (option D). People vary widely in their perceived sense of stress in response to a given life situation, depending on personality, resilient resources, and other factors. One of the interesting aspects of stress in this regard is an apparent U-shaped relationship between the degree of life adversity and a person's sense of satisfaction (option E).

111-4. **The answer is E.** *(Hurst's The Heart, 14th Edition, Chap. 111)* Several mechanisms appear to account for the increased risk associated with low SES. First, low SES is associated with a higher frequency of poor health habits, such as poor nutrition and overeating, smoking, and physical inactivity (option A).[6] Second, the stress associated with low SES (eg, economic hardship, job insecurity) increases the prevalence of depression and other mental status parameters that may in turn increase CVD (option B).[7] In addition, pathophysiologic mechanisms that can promote CVD are also more prevalent in low SES populations, such as more autonomic and metabolic dysfunction (option C).[8,9] Psychological stressors are also potentiated when they occur among individuals with low SES (option D).[10,11] Depression and anxiety are highly comorbid, and when both are present, the likelihood for future clinical event rates is elevated compared to the presence of either emotion alone.[12]

111-5. **The answer is E.** *(Hurst's The Heart, 14th Edition, Chap. 111)* A higher sense of purpose has also been linked to a reduced risk of stroke (option A),[13] future physical disability (option B),[14] and dementia (option C).[15] Purpose in life may be health promoting through a number of mechanisms. Preliminary data suggest that life purpose may provide positive physiological buffering,[16] although the data are scant in this regard. Purpose in life may also serve to promote healthier behaviors and less use of medical services. In addition, purpose in life may be associated with greater resilience, as suggested by a meta-analysis of 70 studies that found that purpose in life was associated with a greater sense of competence, stronger social integration, and more positive affect.[17]

111-6. **The answer is A.** *(Hurst's The Heart, 14th Edition, Chap. 111)* Exercise can favorably affect psychological mood, as shown by cross-sectional studies of community cohorts that have observed fewer depressive symptoms among those who exercise, as well as by longitudinal studies that have demonstrated a lower frequency of subsequent depression among subjects who were physically active at baseline.[18] In addition, a meta-analysis of 25 randomized studies that compared exercise with either standard therapy for depression, placebo, or no treatment found a large treatment effect for reducing depression among those randomized to exercise.[19] The strongest evidence comes from three randomized trials conducted by Blumenthal and colleagues. In each trial, exercise training was as effective as antidepressant medication in the reduction of depressive symptoms (option A).[20-22] Additionally, exercise has been shown to improve executive function and cognitive vitality and appears to provide a protective effect against the development of dementia (option E).[23,24] Further, newer data indicate that exercise serves to reduce the pathophysiologic effects associated with psychosocial risk factors (option B). For instance, studies indicate that physical fitness is associated with reduced heart rate, blood pressure, and cortisol responses to psychosocial stress.[25] Physical fitness can also buffer the relationship between depression and inflammation (option D),[26] reduce the likelihood of impaired glucose metabolism in response to chronic stress,[27] and reduce the effect of chronic stress on telomere length (option C).[28] Finally, exercise can aid in the management of other health behaviors, including diet and sleep.

111-7. **The answer is A.** *(Hurst's The Heart, 14th Edition, Chap. 111)* The management of patients' health behaviors is intrinsically challenging. Poor adherence to medication usage is common, and poor adherence to diet, exercise, and other behavioral suggestions is even more common. Physician management of patients' health behaviors can be addressed according to a three-component model of behavioral change: (1) promoting patients' motivation for initiating behavioral change (option B); (2) helping patients in their execution of behavioral health goals (option C); and (3) helping patients to sustain the long-term practice of new health behaviors (option D).

111-8. **The answer is D.** *(Hurst's The Heart, 14th Edition, Chap. 111)* Even if motivated, lack of goal execution may result from many factors, such as competing priorities, lack of sustained willpower, or lack of know-how in executing behavioral goals. The more time pressure a person feels as a result of daily obligations, the less likely he or she is to regard the importance of health goals. For this reason, it is helpful to capitalize on the inspiration provided by a clinical event or office visit by helping patients to anchor health goals with a committed action plan. The health goal should be specific and measurable. The action plan should be detailed rather than vague and should involve an action step that will be carried forward as a daily commitment, just as a work goal would. For instance, the desire to start exercising is a vague goal. The intention to join a health club is more specific but not specifically measurable. By contrast, the commitment to exercise at the gym three times per week provides a specific and measurable goal that can be anchored in one's daily planning and followed by one's health care team (option D).

111-9. **The answer is D.** (*Hurst's The Heart, 14th Edition, Chap. 111*) Psychosocial interventions within cardiac practice can be organized according to a tiered approach consisting of three basic tiers (Figure 111-1).[3] Depending on severity, various psychosocial risk factors may be addressed directly by physicians without referral to staff or behavioral specialists. The second tier of psychosocial management calls for the referral of patients with greater psychosocial dysfunction to ancillary support staff, such as a physician's own office staff or hospital or community programs. The third tier of psychosocial management involves the referral of patients with moderate to severe psychological dysfunction to appropriate mental health care specialists.

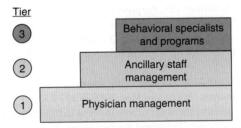

FIGURE 111-1 Clinical management can be facilitated by a tiered approach to behavioral and psychosocial interventions, centered around basic screening and counseling functions that can be performed by the physician (tier 1), with referral of patients to ancillary office staff (tier 2), or by behavioral specialists or organized hospital or community programs (tier 3) when appropriate.

111-10. **The answer is E.** (*Hurst's The Heart, 14th Edition, Chap. 111*) An important advance over the past decade is the increasing recognition that positive psychosocial functioning is protective of health (option A), both because of physiologic buffering and because of its positive impact on health behaviors. The management of health behaviors and psychosocial risk factors is interrelated, and improvement in one arena can enhance the other. An increasing number of techniques and tools have been developed to promote patient motivation and to assist in the execution and long-term maintenance of new health behaviors (option D), as well as to manage psychosocial risk factors in the context of medical practice. However, to date, the translation of these interventions into conventional practice has been relatively modest (option B). Practical barriers, such as the need to develop more affordable interventions, must still be addressed (option C). However, because of the growing frequency of adverse health behaviors in recent decades and because of the high concentration of psychological risk factors within medical populations, interest in integrating the management of psychosocial risk factors into medical practice is growing, and advances are likely to accelerate.

References

1. Cappuccio FP, Cooper D, D'Elia L, et al. Sleep duration predicts cardiovascular outcomes: a systematic review and meta-analysis of prospective studies. *Eur Heart J.* 2011;32:1484-1492.
2. Sofi F, Cesari F, Casini A, et al. Insomnia and risk of cardiovascular disease: a meta-analysis. *Eur J Prev Cardiol.* 2014;21(1):57-64.
3. Rozanski A, Blumenthal JA, Davidson KW, Saab PG, Kubzansky L. The epidemiology, pathophysiology, and management of psychosocial risk factors in cardiac practice: the emerging field of behavioral cardiology. *J Am Coll Cardiol.* 2005;45:637-651.

4. Russ TC, Stamatakis E, Hamer M, et al. Association between psychological distress and mortality: individual participant pooled analysis of 10 prospective cohort studies. *BMJ.* 2012;345:e4933.

5. Rich-Edwards JW, Mason S, Rexrode K, et al. Physical and sexual abuse in childhood as predictors of early-onset cardiovascular events in women. *Circulation.* 2012;126:920-927.

6. Lantz PM, Golberstein E, House JS, Morenoff J. Socioeconomic and behavioral risk factors for mortality in a national 19-year prospective study of U.S. adults. *Soc Sci Med.* 2010;70:1558-1566.

7. Hudson DL, Puterman E, Bibbins-Domingo K, Matthews KA, Adler NE. Race, life course socioeconomic position, racial discrimination, depressive symptoms and self-rated health. *Soc Sci Med.* 2013;97:7-14.

8. Steptoe A, Kunz-Ebrecht S, Owen N, et al. Socioeconomic status and stress-related biological responses over the working day. *Psychosom Med.* 2003;65:461-470.

9. Kumari M, Badrick E, Chadola T, et al. Measures of social position and cortisol secretion in an aging population: findings from the Whitehall II study. *Psychosom Med.* 2010;72:27-34.

10. Redmond N, Richman J, Gamboa CM, et al. Perceived stress is associated with incident coronary heart disease and all-cause mortality in low- but not high-income participants in the Reasons for Geographic and Racial Differences in Stroke study. *J Am Heart Assoc.* 2013;2:e000447.

11. Lazzarino AI, Hamer M, Stamatakis E, Steptoe A. Low socioeconomic status and psychological distress as synergistic predictors of mortality from stroke and coronary heart disease. *Psychosom Med.* 2013;75:311-316.

12. Watkins LL, Koch GG, Sherwood A, et al. Association of anxiety and depression with all-cause mortality in individuals with coronary heart disease. *J Am Heart Assoc.* 2013;2:e000068.

13. Kim ES, Sun JK, Park N, Peterson C. Purpose in life and reduced incidence of stroke in older adults: the Health and Retirement Study. *J Psychosom Res.* 2013;74:427-432.

14. Boyle PA, Buchman AS, Bennett DA. Purpose in life is associated with a reduced risk of incident disability among community-dwelling older persons. *Am J Geriatr Psychiatry.* 2010;18:1093-1102.

15. Boyle PA, Buchman AS, Barnes LL, Bennett DA. Effect of a purpose in life on risk of incident Alzheimer disease and mild cognitive impairment in community-dwelling older persons. *Arch Gen Psychiatry.* 2010;67:304-310.

16. Cohen R, Bavishi C, Rozanski A. Purpose in life and its relationship to all-cause mortality and cardiovascular events: a meta-analysis. *Psychosom Med.* 2016;78:122-133.

17. Pinquart M. Creating and maintaining purpose in life in old age: a meta analysis. *Aging Int.* 2002;27:90-114.

18. Rozanski A. Exercise as medical treatment for depression. *J Am Coll Cardiol.* 2012;60:1064-1066.

19. Mead GE, Morley W, Campbell P, Greig CA, McMurdo M, Lawlor DA. Exercise for depression. *Cochrane Database Syst Rev.* 2009:CD004366.

20. Blumenthal JA, Babyak MA, Moore KA, et al. Effects of exercise training on older patients with major depression. *Arch Intern Med.* 1999;159:2349-2356.

21. Blumenthal JA, Babyak MA, Doraiswamy PM, et al. Exercise and pharmacotherapy in the treatment of major depressive disorder. *Psychosom Med.* 2007;69:587-596.

22. Blumenthal JA, Sherwood A, Babyak MA, et al. Exercise and pharmacological treatment of depressive symptoms in patients with coronary heart disease: results from the UPBEAT (Understanding the Prognostic Benefits of Exercise and Antidepressant Therapy) study. *J Am Coll Cardiol.* 2012;60:1053-1063.

23. Colcombe S, Kramer AF. Fitness effects on the cognitive function of older adults: a meta-analytic study. *Psychol Sci.* 2003;14:125-130.

24. Hamer M, Chida Y. Physical activity and risk of neurodegenerative disease: a systematic review of prospective evidence. *Psychol Med.* 2009;39:3-11.

25. Rimmele U, Zellweger BC, Marti B, et al. Trained men show lower cortisol, heart rate and psychological responses to psychosocial stress compared with untrained men. *Psychoneuroendocrinology.* 2007;32:627-635.

26. Rethorst CD, Moynihan J, Lyness JM, Heffner KL, Chapman BP. Moderating effects of moderate-intensity physical activity in the relationship between depressive symptoms and interleukin-6 in primary care patients. *Psychosom Med.* 2011;73:265-269.

27. Puterman E, Adler N, Matthews KA, Epel E. Financial strain and impaired fasting glucose: the moderating role of physical activity in the Coronary Artery Risk Development in Young Adults study. *Psychosom Med.* 2012;74:187-192.

28. Puterman E, Lin J, Blackburn E, et al. The power of exercise: buffering the effect of chronic stress on telomere length. *PLoS One.* 2010;5:e10837.

CHAPTER 112

Economics and Cost-Effectiveness in Cardiology

Mark J. Eisenberg

QUESTIONS

DIRECTIONS: Choose the one best response to each question.

112-1. According to the Centers for Medicare and Medicaid Services (CMS), what percentage of the United States gross domestic product (GDP) was spent on health care in 2014?

A. 10%
B. 15%
C. 17.5%
D. 21.5%
E. 26%

112-2. Which of the following is *not* a major reason that can be offered to explain why health care spending is expected to keep increasing?

A. Technological innovations that improve medical care
B. Aging of the population
C. Inflation
D. Raised expectations of the public
E. All of the above are reasons to explain increasing health care spending

112-3. Which of the following statements about methods of economic efficiency analysis is *false*?

A. Cost-effectiveness analysis provides an estimate of the relationship between money spent and health benefits produced
B. Similar to cost-benefit analysis, cost-effectiveness and cost-utility ratios have a natural interpretation
C. Cost-benefit analysis requires all incremental health benefits to be converted to their monetary equivalent

D. Cost-effectiveness analysis values all units of survival the same, regardless of who benefits
E. Cost-utility analysis uses patient or social preference weights to adjust survival data

112-4. What cost-effectiveness ratio per life-year (or QALY) saved is typically considered economically attractive in the United States?

A. ≤ $25,000
B. ≤ $50,000
C. ≤ $75,000
D. ≤ $90,000
E. ≤ $100,000

112-5. What was the overall annual US medical spending attributed to heart failure in 2012?

A. $10 billion
B. $15.6 billion
C. $25.8 billion
D. $30.7 billion
E. $40.2 billion

112-6. Which of the following statements about primary and secondary prevention economics is *correct*?

A. The incremental costs of prevention tend to be relatively insensitive to the primary and secondary prevention distinction
B. Secondary prevention costs more than primary prevention
C. Primary prevention is economically efficient
D. Both B and C are correct
E. All of the above are correct

112-7. Which of the following statements about the cost-effectiveness of statins is *correct*?

A. Starting statin therapy in 9.7 million adults and intensifying statin therapy in an additional 1.4 million adults would reduce the number of MIs by 20,000 per year

B. Providing low-cost statin therapy to men over age 44 regardless of lipid levels might be an effective and economically attractive prevention strategy

C. In addition to drug costs, coronary artery disease (CAD) risk level and age affect the economic attractiveness of statin therapy

D. There are a number of important primary prevention trials of statin therapy, but none include prospective assessment of economics

E. All of the above are correct

112-8. The most recent comparison of medicine versus revascularization is the Bypass Angioplasty Revascularization Investigation (BARI) 2D trial, which randomized 2368 patients with type 2 diabetes and stable CAD. Which statement concerning the economics of medicine versus revascularization in this trial is *false*?

A. In the percutaneous coronary intervention (PCI) stratum, at the end of 4 years, PCI costs were higher by $5600 and clinical outcomes were better in the medical arm

B. Extrapolating to a lifetime perspective, total costs for the medical arm were approximately $200 higher than PCI, and life expectancy was shorter

C. The cost-effectiveness ratio for medicine versus PCI was $600 per added life-year

D. In lifetime projections, CABG increased survival by 0.52 life-years per patient at an incremental cost that remained at approximately $20,000

E. The cost-effectiveness ratio for CABG versus medicine was $47,000 per added life-year

112-9. Which of the following questions is *not* one of the major questions of health economics?

A. What long-term effects does this health care service or technology have on health outcomes, and what is the level of evidence supporting the current state of understanding about clinical effectiveness?

B. Is this health care service or technology good value for money?

C. Can we afford this health care service or technology?

D. How publicly accessible is this health care service or technology?

E. All of the above are major questions of health economics

112-10. Which of the following statements about data in health economics is *correct*?

A. A complexity about the concept of cost is that a perspective must always be defined in order to measure and understand costs

B. In most economic analyses, the primary analyses should be done using the societal perspective

C. Measuring and comparing costs across international borders is increasingly important

D. It may make sense to pool resource use data across countries and assign common costs

E. All of the above are correct

ANSWERS

112-1. **The answer is C.** *(Hurst's The Heart, 14th Edition, Chap. 112)* According to the Centers for Medicare and Medicaid Services (CMS), the United States spent 17.5% (option C) of its gross domestic product (GDP) on health care in 2014, amounting to approximately $3 trillion.[1]

112-2. **The answer is E.** *(Hurst's The Heart, 14th Edition, Chap. 112)* Four major reasons can be offered to explain why health care spending is expected to keep increasing: (1) technological innovations that improve medical care[2] (option A)—the care of the cardiovascular patient in 2017 is vastly different (and largely better) than it was in 1980, but innovation in diagnosis and therapy generally increases costs relative to the prior patterns of care, as is reviewed in the second part of this chapter; (2) the aging of the population (option B)—an issue for all developed countries and one that has just begun to manifest itself (the vanguard baby boomers born in 1945 reached retirement age in 2010); (3) inflation (option C), which refers to an increase in the cost of the same good or service (contrasted with an improved medical care service described in the first reason, above); and (4) raised expectations of the public (option D) regarding what medicine can and should offer them when they become ill, in part as a result of the global information revolution created by the Internet and search engines such as Google. Patients are no longer dependent on their doctors to tell them what is possible in a particular medical situation, and there appears to be no limit to the human desire to subdue morbidity and mortality technologically.

112-3. **The answer is B.** *(Hurst's The Heart, 14th Edition, Chap. 112)* *Cost-benefit analysis* requires all incremental health benefits to be converted to their monetary equivalent (option C). As might be imagined, the methods for doing this are controversial because they require answers to some of society's most difficult value questions.[3,4] *Cost-effectiveness analysis* avoids this hornet's nest of difficulty by valuing all units of survival the same, regardless of who benefits (option D). *Cost-utility analysis* modifies this by using utility values (patient or societal preference weights) to adjust the survival data (option E). Thus, survival in a severely disabled state or in severe pain would be valued much less (lower utilities and thus lower calculated QALYs) than survival in good or excellent health. Cost-effectiveness analysis provides an estimate of the relationship between money spent and health benefits produced (option A), but unlike cost-benefit analysis, the cost-effectiveness and cost-utility ratios have no natural interpretation (option B). Thus, benchmarks are needed to help interpret the results of these analyses.

112-4. **The answer is B.** *(Hurst's The Heart, 14th Edition, Chap. 112)* Typically in the United States, a cost-effectiveness ratio of $50,000 or less per life-year (or QALY) saved has been considered economically attractive (option B), whereas values of $100,000 or more per life-year (or QALY) saved have been considered economically unattractive. Apparently the $50,000 figure was initially chosen because it was the cost to keep an end-stage renal failure patient alive on hemodialysis for a year compared to no dialysis. Dialysis is a form of medical care that Congress had guaranteed to fund for all affected renal failure patients, and it thus represents an explicit policy statement by the US federal government (representing "society") of how much it is willing to pay to save a life-year.

112-5. **The answer is D.** *(Hurst's The Heart, 14th Edition, Chap. 112)* The overall annual US medical spending attributed to heart failure in 2012 was approximately $30.7 billion (option D), with 68% attributable to direct medical costs.[5] It must be kept in mind that given the difficulties in identifying heart failure on a population level, these estimates are extremely crude. However, the data are sufficient to conclude that heart failure is common and accounts for a large amount of health care spending. It follows that if we could allocate resources to prevent the disease or, failing that, prevent it from progressing to decompensation, we might improve the health of these patients efficiently and without a massive increase in health care spending.

112-6. **The answer is A.** *(Hurst's The Heart, 14th Edition, Chap. 112)* In both primary and secondary prevention, the general goal is the same: prevent death and morbidity. The risks (ie, the number of available events that need to be prevented) are of course much higher in secondary prevention patients. The incremental costs of prevention, however, tend to be relatively insensitive to the primary and secondary prevention distinction (option A). In fact, a treatment as secondary prevention may have a lower net cost than the same treatment as primary prevention because it may prevent more expensive complications (eg, MIs) and palliative procedures (eg, coronary revascularization). So secondary prevention costs the same or less (option B), and for any relative reduction in major events, it prevents a larger absolute number of complications. Primary prevention is often inefficient economically (option C) because many people with risk factors will never develop disease complications, regardless of how they are treated. For this reason, many studies of primary prevention have tried to identify higher-risk subsets of the at-risk population in which therapy may be more economically and clinically efficient. The use of a multicomponent inexpensive polypill in older adults is an alternate approach to efficient primary prevention targeting intervention at a population level based on simple demographic features.[6,7]

112-7. **The answer is E.** *(Hurst's The Heart, 14th Edition, Chap. 112)* There are a number of important primary prevention trials of statin therapy, but none included prospective assessment of economics (option D). A CHD Policy Model analysis of primary prevention strategies for lipid lowering assessed the cost-effectiveness and public health impact of Adult Treatment Panel III guidelines for targeting statin therapy in persons age 35 to 85 years.[8,9] This analysis found that starting statin therapy in 9.7 million adults and intensifying statin therapy in an additional 1.4 million adults would reduce the number of MIs by 20,000 per year (option A) and the number of CAD deaths by 10,000 per year. Assuming a cost of $2.11 per low-intensity tablet and $2.81 per high-intensity tablet, over 30 years, the cost-effectiveness ratio for full adherence to Adult Treatment Panel III primary prevention guidelines would be $42,000 per QALY. In addition to drug costs, CAD risk level and age affected the economic attractiveness of statin therapy (option C). Hypothetically, providing low-cost statin therapy to men over age 44 regardless of lipid levels might be an effective and economically attractive prevention strategy (option B), although it seems unlikely to be viable on other grounds.[10]

112-8. **The answer is B.** *(Hurst's The Heart, 14th Edition, Chap. 112)* The most recent comparison of medicine versus revascularization is the BARI 2D trial, which randomized 2368 patients with type 2 diabetes and stable CAD.[11] Overall, total mortality (the primary end point) did not differ in the two arms. One interesting feature of the BARI 2D was a prospective definition of a PCI and a CABG subset before randomization. In the CABG subset, major cardiovascular events were reduced by CABG compared to medicine alone. Economic analysis results differed substantially in these two strata.[12] In the PCI stratum, at the end of 4 years, PCI costs were higher by $5600 and clinical outcomes were better in the medical arm (option A). Extrapolating to a lifetime perspective, total costs for the medical arm were approximately $200 higher than PCI, but life expectancy was longer (option B), and the cost-effectiveness ratio for medicine versus PCI was $600 per added life-year (option C). In the CABG stratum, 4-year costs were $20,300 higher for the CABG patients. In the lifetime projections, CABG increased survival by 0.52 life-years per patient at an incremental cost that remained at approximately $20,000 (option D). The cost-effectiveness ratio for CABG versus medicine was $47,000 per added life-year (option E).

112-9. **The answer is D.** *(Hurst's The Heart, 14th Edition, Chap. 112)* Although it is natural to expect that the most important questions for a health economics analysis would deal with some aspect of cost, understanding the clinical effectiveness is actually almost always much more important.[13] The first question of importance regarding a particular health care service or technology is: What long-term effects (both positive and negative) does it have on health outcomes, and what is the level of evidence supporting the current state of understanding about clinical effectiveness (option A)? The second critical health economics question is: Is it good value for the money (option B)? By good value, we basically mean that a given health care service or product can be used to produce a relatively large amount of "health" for relatively little money. The third major question of health economics is: Can we afford it (option C)? This question really represents the intersection of policy and health economics.

112-10. **The answer is E.** (*Hurst's The Heart, 14th Edition, Chap. 112*) A further complexity about the concept of cost is that a perspective (sometimes termed a viewpoint) must always be defined in order to measure and understand costs (option A).[14] For example, if a patient undergoes a successful PCI with a drug-eluting stent and is discharged from the hospital without complications but is readmitted 3 months later with a stent thrombosis, that readmission is a cost from the payer's perspective and from the societal perspective but not from the hospital's perspective or the physician's perspective, unless they are operating in a capitated system. If a patient comes to clinic with chest pain and gets a clinical workup and a stress test, the cost of all that from the patient's perspective (assuming the patient is insured) may simply be his copay. The clinic and society, however, each have different perspectives on that same episode of care. In most economic analyses, the primary analyses should be done using the societal perspective (option B), which is the perspective in which the winner/loser problem described in these examples is minimized. The problem of measuring and comparing costs across international borders is a difficult one that offers no easy solution, but it is increasingly important in the current era of international cardiology mega-trials (option C).[15,16] To the extent that practice patterns are converging around common standards that cross international borders, it may make sense to pool resource use data across countries and assign common costs (option D). However, local variations in price data make it problematic to decide what prices to use in such an exercise.

References

1. Centers for Medicare and Medicaid Services. National health expenditure data—historical, 2015. https://www.cms.gov/research-statistics-data-and-systems/statistics-trends-and-reports/nationalhealthexpenddata/nationalhealthaccount¬shistorical.html. Accessed January 8, 2016.

2. Health Affairs Blog. Spending growth trends: keeping an eye on spending per person. 2015. http://healthaffairs.org/blog/2015/07/28/spending-growth-trends-keeping-an-eye-on-spending-per-person/. Accessed March 13, 2016.

3. Stone D. *Policy Paradox. The Art of Political Decision Making*. 3rd ed. New York: W.W. Norton; 2012.

4. Brazier J, Ratcliffe J, Tsuchiya A, Salomon J. *Measuring and Valuing Health Benefits for Economic Evaluation*. Oxford, UK: Oxford University Press; 2007.

5. Mozaffarian D, Benjamin EJ, Go AS, et al. Heart disease and stroke statistics—2016 update: a report from the American Heart Association. *Circulation*. 2016;133:e38-e360.

6. Wald NJ, Luteijn JM, Morris JK, Taylor D, Oppenheimer P. Cost-benefit analysis of the polypill in the primary prevention of myocardial infarction and stroke. *Eur J Epidemiol*. 2016;31(4):415-426.

7. Webster R, Patel A, Selak V, et al. Effectiveness of fixed dose combination medication ("polypills") compared with usual care in patients with cardiovascular disease or at high risk: a prospective, individual patient data meta-analysis of 3140 patients in six countries. *Int J Cardiol*. 2016;205:147-156.

8. Pletcher MJ, Lazar L, Bibbins-Domingo K, et al. Comparing impact and cost-effectiveness of primary prevention strategies for lipid-lowering. *Ann Intern Med*. 2009;150:243-254.

9. Grundy SM, Cleeman JI, Merz CN, et al. Implications of recent clinical trials for the National Cholesterol Education Program Adult Treatment Panel III guidelines. *Circulation*. 2004;110:227-239.

10. Macchia A, Mariani J, Romero M, et al. On the hypothetical universal use of statins in primary prevention: an observational analysis on low-risk patients and economic consequences of a potential wide prescription rate. *Eur J Clin Pharmacol*. 2015;71:449-459.

11. Frye RL, August P, Brooks MM, et al. A randomized trial of therapies for type 2 diabetes and coronary artery disease. *N Engl J Med*. 2009;360:2503-2515.

12. Hlatky MA, Boothroyd DB, Melsop KA, et al. Economic outcomes of treatment strategies for type 2 diabetes mellitus and coronary artery disease in the Bypass Angioplasty Revascularization Investigation 2 Diabetes trial. *Circulation*. 2009;120:2550-2558.

13. Hlatky MA. Effectiveness is the key to cost-effectiveness. *Circulation*. 2013;127:764-765.

14. Drummond MF, Schulper MJ, Claxton K, Stoddart GL, Torrance GW. *Methods for the Economic Evaluation of Health Care Programmes*. 4th ed. Oxford, UK: Oxford University Press; 2015.

15. Reed SD, Anstrom KJ, Bakhai A, et al. Conducting economic evaluations alongside multinational clinical trials: toward a research consensus. *Am Heart J*. 2005;149:434-443.

16. Manca A, Willan AR. 'Lost in translation': accounting for between-country differences in the analysis of multinational cost-effectiveness data. *Pharmacoeconomics*. 2006;24:1101-1119.

INDEX

Page references followed by *f* indicate figures; those followed by *t* indicate tables.

INDEX

type I collagen, 38, 40
typical AVNRT, 553, 555–556

U

UA. *See* unstable angina
UFH. *See* unfractionated heparin
ultrasonography, 136, 137
unfractionated heparin (UFH), 268, 271, 494, 497, 498
unipolar pacemaker configuration, 588, 591
UNOS status, 473, 475
unstable angina (UA), 235, 237, 238
uremic pericarditis, 699, 701
urinary 5-hydroxyindoleacetic acid levels, 394, 396–397
urinary norepinephrine, SDB and elevated, 505, 508
urine, inspection of, 3, 5

V

VA ECMO. *See* venoarterial extracorporeal membrane oxygenation
vagal maneuvers, for AVNRT treatment, 554, 556
Valsalva maneuver, 382, 384
  square wave blood pressure response to, 467, 469–470
valve of Vieussens, 516, 519
valve stenosis, 79, 81
valvular heart disease
  antithrombotic therapy for, 341–345
  mixed, 347–350
valvular injury, secondary to blunt chest trauma, 694, 696
valvular murmurs, 6
varenicline
  with NRT for smoking cessation, 204, 206
  for smoking cessation, 196, 199–200, 203, 205
variable penetrance, inherited arrhythmias and, 531, 534
variant angina, 254, 258
vasa vasorum, 218, 220, 619, 621
vascular development, 43, 45
vascular smooth muscle
  conversion to synthetic phenotype, 43, 45
  signaling pathways in, 44, 46
vasculitides, coronary arteritis and, 230, 232
vasculogenesis, postnatal, 43, 45
vasodilation, blood pressure and increased, 149, 151
vasodilator SPECT-MPI, for LBBB prediction, 112, 115
vasodilator stress, 119, 123
vasodilator stress nuclear MPI, 113, 115
vasopressin, 611, 613
vasovagal syncope, 536, 538
VEGF inhibitors, hypertension and, 150, 152
vein of Marshall, 26, 28–29, 515, 518

venae cavae, 27
venoarterial extracorporeal membrane oxygenation (VA ECMO), 480, 482
venous insufficiency, 647, 648, 650–651
venous return curves, arteriolar vasodilation and, 33, 33f, 35
venous system, 647, 649
venous thromboembolism (VTE), 493–495, 497–498
venous thrombosis, Virchow's Triad for, 647, 649
venous ulcers, 648, 651, 651t
venous valves, 3, 5
ventricle, 3, 5
ventricular arrhythmias, 362, 364, 535–538
  MI and, 242, 245
ventricular fibrillation (VF), 530, 533
ventricular filling, 32, 34
ventricular interdependence, constrictive pericarditis and, 428, 432
ventricular myocardium, 516, 519
ventricular pacing, 542, 545
ventricular pressure, 32, 34
ventricular septal defect (VSD)
  Eisenmenger syndrome and nonrestrictive, 361, 363
  pulmonary stenosis associated with, 83, 86
  small restrictive, 361, 364
ventricular stiffness, 32, 34
ventricular tachycardia (VT), 522, 525, 530, 533. *See also* catecholaminergic polymorphic ventricular tachycardia
  Chagas disease and, 560, 563
  fascicular, 542, 545, 559, 561
  ICD and, antiarrhythmic drugs for, 560, 562
  ischemic, ECG features of, 559, 561–562
  lidocaine for, 576, 578–579
  "outflow tract," 559, 561
  right ventricular outflow tract, 400, 403, 559, 561
verapamil
  AVNRT treatment and, 554, 556
  pregnancy and, 579t
very-low-density lipoproteins (VLDLs), 189
vessel wall
  biology of, 43–46
  coagulation cascade and, 217, 219
vessels with positive remodeling, 132, 133
VF. *See* ventricular fibrillation
viral myocarditis, 376, 378
  coxsackie-mediated, 407, 409
  LGE and, 98, 98f, 101, 407, 409
  NYHA classes of, 407, 409
Virchow's Triad, for venous thrombosis, 647, 649
vitamin K, 217, 219
VLDLs. *See* very-low-density lipoproteins
von Willebrand disease, 218, 221
von Willebrand factor (vWF), 217, 218, 219, 221

V/Q testing, 493, 496
VSD. *See* ventricular septal defect
VT. *See* ventricular tachycardia
VTE. *See* venous thromboembolism
vulnerable plaque, 279, 281
vWF. *See* von Willebrand factor

W

Waller, Augustus, 5
warfarin, 462, 464, 627, 629, 674, 676
  Barth syndrome and, 388, 390
  for coronary thrombosis, aspirin and clopidogrel with, 180, 184
  mitral valve replacement and, 341, 344
  pregnancy and, 361, 363
  pregnancy with mechanical heart valve and, 342, 344, 345
  VTE and, 494, 498
water hammer pulse, 71
weight loss
  bariatric surgery for, 172, 176
  CVD risk factors and, 172, 175
  hormone secretion following, 171, 173
  medications for, adolescents and, 172, 175–176
  type 2 diabetes and, 172, 175
weight training, 706, 708
Wells score, for DVT diagnosis, 647, 649, 649t
Wenckebach block, 535, 537
WHF. *See* World Heart Foundation
white coat hypertension, 143, 145
Whites, 734t
WHO. *See* World Health Organization
Wolff-Parkinson-White (WPW) syndrome, 541, 542, 544, 545, 578
  ablation for, 537
  AF and, 554, 557
  ECG and, 75, 77
  SCD and, 554, 557
women. *See also* gender
  atherosclerotic plaque erosion and, 241, 244, 723, 725–726
  CABG surgery and, 724, 727
  cigarette smoking and, 724, 726
  coronary blood flow in, 223, 226
  CVD treatment for, 715, 718
  IHD and, 723–727
  MI in, 723, 725
World Health Organization (WHO), 204, 206–207
World Heart Foundation (WHF), 369, 372
worsening renal function (WRF), 469
WPW syndrome. *See* Wolff-Parkinson-White syndrome
WRF. *See* worsening renal function

X

X chromosome, monosomy of, 355, 358
xanthelasmas, FH and, 187, 189

Z

zidovudine, 679, 681
Zoll, Paul, 6